Nutrition & Diet Therapy

FIFTH EDITION

Nutrition & Diet Therapy

FIFTH EDITION

Carroll A. Lutz, MA, RN
Associate Professor Emerita
Jackson Community College
Jackson, Michigan

Karen Rutherford Przytulski, MS, RD
Clinical Dietitian
DaVita
Port Charlotte, Florida

F.A. Davis Company • Philadelphia

F. A. Davis Company
1915 Arch Street
Philadelphia, PA 19103
www.fadavis.com

Printed in the United States of America

Last digit indicates print number: 10 9 8 7 6 5 4 3 2

Acquisitions Editor: Jonathan Joyce
Director of Content Development: Darlene Pedersen
Senior Project Editor: Padraic Maroney
Project Editor: Christina Burns
Cover Design: Carolyn O'Brien

As new scientific information becomes available through basic and clinical research, recommended treatments and drug therapies undergo changes. The author(s) and publisher have done everything possible to make this book accurate, up to date, and in accord with accepted standards at the time of publication. The author(s), editors, and publisher are not responsible for errors or omissions or for consequences from application of the book, and make no warranty, expressed or implied, in regard to the contents of the book. Any practice described in this book should be applied by the reader in accordance with professional standards of care used in regard to the unique circumstances that may apply in each situation. The reader is advised always to check product information (package inserts) for changes and new information regarding dose and contraindications before administering any drug. Caution is especially urged when using new or infrequently ordered drugs.

Library of Congress Cataloging-in-Publication Data

Lutz, Carroll A.
Nutrition & diet therapy / Carroll A. Lutz, Karen Rutherford Przytulski.—5th ed.
p. ; cm.
Other title: Nutrition and diet therapy
Includes bibliographical references and index.
ISBN-13: 978-0-8036-2202-9
ISBN-10: 0-8036-2202-3
1. Dietetics. 2. Diet therapy. 3. Nutrition. I. Przytulski, Karen Rutherford. II. Title. III. Title: Nutrition and diet therapy.
[DNLM: 1. Diet Therapy. 2. Diet. 3. Nutritional Physiological Phenomena. WB 400 L975n 2010]
RM217.L88 2010
613.2—dc22 2010022784

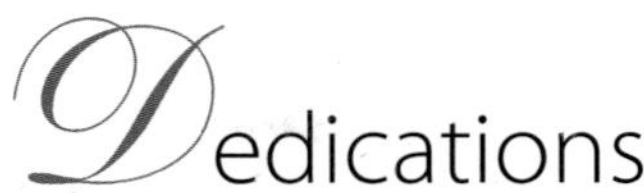

Dedications

To our son, Joe, with love.

—Carroll A. Lutz

To my sister, Anne, her husband, Steve, my nephew, Steven, and my Mother, thanks for all your help.

—Karen R. Przytulski

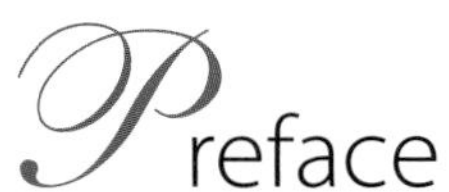reface

The fifth edition of *Nutrition & Diet Therapy* is designed to provide the beginning student with knowledge of the fundamentals of nutrition related to the promotion and maintenance of optimal health. Practical applications and treatment of pathologies with nutritional components are stressed. In addition, basic scientific information is introduced to enable students to begin to understand nutritional issues reported in the mass media. The sequential introduction of material continues to be a unique feature of this text. The authors resist the temptation to introduce concepts and examples of applications before the underlying basic science and vocabulary have been covered. The fifth edition has been extensively updated with new information and reorganized to highlight pertinent facts with bullets and many new tables.

This book was written to meet the educational needs of nursing students, dietetic assistants, diet technicians, and others. Support materials for the student include case studies with examples of care plans and clinical analysis study questions. Critical Thinking Questions follow the care plans and are designed to provoke imaginative thought and to foster discussion. Currently there exists an information explosion related to the science of nutrition. Particularly striking is the evidence showing genetic differences in individuals' metabolism of nutrients. As researchers discover new and more effective treatments for nutrition-related disorders and health maintenance, the ability to think critically becomes increasingly important for professional growth and development. Students need not only to grasp the facts but also to apply the information in a clinical environment. This text has been developed to facilitate acquiring these skills.

The text can be used to teach a complete course in nutrition or as a desk reference for practitioners. The student using this book needs no previous grounding in anatomy, physiology, or medical terminology. Subjects are fully supported by diagrams, illustrations, figures, and tables. Depending upon the curriculum, chapters may be omitted or presented in a different sequence. We recognize that this text contains an immense amount of data and information. We hope this rich store of information permits instructors to adapt the text to the objectives of their courses while at the same time serving as a reference and directory for students satisfying their curiosities or completing solo or group projects whether in preclinical or in clinical courses.

The content of *Nutrition & Diet Therapy,* fifth edition, is organized into three units.

Unit 1, **The Role of Nutrients in the Human Body,** covers basic information on nutrition as a science and how this information is applied to nutritional care. All the essential nutrients are covered, including definitions and descriptions of functions, effects of excesses and deficiencies, and food sources. Nutritional standards, including the Dietary Reference Intakes, are explained and incorporated into discussions of nutrients. Information on the use of food in the body and how the body maintains energy balance completes the unit.

Unit 2, **Family and Community Nutrition,** provides an overview of topics such as nutrition throughout the life cycle, food management, nutrient delivery via oral, enteral, and parenteral routes, and interactions among foods, nutrients, medications and supplements.

Unit 3, **Clinical Nutrition,** focuses on the care of clients with pathologies caused by or causing nutritional impairments. Pathological conditions include diabetes mellitus and hypoglycemia, cardiovascular disease, renal disease, gastrointestinal disease, cancer, and HIV and AIDS. Other pertinent topics include weight control; nutrition in critical care and during stress, and care of the client with a terminal illness.

Special features are used throughout the text to facilitate the teaching and learning process. All of the chapters include the following:

Boxes and Tables contain summaries, assessment tools, commonly prescribed diets employed in Medical Nutrition Therapy, and research findings.

Clinical Applications stimulate the interest of the beginning student by showing how the information is pertinent to providing health care.

Clinical Calculations isolate and explain many of the mathematical calculations that are used in nutritional science.

New—**Dollars & Sense items** feature costs associated with commonly used foods and supplements.

New—**Genomic Gems** highlight links between a person's genetic makeup and utilization of nutrients and dietary substances.

Illustrations reinforce important points in the text or graph statistical data for clarity.

Flowcharts of physiological and pathological processes lead the student to an understanding of the relationship between nutrition and health.

Case Study with a proposed **Care Plan** allow the student to see how the nutrition principles described in the chapter are applied in a specific clinical situation. The case studies were written to incorporate elements that are likely to recur in practice.

New—**Teamwork** ( ) following the care plan illustrates continuing care of a client by various members of the health care team.

Study Aids, Chapter Review Questions and Clinical Analysis Questions, help the student to focus on essential concepts. Answers to the Study Aids questions are printed in the Appendix.

Critical Thinking Questions invite the student to think holistically with compassion and creativity. They can be used as a basis for class discussion.

Bibliography, divided by chapters, supports the text with data sources and introduces the student to the scientific literature.

Glossary of more than 950 entries assists the reader to recall definitions of terms boldfaced in the text.

Appendix serves as a ready source of information for students in class discussions or group assignments.

Electronic Updates as new information becomes available, updates will be posted on the F. A. Davis website accessible under the authors' names and this edition of *Nutrition & Diet Therapy*.

Accompanying the text for instructors who adopt it for their classes are:

Instructors' Guide with suggestions for course organization, classroom activities, and student assignments.

PowerPoint Presentations of more than 650 PowerPoint slides covering all the chapters of the book. These presentations provide a ready source of material to select for classroom use.

Electronic Test Bank containing more than 1,100 questions arranged by chapter.

We believe that *Nutrition & Diet Therapy,* fifth edition, provides the clinical information necessary for a fuller understanding of the relationship between the knowledge about nutrition and diet and its clinical application. This text balances direct explanations of the underlying science with an introduction to the clinical responsibilities of the health care professional.

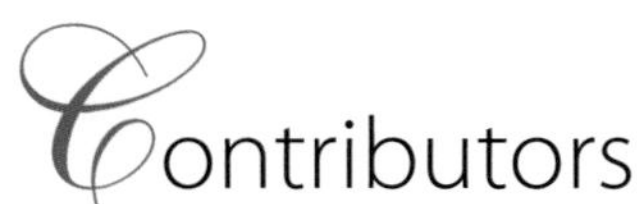

Contributors

Co-Author
Theresa Tomak, RD, CSR
Renal Dietitian
Sparrow Health Systems
Lansing, Michigan
Chapter 19, Diet in Renal Disease

Consultant
Renee Zubay Fife, RN, MSN
Assistant Clinical Professor of Nursing
Purdue University Calumet
Hammond, Indiana

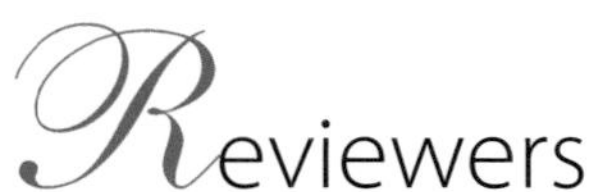

Reviewers

Tara L. Clark, RN, MSN
Assistant Professor of Nursing
Morehead State University
Morehead, Kentucky

Eileen O. Costello, RN, MSN
Dean, School of Health Sciences and Community Service Programs
Mount Wachusett Community College
Gardner, Massachusetts

Joan Cranford, RN, MSN, EdD (c)
Division Chair for Nursing and Health Sciences
Gordon College
Barnesville, Georgia

Amber Derksen, RN, MSN
Assistant Professor
Armstrong Atlantic State University
Savannah, Georgia

Helen C. Estes, RN, MS
Nursing Instructor
Manhattan Area Technical College
Manhattan, Kansas

Catherine Harris, RN, MSN, CEN, CNE
Nursing Faculty
Cape Cod Community College
West Barnstable, Massachusetts

Teresa Johnson, MACTN, RD
Assistant Professor
Troy University School of Nursing
Troy, Alabama

Teresa Kochera, RN, MSN, PCCN
Assistant Professor of Nursing
Macon State College
Macon, Georgia

Jane E. Lucht, BSN, MSEd
Associate Professor
Edgewood College School of Nursing
Madison, Wisconsin

Carol Isaac MacKusick, RN, MSN, CNN
Assistant Professor of Nursing
Clayton State University
Morrow, Georgia

Barbara Maxwell, RN, MSN, MS
Associate Professor of Nursing
SUNY Ulster
Stone Ridge, New York

Rebecca Scarborough, RD, LDN, BSN, MAEd
Clinical Dietitian
Pitt County Memorial Hospital
Greenville, North Carolina

Debra Smith, APRN, MSN, C-PNP
Assistant Professor Nursing
Louisiana State University – Alexandria
Alexandria, Louisiana

Beryl Stetson, RNBC, MSN, LCCE, CLC
Assistant Professor of Nursing
Raritan Valley Community College
Somerville, New Jersey

Ann Tritak, RN, EdD, MA, BSN
Dean, School of Nursing/Associate Professor of Nursing
Saint Peter's College
Jersey City, New Jersey

Acknowledgments

Writing a book, even a fifth edition, is a huge task, requiring the assistance of many people. Our colleagues contributed to this project, sometimes with information and critiques, sometimes just by being supportive.

We would like to thank all the organizations and publishers that gave permission for the use of their materials. The staff at the Jackson Community College Learning Resource Center, especially Marion VanLoo, obtained literature from distant sources through interlibrary loans. Special notice is due to colleagues who shared their expertise including:

William Beiswenger, RN, MA, CDE
Colleen Chadderton, RN, MSN, PNP
Kent Clark, CNSD, RD, provided valuable input for Chapter 24, Nutritional Care of the Terminally Ill
Terri Tomak, RD, CSR, who co-authored Chapter 19, Diet in Renal Disease

Our editorial and production staff at F. A. Davis Company, including Jonathan Joyce, Christina Burns, Padraic Maroney, and Steve Lutrell, shared their knowledge and expertise in all phases of our joint project. Our Developmental Editor, Carol Munson, Production Manager, Sam Rondinelli, and Berta Steiner kept us focused on our common goal of excellence. To all of them go our heartfelt thanks.

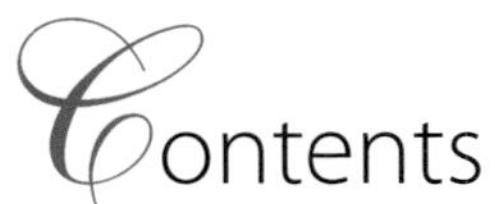

Contents

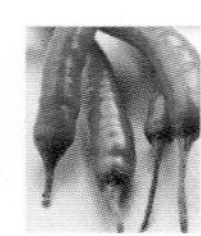

Unit 3

Clinical Nutrition 277

Appendices

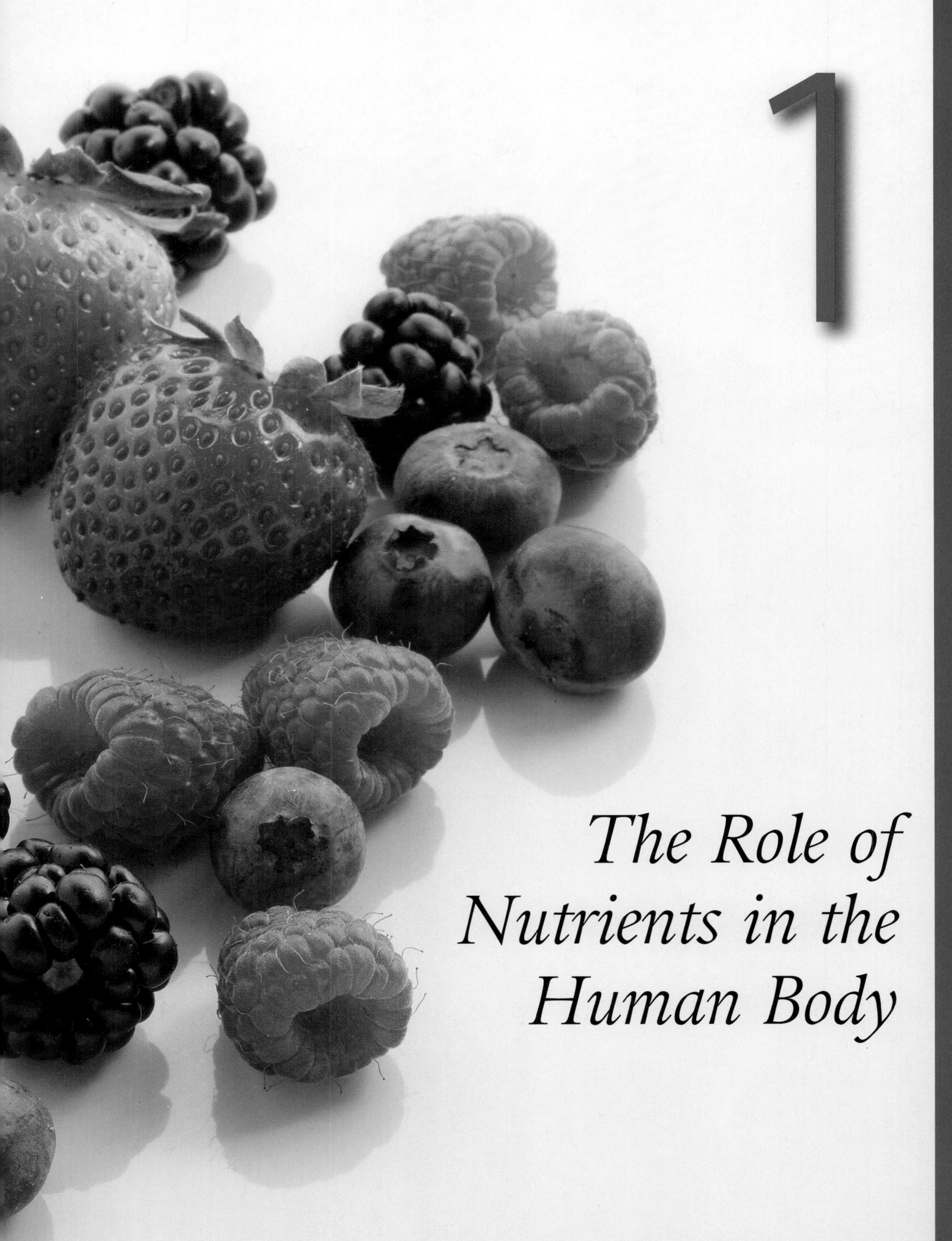

1

The Role of Nutrients in the Human Body

1

An Introduction to Nutrition

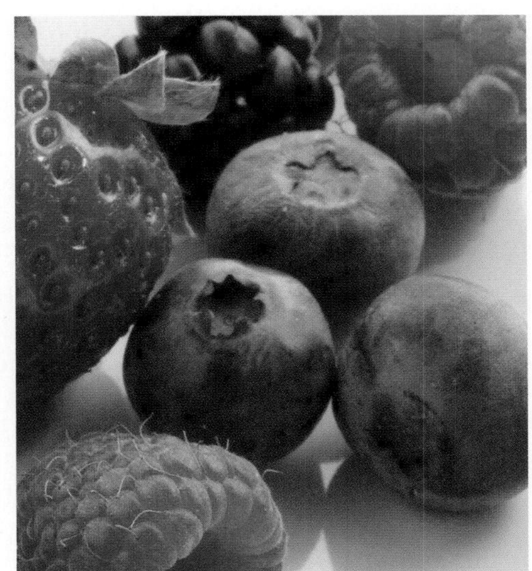

LEARNING OBJECTIVES

After completing this chapter, the student should be able to:

- State the three functions of nutrients.
- Identify the six classes of nutrients.
- Define nutrigenomics.
- Describe the relationship between nutrition and health.
- Discuss the ways in which various health care providers contribute to excellent nutritional care.
- Discuss current Dietary Guidelines for Americans.
- Access www.mypyramid.gov and create a personalized diet plan.

This chapter introduces basic terminology, defines and introduces nutrigenomics, and presents food guides and guidelines. It concludes with a discussion of the roles of various health-care professionals.

Basic Terminology

Understanding nutrition starts with knowing a few basic definitions.

Nutrition

Nutrition is the study of the relationship of humans to food. Many other sciences—biology, chemistry, genetics, economics, educational theory, nursing, medicine, pharmacology, physiology, psychology, and sociology—also contribute to the study of nutrition. These connections suggest the far-reaching implications of good nutrition.

Health

Food and health have always been connected. **Health** is defined as a state of complete physical, mental, and social well-being, not just the absence of disease or infirmity.

Nutrients

Historically, the science of nutrition has been based on the nutrients in food. **Nutrients** are the chemical substances supplied by food that the body needs for growth, maintenance, and repair. Nutrients are divided into six classes:

1. Carbohydrates (often abbreviated as CHO)
2. Fats (lipids)
3. Proteins
4. Minerals
5. Vitamins
6. Water

Each nutrient class is discussed in subsequent chapters.

Nutrients are considered **essential, nonessential,** or **conditionally essential,** depending on whether the body can or cannot manufacture them.

- A nutrient is called essential if the human body requires it and cannot manufacture it in sufficient amounts to meet bodily needs. Thus, essential nutrients must be supplied by foods in the diet. Vitamin C, vitamin A, and calcium are 3 of the more than 40 essential nutrients.
- Nutrients not needed in the diet because the body can make them are called nonessential. For example, the amino acid alanine is a nonessential nutrient because the body can manufacture it from other raw materials.
- A small number of nutrients are classified as conditionally essential. Under most circumstances, a healthy body can manufacture enough of these nutrients; however, in certain situations the body cannot manufature an optimal amount. The amino acid arginine is an example of a conditionally essential nutrient.

Functions of Nutrients

All nutrients perform one or more of the following functions:

1. Serve as a source of energy or heat
2. Support the growth and maintenance of tissue
3. Aid in the regulation of basic body processes

These three life-sustaining functions collectively are part of **metabolism,** the sum of all physical and chemical changes that take place in the body. Nutrients have specific metabolic functions and interact with one another to maintain the body.

SOURCE OF ENERGY

Energy is defined in the physical sciences as the capacity to do work. Energy exists in a variety of forms: electric, thermal (heat), chemical, mechanical, and others.

All food enters the body as chemical energy. The body processes the chemical energy of food and converts it into other energy forms. For example, chemical energy is transformed into electric signals in nerves and into mechanical energy in muscles.

Carbohydrates, fats, and proteins, the nutrients that supply energy, are referred to as the **energy nutrients.** The energy both in foods and in the body is measured in **kilocalories,** abbreviated kcal (see Glossary). Because energy cannot be seen, heard, or felt, it is one of the most difficult biological concepts to understand. For this reason, it warrants its own chapter (see Chapter 6).

GROWTH AND MAINTENANCE OF TISSUES

Some nutrients provide the raw materials for building body structures, and they participate in the continued growth and maintenance of necessary tissues. Water, proteins, fats, and minerals are the nutrient classes that contribute in a major way to building body structures.

REGULATION OF BODY PROCESSES

Some nutrients control or regulate chemical processes in the body. For example, certain minerals and proteins help regulate how water is distributed in the body. Vitamins are necessary in the series of reactions involved in generating energy. Vitamins themselves are not energy sources, but if the body lacks a particular vitamin, it will not produce energy efficiently.

Malnutrition

Ingesting too much or too little of a nutrient can interfere with health and well-being. Each nutrient has a beneficial range of intake; an intake below or above that range is incompatible with optimal health. Thus, **malnutrition** (poor nutrition) occurs when body cells receive too much or too little of one or more nutrients. For example, a single-food diet, such as a grapefruit diet to lose weight, will result in malnutrition if followed for an extended period. To prevent malnutrition, a diet should contain a variety and balance of different foods eaten in moderation.

Phytochemicals and Zoochemicals

The philosophy that food can be health promoting beyond its traditional value as a source of nutrients has gained acceptance among scientists and health professionals. Knowledge of physiologically active food ingredients in animal sources (**zoochemicals**) and plant sources (**phytochemicals**) has expanded our understanding of the role of diet in health. Foods that contain zoochemicals and phytochemicals are sometimes called **functional foods**.

Substances in animal products that have been associated with reduced risk of disease have been identified. For example, fermented dairy products, such as yogurt, that contain probiotics have been shown to improve gastrointestinal health. **Probiotics** are bacteria found in food that reduce the duration of acute diarrhea in children. The positive attributes of yogurt are most pronounced during a course of treatment with antibiotics.

The prefix *phyto-* comes from the Greek word for *plant*. Phytochemicals are nonnutrient food components (food chemicals) that provide medical or health

TABLE 1-1 ■ Selected Functional Foods, Phytochemicals, and Reported Health Benefits

FUNCTIONAL FOODS	PHYTOCHEMICAL(S) IDENTIFIED	REPORTED HEALTH BENEFIT
Tomatoes, Grapefruit	Lycopene	Reduce risk for prostate cancer. Reduce risk for heart disease.
Garlic, Onions, Chives	Allyl sulfides	Reduce risk for stomach and colon cancer. Reduce risk for heart disease.
Soy Products, Legumes, Peanuts	Isoflavones: genistein, diadzein	Reduce risk for breast, prostate, and endometrial cancer. Reduce risk for heart disease. Reduce risk for osteoporosis. May assist in the treatment of menopausal symptoms.
Whole Flaxseed (ground)	Lignans, phytoestrogens	Increase laxation (increased frequency and bulk of feces). May protect against heart disease, cardiac arrhythmia, and stroke. Reduce risk for hormone-sensitive cancers. Favorably affects the immune system by reducing inflammation. May prevent retinopathy in premature infants.
Green Tea	Polyphenols	Reduces risk for gastric, esophageal, and skin cancers. Reduces risk for heart disease.
Broccoli, Cabbage, Brussels Sprouts, Cauliflower, Kohlrabi, Watercress, Turnips	Sulforaphanes, indoles, isothiocyanates	May reduce risk of breast, stomach, and lung cancers. May protect the retina from light-induced oxidative damage. May be responsible for reversing eye damage or macular degeneration in very early stages.
Fruits, Vegetables, Nuts, Tea, Wine, Oregano	Flavonoids	May reduce cancer risk; acts as an **antioxidant.**

benefits, including the prevention or treatment of disease (Table 1-1). Research has shown that phytochemicals can stop a cell's conversion from healthy to cancerous at many different stages of cell division and growth. Phytochemicals also may decrease risk for chronic diseases, such as cardiovascular disease, cancer, and diabetes. It is not known whether each of the more than 400 known phytochemicals produces its reported health benefits by functioning alone or in combination with others. Therefore, most experts advise eating a wide variety of fruits, whole grains, and vegetables and not narrowing intake to particular foods.

Nutrition and Health

Good nutrition is essential for good health and important for physical growth and development, good body composition, and mental development. A person's nutritional state can protect him from or predispose him toward chronic disease. Only recently has it been discovered that nutrition influences our genetic code. See Genomic Gem 1-1. For now, think of the genetic code as "software" that provides instructions to the human body. Medical treatment for many diseases includes diet therapy. Nutrition is thus both a preventive and a therapeutic science.

Genomic Gem 1-1
Nutrigenomics

In April 2003 the Human Genome Project announced that the actual sequence of the human genetic code had been transcribed. In simple terms, the **genetic code** is the human body's software instructions. **Nutrigenomics** is the study of the interaction of foods with specific genes to increase the risk of common chronic diseases (www.medterms.com, 2008).

To visualize the relationship among the human body, genetic code, and diet, think of the body as a machine similar to a personal computer. Software provides directions to the computer; a person's genetic code provides instructions to the body. Just as a personal computer cannot operate without software, the human body cannot operate without instructions from the genetic code. Think of data input by the operator as much like food that is input, or eaten.

For years, scientists have studied the effects of nutrients and phytochemicals on our body's hardware, or structure. Only recently have researchers begun the study of nutrients and phytochemicals on the body's software, or genetic code. Almost everyone has software on their computers that is never used. The human body also has instructions that are similarly never used.

What causes a software program or gene in the human body to be turned on or expressed? Some scientists are beginning to understand the activation is partly due to the food we eat or do not eat. The premise underlying nutrigenomics is that diet's influence on health depends on an individual's genetic makeup (www.medterms.com, 2008). Thus, one person would be more susceptible to the negative effects of a suboptimal diet than another person would be.

Physical Growth and Development

Although genetics determines much of individual growth patterns and heritable potential, malnutrition can delay or prevent individuals from achieving that potential. Without enough calcium, phosphorus, and protein, for example, bones cannot grow properly. Children who are malnourished may never reach their genetic potential for height.

Body Composition

Nutrient intake can affect body composition, which in turn can affect health. The human body is composed of four main types of substances and one minor substance (Fig. 1-1). The four types are:

1. Water
2. Fat
3. Ash
4. Protein

The minor substance is carbohydrate.

One-half to three-quarters of the body is made up of water. A normally active woman has a body fat content between 18% and 22%. A normally active man has a body fat content between 15% and 19%. Body ash, which accounts for approximately 6% of body weight, is the body's mineral content. It includes, for example, the calcium and phosphorus that are constituents of the human skeleton.

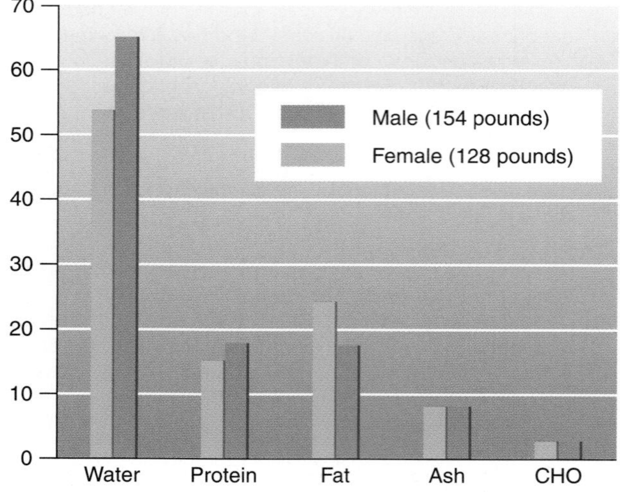

FIGURE 1-1 Approximate body composition of a typical 25-year-old man (154 lb) and woman (128 lb). Note that the typical woman has a higher percentage of body fat than does the typical man. The man has a higher percentage of lean body mass. The percentage of ash content is equal in both sexes. The human body has minimal carbohydrate content.

Approximately 15% of the body's weight is protein; the male body contains more protein than the female body. With age, body composition typically becomes higher in fat and lower in protein. Protein is stored primarily in muscle tissue and organs and forms certain body chemicals. For example, albumin, a protein in the blood, is partly manufactured from dietary protein. When the body loses protein, it is losing muscle tissue, organ mass, the protein stored in body substances, or combinations thereof. Preservation of body protein is necessary for optimal health. A loss of structural body content (heart muscle, kidney, liver, or blood proteins) leads to illness.

A person's body fat and protein content can be modified by food intake, exercise, or both. Exercise increases body protein content by increasing muscle. (Fig. 1-2). Eating too much food (ingesting more calories than the body expends) increases the fat content of the body because fat is stored for future use. Excessive body fat has health consequences.

Mental Health

Researchers continue to find relationships between mental health and diet. For example, adults, teens, and children who experience food insecurity have an increased risk for poor psychological and cognitive (act of knowing) functioning and substandard academic achievement. See Box 1-1 for information on food insecurity.

Even in the short term, diet has been found to enhance mental function. Children who consume less than half of the energy recommended for breakfast have significantly poorer attendance, punctuality, and grades at school than children who eat more for breakfast. Poor eaters also have more behavioral problems. After getting breakfast at school, the attendance, math grades, and behavior of the poor eaters improves (www.nutrition.about.com/od/nutritionforchildren/a/dietandlearning.htm, 2010). Elderly people also have better memory and task performance after consuming carbohydrates (www.eatright.org/public, 2010). Starvation seems to impede concentration.

Box 1-1 ■ *Food Insecurity*

Food insecurity is the limited or uncertain availability of nutritionally adequate and safe foods or uncertain ability to acquire food. Food-insecure mothers of young children often suffer from depression. Their children are more likely to:

- Be suspended from school
- Experience difficulty getting along with others
- Be at an increased risk of suicide (American Dietetic Association, 2006)

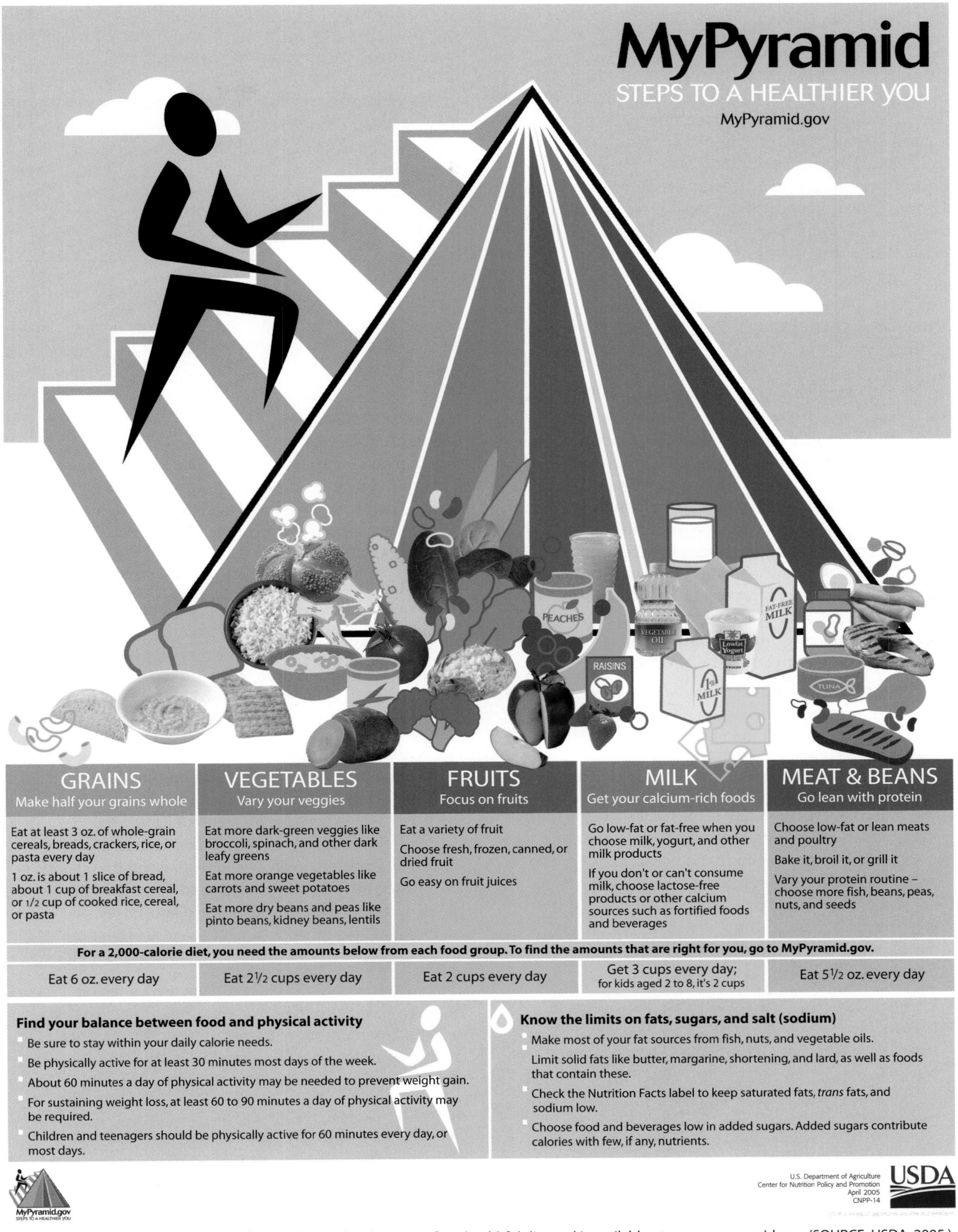

MyPyramid
STEPS TO A HEALTHIER YOU
MyPyramid.gov
PEACHES
VEGETABLE OIL
RAISINS
Lowfat Yogurt
FAT-FREE MILK
1% MILK
TUNA
GRAINS
Make half your grains whole
Eat at least 3 oz. of whole-grain cereals, breads, crackers, rice, or pasta every day
1 oz. is about 1 slice of bread, about 1 cup of breakfast cereal, or 1/2 cup of cooked rice, cereal, or pasta
VEGETABLES
Vary your veggies
Eat more dark-green veggies like broccoli, spinach, and other dark leafy greens
Eat more orange vegetables like carrots and sweet potatoes
Eat more dry beans and peas like pinto beans, kidney beans, lentils
FRUITS
Focus on fruits
Eat a variety of fruit
Choose fresh, frozen, canned, or dried fruit
Go easy on fruit juices
MILK
Get your calcium-rich foods
Go low-fat or fat-free when you choose milk, yogurt, and other milk products
If you don't or can't consume milk, choose lactose-free products or other calcium sources such as fortified foods and beverages
MEAT & BEANS
Go lean with protein
Choose low-fat or lean meats and poultry
Bake it, broil it, or grill it
Vary your protein routine – choose more fish, beans, peas, nuts, and seeds
For a 2,000-calorie diet, you need the amounts below from each food group. To find the amounts that are right for you, go to MyPyramid.gov.
Eat 6 oz. every day
Eat 2½ cups every day
Eat 2 cups every day
Get 3 cups every day; for kids aged 2 to 8, it's 2 cups
Eat 5½ oz. every day
Find your balance between food and physical activity
Be sure to stay within your daily calorie needs.
Be physically active for at least 30 minutes most days of the week.
About 60 minutes a day of physical activity may be needed to prevent weight gain.
For sustaining weight loss, at least 60 to 90 minutes a day of physical activity may be required.
Children and teenagers should be physically active for 60 minutes every day, or most days.
Know the limits on fats, sugars, and salt (sodium)
Make most of your fat sources from fish, nuts, and vegetable oils.
Limit solid fats like butter, margarine, shortening, and lard, as well as foods that contain these.
Check the Nutrition Facts label to keep saturated fats, trans fats, and sodium low.
Choose food and beverages low in added sugars. Added sugars contribute calories with few, if any, nutrients.
MyPyramid.gov
STEPS TO A HEALTHIER YOU
U.S. Department of Agriculture
Center for Nutrition Policy and Promotion
April 2005
CNPP-14
USDA

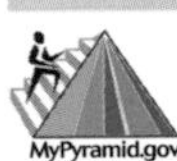

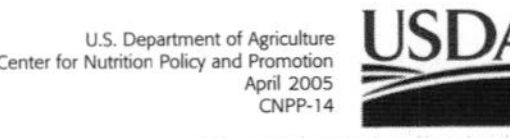

FIGURE 1-2 MyPyramid is one tool used to teach people what to eat for a healthful diet and is available at www.mypyramid.gov. (SOURCE: USDA, 2005.)

Diet as Therapy

A modified diet is often an important component of a client's total health care. Box 1-2 discusses how diets may be modified. For example, diet is an important part of the treatment for metabolic diseases such as diabetes. Special dietary measures may be required to maintain the lives of patients who have chronic heart, kidney, liver, and gastrointestinal diseases. These diets must also consider the effects of medications on nutrients. Adjustments in diet are also necessary in other situations, such as after highly stressful or traumatic events including severe burns, broken bones, and surgery.

Box 1-2 ■ *Modified Diets*

A **modified diet** is one that has been altered to:

- Include more or fewer nutrients
- Effect a change in the texture or consistency of what is ingested
- Restrict the intake of any substance

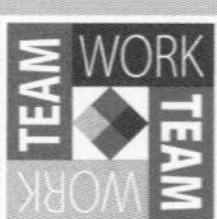

1-1 Health-Care Professionals in Nutrition Delivery

Clients are the focus of the health-care team, and those who participate in their own care are more likely to achieve set goals. Clients are also more likely to change negative behaviors if they believe the benefits of therapy are worth the consequences. When a client accepts his or her medical condition, requests and accepts information, and can describe how learning is best achieved (written instructions, verbal instructions, demonstration, and so forth), a readiness to change becomes apparent. Family members, caregivers, or designated guardians need to be involved in the client's eduction.

A client's health-care team may include more than 15 members. The following are the respective titles and responsibilities of the major members of the health-care team.

Registered Nurses

Registered nurses (RNs) are often the first team members to interview a client, and they communicate important nutritional information such as a client's response to food, including intake and tolerance, to other team members. In addition, they identify and refer clients at high nutritional risk to other team members, and they provide some nutritional information to clients.

Licensed Practical Nurses/Licensed Vocational Nurses

Licensed practical nurses (LPNs) and licensed vocational nurses (LVNs) supervised by RNs feed clients, monitor food consumption, measure intake and output, and record data.

Registered Dietitians

Registered dietitians (RDs) and physicians are responsible for meeting clients' nutritional needs. Dietitians interpret the physician's diet order in terms of clients' food habits and food choices, calculate clients' nutritional requirements, evaluate clients' response to therapeutic diets, and provide in-depth nutrition education and counsel clients. Among team members, the registered dietitian usually has the most education and training in the nutritional sciences.

Clinical Pharmacists

Pharmacists (RPhs) prepare, preserve, and compound medicines and dispense them according to the prescriptions of physicians. They may also counsel clients about food–drug and drug–drug interactions and function as valuable resources for all team members.

Physicians

Physicians are responsible for the diagnosis and treatment of medical conditions. They manage medical care, order laboratory tests, and prescribe medications and diets. Physicians are responsible for communicating the diagnosis and explaining treatment options to clients. Treatment options should always be presented to clients at the same time clients are given bad news. Only the physician or the designee can order diagostic tests, medications, and other treatments.

Dietetic Technicians

Dietetic technicians (DTs) assist dietitians by taking nutrition histories and body measurements, reviewing records, and monitoring clients' food intake. They are often responsible for screening clients for nutritional risk and referring clients at risk to the registered dietitian.

Licensed Speech Pathologists

Speech pathologists treat swallowing disorders along with other nonnutrition-related disorders. Treatment for swallowing disorders may include exercises, positions, and strategies, such as changing food and liquid textures, for easier and safer swallowing.

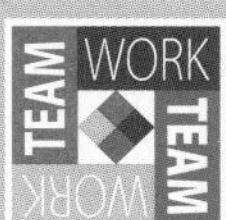

1-1

Health-Care Professionals in Nutrition Delivery—cont'd

Medical Assistants
Medical assistants are responsible for taking vital signs and measuring a client's height and weight. When this information is not available, a complete nutritional assessment is not possible.

Other Health-Care Personnel
Other health-care personnel who may be involved in client care include licensed social workers, medical technologists, nurse practitioners, and psychologists.

Many health-care personnel have advanced training and certification in one specific area. For example, both registered nurses and registered dietitians may elect to obtain Certified Diabetes Educators (CDE) certification.

Identifying a problem, but having insufficient resources to address it, is more likely than having too much assistance from other team members. Many functions of health-care personnel overlap in order to avoid missing a client's problem. See Dollars and Sense 1-1.

Dollars & Sense 1-1

All health-care workers' roles are interconnected. Often co-workers cannot function efficiently unless someone else has done their assigned duties in a timely fashion. For example, the dietitian cannot accurately estimate a client's nutritional needs without an accurate height. The physican is hesitant to order a tube feeding without the dietitian's recommendations or the pharmacist will not mix a solution without a client's weight. This can have a significant impact on the cost of health care.

Dietary Guidelines and Food Guides

Worldwide, many governments have published well-researched and practical dietary and food guidelines. This text discusses only the U.S. recommendations; however, other governments have published equally reliable educational tools.

United States Dietary Guidelines

The U.S. Departments of Agriculture and Health and Human Services have jointly published Dietary Guidelines for Americans every 5 years since the 1980s. The current guidelines for health promotion were published in 2010. The *Dietary Guidelines for Americans 2010,* based on the latest scientific and medical information, are intended for use by government policymakers, nutrition educators, and health providers. For example, the Guidelines would be used to write menus for school lunch programs, nursing home residents, and prisoners.

The Guidelines provide advice for people 2 years and older about how proper dietary habits can promote health and reduce risk for major chronic diseases. They are intended to evaluate several days' intake of food, not to evaluate individual food items or a single meal or day's intake. In addition, do not apply to individuals who have diseases or conditions that alter normal nutritional requirements. Clinical Application 1-1 summarizes the key recommendations for the general population.

The Food Guide Pyramid

The *Dietary Guidelines* form the foundation for the Food Guidance System (www.MyPyramid.gov), which presents the nutrition science in a consumer-friendly way and helps people apply the science to their own lives (www.health.gov/dietaryguidelines).

In 2005, the U.S. Department of Agriculture created MyPyramid, which includes healthful diet choices balanced with appropriate activity (Fig. 1-2). MyPyramid groups foods into six categories based on similar nutrient content. For example, foods in the milk group are high in calcium, riboflavin, and protein. Each food group supplies some but not all of the essential nutrients, thus some foods from each group should be eaten daily. The groups are:

1. Grains
2. Vegetables
3. Fruits
4. Oils
5. Milk
6. Meat and beans

In addition to the MyPyramid graphic, the United States Department of Agriculture (USDA) developed the USDA Food Guide 2005. This guide divides food into seven major groups and provides information on the most notable nutrients from each group, sorts them by nutrient density, and serving equivalents. A copy of this food guide is available at www.dietaryguidelines.gov.

1-1

2010 Dietary Guidelines Executive Summary

Eating and Physical activity patterns that are focused on consuming fewer calories, making informed food choices, and being physically active can help people attain and maintain a healthy body weight, reduce the risk of chronic disease, and promote overall health. The Dietary Guidelines for Americans, 2010 exemplifies these strategies through recommendations that accommodate the food preferences, cultural traditions, and customs of many diverse groups who live in the United States.

Dietary Guidelines for Americans is revised and updated if necessary, every 5 years. The U.S. Department of Agricultural (USDA) and U.S. Department of Health and Human Services (HHS) jointly create each edition.

Dietary Guidelines recommendations traditionally have been intended for healthy Americans ages 2 years and older. However, Dietary Guidelines for Americans 2010, is being released at a time of rising concern about the health of the American population. Poor diet and physical activity are the most important factors contributing to an epidemic of overweight and obesity affecting men, women, and children in all segments of our society. Even in the absence of overweight, poor diet, and physical inactivity are associated with the major causes of morbidity and morality in the United States. Therefore, the Dietary Guidelines for Americans, 2010 is intended for Americans 2 years and older, including those at increased risk of chronic disease.

Dietary Guidelines for Americans, 2010 also recognizes that in recent years nearly 15 percent of American households have been unable to acquire adequate food to meet their needs. This dietary guidance can help them maximize the nutritional content of their meals. Many other Americans consume less than optimal intake of certain nutrients even though they have adequate resources for a healthy diet.

The intent of the Dietary guidelines is to summarize knowledge about individual nutrients and food components into a interrelated set of recommendations for healthy eating that can be adopted by the public. Taken together, the Dietary Guidelines recommendations encompass two over arching concepts:

MAINTAIN CALORIE BALANCE OVER TIME TO ACHIEVE AND SUSTAIN A HEALTHY WEIGHT

People who are most successful at achieving and maintaining a healthy weight do so through continuing attention to consuming only enough calories from food and beverages to meet their needs and by being physically active. To curb the obesity epidemic and improve healthy, many Americans must decrease the calories they consume and increase the calories they expend through physical activity.

FOCUS ON CONSUMING NUTRIENT-DENSE FOODS AND BEVERAGES

Americans currently consume too much sodium and too many calories from solid fats, added sugars, and refined grains. These replace nutrient-dense foods and beverages and make it more difficult for people to achieve recommended nutrient intake while controlling calorie and sodium intake. A healthy eating pattern limits intake of sodium, solid fats, added sugars and refined grains and emphasizes nutrient dense foods and beverages – vegetables, fruits, whole grains, fat-free or low-fat milk products, seafood, lean meats and poultry, eggs, beans and peas, and nuts and seeds.

The following are the Dietary Guidelines for Americans 2010 Key Recommendations:

BALANCING CALORIES TO MANAGE WEIGHT

- Prevent and/or reduce e overweight and obesity through Improved eating and physical activity behaviors
- Control total calorie intake to manage body weight,. For people who are overweight or obese, this will mean consuming fewer calories from foods and beverages
- Increase physical activity and reduce time spent in sedentary behaviors.
- Maintain appropriate calorie balance during each stage of life-childhood, adolescence, adulthood, pregnancy, and breastfeeding, and older age.

FOOD AND FOOD COMPONENTS TO REDUCE

- Reduce daily sodium intake to less than 2,300 milligrams (mg) and further reduce intake to 1,500 mg among persons who are 51 and older and those of any age who are African American or have hypertenstion, diabetes, or chronic kidney disease. The 1,500 mg recommendations applies to about half of the U.S. population, including children, and the majority of adults.
- Consume less than 10 percent of calories from saturated fatty acids by replacing them with monounsaturated and polyunsaturated fatty acids.
- Keep *trans* fatty acid consumption as low as possible by limiting foods that contain synthetic sources of *trans* fats, such as partially hydrogenated oils, by limiting solid fats.
- Reduce the intake of calories from solid fats and added sugars.
- Limit the consumption of foods that contain refined grains, especially refined grain foods that contain solid fats, added sugars, and sodium.
- If alcohol is consumed, it should be consumed in moderation-up to one drink per day for woman and two drinks per day for men-and only by adults of legal drinking age.

Foods and Nutrient to Increase-Individuals should meet the following recommendations as part of a healthy eating pattern while staying within their caloric needs.

- Increase fruit and vegetable intake
- Eat a variety of vegetables, especially dark green and red and orange vegetables and beans and peas
- Consume at least half of all grains as whole grains. Increase whole grain intake by replacing refined grains with whole grains.
- Increase intake of fat-free or low-fat milk, and milk products, such as milk, yogurt, cheese, or fortified soy beverages.
- Increase the amount and variety of seafood consumed by choosing seafood in place of some meat and poultry.
- Replace protein foods that are higher in solid fats with choices that are lower in solid fats and calories and/or sources of oils.
- Choose foods that provide more potasssium, dietary fiber, calcium, and vitamin D, which are nutrients of concern in American diets. These foods include vegetables, fruits, whole grains, and milk and milk products.

Clinical Application—cont'd 1-1

BUILDING HEALTHY EATING PATTERNS

- Select an eating pattern that meets nutrient needs over time at an appropriate calorie level.
- Account for all foods and beverages consumed and assess how they fit within a total healthy eating pattern.
- Follow food safety recommendations when preparing and eating foods to reduce the risk of foodborne illnesses

RECOMMENDATIONS FOR SPECFIC POPULATION GROUPS

Women capable of becoming pregnant:

- Choose foods that supply heme, iron, which is more readily absorbed by the body, additional iron sources, and enhancers of iron absorption such as vitamin C rish foods.
- Consume 400 micrograms (mcg) per day of synthetic folic acid (from fortified foods and/or supplements) in addition to food forms of folate from a varied diet.

Women who are pregnant or breastfeeding

- Consume 8 to 12 ounces of seafood per week from a variety of seafood sources.
- Due to their high methyl mercury content, limit white (albacore) tuna to 6 ounces per week and do not eat the following 4 types of fish: tilefish, shark, swordfish, and king mackerel.
- If pregnant. Take an iron supplement, as recommended by an obstetrician or other health care provider

Individuals ages 50 years and older

- Consume foods fortified with vitamin B 12, such as fortified cereals, or dietary supplements.

SOURCE: *Dietary Guidelines for Americans, 2010.*
http://www.cnpp.usda.gov/DietaryGuidelines.htm

Keystones

- Nutrition is the science of food.
- Nutrients provide fuel, support tissue growth and maintenance, and regulate body processes.
- A nutrient is called essential if the body requires it and cannot manufacture it in sufficient amounts to meet bodily needs.
- Phytochemicals and zoochemicals are chemical constitutents in food that have also been found to play major roles in good health.
- Nutrigenomics is the study of how nutrition influences the body's software, or genetic code.
- Health is a state of complete physical, mental, and social well-being, not just the absence of disease or infirmity. Optimal health is not possible with an inferior diet.
- The principles of nutrition are applied by the health-care team to promote health and treat many diseases.
- A balanced diet is vital for physical growth and development, optimal body composition, mental development, and disease prevention.
- The *Dietary Guidelines* are based on the lastest scientific information.
- The MyPyramid food guidance system was developed to help consumers make wise food choices and is based on the *Dietary Guidelines for Americans*.
- USDA Food Guide 2005 provides detailed information on how to select nutritious foods wisely.

Chapter Review

1. Women's bodies normally contain more ___ and less ___ than men's bodies.
   a. Carbohydrate, protein
   b. Fat, protein
   c. Protein, ash
   d. Water, fat
2. Malnutrition occurs as a result or part of:
   a. The aging process
   b. A low income
   c. Infirmity
   d Overnutrition
3. Which of the following is not one of the traditional groups of nutrients?
   a. Zoochemicals
   b. Vitamins
   c. Minerals
   d. Proteins
4. An example of an energy nutrient is:
   a. Water
   b. Fat
   c. Vitamins
   d. Minerals
5. The health-care team member who specializes in swallowing disorders is a:
   a. Registered nurse
   b. Physician
   c. Speech therapist
   d. Medical assistant

Clinical Analysis

1. Mrs. A believes she can cleanse her body of toxic compounds by abstaining from all food for 10 days. You should:
   a. Tell Mrs. A she needs to drink extra fluids for this approach to succeed.
   b. Ignore Mrs. A because you think she will not listen to you.
   c. Pretend to agree with Mrs. A. because you do not want to make her angry.
   d. Explain to Mrs. A the importance of variety, balance, and moderation in the diet.
2. Mr. and Mrs. J are members of a local fitness club and have recently had their body fat content analyzed. Mr. J expresses concern because his wife's body fat content (20%) is higher than his body fat content (15%). He asks, "Why is there a difference?" An appropriate response would be:
   a. A normally active woman has a body fat content between 18% and 22%.
   b. A normally active woman has a body fat content between 15% and 19%, so his wife should exercise more.
   c. A person's body fat content is not that important.
   d. If his wife would increase her protein intake, her body fat content would decrease.
3. The health-care educator is talking to Ms. S about her excessive weight gain. Which of the following is incorrect to say?
   a. For some people, 60 to 90 minutes of moderate to vigorous physical acitivity each day is often necessary to manage body weight.
   b. It is important to eat foods high in nutrient-density during weight loss.
   c. Milk chocolate is a good subsitute for milk because it is in the same food group.
   d. As most people get older it is important to have small decreases in food and beverage intake and increased physical activity to prevent weight gain.

2

Individualizing Client Care

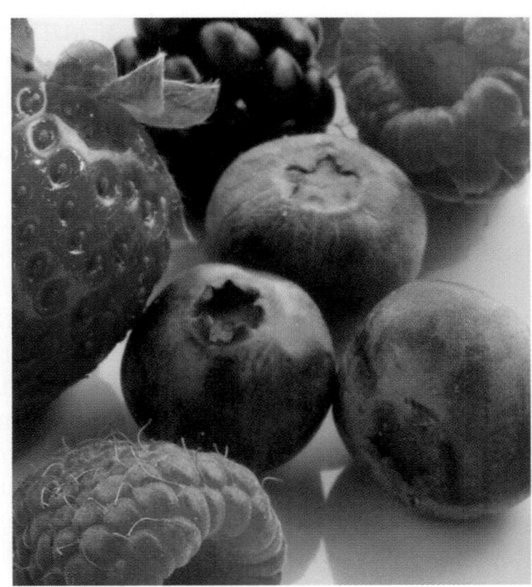

LEARNING OBJECTIVES

After completing this chapter, the student should be able to:

- Define the terminology used in nutrition assessment.
- Describe methods of nutrition assessment.
- Demonstrate the use of three techniques to analyze dietary status.
- Describe the dietary exchange system and identify the exchange lists of foods.
- Identify components of the health belief systems that affect the nutrition of large cultural groups.
- Explain the components of various religious customs that affect individual food intake.
- Discuss strategies to provide culturally competent nutritional care.

This chapter introduces the terminology and methodology used for measuring and evaluating nutritional status. Because cultural traditions influence the way that people regard certain foods and the effects of those foods on health, the last section of this chapter covers culturally competent care.

Fictional case studies throughout this book integrate the steps of the nutritional care process: **assessment** or data collection, **analysis** yielding a **diagnosis, planning** for desired outcomes, **implementation** of the plan, and **evaluation.**

Terminology

Nurses and dietitians have defined the terminology used in the practice of their professions. Knowledge of this terminology will help students understand the clinical examples in the remaining chapters.

Standardized Languages

Computerized information systems hold great potential for collecting and analyzing data pertaining to health care. For the system to work, however, the data must be in an appropriate form. Words must have standardized meanings regardless of the health-care setting. Institutions have adapted various standardized languages to incorporate health-care providers' documentation in an electronic patient record.

Nutritional Terms

Nutritional status refers to the body's condition as it relates to the intake and use of nutrients. All members of the health-care team have roles in the effective evaluation of a client's nutritional status.

Dietary status describes what a client has been eating. Although a client's dietary status may be adequate, his or her nutritional status may be poor. An evaluation of a client's dietary status can help to determine the reason for this poor nutritional status, or it may rule out poor diet as the source of the client's problem.

Two levels of methodology are commonly used to identify clients at nutritional risk. Box 2-1, a validated screening tool, is an example of the first level of nutritional care, screening, used to quickly identify persons at nutritional risk.

A nutritional screening should be brief enough that the information can be gathered in a short time. The time to administer the tool presented in Box 2-1 may be extremely brief because if one factor is found to be present, the screening is stopped and the client is declared at nutritional risk and referred to a dietitian.

More comprehensive than screening, a nutritional assessment is the second level of methodology. A **nutritional assessment** is the evaluation of a client's nutritional status (nutrient stores) based on a physical examination, **anthropometric measurements,** laboratory data, and food intake information. Many members of the health-care team are involved in a comprehensive nutritional assessment, including the physician, dietitian, nurse, social worker, and laboratory staff.

Because it requires many resources, this second level of nutritional care is usually completed only in the cases of clients at high nutritional risk. For example, a surgeon may order a comprehensive nutritional assessment before surgery to determine whether the client could tolerate a procedure better after nutritional rehabilitation.

Assessment

The first and most basic step of the nutritional care process is assessment. An organized and systematic search for pertinent subjective and objective data (Table 2-1) creates a sound foundation upon which to build health care.

Subjective Data

Subjective data as they relate to nutrition include the client's history from an interview or questionnaire. When more detailed food intake information is required, one of the five techniques listed in Table 2-2 may be used. Some of the advantages and disadvantages of each are given. For sample assessment tools, see DavisPlus.

Neither reported dietary intake nor any other item of assessment data is suitable to use as the sole criterion of nutritional status.

Box 2-1 ■ *Admission Nutrition Screening Tool*

A. Diagnosis

If the patient has at least ONE of the following diagnoses, circle and proceed to section E to consider the patient AT NUTRITIONAL RISK and stop here.

Anorexia nervosa/bulimia nervosa
Malabsorption (celiac sprue, ulcerative colitis, Crohn's disease, short bowel syndrome)
Multiple trauma (closed-head injury, penetrating trauma, multiple fractures)
Decubitus ulcers
Major gastrointestinal surgery within the past year
Cachexia (temporal wasting, muscle wasting, cancer, cardiac)
Coma
Diabetes
End-stage liver disease
End-stage renal disease
Nonhealing wounds

B. Nutrition Intake History

If the patient has at least ONE of the following symptoms, circle and proceed to section E to consider the patient AT NUTRITIONAL RISK and stop here.

Diarrhea (>500 mL 2 days)
Vomiting (>5 days)
Reduced intake (<½ normal intake for >5 days)

C. Ideal Body Weight Standards

Compare the patient's current weight for height to the ideal body weight chart. If at <80% of ideal body weight, proceed to section E to consider the patient AT NUTRITIONAL RISK and stop here.

D. Weight History

Any recent unplanned weight loss? No _______ Yes _______
Amount (lb or kg) _______
If yes, within the past _______ weeks or _______ months ____
Current weight (lb or kg) _______
Usual weight (lb or kg) _______
Height (ft, in., or cm) _______

Find percentage of weight lost:

$$\frac{\text{Usual Wt} - \text{Current Wt}}{\text{Usual Wt}} \times 100 = \%\ \text{Wt Loss}$$

Compare the % wt loss with the chart values and circle appropriate value

Length of time	Significant (%)	Severe (%)
1 week	1–2	>2
2–3 weeks	2–3	>3
1 month	4–5	>5
3 months	7–8	>8
5+ months	10	>10

If the patient has experienced a significant or severe weight loss, proceed to section E and consider the patient AT NUTRITIONAL RISK.

E. Nurse Assessment

Using the above criteria, what is this patient's nutritional risk? (check one)

_______ LOW NUTRITIONAL RISK
_______ AT NUTRITIONAL RISK

From Kovacevich et al. (1997, p 22), with permission.

TABLE 2-1 ■ Sample Subjective and Objective Nutritional Data

SUBJECTIVE	OBJECTIVE
Usual diet and fluid intake	Accurate actual height and weight
Number of meals per day	Body build or frame
Last meal: time, foods, beverages, and amounts	Skin **turgor** and/or dryness
Food and nutrient supplements	Condition of teeth and gums
Appetite	Hair quantity and quality
Problems with digestion and/or elimination	Body fat measurements
Allergies or food intolerances	Complete blood count
Usual alcohol consumption	Serum albumin
Chewing and swallowing problems	Serum electrolytes
Use of dentures	
Usual weight and recent changes	
Likes and dislikes	

Objective Data

A physical examination can include general appearance, anthropomorphic measurements, and laboratory or other diagnostic tests.

General Appearance

Well-nourished people generally look healthy and usually have an optimistic perspective. Table 2-3 compares the appearance of a well-nourished individual with that of an individual who is less well nourished. A person need not display all of the abnormal signs listed to be regarded as malnourished.

Anthropometric Data

For clinical purposes, body size, weight, and proportions are determined by **anthropometry,** the science

TABLE 2-2 ■ Commonly Used Techniques to Obtain Food Intake Information

TECHNIQUE	ADVANTAGES	DISADVANTAGES
Comparison With the MyPyramid Model Health-care provider asks client what he or she eats and compares this reported food intake with MyPyramid Model.	Can be used to screen many clients quickly. Requires a minimally trained interviewer.	Is not comprehensive. May overlook some clients who would benefit from nutritional care.
Food Frequency Questionnaire Health-care provider requests client fill out a questionnaire asking about **usual food intake** during specified times, such as "What do you usually eat for breakfast?"	Questionnaire can be tailored to particular nutrients of interest (e.g., lactose, gluten). May assess food usage for any length of time: day, week, month, weekends versus weekdays, summer versus winter, etc. Initial client contact does not require a highly trained interviewer.	May require special resources (e.g., computerized database) to evaluate the information collected. Provides limited information on a client's food behaviors such as shopping and preparation, meal spacing, length of usual mealtime, etc.
Food Records Health-care provider asks client to record his or her food intake for a specified length of time (1, 3, or 7 days).	A motivated client will provide reasonably accurate information. Research shows some clients will change their food habits while keeping a food record; therefore, this technique works well when a behavior change is desired.	A less highly motivated client will "forget to keep" part or all of the food record or record questionable amounts. Conversely, this technique could yield inaccurate data to determine a client's actual dietary and/or nutritional status. May require special resources (e.g., a computerized database) to evaluate the information obtained. Requires a follow-up visit to review the evaluated food records. Analysis of data is time-consuming.
24-Hour Dietary Recall Health-care provider asks client what he or she has eaten during the previous 24 hours.	Is fairly simple. Interviewer should be trained not to ask leading questions.	Yields limited information. The previous 24 hours may not have been usual for the client. Typically, clients may not remember what they ate and the amounts they ate. Estimates of amounts are frequently inaccurate.
Diet History Health-care provider conducts an in-depth interview to obtain information about usual food intake, drug and medication usage, alcohol and tobacco use, financial and physical ability to obtain food, special dietary needs, food allergies and intolerances, weight history, cultural and religious preferences that may influence food selection, ability to chew and swallow foods, previous dietary instructions received, client knowledge about nutrition, and elimination patterns.	Is comprehensive. Requires a highly trained interviewer, usually a dietitian. An analysis of the results obtained can usually be provided on the same day the information is collected. Is a good technique for high-risk clients when information is needed to evaluate the need for nutritional support and the likelihood of dietary prescriptions being implemented.	Is highly dependent on the willingness of the client to reveal information to the interviewer. Client must be a good historian. Is time-consuming.

TABLE 2-3 ■ General Appearance as an Indicator of Nutritional Status

	NORMAL	ABNORMAL
Demeanor	Alert, responsive Positive outlook	Lethargic Negative attitude
Weight	Reasonable for build	Underweight Overweight, obese
Hair	Glossy, full, firmly rooted Uniform color	Dull, sparse; easily, painlessly plucked
Eyes	Bright, clear, shiny	Pale conjunctiva Redness, dryness
Lips	Smooth	Chapped, red, swollen
Tongue	Deep red Slightly rough One longitudinal furrow	Bright red, purple Swollen or shrunken Several longitudinal furrows
Teeth	Bright, painless	Caries, painful, mottled, or missing
Gums	Pink, firm	Spongy, bleeding, receding
Skin	Clear, smooth, firm, slightly moist	Rashes, swelling Light or dark spots Dry, cracked
Nails	Pink, firm	Spoon shaped or ridged Spongy bases
Mobility	Erect posture Good muscle tone Walks without pain or difficulty	Muscle wasting Skeletal deformities Loss of balance

of measuring the body. Such measurements are used to determine growth, body composition, and nutritional status. The body's energy and protein stores also can be derived from these measurements.

The collection of anthropometric data on height and weight—**triceps skinfold,** midarm circumference, abdominal circumference, and waist and hip measurements—is described briefly in the following sections. Other measurements may also be selected.

HEIGHT AND WEIGHT

Height may be measured in inches or centimeters. Adults and older children are measured standing with head erect; infants and young children are measured lying on a firm, flat surface.

Weight may be recorded in pounds or kilograms. The agency policy regarding calibration of the scale should be followed. Each time the client is weighed, it should be on the same scale at the same time of the day, and the client should be wearing the same kind of clothing.

TRICEPS SKINFOLD

The measurement of subcutaneous tissue over the triceps muscle in the upper arm provides an estimate of the amount of body fat. The **triceps skinfold** measurement helps to differentiate between a person who is heavy because of muscle mass and one who is heavy because of excess fat.

The ability to take accurate measurements requires practice. Typically research designs require the same researcher to take all measurements and record the average of two or three values at each site. Body areas other than the triceps can also be used to measure skinfolds. Although dietitians usually take skinfold measurements, other health-care providers need to be able to answer clients' questions regarding the procedure and the information obtained from it.

MIDARM CIRCUMFERENCE

Because 50% of the body's protein stores are located in muscle tissue, the circumference (circumference is the outside edge of a circle) of the midarm provides information about body protein stores. The upper arm is measured between the shoulder and the elbow. The **midarm circumference** measurement is easily obtained and can be used to monitor a client's progress.

BODY FRAME SIZE

Wrist measurement is one method of categorizing a person's frame that requires no tools or references. Have the client wrap the thumb and middle finger of one hand around the smallest part of the opposite wrist. The body frame size is designated:

- Small if the digits overlap by 1 centimeter or more
- Medium if the thumb and middle finger touch
- Large if the gap between digits is 1 centimeter or more.

An alternate method requiring measurements is shown in Clinical Calculation 2-1.

ABDOMINAL CIRCUMFERENCE

The measurement of the abdomen, in inches or centimeters, is often taken at the umbilicus (belly button). **Abdominal circumference (girth)** provides information when an individual is accumulating fluid in the abdominal cavity, a condition called **ascites.** Girth is also measured to monitor growth of a fetus or of abnormal tissue within the abdomen.

WAIST AND HIP MEASUREMENTS

Within an agency, a standard procedure should be used for waist and hip measurements. With the person standing, the waist is measured at the narrowest site and the hips are measured at the greatest circumference. The tissue should not be compressed.

BODY DENSITY MEASURES

Muscle and fat tissue have different rates of metabolism. Therefore, the proportions of each in the body

Clinical Calculation 2-1

Measure the smallest part of the wrist between the wrist bones and the hand. If the person's height is not known, measure him or her, in feet and inches, without shoes. Taking that information, look at the chart below. Find the person's height on the left and wrist size at the bottom, and compare the shaded area with the boxes at the bottom. As an example, find the frame size of a person who is 5 ft 4 in. and has a wrist circumference of 6¼ in. (The person has a medium frame.)

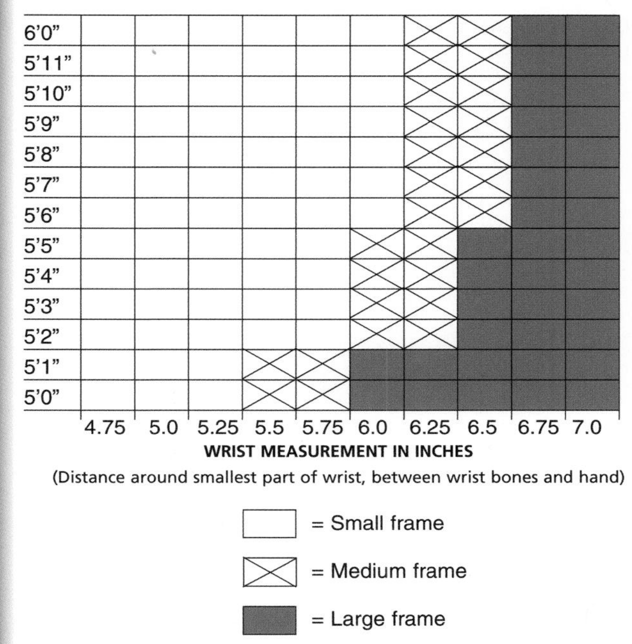

influence whether a person is overweight. These proportions can be determined by several techniques, including underwater weighing, dual-energy x-ray absorptiometry, and bioelectrical impedance.

Underwater weighing compares the person's scale weight with his or her weight underwater. After correcting for lung volume, the examiner calculates the proportion of body fat. Underwater weighing provides the most accurate assessment of the amount of fat in the body. It is not easily determined, however. Even in research studies, several measurements must be taken and averaged to obtain a value that minimizes error. Because the technique is cumbersome and time consuming and requires special equipment, its main use is in research.

In **dual-energy x-ray absorptiometry (DEXA),** two x-ray beams are passed through the body. The amount of energy detected after the beams pass through the body varies with bone, fat, and muscle tissue. DEXA has been validated against underwater weighing and is another research tool (Daniels, Khoury, and Morrison, 1997). In clinical practice, DEXA is used to measure bone mineral density as an indicator of conditions marked by bone loss, such as osteopenia and osteoporosis (see Chapter 8). A screening test to determine a person's level of risk for those conditions can be conducted with an **ultrasound bone densitometer** that involves no radiation exposure.

In the **bioelectrical impedance test,** electrodes on the extremities are stimulated. The greater electrolyte content and conductivity of the body's **fat-free mass** is compared with that of fat or bone. Tissues rich in water and electrolytes allow an electrical current to pass with greater ease than do denser fat and bone (Heymsfield, Nunez, and Pietrobelli, 1997). Measurements are not painful and usually are not felt because the frequencies used do not stimulate nerves and muscles (Jacobs, 1997).

Body composition is predicted in the bioelectrical impedance test from a measure of total body water. The client's fat-free mass is predicted, and his or her percentage of body fat is determined by comparing body weight with the predicted fat-free mass. The three measurements obtained are percentage of:

1. Body water
2. Lean body mass
3. Body fat

Bioelectrical impedance tends to overestimate percentage of body fat in lean subjects and underestimate it in obese persons (Sun et al., 2005). However, bioelectrical impedance spectroscopy correctly estimated average fat free mass in healthy 75-year-old Swedes (Tengvall et al., 2009). Because bioelectrical impedance is based on total body water, any factors disturbing water balance may alter the results. Examples are diuretic use, excessive sweating, hemodialysis, premenstrual edema, and alcohol consumption within the 24 hours before the test.

Laboratory Tests

Laboratory tests analyze body fluids and excretions. These data include results from blood, urine, and stool tests. From these tests, much information can be obtained concerning what a person has eaten, what his or her body has stored, and how the body is using nutrients.

Blood can be analyzed for glucose, protein, or fat content. Vitamin and mineral status can be determined directly by examining the blood or indirectly by examining enzymes related to the vitamin or mineral. Many experts doubt, however, that vitamin or mineral body stores can be accurately determined by blood samples. The uncertainty lies in whether the nutrient in the blood reflects body stores, a transport form of the nutrient, or the amount in one specific body compartment.

Good clinical judgment must be used in selecting tests and interpreting results. Reliance upon a single test or single reading is not recommended.

Analysis

The health-care provider uses subjective or objective data or both to identify the level of the client's wellness regarding nutrition. The client's physical findings are compared with standard nutritional parameters. His or her dietary intake is compared to that recommended for his or her age and activity level.

Basic Nutritional Parameters

Commonly used standards include height–weight tables, body mass index, and waist measurements.

Height–Weight Tables

Many height–weight tables are currently in use, each based on a different underlying assumption. Table 2-4

TABLE 2-4 ■ Metropolitan Life Insurance Company Height–Weight Table

MEN (INDOOR CLOTHING†)								
HEIGHT (IN SHOES*)			SMALL FRAME		MEDIUM FRAME		LARGE FRAME	
Feet	Inches	Centimeters	Pounds	Kilograms	Pounds	Kilograms	Pounds	Kilograms
5	2	157.5	128–134	58.2–60.9	131–141	59.5–64.1	138–150	62.7–68.2
5	3	160.0	130–136	59.1–61.8	133–143	60.4–65.0	140–153	63.6–69.5
5	4	162.6	132–138	60.0–62.7	135–145	61.4–65.9	142–156	64.5–70.9
5	5	165.1	134–140	60.9–63.6	137–148	62.3–67.2	144–160	65.5–72.7
5	6	167.6	136–142	61.8–64.5	139–151	63.2–68.6	146–164	66.4–74.5
5	7	170.2	138–145	62.7–65.9	142–154	64.5–70.0	149–168	67.7–76.4
5	8	172.7	140–148	63.6–67.2	145–157	65.9–71.4	152–172	69.1–78.2
5	9	175.3	142–151	64.5–68.6	148–160	67.2–72.7	155–176	70.5–80.0
5	10	177.8	144–154	65.5–70.0	151–163	68.6–74.1	158–180	71.8–81.8
5	11	180.3	146–157	66.4–71.4	154–166	70.0–75.5	161–184	73.2–83.6
6	0	182.9	149–160	67.7–72.7	157–170	71.4–77.3	164–188	74.5–85.5
6	1	185.4	152–164	69.1–74.0	160–174	72.7–79.1	168–192	76.4–87.3
6	2	188.0	155–168	70.5–76.4	164–178	74.5–80.9	172–197	78.2–89.5
6	3	190.5	158–172	71.8–78.2	167–182	75.9–82.7	176–202	80.0–91.8
6	4	193.0	162–176	73.6–80.0	171–187	77.7–85.0	181–207	82.3–94.1
WOMEN (INDOOR CLOTHING†)								
HEIGHT (IN SHOES*)			SMALL FRAME		MEDIUM FRAME		LARGE FRAME	
Feet	Inches	Centimeters	Pounds	Kilograms	Pounds	Kilograms	Pounds	Kilograms
4	10	147.3	102–111	46.4–50.0	109–121	49.5–55.0	118–131	53.6–59.5
4	11	149.9	103–113	46.8–51.4	111–123	50.0–55.9	120–134	54.5–60.9
5	0	152.4	104–115	47.3–52.3	113–126	51.4–57.2	122–137	55.5–62.3
5	1	154.9	106–118	48.2–53.6	115–129	52.3–58.6	125–140	56.8–63.6
5	2	157.5	108–121	49.1–55.0	118–132	53.6–60.0	128–143	58.2–65.0
5	3	160.0	111–124	50.5–56.4	121–135	55.0–61.4	131–147	59.5–66.8
5	4	162.6	114–127	51.8–57.7	124–138	56.4–62.7	134–151	60.9–68.6
5	5	165.1	117–130	53.2–59.0	127–141	57.7–64.1	137–155	62.3–70.5
5	6	167.6	120–133	54.5–60.5	130–144	59.0–65.5	140–159	63.6–72.3
5	7	170.2	123–136	55.9–61.8	133–147	60.5–66.8	143–163	65.0–74.1
5	8	172.7	126–139	57.3–63.2	136–150	61.8–68.2	146–167	66.4–75.9
5	9	175.3	129–142	58.6–64.5	139–153	63.2–69.5	149–170	67.7–77.3
5	10	177.8	132–145	60.0–65.9	142–156	64.6–70.9	152–173	69.1–78.6
5	11	180.3	135–148	61.4–67.3	145–159	65.9–72.3	155–176	70.5–80.0
6	0	182.9	138–151	62.7–73.6	148–162	67.3–73.6	158–179	71.8–81.4

*Shoes with 1-in. heels.

†Allow 3 lb.

NOTE: The weights presented are those associated with the lowest mortality. They are not necessarily the weights of which people are healthiest, perform their jobs optimally, or even look their best.

SOURCE: Reprinted courtesy of Met Life Insurance Company, Statistical Bulletin, 1983, with permission.

shows the Metropolitan Life Insurance table, which lists weights for height based on the lowest mortality (but it is not certain that the specified weights in this table are equated with maximum health). A reliable height–weight table should stipulate allowable shoe heel height and the weight of clothing. The information from height–weight tables is used to calculate a person's percentage of **healthy body weight (HBW).** If a range of weights is given, the midpoint of the range is used. Clinical Calculation 2-2 illustrates the process.

Body Mass Index

The **body mass index (BMI)** is derived from weight and height (BMI = weight in kilograms divided by (height in meters)^2). It can also be calculated with reasonable accuracy using common American measures as shown below.

1. Multiply weight in pounds by 705.
2. Divide the result by height in inches.
3. Divide the second result by height in inches.

BMI was designed to provide a measure of weight independent of height. Although the BMI has been used as an indicator of obesity, it fails to distinguish **adipose tissue** from muscle or water weight.

Chapter 16 contains a table listing BMIs for weights at various heights. In general, the following classifications are used:

- BMI of 18 or less: Underweight
- BMI of 19 to 24: Normal
- BMI of 25 to 29: Overweight
- BMI of 30 to 39: Obese
- BMI of 40 or greater: Morbidly obese

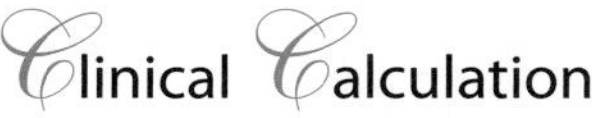

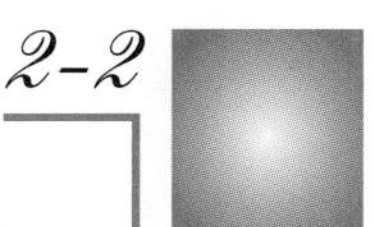

Percent Healthy Body Weight

The formula for calculating percent healthy body weight (HBW) is:

$$\frac{\text{Client's Wt}}{\text{Weight from Table}} \times 100 = \text{Percent Healthy Body Wt}$$

For example, according to the height–weight table (Table 2-4), a 5 ft 5 in. woman with a medium frame has a range of 130 to 144 lb, including 3 lb of clothing. Assuming she is 5 ft 5 in. barefoot, the table is entered at 5 ft 6 in. to allow for 1-in. heels. The midpoint of the range is 137 lb.

If the woman weighed 137 lb, her HBW would be 100%. If she weighed 159 lb, her HBW would be 116%, calculated as follows:

$$159 \text{ lb}/137 \text{ lb} \times 100 = 116\%$$

Someone with 90% HBW is considered underweight. A person at 111–119% HWB is overweight. A person at 120% HWB or greater is obese.

Waist Measurements

Waist circumferences of more than 40 inches in men and 35 inches in women are related to increased risk of cardiovascular disease. Similarly, waist-to-hip ratios (WHR) greater than 0.8 in women and greater than 0.95 in men indicate increased risk of problems related to obesity. To attain **waist-to-hip ratio (WHR),** the waist measurement is divided by the hip measurement.

The chances of developing health problems are increased when a person is overly fat. Excess body fat is correlated with cardiovascular disease, the most common form of diabetes, certain cancers, and other illnesses.

Analysis of a Client's Dietary Intake

A client's reported or recorded food intake can be grouped according to the classifications in MyPyramid, or individual foods can be analyzed using a table of food composition or a computerized diet analysis program.

Analysis by Food Groups

A simple method of comparing a client's reported intake with that recommended for him is to focus on the food groups found in MyPyramid as described in Chapter 1. Errors might occur if amounts consumed are estimated rather than measured.

Analysis of Nutrients

More detailed information can be obtained by examining foods for their component nutrients and comparing the client's data to Dietary Reference Intakes (described later). This process can be performed manually or electronically.

The U.S. Department of Agriculture (USDA) publishes a food composition table entitled Nutritive Values of the Edible Part of Foods (abridged in DavisPlus). The entire database can be searched at http://www.nal.usda.gov/fnic/foodcomp/search.

Many computer software programs are available for comparing an individual's nutrient intake with that recommended for someone of the same age and gender. Some of the programs include height, weight, and activity level.

Whether analyzed manually or electronically, care must be taken when selecting food items. For example, selection of "orange juice concentrate" instead of "orange juice" will skew the analysis.

Regardless of the process used, the information gained needs correct interpretation. The only scientifically correct statement to be made is that the intake for a given period does or does not meet the RDA. It is inappropriate to base a judgment of nutritional or dietary status solely on a comparison to the RDA.

Planning

Having assessed and analyzed a client's nutritional status, the next step is to plan a strategy that addresses identified problems to treat or strengths to reinforce. The strategy may include referral to a dietitian.

Determine the Best Provider

A fundamental decision during planning is whether to treat the client's nutritional problems within the nursing department or the dietary department. When the nurse chooses to treat the client's nutritional problems, the nurse and client must prioritize the problems and select acceptable interventions. Making one or two changes may be easier for the client to sustain than overhauling the client's entire diet. For that reason, selecting the interventions most likely to make a major difference in the client's health status is important.

A nurse is likely to refer the client to a dietitian if the nutritional problem is severe or complex. A lack of nursing time and resources also may necessitate a referral. The referral system has two functions:

1. Ensuring comprehensive care
2. Increasing awareness of the need for and benefits of nutritional services

Dietary Reference Intakes

Additional standards used to plan nutritional care are the Dietary Reference Intakes (DRIs). Part of the DRIs are the Recommended Dietary Allowances. When first promoted, the Recommended Dietary Allowances (RDAs) focused on preventing deficiency diseases. Recent research supports a role for certain nutrients in reducing the risk of chronic diseases. This information was included in the new standards for North America (National Academy of Sciences, 1997a, 1997b, 1997c). In addition to RDAs for vitamins and minerals, DRIs have been established for the macronutrients (carbohydrate, fat, and protein) and for water and electrolytes.

Dietary Reference Intakes (DRIs) are composed of five nutrient-based reference values that can be used for assessing and planning diets for groups according to life-stage and gender. The DRIs are intended to apply to the healthy general population and refer to average daily intakes for one or more weeks. The components of the DRIs are:

- **Estimated Average Requirements (EARs)**: Intake that meets the estimated nutrient needs of 50% of the individuals in the defined group. EAR is used to set the RDA and to assess or plan the intake of groups.
- **Recommended Dietary Allowances (RDAs)**: Intake that meets the needs of 97% to 98% of individuals in the defined group. RDA is intended for use as a goal for daily intake by individuals, not for assessing the adequacy of an individual's nutrient intake.
- **Adequate Intakes (AIs):** Average observed or experimentally determined intake that appears sufficient to meet individuals in the stated group. AI is used if an EAR or RDA cannot be set because of lack of information.
- **Acceptable Macronutrient Distribution Range (AMDR):** Percentage of kilocalories (see Chapter 6 for information on kilocalories) from carbohydrate, fat, and protein associated with reduced risk of chronic disease while still providing sufficient intake of essential nutrients. Only the AMDR for protein has been set with the certainty of the RDA. See Appendix A. Figure 2-1 illustrates a single meal that complies with the AMDR.

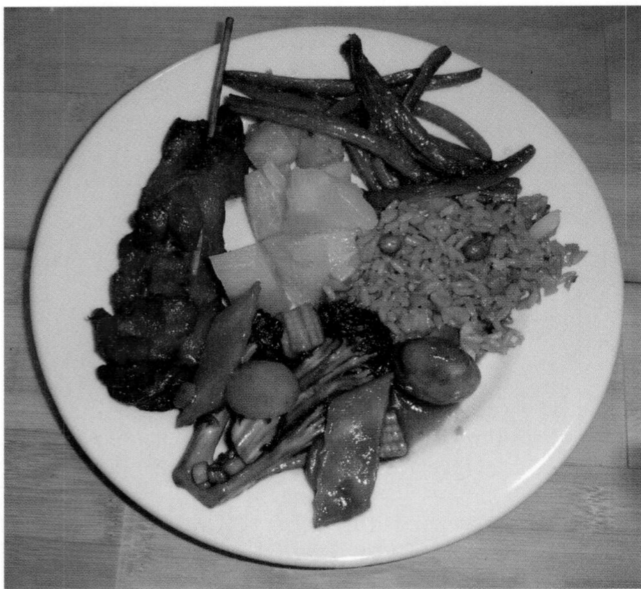

FIGURE 2-1 A plate from a Chinese buffet shows an acceptable distribution of macronutrients; however, the AMDRs and all the DRIs are recommendations for a week or longer.

- **Tolerable Upper Intake Levels (ULs):** Highest average daily intake by an individual that is unlikely to pose risks of adverse health effects in 97% to 98% of individuals in the defined group. Ordinarily the UL refers to intake from food, fortified food, water, and supplements; exceptions are footnoted in the table in Appendix A.

Because the RDAs and AIs represent the quantities of nutrients found in typical diets in the United States and Canada, caregivers must adjust their planning for clients who take supplements or follow very unusual diets. Similarly, clients with special needs may exceed the ULs as the use of higher levels of nutrients for specific purposes under the supervision of a health professional is beyond the scope of the ULs (Yates, 2006).

Table 2-5 compares and gives examples of these components of the DRIs. The Dietary Reference Intakes are listed in Appendix A.

Implementation

After assessment, diagnosis, and planning, the next step is implementation. It may take time and patience to select appropriate interventions for an individual client or family. Eating wisely or unwisely involves choices every day that affect the budget as well as health. See Dollars and Sense 2-1.

A given diet prescription may be implemented in various ways, but finding the approach a client will use faithfully is not only a challenge but also the key to success. Two food-based interventions include (1) MyPyramid and (2) the American Diabetes and Dietetic Associations' Exchange Lists.

TABLE 2-5 ■ Dietary Reference Intake Components

DRI	PERCENTAGE OF HEALTHY POPULATION INCLUDED	USE	EXAMPLES
EAR	50	Set RDAs Assess/plan for groups	Not applicable to individuals
RDA	97–98	Goal for individual daily intake	290 µg of iodine for lactating women
AI	Unknown	Goal for individuals Tentative goals for groups	Vitamin D amounts for all Most nutrients for infants
UL	97–98	Monitor potential excesses	45 mg of iron for all older than 14 years of age
AMDR	Not specified	Suggested allocation of kilocalories to optimize health	Protein should contribute 10%–35% of daily kilocalories for adults

Dollars & Sense 2-1

Choosing Snacks Wisely

Veggies as snacks are not only healthier than salty munchies, but also less costly and less kilocalorie dense.

Item	Price	Serving Size	Kilocalories	Cost/Serving
Potato chips, national brand	$3.99/9.5 oz	1 oz, about 11 chips	160	$0.42
Baby cut carrots, store brand	$1.69/lb	3 oz, about 13 carrots	35	$0.32

MyPyramid

In this strategy, amounts of foods are given in household measures rather than in servings, which could vary from person to person and permit overconsumption. For clients who wish to use it, the USDA interactive Web site permits tracking of a person's progress at http://www.mypyramidtracker.gov/.

American Diabetes and Dietetic Associations' Exchange Lists

Few foods contain just one nutrient but can be sorted into equivalent groups to simplify choices. The ADA **Exchange Lists,** published jointly by the American Diabetes and Dietetic Associations, are used to calculate a client's food intake, to educate a client about nutrition and meal planning, and to counsel a client about food choices. The lists are sometimes used to label frozen prepared meals. In addition, it is possible to approximate a client's carbohydrate, fat, protein, and kilocalorie intake with exchange lists.

The system is composed of six exchange lists of foods grouped by nutrient composition. For example, corn is on the starch list because it is closer in composition to a slice of bread than to green beans. The six basic lists are:

1. Starch
2. Fruit
3. Milk in three groups: skim, low fat, and whole
4. Vegetable
5. Meat in four groups: very lean, lean, medium fat, and high fat
6. Fat in three groups: monounsaturated, polyunsaturated, and saturated

Table 2-6 identifies typical foods in each exchange list. In addition, some foods are considered "free" and are permitted in large amounts because they contain little energy (few kilocalories). Free foods are on a separate list. Some free foods have limitations on the amount to be consumed in a day or at one time. In addition, combination foods (soups, casseroles) and selected fast foods appear on separate lists. An adaptation of the exchange list appears in Appendix B.

Table 2-7 displays the amount of carbohydrate, protein, fat, and kilocalories (energy) for one exchange on each list. As the table shows, one exchange on the fruit list is not equal to one exchange on the fat list. To use this method of meal planning correctly, clients must choose the correct number of items from each appropriate list.

In this context, ***exchange*** means a defined quantity of food within a list that can be interchanged with other foods in the same list. For example, one bread exchange is a single slice (a defined quantity); it might be exchanged, or swapped, with one-half a hamburger roll. In other words, individual food items within an exchange list are essentially equal in nutrient composition and can thus be exchanged, or swapped, for each other.

Portion sizes in the lists for various items have been adjusted to make each exchange approximately equal. Table 2-8 shows items equal to one starch exchange. Clearly, puffed cereal would be more filling than rice.

TABLE 2-6 ■ Typical Foods in Each Exchange List

EXCHANGE LIST	FOOD ITEMS
Starch	Cereals, grains, pasta, dried beans, peas, lentils, starchy vegetables, bread, crackers
Meat	Beef, pork, veal, poultry, fish, wild game, cheese, eggs, tofu, peanut butter
Fruit	Fresh, frozen, or unsweetened canned fruit; dried fruit; fruit juice
Vegetable	Raw or cooked nonstarchy vegetables, vegetable juices
Milk	Milk, yogurt, evaporated milk, powdered milk
Fat	Avocado, margarine, mayonnaise, nuts, seeds, oil, salad dressing, bacon, coconut, powdered coffee whitener, cream, sour cream, whipped cream, cream cheese

Adapted from: American Diabetes Association and American Dietetic Association (1995).

Using the Exchange Lists

Exchange lists can be adapted for any prescribed kilocalorie, protein, fat, or carbohydrate level. A specific meal plan for a client should be given with the exchange lists.

A meal plan is a food guide that shows the number of choices or exchanges the client should eat at each meal or snack. Table 2-9 illustrates meal plans for two different kilocalorie levels. The table also illustrates how the exchanges might be distributed among meals.

In summary, exchange lists and meal plans:

- Provide food choices that necessitate minimal calculation
- Control the distribution of nutrients throughout the day

TABLE 2-8 ■ Examples of One Starch Exchange

Puffed cereal	1½ cups
Bread	1 slice
Corn, whole kernel	½ cup
Rice, cooked	⅓ cup

Adapted from American Diabetes Association and American Dietetic Association (1995).

TABLE 2-7 ■ Energy Composition of the Six Exchange Lists

EXCHANGE LIST	CARBOHYDRATE (GRAMS)	PROTEIN (GRAMS)	FAT (GRAMS)	KILOCALORIES
Starch	15	3	0–1	80
Meat				
Very lean	0	7	0–1	35
Lean	0	7	3	55
Medium fat	0	7	5	75
High fat	0	7	8	100
Vegetable	5	2	0	25
Fruit	15	0	0	60
Milk				
Skim	12	8	0–3	90
2%	12	8	5	120
Whole	12	8	8	150
Fat (all)	0	0	5	45

SOURCE: The exchange lists are the basis of a meal planning system designed primarily for people with diabetes and others who must follow special diets. The exchange lists are based on principles of good nutrition that apply to everyone. © With permission 1995 American Diabetes Association and American Dietetic Association.

TABLE 2-9 ■ 1500- and 1800-kcal Meal Plan Using Exchanges for 1 Day

	1500 KCAL	1800 KCAL
Starch	7	7
Meat, lean	1	3
Meat, medium	3	3
Vegetable	4	5
Fruit	3	5
Milk, skim	2	2
Fat	6	7

DISTRIBUTION OF EXCHANGES THROUGHOUT THE DAY

1500-kcal Meal Plan

	Breakfast	Lunch	Dinner	Snack
Starch	2	2	2	1
Meat, lean	0	1	0	0
Meat, medium	0	0	3	0
Vegetable	0	2	2	0
Fruit	1	1	1	0
Milk, skim	1	0	0	1
Fat	2	2	2	0

Evaluation

After implementing a nutritional plan, the health-care provider and the client decide to what extent the objective has been met. If progress has been unsatisfactory, they explore the reasons, such as unrealistic expectations, not enough time elapsed, or interventions not appropriate or not implemented.

A diet can be measured against three criteria:

1. Balance; a **balanced diet** includes sufficient foods daily from each of the five major food groups (grains, vegetables, fruits, milk, and meat & beans).
2. Moderation; moderation means avoiding too much or too little of any one food or food group.
3. Variety; a varied diet contains many different foods within each major food group.

Documenting Nutritional Care

Agencies specify the format for documentation. One commonly used system is using SOAP notes. The letters stand for:

S : Subjective data (explained earlier)
O: Objective data (explained earlier)
A: Analysis or diagnosis based upon S and O data
P : Plan of action or treatment.

Within an agency, the client's problems may be numbered sequentially and each SOAP note is numbered to correspond to a specific problem. In other systems, each encounter with the client is treated separately.

Documentation of services provided is a basic requirement for all health-care providers. Employing a universal format facilitates communication among providers of various disciplines. The Teamwork Notes following the Case Studies in this text are written in the SOAP format.

Impact of Culture on Nutrition

Culture refers to human attitudes, beliefs, and customs shared by members of a particular group that guide their thoughts and actions. Although nation of origin, ethnic identity, and religious affiliation are prime examples of culture, other alliances such as colleges, corporations, professions, political parties, and service clubs also imbue people with values and behavioral norms.

Health practices draw together people of similar habits, such as athletes or vegetarians. Thus, some aspects of culture are passed on from birth, but other aspects are voluntarily selected. All aspects of culture, including the family's food ways, ethnicity, and religion, may influence an individual's food choices. Figure 2-2 shows a multigenerational birthday party shaped in part by culture.

Even among individuals of similar cultural heritage, differences exist. Dietary preferences, for example, differ among people of Hispanic descent from such diverse places as Cuba, Puerto Rico, and Mexico. Just because a person belongs to a certain ethnic or

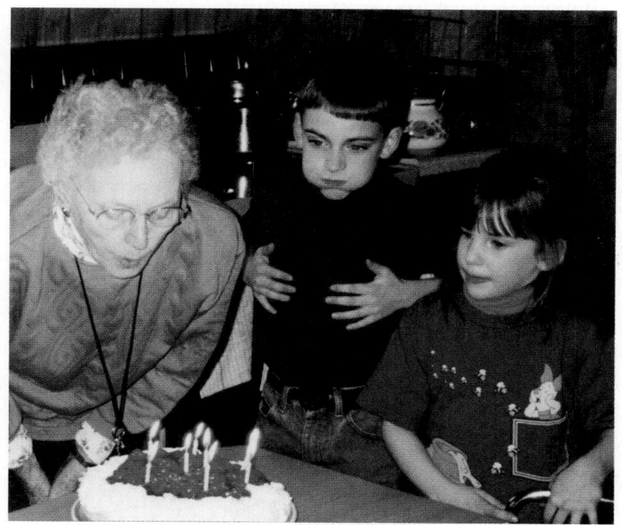

FIGURE 2-2 Many cultures have their own ways to observe life's milestones: births, birthdays, weddings, deaths. These children are sharing a birthday tradition with their 88-year-old great-grandmother.

religious group does not mean that he or she has adopted its traditional lifestyle and practices.

Caution is advised before replacing traditional food preparation techniques that have succeeded for generations; changes can sometimes cause disease. For example, botulism outbreaks were traced to substituting plastic bags for clay pots in preparing a Native American dish in Alaska and to substituting similar bags for waxed paper and wooden crates to ship smoked fish in Michigan. The plastic bags excluded air and permitted the botulism organism to produce its toxin. And mad cow disease spread after changes in feed production in England.

Ethnocentrism

The belief that one's own group's view of the world is superior to that of others is **ethnocentrism.** Historically, the dominant cultural group in the United States has been white descendants of northern Europeans who are middle class and Protestant. As a result, our health-care system reflects the important values of this culture:

- Education
- Work
- Punctuality
- Independence
- A future orientation

Health-care providers have tried, often unsuccessfully, to deliver this version of health care to clients without regard to the clients' cultures. Hence, clients who failed to achieve goals imposed on them were labeled "noncompliant." Clients unable to communicate in the dominant culture's language were defined as having "altered communication."

Acculturation

The process of adopting the values, attitudes, and behavior of another culture, **acculturation,** typically puts people at risk in their overall health. For example, among women of Mexican descent, lifetime residents of the United States were 2.4 times more likely to stop breastfeeding and 1.5 times more likely to stop exclusive breastfeeding than immigrants who had lived in the United States for five years or less (Harley, Stamm, and Eskenazi, 2007). Breastfeeding is the preferred method of infant nourishment but perhaps is perceived as old-fashioned by new residents of the United States. (See Chapters 10 and 11.)

Another adverse effect of acculturation is seen in the increase in various diseases in native populations. A major disease affecting widely scattered indigenous populations undergoing acculturation is type 2 diabetes mellitus. The world's highest incidence of the disease occurs in Pima Indians. In Australia, native people have 17 times the death rate from diabetes as that of non-indigenous persons (Shannon, 2002). Adopting the modern lifestyle, including dietary changes leading to obesity, is credited with worsening health status of native peoples.

Culturally Competent Care

Knowledge and acceptance of and respect for other cultures underpin culturally competent care. Even though health-care providers cannot be experts on every cultural group they encounter, they can develop an openness to learning the client's perspective. The goal is a treatment plan that successfully blends the client's cultural beliefs with the practices of modern medicine. Clinical Application 2-1 illustrates the adaptation of diabetic teaching to Native American mythology.

Food Preferences of Ethnic Groups

Food items considered appropriate for human consumption vary widely by culture and reflect economic and geographic constraints. Rituals of preparation may be culturally determined and allocation of food resources within a household may reflect the culture's values. Ethnic identity is important in determining staple foods, meal structure, and traditional holiday feasts.

Familiarity of cuisine may aid adaptation to unfamiliar circumstances. Among international postgraduate students in England, eating together was a

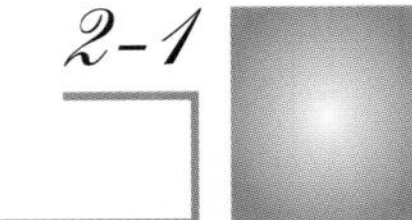

Using Ojibway Mythology in Diabetic Teaching

A Toronto program capitalized on Ojibway mythology to provide diabetes self-care instruction. The program was organized at the request of Native Canadians and included day-long educational workshops conducted by an elder. All participants sat in a circle, which confers equal status on every individual and represents harmony with nature.

The beginning focus was on Nanabush, a legendary teacher of the Ojibway who symbolizes moderation and balance. Traditional narratives show him conversing with Diabetes. The moral of the story is to learn about "Diabetes," to live with him, and to control one's life through spiritual strength. Workshop activities included exercise breaks and a buffet lunch that allowed participants to choose their meals.

Practitioners learned that avoiding a rigid diet prescription would enhance the individual's freedom, which was highly valued among the Ojibway (Hagey, 1984).

popular leisure activity, with food of home the most popular menu. Eating home country food offered emotional as well as physical sustenance (Brown, Edwards, and Hartwell, 2010).

In addition, certain foods may be culturally endorsed treatments for disease. For example, many cultures espouse variations of the "hot/cold" systems described below under Hispanic Americans and Chinese Americans. Also, foods traditionally given to children when they are sick may bring comfort to ill adults as well.

The following brief summaries describe traditional foods of five cultural groups and suggest possible applications for adapting nutritional needs to accommodate these preferences.

African Americans

Traditional African American cuisine started with the necessity of making do with ingredients available to slaves. One-pot dinners serve to tenderize meat and flavor vegetables. These stews often contain pork and greens such as dandelion, turnip, and collards. Other foods often served are dried beans, sweet potatoes, rice, grits, cornbread, and specialty gravies (red-eye, sausage, or cream).

Soul food signifies a shared heritage and loving preparation, not just favorite and familiar foods. African Americans who choose this type of food should be encouraged to use beans, rice, and sweet potatoes but to cook without a lot of fat, such as by steaming. Traditional foods can be prepared by baking, braising, broiling, or grilling instead of frying. Fat-free broths can be substituted for rich gravies.

Hispanic Americans

The dietary pattern covered in this section is that of Mexican Americans. Table 2-10 lists characteristic foods consumed by Puerto Rican and Cuban people

TABLE 2-10 ■ Characteristic Eating Patterns of Selected Cultural Groups

GROUP	GRAINS AND STARCHES	FRUITS	VEGETABLES	MEATS AND MEAT SUBSTITUTES	MILK AND MILK SUBSTITUTES	TO DECREASE FAT
LATINO						
Mexican	Tortillas, corn products, potatoes, corn		Chili peppers, tomatoes, onions, beets, cabbage, pumpkins, string beans	Meat, poultry, eggs; pinto, calico, garbanzo beans	Cheese; milk seldom consumed	Encourage: ■ Salsa as dip or topping ■ Baked corn tortillas, especially stuffed with chicken to make tamales, tostados, or enchiladas
Puerto Rican	Plantains (starchy vegetable that looks like a large banana), Puerto Rican bread (resembles Italian bread), rice, viands (starchy vegetable whose roots and tubers are peeled, boiled, and eaten as a side dish)	Guava, canned peaches, pears, fruit cocktail	Beets, eggplant, carrots, green beans, onions	Legumes (especially red kidney beans), eggs, pork, chicken, cod, fish, pigeon, peas, garbanzo beans	Flan (custard); milk seldom consumed	■ Rice with chicken or beans ■ Reduced-fat cheeses Discourage: ■ Fried tortillas ■ Sour cream and regular cheese as toppings ■ Refried beans that are cooked in lard ■ Deep-fried foods such as chimichangas
Cuban	Rice		Green peppers, onions, tomatoes	Black beans, pork, chicken, chorizo (a highly seasoned sausage)	Milk seldom used	
ITALIAN	Pasta, yeast breads, starchy root vegetables		Green peppers, onions, tomatoes	Spiced sausages, fish, tomato-based meat sauces	Cheese; milk seldom consumed (high incidence of lactose intolerance)	Encourage: ■ Salad with no-fat dressing ■ Minestrone soup ■ Pasta with tomato or clam sauce ■ Grilled meat or seafood Discourage: ■ White sauces made with cream, butter, or cheese ■ Breaded and fried meats and vegetables ■ Sausages and other fatty meats such as prosciutto (spiced ham)

continued

TABLE 2-10 ■ Characteristic Eating Patterns of Selected Cultural Groups (Continued)

GROUP	GRAINS AND STARCHES	FRUITS	VEGETABLES	MEATS AND MEAT SUBSTITUTES	MILK AND MILK SUBSTITUTES	TO DECREASE FAT
SOUTHERN BLACK AMERICAN	Cornbread, biscuits, white bread, butter beans, corn, sweet potatoes, grits, rice, white potatoes, yams	Melons, bananas, peaches	Kale, collards, mustard greens, okra, tomatoes, cabbage, summer squash	Catfish, pork, chicken, black-eyed peas, other dried beans and peas	Buttermilk, evaporated milk, ice cream (high incidence of lactose intolerance)	Encourage: ■ Baked fish and chicken ■ Steamed vegetables ■ Fresh melon ■ Grilled foods
ASIAN **Southern Chinese**	Rice	All	Mushrooms, bean sprouts, Chinese greens, bok choy	Beef, pork, poultry, seafood	Limited except for ice cream	Encourage: ■ Hot and sour soup; wonton soup ■ Steamed (not fried) dumplings
Northern Chinese	Wheat, millet seed used in noodles, bread, dumplings		Chinese greens, bamboo, alfalfa sprouts, bok choy	Beef, poultry, seafood, eggs, tofu, soybeans	None (high incidence of lactose intolerance among all Chinese)	■ Lightly stir-fried chicken or seafood ■ Steamed whole fish ■ Steamed vegetables and steamed rice
Japanese	Rice, most other complex carbohydrates		All	Fish, beef, pork, eggs, poultry, shellfish, soybean products	None (high incidence of lactose intolerance)	Discourage: ■ Egg rolls ■ Crispy fried noodles ■ Fried rice ■ Deep-fried entrees ■ Spareribs ■ Tempura
Asian Indian	Rice, wheat, millet, barley, maize, ragi (Old World cereal grain)	Mangoes, bananas	Cabbage, cauliflower, onions, chilies, tomatoes, potatoes, green leafy vegetables, okra, green beans, root vegetables	Legumes, nuts (Many vegetarians depending upon region)	Yogurt, buttermilk, milk added to coffee and tea	Encourage: ■ Broiled, poached, or steamed lean meats and poultry if nonvegetarian and religious practice permits ■ Steamed, stir fried, baked, or roasted vegetables ■ Olive oil, canola oil ■ Low-fat dairy products Discourage: ■ Deep fried breads and snacks ■ Coconut oil
EUROPEAN **Middle Eastern**	Pita bread, rice, couscous, bulgur wheat	Figs, peaches, dates	Grape leaves, tomatoes, peppers, olives, eggplant, onions, squash, fennel, okra, peas	Lamb, chicken, goat, legumes, fish, squid	Yogurt, feta cheese	Encourage: ■ Baked or grilled lean meats and vegetables, legumes ■ Fresh fruit ■ Yogurt dressings Discourage: ■ Fried meats and fish, excess cheese, butter between layers of phyllo (pastry) ■ Sour cream
Northern European	Dark breads, wheat breads, potatoes	All	All, especially onions, carrots, beans	Beef, pork, poultry, fish, shellfish, eggs, sausages	All cheese and milk products	Encourage: ■ Broiled, poached, or steamed lean meats ■ Wine- and tomato-based sauces ■ Consommé Discourage: ■ Creamed soups and sauces ■ Sausages ■ Whole milk and whole-milk products ■ Fried potatoes ■ Sour cream

TABLE 2-10 ■ Characteristic Eating Patterns of Selected Cultural Groups (Continued)

GROUP	GRAINS AND STARCHES	FRUITS	VEGETABLES	MEATS AND MEAT SUBSTITUTES	MILK AND MILK SUBSTITUTES	TO DECREASE FAT
NATIVE AMERICAN	Corn, wild oats and rice, Indian biscuits (Bannock bread)	Wild berries, choke cherries, black cherries, crab apples	Wild rhubarb, Indian celery, wild mushrooms and roots	Game, seafood, acorns, hazelnuts, pine nuts	Few used (high incidence of lactose intolerance)	Encourage: ■ Game with visible fat removed ■ Broiled, poached, or steamed meats Discourage: ■ Excessive fish oil ■ Fried food ■ Lard in cooking

as well as other ethnic groups. The table also suggests means of decreasing fat intake.

Corn is the staple crop of Mexico. Vegetables and meat characteristically are incorporated into a main dish and served with salsa. Foods are typically stewed or fried in oil or lard. Fruits are popular. Sweet foods, such as yeast pastries, are common in the traditional Mexican diet, and sugar is commonly added to foods.

A health belief that may influence a Mexican American's food choices is the hot–cold system. Illness and physiological conditions are categorized as "hot" or "cold." Foods of the opposite category are eaten in an attempt to return balance to the body. Because these categories vary widely from region to region, it is best simply to ask clients what foods they would like to eat.

The traditional Mexican diet can be adapted to the recommendations of the Dietary Guidelines with some changes in preparation. Beans can be boiled, for example, instead of refried; beef can be grilled instead of fried; diet drinks can be substituted for lemonade or soda. The starches and fruits that are part of the Mexican American diet can still be used.

Native Hawaiians

Before the arrival of Westerners, native Hawaiians consumed a diet based on taro (a starch root similar to potato), sweet potatoes, breadfruit, fruit, greens, and seaweed. Fat content was approximately 10% of kilocalories. Foods were eaten raw or steamed.

Adopting a Western diet has been detrimental to native Hawaiians' health. Among all of the population groups in the United States, the prevalence of obesity among native Hawaiians is second only to that of the Pima Indians. Longevity is greater in Hawaii than in any other state, except among native Hawaiians, who have the shortest lifespan of the ethnic groups.

An experimental diet was introduced to native Hawaiians to determine whether short-term dietary changes could alter their risk factors for cardiovascular disease. At the start, these individuals had an average BMI of 39.6. All of the food was provided in two on-site meals and take-home snacks. The evening meal included a cultural or health education session.

During the 3-week experiment, the participants were encouraged to eat as much of the traditional Hawaiian foods as they wanted but limited amounts of fish and chicken. Participants' average energy intake decreased 41% and their serum cholesterol decreased 14% (Shintani et al., 1991). An average weight loss of 15.1 pounds was maintained for an average of 2.8 years of follow-up (Shintani et al., 1999).

As detailed in later chapters, total fat and cholesterol intakes are linked to an increased risk of chronic disease. For these native Hawaiians, adopting an ancestral diet dramatically altered risk factors for diabetes mellitus and heart disease. Some of the program's success was attributed to inspiring pride in their heritage, but another theory is presented in Genomic Gem 2-1.

Genomic Gem 2-1
Ancestral Foods

Much about the occurrence of diseases is still unknown, particularly why some populations seem to be more at risk than others and why certain dietary practices are more protective of some people than others. Perhaps the correct combination of genetic, cultural, and socioeconomic factors is needed to achieve the desired health benefit.

If the metabolism of a group of people evolved to work optimally on an ancestral diet rather than with a modern diet, possibly the **alleles** that are associated with increased disease risk may be silenced in the presence of the more ancestral and traditional diet and lifestyle (Ordovas, Kaput, and Corella, 2007).

Chinese Americans

As throughout the world, Chinese cooking is based on the availability of foodstuffs. Wheat is produced in northern China, where noodles and dumplings are a major part of the cuisine, whereas rice grown in the south is the staple grain of that area.

Cooking technique involves cutting meats into bite-sized pieces in the kitchen. Experience with diseases resulting from poor sanitation led to avoidance of cold water and raw fruits and vegetables. Fruits and vegetables are cooked quickly to retain a crisp texture.

Chinese medicine views sickness as an imbalance between *yin* and *yang* forces, a system that some compare to the parasympathetic and sympathetic nervous systems. Certain illnesses, foods, and medicines are categorized as *yin* or *yang*. *Yin,* or cold, foods include pork, most vegetables, boiled foods, foods served cold, and white foods. *Yang,* or hot foods, include beef, chicken, eggs, fried foods, foods served hot, and red foods. Noodles and soft rice are neutral, neither *yin* nor *yang*.

To maintain fluid intake, Chinese Americans prefer hot tea to ice water. Dairy products are rarely used. A caregiver interested in increasing a Chinese American's calcium intake would probably achieve better results advocating green leafy vegetables or tofu rather than milk.

Family members may cook food at home to provide the hospitalized client with hot or cold foods. Because *yin* and *yang* cover various categories of foods, cooking methods, and colors, the perceptive nurse or dietitian can suggest items or procedures that also fit the diet prescribed by Western medicine. Clinical Application 2-2 relates such a case.

Clinical Application 2-2

Bridging *Yin* and *Yang* Beliefs and the Germ Theory of Disease

A Chinese infant experienced repeated bouts of diarrhea. Several tests were performed, and changes were made in the child's formula to no avail. Finally, a nurse made a home visit. She discovered several bottles of home-prepared formula on the windowsill, while others were in the refrigerator. The family lived in a New York apartment without air-conditioning, and it was midsummer.

When the nurse asked about the procedure used to store the formula, the mother stated that childbirth is regarded as a cold condition, so she should avoid cold. Her husband, therefore, removed the day's bottles from the refrigerator before he left for work every morning so the bottles would be warm for the mother's condition.

The nurse explained that storing the formula at room temperature permitted bacteria to grow in it and that these organisms were causing the baby's diarrhea. Together, the mother and nurse searched for another procedure to bridge the cultural belief and the germ theory of disease. The mother decided to don a coat, hat, and gloves before opening the refrigerator to retrieve each bottle at feeding time. The nurse wisely guided the mother to a solution that left the mother's belief system intact, and the infant's diarrhea was cured (Jackson, 1993).

Jewish Americans

Orthodox Jews interpret dietary laws stringently. These are the three key characteristics of strict kosher food preparation:

1. Only designated animals may be eaten.
2. Some of those animals must be ritually slaughtered and dressed.
3. Dairy products and meats must not be eaten at the same meal.

Separate cooking and serving utensils are used for dairy meals and meat meals. Fruits, vegetables, and starches need no special preparation and can be served with either meat or dairy meals.

When a preplanned kosher meal is unavailable, a cottage cheese fruit plate is a good choice for an Orthodox Jew. The cottage cheese should be transferred to a paper plate with new disposable plastic utensils because neither the plate nor the utensils used can have ever touched meat. If bread or crackers are served, labels must indicate that they contain no meat products.

Food Restrictions by Religious Customs

Certain religious practices may promote healthy lifestyles. Among Thai persons with type 2 diabetes, higher scores for Buddhist values were significantly correlated with better medication self-care and better dietary self-care than among those with lower scores (Sowattanangoon, Kochabhakdi, and Petrie, 2008).

Table 2-11 lists selected religious customs that affect food intake, but practices change with locale and over time. Individuals also vary in the extent to which they implement dietary restrictions.

TABLE 2-11 ■ Selected Religious Customs That Affect Food Intake

RELIGION	RESTRICTED FOODS AND BEVERAGES
Buddhism	1. All meat
Catholicism	1. Meat prohibited by some denominations on holy days such as Good Friday and Ash Wednesday 2. Alcoholic beverages by some denominations
Hinduism	1. Beef, pork, and some fowl
Islam	1. All pork and pork products 2. All meat must be slaughtered according to ritual letting of blood. 3. Carnivorous animals, birds of prey, and land animals without external ears 4. Blood and blood byproducts 5. Alcohol and intoxicants
Orthodox Judaism	1. All pork and pork products 2. All fish without scales and fins 3. Dairy products should not be eaten at the same meal that contains meat and meat products. 4. All meat must be slaughtered and prepared according to Biblical ordinances. Since blood is forbidden as food, meat must be drained thoroughly. 5. Bakery products and prepared food mixtures must be prepared under acceptable kosher standards. 6. Leavened bread and cake are forbidden during Passover.
Seventh-Day Adventist	1. All pork and pork products 2. Shellfish 3. All flesh foods (some members) 4. All dairy products and eggs (some members) 5. Blood 6. Highly spiced foods 7. Meat broths 8. All alcoholic beverages 9. Coffee and tea

Keystones

- Nutritional care begins with assessment followed by analysis, planning, implementation, and evaluation.
- Nutritional diagnoses are derived by comparing the client's assessment with nutritional standards.
- Dietary Reference Intakes define nutrient intakes suitable for healthy people in specific life-stage and gender groups.
- Exchange lists categorize foods according to similar nutrient composition and may be used to teach a client about healthful eating.
- Culture influences lifestyles including food choices and nutritional care.
- Health-care providers should ask clients about their dietary preferences and work those into the nutritional care plan.

CASE STUDY 2-1

A student in a beginning nutrition course is showing a friend the textbook. "You could help me improve my diet," the friend says. "I know I am not eating right." At the time, the friend was eating a chocolate bar. She described herself as 18 years old and sedentary. The student asks the friend to list what she had eaten during the past 24 hours. From the friend's list, the student gathers the following data:

Breakfast: 8 ounces of orange juice, 2 cups of black coffee
Lunch: 8 ounces of fruit yogurt and 6 square graham crackers
Midafternoon snack: Mr. Goodbar
Dinner: 3-ounce boneless pork chop, 2 cups of green salad, 2 tablespoons low-calorie French dressing, 12 ounces of diet Coke

Comparing the friend's intake to the tables for 18-year-old women available at MyPyramid, the student finds her friend's intake should be 1800 kilocalories distributed as follows:

	Friend's Intake	MyPyramid
Oils	½ tsp	5 tsp
Milk	1 cup	3 cups
Meat and beans	3 oz	5 oz equivalents
Vegetables	1 cup	2½ cups
Fruits	1 cup	1½ cups
Grains	3 oz equivalents	6 oz equivalents
Discretionary kilocalorie allowance	267	195

In this situation, the student probably would not formalize a nutritional care plan for the friend, but the following plan illustrates the thought process involved in developing a care plan for this case.

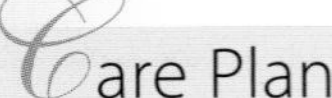

Care Plan

Subjective Data

Expressed need for instruction in healthy diet. Twenty-four hour recall shows fewer than the recommended MyPyramid intake for all food groups but excessive discretionary kilocalories.

Objective Data

Observed eating a chocolate bar at 3 P.M.

Analysis

Self-reported need to improve nutrition

Plan

DESIRED OUTCOMES EVALUATION CRITERIA	ACTIONS/INTERVENTIONS	RATIONALE
Friend will keep a food record for 3 days.	Instruct friend to list everything she eats or drinks for 3 days.	Food record will gather facts about the friend's food intake to use as an instructional tool.
Friend will read the section on MyPyramid in student's textbook by this evening.	Lend friend textbook to read.	Providing literature utilizes expert opinion to reinforce student's teaching. Reading and seeing illustrations elicits active participation and employs senses other than hearing.
Friend will meet with student in 4 days to compare food record to MyPyramid and design a plan of action.	Meet with friend in 4 days to sort and analyze food record data. Provide apples at meeting to model healthy snack food.	Setting follow-up visit just after food record is completed; will maintain the friend's interest. Modeling desirable behavior is a technique to encourage change.

After 4 days, the two friends met in the college library to access MyPyramid on the Internet. The friend says she has not been keeping the requested food diary. "I'm hopeless. I'll never be able to change," she moans. ■ Undaunted, the nutrition student suggests they input the day's intake that the friend reported 4 days earlier. They agreed that "It's someplace to start." However, the friend balked at sharing her weight with the student for the opening screen of MyPyramid. ■ At that point, thinking her friend required more professional help than her friendship could provide, the student recommended the free clinic run by the college's nursing department.

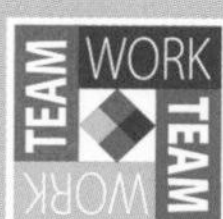

2-1

Clinic's Notes

The following Clinic's Notes are representative of the documentation found in a client's medical record.

Subjective: Requesting assistance with diet planning. Shared dietary recall from last week. Not inclined to keep food diary. Denies chronic illness. Has attempted weight control on her own with little success due to splurging on sweets. Recognizes need for lifestyle changes as well as dietary improvement. Unsure of social support for lifestyle changes.

Objective: Ht 5 ft; 4 in. Wt 163 lb BMI 28. VS WNL (Vital signs within normal limits)

Analysis: Overweight due to unbalanced diet and sedentary lifestyle.

Plan: Instruct in basic nutrition. Suggest private use of MyPyramid site to track diet. Recommend participation in daily walking group that meets in Physical Education Department. Follow-up visit in 1 week.

Critical Thinking Questions

1. When the student met with the friend after 4 days, what other options might have been chosen instead of referral to the nursing clinic?
2. You have a friend or relative who displays food intake similar to that described in Case Study 2-1. You care deeply for this person. How might you approach the subject of healthy eating if the person does not ask for assistance?
3. In what way has geography impacted ethnic eating patterns listed in Table 2-10? In what way has geography affected the typical diet in the United States?

Chapter Review

1. Which of the following techniques is used to estimate the body's protein stores?
   a. Estimating body frame size
   b. Measuring midarm circumference
   c. Calculating the body mass index
   d. Determining triceps skinfolds
2. Which of the following techniques used to assess food intake would yield the most comprehensive information?
   a. 24-Hour diet recall
   b. Diet history
   c. Food frequency questionnaire
   d. Food records
3. Which statement about the use of the ADA exchange lists is true?
   a. Two starch exchanges can be substituted for two meat exchanges.
   b. Exchange lists are used to calculate an individual's RDA.
   c. An exchange is a defined quantity of food on a particular list.
   d. Calculating the permitted exchanges requires paper and pencil or a calculator.
4. Which of the following is true of the traditional Chinese *yin* and *yang* health belief system?
   a. A cold, or *yin*, condition is balanced by consuming hot, or *yang*, foods.
   b. A hot condition is flushed with large quantities of cold water.
   c. Rice is considered magical and is consumed at every meal.
   d. *Yang*, or hot, foods include only foods served hot.
5. Which of the following adheres to strict kosher regulations?
   a. Avoiding cheese and cheese products
   b. Eating only certain cuts of pork
   c. Keeping separate utensils and dishes for meat and dairy meals
   d. Serving lobster, clams, and shrimp only on festive occasions

Clinical Analysis

1. Ms. G has just been diagnosed with type 2 diabetes. She is a Native American who has left her reservation for employment in town. Which of the following actions by the nurse shows respect for Ms. G's culture?
   a. Instructing her to increase her intake of vegetables
   b. Telling her to lose weight and avoid alcohol and fast-food restaurants
   c. Giving Ms. G an instruction sheet based on the ADA exchange system
   d. Asking Ms. G how she "sees" or perceives diabetes in her life

2. Mr. P is a 65-year-old man, recently widowed, whose physician is recommending weight loss. Mr. P has had little experience with grocery shopping or cooking. Which of the following systems for instructing Mr. P would the nurse select to offer the best chance of success?
   a. A computerized diet analysis program
   b. MyPyramid
   c. The ADA exchange lists
   d. The RDA/AI tables

3. Ms. E attended a community health fair where she entered her recalled intake for the previous 24 hours into a computer for analysis. On the basis of the printout she was given, she now thinks she should begin taking vitamin and mineral supplements. A friend who is a nurse correctly bases her advice on the following:
   a. A 1-day diet recall is inadequate data on which to base supplementation.
   b. A hand recalculation should be done to verify the accuracy of the computer printout.
   c. The RDAs on which computer programs are based are intended for only the 50% of the population who are obsessed with health.
   d. Undoubtedly, the operators of the computer at the fair had a product to sell: "Let the buyer beware."

3

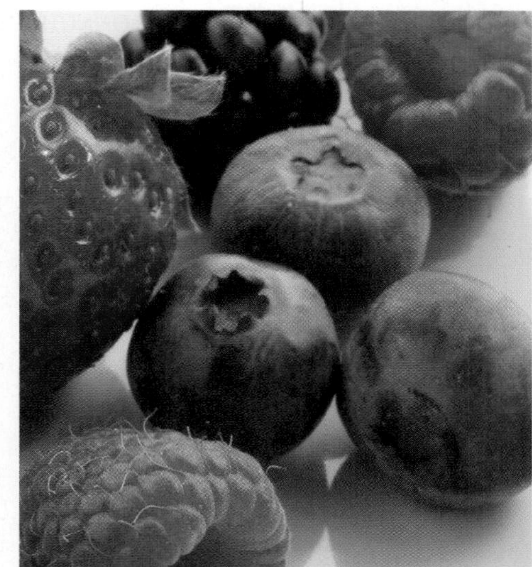

Carbohydrates

LEARNING OBJECTIVES

After completing this chapter, the student should be able to:

- Describe the types of carbohydrates, identify food sources of each, and indicate their functions in the body.
- List the major functions of carbohydrates and methods by which the body stores them.
- Discuss dietary fiber and list its functions; identify dietary food sources.
- Describe the relationship between carbohydrates and dental health.
- List the carbohydrate content (in grams) of each appropriate exchange list.
- Discuss dietary recommendations relating to fiber, added sugar, and total carbohydrate intake.

Carbohydrates, fats, and proteins all meet the body's basic energy needs. Carbohydrates, however, are recommended as the major source of energy because they break down rapidly and are therefore readily available for use. This chapter defines basic terminology related to carbohydrates and discusses the body's use of carbohydrates and the way carbohydrates relate to the other energy nutrients.

Green plants manufacture carbohydrates during a complex process called **photosynthesis.** In this process, carbon dioxide from the air and water from the soil are transformed into sugars and **starches.** Sunlight and the green pigment **chlorophyll** are necessary for this conversion. All the food we eat is a product of photosynthesis. If this process did not occur, the whole food chain would collapse and life would cease. Figure 3-1 illustrates this amazing process.

Based on their chemical structure, carbohydrates are divided into two major groups: sugars and starches. Sugars have a simple structure; starches are more complex. Therefore, sugars are often called **simple carbohydrates,** and starches are called **complex carbohydrates.**

Composition of Carbohydrates

Understanding the composition of carbohydrates involves understanding three structures: molecule, element, and atom:

1. A **molecule** is the smallest quantity into which a substance may be divided without loss of its characteristics. For example, the formula for water is H_2O. If the hydrogen atoms are pulled from the oxygen atom, the resulting products are hydrogen and oxygen, which bear no resemblance to water. Molecules are made of elements. In the case of water, H_2O, the elements are hydrogen and oxygen.
2. An **element** is a substance that cannot be separated into simpler parts by ordinary means.
3. An **atom** is the smallest particle of an element that retains its physical characteristics.

Sunlight
Carbon Dioxide
Enters the Plant
Oxygen Released
Carbohydrate
Produced
6H2O + 6CO2 = C6H12O6 + 6O2
water + carbon dioxide = carbohydrate + oxygen

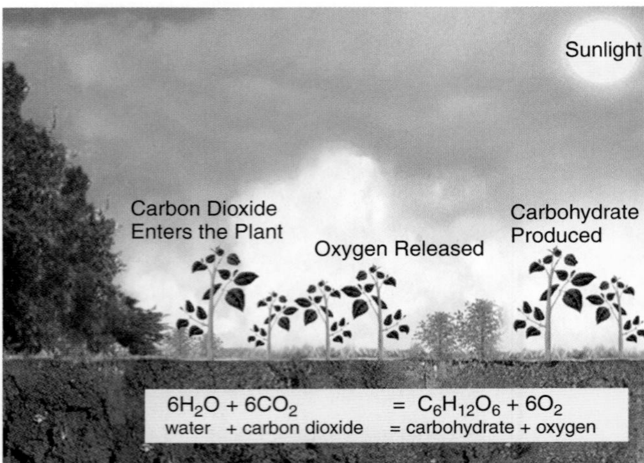

FIGURE 3-1 Photosynthesis is a vital process that transforms carbon dioxide and water into carbohydrates.

Basic Terminology

Carbohydrates are composed of the elements carbon, hydrogen, and oxygen. The ratio of hydrogen to oxygen is the same as that for water: two parts of hydrogen to one part of oxygen. The simplest carbohydrates have the formula $C_6H_{12}O_6$. Carbohydrates in general are frequently abbreviated CHO.

Simple carbohydrates (sugars) include monosaccharides and disaccharides (*mono-* means one, *di-* means two, and *-saccharide* means sweet). Starches are called **polysaccharides.**

Simple Carbohydrates

Simple carbohydrates are of two types: monosaccharides and disaccharides:

1. A **monosaccharide** contains one molecule of $C_6H_{12}O_6$.
2. A **disaccharide** is composed of two molecules of $C_6H_{12}O_6$ joined together (minus one unit of H_2O).

When the body joins two monosaccharide molecules, a molecule of water is released in the process.

Monosaccharides

Monosaccharides are the building blocks of all other carbohydrates. The three monosaccharides of importance in human nutrition are glucose, fructose, and galactose. Note the -ose ending in the name of each of these sugars. All monosaccharides and disaccharides end with the letters -ose.

Glucose

The monosaccharide glucose in the body is commonly called blood sugar. It is the major form of sugar in the blood. Normal **fasting blood sugar (FBS)** is 70 to 125 milligrams per 100 milliliters of serum or plasma (www.care.diabetesjournal.org). Regardless of the form of sugar consumed, the body readily converts it to glucose. Glucose is present in only small amounts in some fruits and vegetables and is moderately sweet.

Another name for glucose is **dextrose (abbreviated D).** Clients in health-care facilities often receive intravenous feedings. **Intravenous** simply means within or into a vein. The most common intravenous feeding is D_5W (5% dextrose in water), used primarily to deliver fluids to the client.

Fructose

Found in fruits and honey, fructose is commonly referred to as honey sugar. It is the sweetest of all the monosaccharides. Fructose is used extensively in soft drinks, canned foods, and various other processed foods. Relatively new on the list of food sweeteners is high-fructose corn syrup (HFCS). This syrup is very sweet because the cornstarch has been treated with an enzyme that converts some of the naturally present glucose to the sweeter fructose. The human body readily converts fructose to glucose.

Galactose

The monosaccharide galactose comes mainly from the breakdown of the milk sugar lactose. Yogurt and unaged cheese may contain free galactose. It is the least sweet of all the monosaccharides. The body converts galactose into glucose after ingestion.

Disaccharides

When two monosaccharides are linked, a disaccharide is formed. The three important disaccharides are:

1. Sucrose
2. Lactose
3. Maltose

Sucrose

The most prevalent disaccharide, sucrose, is ordinary white table sugar made commercially from sugar beets and sugar cane. Brown, granulated, and powdered sugars are all forms of sucrose. Sucrose is also found in molasses, maple syrup, and fruits. The two monosaccharides joined to form sucrose are glucose and fructose. See Box 3-1 for more information on

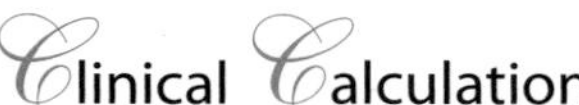
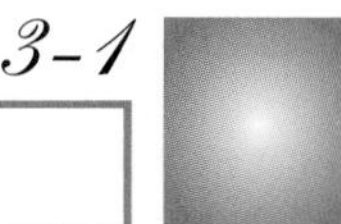

Converting Grams of Sugar into Teaspoons of Sugar

An added sugar intake of 60 grams does not mean much to average American consumers, because most Americans are not familiar with the metric system. Food labels use the metric system to list the nutritional content of a product. To enhance understanding of label reading, let us convert grams of sugar into teaspoons. One teaspoon of sugar contains 4 grams of CHO. Therefore, 60 grams of sugar is equal to 15 teaspoons.

sugar in the U.S. diet. Clinical Calculation 3-1 provides information on converting grams of sugar into teaspoons of sugar.

For an optimum diet, the Food and Nutrition Board of the National Academy of Sciences suggests that the *maximum* intake of added sugar not exceed 25% of calorie intake. Distinguished from the natural sugars such as lactose in milk and fructose in fruits, added sugars are those incorporated into foods and beverages during production. Major sources of added sugar include:

- Candy
- Soft drinks
- Fruit drinks
- Pastries
- Other sweets (Food and Nutrition Board Institute of Medicine, Food and Nutrition Board, 2002)

Lactose

Because lactose occurs naturally only in milk, it is commonly referred to as milk sugar. Lactose is the least sweet of the disaccharides. The two monosaccharides that make up lactose are glucose and galactose.

Box 3-1 ■ *Added Sugar in the U.S. Diet*

Most nutrition experts agree that sugar in appropriate amounts is not a health detriment. Aside from dental caries, the major concern of researchers is the reduced intake of essential micronutrients when sugar in the diet displaces more nutritious items such as milk.

What is an appropriate amount of added sugar in a healthful diet? According to the *Dietary Guidelines for Americans 2005*, added sugar along with alcohol and higher fat choices are part of the discretionary kcal group. The *USDA Food Guide* includes a table clearly indicating the total number of discretionary kcal recommended for 12 different kcal levels. For example, on a 2000-kcal diet only 267 kcal are discretionary kilocalories.

Currently, the largest contributor of added sugar in the diet is sweetened carbonated beverages and other sweetened beverages, which provide 37% of added sugars (Bachman, 2008). The second largest contributor is table sugar and candy at 16.1% (USDA, 2005).

Maltose

Maltose is a double sugar that occurs primarily during starch digestion. The disaccharide maltose is produced when the body breaks starches into simpler units. Smaller amounts of this disaccharide are present in malt, malt products, beer, some infant formulas, and sprouting seeds. Maltose consists of two units of glucose.

Sugar in Foods

How much sugar is in a food product can be found on its label. The total amount of sugar in grams can be found on the Nutrition Facts portion of the label. Sugar is both present naturally in foods and added to foods. For example, fruits contain fructose.

The federal government regulates the use of terms such as *sugar free, reduced sugar, less sugar* for food products that have added sugar. Terms such as those can be located anywhere on the package's label. Table 3-1 lists the standards, or definitions, for legally defined label descriptors.

Sugar Alcohols

Some food products contain ***sugar alcohols.*** Sugar alcohols have various names, such as sugar replacers, polyols, nutritive sweeteners, and bulk sweeteners. Lactitol, maltitol, isomalt, sorbitol, xylitol, and mannitol are all sugar alcohols (also called sugar replacers) and currently are approved for use in the United States.

Sugar alcohols are commonly used on a one-for-one replacement basis for sugars in recipes. For example, 1 cup of sugar would be replaced with 1 cup of isomalt in a recipe. Sugar alcohols add not only sweetness but also bulk to recipes. Sugar alcohols have the following characteristics:

- Generally do not promote tooth decay
- Commonly have a cooling effect on the tongue

TABLE 3-1 ■ Approved Definitions for Food Label Terms

TERM	STANDARD
Sugar-free	Contains less than ½ gram of sugars per serving
Reduced sugar or less sugar	At least 25% less sugar or sugars per serving than a standard serving size of a traditional food
No added sugar or without added sugar	No sugars added during processing or packing, including ingredients that contain sugar, such as juice or dry fruit
Low sugar	May not be used as a claim on a food label

- Are slowly and incompletely absorbed from the intestine into the blood
- May have a laxative effect for some people if consumed in excess

Intense Sweeteners

Intense sweeteners, unlike sugar replacers, do not add bulk or volume to a food product; they add only sweetness. They are 150 to 500 times as sweet as sugar and are mostly artificial, or synthetic. Intense sweetener is still relatively new terminology for nonnutritive sweeteners (artificial sweeteners) such as aspartame, saccharin, and sucralose. Table 3-2 discusses intensive sweeteners in more detail.

Complex Carbohydrates

Chemically complex carbohydrates are called **polysaccharides.** *Poly-* means many, and polysaccharides consist of many molecules of $C_6H_{12}O_6$ joined and many molecules of water released in the process. Polysaccharides can be composed of various numbers of monosaccharides and disaccharides. The three types of complex carbohydrates of nutritional importance are starch, glycogen, and fiber. Table 3-3 summarizes the composition of carbohydrates.

Starch

Starch, the major source of carbohydrate in the diet, is found primarily in grains, starchy vegetables, and legumes and in foods made from grains—cereals, breads, and pasta. Box 3-2 lists the many kinds of legumes available. Strictly speaking, all starches yield simple sugars on digestion; starchy foods are mostly low in fat and high in carbohydrates, and some starchy foods have the advantage of containing much fiber (discussed later).

Glycogen

The polysaccharide ***glycogen*** is commonly called ***animal starch*** because it is found in liver and muscle tissue. Although it is not a significant source of dietary carbohydrate, glycogen is crucial to the function of the human body. Glycogen is continually broken

TABLE 3-3 ■ Composition of Carbohydrates

Elements	C (carbon) H (hydrogen) O (oxygen)
Molecule	$C_6H_{12}O_6$
Monosaccharide (simple)	One unit of $C_6H_{12}O_6$
Disaccharide (simple)	Two units of $C_6H_{12}O_6$ minus one unit of H_2O
Polysaccharide (complex)	Many units of $C_6H_{12}O_6$ minus many units of H_2O

Box 3-2 ■ *Legumes*

Legumes include these dried peas and beans:

- Black beans
- Pinto beans
- Kidney beans
- Navy beans
- Soybeans
- Black-eyed peas
- Split peas
- Yellow peas
- Chick peas (garbanzo)
- Lentils

TABLE 3-2 ■ Artificial Sweeteners

ARTIFICIAL SWEETENER	TRADE NAME	COMMENTS
Aspartame	Nutrasweet®	Used in sweetened products such as puddings, gelatins, frozen desserts, yogurt, hot cocoa mixes, powdered soft drinks, carbonated beverages, teas, breath mints, chewing gums, some vitamins, and cold preparations. Also used as a tabletop sweetener. Reviewed by such regulatory agencies as the Centers for Disease Control (CDC) and Food and Drug Administration (FDA) and found to be safe. Should not be used by individuals with a rare genetic disease called phenylketonuria (PKU) (www.aspartame.org)
Saccharin	Equal®	Artificial sweetener.
	Sweet'N Low®	Carbonated beverages, toothpaste, cold remedies, dietetic puddings, cakes, cookies.
	Sugar Twin®	Saccharin was banned in Canada in 1977. The U.S. Food and Drug Administration also proposed a ban on saccharin, but Congress passed a moratorium on the ban. Although high doses of saccharin were shown to cause bladder cancer in male rats, numerous human studies have shown no association between saccharin and cancer at human levels of consumption.
Sucralose	Splenda®	Only noncaloric sweetener made from sugar. Approved for use by the Food and Drug Administration (FDA).
Stevia	Stevia	Natural alternative sweetener that is classified as an herb. It is sold as a dietary supplement. Stevia has not undergone the FDA approval process as a sweetener.

down and built up to provide immediate fuel for muscle action. Glycogen represents the body's carbohydrate stores. Liver glycogen helps sustain blood glucose levels during sleep.

The typical human body has an available store of glucose in the form of glycogen for about one day's energy needs. Because the body's ability to store carbohydrate in the form of glycogen is limited, an adequate intake of dietary carbohydrates is essential. When glycogen is stored, water is also stored. Each glycogen molecule attracts many molecules of water because of the way the elements are arranged. When glycogen stores are completely filled, the average person weighs about 4 pounds more than when glycogen stores are empty.

Dietary Fiber

Dietary fiber refers to foods, mostly from plants, that the human body cannot break down to digest, and, therefore, eliminates in intestinal waste. Sometimes called roughage or bulk, fiber adds almost no fuel or energy value to the diet, but it does add volume. Bulk fills the stomach, and most experts believe a full stomach contributes to a feeling of satisfaction so further eating ceases.

The recommended daily adequate intake (AI) for fiber is as follows (Food and Nutrition Board, 2005):

- Men 50 years and younger: 38 grams
- Women 50 years and younger: 25 grams
- Men older than 50: 30 grams
- Women older than 50: 21 grams

In the United States, the average person consumes less than the recommended amount of dietary fiber, and few people consume the recommended levels. Recent research indicates the average fiber intake for U.S. adults is only 15 grams per day (USDA, 2005). Whole grains are an excellent source of dietary fiber. Dollars and Sense 3-1 provides a recipe for an economical, easy-to-prepare oatmeal dish.

Eating too much fiber can cause problems. Much evidence suggests that eating more than 50 grams of fiber a day can interfere with mineral absorption, which can lead to problems such as anemia and osteoporosis. Healthy people should achieve a desirable fiber intake by consuming fiber-rich fruits, vegetables, legumes, and whole-grain cereals which also provide minerals, vitamins, and phytochemicals—instead of adding fiber concentrates (such as psyllium) to their diet.

Fiber is classified as either soluble or insoluble. **Solubility** is the ability of one substance to dissolve in another. For example, oil does not dissolve in water, so oil is insoluble in water. Insoluble fiber does not dissolve in water; whereas soluble fiber does. Soluble fiber and insoluble fiber react differently in the body and are needed for different reasons.

$ Dollars & Sense 3-1

Versatile Oatmeal

Plan your meals around whole grains. Start with brown rice, whole grain pasta, barley, or oatmeal and add other ingredients as your budget allows. For example, top the grains with seasonal vegetables or fruits or stir them in.

Pack several containers of this economical, easy-to-fix lunch or dinner for those super busy times.

¼ cup quick or regular oats (½ cup oats if kcal needed)
1 tablespoon chopped walnuts
1 tablespoon raisins or other dried fruit such as dried cranberries
½ teaspoon ground flaxseeds
1 tablespoon soy nuts
1 teaspoon brown sugar (optional)
½ cup nonfat milk or water (1 cup nonfat milk, if kcal needed)

Place the oats, walnuts, raisins or other dried fruit, flaxseeds, soy nuts, sugar, and milk or water in a small microwaveable bowl. Microwave on high for 1 to 1½ minutes or until desired consistency is achieved. Top with fresh blueberries or other seasonal fruit.

Makes 1 serving.

SOLUBLE FIBER

Sources of soluble fibers include beans, oatmeal, barley, broccoli, and citrus fruits; oat bran is a particularly good source of soluble fiber. Soluble fibers dissolve in water and thicken to form gels. The reported health benefits of soluble fibers include reduced cholesterol levels, regulated blood sugar levels, and weight loss (by helping dieters control their appetites).

INSOLUBLE FIBER

Examples of sources of insoluble fibers include the woody or structural parts of plants, such as fruit and vegetable skins, and the outer coating (bran) of wheat kernels. Insoluble fibers have been reported to promote regularity of bowel movements and reduce the risk of diverticular disease and some forms of cancer. Table 3-4 lists the food sources of each type of fiber and their reported health benefits.

Functions of Carbohydrates

Carbohydrates play the following roles in the body:

- Provide fuel
- Spare body protein
- Help prevent ketosis
- Enhance learning and memory processes

TABLE 3-4 ■ Foods and Reported Benefits of Fiber

	INSOLUBLE FIBER	SOLUBLE FIBER
Solubility	Does not dissolve in water	Dissolves in water
Food Sources	Wheat bran Corn bran Vegetables Nuts Fruit skins Some dry beans*	Oatmeal Oat bran, barley Some fruits such as apples, oranges Broccoli Some dry beans*
Reported Benefit	Promotes regularity May help reduce risk of some forms of cancer May reduce risk of diverticular disease	May help reduce cholesterol levels May assist in regulating blood sugar levels May promote weight loss by increasing **satiety**†

*Current laboratory methods to assay soluble fiber content of individual foods are imprecise. This is the subject of much research.
†Satiety is defined as the sensation of fullness after eating.

Provide Fuel

Carbohydrates, fats, and proteins provide the body's energy needs. **Energy** is the capacity to do work. To understand the concept of energy, think of the human body as a machine. Just as gasoline is a car's fuel, so carbohydrates, proteins, and fats are the human machine's fuel. Without fuel, a car powered by gas ceases to operate. Without fuel sources over an extended time, the human machine dies from starvation. Just as a person cannot efficiently substitute something other than gasoline to fuel a car with a gasoline engine, a person cannot efficiently substitute something other than carbohydrate, protein, and fat for fuel in the human body.

Carbohydrate is a primary source of fuel for the brain, other nervous tissue, and the lungs. Because the brain cannot store carbohydrate, it must have an uninterrupted, ongoing source of carbohydrate, the minimum requirement of which is determined by the brain's need for glucose (Gottschlich, 2007). Although the amount of dietary carbohydrate that provides optimal health in humans is unknown, strong evidence exists that a minimum of 50 grams of carbohydrates per day is necessary for adequate (though not optimal) brain and body function.

Spare Body Protein

When we eat too few carbohydrates, our bodies suffer. We must have a continuous supply of glucose for all cells to function, particularly those of the central nervous system. Remember that our glycogen stores are limited. But the body can convert protein to glucose. Therefore, the body will break down internal protein stores (muscle tissue) before fat stores if carbohydrate intake is inadequate. An adequate supply of dietary carbohydrates spares body protein stores from being partially converted into glucose and allows protein to be used for growth and repair of body tissue. This principle has important ramifications, which are discussed throughout the text.

Help Prevent Ketosis

A balanced intake of energy nutrients is vital. If carbohydrate intake is too low, the body will break down both stored fat and internal protein to meet its fuel needs. The body cannot handle the excessive breakdown of stored fat because the body lacks the necessary equipment. As a result, partially broken-down fats accumulate in the blood in the form of ketones, and the person is said to be in a state of **ketosis.** Survival is possible on a very low carbohydrate diet, but good health is not.

Fatigue, nausea, and lack of appetite are some of the undesirable consequences of ketosis. Coma and death have occurred in severe cases. The presence of ketosis is easily determined by testing for the presence of acetone or diacetic acid in the urine. **Acetone** and **diacetic acid** are ketone bodies. Fifty grams of carbohydrate each day is usually enough to prevent ketosis.

Enhance Learning and Memory

Considerable evidence exists that blood glucose concentrations regulate neural and behavioral processes. Glucose enhances learning and memory in humans throughout the life cycle. Findings across many laboratories demonstrate that glucose consumed early in the morning facilitates specific forms of cognitive function, particularly verbal declaration memory (intentional memory for words and narratives). Children score higher on tests when they eat breakfast. Improvements include both enhanced memory and retrieval of information from long-term memory. Glucose enhanced cognitive function in elderly test subjects who had some mild age-related memory deficits (Korol, 2002).

Health and Carbohydrates

The kinds of carbohydrates eaten are important to health. Epidemiological data support the association between a high intake of vegetables and fruits and low risk of chronic disease. Legumes are low in fat and are excellent sources of protein, dietary fat, micronutrients, and phytochemicals. Numerous studies have linked regular consumption of whole grains with a lower risk of certain cancers and heart disease. Many nutrition experts attribute these health benefits to the fiber contained in whole grains.

Sugary foods also often displace other more nutritious foods in the diet. For example, carbonated beverages may be consumed instead of milk and fruit juices. Although too much sugar can lead to undesirable weight gain, in moderate amounts it can be used to make nutritious foods more appealing and increase a person's desire to eat them.

Consumption Patterns

Most of the world's population subsists primarily on carbohydrates. Foods rich in carbohydrates are easily grown in most climates, are low in cost, and are easily stored. Many carbohydrates do not require refrigeration or electricity, and their shelf life may stretch to years. In Asia, where rice is a dietary staple, carbohydrates provide as much as 80% of the fuel in the diet. In the United States population as a whole, the largest source of added sugar is regular soft drinks, which accounts for one-third of intake.

The most recent nationwide data on dietary intakes are based on the United States Department of Agriculture's (USDA) Continuing Survey of Food Intake by Individuals. Findings included these statistics:

- U.S. adults averaged only one serving per day of whole grains.
- 2% of adults consumed no whole grain.
- Consumption of milk decreased by 16% since the late 1970s, whereas consumption of carbonated soft drinks increased by 16%.
- Only 54% of individuals ate fruit on a given day (USDA, 2005).

Dental Caries

Several studies have shown a relationship between carbohydrate consumption and dental caries. Dental caries is the gradual decay of the teeth. A dental cavity is a hole in a tooth caused by dental caries. Dental caries results from the interaction of four factors: a genetically susceptible tooth, bacteria, carbohydrate, and time. All four must occur simultaneously for a cavity to form, as Figure 3-2 illustrates. Some people are more genetically susceptible to caries than other people, as Genomic Gem 3-1 discusses.

Genomic Gem 3-1
Caries

Genetic susceptibility is an individual's likelihood of developing a given trait as determined by heredity. We cannot control our genetic susceptibility for cavities, and bacteria are always present in our mouths and difficult to eliminate. However, we can control the length of time carbohydrate-containing foods are in our mouths and the kinds of carbohydrates we eat.

Risk Factors for Cavity Formation

Bacteria, carbohydrate-containing foods, and the length of time that teeth are exposed to sugars influence cavity formation. Bacteria normally present in the mouth interact with dietary carbohydrates and produce acids. The acids, not the sugar, cause decay. All types of sugars can promote cavity formation, including fructose, glucose, maltose, lactose, and sucrose.

A strong relationship exists between the length of time sugars are present in the mouth and the development of caries. For example, sticky foods such as caramels and raisins, which adhere to the tooth surface for long periods, are more likely than other foods to lead to tooth decay in susceptible people. Sipping sweetened beverages continually throughout the day can lead to tooth decay.

Eating Right to Prevent Cavities

Certain foods may help counteract the effects of the acids produced by oral bacteria. Aged cheese (cheddar, Swiss, blue, Monterey jack, Brie, Gouda), as well as processed American cheese, may inhibit tooth decay. Cheese stimulates the production of saliva. Chewing fibrous foods such as apples or celery stimulates the production of generous amounts of saliva. Saliva helps clear the mouth of food and counteracts acid production. Because saliva production is increased during a meal, sugars eaten with a meal are less likely to cause decay than those eaten between meals.

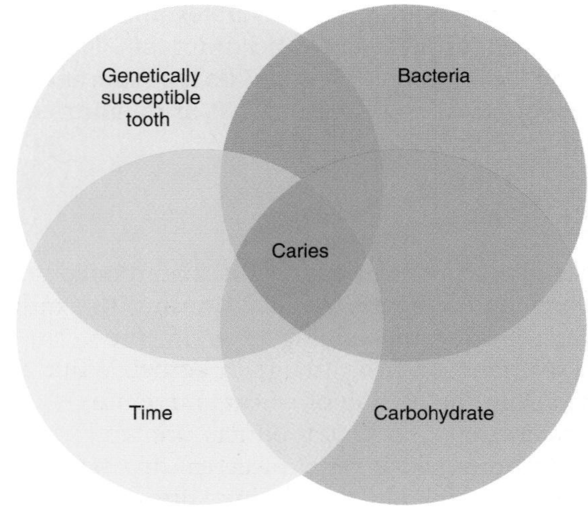

FIGURE 3-2 Interactions necessary for dental cavity formation.

Food Sources

Carbohydrates fall into two general groups: sugars and starches. All starches contain fiber; however, all starches do not provide equal amounts of fiber.

3-1

Clinical Application

Nursing-Bottle Syndrome

Nursing-bottle syndrome is a dental condition caused by the frequent and prolonged exposure of an infant's or young child's teeth to liquids containing sugars. Milk, formula, fruit juice, and other sweetened drinks can all cause rampant dental cavities.

Typically, nursing-bottle syndrome occurs when a caretaker habitually puts a baby to bed with a bottle of milk, juice, or other sweetened liquid. During sleep, the flow of saliva decreases, which allows liquids from the nursing bottle to pool around the teeth, undiluted for extended periods. Parents need to be cautioned against this practice.

The main ways to maintain oral health include these steps:

- Reduce consumption and especially frequency of food and drink containing sugar.
- Consume sugar only as part of a meal.
- Snacks and drinks should be sugar-free.
- Avoid frequent consumption of acidic drinks.

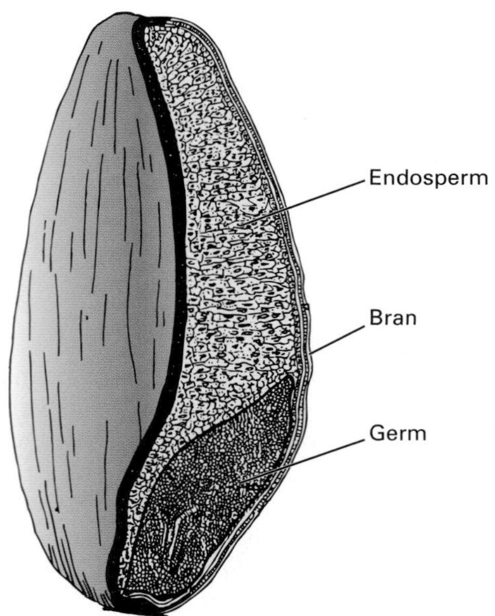

FIGURE 3-3 The most nutritious parts of wheat germ are the bran and endosperm, which are removed during the milling of grain.

Sugars

Table sugar contains approximately 4 grams of carbohydrates per teaspoon. When determining a person's sugar consumption, we consider not only the simple sugars such as honey, jam, and jelly but also the sugars present in carbonated beverages, ice cream, sherbet, cakes, pies, cookies, and donuts. The new sugar replacers contain on average about 2 grams of carbohydrate per teaspoon.

Starches

Starches are complex carbohydrates and are important sources of fiber and other nutrients. Figure 3-3 illustrates a typical cereal grain. Its main parts are the germ, bran, and endosperm. Most of the nutrients in cereal are in the bran and germ.

Whole Grains

Whole grains are more nutritious than refined grains, in which nutrients are removed during the **milling** process. During the milling of grain, the germ and bran are removed from the grain kernel. White flour results from the milling of wheat and white rice from the milling of rice. Oat products are not normally milled. The nutritive value of cereal depends on the amount of bran and germ retained during the milling process. For this reason, the use of whole grains should be encouraged whenever possible. Examples of whole grains include:

- Cornbread made from whole ground cornmeal
- Ground cornmeal
- Cracked wheat bread
- Oatmeal and oatmeal bread
- Pumpernickel bread (when made from whole grain flours)
- Rye bread (when made from whole grain flours)
- Whole-wheat bread
- Breads made from bran
- Barley
- Graham crackers

Carbohydrate Counting

In health care, carbohydrate counting helps teach clients about the carbohydrate content of foods and healthful portion sizes. According to one study, portion sizes and energy intake have increased markedly between 1977 and 1998 for food consumed at fast-food restaurants and in the home (Nielson and Popkin, 2003). A serving is not the amount commonly eaten but a defined amount of a particular food according to nutrition experts.

Because of the large number of defined portion sizes in the American Diabetic and Dietetic Associations exchange lists for menu planning (ADA, 2007) and the widespread use of this meal-planning system throughout health care, this text uses Exchange Lists. One serving or exchange of milk, fruit, grain, cereal, bread, or starchy vegetable is considered to be 15 grams of carbohydrate.

Eating too much of any of the energy nutrients can result in an unhealthful weight gain. Perhaps no other concept is more important to understanding nutrition than healthful portion sizes.

Exchange List Values

Exchange lists were introduced in Chapter 2. This section focuses on exchange lists that contain carbohydrates. Exchanges that include carbohydrates are the starch/bread, vegetable, fruit, and milk lists.

Starch/Bread Exchange List

One American Dietetic Association/American Diabetes Association (ADA) exchange of starch contains approximately 15 grams of carbohydrates. For example, each of the food items in Figure 3-4 is equal to one starch exchange. Some foods are higher in fiber than other foods. See Table 3-5.

Vegetable Exchange List

Raw and cooked vegetables are also good sources of carbohydrates. Vegetables contain between 2 and 3 grams of fiber per serving. One vegetable exchange

TABLE 3-5 ■ Selected Starch Exchanges

Bran cereal*	½ cup
Cooked cereal	½ cup
Ready-to-eat, unsweetened cereal	¾ cup
Sugar-frosted cereal	½ cup
Beans and peas (cooked)*	⅓ cup
Corn, whole kernel	½ cup
Potato, baked	1 small (3 oz)
Whole-wheat bread	1 slice (1 oz)

General rule: ½ cup of cereal, grain, or pasta or 1 oz of a bread product is equal to one starch exchange.
*Higher in fiber.

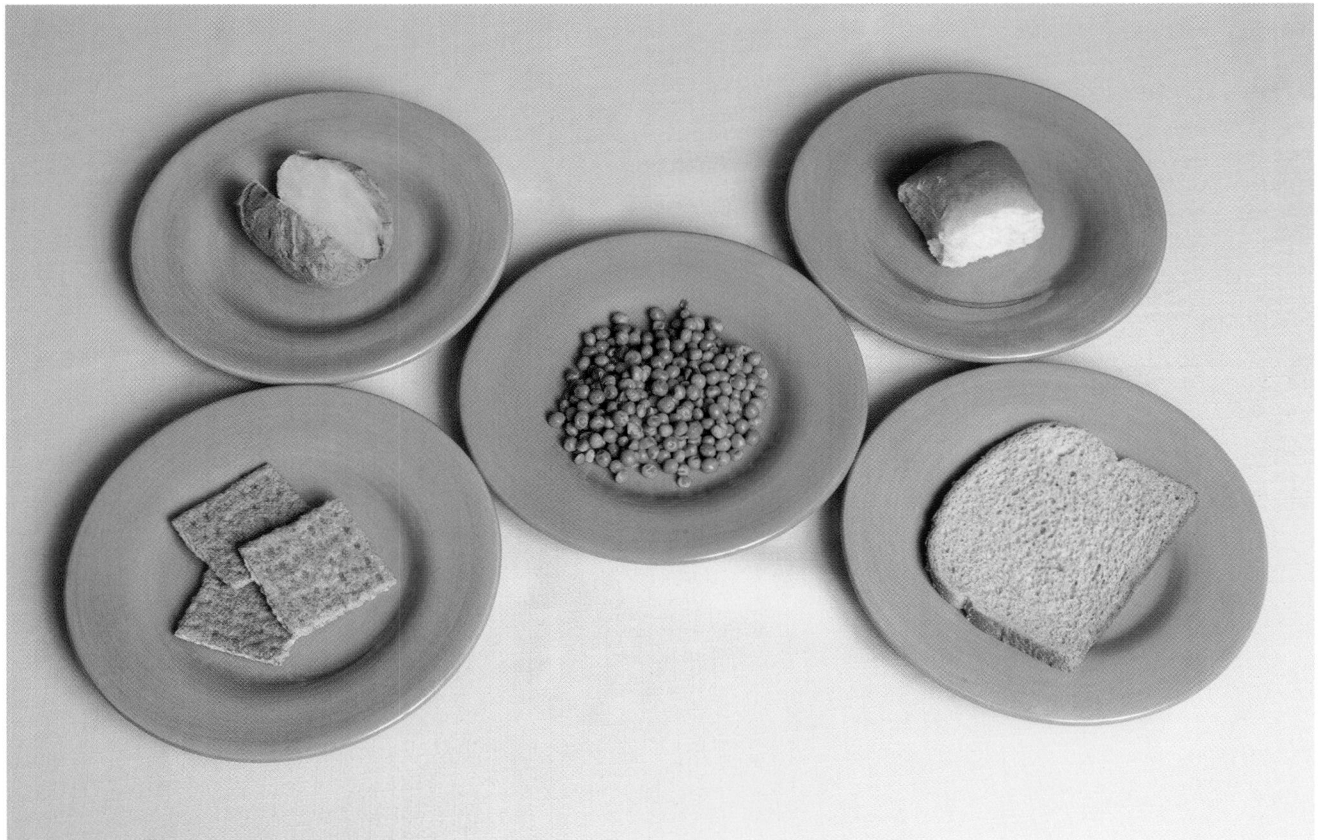

FIGURE 3-4 Each of these foods is equal to one starch exchange and contains about 15 grams of carbohydrates.

contains approximately 5 grams of carbohydrate. One-half cup of cooked vegetable or one cup of raw vegetables equals one vegetable exchange. Vegetables also contribute vitamins and minerals to the diet.

Fruit Exchange List

Fruits are another source of carbohydrates. One ADA exchange of fruit contains approximately 15 grams of carbohydrates (Table 3-6). Many fruits are excellent sources of fiber and contain vitamins and minerals. Figure 3-5 illustrates one serving or exchange of fruit.

TABLE 3-6 ■ Selected Fruit Exchanges

Apple (raw, 2 in across)	1 apple
Banana (small)	1 banana
Blueberries*	¾ cup
Grapefruit (medium)	½ grapefruit
Nectarine, small	1 nectarine
Strawberries (raw whole)*	1¼ cup
Prunes (dried)*	3 medium
Orange (2½ in across)	1 orange
Orange juice	½ cup

*Contains 3 g or more of fiber.

Milk Exchange List

Milk, with its lactose content, is an important source of carbohydrates. One cup of milk contains 12 grams of carbohydrates. Skim, whole, and 2% milk all contain approximately the same amount of carbohydrates. Box 3-3 lists milk equivalents.

Dietary Recommendations

The Food and Nutrition Board of the National Academy of Sciences, Institute of Medicine issued dietary recommendations for carbohydrates in 2005. To meet the body's daily energy and nutritional needs while minimizing risk for chronic disease, adults should get 45% to 65% of their kcalories from carbohydrates.

The committee reasoned that because carbohydrates, fat, and protein all serve as energy sources and can substitute for one another to some extent to meet kilocalorie needs, the recommended ranges for consuming energy nutrients should be useful and flexible for dietary planning, hence the wide 45% to 65% range. The ranges for children are similar to those for adults in respect to carbohydrates.

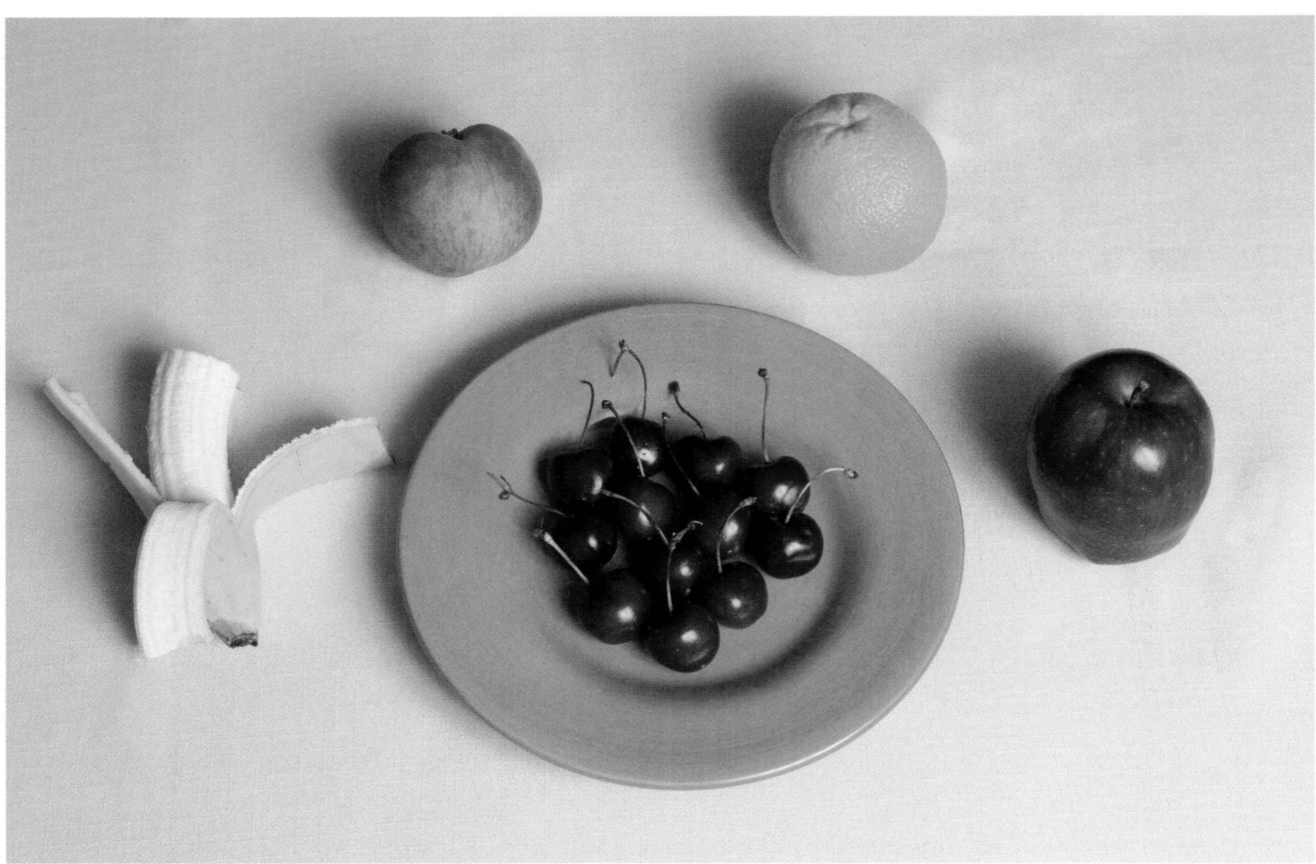

FIGURE 3-5 Each of these foods is equal to one fruit exchange.

Box 3-3 ■ *Milk Equivalents*

Each of the following is equal to one exchange.

- Eight ounces of plain low-fat yogurt (with added nonfat milk solids)
- ⅓ cup dry nonfat milk
- ½ cup evaporated milk
- 1 cup of buttermilk

The RDA for children older than 1 year of age and most adults younger than 70 years of age is 130 grams of CHO/day. The RDA is 175 grams of CHO per day for pregnant women and 210 grams per day for lactating women. In addition, added sugars should comprise no more than 25% of total kcalories eaten. This suggested maximum stems from evidence that people with diets high in added sugars have lower intakes of essential nutrients.

Keystones

- Carbohydrates are composed of sugars and starches.
- The average American's intake of sugars is considered excessive, whereas the intake of starches is considered low.
- Many Americans would benefit from increasing their fiber intake through the consumption of more whole-grain starches, fruits, and vegetables.
- Dietary carbohydrates promote tooth decay in susceptible individuals.
- The ADA exchange lists that contain carbohydrates are the starch, vegetable, fruit, and milk lists.
- Strong evidence exists that a minimum of 50 grams of carbohydrates per day is necessary for adequate (though not optimal) brain and body function.
- When there is no or little carbohydrate in the diet and the body uses protein or fat as a fuel source, the body in effect cannibalizes itself for glucose. Muscle and organ mass is lost in the process.
- The RDA for CHO is 130 grams of carbohydrates a day. Pregnant and lactating women have a higher RDA for CHO.

CASE STUDY 3-1

K. L. is a 19-year-old college student. He is interested in bodybuilding and spends much of his time on strength conditioning. He lifts weights or uses the Stairmaster (an aerobic conditioning machine) daily. He is 6 ft tall and weighs 175 lb. For the past 3 weeks, he has been drinking a powdered protein supplement (that contains no carbohydrate) instead of eating the dorm food, which he states "isn't any good anyway." He also takes a high-stress vitamin and mineral tablet. He arrived at the clinic today with complaints of fatigue, nausea, a lack of appetite, lightheadedness, and memory loss. His urine tested positive for ketones. The client is willing to talk to a registered dietitian.

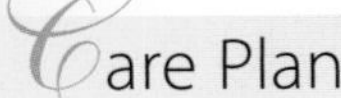

Care Plan

Subjective Data

The client has chosen not to eat any foods that contain carbohydrates for approximately 3 weeks.

Objective Data

Urine positive for ketones

Analysis

Inadequate intake of CHO, related to erroneous ideas about healthy eating as evidenced by verbal statements that he has not been eating CHO-containing foods and by urine positive for ketones.

(Continued on the following page)

CASE STUDY *(Continued)*

Plan

DESIRED OUTCOMES EVALUATION CRITERIA	ACTIONS/INTERVENTIONS	RATIONALE
Client will state one reason why he needs CHO by the end of the appointment.	Encourage client to consume foods from the Food Pyramid, including milk, starches, fruits, and vegetables. Refer to the dietitian for instruction on normal nutrition and protein needs for athletes.	Explaining why carbohydrates are necessary in the diet may motivate the client to eat carbohydrates. Milk, vegetables, fruits, and starches are all good sources of CHO. The nurse may need to educate the client about dietary sources of carbohydrates.
Schedule the client for a return visit in 1 week. Client will keep a food record for the dietitian.	On next visit, ask client to demonstrate knowledge gained. (For example, "How many servings of starch, fruits, and vegetables do you need daily?") Test the urine for ketones at the next visit.	

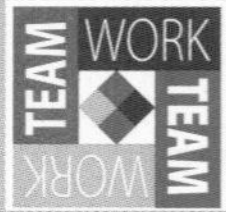

3-1

Dietitian's Note

The following Dietitian's Notes are representative of the documentation found in a client's medical record.

Dietitian's Notes

Subjective: Client states he wants to be able to lift more weight. Food records for 4 days show an average daily intake of 18 meats, 12 fats, 1 starch, 1 fruit, and 1 vegetable, and 1 low-fat milk. Client states he has just recently added starch, fruit, and milk to his diet per nurse's recommendation. Patient continues to complain of fatigue and constipation. He finds it difficult to concentrate and study.

Objective: Ketones in urine, weight 175 lb (81 kg) height: 6 ft

Analysis: Ideal body weight 178 ± 10%; estimated protein needs 81–97 grams. Estimated kcal need based on 81 kg and 25–35 kcal/kg = 2025–2835; Food records show an approximate intake of 2111 kcal and 25% protein, 66% fat, and 8% carbohydrate.

Inadequate carbohydrate intake related to food and nutrition-related knowledge deficit as evidenced by ketone smell on breath, complaints of fatigue and difficulty concentrating, and food records.

Client appears open to learning and prefers written and oral instructions.

Plan

1. Client to substitute CHO kcal for fat kcal by eliminating bacon, olives, soy nuts, and fatty meats from diet.
2. Client agreed to try adding 3 cups low-fat milk, 4 vegetables, 3 fruits, and 6 whole grains to diet.
3. Appointment scheduled for follow-up in 1 week.
4. Copy of Food Pyramid given to client.

Critical Thinking Questions

1. At the client's next visit, what would you do if the food records showed a recorded carbohydrate intake of only 30 grams for most days? What if the client said, "I don't want to eat any more because I feel better"?
2. At the next client visit, what would you do if the food records showed that the client ate only sugar to increase his carbohydrate intake because "Sugar is a quick energy food"?

Chapter Review

1. Which of the following is a disaccharide?
   a. Glucose
   b. Lactose
   c. Fructose
   d. Galactose
2. A healthy adult needs ___ grams of fiber each day.
   a. 5 to 11
   b. 12 to 20
   c. 21 to 38
   d. More than 50
3. Twelve grams of simple carbohydrate is equal to ___ teaspoon(s) of sugar.
   a. 1
   b. 2
   c. 3
   d. 8
4. One slice of bread contains approximately ___ grams of carbohydrates.
   a. 5
   b. 8
   c. 10
   d. 15
5. Which of the following may cause diarrhea?
   a. A medication that contains sorbitol
   b. A lack of dietary fiber
   c. A lack of exercise
   d. An insufficient fluid intake

Clinical Analysis

1. Ms. C is concerned about the dangers associated with the consumption of artificial sweeteners and wants to know if they are safe. As a health-care worker, it is appropriate for you to:
   a. Ignore Ms. C's comments because you think she is overly concerned.
   b. Assure her that the government wouldn't allow a food or herbal product to be sold if it was hazardous to her health.
   c. Explain to her that no food is guaranteed to be 100% safe, and it is best to avoid artificial sweeteners if she is not comfortable with these products.
   d. Refer her to the local health food store.
2. Mr. J claims he is trying to lose weight, and his urinalysis shows that his urine contains ketones (ketonuria). You should ask him:
   a. When he ate last
   b. How much milk, fruit, and starch he usually eats
   c. What else he usually eats
   d. All of the above
3. Mr. P complains of constipation. As his nurse, you would like to teach him to eat more insoluble fiber to help alleviate his discomfort. You should encourage the intake of:
   a. Wheat and corn bran, nuts, fruit skins, and dried beans
   b. Eggs, cheese, and chicken
   c. Milk, yogurt, and ice cream
   d. Oatmeal, barley, and broccoli

4

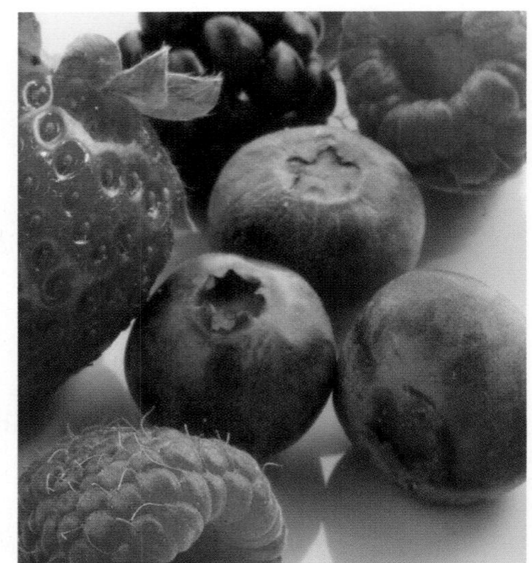

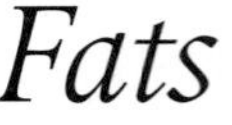

Fats

LEARNING OBJECTIVES

After completing this chapter, the student should be able to:

- Identify how fats are classified and discuss their physical properties.
- List the major functions of fats both in the diet and in the body.
- Discuss the relationships to health of cholesterol, saturated fat, polyunsaturated fat, *trans*-fatty acids, and monounsaturated fat.
- List three current recommendations of the Food and Nutrition Board of the National Research Council that pertain to fat.
- Correctly read food labels and identify the amounts and kinds of fats in foods.

This chapter presents an introduction to lipids for students without a chemistry background. Chapter 18 expands on this chapter and discusses clinical nutrition in more detail. The descriptive name for fats of all kinds, lipids, is used in clients' medical records. **Lipids** include true fats and oils as well as related fat-like compounds such as **lipoids** and **sterols.** Fats and oils are present in the body and in foods. Fats are typically thought of as solids, whereas oils are regarded as liquids. For example, the body produces oil adjacent to hair. Not as readily apparent to some people is the layer of fat beneath the skin, which is solid. At room temperature, dietary fats such as lard and butter are solid, whereas corn and olive oils are liquid.

Lipids are **insoluble** in water and are greasy to the touch. When two insoluble substances are mixed together, they separate readily, such as vinegar and oil. You can shake the vinegar and oil combination repeatedly, but it will still separate after the agitation stops.

Basic Terminology

Lipids are composed of the elements carbon, hydrogen, and oxygen. These are the same three elements that make up carbohydrates, but the proportion of oxygen to carbon and hydrogen is lower in fats (the implications of which are discussed later). The basic structural unit of a true fat is one molecule of **glycerol** joined to one, two, or three fatty acid molecules. Glycerol is thus the backbone of a fat molecule.

A **fatty acid** is composed of a chain of carbon atoms with hydrogen and a few oxygen atoms attached. The fatty acid chains joined to the glycerol molecule vary in length (depending on the number of carbon atoms present) and composition. The different taste, smell, and physical appearance of each fat results from the variety of fatty acids and their physical arrangement in the fat molecules. Beef fat tastes, smells, and looks different from that of chicken mostly because of the difference in fatty acid composition. All fats contain fatty acids.

A fat can have from one to three fatty acids, and the number of fatty acids a fat contains has important implications for both diet and health.

Monoglycerides and Diglycerides

When a single fatty acid is joined to a glycerol molecule, the resulting fat is called a **monoglyceride**. When two fatty acids are joined to a glycerol molecule, the fat is called a **diglyceride**. The terms monoglyceride and diglyceride are commonly seen on food labels.

Triglycerides

When three fatty acids are joined to a glycerol molecule, a **triglyceride** is formed. Most of the fat found in our diets and in the body is in the form of triglycerides. Excess triglycerides are stored in the specialized **adipose cells** that make up adipose tissue. The human body has a virtually unlimited capacity to store fat. Figure 4-1 illustrates the structure of monoglycerides, diglycerides, and triglycerides.

Length of Fatty Acid Chain

Fatty acids vary in the length of their fatty acid chains: Each chain is determined by the number of carbon atoms present, which can vary from 2 to 24. The length of the chain determines how the body transports the fat in the body, as fatty acid chains of short length (<6 carbon atoms) and medium length (8–12 carbon atoms) are processed differently than longer chains are. The chain length has dietary implications in many diseases. For example, in certain diseases of malabsorption, the client cannot tolerate foods with long-chain fatty acids. This problem is discussed in more detail in later chapters.

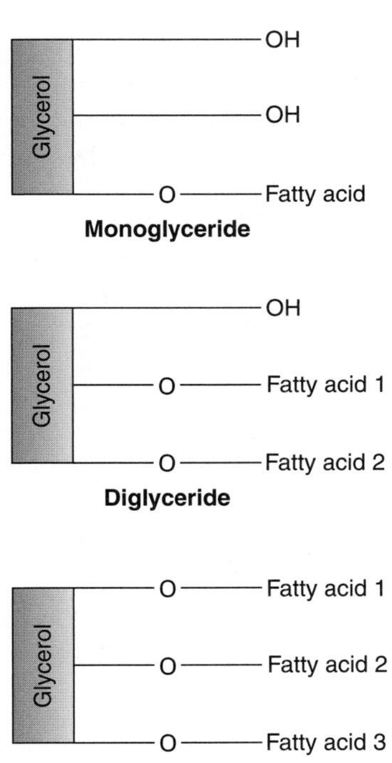

FIGURE 4-1 Monoglycerides, diglycerides, and triglycerides. A monoglyceride has one fatty acid attached to the glycerol molecule, a diglyceride has two fatty acids attached to the glycerol molecule, and a triglyceride has three fatty acids attached to the glycerol molecule.

Degree of Saturation

The terms *saturated, unsaturated, monounsaturated,* and *polyunsaturated* have become household words. *Trans-fatty acid* is a more recent addition to this list. Consumers and clients ask sophisticated questions about fats and expect health-care professionals to define and explain the terminology. Technically, all of these terms refer to the chemical structure of fatty acids, based on the degree or nature of the hydrogen atom saturation.

The degree of saturation of a fatty acid depends on the extent to which hydrogen is joined to the carbon atoms present. A **saturated fatty acid** is filled with as many hydrogen atoms as the carbon atoms can bond with and has no double bonds between carbons. In this case, a **double bond** describes the type of chemical connection between two neighboring carbon atoms, each lacking one hydrogen atom. In an **unsaturated fatty acid,** the carbon atoms are joined together by one or more of such double bonds.

Wherever a double bond occurs, another hydrogen atom could potentially join the chain. In other words, the fatty acid chain is lacking hydrogen atoms and is thus less saturated than a chain that is completely filled. A fatty acid with only one carbon-to-carbon double bond is **monounsaturated.** A fatty acid with more than one carbon-to-carbon bond is **polyunsaturated.** See Figure 4-2 for a structural comparison of saturated, monounsaturated, and polyunsaturated fatty acids.

In addition to the fats in the body, the fats found in foods are combinations of saturated and unsaturated fatty acids. They are designated as follows:

- Saturated fat: Composed mostly of saturated fatty acids
- Unsaturated fat: Composed mostly of unsaturated fatty acids
- Monounsaturated fat: Composed mostly of monounsaturated fatty acids
- Polyunsaturated fat (PUFA): Composed mostly of polyunsaturated fatty acids
- *Trans*-fatty acids: Composed of partially hydrogenated fatty acids

Figure 4-3 shows the mixtures of fatty acids in dietary fats.

Saturated

Saturated (no carbon-to-carbon double bonds)

Unsaturated

Monounsaturated (one carbon-to-carbon double bond)

Polyunsaturated

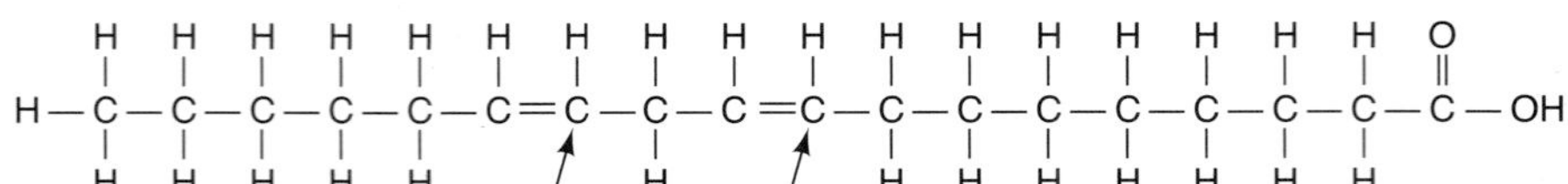

Polyunsaturated (more than one carbon-to-carbon double bond)

FIGURE 4-2 Saturated, monounsaturated, and polyunsaturated fatty acids. A saturated fatty acid has no carbon-to-carbon double bonds. A monounsaturated fatty acid has one carbon-to-carbon double bond. A polyunsaturated fatty acid has more than one carbon-to-carbon double bond.

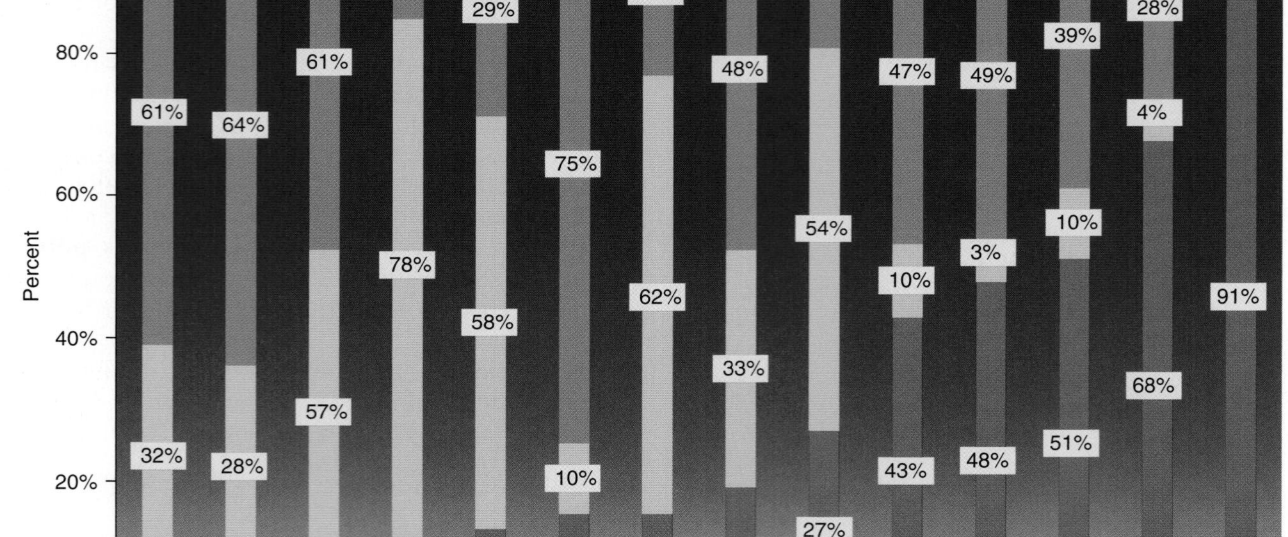

FIGURE 4-3 Comparison of fatty acid composition of edible fats, oils, and flaxseed. The oil with the highest monounsaturated fat content is olive oil. The oil with the lowest saturated fat content is canola.

Physical Properties and Food Sources

Terms such as saturated fats, unsaturated fats, and hydrogenation are commonly used. This section of the text introduces these terms and discusses food sources.

Saturated Fats

Saturated fats, which are likely to be solid at room temperature, are usually found in animal products such as meat, poultry, and whole milk. The exceptions are tropical coconut and palm-kernel oils and cocoa butter, which are vegetable sources of saturated fat. See Tables 4-1 and 4-2 for a more complete list of foods containing saturated fat.

Saturated fats are more chemically stable than unsaturated fats. For this reason, saturated fats become rancid very slowly because the chemical bond between carbon and hydrogen is very stable. A rancid fat has an offensive odor and taste caused by the partial chemical breakdown of the fat's molecular structure. Consumers usually discard **rancid** foods because of the highly offensive odor.

Products made with saturated fats have a fairly long shelf life (the time a product can remain in storage without deterioration) because the fat in the product is fairly stable. However, saturated fats have been targeted for reduction in the average American's diet by health authorities because these fats have unhealthful effects when ingested in excess of the body's needs.

Unsaturated Fats

Unsaturated fats are likely to be liquid at room temperature and of plant origin; they tend to become rancid more quickly than saturated fats. The double carbon bonds in unsaturated fatty acids are very unstable and therefore easily broken. For this reason, many convenience products have traditionally been made with saturated fats to lengthen their shelf life. The food industry is changing this practice; increasingly, more convenience products are made with unsaturated fats. Examples of unsaturated fats are corn, cottonseed, safflower, soybean, and sunflower oils. See Table 4-3 for a more complete list of unsaturated fats.

TABLE 4-2 ■ Selected Foods High in Cholesterol and/or Saturated Fat

FOOD	AMOUNT	CHOLESTEROL (MG)	SATURATED FAT (MG)
Liver	3 oz	410	2.4
Cream puff	1	228	10.0
Baked custard	1 cup	213	7.0
Egg, hard cooked	1	215	5.0
Waffles, homemade	2	204	8.0
Coconut custard pie	1 piece	183	8.0
Cheesecake	3.25 oz	170	10.0
Shrimp, boiled	6 large	167	0.2
Eggnog, commercial	1 cup	149	11.0
Bread pudding/raisins	1 cup	142	4.5
Whole milk	1 cup	124	5.0
Ground beef, 21% fat	3 oz cooked	76	7.0

TABLE 4-3 ■ Food Sources of Unsaturated Fats

FOODS HIGH IN MONOUNSATURATED FATTY ACIDS	FOODS HIGH IN POLYUNSATURATED FATTY ACIDS
Canola, olive, peanut oils	Corn, cottonseed, mustard seed, safflower, sesame, soybean, and sunflower seed oils
Almonds, avocados, cashews, filberts, olives, and peanuts	Halibut, herring, mackerel, salmon, sardines, fresh tuna, trout, whitefish

TABLE 4-1 ■ Food Sources of Saturated Fats

Meat products	Visible fat and marbling in beef, pork, and lamb, especially in prime-grade and ground meats, lard, suet, salt pork
Processed meats	Frankfurters Luncheon meats such as bologna, corned beef, liverwurst, pastrami, and salami Bacon and sausage
Poultry and fowl	Chicken and turkey (mostly beneath the skin), Cornish hens, duck, and goose
Whole milk and whole-milk products	Cheeses made with whole milk or cream, condensed milk, ice cream, whole-milk yogurt, all creams (sour, half-and-half, whipped)
Plant products	Coconut oil, palm-kernel oil, cocoa butter
Miscellaneous	Fully hydrogenated shortening and margarine, many cakes, pies, cookies, and mixes

Hydrogenation

Commercial food processing frequently involves hydrogenation—adding hydrogen to a fat of vegetable origin (unsaturated) to either extend the fat's shelf life or make the fat harder. This process of adding hydrogen to a fat is called **hydrogenation**. If only some of the fat's double bonds are broken by the hydrogenation, the product becomes partially hydrogenated. If all of the double bonds are broken, the product becomes completely hydrogenated.

Completely hydrogenated fats are highly saturated fats; that is, they have no carbon-to-carbon double bonds. For example, a completely hydrogenated corn oil is closer to lard in saturation than a partially hydrogenated corn oil. All vegetable spreads, such as corn oil margarine, have been hydrogenated to some extent. If these spreads had not been hydrogenated, they would be liquids (except for the saturated tropical oils). Clients are usually advised to avoid products that contain completely hydrogenated fats when the therapeutic goal is to decrease saturated fat intake.

A health consequence of hydrogenation is the formation of ***trans*-fatty acids.** *Trans*-fatty acids are produced by the partial hydrogenation of unsaturated vegetable oils. As illustrated in Figure 4-4, a *cis* configuration double bond between carbon atoms in a fatty acid has a kink or bend. A *trans* configuration double bond between carbon atoms in a fatty acid is straighter.

During hydrogenation, many of the fatty acids are converted from the *cis* to the *trans* configuration. Evidence indicates that the *trans* configuration is detrimental to health. If the dietary goal is to decrease consumption of *trans* fatty acids, the client must decrease consumption of hydrogenated foods. Foods that may be high in *trans* fatty acids include:

- Commercially baked goods
- Fried foods in restaurants

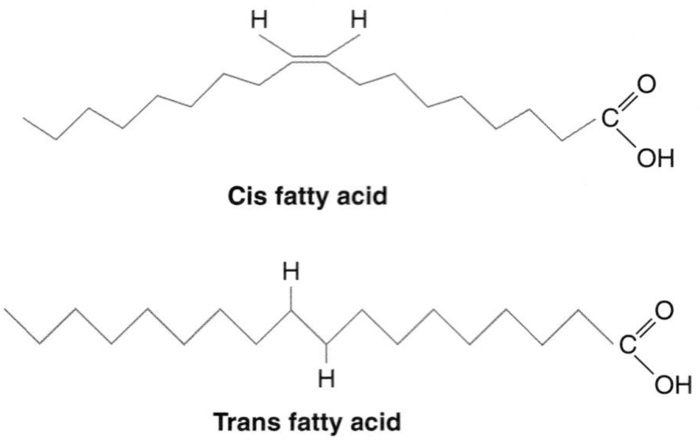

H H O C OH

Cis fatty acid

H O C H OH

Trans fatty acid

FIGURE 4-4 A *cis* fatty acid and a *trans* fatty acid. Whenever there is a change from *cis* to *trans* configuration in a fatty acid, the three-dimensional shape of the molecule is altered.

- Hard margarines and shortenings
- Crackers
- Biscuit and some cake mixes
- Some candy
- Animal crackers and cookies
- Frozen waffles and pancakes
- Microwave popcorn

The food industry is currently in the process of reformulating many of these products to decrease their *trans*-fatty acid content.

Functions of Fats

Lipids are important in the diet and serve many functions in the human body.

Fats in Food

Fats serve several functions in food including serving as a fuel source and acting as a vehicle for fat-soluble vitamins.

Fuel Source

Fats are the major dietary source of fuel. Because fats have proportionately more carbon and hydrogen and less oxygen than carbohydrates, fats have a greater potential for the release of energy. In practical terms, this means that fats are a concentrated source of fuel or kcalories.

Fats furnish more than twice as many kcalories, gram for gram, as carbohydrates. Each gram of fat yields 9 kcalories, so 1 teaspoon of fat, which is equivalent to 5 grams of fat, yields 45 kcalories. Compare these numbers with those for carbohydrates, each gram of which yields only 4 kcalories. A teaspoon of sugar contains 4 grams of carbohydrates and therefore yields only 16 kcalories.

Vehicle for Fat-Soluble Vitamins

In foods, fats act as a vehicle for vitamins A, D, E, and K. In the body, fats assist in the absorption of these fat-soluble vitamins.

Satiety Value

Fats also contribute flavor, satiety value, and palatability to the diet. They supply texture to food, trap and intensify its flavor, and enhance its odor. Satiety is a person's feeling of fullness and satisfaction after eating. Fat contributes to the sensation of satisfaction because it leaves the stomach more slowly than carbohydrates.

Consider for a moment the sensations felt when eating 2 cups of ice cream versus 2 cups of chopped apples. Ice cream has a high fat content, and apples have no fat. An individual may feel full after eating 2 cups of apples but complain of a bloated feeling and a lack of gratification. Satiety is feeling full, completely satisfied, and that enough or too much food has been eaten.

Sources of Essential Fatty Acids

An essential nutrient is one that must be supplied by the diet because the body cannot manufacture it in sufficient amounts to prevent disease. Fat contains the essential fatty acids linoleic, arachidonic, and linolenic. Linolenic acid is subdivided into two groups, alpha and gamma. Figure 4-5 shows the pathways of these fatty acids.

Although the body can manufacture gamma-linoleic (-linolenic) acid and arachidonic acid from linoleic acid, all three of these fatty acids are now considered essential. Linoleic is called an omega-6 fatty acid. Omega is the last letter in the Greek alphabet and is used by chemists for naming fatty acid classes by their chemical structure. The six designation means that the first double bond is located six carbons down the chain (counting from the omega end).

Linoleic acid strengthens cell membranes and has a major role in the transport and metabolism of cholesterol. The omega-6 fatty acids together prolong blood-clotting time, hasten fibrolytic activity, and are involved in the development of the brain. **Prostaglandins,** compounds with extensive **hormone-**like actions, require arachidonic acid for synthesis.

Another name for alpha-linolenic fatty acid is omega-3 polyunsaturated fatty acid (PUFA). The omega-3 PUFA has a variety of biological effects that may influence the risk of cardiovascular disease and reduce the risk of incident Alzheimer disease (http://en.wikipedia.org/wiki/omega-3-fatty-acid, 2010). More of this research is discussed in Chapter 18 on cardiovascular disease.

Linoleic acid deficiency was first observed in the medical community during the middle of the 20th century with the introduction and widespread use of infant baby formulas. Initially, the formulas were deficient in linoleic acid and infants subsequently fed formula developed dry and flaky skin. When linoleic was added to formula recipes, the infants' symptoms ceased. Currently, all infant formulas contain linoliec acid (Wiese, Hansen, and Adam, 1958).

Linoleic acid deficiency was again observed in the early 1970s in hospitalized clients fed exclusively with intravenous fluids containing no fat. Symptoms included scaly skin, hair loss, impaired wound healing, increased susceptiblity to infection, and immune dysfunction. When lipids were introduced into intravenous feedings, such symptoms ceased.

Fats in the Body

Fat serves six major functions in the human body:

1. Supply fuel to most tissues
2. Function as an energy reserve
3. Insulate the body
4. Support and protect vital organs
5. Lubricate body tissues
6. Form an integral part of cell membranes

Fuel Supply

Fat serves as a fuel that supplies body tissues with needed energy.

Fuel Reserve

Fat also functions as the body's main fuel or energy reserve. Excess kcalories consumed are stored in

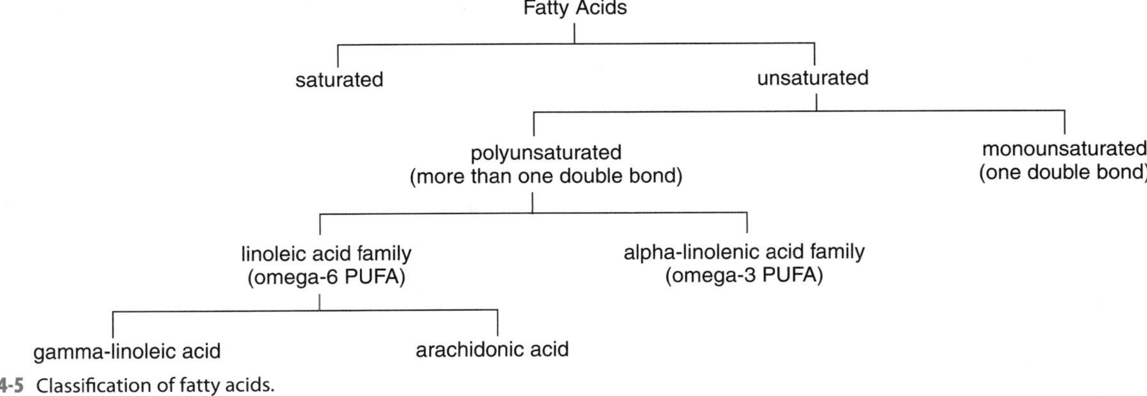

FIGURE 4-5 Classification of fatty acids.

specialized cells called adipose cells. When an individual does not eat enough food to meet the energy demands of the body, the adipose cells release fat for fuel.

Lubrication

Fats also lubricate body tissue. The human body manufactures oil in structures called sebaceous glands. Secretions from the sebaceous glands lubricate the skin to retard loss of body water to the outside environment.

Organ Protection

Fatty tissue cushions and protects vital organs by providing a supportive fat pad that absorbs mechanical shocks. Examples of organs supported by fat are the eyes and kidneys.

Insulation

The subcutaneous layer of fat beneath the skin helps to insulate the body by protecting it from excessive heat or cold. A sheath of fatty tissue surrounding nerve fibers provides insulation to help transmit nerve impulses.

Cell Membrane Structure

Fat serves as an integral part of cell membranes and in this capacity plays a vital role in drug, nutrient, and metabolite transport and provides a barrier against water-soluble substances.

Cholesterol

Cholesterol is not a true fat but belongs to a group called sterols. Cholesterol is a component of many of the foods in our diet. In addition, the human body manufactures about 1000 milligrams of cholesterol a day, mainly in the liver. See Genomic Gem 4-1. The liver also filters out excess cholesterol and helps to eliminate it from the body.

Functions

Cholesterol has several important functions. It is:

1. A component of bile salts that aid digestion
2. An essential component of all cell membranes
3. Found in brain and nerve tissue and in the blood

Genomic Gem 4-1

Client Response to Dietary Modification

A great deal of evidence indicates a relationship between cholesterol intake (especially one component of cholesterol called low-density liopoprotein cholesterol) and increased risk of coronary heart disease. In addition, increasing evidence shows genetic factors influence a person's response to both increases or decreases in cholesterol intake. For example, one study found defects in two different genes can lead to markedly increased absorption of both cholesterol and plant sterols (Food and Nutrition Board, 2005).

Another gene has been found to attenuate the plasma cholesterol response to dietary cholesterol in diets high in polyunsaturated fat but not in diets high in saturated fat (Food and Nutrition Board, 2005). These studies have been done in animals, but to date such human data are lacking. The goal of this research is to be able to predict exactly what factors will lead to a disease in a particular individual. Genetics is the branch of biology that studies heredity and variation in both plants and aninals. Genetics may also explain why one client may respond to diet modification while another client may not respond.

Cholesterol is also necessary for the production of several hormones, including:

- Cortisone
- Adrenaline
- Estrogen
- Testosterone

A **hormone** is a substance produced by the endocrine glands and secreted directly into the bloodstream. Hormones stimulate functional activity of organs and cells or stimulate secretion of other hormones to do so.

Food Sources

Cholesterol is present in the foods we eat. In fact, many of the products sold in supermarkets are targeted to shoppers interested in controlling their blood cholesterol levels through diet. Cholesterol occurs naturally in all animal foods and is produced only in liver tissue. When we ingest animal products, we also ingest the cholesterol the animal made. For this reason, the American Heart Association advocates the consumption of low-fat or nonfat dairy products, fish, legumes, poultry, and lean meats (Pearson et al., 2002).

Table 4-2 lists selected foods high in cholesterol. Note that one egg supplies about 215 milligrams of cholesterol. Eggs are the major contributor of cholesterol into the average American's diet. The American

Heart Association recommends that consumers limit their intake of egg yolks to no more than four per week.

The current thinking among most nutrition experts is that total diet should be evaluated for risk prevention. An overall healthy eating pattern that includes fruits, vegetables, and grains is important for risk reduction. No one food, even if it contains cholesterol, is unhealthy if eaten in appropriate amounts.

Fat Intake as a Worldwide Concern

The combination of underweight in children and overweight in adults, frequently coexisting in the same family, is a new phenomenon in developing countries undergoing nutrition transition (Caballero, 2005). Changes in diet, food availability, and lifestyle are all components of transition as countries modernize. However, obesity in adults has been linked to the availability of cheap energy-dense foods (including those from street vendors and fast-food restaurants) that facilitate the consumption of more fat. In addition, the introduction of low-cost vegetable oils from industrialized countries greatly increases the amount of fat in the average diet.

Healthier foods, including fruits and vegetables, are usually more expensive and not available to the world's poorest people. Many health experts believe messages should focus on the benefits of increasing fruit and vegetable intake, improving overall diet quality, and increasing physical activity (Doak et al., 2005). However, education does not address the reality that much of the world's population cannot afford a quality diet and more fruits and vegetables.

Dietary Recommendations Concerning Fat

The National Academy of Science report on Dietary Reference Intakes for Macronutrients issued guidelines pertaining to fats in 2005 (Food and Nutrition Board, Institute of Medicine, 2005). Box 4-1 discusses the acceptable macronutrient distribution range (AMDR) for fats.

Before this recommendation, most government health authorities and professional groups recommended that the fat content of the U.S. diet not exceed 30% of kcaloric intake. The rationale for the change is that carbohydrates, fat, and protein all serve as fuel sources and can substitute for one another to some extent to meet fuel needs. Therefore, the recommended ranges for consuming these nutrients should be useful and flexible for dietary planning (Food and Nutrition Board, Institute of Medicine, 2005). Table 4-4 lists the recommended ranges in grams of fat for various kcalorie levels. See Clinical Calculation 4-1 as well.

The Food and Nutrition Board of the Institute of Medicine stated that saturated fat and cholesterol provide no known beneficial role in preventing

Box 4-1 ■ *AMDR for Fats*

A range of intake for a particular energy source that is associated with a reduced risk of chronic disease and that provides adequate intakes of essential nutrients is called the acceptable macronutrient distribution range (AMDR) (Hise and Brown, 2007). The AMDR for adults is 20%–35% of kcalories from fat. The AMDR for infants and young children is 25%–40% of kcalories from fat.

TABLE 4-4 ■ Recommended Range of Fat Intake at Selected Kilocalorie Levels

KCALORIE LEVEL	TOTAL FAT (GRAMS)
1200	26–46
1500	33–58
1600	35–62
1800	40–70
2000	44–78
2200	49–85
2400	53–93
2500	55–97

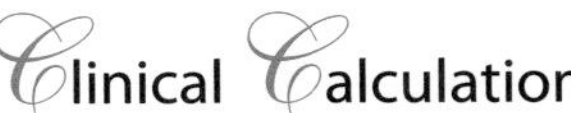

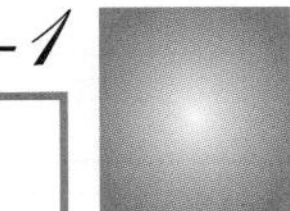

4-1

Percent of Kcalories from Fat

The following formula can be used to determine the percentage of kcalories from fat in many packaged foods:

Kcalories from
fat per serving/Kcalories* × 100 =
Percent kcalories from fat per serving

Example: kcalories from fat = 30
kcalories per serving = 90
% kcalories from fat = 30%

*Food labeling regulations require manufacturers to list both the number of kcalories in a serving and the number of kcalories from fat.

chronic diseases and are not required at any level in the diet. However, the complete elimination of saturated fat and cholesterol from the diet would make it very difficult to meet other nutritional guidelines. Some monounsaturated and polyunsaturated fatty acids are required to provide the essential fatty acids. See Box 4-2 and Dollars and Sense 4-1.

The committee was also asked to address the subject of *trans*-fatty acids. The committee concluded that because *trans*-fatty acids are not essential and provide no known health benefits, there is no safe level for *trans*-fatty acids in the diet. People should eat as little of them as possible while consuming a nutritionally adequate diet.

Dietary Fat Intake and Health

Fat plays a key role in diet and health. A diet too low in fat not only lacks satiety and palatability but also may lack adequate levels of the essential fatty acids; a diet with excessive fat may result in increased risk of disease.

Dietary Fat

A diet that has an appropriate balance of fat and carbohydrate is important for optimal health. Chronic consumption of either a low-fat high-carbohydrate or a high-fat low-carbohydrate diet may result in the inadequate intake of nutrients (Food and Nutrition Board, 2005). A diet too low in fat not only lacks satiety and palatability but also may lack adequate levels of the essential fatty acids, zinc, and certain B vitamins (Food and Nutrition Board, 2005). Excessive dietary fat has been associated with an increased risk of cardiovascular disease, the development of obesity and diabetes, and an increased risk of certain cancers.

One major issue concerning kcalorie distribution is whether eating a high-fat diet predisposes a person to becoming overweight or obese. Some experts argue that it is far from proven that eating low-fat foods automatically helps individuals keep off excess weight.

The food industry has cut the amount of fat in foods, such as reduced-fat cakes, cookies, ice cream, luncheon meats, and salad dressings. Yet Americans are still becoming heavier. Many experts attribute

Box 4-2 ■ *Essential Fatty Acids*

AI for Essential Fatty Acids for Adults 19–51 Years Old*		Kind	Food Sources
Men Women	17 grams 12 grams	Omega-6 fatty acids Linoleic acid	■ Vegetable oils such as safflower, corn, soybean, cottonseed ■ Poultry fat ■ Nuts and seeds
Men Women	1.6 grams 1.1 grams	Omega-3 fatty acids Linolenic acid	■ Human milk ■ Fatty fish ■ Vegetable oils such as soybean, flax, canola ■ Wheat germ ■ Soybeans

*Refer to DRI tables for other age groups.

$ Dollars & Sense 4-1

Dietary Guidelines for Fat

The *Dietary Guidelines for Americans 2005*, American Heart Association, and The National Heart, Lung, and Blood Institute (NHLBI) recommend that most dietary fats come from sources of polyunsaturated and monounsaturated fatty acids. One way to obtain these fats is to incorporate nuts in the diet.

Nuts also provide other essential nutrients such as linolenic acid, vitamins A and E, magnesium, dietary fiber, copper and zinc. Many nuts are also high in phytonutrients.

The best method of incorporating nuts into the diet on a daily basis is to practice good portion control. For example, an exchange or serving of nuts contains about 5 grams of fat and 45 kcalories. One pound of shelled pistachios may appear to be expensive but if eaten in exchange serving sizes of 16 nuts (roughly one tablespoon), that pound should yield 60 servings.

this weight gain to substituting sugar and refined carbohydrates for fat. Other experts think dietary fat content is a risk factor for weight gain (Blundell and Stubbs, 2004).

A healthy choice is to substitute vegetables and whole grains for fat as all carbohydrates are not equal in the promotion of health.

Monounsaturated Fats

The health benefits of monounsaturated fatty acids have been a better-understood phenomenon. Most health educators recommend increasing intake of monounsaturated fats while decreasing intake of saturated and polyunsaturated fats. Evidence suggests that individuals with a high intake of monounsaturated fats, a low intake of saturated fats, and a low total fat intake may have a decreased risk of coronary heart disease.

Monounsaturated fats are found in canola, olive, and peanut oil. Many nutrition experts advocate the consumption of fats derived from plant sources, such as those shown in Figure 4-6 because those foods also contribute fiber, antioxidants, and phytochemicals to the diet.

Polyunsaturated Fats

The average healthy American should not increase his or her intake of polyunsaturated fat. At very high levels of polyunsaturated fat intake, animal studies consistently show an increase in colon and mammary cancers. Observations in humans have shown that a polyunsaturated fat intake of less than 10% of kcalories does not increase the population's risk of cancer.

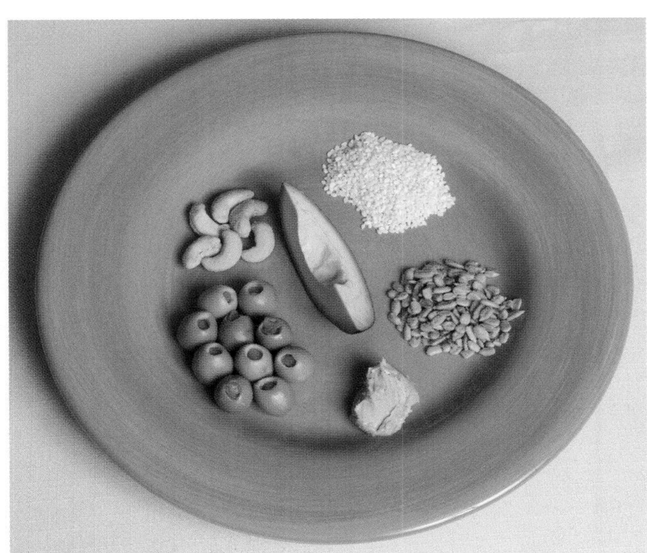

FIGURE 4-6 Plant sources of fats include avocado, nuts, olives, peanut butter, and some seeds such as sesame and flax.

Body Fat

Both the amount of body fat a person carries and its distribution on the body are related to health risk. Many experts feel that the ratio of body fat to total weight is more important than total weight. Healthy ranges for body fat are 15% to 19% for men and 18% to 22% for women. A high percentage of body fat has been associated with increased risk of disease, even when total body weight is normal.

The location of excess body fat is also important. Excessive fat on the lower body, specifically on the hips and thighs, seems to be less dangerous than excessive fat on the abdomen and upper body, which is associated with a much higher risk of diseases such as cancer, heart disease, and diabetes. The exchange lists in the next section can be used to assist in planning meals low in fat and teach clients about food composition.

Exchange Lists

Exchange lists can be used to learn food composition and portion control and assist in planning lower-fat meals. For example, many people do not know that sugar and fruit contain no fat and oil contains no carbohydrate. Exchange categories that include fat are the milk, meat, and fat lists. The amount of fat in one exchange of meat or milk varies within the list. Some foods not listed on the exchange lists are also high in fat. Many of these foods may be found in the nutritive values of foods tables (see "Caffeine and Nutritive Values of Foods" on DavisPlus.com).

Milk Exchange List

The fat content of milk varies according to the type of milk—whole, 2%, 1%, or nonfat. Table 4-5 shows the grams of fat and percentage of kcalories from fat in one milk exchange for each kind of milk. Although whole milk and 2% milk contain saturated fat and

TABLE 4-5 ■ Grams of Fat in One Milk Exchange

TYPE	FAT (GRAMS)	PERCENTAGE OF KCALORIES FROM FAT
Whole milk	8	48
2% (low fat)	5	38
Nonfat milk	Trace	<1

cholesterol, the protein, carbohydrate, vitamin, and mineral contents of whole, 2%, 1%, and nonfat milk are comparable. Nonfat milk contains only a trace of fat and is thus a nutritional bargain.

Meat and Meat Substitute Exchange List

The meat exchange list is divided into four subgroups:

- *One very lean* meat exchange contains less than 1 gram of fat.
- *One lean* meat exchange contains 3 grams of fat.
- *One medium*-fat meat exchange contains 5 grams of fat.
- *One high*-fat meat exchange contains 8 grams of fat.

Table 4-6 lists selected food examples from each of the meat exchanges.

Many clients have misconceptions about meat. Some clients avoid all red meat because they think it contains excessive fat. In fact, some beef and pork products are not excessively high in fat. Many consumers are not aware of the lean cuts of beef or pork. Conversely, not all fish and poultry items are lean meat exchanges. Nurses and other health educators can help clients by providing correct information about meats.

Different methods of food preparation can greatly influence the fat content of meats. Those that are baked, broiled, grilled, or roasted contain fewer kcalories than fried versions. Some clients have the misconception that if they eat only lean meats, they can eat

TABLE 4-6 ■ Examples of Very Lean, Lean, Medium-Fat, and High-Fat Meat Exchanges

Each of the following is one very lean meat exchange and contains less than 1 gram of fat:		
Poultry	Chicken or turkey (white meat, no skin)	1 oz
Fish	Fresh or frozen cod, flounder, haddock	1 oz
Game	Venison	1 oz
Cheese	Nonfat cottage cheese Fat-free cheese	¼ cup 1 oz
Other	Egg whites Hot dogs with less than 1 g of fat Egg substitute	2 1 oz ¼ cup
Each of the following is one lean meat exchange and contains 3 grams of fat:		
Beef	Round, sirloin, or flank steak	1 oz
Fish	Salmon (fresh or frozen)	1 oz
Pork	Tenderloin	1 oz
Veal	Lean chop or roast	1 oz
Poultry	Chicken, dark meat, no skin	1 oz
Game	Goose, no skin	1 oz
Cheese	4.5% fat cottage cheese Cheeses with less than 3 g of fat per oz	¼ cup 1 oz
Other	Hot dogs with less than 3 g of fat per oz Processed lunch meat with less than 3 g of fat per oz	1 oz 1 oz
Each of the following is one medium-fat meat exchange and contains 5 grams of fat:		
Beef	Ground beef, corned beef	1 oz
Pork	Chops	1 oz
Poultry	Chicken, dark meat, with skin	1 oz
Fish	Any fried fish product	1 oz
Cheese	Mozzarella	1 oz
Other	Egg (high in cholesterol) Tofu	1 ½ cup
Each of the following is one high-fat meat exchange and contains 8 grams of fat:		
Pork	Spareribs, pork sausage	1 oz
Cheese	All regular cheeses such as cheddar, Swiss, and American	1 oz
Other	Bologna Knockwurst, bratwurst Bacon	1 oz 1 oz 3 slices

large quantities prepared in any manner. But preparation really does count. For example, a 3-ounce breaded fried chicken breast contains more fat than a grilled hamburger patty.

Meat exchanges are usually 1 ounce, but a usual portion is 3 ounces, about half a chicken breast. Table 4-7 shows the total fat content of three meat exchanges. Typically, Americans eat large amounts of meats such as prime rib (from 6-ounce to 16-ounce servings). Therefore, teaching clients about meat portion sizes is usually indicated when the goal is to decrease fat intake and decrease total kcalorie intake.

Whether the meat is classified as a very lean, lean, medium-fat, or high-fat meat exchange, the grams of fat in each exchange are calculated based on the following assumptions:

- Visible fat on meat is not consumed.
- Meat is weighed after cooking.
- Meat is cooked by a low-fat method—baked, boiled, broiled, grilled, or roasted (unless otherwise indicated).

Since 1994 food-labeling regulations have allowed two definitions for the fat content labeling of meat, poultry, seafood, and game meats: *lean* and *extra lean.*

- *Lean* can be used on meat, poultry, seafood, or game meat products only if the product contains less than 10 grams of fat, less than 4.5 grams of saturated fat, and less than 95 milligrams of cholesterol per 100-gram serving (3½ ounces). The legal term *lean* thus equals the ADA exchange list definition for a lean meat exchange.
- *Extra lean* can be used only if the product contains less than 5 grams of fat, less than 2 grams of saturated fat and *trans* fat combined, and less than 95 milligrams of cholesterol per serving and per 100 grams (3½ ounces).

Some clients may choose not to eat animal products. Health-care workers should always accommodate their client's religious, ecological, and ethical beliefs and values. See Appendix B for brief exchange list information, which includes some meat substitutes. Many low-fat meat substitutes including dried beans, peas, and lentils are not derived from animals. Medium-fat vegetarian meat exchanges include soymilk, tempeh, and tofu. Peanut butter, which contains 8 grams of fat per exchange (2 tablespoons), is a high-fat meat exchange.

TABLE 4-7 ■ Total Fat in Three Meat Exchanges

MEAT	SUBGROUP	GRAMS OF FAT/ EXCHANGE	GRAMS OF FAT PER SERVING
Cod	Very lean	1	3
Sirloin steak	Lean	3	9
Hamburger patty, broiled*	Medium fat	5	15
Spareribs†	High fat	8	24

*About 4 oz raw.
†Boneless.

Fat Exchange List

Each fat exchange provides 5 grams of fat. Figure 4-7 illustrates three fat exchanges. The fat list is subdivided into two groups: unsaturated fats (monounsaturated and polyunsaturated) and saturated fats. Table 4-8 lists selected exchanges from each group.

Additional Food Sources of Fat

It is important to advise clients that snack foods, including crackers, cakes, pies, donuts, and cookies, may be high in both total fat and *trans*-fatty acids. Often, potato chips, gravies, cream sauces, soups, pizza, tacos, and spaghetti are high in fat. Microwave popcorn is higher in fat than air-popped popcorn (without added fat).

Consumers who desire low-fat foods need not avoid eating out, but they do need to make wise food choices, especially if they eat most meals in restaurants. Many of the specialty fast-food hamburgers are high in fat; therefore, a small hamburger is the best burger choice. A small side salad with low-fat dressing is a better low-fat choice than French fries. Nonfat milk is lower in fat than either a milkshake or whole milk. A grilled chicken breast salad with a fat-free dressing is also a good choice. See Box 4-3.

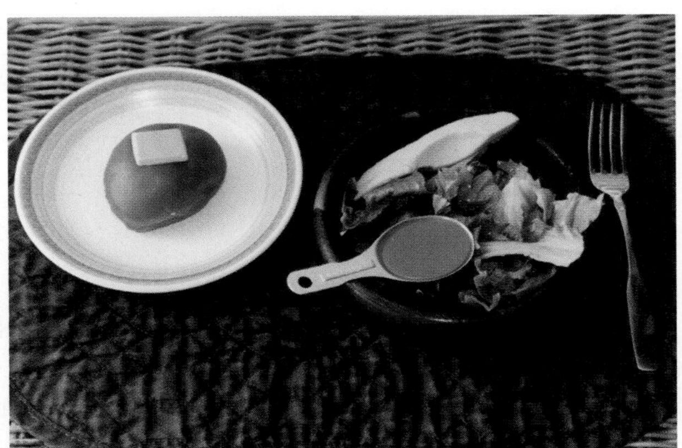

FIGURE 4-7 One teaspoon of margarine, one tablespoon of regular French dressing, and ⅛ of an avocado are each equal to one fat exchange and contains about 5 grams of fat.

Plant Stanols and Sterols

Foods that contain plant stanols and sterols have been shown to reduce blood cholesterol levels (USDA, 2000). Plant sterols and stanols work by blocking dietary cholesterol's entrance into the body. Foods that contain plant stanols and sterols include certain margarine spreads and salad dressings. Benecol®, Take Control®, and Smart Balance® are brand names currently available in grocery stores. Minute Maid Premium Heart Wise® orange juice was the first orange juice to contain plant sterols.

TABLE 4-8 ■ Examples of Monounsaturated, Polyunsaturated, and Saturated Fat Exchanges

Each of the following is one fat exchange high in monounsaturated fatty acids and contains 5 g of total fat:	
Olives	5 large
Canola oil	1 tsp
Peanut butter	2 tsp
Pecans	4 halves
Each of the following is one fat exchange high in polyunsaturated fatty acids and contains 5 grams of total fat:	
Margarine, stick or tub	1 tsp
Mayo, regular	1 tsp
Corn oil	1 tsp
English walnuts	4 halves
Each of the following is one fat exchange high in saturated fatty acids and contains 5 grams of total fat:	
Bacon	1 slice (20 slices/lb)
Butter, stick	1 tsp
Cream cheese, regular	1 tbsp (½ oz)
Cream cheese, reduced-fat	2 tbsp (1 oz)
Sour cream, regular	2 tbsp
Sour cream, reduced-fat	3 tbsp

Box 4-3 ■ *Food Label Terms*

Food labeling regulations spell out what terms may be used to describe the level of fat in a food and how the labels can be used. Theses are the terms:

- *Fat-free* on a food label means that the food contains no more than 0.5 grams of fat per serving. Synonyms for *free* include *without, no,* and *zero. Nonfat* is another synonym for *fat-free.* These terms legally can be used on a food label only if the product contains no amount of—or only trivial or "physiologically inconsequential" amounts of—fat, saturated fat, and cholesterol.
- *Low-fat* is legally defined as a food that contains no more than 3 grams of fat in a serving.
- *Low saturated fat* is legally defined as a food that contains no more than 1 gram of saturated fat per serving.
- *Low cholesterol* is defined as a food that contains less than 20 milligrams of cholesterol per serving. Synonyms for *low* include *little, few,* and *low source of.*

In addition, serving sizes listed on food labels are standardized to make nutritional comparisons of similar products easier.

Keystones

- The group name for all fats is lipids.
- Hydrogen, oxygen, and carbon are the primary elements in fats.
- Gram for gram, fats contain more than twice the kcalories of carbohydrates.
- Fats are labeled according to the amount and type of fatty acids they contain as saturated, unsaturated, monounsaturated, polyunsaturated and *trans*-fatty acids.
- Fats serve many important functions in our diets and our bodies.

Keystones—cont'd

- A balanced intake of carbohydrate and fat is essential for optimal health. Excess fats in our diets are associated with cardiovascular disease, obesity and diabetes, and some types of cancer.
- Cholesterol is a fat-like substance that is present in animal food sources and produced by the human body.
- Many Americans would benefit from decreasing their intake of cholesterol, *trans*-fatty acids, and saturated fat.
- The National Academies of Science on Dietary Reference Intakes for Macronutrients recommends that adults consume between 20% and 35% of their kcalories from fat (Food and Nutrition Board, 2005).
- *Dietary Guidelines for Americans* recommends a saturated fat intake of less than 10% of kcalories and dietary cholesterol intake of less than 300 milligrams per day.
- The ADA exchanges that contain fat are the milk, meat, and fat lists.

CASE STUDY 4-1

Mr. D had a physical examination by his family physician, who also treated the client's brother and his father. His father had died of a stroke and his 35-year-old brother recently had a myocardial infaction (heart attack). The physcian noted several xanthomas around his eyes. His height is 5 feet 6 inches and his weight is 180 pounds. The client reports consuming frequent or large portions of high-fat foods. The client agreed to speak with the student nurse directly after the appointment. The student is doing a practicum in the doctor's office. The registered nurse supervising the student nurse (Mike) requested that he do the following:

1. Schedule the client for follow-up with the physician
2. Develop a nursing care plan that addresses the client's nursing problem to complement the medical diagnosis.

As the student was assigned only one client, he had the time to complete his assigned tasks in greater detail than a nurse normally would. As the student did not have a computer data program available, it took him several hours to complete this assignment.

Mike, the student nurse, scheduled the follow-up appointment with the physician for 2 days later (just before the client was leaving for his cruise). Mr. D was instructed by the student to write down all food he consumed for 1 day before the appointment. The client was advised to choose a typical day to record his food intake to provide a more accurate analysis of his usual diet.

Two Days Later

Mr. D arrived on the appropriate day and handed his food record to the student for review. Mike calculated the grams of fat in Mr. D's food record based on a combination of ADA exchanges and a table of food composition. Mr. D's food record and Mike's calculations are below.

The physician has just seen the client at his follow-up appointment and reviewed Mr. D's food record and Mike's calculations. Mr. D's total cholesterol was 350 mg/dL (normal for laboratory test is < 200 mg/dL). His low-density lipoprotein (LDL) cholesterol was elevated to 150 mg/dL (normal for laboratory test is <100 mg/dL).

Mr. D told the doctor "I cannot understand why my cholesterol is elevated. My weight is stable. I always select the salad bar for lunch, avoid sweets, and drink low-fat milk." The client agreed to meet with the dietitian after his cruise.

(Continued on the following page)

CASE STUDY *(Continued)*

11:00 A.M.	
Food	*Grams of Fat*
Salad Bar	
Assorted vegetables and lettuce	0
4 tbsp blue cheese dressing (cup)	20 (4 fats)
4 oz shredded cheese	32 (4 high-fat meat)
1 oz diced ham	3 (1 lean meat)
1 cup potato salad	14*
Dinner roll	0
4 tsp butter	20 (4 fat)
1 cup clam chowder	7*
7:00 PM Restaurant	
Food	*Grams of Fat*
4 oz hamburger, checked weight	20 (4 medium-fat meats)
2 oz cheese	16 (2 high-fat meat)
2 tbsp mayo	30 (6 fats)
Bun	0
6 onion rings	15*
Tossed salad	0
4 tbsp blue cheese dressing	20 (4 fats)
11:00 PM Home	
Food	*Grams of Fat*
1 cup 2% milk	5
1 orange	0
Total fat for the day	202 g of fat

*Values obtained from a table of food composition.

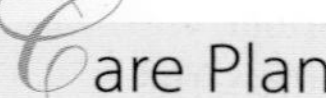

Care Plan

Subjective Data

Admitted knowledge deficit. Food record for 1 day contained 202 grams of fat.

Objective Data

Cholesterol level: 350 mg/dL and LDL level was 150; height: 5 ft, 6 in.; weight: 160 lb

Analysis

Client's dietary intake of cholesterol is related to elevated blood cholesterol levels.

Plan

DESIRED OUTCOMES EVALUATION CRITERIA	ACTIONS/INTERVENTIONS	RATIONALE
Client will keep a food record for one day.	Instruct the client on the recording of his food intake.	Keeping food records will remind the client of the importance of decreasing his or her fat intake. Reviewing them with the client permits positive reinforcement and correction of misperceptions.
Client will decrease his fat intake by 50%.	Encourage client to first cut the major sources of fat in his diet: salad dressings and cheese.	50% of client's fat intake is from cheese, mayo, and salad dressings.
Encourage the client to meet with the dietitian after his cruise.	Offer the client a referral to the dietitan so that his estimated nutritional needs can be calculated and receive tips on long-term compliance.	A student cannot be expected to follow client long term.
	Tell the client to call the nurse if he is having trouble interpreting dietary instructions at home.	Offers the client support between visits.

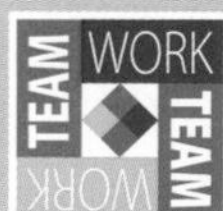

4-1

Dietitian's Note

The following dietitian's notes are representative of the type of documentation found in the narrative portion of a client's medical record.

Six weeks later

Subjective: Met with the client and his significant other. Although the client has made a recent change to substitute fat-free mayo and salad dressings for regular dressings, he was not able to give up cheese. Admits to sedentary lifestyle. The 24-hour dietary recall cross-checked with a food frequency showed a three-meal-per-day pattern with a salad for lunch and the evening meal in a restaurant.

Objective: Most recent cholesterol was 330 mg/dL and LDL was 142 mg/dL. Height: 5 ft 6 in.; weight 158 lb.

Analysis: Ideal body weight at 106 lb for the first 5 ft and 6 lb for each additional inch = 128–156. Estimated kcaloric need at 10–11 kcal/lb at 156 lb (maximum body weight) = 1560–1760 kcal. Maximum recommended kcal from fat at 35% of total kcalories = 546 to 616 kcal and 60–68 grams. Clients estimated fat intake from 24-hour recall and food frequency showed an intake of 110–115 grams of fat.

Excessive fat intake as evidenced by food and nutrition-related knowledge and elevated cholesterol (330) and LDL (142) and reported food intake.

Plan

1. Encourage client to attend group class "Healthy Heart."
2. Monitor weight and blood lipid levels.
3. Recommend the client substitute nonfat cheese for regular cheese and consider packing his lunch.
4. Encourage the client to record his food intake 3 days per week.
5. Congratulate the client on his recent weight loss and slight drop in his blood lipid levels.

Critical Thinking Questions

1. Do you think this client will respond to diet therapy? What would you do if after 3 months a client's food diary shows greatly reduced dietary fat but his or her cholesterol has not dropped? The physician would probably decide to prescribe medication to lower the cholesterol. How would you explain this therapy to the client?
2. What would you do if, at the following visit, the food diary shows that the client has returned to his former eating habits, thinking fat consumption no longer matters because he is taking medication?

Chapter Review

1. Monoglycerides and diglycerides are names of lipids commonly seen:
   a. In clients' medical records
   b. On laboratory reports
   c. On food labels
   d. On clients' skin
2. Cholesterol is found:
   a. Only in saturated fats
   b. Only in foods of animal origin
   c. Mostly in eggs
   d. Only in triglycerides
3. Saturated fats are:
   a. Liquid at room temperature
   b. More likely to become rancid than other types of fats
   c. Primarily of animal origin
   d. Composed of many double carbon bonds
4. According to most health authorities, the average American would benefit by increasing his or her intake of which of the following fats while decreasing intake of other fats?
   a. Corn oil
   b. Olive oil
   c. Safflower oil
   d. Lard
5. One ounce of very lean meat contains 1 gram of fat and 35 kcalories. What percentage of kcalories comes from fat?
   a. 9
   b. 20
   c. 26
   d. 49

Clinical Analysis

1. Mrs. S, 50 years old, has a cholesterol level of 233 mg/dL. She weighs 125 lb and is 5 ft, 5 in. tall. The dietitian has estimated her body fat content to be 35%. When taking a nursing history, the nurse asks Mrs. S if she eats any foods that may be related to her elevated cholesterol level. Which of the following groups of foods are most related to an elevated cholesterol level?
   a. Vegetable oils such as corn, cottonseed, and soybean
   b. Fruits and vegetables
   c. Starches such as bread, potatoes, rice, and pasta
   d. Animal fats such as butter, meats, lard, and bacon

2. Mr. B buys as many low-fat foods as possible. He eats fat-free muffins for breakfast, eats low-fat brownies or cookies for lunch each day, uses only fat-free ice cream, and buys fat-free salad dressings. He eats very little meat and chooses fat-free dairy products. He wonders why he hasn't lost more weight. The best advice is to encourage him to:
   a. Consider the amount of soda and sugar he consumes
   b. Eat even less meat
   c. Consume fewer dairy products
   d. Quit trying to lose weight

3. When Mrs. L describes her regular intake of foods, you observe that her diet is especially low in monounsaturated fats. Which of the following oils would you recommend be used in place of corn oil to increase her intake of monounsaturated fats?
   a. Sunflower seed
   b. Soybean
   c. Olive
   d. Cottonseed

5

Protein

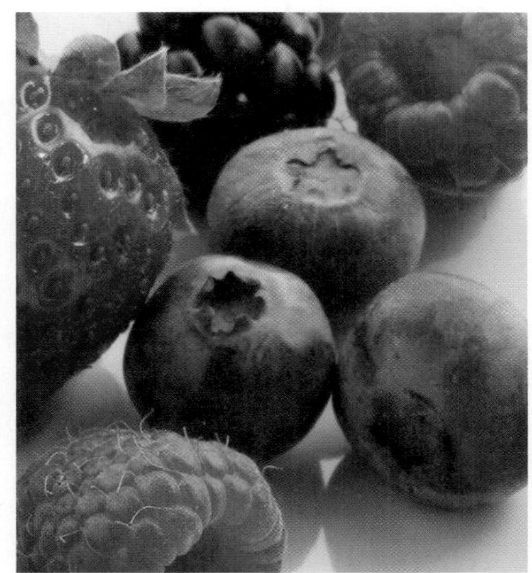

LEARNING OBJECTIVES

After completing this chapter, the student should be able to:

- Discuss the functions of proteins in human health and illness.
- Explain the difference between complete and incomplete proteins and give examples of food sources of each.
- Define anabolism and catabolism and list possible anabolic and catabolic conditions.
- List the grams of protein in each exchange list containing significant amounts of protein.
- Design a daily meal plan with adequate protein intake for a healthy adult.
- Prepare an outline of topics to discuss with a client consuming a vegan diet.

Along with carbohydrate and fat, protein is an energy nutrient, but in many ways it is paramount. Even the term *protein,* which is derived from the Greek *proteos,* means primary or taking first place. Protein makes unique contributions to the body's health that cannot be duplicated by carbohydrate or fat. This chapter covers the functions, composition, and dietary sources of protein, plus clinical implications of dysfunctional protein metabolism.

Protein can also be used as an auxiliary source of energy if kilocaloric intake is inadequate. As is true of carbohydrates and fats, protein eaten in excess can contribute to body fat stores.

Proteins are the building blocks of the body's tissues and organs. Almost half the dry weight of the body's cells is protein. It is second only to water in amounts present in the body. Descriptions of some of the tissues composed of protein appear in Box 5-1.

Composition of Proteins

To understand the functions of protein in the body, it is necessary first to comprehend their basic structure: their chemical elements and the arrangement of those elements.

Proteins are composed of four elements:

1. Carbon
2. Hydrogen
3. Oxygen
4. Nitrogen

These elements are arranged in building blocks called amino acids. Nitrogen is the element that distinguishes the structure of proteins from that of carbohydrates and fats as described in previous chapters. Sometimes, sulfur and other elements also form part of the protein molecule.

Box 5-1 ■ *Examples of Proteins in the Human Body*

People need a steady intake of protein for normal body maintenance because most cells require periodic replacement. Even bone tissue undergoes change in healthy adults. However, the body cannot effectively repair tooth enamel destroyed by decay, hence the need for dental restoration, or fillings. When a person is growing or has diseased or injured tissue to repair, the need for protein is even greater than usual.

Scar Tissue

Wound healing requires proteins. Many blood clotting factors, such as the protein prothrombin, form a blood clot. The fibrin threads that form the mesh to hold the scar tissue in place are composed of protein. Low serum protein levels have been significantly associated with prolonged healing (Dwyer et al., 2005; Liu et al., 2007).

Hair

Hair cells are dead. Hence, haircuts do not hurt. The new growth of hair does require protein building blocks, however. One sign of malnutrition is hair that can be easily and painlessly plucked.

Blood Albumin

Albumin is a transport protein that carries nutrients or elements. In addition to carrying substances to body cells, albumin has functions relating to water balance (see Chapter 8) and plays a significant role in medication absorption and metabolism (see Chapter 15).

Hemoglobin

Another transport protein, **hemoglobin,** is the oxygen-carrying part of the red blood cell. The **globin** part of this molecule is a simple protein.

Box 5-2 exemplifies the importance of a diet adequate in protein along with correct food processing techniques.

Amino Acids

Amino acids are linked by **peptide bonds** in an exact order to make a particular protein. A chain of two or more amino acids joined together by peptide bonds is called a **polypeptide**. A single protein may consist of a polypeptide comprising from 50 to thousands of amino acids. Scientists have estimated that the human body contains up to 50,000 different proteins, of which only about 1000 have been identified. Thus, an enormous variety of combinations is possible.

Think of the elements as the letters of the alphabet and amino acids as words. The letters (the elements) can make countless words (amino acids). Words put into a certain order make up sentences that have a specific and unique meaning. In this comparison, a sentence is a protein. Each protein has a specific and unique sequence of amino acids. To complete the analogy of language to anatomy, see Table 5-1.

Animal and vegetable proteins that we eat are disassembled in the digestive process into component amino acids. They are then reassembled to form human proteins (see Chapter 9). Precision is necessary to manufacture proteins. A slight error in the construction of a protein, such as occurs in sickle cell disease, can have severe consequences (see Clinical Application 5-1).

Twenty-three amino acids have been identified as important to the body's metabolism. These amino acids are classified as essential, conditionally (or acquired) essential, or nonessential.

Box 5-2 ■ *Cyanide in Food*

In parts of Africa, a staple of the diet is flour made from bitter cassava root—a hardy, drought-resistant plant that thrives in poor soil and produces cyanide as a defense mechanism. If the roots are not adequately processed and a person's diet is low in sulfur-containing amino acids (methionine and cysteine) that the body uses to detoxify the cyanide, a permanent, but not progressive, paralytic disease of the legs called **konzo** can result (Diasolua Ngudi, Kuo, and Lambein, 2002).

Varieties of the plant are also grown in Central and South America and the South Pacific. Different cultures have designed various means to decrease the cyanide in the plant before consuming the product. In Africa, the main methods involve drying the roots and efforts are ongoing to promote the correct drying procedure among the populace (Denton, 2007).

TABLE 5-1 ■ Comparison of Language and Anatomy

COMPONENT OF LANGUAGE	COMPONENT OF ANATOMY
Letters	Elements
Word	Amino acid
Sentence	Protein
Paragraph	Cell
Chapter	Tissue
Book	Organ
Books on a subject	System
Library	Human body

Essential Amino Acids

An amino acid is classified as essential if the body is unable to make it in sufficient amounts to meet metabolic needs. All **essential amino acids** must be available in the body simultaneously and in sufficient

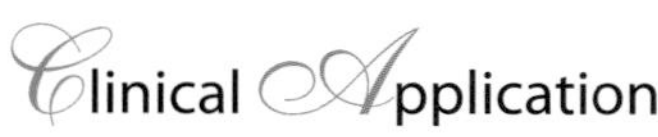
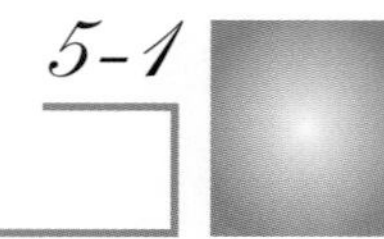

Clinical Application 5-1

Sickle Cell Disease

Hemoglobin (Hgb) consists of 146 amino acids combined in a specific order. In the hemoglobin of a person with sickle cell disease, one amino acid, glutamic acid, has been replaced by valine at one specific location on the protein chain.

In sickle cell disease the body has 99.3% of the amino acids in the correct sequence in the red blood cell, but early death can result from the 0.7% error. Sickle cell disease, an **autosomal recessive** disease, is most common among black people but also occurs in Mediterranean people, affecting approximately 1 in 350 African American newborn infants each year (Bonds, 2005). To have the disease, an individual has to be **homozygous** for the defective gene. One who is **heterozygous** is a carrier of the trait.

In sickle cell disease the red blood cells (RBCs) have a lifespan of 10–12 days compared with the normal 120 days, leading to chronic anemia. In addition, the RBCs become rigid and crescent-shaped. These abnormal cells tend to clump together and block small blood vessels in many different organs, leading to strokes, acute chest syndrome (a life-threatening, pneumonia-like illness), and pain crises (Fig. 5-1).

The only cure is a bone marrow transplant from a compatible donor (Chang, Ye, and Kan, 2006), but research is ongoing in gene therapy, including a clinical trial in Paris (Bank, 2008).

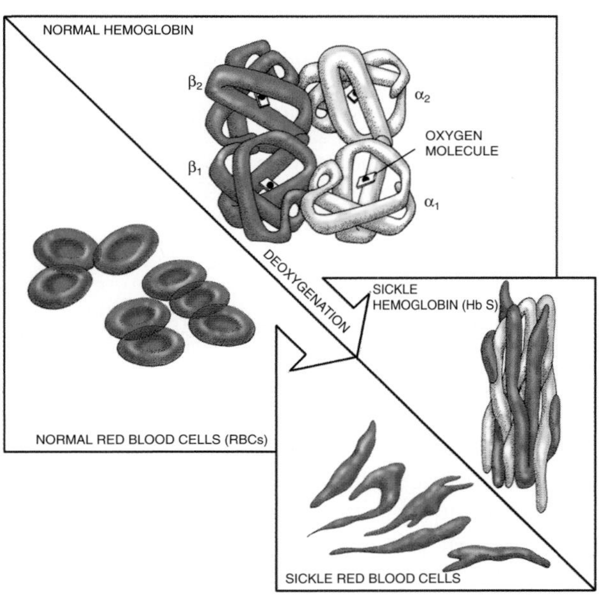

FIGURE 5-1 Normal red blood cells (RBCs) and hemoglobin (Hgb) compared with those in sickle cell anemia. (Reprinted from Venes, D [ed]: *Taber's cyclopedic medical dictionary*, ed 21. FA Davis, Philadelphia, 2010, p 119, with permission.)

quantity for the synthesis of body proteins (Fig. 5-2). These amino acids may come from recently ingested food or from the body's own cells as they age and are broken down and replaced. Approximately 340 grams of amino acids enter the free pool each day, but only about 90 grams are derived from the diet (Matthews, 2006).

A person's physiological state influences the need for essential amino acids. Thus, for infants and young children, 30% of the protein requirement should be constituted of essential amino acids. That figure drops to 20% in later childhood and to 11% in adulthood (Matthews, 2006).

Special preparations that the body converts to six of the essential amino acids are available but not for lysine, histidine, and **threonine.** For this reason, some authorities list only those three amino acids as totally indispensable (Gropper, Smith, and Groff, 2009).

Conditionally (Acquired) Essential Amino Acids

Other amino acids are conditionally essential or can become essential, depending on the biochemical needs of the body and the health of its organs. For example, cysteine and proline are indispensable for premature infants. In phenylketonuria (PKU; see Clinical Application 5-2) tyrosine becomes essential because normally it is produced from phenylalanine by the same enzyme that is lacking in PKU clients (Gropper, Smith, and Groff, 2009).

Nonessential Amino Acids

Nonessential amino acids are those that the body ordinarily can build in sufficient quantities to meet its needs. Typically, they are derived from other amino acids. Nonessential amino acids are necessary for good health, but under normal conditions, adults do not have to obtain them from food. Table 5-2 lists the amino acids that have been classified as essential, conditionally and/or acquired essential, and nonessential.

Functions of Proteins in the Body

Protein serves six major functions in the body, as shown in Table 5-3.

Provision of Structure

Proteins provide much of the body's mass. Contractile proteins, actin and myosin, are found in muscles. Fibrous proteins, such as collagen, elastin, and keratin, are found in blood vessels, bone, cartilage, hair, nails, tendons, skin, and teeth.

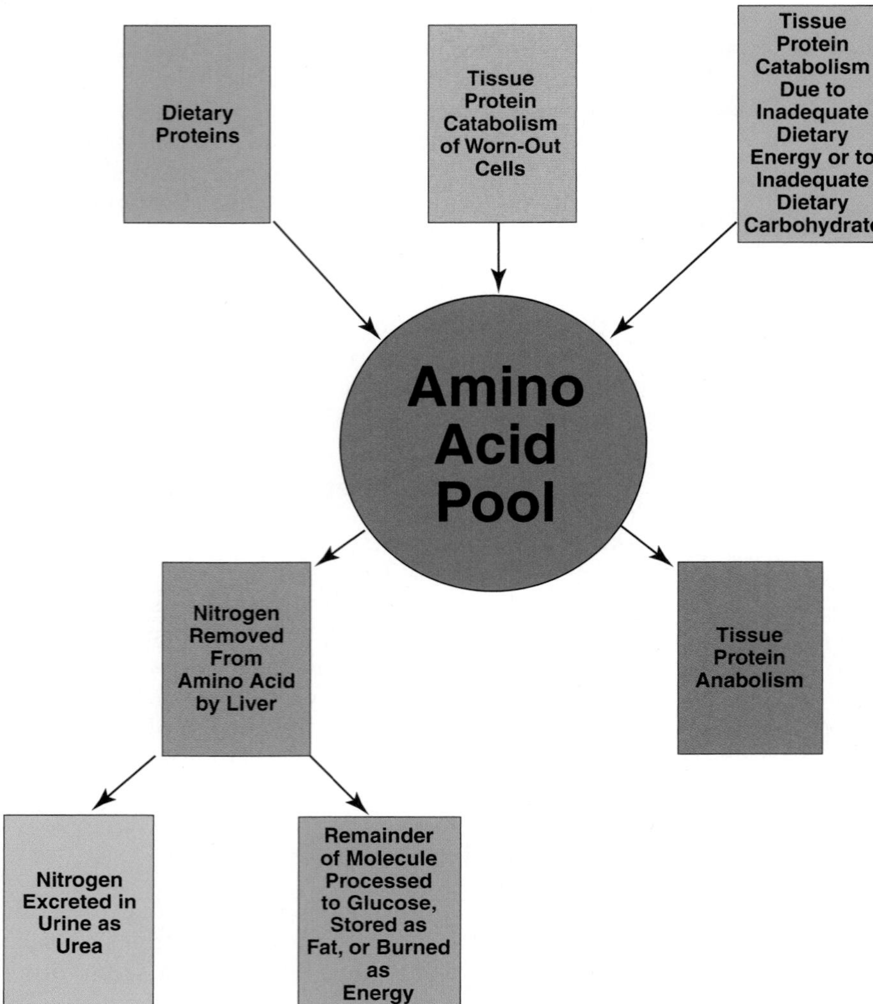

FIGURE 5-2 Anabolism/catabolism of protein. The body obtains amino acids from dietary protein and the catabolism of body tissue, enzymes, and secretions. The body uses amino acids to build new tissue or for immediate or future energy use. Every meal or snack does not have to contain every essential amino acid to permit anabolism. To maximize an adult's health, all essential amino acids should be supplied in adequate amounts by diet daily or at least every 2 to 3 days.

Maintenance and Growth

Because protein is a part of every cell (half the dry weight), adults as well as growing children require adequate protein intake. As cells of the body wear out, they must be replaced.

Anabolism and Catabolism

Anabolism is the building up of tissues as occurs in growth or healing. **Catabolism** is the breaking down of tissues into simpler substances that the body can reuse or eliminate.

Both processes occur simultaneously in the body. For example, tissue proteins are constantly being broken down into amino acids, which are then reused for building new tissue and repairing old tissue. Anabolism and catabolism, however, are not always in balance; at times, one process may dominate the other.

Nitrogen Balance

Foods or artificial feedings containing protein are the body's only external sources of nitrogen. Nitrogen is excreted in the urine, feces, and sweat and is sometimes lost through bleeding or vomiting. A person is in nitrogen equilibrium or nitrogen balance when the amount of nitrogen taken in equals the amount excreted (Clinical Calculation 5-1). A healthy adult at a stable body weight is usually in nitrogen equilibrium. Under certain circumstances, however, nitrogen balance may be either positive or negative.

POSITIVE NITROGEN BALANCE

A person consuming more nitrogen than he or she excretes is in positive **nitrogen balance.** The body is building more tissue than it is breaking down, a desirable state during periods of growth such as infancy, childhood, adolescence, and pregnancy.

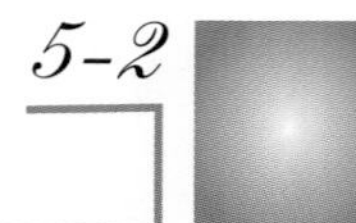

Clinical Application 5-2

Phenylketonuria Overview

Persons with **phenylketonuria (PKU)** are unable to convert the essential amino acid **phenylalanine** to tyrosine because the enzyme *phenylalanine hydroxylase* is lacking or defective. Phenylalanine occurs in all protein foods, including milk. Once feedings start, affected infants are at risk of accumulating high blood levels of phenylalanine and consequent mental retardation.

In the United States, screening tests performed 24–48 hours after birth, using a few drops of blood from an infant's heel, are mandated by all states. If a test is done before the infant is 24 hours old, retesting is recommended at 1–2 weeks of age to ensure adequate intake of milk to cause a reaction.

Lifelong dietary restriction of phenylalanine is the standard treatment. Because phenylalanine is an essential amino acid, small amounts of breast milk or infant formula are given to provide just the amounts of phenylalanine the infant needs and can use for growth and metabolism without excessive accumulation. Special phenylalanine-free formulas provide the remaining amino acids. Later solid foods may include fruits, vegetables, and some cereals but no high-protein foods.

The artificial sweetener **aspartame** (Equal®, NutraSweet®), which is composed of aspartic acid and phenylalanine, bears a warning label regarding PKU. This disease requires frequent monitoring that should be provided by specialists in this field.

Until the 1980s, restrictions were relaxed as the client grew, so that now pregnant women with PKU may be eating protein foods during the 8 weeks after the woman's last menstrual period—a critical developmental period for the central nervous system and heart. Consequently, their infants may be born with microcephaly, mental deficiency, and congenital heart disease. Because most of these infants have not inherited PKU but instead were injured by their mothers' high blood levels of phenylalanine, even the rigorous standard treatment for PKU cannot help them.

Tragically, 75% of women with PKU are not in metabolic compliance when they become pregnant (Gambol, 2007). A world literature review showed that since 1990, 60 women with previously undiagnosed PKU, most with relatively normal intellectual function, produced 119 offspring, virtually all profoundly damaged. Even among women with diagnosed PKU, up to 10% in the reproductive age group have been lost to follow-up (Hanley, 2008). Careful history-taking may reveal a family history of mental retardation or the fact that a woman was on a special diet as a small child and thus may need to have phenylalanine levels tested and PKU treatment resumed before attempting pregnancy.

The FDA has approved *sapropterin dihydrochloride* to be used with dietary restriction to treat PKU in clients who have some *phenylalanine hydroxylase* activity (US Food and Drug Administration, 2007). As an indication of the complexity of PKU, one study identified 57 mutations in the *phenylalanine hydroxylase* gene presumed to be associated with responsiveness to the drug (Zurfluh et al., 2008). One woman with such a mutation was treated with the drug and diet during pregnancy with a resulting normal infant (Koch, Moseley, and Guttler, 2005). For other information on genetic implications of PKU, see Genomic Gem 5-1.

Genomic Gem 5-1

Phenylketonuria

An autosomal recessive disorder, PKU occurs most commonly in whites for whom the incidence is about 1 in 10,000 births (Merck Manual, 2008). The phenylalanine hydroxylase gene on chromosome 12 has more than 400 known mutations permitting more than 10,000 genotypic combinations. Because of the complexity, carrier screening, although possible, is imprecise and impractical (Gambol, 2007). Researchers are attempting to genetically engineer the defective enzyme and to devise gene therapy techniques (March of Dimes, 2007).

TABLE 5-2 ■ Essential, Conditionally and/or Acquired Essential, and Nonessential Amino Acids

ESSENTIAL	CONDITIONALLY AND/OR ACQUIRED ESSENTIAL*	NONESSENTIAL
Histidine	Arginine	Alanine
Isoleucine	Cysteine*,†,‡	Asparagine
Leucine	Glutamine	Aspartic acid
Lysine	Proline	Glutamic acid
Methionine‡	Tyrosine	Glycine
Phenylalanine		Serine
Threonine		
Tryptophan		
Valine		

*Gropper, Smith, and Groff (2009). Classification varies in references.
†Also called cystine.
‡Sulfur-containing amino acids.

TABLE 5-3 ■ Functions of Protein

FUNCTION	EXAMPLE
Provide structure	Muscle mass
Maintain and build cells	Hair growth
Regulate body processes	Glucagon (actions opposite those of insulin)
Produce immunity	Antibodies
Substitute as fuel	If adequate carbohydrate and fat are lacking
Maintain blood volume and pressure	Albumin draws fluid back into capillaries from interstitial (between the cells) spaces

NEGATIVE NITROGEN BALANCE

A person consuming less nitrogen than he or she excretes is in negative nitrogen balance. Such a person is receiving insufficient protein, and the body is breaking down more tissue than it is building. Situations marked by negative nitrogen balance include undernutrition, illness, and trauma. Even healthy volunteers lose muscle tissue when confined to bed for weeks. Appropriate nutritional supplementation not only can preserve skeletal muscle but also can minimize functional losses

5-1

Clinical Calculation

Nitrogen Balance Studies

To calculate a client's nitrogen balance, the dietitian compares the amount of nitrogen in the foods the client consumes with the amount of nitrogen excreted in the urine. Other potential losses are estimated.

Protein is approximately 16% nitrogen, so the amount of protein consumed (in grams) is multiplied by 0.16. Thus, a person who ingests 50 grams of protein has a nitrogen intake of 8 grams. If he is in nitrogen equilibrium, he would be expected to excrete or lose 8 grams of nitrogen.

due to prolonged inactivity (Ferrando, Paddon-Jones, and Wolfe, 2006).

Clients who receive inadequate food, sometimes for days, because of treatments or diagnostic tests are at risk for malnutrition. An alert health-care provider intervenes in such cases to rearrange meal schedules or obtain food supplements.

Institutionalized clients are susceptible to **protein-energy malnutrition (PEM),** also termed **protein-calorie malnutrition (PCM),** when they are unable to feed themselves. In the developed world, PEM most often accompanies a disease process. **Lean body mass,** chiefly skeletal and visceral muscle, is the critical element that is lost in PEM.

Two subtypes of PEM are marasmus and kwashiorkor. **Marasmus** occurs when the victim consumes too few kilocalories and insufficient protein. The person appears to be wasting away. Marasmus is commonly seen in children in developing countries, but it also occurs in debilitating diseases such as cancer or AIDS.

Kwashiorkor classically occurs in a child shortly after weaning from breast milk. The child receives more kilocalories than one with marasmus but not enough protein to support growth. Clinically, he or she may look chubby, especially in the abdominal area, but the cause of this swelling is fluid retention, not fat (Fig. 5-3). Kwashiorkor is **endemic** in areas where the staple diet has a low protein to energy ratio.

Clinical Application 5-3 presents a firsthand account of the desperate situation of people in a developing country. Although rare, kwashiorkor also occurs in industrialized nations, not because of lack of food but because of parental ignorance about nutrition. In recent reports, three children developed kwashiorkor after subsisting mainly on a rice beverage with inadequate protein content (Carvalho et al., 2001; Katz et al., 2005). Kwashiorkor even has been documented in a child abuse fatality case for which the parents were imprisoned (Piercecchi-Marti et al., 2006).

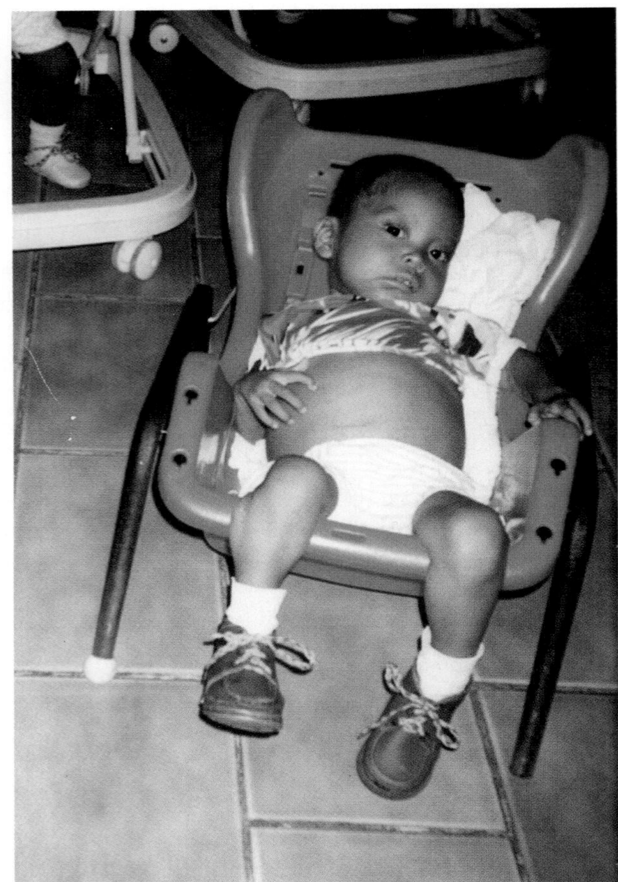

FIGURE 5-3 A child with kwashiorkor at the Nutrition Rehabilitation Center in San Carlos, Bolivia.

Regulation of Body Processes

Protein contributes to the regulation of body processes. Hormones and enzymes are prime examples. Table 5-4 lists some of these regulators and gives examples of each. Nucleoproteins, also containing protein, are essential to normal body functioning.

Hormones

Hormones are chemicals secreted by various organs to regulate body processes. Hormones are secreted directly into the bloodstream rather than into a duct or an organ. **Insulin** and **glucagon** are two important hormones that help control glucose metabolism. Growth hormone regulates cell division and protein synthesis.

Enzymes

Enzymes are crucial to many body processes, such as digestion. The breakdown of foods in the stomach and small intestine involves enzymes, which act as

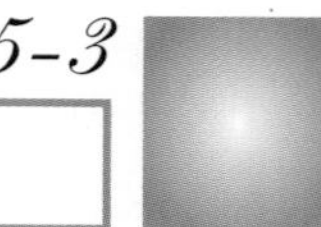

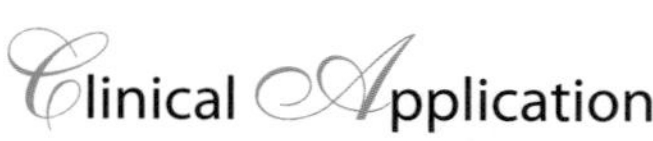

5-3 Clinical Application

Letters From Valle de Sacta, Bolivia

By Constance O'Connor BSN, RN

Your letter arrived January 17th, the first mail since a week before Christmas. Mail here is an event ... no TV, no newspapers. Shortwave BBC is about it for input. Much of what I do is aimed at keeping us healthy, such as ironing all line-dried clothes to get rid of any tiny insects or larvae. All fruits and vegetables are washed in chlorine bleach solution before use. Water we consume is either bottled or boiled for 20 minutes.

The people here are very poor, most living out in the bush, clearing land to grow bananas, pineapples, oranges, lemons, and coca. They usually construct a two-story hut on stilts so they can get out of the water with the rains. There are half-walls, if any, no screens, no toilets, rarely a well. It is a hard life. Few people survive past 55 and many children die at birth or in the first year.

Statistics are hard to obtain, as reporting even of births and deaths is minimal. A study done in our area in 1998 found 38.9% of children younger than 5 years of age suffered from chronic malnutrition, and 0.6% from acute malnutrition.

One acute case we saw, an 18-month-old boy, was so jaundiced and had such swelling in his lower extremities, we thought he had a kidney or liver problem. We did get care for him and learned the doctors here call that edema "the edema of hunger." These parents were motivated to get treatment as their first child died at 18 months with the same symptoms. When we visited a center for disnutrition about 50 miles from us, we learned that of the 54 children there, all younger than 3 years old, 21 had kwashiorkor.

Today I am taking a 3-year-old child to a malnutrition center about a 3-hour drive from us, hoping that it is not too late to save her life. The parents refused care for her up to this point though our pueblo elders, neighbors, and other family members pleaded with them. She has protein-energy malnutrition with kwashiorkor syndrome.

We personally pay for the children we send to these centers. Obviously, if the parents had money their children would not be starving. Most poor parents just accept that the children will die. They will dress them in their nicest clothes, hold them almost constantly during this dying process, and bury them soon after death. No funeral, no coffin.

Malnutrition is a factor in many of the measles, pneumonia, shigellosis, staphylococcal disease, and of course, tuberculosis cases Jim and I care for here. On our first Christmas here we were in the middle of a yellow fever outbreak. I have had to cope with children dying from malnutrition, dehydration, infections that did not get treated in time. I think I will always see their faces.

I hope to see you in March when I'm home begging for medicines and supplies. Many thanks for your letters.

catalysts (chemicals that influence the speed at which a chemical reaction takes place but do not actually enter into the reaction). Chapter 9 details the enzymes listed in Table 5-4. Without the aid of enzymes, many of the processes in the body would proceed too slowly to be effective.

TABLE 5-4 ■ Examples of Regulators of Body Processes

REGULATOR	EXAMPLES	SOURCE	ACTION
Hormones	Growth hormone	Anterior pituitary	Increases transport of amino acids into cells Increases rate of protein synthesis.
	Glucagon	Pancreas	Increases use of fats and amino acids for energy.
Enzymes	Lipase	Pancreas	Breaks down emulsified fats into fatty acids and glycerol.
	Peptidase	Small intestine	Splits polypeptides into amino acids.
	Sucrase	Small intestine	Splits sucrose into glucose and fructose.

An enzyme provides a place (its surface) for two substances to meet and react with each other. The new substance is then released and the enzyme catalyzes a new reaction. If it were not for enzymes, the two substances would be less likely to encounter one another, and basic body functioning would be impossible.

The lack of an effective enzyme can have devastating effects on health. Such a condition is addressed in Clinical Application 5-2.

Nucleoproteins

Nucleoproteins are regulatory complexes that include proteins. These complexes are located in the cell nucleus, where they direct the maintenance and reproduction of the cell. **Deoxyribonucleic acid (DNA)** and **ribonucleic acid (RNA)** are nucleoproteins that control the protein synthesis in the cell.

A **gene** is a part of the DNA that carries the code to direct the synthesis of a single protein. The kinds of proteins the cell makes vary with the nature of the cell, for example, whether an intestinal or skin cell or an ovum or sperm cell.

Immunity

A protein called an **antibody** is produced in the body in response to the presence of a foreign substance or a substance that the body senses to be foreign. Antibodies provide **immunity** to certain diseases and other toxic conditions. A specific antibody is created for each foreign substance.

If a person is exposed to a certain kind of disease-producing organism, the body designs an antibody that neutralizes the harmful effects of only that particular species or strain of organism. For some diseases, once the body has produced many copies of a given antibody, it can respond quickly to another attack, making the individual immune to that disease.

Circulation

The main protein in blood is albumin. It helps to maintain blood volume by drawing fluid back into the veins from body tissues. Thus, it plays a major role in maintaining blood pressure. In addition, some proteins aid in maintaining the body's acid–base balance. This buffering action is described in Chapter 8.

Some proteins serve as transport vehicles for nutrients or drugs, such as the proteins that attach to fats to become lipoproteins for moving lipids in the bloodstream. Drugs bind with albumin in the bloodstream. The term *protein-bound* refers to the portion of a drug dose that is inactive because it is attached to albumin. Chapter 15 elaborates on this process and its implications.

Energy Source

Glucose is the most efficiently used source of energy, but fat and protein can be adapted as backup sources. Most other body systems use fat for energy more readily than the nervous system does. When the body has insufficient glucose available for nervous system energy needs (as in a carbohydrate dietary deficit of longer than 12 hours), the body will utilize body protein tissue to meet the energy needs of the brain and spinal cord.

Thus, adequate carbohydrate intake is necessary to:

1. Spare protein for its unique contribution to tissue building
2. Avoid the undesirable consequences—ketosis and muscle loss—of obtaining energy from the less efficient sources: fat and protein

The amount of energy obtained from a gram of protein is the same as the amount obtained from a gram of carbohydrate: 4 kilocalories. Loss of about 30% of body protein is likely to be fatal due to reduced muscle strength for breathing, impaired immune function, and decreased organ function (Matthews, 2006).

Classification of Food Protein

Few foods are composed solely of protein. The white of an egg comes close, with 80% of its kilocalories derived from protein. Most foods contain various combinations of protein, fat, and carbohydrates. Some foods, however, are better sources of protein than others.

Protein foods are classified by the number and kinds of amino acids they contain:

- **Complete proteins** are foods that supply all nine essential amino acids in sufficient quantity to maintain tissue and support growth.
- **Incomplete proteins** lack one or more of the essential amino acids.

Complete Protein

With few exceptions, single foods containing complete protein come from animal sources such as meat, poultry, fish, eggs, milk, and cheese. Although gelatin is an animal product, it is an incomplete protein because it lacks the essential amino acid tryptophan. Soybeans are one plant source of complete protein that is processed into several products.

Meat and milk products are both good sources of complete protein. An adult requiring 2000 kilocalories per day following MyPyramid would consume the equivalent of 5½ ounces from the meat group and three cups of milk daily. MyPyramid categorizes cheese with milk, whereas the exchange-group system places it with meat.

Each exchange of meat contains 7 grams of protein regardless of the amount of fat. All beef is not high in fat, just as all fish and poultry is not low in fat. Figure 5-4 shows a 3-ounce portion of beef tenderloin equal to three lean meat exchanges providing 21 grams of protein.

Each milk exchange furnishes 8 grams of protein but the lists are subdivided into very low fat, low fat, and whole milk sections. All of these milk exchanges offer equal protein nutrition, but are not nutritionally equivalent because their fat content varies.

Incomplete Protein

Plant foods that contain protein lack sufficient amounts of one or more of the essential amino acids. Thus, the protein of plants is called incomplete but the term *incomplete* does not mean these foods are undesirable. Different types of plant foods can be combined to provide all the essential amino acids. Grains, vegetables, legumes, nuts, and seeds contain incomplete protein.

The vegetable and starch/bread exchanges are sources of incomplete protein. A vegetable exchange contains 2 grams of protein. One starch/bread

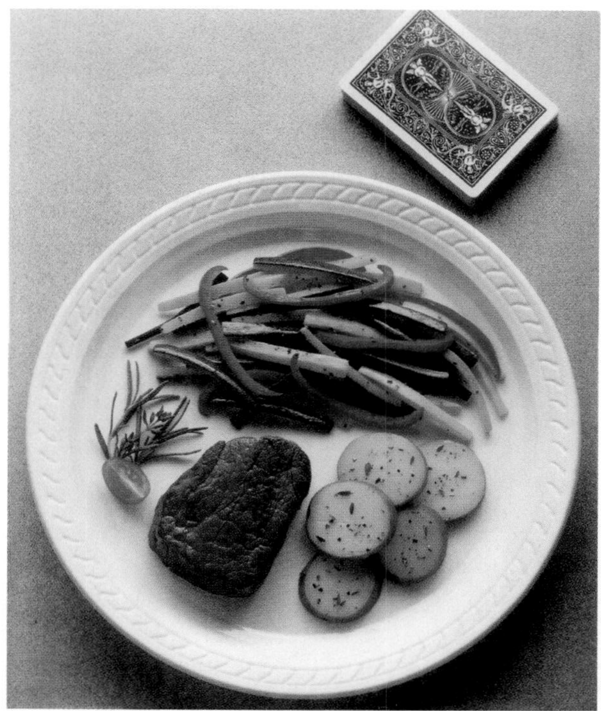

FIGURE 5-4 The 3-oz beef tenderloin pictured equals three lean meat exchanges. A standard deck of playing cards is shown for size comparison. (From the National Live Stock and Meat Board, 444 North Michigan Ave, Chicago, IL 60611, with permission.)

exchange contains 3 grams of protein. It is important to note the size of the item; specialty bagels and muffins may be much larger than the referenced item on the exchange list. Table 5-5 summarizes the protein content of the exchange lists.

Limiting Amino Acids and Complementation

Plants are classified as incomplete protein sources because they lack one or more essential amino acids. This undersupplied amino acid is called the **limiting amino** acid. In cereal grains, the limiting amino acid is **lysine;** in legumes, it is **methionine.**

Based on animal studies, the principle of **complementation** was promoted, recommending every meal contain a combination of plant foods that provide all the essential amino acids. Later human studies showed that adults are adequately nourished by consuming assorted plant proteins throughout the day. As shown in Figure 5-2, supplying the amino acid pool is a dynamic process, not completely dependent upon diet.

Young children showed less effective use of protein if the complementary protein was fed at intervals greater than 6 hours, but this is an unusually long time between meals or snacks for young children (Johnston and Sabate, 2006).

TABLE 5-5 ■ Grams of Protein per Exchange

EXCHANGE	GRAMS OF PROTEIN	EXAMPLES
Milk	8	
Very low fat		1 cup 1% milk
Low fat		1 cup 2% milk
Whole milk		½ cup evaporated whole milk
Meat	7	
Very lean		1 oz white meat chicken w/o skin
Lean		1 oz boiled ham
Medium fat		1 egg
High fat		1 oz cheddar cheese
Starch/Bread	3	1 slice of bread
		½ bagel (1 oz)
		½ cup cooked cereal
		1 small potato
		⅓ cup baked beans
		½ cup corn
Vegetable	2	½ cup cooked broccoli
		1 cup raw carrots

Adapted from: American Diabetes Association and American Dietetic Association (1995).

Vegetable Sources of Protein

For vegetarians or other individuals who limit their intake of animal foods, **legumes** are an important protein source. Legumes are plants having roots containing **nitrogen-fixing bacteria** that lock nitrogen into the plant's structure, thus increasing its nitrogen content.

Commonly consumed legumes are peas, beans, lentils, and peanuts. Not all peas and beans are legumes. Figure 5-5 compares the protein content of peas, beans, and nuts. Many legumes are not only low in fat but also high in fiber.

Box 5-3 locates some legumes and nuts in the exchange lists.

Textured vegetable protein products made from soybeans, peanuts, and cottonseed can enhance the vegetarian diet. The protein is spun into fibers and flavored, colored, and shaped for use as a meat substitute. In their natural form, plant proteins are less digestible than animal proteins, but well-processed soybean isolates are as digestible as egg protein (Johnston and Sabate, 2006).

Vegetarianism

There are many degrees of vegetarianism, depending on the beliefs of the individual or family. Some vegetarians eat fish or poultry occasionally. Clinical Application 5-4 distinguishes various vegetarian diets. The more restrictive the diet, the more care is required to ensure adequate nutrition.

Pregnant women, infants, children, and elderly people who are vegetarians may need special assessment

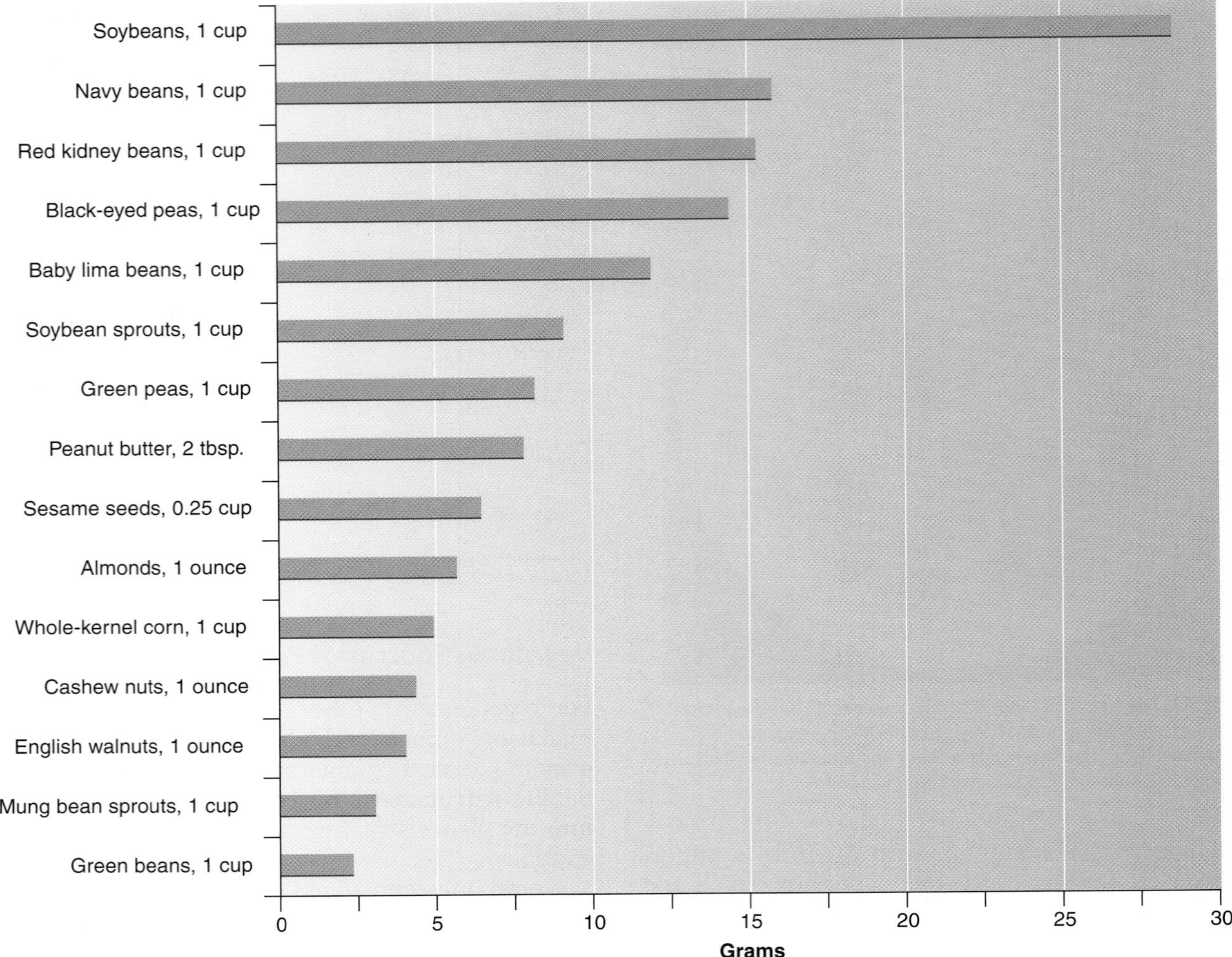

FIGURE 5-5 Protein content of selected plant foods. Notice that all foods named peas or beans are not legumes. Green beans offer just 2 grams of protein, whereas navy beans contain 16 grams.

Box 5-3 ■ *Exchanges of Some Plant Proteins*

Dried beans, peas, and lentils appear on a separate exchange section in the starch/bread list. They are counted as:

- 1 starch/bread *plus*
- 1 very lean meat exchange.

Nuts appear on the fat exchange list. One exchange equals

- Six cashews or
- 10 peanuts.

Peanut butter appears on two exchange lists:

- High-fat meat *and*
- Monounsaturated fat.

Adapted from: American Diabetes Association and American Dietetic Association (1995).

and instruction in the use of fortified foods and supplements.

Embracing a healthful vegetarian lifestyle encompasses more than just eliminating foods derived from animals. It is necessary to find appropriate substitutes for the nutrient-dense animal products. Many traditional regional or ethnic dishes combine a grain with a legume. For example:

- A peanut butter sandwich
- Baked beans with brown bread
- A bean burrito

Similarly, eliminating meat does not necessarily decrease fat intake. Vegetable oils and cheeses used in sauces to enhance flavor are high in fat.

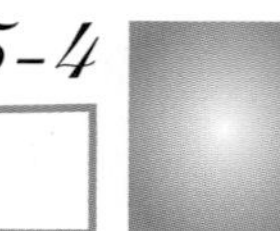

5-4

Clinical Application

Vegetarian Diets

Vegetarians practice different degrees of strictness. From most liberal to most restrictive, the vegetarian diets are ovolactovegetarian, lactovegetarian, ovovegetarian, and strict vegetarian or vegan. The prefixes *ovo-* and *lacto-* mean eggs and milk, respectively. Persons following macrobiotic diets consume unrefined/unprocessed grains, small amounts of fruits, vegetables, and legumes, and sometimes milk products. A fruitarian consumes only raw fruits, nuts, seeds, and berries.

Foods Chosen in the Various Vegetarian Diets

	MEAT, FISH, POULTRY	DAIRY PRODUCTS	EGGS
Ovolactovegetarian	No	Yes	Yes
Lactovegetarian	No	Yes	No
Ovovegetarian	No	No	Yes
Strict vegetarian (vegan)	No	No	No

Nutrients Vegetarians May Need to Obtain From Supplements or Designated Food Sources

NUTRIENT	SITUATION TO CONSIDER SUPPLEMENTATION
Vitamin B_{12}	Individuals consuming few or no animal products
Vitamin D	Individuals consuming few or no animal products; Vitamin D_2 may be preferred source (see Chapter 7)
Calcium	Individuals not consuming dairy products
Omega-3 fatty acids (Kris-Etherton and Skulas, 2005)	Individuals consuming few or no animal products: algae-based **DHA** supplement in cellulose capsules; **ALA** from flaxseed oil, ground flaxseed, walnuts, or canola oil

Usually hospital or care facility dietitians can provide balanced vegetarian diets. Rather than expect the client to select acceptable items from a general menu, it is better to inform the dietitian of the client's wishes.

Dietary Reference Intakes

Dietary reference intakes are provided in Appendix A.

The RDAs for protein assume adequate intake of the other energy nutrients. See Appendix A and

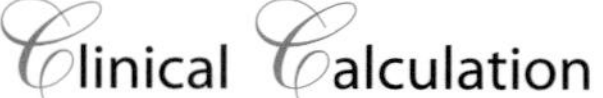
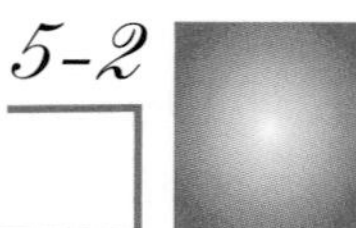

5-2

Clinical Calculation

Individualized Protein Requirement

The standard on which the RDA is based is 0.8 grams of protein per kilogram of body weight.

$$\frac{\text{Weight in pounds}}{2.2} = \text{Weight in kilograms} \times 0.8 = \text{protein RDA in grams}$$

$$\frac{\text{154 pounds}}{2.2} = 70 \text{ kg} \times 0.8 = 56 \text{ grams of protein}$$

Clinical Calculation 5-2. Higher intakes may be prescribed for elderly clients and athletes. (See Chapters 12 and 15.)

Wise Protein Choices

Some protein foods are much less expensive than others. Dollars and Sense 5-1 lists equivalent sources of 10 grams of protein by price. Typical regular prices of nationally advertised brands were used, except for bread, cottage cheese, eggs, milk, and steak. Substituting store brands, buying on sale, and using home-prepared foods lessen the cost.

High-protein diets have some experts concerned about:

- Stress on the liver and kidneys as those organs convert amino acids to glucose and excrete the waste products
- Possible bone loss if calcium, fruit, and vegetable intakes are low (Gropper, Smith, and Groff, 2009)

Environmentally and socially conscious consumers may choose to decrease the amounts of animal proteins they ingest to conserve resources. Meat production requires many pounds of plant protein that they believe could be better used to feed people directly.

Dollars & Sense 5-1

Comparative Sources of 10 Grams of Protein

Food	Portion	Kcalories	Price/Amount	Cost/10 gram of Protein
Tuna, canned in water	1.4 oz	46	$0.76/6 oz	$0.14
Peanut butter	2.5 tbsp	238	$1.99/16.3 oz	$0.17
1% milk	1¼ cups	128	$3.09/gal	$0.24
American cheese	1.7 oz	177	$4.49/2 lb	$0.24
Large eggs, poached	1.7	133	$2.08/doz	$0.29
Cottage cheese, 2% low fat	⅓ cup	65	$3.99/24 oz	$0.43
Bologna	2.9 oz	261	$2.19/12 oz	$0.53
Cracked wheat bread	5 slices	325	$3.19/24 oz	$0.59
Boneless sirloin steak, lean only	1.2 oz	66	$8.99/lb	$0.65
Bean soup, condensed, prepared with water	1¼ cups	215	$1.67/11.5 oz	$0.83

Keystones

- Protein contributes to body structure, tissue maintenance and growth, the regulation of body processes, immunity, the circulation of blood and nutrients, and if necessary, to energy needs.
- The building blocks of proteins are amino acids that contain nitrogen in addition to carbon, hydrogen, and oxygen. Complete protein foods contain all essential amino acids in amounts sufficient to support growth and usually come from animal sources, especially the meat and milk groups.
- Incomplete protein foods are grains, vegetables, legumes, nuts, and seeds. A person who eats a grain product and a legume at the same meal, however, is likely to receive all essential amino acids at that meal.
- Overall balance in intake of protein foods is more important than individual meals for most healthy adults.
- Protein provides 4 kilocalories per gram.
- Milk exchanges provide about 8 grams of protein, meat exchanges 7 grams, bread/starch exchanges 3 grams, and vegetable exchanges 2 grams.

CASE STUDY 5-1

Mrs. F is a 72-year-old widow who eats independently in her family homestead. Her usual meals are tea and toast for breakfast, canned fruit and a muffin for lunch, and frozen potpie or canned hash for dinner. She complains that she has been having trouble chewing with her old dentures and has not been eating as much food as she usually does. She does not like milk.

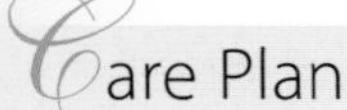

Care Plan

Subjective Data

Food deficit as evidenced by usual food intake information ■ Has trouble chewing. ■ Does not like milk.

Objective Data

Height: 5 ft 4 in. in stocking feet ■ Weight: 109 lb ■ Wrist measurement: 5.25 in. ■ Loose-fitting dentures

Analysis

Inadequate intake of protein and kilocalories, related to difficulty chewing, as evidenced by stated usual intake of 28 to 32 grams of protein per day and body weight 7% under minimum for height and frame

CASE STUDY *(Continued)*

Plan

DESIRED OUTCOMES EVALUATION CRITERIA	ACTIONS/INTERVENTIONS	RATIONALE
Client will gain 1 lb per week during the next 2 weeks.	Encourage easily chewed sources of complete protein: cheese, eggs, ground meat, and fish.	Complete protein foods contain all essential amino acids necessary for tissue building.
Client will increase her total protein intake by 14–18 grams per day.	Create a model meal plan with Mrs. F using the Exchange Group system to count grams of protein.	Mrs. F's RDA is 46 grams of protein. The meal plan she described in her history contains only 28–32 grams depending on dinner selection.
Client will call for dental appointment within next 2 weeks.	Explore sources of financial assistance for dental care if necessary or refer to social worker.	Better fitting dentures would permit Mrs. F a wider variety of foods.

When following up after 2 weeks, the nurse finds that Mrs. F has gained one-half pound instead of 2 as set in the desired outcome. She has increased her intake of eggs and cheese as instructed but says she feels full before finishing her meal. She has not made a dental appointment. Her dentist retired and she is embarrassed to have to negotiate payment with a new one. The nurse refers the client to the agency social worker.

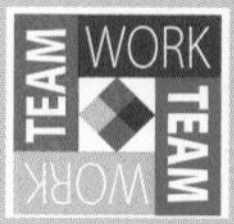

5-1

Social Worker's Notes

The following Social Worker's Notes are representative of the documentation found in a client's medical record.

Subjective: *Client's resources are mainly Social Security payments. She does not have dental insurance.*

Objective: *Demonstrable ill-fitting dentures.*

Analysis: *Financial issues preclude private dental care.*

Plan: *Refer to Family Health Center dental clinic.*

Critical Thinking Questions

1. What other food groups or nutrients are lacking in Mrs. F's usual diet? Would you have given any of them a higher priority than protein? Why or why not?
2. Speculate on the reasons Mrs. F has developed her present meal pattern. What additions could you make to the care plan to improve her nutritional intake?
3. If Mrs. F added one egg and one ounce of Swiss cheese per day without changing the other components of her meal plans, to what extent would she have met her protein needs? What additional interventions would you suggest?

Chapter Review

1. For which of the following functions of protein can other nutrients be substituted?
   a. Energy source
   b. Immunity
   c. Maintenance and growth
   d. Regulation of body processes
2. Which of the following foods is a complete protein?
   a. Baked beans
   b. Broccoli
   c. Beef kabobs
   d. Bread sticks
3. If a person has difficulty purchasing meat to serve every day, which of the following foods should the nurse suggest as offering the best source of protein?
   a. Bran muffins with raisins
   b. Red beans and rice
   c. Green bean, onion, and mushroom casserole
   d. Sweet potatoes and cornbread
4. How much protein would a person receive from a glass of milk?
   a. 7 grams
   b. 8 grams
   c. 14 grams
   d. 21 grams
5. Which of the following people would the nurse treat as being in a catabolic state?
   a. Adolescent boy who is into bodybuilding
   b. Lactating mother
   c. Pregnant woman in the second trimester
   d. Surgical client, first day after a stomach resection

Clinical Analysis

Mr. P, a 65-year-old man, widowed for 6 months, has been referred to your home health agency for assistance in managing his nutritional intake. He has lost 10 pounds over the past 6 months. A physical examination within the past month revealed no disease processes requiring treatment.

1. In assessing Mr. P, which of the following data would the nurse gather first?
   a. List of current medications the client takes
   b. Blood protein levels analyzed during the recent physical examination
   c. A description of the procedure Mr. P uses to weigh himself
   d. Dietary recall of Mr. P's food and fluid intake
2. Which of the following plans would be most appropriate to increase Mr. P's protein consumption immediately?
   a. Refer client to nutrition education program.
   b. Have Mr. P apply for home-delivered meals.
   c. Recommend that Mr. P supplement his meals with one of the milk-based liquid breakfast products.
   d. Suggest to Mr. P that he sign up for cooking lessons at the local high school or community college.
3. Which of the following outcomes would indicate achievement of the nutritional objective for Mr. P?
   a. A gain in weight of 2 pounds in 2 weeks
   b. An invitation to the nurse to join him for a dinner he has learned to cook
   c. A report by Mr. P that he is eating better
   d. A visual inspection of Mr. P's refrigerator revealing fresh meat and milk products in abundance.

6

Energy Balance

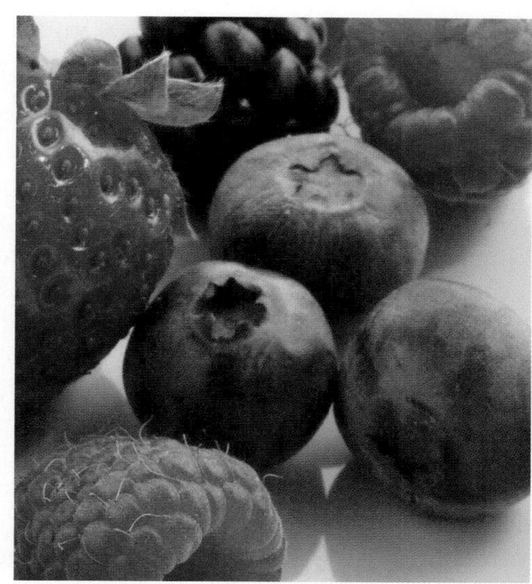

LEARNING OBJECTIVES

After completing this chapter, the student should be able to:

- Describe energy homeostasis. List two reasons the body needs energy.
- Describe how energy is measured both in foods and in the human body.
- Discuss the effect of body composition on energy output.
- Name the energy nutrient that has the highest kilocalorie density and identify two substances usually found in foods with a low kilocalorie density.

A complete understanding of the human body's energy balance system eludes experts. In approximately 40% of the U.S. population, the human body regulates energy intake and expenditure automatically to maintain an **energy balance.** This balance occurs even when the amount of energy needed varies and food intake is erratic. The body can also compensate during food restriction or starvation by conserving energy. Maintenance of a reduced or elevated body weight is associated with compensatory changes in energy expenditure, which oppose the maintenance of a body weight that is different from the usual body weight.

Most experts agree that the human body's energy balance system is the most complex of all the biological systems. However, during the past 2 years we have learned more about the human energy balance system than in all the previous years combined. This text provides an introduction to this fascinating research.

A basic understanding of what is known about energy balance is necessary for understanding energy imbalance. This chapter, therefore, focuses on energy balance (Chapter 16 on weight management focuses on energy imbalance), and in particular on the effects of energy intake and expenditure on energy balance. Topics include:

- Energy measurements
- Factors influencing the body's energy need
- Energy consumption patterns
- The kilocaloric content and nutrient density of foods
- Energy allowances
- Current recommendations concerning energy consumption

Homeostasis and Survival

The human body seeks homeostasis—that is, equilibrium, or balance. Homeostasis, in terms of energy balance, occurs when the number of kilocalories eaten equals the number used to produce energy. An individual who maintains a stable body weight is usually in energy balance.

However, the human body has developed biological mechanisms allowing it to survive at the cost of maintaining energy balance. Throughout human history, periods of feast or famine were common. The human body developed numerous redundant systems to safeguard against death by starvation. In the event that one metabolic pathway malfunctioned, another evolved to compensate. However, in modern times—when food is often plentiful—these evolutionary survival mechanisms have proved to be a detriment for many people. This disadvantage is evident by the increasing number of people who are overweight or obese.

Energy Intake

The typical adult eats 500,000 to 850,000 kilocalories per year. Eating an excess of only 1% or 15 extra kilocalories per day would result in a weight gain of 1.5 pounds per year—the kilocalories in ⅓ teaspoonful of butter or a quarter of a small apple. Individuals at a stable, healthy weight give little thought to the amount of food that they eat each day, yet their body weight remains constant.

Eating appears to be a voluntary act influenced by the external environment, but it is regulated internally as well. The internal regulation of energy balance involves the gastrointestinal tract, the endocrine system, the brain, and body fat stores. Physiologic regulation is evidenced by the constancy of body weight in adults and the fact that, after weight gain or loss, this constant body weight is reestablished. Over the long term, food energy intake is regulated to balance energy expenditure. See Box 6-1 for a discussion on appetite and hunger.

Energy Expenditure

Energy expenditure, which varies daily, is measured by the number of kilocalories used to meet the body's demand for fuel. A person uses many more kilocalories to run a marathon than to sleep. Physical activity expends energy.

Adaptive Thermogenesis

Energy expenditure frequently adapts to large increases or decreases in food intake of several days' duration by means of a process called **adaptive thermogenesis**. Adaptive thermogenesis is one example of how the human body evolved to cope with feast-or-famine conditions. Energy expenditure decreases during food restriction or starvation. Kilocalories are burned more efficiently. Adaptive thermogenesis causes an individual trying to lose weight either to lose at a slower rate or to stop losing weight. As a result, losing weight is difficult for many people but not impossible.

However, overeating for several days will cause an increase in energy expenditure. Energy expenditure has been found to be higher than predicted during the refeeding of previously starved patients, especially within the first week (Hoffer, 2006).

Box 6-1 ■ *Appetite versus Hunger*

Appetite is different from hunger.

Appetite is a strong desire for food or a pleasant sensation, based on previous experience, that causes one to seek food for taste and enjoyment.

Hunger is a sensation that results from a lack of food, characterized by a dull or acute pain around the lower part of the chest. A truly hungry person will most likely eat anything and take drastic action to acquire food.

Unfortunately, eating is not always the result of hunger. People eat or do not eat in response to stress, time of day, boredom, physical activity, and other reasons. In short, people can override the internal biological signals for eating.

Measuring Energy

Both the energy (fuel) foods contain and the amount of energy the body uses can be measured. The methods used to measure energy are fairly universal.

Units of Measure

The energy content of food is measured in kilocalories and increasingly in joules.

A **kilocalorie (abbreviated kcalorie or kcal),** is the amount of heat required to raise 1 kilogram of water 1°C. Non–health-care professions often call kilocalories *calories.* In chemistry, a calorie is the amount of heat required to raise 1 gram of water 1°C. One kilocalorie, as used in the nutritional sciences, contains 1000 times as much energy as 1 calorie used in chemistry. Understanding the difference is important. *Kilocalorie or kcal or kcalories* are the terms used throughout this text because these terms are used in the medical literature, including patients' medical records. Using kcalories for nutritional measurement eliminates the large numbers that using the chemical term would necessitate. This is a confusing concept because food labels use the term calories incorrectly.

The **joule** is another unit used to measure energy. One **kilojoule** is the amount of energy required to move a mass of 1 kilogram with an acceleration of 1 meter per second. The kilojoule is equal to 0.239 kilocalorie; a kilocalorie equals 4.184 kilojoules.

Energy Nutrient Values

The energy nutrients are carbohydrates, fat, and protein. Alcohol (ethanol) also yields energy. A food's kcalorie value is determined by its content of protein, fat, carbohydrates, and alcohol.

- 1 gram of carbohydrate equals 4 kilocalories (or 17 kilojoules)
- 1 gram of protein equals 4 kilocalories (or 17 kilojoules)
- 1 gram of fat equals 9 kilocalories (or 37.6 kilojoules)

- 1 gram of alcohol equals 7 kilocalories (or 29.3 kilojoules).

Water, fiber, vitamins, and minerals do not provide kilocalories. Clinical Calculation 6-1 demonstrates how to determine the energy content of a food item.

Determining Energy Values

Energy, whether in foods or the body, is measured as a form of heat.

Foods

The energy content of individual foods is measured by a device called a bomb calorimeter, illustrated in Figure 6-1. A bomb calorimeter is an insulated container that has a chamber in which food is burned. The amount of heat (kcalories) produced by the burning of the food is determined by the change in the temperature of a measured amount of water that surrounds the chamber. All energy in food is in the form of chemical energy. In a bomb calorimeter, the chemical energy stored in the food sample is transformed into heat energy. The following equation may facilitate understanding of this concept:

Protein + oxygen = heat energy + water + carbon dioxide

(Carbohydrate or fat may be substituted for protein in the equation.)

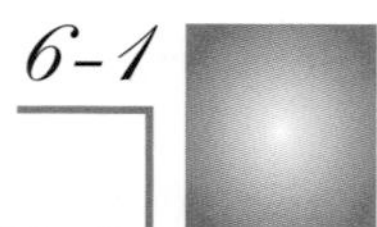

Clinical Calculation 6-1

Calculating the Energy Content of a Food Item

If you know the carbohydrate, fat, and protein content of a food item, you can readily calculate the food's kcalorie content. Two examples are shown below. One starch exchange contains 3 grams of protein and 15 grams of carbohydrate. Adding the protein and carbohydrate content in the starch exchange equals 18.

	Carbohydrate (grams)		Protein (grams)		Fat (grams)		Total (grams)
One starch exchange	15	+	3	+	0	=	18

Each gram of carbohydrate and protein has 4 kcal, so to obtain the kcalorie content of the starch exchange, multiply 4 by 18. Thus, one starch exchange has 72 kcal.

One fat exchange contains 5 grams of fat.

	Carbohydrate (grams)		Protein (grams)		Fat (grams)		Total (grams)
One fat exchange	0	+	0	+	5	=	5

A gram of fat has 9 kcal. To obtain the kilocaloric content of one fat exchange, multiply 5 by 9. Thus, one fat exchange contains 45 kcal.

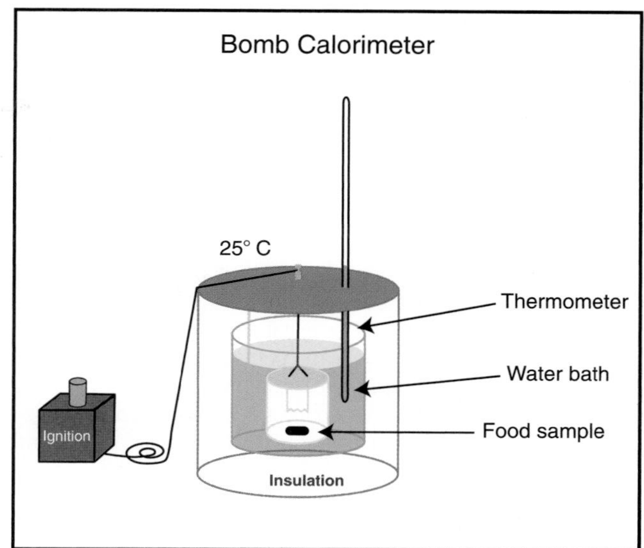

FIGURE 6-1 Illustration of a bomb calorimeter. The food sample is ignited and burned. The heat produced is absorbed by the known volume of water in the surrounding section. Change in temperature provides a measure of the heat produced.

The Human Body

A process similar to the combustion of food in the bomb calorimeter occurs in the body. The amount of energy the human body uses can be measured directly or indirectly.

Direct measurement of energy used by the human body requires expensive equipment that is used only in scientific research. Energy is measured directly by placing a person in an insulated heat-sensitive chamber and measuring the heat emitted by the body.

Indirect measurement of energy (also called indirect calorimetry) is discussed in Clinical Application 6-1.

Components of Energy Expenditure

The human body requires energy to meet its resting energy expenditure needs, to satisfy its physical activity requirements, and to process nutrients. Resting energy expenditure, which includes all involuntary activities, is the kcalories a person burns under controlled conditions and lying comfortably. Voluntary physical activity includes the energy needed for voluntary activities—which are consciously controlled, such as running, walking, and swimming. The third component of energy expenditure is the

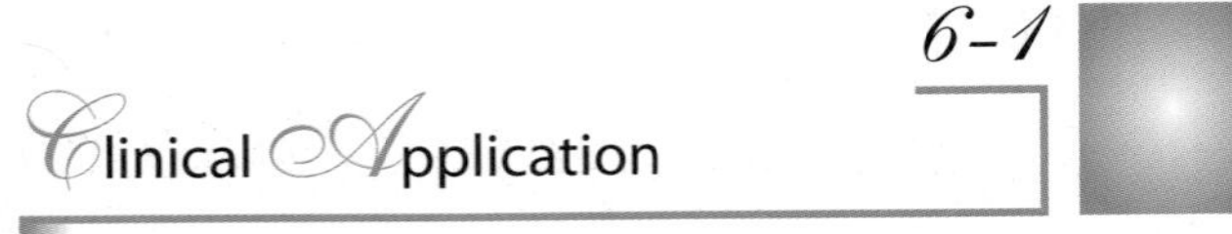

Measurement of REE by Indirect Calorimetry

Two techniques indirectly measure resting energy expenditure. One method measures the amount of carbon dioxide exhaled and the amount of oxygen inspired for a given period of time. From these data, the number of kcalories expended can be calculated. The device used to compute the intake of oxygen and output of carbon dioxide is called a respirator or metabolic machine. A health-care worker is most likely to observe this procedure in the intensive care unit of an acute care hospital. The second, less expensive method to measure REE is relatively new and measures only the amount of oxygen consumed. Using these data, the machine calculates the client's REE. The manufacturer of this machine claims it will be useful for determining the REE for routine nutritional assessment services and for clients on weight-management programs (www.korr.com).

energy expended to digest, absorb, transport, and utilize nutrients.

Resting Energy Expenditure

Resting energy expenditure represents the energy expended or used by a person at rest. In most people, resting energy expenditure (REE) requires more total kcalories than physical activity. Clinical Application 6-1 discusses the measurement of REE in clients. The term REE is generally associated with the use of a respirometer or a device that measures oxygen consumption. The kcalories necessary to support the following contribute to resting energy expenditure:

- Contraction of the heart
- Maintenance of body temperature
- Repair of the internal organs
- Maintenance of cellular processes
- Muscle and nerve coordination
- Respiration (breathing)

REE accounts for approximately 66% of most people's total energy requirements. Body composition influences resting energy expenditure. Individuals of similar age, sex, height, and weight with a higher percentage of muscle (lean body mass) have a higher REE than those with less muscle. It takes more energy, or kcalories, to support lean body mass (protein) than to support body fat. Muscle tissue requires more kcalories than does fat tissue, even when muscle tissue is resting. Therefore, the higher a person's body protein content, the more kcalories he or she can eat and still maintain a stable body weight.

Age

REE varies with lean body mass, which varies with age. The highest rates of energy expenditure per pound of body weight occur during infancy and childhood. In adults, REE declines about 2% per decade because of a decline in lean body mass. The result is a reduced need for kcalories. Individuals can slow the decline in lean body mass somewhat by increasing their exercise. An individual who fails either to decrease kilocaloric intake to compensate for this reduced need or to increase physical activity may experience a slow weight gain. Hence, the "middle-age spread."

Sex

Differences in body composition between men and women occur as early as the first few months of life. The differences are relatively small until the child reaches age 10. During adolescence, body composition changes radically. Men develop proportionately greater muscle mass than women, who deposit fat as they mature. Consequently, REE differs by as much as 10% between men and women.

Growth

Human growth is most pronounced during the growth spurts that take place before birth and during infancy and puberty. Kcalories required per kilogram of body weight are highest during these growth spurts because the kilocaloric cost of anabolism is greater than the kilocaloric cost of catabolism.

Body Size

People with large bodies require proportionately more energy than smaller ones. A tall individual uses more energy because he or she has a greater skin surface through which heat is lost than does a shorter person. A shorter person also has less muscle tissue or lean body mass than a taller person.

Most health-care professionals are surprised at the large volume of food needed to maintain a tall male's body weight (greater than 6 feet tall) and how small a volume of food is needed to maintain weight in a short female (less than 5 feet tall). In proportion to total body weight, the infant has a large surface area, loses more heat through the skin, and therefore has a proportionately high REE.

Climate

Climate affects REE because kcalories are needed to maintain body temperature. This fact pertains to extreme differences in external temperatures, whether cold or hot. In the United States and Canada, most people do not need to eat more kcalories during colder months because most living environments range from 68°F to 77°F. Outside, people usually protect themselves from extreme cold and shivering, which causes an increase in REE, by wearing warm clothes.

Genetics

REE is strongly influenced by individual genetic patterns; see Genomic Gem 6-1.

Thermic Effect of Food

After a meal, the heat produced by the body is called the **thermic effect of food** (TEF). An older term for this energy cost is specific dynamic action (SDA). Energy is needed to chew, swallow, digest, absorb, and transport nutrients. Metabolism increases after eating. As metabolism increases, more kcalories are used.

The consumption of protein and carbohydrates results in a larger thermic effect than the consumption of fat. Fat is metabolized efficiently, with only 4% wastage, compared to 25% wastage when carbohydrate is converted to fat (Mahon and Escott-Stump, 2007). If an individual eats as many kcalories from carbohydrate or protein as from fat, he or she will store fewer of the nonfat kcalories as body fat.

Kcalories do count, however, regardless of the source. Consumers need to read food labels carefully. Sometimes a regular version of a food may actually contain fewer kcalories than the fat-free or reduced-fat version. For example, a regular fig cookie contains 50 kcalories, and one fat-free version contains 70 kcalories. One-half cup of regular ice cream contains 180 calories, and the same amount of one kind of reduced-fat ice cream contains 190 kcalories. Sometimes consumers are under the illusion that because the food they are eating is low-fat, they can eat unrestricted amounts and maintain body weight (see Dollars and Sense 6-1).

Genomic Gem 6-1
Resting Energy Expenditure

REE is strongly influenced by individual genetic patterns. Each person appears to be programmed with a need to burn a certain number of kcalories to maintain energy balance. This fact becomes apparent to health-care workers when counseling two very similar clients. Both clients may be of the same sex, of equal weight, perform similar types of physical activity, and have about the same body fat content. Yet each client may need to eat a different number of kcalories to maintain a stable body weight. Many individuals have little control over the number of kcalories required to meet the needs of REE.

Physical Activity

For most of the world's population, physical activity uses fewer kcalories than those required for resting energy expenditure. Very few people are active enough to burn more kcalories as a result of physical activity than as a result of their resting energy expenditures; however, some very active individuals do expend more kcalories as a result of physical activity (Fig. 6-2). For

Dollars & Sense 6-1
Kcalorie Control

Kcalorie control = Portion control = Fewer dollars spent at the grocery store.

Here's why: Some nutrients are needed daily because the body is unable to store them. Vitamin C is one example. Orange juice is high in vitamin C and is best consumed in ½ cup serving sizes to meet the daily need for vitamin C. If a food purchaser drinks an entire quart of orange juice daily, he or she will need to buy this item frequently.

Because fruits and fruit juices are becoming increasingly more expensive, think of expensive food items primarily as sources of nutrients to be eaten in recommended serving sizes.

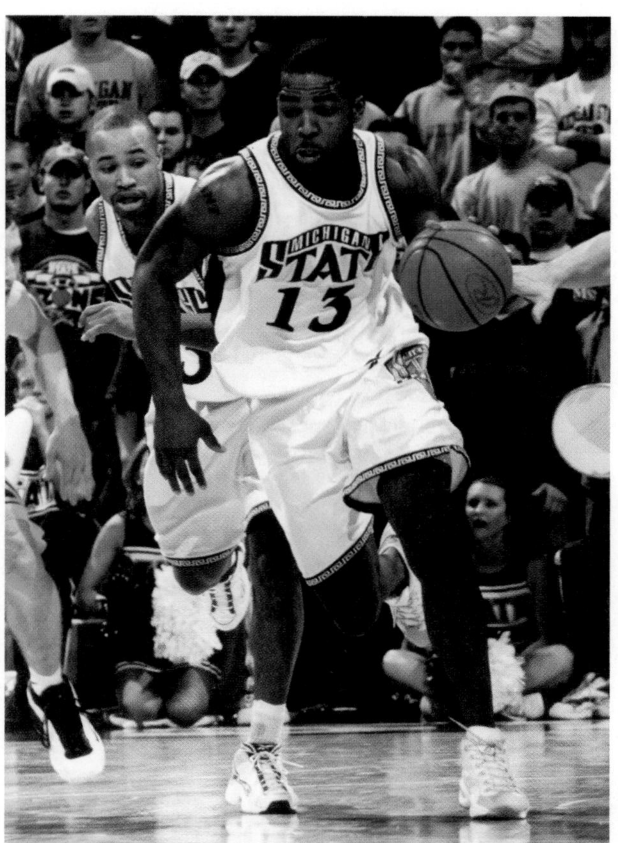

FIGURE 6-2 A trained athlete may burn more kcalories as a result of physical activity than as a result of resting energy expenditure. (Courtesy of Kevin Fowler, Sports Information, Michigan State University.)

example, professional athletes may burn a large number of kcalories as a result of training and engaging in competition.

As Table 6-1 shows, the intensity and duration of any physical activity enormously influences kcalorie expenditure. For example, a 180-pound man who trains by weight lifting will expend almost 600 kcalories in a 1-hour training session. The energy cost of physical activity is frequently referred to as the thermic effect of exercise (TEE).

Daily fluctuations in physical activity can greatly influence an individual's energy requirements (Table 6-2). For example, a 154-pound man of normal weight may require only 2002 kcalories on a very sedentary day and as many as 2772 kcalories on a very active day. A 128-pound woman of normal body weight may require only 1664 kcalories on a very sedentary day and as many as 2304 kcalories on a very active day.

Table 6-3 describes a method to estimate energy needs that includes both those needed for REE and activity. This method to estimate kcaloric need is often used in wellness programs to give clients some idea of their approximate energy need. The most accurate method for determining a client's kcalorie requirement is to monitor both food intake and body weight over time. Sometimes in clinical settings, obtaining weight and food intake information is impossible during a client's assessment. In the critical care chapter, we provide a formula that takes into account age, sex, weight, and height for estimating kcal need.

Thermic Effect of Exercise

Energy expended during exercise is only a portion of the total energy cost of physical activity. Exercise may also affect both resting energy expenditure (REE) and the thermic effect of exercise (TEF). Some clients' REE increases for up to 48 hours after exercise. Although the exact reason for this increase is unknown, the most plausible explanation is that glycogen stores need to be refilled. Because exercise depletes glycogen stores, energy is used to refill these stores during the postexercise.

TABLE 6-1 ■ Kcalories Expended in 30 Minutes

ACTIVITY	KCALORIES EXPENDED BY A 140-POUND PERSON	KCALORIES EXPENDED BY A 180-POUND PERSON
Sitting quietly	39	51
Walking	228	291
Running	396	510
Jogging	324	417
Cycling	192	246
Gardening	177	225
Golf (pull/carry clubs)	162	210
Golf (power cart)	75	96
Swimming (crawl, moderate pace)	270	348
Social dancing	192	246
Weight training	228	294

SOURCE: United States Department of Agriculture (USDA), www.mypyramidfoodintakepatterncalorielevels.com.

TABLE 6-2 ■ Energy Needs Based on Weight and Activity

ENERGY NEEDS IN KCALORIES PER POUND OF BODY WEIGHT			
	Sedentary*	Moderately Active†	Very Active‡
Overweight	9–11	13	16
Normal weight	13	16	18
Underweight	13	18	18–23

*Patients with severely limited mobility.
†Active students, sales clerks, many farm workers.
‡Full-time athletes, unskilled laborers, Army recruits.
SOURCE: Adapted from United States Department of Agriculture (2008). www.mypyramidfoodintakepatterncalorielevels.com.

Adaptive Response to Exercise

An individual with well-developed muscles performs more efficiently—uses fewer kcalories to perform a given amount of physical work—than an individual with less well-developed muscles. As exercise is repeated, the body learns how to get the job done with the least effort (the body's adaptive response to exercise). If an individual has a weight loss due to increased exercise, he or she will eventually use fewer kcalories to do a specific activity. This is the reason body builders need to continually increase the amount of weight lifted to achieve maximum results. Lighter people require fewer kcalories for a given amount of exercise than heavier people do; it takes fewer kcalories to move a smaller mass than a larger one.

Although heavier people, who move more weight, burn more kcalories than lighter people when they exercise, a heavy body is a disincentive for movement and physical activity. Heavier people tend to do fewer energy-demanding activities. This disincentive has been attributed to mechanical problems—including arthritis, arthralgia (pain in a joint), low back pain, chest and wall diaphragm restriction, incontinence, obstructive sleep apnea, and cellulites—associated with increased body weight (Swinburn, 2004).

Exercise and Appetite

Many exercise researchers think that exercise decreases appetite—that is, a person may be satisfied with less food after exercise. Some types of exercise

TABLE 6-3 ■ Dietary Reference Intake Values for Energy for Active Individuals

		ACTIVE PAL EER (kcal/day)	
LIFESTYLE GROUP	CRITERION	Male	Female
Infants			
0–6 mo	Energy expenditure + energy deposition	570	520 (3 mo)
7–12 mo	Energy expenditure + energy deposition	743	676 (9 mo)
Children			
1–2 yr	Energy expenditure + energy deposition	1046	992 (24 mo)
3–8 yr	Energy expenditure + energy deposition	1742	1642 (6 yr)
9–13 yr	Energy expenditure + energy deposition	2279	2071 (11 yr)
14–18 yr	Energy expenditure + energy deposition	3152	2368 (16 yr)
Adults			
>18 yr	Energy expenditure	3067*	2403* (19 yr)
Pregnant women			
14–18 yr	Adolescent female EER + change in TEE + pregnancy energy deposition		
First trimester		2368 (16 yr)	
Second trimester		2708 (16 yr)	
Third trimester		2820 (yr)	
19–50 yr	Adult female EER + change in TEE + pregnancy energy deposition		
First trimester		2403 (19 yr)	
Second trimester		2743 (19 yr)	
Third trimester		2855 (yr)	
Lactating women			
14–18 yr	Adolescent female EER + milk energy output – weight loss		
First 6 mo		2698 (16 yr)	
Second 6 mo		2768 (16 yr)	
19–50 yr	Adult female EER + milk energy output – weight loss		
First 6 mo		2733 (19 yr)	
Second 6 mo		2803 (19 yr)	

*Subtract 10 kcal/day for men and 7 kcal/day for women for each year above 19.
For healthy active Americans and Canadians at the reference height and weight.
PAL, physically active level; EER, estimated energy requirement; TEE, total energy expenditure.
Data compiled from Institutes of Medicine of The National Academies Press. Food and Nutrition Board, Institute of Medicine, National Academies. (A Report of the Panel on Macronutrients, Subcommittes on Upper Reference Levels of Nutrients and Interpretation and Uses of Dietary Reference Intakes, and the Standing Committee on Scientific Evaluation of Dietary Reference Intakes. Reprinted with permission from the National Academies Press, Copyright 2005, National Academy of Sciences.)

release a chemical in the brain called beta-endorphin. Beta-endorphin has an effect similar to that of natural morphine; it produces a state of relaxation. In effect, exercise can be a safe substitute for overeating in some individuals who eat to decrease stress and tension. On the other hand, an individual with a severe eating disorder may exercise compulsively to relax.

Aerobic Exercise

Aerobic exercise is any activity during which the energy metabolism needed is supported by the amount of increase in oxygen inspired. Aerobic exercises increase physical fitness and involve large muscle groups. Vigorous workouts that last at least 30 minutes require an increase in the amount of oxygen inspired. Box 6-2 provides examples of aeròbic exercise. Aerobic exercise provides many health benefits, including:

- Decreased risk of cardiovascular disease
- Improved blood sugar control for people with diabetes
- Decreased risk of obesity
- Reversal or prevention of varicose veins
- Decreased risk of osteoporosis
- Improved quality of sleep
- Improved hypertension control

Box 6-2 ■ *Examples of Aerobic Exercise*

These are some popular forms of aerobic exercise:

Fast walking
Cycling
Swimming
Skating
Jumping rope
Dancing
Hiking
Jogging
Rowing

Anaerobic Exercise

Exercise during which energy is provided without an increase in the use of inspired oxygen is **anaerobic**

exercise. Short bursts of vigorous activity, such as resistance or muscle strength training (e.g., weight lifting), are forms of anaerobic exercise. Anaerobic exercise allows for:

- Muscle toning
- The building of muscular strength and endurance
- Building of bone mass.

This kind of training provides added strength and toughness, which help to reduce injury during aerobic exercise; prevents lower back problems; and allows for a more muscular appearance.

Diet and Activity

A healthy lifestyle depends on much more than diet. Physical activity makes a vital contribution to health, function, and performance. The greatest benefit derived from physical activity is gained when a person moves from sedentary to moderate levels of activity. The combination of a balanced diet and regular physical activity has a stronger effect on energy balance than either strategy alone.

Every adult should engage in 60 minutes or more of moderate-intensity physical activity on most, preferably all, days of the week—that is, a total of 60 minutes per day of brisk walking, stair climbing, calisthenics, heavy gardening, or dancing. The activity need not be continuous but may be broken up into short sessions. For example, six brisk 10-minute walks would meet the minimum requirement. A person performing these activities for 60 minutes expends 400 total kcalories (see Fig. 6-3). Some health benefits can be achieved with a minimum of 30 minutes of moderate-intensity physical activity on most days of the week; however, this is insufficient to maintain energy balance in most people.

Energy Intake

Between 2005 and 2006, the mean reported energy intakes for men ages 20 to 59 was 2597 to 2821 kcalories per day (USDA, 2007). The mean reported energy intakes for women aged 20 to 59 was between 1718 to 1959 kcalories per day (USDA, 2007). The average reported intakes for women are of special concern because of the difficulty in incorporating all nutrients at recommended levels in a diet so low in kcalories. The average woman's need to increase energy output or physical activity is well documented.

Many experts attribute increased obesity to decreased energy expenditure. America is becoming an increasingly sedentary society. The current recommendation is that the average person increase physical activity rather than decrease kcalorie intake below their estimated energy requirements (EER) to achieve energy balance. If the average reported intakes for both sexes are compared to the EER, the need for more physical activity in most people becomes very clear. For specifics, refer to the DRIs inside the cover.

Kilocaloric Density of Foods

Some foods are more kilocalorically dense than other foods. Density is the quantity per unit volume of a substance. **Kilocaloric density** refers to the kcalories contained in a given volume of a food. Foods with a high water and fiber content tend to have a lower kcaloric density. Fruits and vegetables such as lettuce, watermelon, and celery are high in water content and low in kcalories. A given volume of grapes has fewer kcalories than an equal volume of raisins because grapes contain more water than raisins.

Fats or foods high in fat have the highest kcaloric density (Fig. 6-4). Whole-milk products, high-fat meat exchanges, fat exchanges, and foods made with these ingredients all contain appreciable amounts of fat. Box 6-3 lists several tips for decreasing the kcaloric density of a diet.

Nutrient Density of Foods

Kilocaloric content alone should not be the criterion to decide whether to include a food in one's diet. The nutrient density of a food—the concentration of nutrients in a food compared with the food's kilocaloric content—is also an important consideration. If a food is high in kcalories and low in nutrients, the nutrient density of the food is low. **Empty kcalories** means that the food contains kcalories and almost no nutrients; table sugar is an example of such a food. If a food is low in kcalories and high in nutrients, the nutrient density of the food is high.

Cantaloupe is an example of a food with a high nutrient density—it is low in kcalories and high in vitamin C and contains a moderate amount of vitamin A. Skim milk and whole milk are similar in nutrient content; both types of milk contain about the same amounts of protein, calcium, vitamin D, and riboflavin. Eight ounces of skim milk provides about 90 kcalories compared with 150 kcalories in 8 ounces of whole milk. Skim milk thus has a higher nutrient density than whole milk.

In 2005, the federal government issued the Dietary Reference Intake (DRIs) for Estimated Energy Requirements (EER) Values for Energy for Active Individuals. See Table 6-4. Note that the values for pregnant and lactating women are higher than for nonpregnant and nonlactating women.

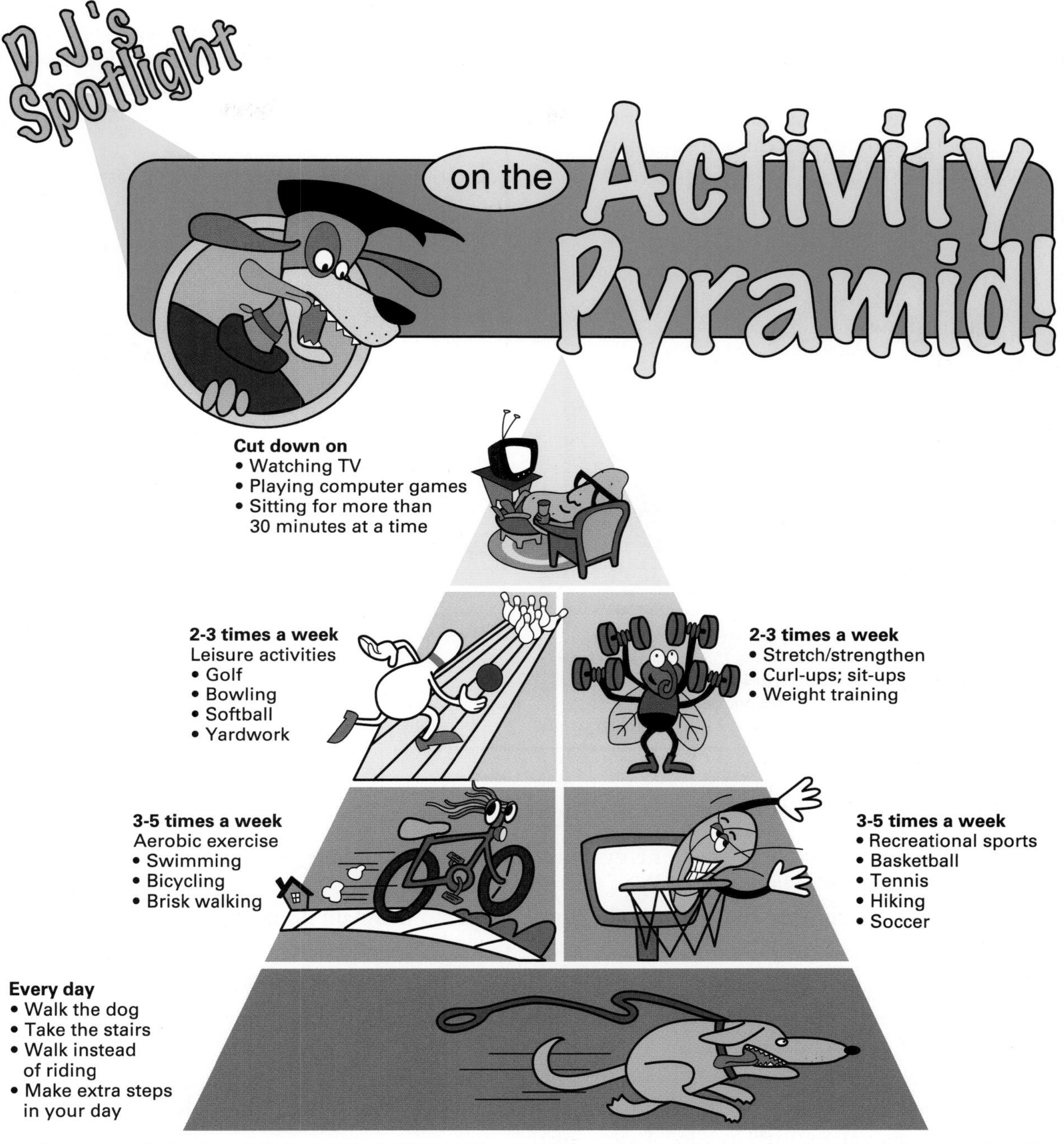

FIGURE 6-3 The President's Council Activity Pyramid for Children. Children should have some activity every day, vigorous activity two to three times a week, and minimal sedentary activity such as watching television and playing computer games. (www.thepresident'scouncilactivitypyramidforkids.com)

Dietary Recommendations

All the major national health organizations recommend that individuals maintain a healthy body weight. The American Heart Association recommends maintaining a healthy body weight to decrease the risk of heart and circulatory diseases. The American Cancer Society cites numerous studies suggesting that lower kilocaloric intake may lower an individual's risk of cancer. Most individuals would benefit by monitoring their weight and increasing their energy expenditure or decreasing their energy intake as necessary to maintain a healthy body weight.

The Food and Nutrition Board of the National Academy of Sciences (NAS) revised their guidelines on energy nutrient distribution in 2002/2005. Table 6-4 compares the 1996 guidelines to the 2005 guidelines. The rationale for the change is that carbohydrate and fat are both energy sources and can substitute for one another to some extent.

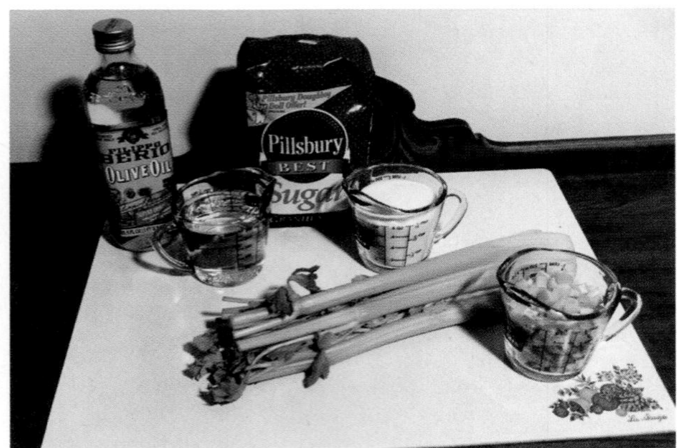

FIGURE 6-4 One cup of celery contains 17 kcalories, 1 cup of sugar contains 770 kcalories, and 1 cup of oil contains 1925 kcalories. Celery is the least kcalorically dense of the foods pictured, and oil is the most dense. Sugar is between celery and oil in kcaloric density.

Box 6-3 ■ *Tips for Decreasing the Kilocaloric Density of a Diet*

- Use low-fat or nonfat dairy products including skim milk, cheese, and yogurt.
- Brown meats by broiling or cooking in nonstick pans with little or no fat. Avoid fried foods.
- Chill soups, stews, sauces, and broths. Lift off and discard hardened fat.
- Trim all visible fat from meat before cooking.
- Use water-packed, canned foods such as fruits and tuna.
- Use fresh fruits and vegetables often. Try to eat at least 2½ cups of these foods each day.
- Use low-kcalorie salad dressings.
- When you eat out, do not look at the menu. Instead, have an idea of what you would like to eat before you arrive at the restaurant. Explain to the waitress or waiter what you would like to eat.
- Eat smaller portion sizes of all foods, but particularly sandwiches.
- Limit consumption of sweetened carbonated beverages and other empty kcalorie foods.

TABLE 6-4 ■ National Academy of Sciences Guidelines

	1996	2005
Kcalories from CHO	50% or more	45%–65%
Kcalories from fat	30% or less	20%–35%
Kcalories from protein	10%–35%	10%–35%

Keystones

- Energy balance exists when energy intake equals energy output. A person whose body weight remains stable is usually in energy balance.
- A person's appetite can overrule the body's ability to maintain homestasis.
- A hungry person will most often be willing to eat almost anything.
- When an individual is not in energy balance, he or she is gaining or losing weight.
- The most accurate method for determining kcalorie need is to monitor both food intake and body weight over time.
- Foods high in water and fiber (fruits and vegetables) are low in kilocaloric density.
- Foods high in fat (fatty meats, oils, spreads, salad dressings, and food made with those ingredients) are high in kilocaloric density.
- Foods that are low in kcalories and contain substantial amounts of one or more nutrients are high in nutrient density.
- The recommended range of energy nutrient intake is:
  - 45% to 65% for carbohydrate
  - 20% to 35% for fat
  - 10% to 35% for protein
- The current recommendation is that individuals who gain weight while consuming their energy EER should increase their activity to maintain energy balance.
- Most Americans are eating too much of one, two, or three of the energy nutrients to maintain energy balance.

CASE STUDY 6-1

The Fairview Nursing Home holds a weekly client care conference. Nursing care plans for all of the facility's residents are reviewed on a rotating basis, with each client's nursing care plan reviewed once every 3 months. All members of the health-care team are often present at the conference. Team members include the administrator, the physician, the director of nursing, the staff nurse, the nursing assistant, the activities director, the social worker, the dietitian, and the client or a family member representing the client.

Mr. G has been experiencing a slow weight gain. His weight history follows:

2/08	169 lb (77 kg)
6/08	172 lb (78 kg)
9/08	175 lb (80 kg)
12/08	180 lb (82 kg)
03/09	183 lb (83 kg)

Mr. G is 5 ft 8 in. tall and 79 years old. He is alert, feeds himself, and has normal bowel and bladder function. Mr. G walks to the dining room three times a day. His favorite activity is watching television. He has good dentition and is on a regular diet. According to the appetite records kept by the nurse's aide, Mr. G's intake is good to excellent. He accepts all of the major food groups. He admits to overeating at social activities, especially those sponsored by the facility in the evenings. Mr. G is concerned with his slow weight gain but claims he does not know what to do. To address the slow weight gain problem, the health-care team and Mr. G developed the following nursing care plan.

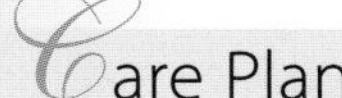

Care Plan

Subjective Data

Client expressed concern about his slow weight gain.

Objective Data

Height is 5 ft, 8 in. Weight:
2/08 169 lb ■ 03/09 183 lb

Analysis

Weight gain related to sedentary activity level and eating in response to external cues.

Plan

DESIRED OUTCOMES EVALUATION CRITERIA	ACTIONS/INTERVENTIONS	RATIONALE
Client will select fresh fruits at social activities.	Request Foods and Nutrition Department to serve fresh fruit at social functions.	Replacing kilocalorically dense cakes, pies, and cookies with fresh fruit will promote weight maintenance.
Refer client to registered dietitian (RD)	Reinforce dietitian's teaching.	The dietitian will generally be able to spend more time with client than the floor nurse.
Refer client to activites director	Reinforce activites director's teaching.	The activites director will be able to discuss opportunities to exercise with client as well as order appropriate foods for activites.

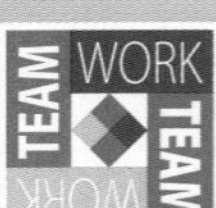

6-1

Dietitan's Notes

The following Dietitian's Notes are representative of the documentation found in a client's medical record.

Subjective: Client states he would like to lose weight but can't resist treats served at social functions. Loves cakes, pie, donuts, and cookies and admits to lack of self-control. Client would appreciate having more healthful snacks available at social functions. Admits to being unaware of what he actually eats everyday. Admits he avoids body movement.

Objective: Height 5 ft 8 in. 02/08 weight 169 lb, 03/09 weight 183 lb Appetite records show a food intake of 100% of all food served plus second portions.

Analysis: Ideal body weight 148 to 180 lb

Estimated kcal needs at 12 kcal/pound = 2280 (between sedentary and moderately active).

Excessive energy intake related to failure to adjust for lifestyle changes and decreased metabolism as evidenced by body weight and client history. Client expressed verbal desire to manage his weight (American Dietetic Association, 2008).

Plan:

1. Client will keep a food record for 3 out of every 7 days to enable him to be more conscious of food choices (self-monitor behavior). Will evaluate food records for 2 weeks.
2. Client's goal is to maintain weight and perhaps lose a few pounds.
3. Will encourage activites director to order fresh fruit at facility functions and evaluate client for physical activity opportunities.

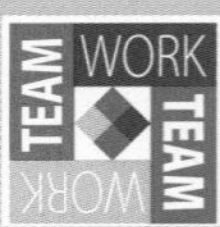

6-2

Activity Director's Note

The following Activities Director's Notes are representative of the documentation found in a client's medical record.

Met with client and discussed activites calendar including those with an exercise component. Will order a fresh fruit option at social activites that serve food.

Critical Thinking Questions

1. What would you do at the next client care conference if Mr. G changed his mind about weight control and said, "All I have left in life is food. I don't want to lose weight"?
2. What would you do at the next client care conference if Mr. G had done everything asked but only managed to maintain his weight.

Chapter Review

1. The components of energy expenditure are:
   a. Mental activity and physical activity
   b. Thermic effects of exercise and foods
   c. Resting energy expenditure, physical activity, and to a lesser extent the thermic effect of foods
   d. Thermic effect of foods, physical activity, and thermic effect of exercise
2. Energy homeostasis exists when:
   a. Kcalories from food intake equal kcalories used for energy expenditure.
   b. Kcalories used for physical activity equal kcalories used for energy expenditure.
   c. An individual is gaining weight.
   d. Kcalories from food intake equal kcalories used for resting energy expenditure.

Chapter Review—cont'd

3. A kilocalorie is used to measure both:
   a. Weight and percentage body fat
   b. Height and weight
   c. The units of energy used in the body and contained in foods
   d. Leanness and body-fat content
4. Kilocalories required per kilogram of body weight are highest during:
   a. Starvation
   b. Growth
   c. Weight loss
   d. Old age
5. Which of the following foods is the most kilocalorically dense?
   a. 1 cup of sugar
   b. 1 cup of celery
   c. 1 cup of skim milk
   d. 1 cup of margarine

Clinical Analysis

1. Monitoring a resident's weight is a government requirement in long-term care facilities. The goal is to prevent a slow weight loss, which, over time, can have health consequences. Mr. I, resident of Sunnybrook Nursing Home, has been experiencing an undesirable slow weight loss. His weight history is as follows:

Feb	180 lb (82 kg)
June	175 lb (80 kg)
Oct	170 lb (77 kg)

   As Mr. I's nurse, you should first:
   a. Encourage Mr. I to eat only twice a day
   b. Call the doctor
   c. Wait for the next client care conference to act on this problem
   d. Monitor Mr. I's food intake and physical activity
2. A teacher noticed that many students in her fifth grade class were overweight. As a school project, the class kept food records for 3 days. A computer software program analyzed the records. Many students were eating less than their recommended dietary allowance for kcalories but gaining weight nonetheless (a common problem among our nation's young). The teacher asked the class by a show of hands what they did after school and on weekends. Many of the same children who were overweight raised their hands when asked if they played mostly video games and watched television when not in school. The teacher shared this information with the school nurse and asked her to speak to the class. The school nurse correctly decided that:
   a. The teacher is overly concerned, because the percentage of overweight students approximates the percentage of overweight adults in the community.
   b. The computer program must be in error.
   c. All the students need to increase their total intake, including foods from the major food groups.
   d. Many students would benefit from an increase in physical activity.
3. A client appears to be totally concerned with the kilocaloric density of foods and not at all concerned with the nutrient density of foods. You need to encourage the consumption of both types of foods. Which of the following behaviors do you need to discourage?
   a. The substitution of skim milk for 2% milk
   b. The avoidance of all meat, fish, and poultry
   c. The inclusion of dark green and yellow fruits and vegetables in the diet
   d. The inclusion of whole grains in the diet

7

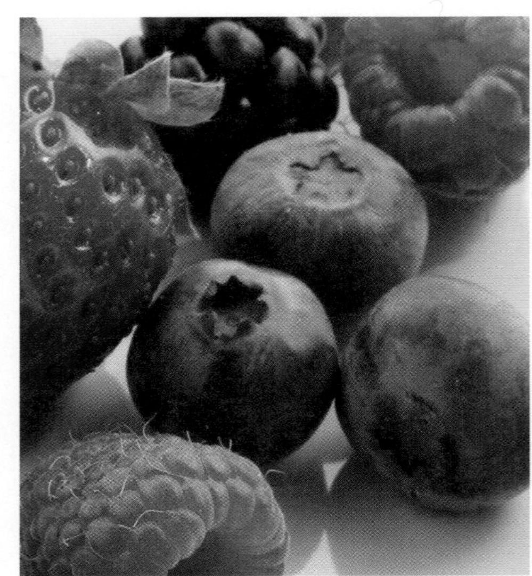

Vitamins

LEARNING OBJECTIVES

After completing this chapter, the student should be able to:

- Differentiate between fat- and water-soluble vitamins.
- State the functions of each vitamin discussed in the chapter.
- Name three good food sources for each vitamin cited in the chapter.
- List diseases caused by specific vitamin deficiencies and identify associated signs and symptoms.
- Describe the prudent use of vitamin supplements.

The importance of vitamins was first recognized by the effects of their absence. Some deficiency diseases have been known for centuries, but it was not until the early 20th century that vitamins were isolated in the laboratory. This chapter considers the importance of vitamins in the body and diet, the general functions of vitamins, the classification of vitamins, and the use of vitamin supplements. It also includes information on metabolism, functions, sources, deficiencies, toxicities, and factors affecting stability.

The Nature of Vitamins

Vitamins are organic substances needed by the body in small amounts for normal metabolism, growth, and maintenance. Organic substances are derived from living matter and contain carbon. Vitamins are not sources of energy, and they do not become part of the structure of the body. Vitamins act as regulators or adjusters of metabolic processes and as **coenzymes** (substances that activate enzymes) in enzymatic systems.

Specific Functions

Vitamin functions are specific. With few exceptions, bodily processes do not permit substitutes. Thus, vitamins are similar to keys in a lock. All the notches in a key have to fit the lock or the key will not turn. Overall, one vitamin cannot perform the functions of another. If a person does not consume enough vitamin C, for instance, taking vitamin D will not correct the deficiency. Vitamin D is the wrong key for that lock.

Classification

A major distinguishing characteristic of vitamins is their solubility in either fat or water. This physical property is used to classify vitamins and is also significant for storage and processing of foods that contain vitamins and for the utilization of the vitamins in the body. Vitamins A, E, D, and K are fat-soluble. The eight B-complex vitamins and vitamin C are water-soluble. See Table 7-1 for the 13 traditionally recognized vitamins. Choline, not a vitamin by strict definition but recently added to the Dietary

TABLE 7-1 ■ Classification of Vitamins	
FAT SOLUBLE	**WATER SOLUBLE**
Vitamin A	Vitamin C
Vitamin D	Thiamin
Vitamin E	Riboflavin
Vitamin K	Niacin
	Vitamin B_6
	Folic acid
	Vitamin B_{12}
	Biotin
	Pantothenic acid

Reference Intake (DRI) list, appears near the end of the chapter.

Dietary Reference Intakes

The amounts of vitamins recommended in the United States to meet the needs of almost all healthy individuals are listed by age and physiological status in Appendix A. Recommended amounts vary in other countries.

Vitamins A, D, and E historically have been measured in International Units, a dosage amount that still appears on some labels. The Recommended Dietary Allowances (RDAs) and Adequate Intakes (AIs), however, are listed in the metric system: **micrograms** and milligrams. There are no generic units that can be converted directly to the metric system. The amount designated by a unit is specific for each vitamin. The formulas to convert **International Units** to the metric system are given in Clinical Calculation 7-1.

Fat-Soluble Vitamins

More or less of a vitamin may be retained in a food, depending on the methods of processing and storing. Compared with water-soluble vitamins, the fat-soluble vitamins A, D, E, and K are more stable and more resistant to the effects of oxidation, heat, light, acidity, and alkalinity. See Box 7-1 for an explanation of oxidation.

Sources of the fat-soluble vitamins with examples of foods containing the RDA/AI of each are given in Table 7-2. A summary of factors affecting stability of vitamins appears as Table 7-3.

Fat-soluble vitamins are absorbed from the intestine in the same way as fats, and like fats, they can be stored in the body, giving the potential for health problems due to excessive intake. Toxicity from vitamins A and D can be fatal.

Clinical Calculation 7-1

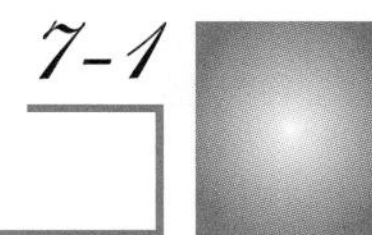

The Elusive International Unit

Formerly, fat-soluble vitamins were measured in International Units (IU), as defined by the International Conference for Unification of Formulae. *A unit of vitamin A is not an equal measure of vitamin D or of vitamin E.* Because that system still appears in laws, on labels, and in research reports, the formulas to convert International Units to metric measures are given below. These equivalents incorporate recent changes in the calculation of provitamin A.

VITAMIN A*
Animal Foods: 3.3 IU = 1 microgram of **Retinol Activity Equivalents (RAEs)**
Plant Foods: 20 IU = 1 microgram of RAE (Conversion Factors, 2006)

VITAMIN D
40 IU = 1 microgram of cholecalciferol

VITAMIN E
Natural form: 1.5 IU = 1 milligram of alpha-tocopherol†
Synthetic form: 2.2 IU = 1 milligram of alpha-tocopherol†

*A vitamin A calculator is available at http://www.nutrisurvey.de/vac/vac.htm.
†Traber (2006).

Box 7-1 ■ *Oxidation*

The process by which a substance combines with oxygen is called **oxidation.** Several substances can be destroyed by oxidation, including vitamin E, provitamin A, and vitamin C. Some molecules become very unstable when they are oxidized. Their accelerated movements can damage nearby molecules.

Vitamin A

For DRIs, see Appendix A. For food and other sources, see Table 7-2. To investigate the vitamin content of a particular item, see "Caffeine and Nutritive Values of Foods" on DavisPlus. For stability information, see Table 7-3.

Vitamin A comes in two forms: preformed vitamin A (**retinol**) and **provitamin A** (found in **beta-carotene** and other **carotenoids,** 50 of which have some provitamin A activity). A **preformed vitamin** is already in a complete state in ingested foods whereas a **provitamin** requires conversion in the body to be in a complete state. Provitamin A is converted to retinol in the intestine. The term *precursor* is often used interchangeably with the term *provitamin*. A **precursor** is a substance from which another substance is derived.

Absorption, Metabolism, and Excretion

Of preformed vitamin A, 70% to 90% is absorbed if consumed with at least 10 grams of fat, but less than 5%

TABLE 7-2 ■ Fat-Soluble Vitamins

VITAMIN	ADULT RDA/AI AND FOOD PORTION CONTAINING IT	FUNCTIONS	DEFICIENCY DISEASE	SIGNS AND SYMPTOMS OF DEFICIENCY	SOURCES
A	700–900 μg 5 or 6 medium raw baby carrots	Dim light vision Differentiation of epithelial cells	Night blindness Xerophthalmia	Night blindness Sore throat, sinus trouble, ear and mouth abscesses Dry and thick outer covering of eye Blindness	*Preformed:* Liver Egg yolk Fortified milk *Provitamin:* Carrots Sweet potatoes Squash Apricots Cantaloupe Spinach, Collards Broccoli, Cabbage
D	5–15 μg 2–6 cups fortified milk	Increases intestinal absorption of calcium Stimulates bone production Decreases urinary excretion of calcium	Rickets Osteomalacia	Bowlegs, knock-knees, misshapen skull Tetany in infants Soft fragile bones, especially of spine, pelvis, lower extremities	Sunlight on skin Fortified milk Cod liver oil Herring, Salmon, Sardines
E	15 mg 3 tbsp safflower oil	Antioxidant Protects polyunsaturated fatty acids in red blood cell membranes from oxidation in lungs	No specific term	Neurological problems Anemia in premature infants	Vegetable oils, especially canola, olive, sunflower, and safflower Whole grains, Wheat germ Fortified ready-to-eat cereals Nuts Leafy vegetables
K	90 to 120 μg 10 raw broccoli flowerets	Used in manufacture of several clotting factors, including prothrombin Assists vitamin D to synthesize a regulatory bone protein	No specific term	Prolonged clotting time	Broccoli Brussels sprouts Cabbage, Collards Salad greens Spinach Synthesis in intestine

TABLE 7-3 ■ Factors Affecting Stability of Vitamins

	STABLE TO				
Vitamin	**Oxygen**	**Heat**	**Light**	**Acids**	**Alkalies**
Fat Soluble					
A	No	Yes	No	No	*
D	Yes	Yes	Yes	*	*
E	No	Yes/No†	No	Yes	No
K	No	No	No	No	No
Water Soluble					
C	No	No	No	Yes	No
Thiamin	No	No	No	Yes/No‡	No
Riboflavin	Yes	Yes	No	Yes	No
Niacin	Yes	Yes	Yes	Yes	Yes
B_6	No	No	No	Yes	No
Folate	No	No	No	No	Yes
B_{12}	No	Yes	No	No	No

*Data unavailable.
†Frying destroys.
‡Destroyed by tannic and caffeic acid; protected by ascorbic and citric acid.

of carotene is absorbed from raw vegetables (Gropper, Smith, and Groff, 2009). Vitamin A is transported bound to a retinol-binding protein. This complex is too large for the kidney to filter, so it is retained in the body. Consequently, poor protein status interferes with the transportation and usage of vitamin A. About 40% of vitamin A metabolites are excreted via the bile in feces and about 60% in urine (Gropper, Smith, and Groff, 2009).

Up to a year's supply of vitamin A is stored in the body, 85% of it in the liver. Excessive carotene is stored in adipose tissue, giving fat a yellowish tint, but it is apparently harmless for most people. (See Vitamin A Toxicity in this chapter and Chapter 21 for information on exceptional situations.)

Functions

Several crucial body functions depend on vitamin A, or retinol: vision, bone growth, and maintenance of epithelial tissue. In addition, provitamin A serves as an antioxidant. (See Vitamin E in this chapter.)

VISION

In many ways, a camera mimics the eye: Both have a dark layer to keep out excess light, a lens to focus light, and a light-sensor. In the eye, the sensor is a light-sensitive layer at the back of the eye, called the **retina.** In the retina, light rays are changed into electrical impulses that travel along the **optic nerve** to the back of the brain. The vitamin A metabolite retinol is part of a chemical in the retina responsible for this electrical conversion. The body can synthesize this chemical, **rhodopsin** (or visual purple), only if it has a supply of vitamin A.

When the eye is functioning in dim light, rhodopsin is broken down into a protein **(opsin)** and vitamin A. In darkness or during sleep, opsin and vitamin A reunite to become rhodopsin. Figure 7-1 shows this reaction. The body can keep reusing the vitamin A, but some of the vitamin is depleted during each visual cycle so that a dietary deficiency produces **night blindness,** or impaired dim-light vision. Clinical Application 7-1 relates a practical method for conserving rhodopsin for night vision.

MAINTAINING EPITHELIAL TISSUE

Epithelial tissue covers the body and lines the organs and passageways that open to the outside of the body. Skin is epithelial tissue, as are the surface of the eye and the lining of the gastrointestinal tract. Epithelial tissue has a protective function, often producing mucus to wash out foreign materials. Vitamin A helps to keep epithelial tissue healthy by aiding the differentiation of specialty cells. This function, control of gene expression, has led some scientists to believe that vitamin A may play a role in cancer prevention. See Clinical Application 7-2 for more information on vitamin A and cancer.

Retinal + Opsin —Sleep→ Rhodopsin

Rhodopsin —Dim Light Vision→ Retinal + Opsin

FIGURE 7-1 Vitamin A and the protein opsin combine during sleep to form rhodopsin. When we need to see in dim light, the rhodopsin breaks down into vitamin A and opsin.

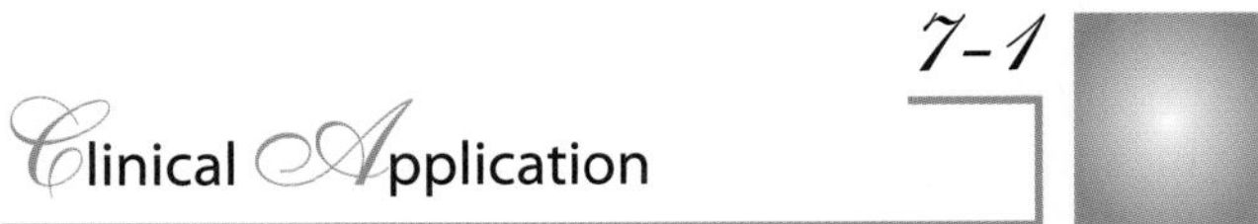

Red Light Conserves Rhodopsin

Red light breaks down rhodopsin more slowly than do other wavelengths of light. Therefore, aviators spend time in a red-lit room before flying at night. In the presence of red light, a build-up of rhodopsin occurs in the rods of the retina and enhances vision in dim light. For this reason, navigational instruments and some automobile dashboards use red light.

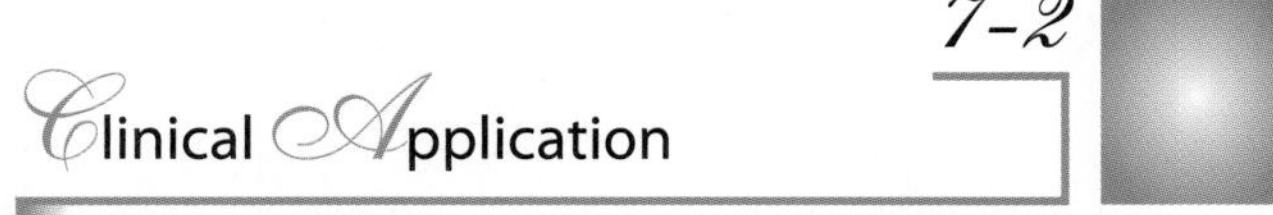

Vitamin A and Cancer

Cancers begin with abnormal differentiation and rampant proliferation of cells. Vitamin A plays a hormone-like role in normal cell differentiation throughout the body. The provitamin also functions as an antioxidant to neutralize **free radicals**. These highly reactive atoms or molecules can damage DNA, with resultant abnormal cell growth.

OTHER FUNCTIONS

Vitamin A participates in bone metabolism so that deficiency causes unusual deposition of bone and excessive amounts cause loss of bone structure. Vitamin A affects body fat reserves through the development and metabolism of adipose tissue and through adaptive thermogenesis, which dissipates some of the food energy as heat instead of storing it as fat (Bonet et al., 2003). Vitamin A also contributes to immunity, to blood formation, and to normal reproduction but less is understood about the physiology involved in those areas.

Deficiency

Even though vitamin A is stored in the body, deficiencies can occur. In developing countries, approximately 127 million preschool-aged children and 7 million pregnant women are vitamin A deficient (West, 2003).

Vitamin A deficiency in the United States is most often due to disease. For example, clients with long-lasting infectious disease, fat absorption problems, or liver disease are at risk of vitamin A deficiency. Vitamin A deficiency after **bariatric surgery** is a well-documented complication. Its main symptom is nightblindness. Prevention of deficiencies requires lifelong vitamin supplementation after these surgeries (Stroh et al., 2010).

SIGNS AND SYMPTOMS

Lack of vitamin A as retinol causes night blindness. In this condition, the resynthesis of rhodopsin is too slow to allow quick adaptation to dim light. Worldwide, 6 million women are afflicted with night blindness during pregnancy (West, 2003).

All epithelial tissue suffers because of vitamin A deficiency. The most serious effect is the thickening of the epithelial tissue covering the eye. **Xerophthalmia,** an abnormal thickening and drying of the outer surface of the eye, is a leading cause of blindness in some developing countries. Figure 7-2 shows a characteristic

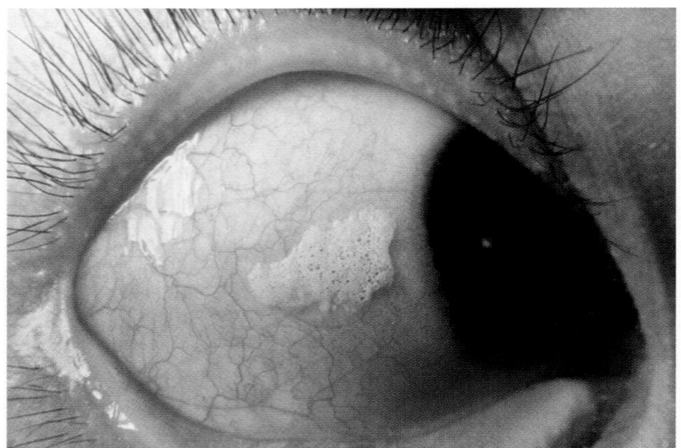

FIGURE 7-2 Bitot spot, a triangular shiny gray spot on the conjunctiva seen in vitamin A deficiency. (From McLaren and Frigg [2001]. Reproduced with permission of Sight and Life.)

lesion. Globally, 4.4 million preschool children have xerophthalmia (West, 2003).

TREATMENT AND PREVENTION

Active corneal xerophthalmia is a medical emergency demanding high-dose vitamin A treatment. High doses are also recommended for infants and young children with xerophthalmia, severe malnutrition, or measles (Ross, 2002). The World Health Organization (WHO) recommends two daily doses of vitamin A for children with measles living where deficiency is common, a practice associated with a reduced risk of mortality in children younger than 2 years old (Huiming, Chaomin, and Meng, 2005).

Prevention of vitamin A deficiency involves multiple strategies: breast feeding, vitamin A supplementation, fortification of foods, and diet diversification, often in combination. An international humanitarian effort to eliminate vitamin A deficiency by DSM Nutritionals provides free vitamin A capsules as well as free educational materials (wall posters, books, videos, Power Point slides) in English, French, German, Spanish, and other languages. Sight and Life is based at P.O. Box 2116, CH 4002 Basel, Switzerland or can be accessed via the Internet.

Sources and Interfering Factors

Preformed vitamin A (retinol) is found in animal foods such as liver, egg yolk, and fortified milk products. The body converts the provitamin A carotenoids present in fruits and vegetables to retinol. The best-utilized sources are ripe colored fruits and cooked yellow tubers, followed by dark green leafy vegetables.

Carotene, a yellow pigment found mostly in fruits and vegetables, is readily visible in yellow and orange foods such as carrots, sweet potatoes, squash, apricots, and cantaloupe. Although not as noticeable because chlorophyll masks the yellow color, carotene is also present in dark leafy green vegetables, including spinach, collards, broccoli, and cabbage.

Vitamin A is fairly stable to heat, but sunlight, ultraviolet light, air, and oxidation easily destroy it. Carotene content of a species of vegetable can vary with the vegetable's maturity, handling, and preparation. Carrots packaged in plastic bags are better protected from light and air than the bouquets secured by a rubber band. **Beta-carotene** is more available to the body in carrots cooked with a small amount of fat than in raw carrots, an exception to the general rule that cooking depletes vitamins.

Toxicity

Although most other vitamin toxicities are a result of supplementation, hypervitaminosis A can be caused by foods. Fetal malformations can be caused by either deficiency or excess of vitamin A. In addition, vitamin A derivatives are often prescribed to control severe acne. The hazards to the fetus from vitamin A excesses are described in Chapter 10.

CAROTENEMIA

Beta-carotene is recognized by the Food and Drug Administration as Generally Recognized as Safe (**GRAS**) as a dietary supplement and a colorant. Nevertheless carotene can be consumed to excess, causing **carotenemia.** The person's skin becomes yellow, first on the palms of the hands and the soles of the feet. The whites of the eyes do not become yellow, however, as they do in people with **jaundice** caused by liver disease. Carotenemia has occurred in infants fed too much squash and carrots. The skin returns to normal within 2 to 6 weeks after stopping the excessive intake.

The assumption that carotene is harmless has been challenged by studies in which beta-carotene supplementation was associated with increased occurrence of lung cancer (see Chapter 21).

HYPERVITAMINOSIS A

Vitamin A toxicity is called **hypervitaminosis A.** Symptoms of vitamin A toxicity are similar to those of a brain tumor, such as headaches and blurred vision and other signs of increased pressure within the skull. Other symptoms include pain in the bones and joints, dry skin, and poor appetite. Some clients have developed symptoms after consuming beef liver once or twice a week. A case of idiopathic intracranial hypertension was attributed to consumption of 2 to 3 pounds of raw baby carrots per week for 16 months (Donahue, 2000).

Self-prescribed vitamin A supplements also have produced liver disease. For one such client, the liver signs and symptoms did not appear until 24,700 International Units daily for 17 years and 270,000 IU daily for 1 year had been ingested (Miksad et al., 2002). Another client died after consuming 25,000 IU (2.5 times the UL) daily for 6 years (Kowalski et al., 1994).

Experts are concerned that intake from preformed sources of vitamin A often exceeds the RDA for adults, especially in developed countries. Osteoporosis and hip fracture are associated with preformed vitamin A intakes that are only twice the current RDA (Penniston and Tanumihardjo, 2006).

One hazard of excessive vitamin A intake is unique to the Arctic. Polar bear liver has made both men and dogs sick. A 3-ounce serving contains 394 times the RDA for men. Other Arctic game poses similar hazards.

Vitamin D

For DRIs, see Appendix A. In 2008, the American Academy of Pediatrics recommended that all infants, children, and adolescents receive a daily intake of 400 IU of vitamin D beginning in the first few days of life (Wagner and Greer, 2008). For food and other sources, see Table 7-2. To investigate the vitamin content of a particular item, see the Internet site of the United States Department of Agriculture at http://www.nal.usda.gov/fnic/foodcomp/search/. For stability see Table 7-3.

Recently, **vitamin D,** which promotes bone growth, has come to be regarded as a hormone rather than a vitamin because of the way it works. Vitamin D receptors have been found in more than 30 organs not usually associated with bone metabolism such as lung and muscle (Gropper, Smith, and Groff, 2009).

Absorption, Metabolism, and Excretion

Two forms of vitamin D are metabolically active. Vitamin D_2, **ergocalciferol,** is formed when ergosterol (provitamin) in plants is irradiated by sunlight. Vitamin D_3, **cholecalciferol,** is formed when 7-dehydrocholesterol (another provitamin) in the skin of animals or humans is irradiated by ultraviolet light or sunlight.

Both forms are absorbed into the blood. About 50% of dietary vitamin D_3 is absorbed, most rapidly in the duodenum but the greatest amount in the distal small intestine (Gropper, Smith, and Groff, 2009). Intestinal absorption of vitamin D decreases with age, as does the capacity of the skin to synthesize cholecalciferol. Like other fat-soluble vitamins, it is transported in the blood bound to protein. The liver alters the vitamin to **calcidiol,** an inactive form of vitamin D. By enzyme action, the kidney converts the calcidiol to **calcitriol,** the active form of vitamin D. Figure 7-3 diagrams the path of these processes.

Functions

Vitamin D has long been recognized as essential to proper bone metabolism. Recent findings suggest a role in preventing a wide range of chronic diseases.

BONE METABOLISM

Vitamin D promotes normal bone mineralization by stimulating:

- DNA to produce transport proteins to increase intestinal absorption of calcium and phosphorus
- Bone cells to build and maintain bone tissue with calcium and phosphorus
- The kidneys to return calcium to the bloodstream rather than excreting it in the urine.

An opposite effect is caused by **parathyroid hormone** that is secreted in response to a low serum calcium level. Parathyroid hormone causes the catabolism of bone to raise the serum calcium level. The body's priority goal is maintenance of correct serum calcium for blood clotting, nerve function, and muscle contraction. Without this mechanism to sustain vital functions, a person would not live long enough to develop rickets, the bone disease of vitamin D deficiency.

POSSIBLE PREVENTION OF CHRONIC DISEASES

Although clear mechanisms have not been delineated, vitamin D intake may partly explain the north–south disparity in the occurrence and prognosis of many diseases. For instance:

- Death rates for both colon and breast cancer tend to be lower in sunny areas and higher in areas with less winter sunlight (Garland et al., 2006).
- At the equator, multiple sclerosis occurrence is near zero (Mark and Carson, 2006) but there is a multifold increase in incidence with distance from the equator (Munger et al., 2006).
- Ultraviolet radiation reduces the incidence of viral respiratory infections, as does cod liver oil. That finding may also explain the seasonality of influenza epidemics (Cannell et al., 2006).
- A multivitamin containing the adult AI of vitamin D can reduce the risk of multiple sclerosis and rheumatoid arthritis by 40% to 50% (Holick, 2006).

Other experts await clinical trials to prove the link between vitamin D and chronic diseases (Bouillon, Norman, and Lips, 2007; Wolpowitz and Gilchrest, 2006). Much remains to be determined about vitamin

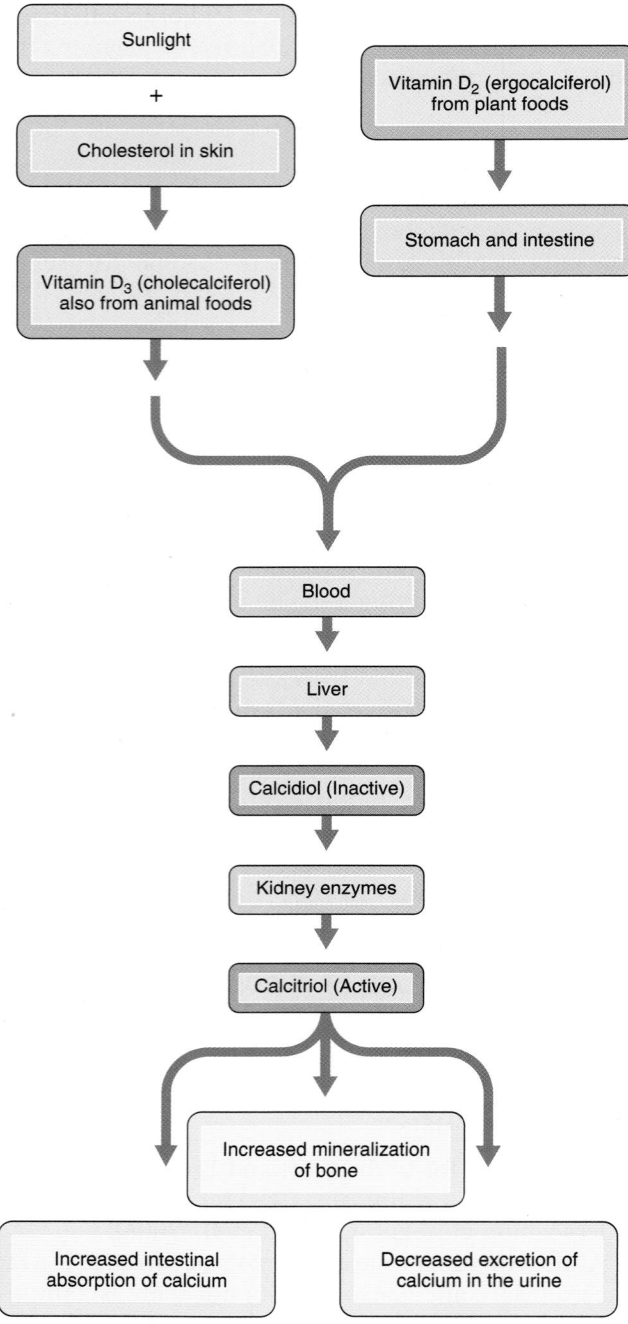

FIGURE 7-3 Vitamin D, whether from food or synthesis in the skin, is metabolized by the liver and the kidneys to its active form.

D's actions in cell differentiation and immune system functioning. See Genomic Gem 7-1.

Deficiency

Lack of sunshine or vitamin D, chronic liver or kidney disease, and rare genetic disorders cause vitamin D deficiency. Children whose bones are still growing are most vulnerable to this deficiency.

Genomic Gem 7-1

Vitamin D and Tuberculosis

Compared with Caucasians, African Americans have increased susceptibility to tuberculosis and suffer from more severe cases of the disease. Because of their dark skins, African Americans also have decreased serum levels of vitamin D.

Recent research has shown that stimulation of **macrophages** induces an enzyme that catalyzes the conversion of calcidiol to calcitriol. Research also shows that **monocytes** possess a vitamin D receptor that triggers induction of at least one antimicrobial peptide effective against the tubercle bacillus. Although not the only mechanisms at work in resisting microbes, polymorphisms in vitamin D receptors may contribute to susceptibility to tuberculosis. The research also sheds light on the success in southwestern sanitariums, before the advent of antibiotics, of using sun exposure to treat tuberculosis (Liu et al., 2006).

RICKETS

Vitamin D deficiency in children is called **rickets.** Although nutritional rickets is preventable, it still occurs in the United States. Cases of rickets in dark-skinned children being breast fed but not receiving vitamin D supplements were reported in New England (Fitzpatrick et al., 2000), north Texas (Shah et al., 2000), North Carolina (Kreiter et al., 2000), and Georgia (CDC, 2001). A 17-month-old child with advanced rickets had received a vegan diet and an unfortified soy beverage after weaning from the breast at ten months of age (Carvalho et al., 2001). To prevent such deficiency diseases or to diagnose them early, health-care providers should assess the client's total situation and not just focus on the immediate reason for the visit.

Rickets can occur without Vitamin D deficiency. Children in equatorial Africa exposed to plenty of sunshine have developed rickets due to lack of dietary calcium and were cured by calcium supplementation alone (Wolpowitz and Gilchrest, 2006).

OSTEOMALACIA

Vitamin D deficiency in adults is called **osteomalacia.** This deficiency disease occurs most often in women who have insufficient calcium intake and little sunlight exposure. It occurs frequently among those who are pregnant or lactating.

Environmental causes for osteomalacia are similar to those for rickets. And people with low exposure to sunlight are at increased risk: cloistered nuns, office workers, residents of smoggy areas, and institutionalized elderly people.

Because of the complex processes involved in vitamin D metabolism, liver or kidney disease can lead to bone deterioration. Chronic kidney failure has caused osteomalacia because of the inability of the kidneys to convert vitamin D to its active form. Clients with kidney disease are commonly prescribed pharmaceutical vitamin D supplements.

SIGNS AND SYMPTOMS

Children with rickets have soft, fragile bones. Classic deformities include bowlegs, knock knees, and misshapen skulls. Vitamin D deficiency may cause **tetany** in infants due to low levels of blood calcium. One such 4-month-old child was admitted in seizures and respiratory arrest (Lamb, 1999).

Adults with osteomalacia also have increasing softness of the bones, causing deformities due to loss of calcium. The bones most commonly affected are those of the spine, pelvis, and lower extremities.

DRIs and Sources

The AIs for vitamin D assume inadequate exposure to sunlight (National Institutes of Health, 2008). Many experts believe vitamin D's AI and the UL are set too low. See Box 7-2.

Two sources of vitamin D are readily available to most people: synthesis by the body and fortified milk, which is readily available in the United States.

SUNLIGHT

A major source of vitamin D is the body itself. Vitamin D is manufactured in the skin. Children with low dietary intakes may escape rickets if their exposure to sunlight is adequate, but a 70-year-old whose skin loses about 75% of its ability to manufacture vitamin D may be at risk of deficiency (Holick, 2007).

Box 7-2 ■ *Proposals to Raise the DRIs for Vitamin D*

One difficulty with setting an RDA for vitamin D is the multiple sources of the vitamin. Some people, particularly outdoor workers, may achieve optimal serum levels without supplements. Conversely, some healthy adults require vitamin D in amounts that might be adverse to others (Vieth, 2006) and therefore may not receive optimal amounts. For instance, the age-related decline in synthesis by the skin and the present UL are barriers to implementing strategies to optimize vitamin D status in the elderly (Heaney, 2006). Proposals from experts to raise the AIs and the ULs have appeared in the literature (Bischoff-Ferrari et al., 2005, 2006; Hathcock et al., 2007; Heaney, 2006; Vieth, 2007) but have not yet been incorporated into the DRIs. Setting AIs and ULs for vitamin D is difficult because few foods are natural sources of the vitamin; therefore, fortification and supplementation are necessary at any level. However, intake from multiple artificial sources should be monitored to avoid toxicity.

For desirable blood levels of vitamin D, individuals must expose their arms, shoulders, and back without sunscreen to sunlight between 11 A.M. and 2 P.M. for 15 minutes in summer and 20 minutes in spring and fall. In the Northeastern United States, however, from November through March, the sun's rays are inadequate to synthesize vitamin D. Exposure of the face is not recommended because precancerous actinic keratoses are related to sun exposure. As a result, fair-skinned or sun-sensitive persons should use oral supplements rather than relying on skin synthesis of vitamin D (Garland et al., 2006). The body regulates skin synthesis of vitamin D to avoid overdosing from this source.

FOOD

For people not exposed to sunshine, food sources of vitamin D become increasingly important. In the United States, the major food source of vitamin D is fortified milk. Milk is the ideal food to link with vitamin D because it also contains calcium and phosphorus, which are necessary for bone anabolism. See Box 7-3 and Clinical Application 7-3 on the **fortification** of foods. For other food sources, see Table 7-2.

SUPPLEMENTS

Historically, the means to obtain vitamin D was cod liver oil, which contains 400 to 1000 IU (10 to 25 micrograms) of vitamin D_3 per teaspoonful (Holick, 2007). Although a natural product, cod liver oil is a supplement, not a food. The form that many vegans prefer is vitamin D_2 because of its plant origin, but D_2 is shorter acting and has only one-third the potency of D_3 when administered as a single large dose and followed for 28 days (Armas, Hollis, and Heaney, 2004). When smaller doses were administered daily, however, vitamin D_2 was found as effective as vitamin D_3 in maintaining serum levels of vitamin D (Holick et al., 2008).

Interfering Factors

Little special handling of foods is necessary but a high-fiber diet interferes with the vitamin's absorption.

Box 7-3 ■ *Enrichment and Fortification*

Enrichment is the replacing of nutrients lost in processing or during storage. Enriched flour is an example. Not all the nutrients are replaced; therefore, whole grain products are recommended.

Fortification is the addition of nutrients not normally present in a given food to increase its nutritional value, for example, vitamins A and D in milk.

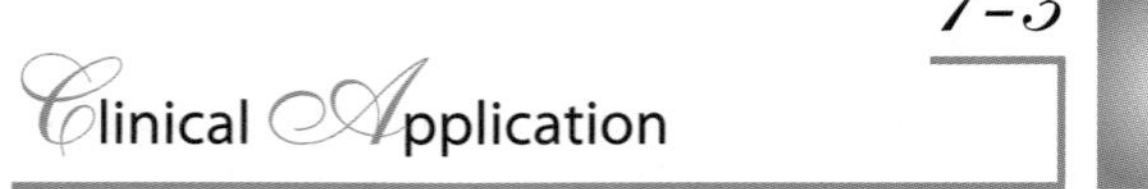

Fortification of Foods: Use and Misuse

Fortification is the addition of nutrients to foods in amounts greater than normally present. Many cereals are fortified with vitamins and minerals not normally found in grains. Almost all of the milk supply in the United States is fortified but other dairy products usually are not (National Institutes of Health, 2008). Occasionally, intentions are better than practices. Between 1985 and 1991, 56 cases of hypervitaminosis D were identified in Massachusetts. Two individuals died as a result and nine were discharged from the hospital with residual effects. Although state law required an upper limit of 500 IU (12.5 micrograms) of vitamin D per quart, the implicated dairy's milk exceeded this by 70–600 times (Blank et al., 1995).

Even without considering errors in processing, experts are concerned that voluntary fortification of multiple foods by the producers could lead to excessive intakes. Currently, foods permitted to be fortified with vitamin D include milk products, cereals, and fruit juices and drinks. Maximum levels of added vitamin D are specified by law (National Institutes of Health, 2008).

Abnormalities of absorption such as diarrhea, fat malabsorption, and biliary obstruction also may lead to vitamin D deficiency.

Toxicity

Because vitamin D is stored in the body, it is possible to ingest too much. Vitamin D from supplements or even foods can be hazardous to health.

DOSAGE

More than any other vitamin, a high consumption of vitamin D is likely to cause toxicity from excess. Doses of 10,000 IU daily for several months have caused hypercalcemia and calcification of soft tissues (Gropper, Smith, and Groff, 2009). Even though 400 IU vitamin D_3 with 1000 mg of calcium carbonate daily over an average of 7 years increased hip bone density, it did not reduce hip fractures and did increase the risk of kidney stones (Jackson et al., 2006).

Infants and children face increased risk from multiple fortified foods and supplements. For example, a 16-month-old previously healthy boy presented to the emergency department with refractory hypercalcemia due to an overdose of an over-the-counter vitamin supplement. He was successfully treated, but the case highlights the potential danger of giving children high-dose vitamin supplements (Chatterjee and Speiser, 2007).

SIGNS AND SYMPTOMS

Clinical manifestations of hypervitaminosis D include loss of appetite, nausea, vomiting, polyuria, muscular weakness, and constipation. More serious consequences of vitamin D overdose result from calcium deposits in the heart, kidneys, and brain.

Vitamin E

For DRIs, see Appendix A. For food and other sources, see Table 7-2. To investigate the vitamin content of a particular item, see the Internet site of the United States Department of Agriculture at http://www.nal.usda.gov/fnic/foodcomp/search/. For stability, see Table 7-3.

Much less is known about vitamin E than about vitamins A and D. No particular disease is caused by vitamin E deficiency but the vitamin has broad functions in the body. More information on interpretation of research findings is provided in Chapter 21.

Absorption, Metabolism, and Excretion

The primary site of absorption of vitamin E is the **jejunum,** where fat and bile are required for optimal uptake. Excretion is via bile in the feces. More than 90% of the body's vitamin E is stored as droplets in adipose tissue (Traber, 2006). Maximum transfer of vitamin E across the placenta occurs just before term delivery. The significance of this phenomenon will become clearer in the sections on vitamin E deficiency and on premature infants in Chapter 11.

Functions

The major function of vitamin E is to protect the integrity of cell membranes. To do this, vitamin E serves as an **antioxidant** by accepting oxygen instead of allowing other molecules to become unstable. In this role, vitamin E protects provitamin A and unsaturated fatty acids from oxidation. It also preserves the stability of the polyunsaturated fatty acids in the red blood cell membranes, protecting them from oxidation in the lungs. The vitamin E in lung cell membranes provides an important barrier against air pollution.

Oxidation has been suspected of contributing to cataract formation and macular degeneration of the retina. If true, antioxidants could conceivably help prevent these eye conditions. The situation, however, is complex. See Genomic Gem 7-2.

Vitamin E has also been investigated in neurodegenerative diseases associated with oxidative stress, but the research results have been generally disappointing. Available data do not support supplementation with

Genomic Gem 7-2
Nutrition and Eye Disease

Although observational studies have generally confirmed a protective role for antioxidants in foods (van Leeuwen et al., 2005) or supplements, intervention trials did not limit risk for cataracts or macular degeneration (Chiu and Taylor, 2007). Research in the United States supporting the effectiveness of high-dose antioxidant and zinc supplementation in halting the progression of macular degeneration in selected individuals has not been confirmed in other countries (Evans, 2006).

Nutrition-related risk factors for macular degeneration are:

- Obesity
- High dietary intake of vegetable fat
- Low dietary intake of antioxidants and zinc

On the other hand, a high dietary intake of omega-3 fatty acids and fish was shown to decrease risk of the more severe form of age-related macular degeneration (Jager, Mieler, and Miller, 2008).

Recent research has identified genes involved in lipid metabolism and in innate immunity to the risk of macular degeneration and a particular chromosome to cortical cataract (Delcourt, 2007). Learning more about these factors may help to target nutritional interventions to prevent eye diseases to persons most likely to benefit. Meanwhile, the advice given in the Dietary Guidelines is still valid.

vitamin E to prevent cardiovascular disease, cancer (Pham and Plakogiannis, 2005a), Parkinson's disease, or Alzheimer's disease (Pham and Plakogiannis, 2005b). Additional information on vitamin E and neurological diseases is provided in Chapter 12.

Deficiency

Usually resulting from fat malabsorption disorders or genetic defects in the metabolism of vitamin E, deficiency produces hemolytic anemia and degenerative neurological problems (Gropper, Smith, and Groff, 2009). The latter may take 10 or 20 years to become symptomatic in adults (Traber, 2006). Premature infants with inadequate reserves of vitamin E develop anemia. Without sufficient vitamin E, the membranes of the red blood cells break down easily when exposed to oxygen or an oxidizing agent.

Sources, Stability, and Interfering Factors

The need for vitamin E increases as the intake of polyunsaturated fatty acids (PUFAs) increases. The best natural source of vitamin E is vegetable oil, and the vegetable oils highest in alpha-tocopherol are the ones high in monounsaturated fatty acids, such as canola, olive, sunflower, and safflower oils (see Chapter 4). In contrast, corn and soybean oils have a greater proportion of gamma-tocopherol, which no longer is counted as contributing to vitamin E intake (Gropper, Smith, and Groff, 2009). See Table 7-2.

Vitamin E is fairly stable on exposure to heat and acid. Normal cooking temperatures do not destroy it, but frying does. Persons who limit fat in their diets are likely limiting their vitamin E intake also.

Toxicity

Toxicity from natural vitamin E from food is unknown. Excessive supplemental vitamin E can cause gastrointestinal symptoms, muscle weakness, double vision, and increased bleeding tendencies. Thus clients taking anticoagulant drugs should not exceed the UL for vitamin E. Clinical Application 7-4 describes an unusual client with vitamin E toxicity.

Vitamin K

For DRIs, see Appendix A. For food and other sources, see Table 7-2. To investigate the vitamin content of a particular item, see the Internet site of the United States Department of Agriculture at http://www.nal.usda.gov/fnic/foodcomp/search/. For stability, see Table 7-3.

Vitamin K is frequently prescribed as a medication and impacts the effectiveness of the commonly prescribed anticoagulant warfarin. Instructions regarding

Clinical Application 7-4
Vitamin E Toxicity

A client was admitted to the hospital for **narcolepsy,** a disorder characterized by recurrent, uncontrollable, brief periods of sleep from which the individual is easily awakened. This client would fall asleep while driving his car.

Narcolepsy can be a sign of uremia, hypoglycemia, diabetes, hypothyroidism, increased intracranial pressure, tumors of the brain stem or hypothalamus, or absence epilepsy. If all of these causes are ruled out, the medical diagnosis is either classical or independent narcolepsy.

During her assessment, the dietitian discovered one unusual nutritional practice: After a clerk in a health foods store had recommended vitamin E, the client had begun and continued to take this supplement. The dietitian investigated vitamin E's adverse effects and suggested to the physician that the narcolepsy could be caused by excessive vitamin E. After the client discontinued taking vitamin E, the narcolepsy disappeared.

In this case, a thorough nutritional assessment and an inquiring attitude eliminated the need for extensive diagnostic tests.

food intake for clients taking warfarin are given in Chapter 15.

Absorption, Metabolism, and Excretion

Two forms of vitamin K can meet the body's needs. Vitamin K_1, or **phylloquinone,** is found in plant foods. Vitamin K_2, or **menaquinone,** is synthesized by intestinal bacteria. A synthetic, water-soluble pharmaceutical form of vitamin K_1, **phytonadione,** can be administered orally or by injection. The intravenous route is used rarely and requires extreme caution because of life-threatening reactions.

Phylloquinone is absorbed primarily in the jejunum, and menaquinone is absorbed in the distal small intestine and the colon. Absorption and utilization of menaquinone vary considerably from person to person. Within the body, vitamin K is found in large amounts in the liver and in lesser amounts in other tissues; the total amount in the body is estimated to be only 50 to 100 micrograms. Turnover of vitamin K in the body occurs every 2.5 hours. Unused vitamin K is excreted in urine and feces via bile (Gropper, Smith, and Groff, 2009).

Functions

The actions of vitamin K in blood clotting have been known and used clinically for a long time. Recently, a protein has been identified in bone that depends on vitamin K. Vitamin K participates with vitamin D in synthesizing this bone protein, which helps to regulate serum calcium levels. In addition, vitamin K–dependent proteins have been found in brain, heart, kidney, liver, lung, and spleen although the mode of action remains to be discovered (Gropper, Smith, and Groff, 2009).

BLOOD CLOTTING

Vitamin K is necessary for the liver to make factors II (**prothrombin**), VII, IX, and X. Three additional coagulation proteins are vitamin K dependent. These factors and proteins plus calcium are key links in the chain of events producing a blood clot.

BONE METABOLISM

Vitamin K influences bone metabolism by facilitating the synthesis of **osteocalcin,** a hormonally regulated calcium-binding protein made almost exclusively by the bone-building cells called **osteoblasts**.

Deficiency

Individuals at risk of vitamin K deficiency include newborn infants as well as adults who avoid green leafy vegetables or are undergoing long-term antibiotic therapy. Clients with malabsorption syndromes are also at risk. Careful assessment of dietary factors in these clients is warranted.

The intestinal tract of a newborn infant is sterile. For this reason, the baby is unable to produce vitamin K until the intestine is colonized with bacteria from the infant's environment, usually within 24 hours. To prevent bleeding that can be severe, a dose of vitamin K is usually given to the infant immediately after birth.

Deficiencies, uncommon in healthy adults, have been associated with disease and with drug therapy. For example, fat absorption problems may hinder vitamin K absorption, resulting in prolonged blood clotting time. In addition, antibiotics, which kill normal bacteria—some of which produce vitamin K—along with the infectious organisms can cause low levels of vitamin K.

Sources

The human body is capable of manufacturing some vitamin K, and many common foods contain adequate amounts.

INTESTINAL SYNTHESIS

The amount of bacterially produced vitamin K that is absorbed and utilized varies from one individual to another. Nevertheless, bacterial synthesis alone will not maintain adequate vitamin K status in healthy children or adults (Gropper, Smith, and Groff, 2009).

FOOD SOURCES

Green leafy vegetables and vegetables of the cabbage family are the best sources of vitamin K. See Table 7-2. Controlling intake of vitamin K is part of the treatment plan for clients receiving a common anticoagulant drug, warfarin (see Chapter 15).

Stability and Interfering Factors

Vitamin K is susceptible to destruction by light and heat (Gropper, Smith, and Groff, 2009) and is unstable in the presence of oxygen, alkalis, and strong acids. In addition, overconsumption of vitamins A and E can interfere with the absorption and metabolism of vitamin K. The anticoagulant **warfarin** interferes with the liver's use of vitamin K, but that is the desired effect of the medication.

Toxicity

The naturally occurring forms of vitamins K_1 and K_2 have not been associated with adverse effects, but caution is warranted, particularly if high doses are taken. Phytonadione, the pharmaceutical preparation of vitamin K_1, causes fewer adverse effects than earlier, stronger formulations but because of life-threatening reactions, intravenous administration is not recommended except in emergencies. As always, special care must be taken when administering any medication, including vitamin K, to infants.

Table 7-2 summarizes the fat-soluble vitamins. See Clinical Application 7-5 for a description of two conditions that mimic deficiencies of fat-soluble vitamins.

Water-Soluble Vitamins

Vitamins that dissolve in water are vitamin C, or **ascorbic acid,** and the B vitamins, including **thiamin, riboflavin, niacin,** vitamin B_6, **folate,** vitamin B_{12}, **pantothenic acid,** and **biotin.** Information on choline, strictly speaking not a vitamin, follows biotin.

Vitamin C

For DRIs, see Appendix A. For food and other sources, see Table 7-4. To investigate the vitamin content of a particular item, see "Caffeine and Nutritive Values of Foods" on DavisPlus. For stability, see Table 7-3.

Most animals manufacture vitamin C in their livers. Humans, along with other primates, guinea pigs, some birds, and fruit-eating bats, cannot synthesize vitamin C. Humans have an inactive form of an encoding gene for the last enzyme in the chain reaction for vitamin C synthesis and therefore must obtain vitamin C from the diet (Li and Schellhorn, 2008).

7-5

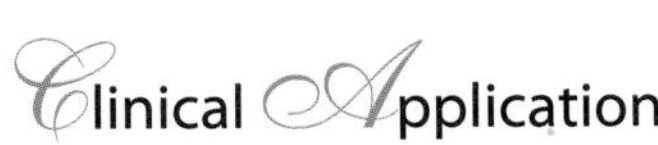

Conditions Mimicking Fat-Soluble–Vitamin Deficiencies

PROTEIN DEFICIENCY

Water and fat do not mix. To circulate fats in the water-based blood, the liver attaches fat-soluble vitamins to protein carriers. Sometimes a protein deficiency hinders the use of the fat-soluble vitamins.

ZINC DEFICIENCY

A zinc-containing protein carries vitamin A from storage in the liver to tissues. For this reason, a zinc deficiency can mimic a vitamin A deficiency.

Absorption, Metabolism, and Excretion

Vitamin C is absorbed from the small intestine. The pituitary and adrenal glands have the highest concentrations of vitamin C, but the greatest total amount is found in the liver.

As the amount of vitamin C consumed increases, the proportion of the vitamin absorbed decreases. Nearly complete absorption occurs at low doses but of a 1250-milligram dose, only 50% is absorbed, and nearly all of it is excreted in the urine (Levine, Katz, and Padayatty, 2006).

Functions

Vitamin C has diverse functions in the body. It contributes to wound, burn, and fracture healing, serves as an antioxidant, enhances the absorption of iron, and assists in the synthesis of hormones and neurotransmitters.

COLLAGEN SYNTHESIS

Vitamin C is necessary in the formation of **collagen,** the strong fibrous protein in connective tissue. Bone, skin, blood vessels, soft dental structures, and scar tissue all contain collagen. Without vitamin C, collagen molecules are inadequately cross-linked, resulting in weak tissue.

ANTIOXIDANT

Vitamin C is a powerful antioxidant. By preventing the uptake of oxygen by other molecules, it deters the destruction of tissue by unstable molecules.

IRON ABSORPTION

Vitamin C facilitates iron absorption by acting with hydrochloric acid to keep iron in the more absorbable **ferrous** form. Four ounces of orange juice, for instance, nearly quadruples the iron absorbed from the plant foods eaten with it.

OTHER FUNCTIONS

High concentrations of vitamin C are found in the **adrenal glands.** These are the organs that secrete adrenalin, the "fight-or-flight" hormone, in times of stress. Vitamin C also aids in the synthesis of norepinephrine and **serotonin.**

Deficiency

Until the 17th century, sailors on long voyages often died of **scurvy** due to lack of vitamin C. Citrus fruit was issued as a preventive measure, leading to the term "limey" for a British sailor. Scurvy develops within 3 months after vitamin C is eliminated from

TABLE 7-4 ■ Water-Soluble Vitamins

VITAMIN	ADULT RDA AND FOOD PORTION CONTAINING IT	FUNCTIONS	DEFICIENCY DISEASE	SIGNS AND SYMPTOMS OF DEFICIENCY	SOURCES
C Ascorbic Acid	75–90 mg 0.75–1 cup of orange juice, prepared from frozen concentrate	Formation of collagen Antioxidant Facilitation of iron absorption	Scurvy	Bleeding mucous membranes Poor wound healing or reopening of scars Softened ends of long bones Teeth loosen, may fall out Death due to internal hemorrhage	Citrus fruit and juice Broccoli, Brussels sprouts Green and red peppers Cantaloupe, Strawberries Kiwi fruit Papayas
B_1 Thiamin	1.1–1.2 mg 3.6 oz pork chop, lean only	Coenzyme in CHO and amino acid metabolism	Beriberi	Anorexia, Weight loss, Muscle weakness and wasting Peripheral neuropathy Right heart failure Wernicke's encephalopathy	Pork Black beans, Black-eyed peas Wheat germ Fortified cereals
B_2 Riboflavin	1.1–1.3 mg 2.4–2.8 cups nonfat milk	Coenzyme in protein metabolism	Aribinoflavinosis	Lesions on lips and in mouth Seborrheic dermatitis Normochromic, normocytic anemia	Milk and dairy products Eggs Meats, especially liver Fortified cereals
B_3 Niacin	14–16 mg niacin equivalents 3.7–4.2 oz water-packed tuna	Coenzyme in energy production Participant in synthesis of fatty acids and steroid hormones	Pellagra	Bilaterally symmetrical dermatitis on face, neck, hands, and feet Diarrhea Dementia	Chicken breast Liver Tuna Other meats, fish, poultry Whole, enriched, or fortified grains Coffee Tea
B_6 Pyridoxine	1.3–1.7 mg 2.6 bananas	Coenzyme in metabolism of amino acids	No specific term	Mouth lesions Sleepiness, fatigue Hypochromic, microcytic anemia Convulsions in infants	Sirloin steak Salmon Chicken breast Whole grains, fortified cereals Orange-flavored breakfast drinks Bananas Nuts
Folate Folic Acid	400 µg 7.5 tbsp wheat germ	Essential to the formation of DNA Participant in formation of heme	No specific term	Fatigue Weakness Shortness of breath Palpitations Megaloblastic anemia	Liver Dried peas, beans, lentils Wheat germ, Peanuts Asparagus Endive Lettuce Brussels sprouts Broccoli Spinach Fortified grain products
B_{12} Cyanocobalamin	2.4 µg 3.2 oz cooked lean beef	Synthesis of DNA, RNA, metabolism of amino and fatty acids Synthesis and maintenance of myelin	Pernicious anemia (lack of intrinsic factor, not dietary)	Fatigue Pallor Shortness of breath Palpitations Megaloblastic anemia Numbness and tingling of extremities Abnormal gait Possible memory loss Dementia	Meat Fish Poultry Milk Cheese Eggs Nutritional yeast Vitamin B_{12}-fortified soymilk or tofu

the diet, but a genetic component has also been suggested. See Genomic Gem 7-3.

SIGNS AND SYMPTOMS

Early signs of scurvy are tender, sore gums that bleed easily and small skin hemorrhages due to weakened blood vessels. The late manifestations of scurvy relate to the breakdown of collagen. Wound healing is delayed; even healed scars may separate. The ends of long bones soften and become malformed and painful, and fractures appear. Teeth loosen in their sockets and fall out. Hemorrhages occur about the joints, stomach, and heart.

Untreated scurvy often progresses to sudden death, probably from internal bleeding.

Diagnosis is based on history and physical examination, confirmed by serum ascorbic acid findings. Relief of symptoms upon administration of ascorbic acid is diagnostic as well as curative (Bingham, Kimura, and Imundo, 2003).

TREATMENT

Moderate doses of vitamin C, 100 milligrams three times a day, will cure scurvy. Because scurvy can be fatal, treatment should not be delayed to await laboratory confirmation (Levine, Katz, and Padayatty, 2006).

RISK FACTORS AND CONTEMPORARY CASES

Case reports still appear in medical journals describing scurvy in developed countries:

- An elderly, alcoholic woman diagnosed in an emergency room—Utah (Stephen and Utecht, 2001)
- A 54-year-old rural Appalachian man who twice developed scurvy by subsisting on cooked foods—Virginia (Levin and Greer, 2000)
- A 49-year-old man with a spinal cord injury, limited transportation, and alcohol abuse—Florida (Harrow et al., 2003)
- A 43-year-old man who eliminated fruits and vegetables from his diet—Massachusetts (Pangan and Robinson, 2001)
- A 16-year-old boy who ate no fruits or vegetables after a bout of diarrhea 7 months earlier—New York (Bingham, Kimura, and Imundo, 2003)
- A 9-year-old boy with a restricted eating pattern—Australia (Akikusa, Garrick, and Nash, 2003)
- A 9-year-old developmentally delayed girl with extremely limited food preferences—Canada (Weinstein, Babyn, and Zlotkin, 2001)
- A 5-year-old boy who refused fruits, vegetables, juices, and chewable vitamin tablets for 5 months—Tennessee (Tamura et al., 2000)

Six of those clients presented with musculoskeletal complaints, and five of them underwent extensive testing before the diagnosis was made. Nutritional assessment entered late in the diagnostic process. In the case of the 5-year-old, the authors suggested that underlying psychiatric disorders in the client or the family merited assessment. Expanding the assessment to include the social situation might uncover persons at increased risk for vitamin C deficiency.

Three foods that are high in both vitamins A and C are shown in Figure 7-4.

Stability and Preservation

Boiling vegetables may decrease vitamin C content by 50 to 80% (Li and Schellhorn, 2008). Orange juice from frozen concentrate contains more vitamin C than ready-to-drink juices. The frozen concentrates have 86 milligrams per cup when prepared and 39 to 46 milligrams per cup after 4 weeks of storage. In contrast, ready-to-drink juices have 27 to 65 milligrams per cup on opening and 0 to 25 milligrams at expiration 4 weeks later (Johnston and Bowling, 2002).

> **Genomic Gem 7-3**
>
> **Possible Genetic Susceptibility to Scurvy**
>
> Modern laboratory techniques reveal that vitamin C intake explains only 17% of the variance in vitamin C serum levels. A possible partial explanation may be related to variances in a plasma protein, haptoglobin, that exists in three **phenotypes:** Hp 1-1, Hp 1-2, and Hp 2-2. Individuals in the last group show the least stability of vitamin C in their serum. Further, lower serum ascorbic acid levels have been observed in European and Chinese persons with the Hp 2-2 phenotype. During explorations and wars, Asians had a higher mortality rate from scurvy than Europeans whose death rate roughly parallels the frequency of the Hp 2-2 phenotype in European populations.
>
> Thus scurvy may have a genetic component but the availability and activity of vitamin C could impact many more common diseases in the 21st century. In particular, oxidative stress is a feature of cardiovascular disease (see Chapter 18) where the Hp 2-2 phenotype is overrepresented in whites diagnosed with it (Delanghe et al., 2007).

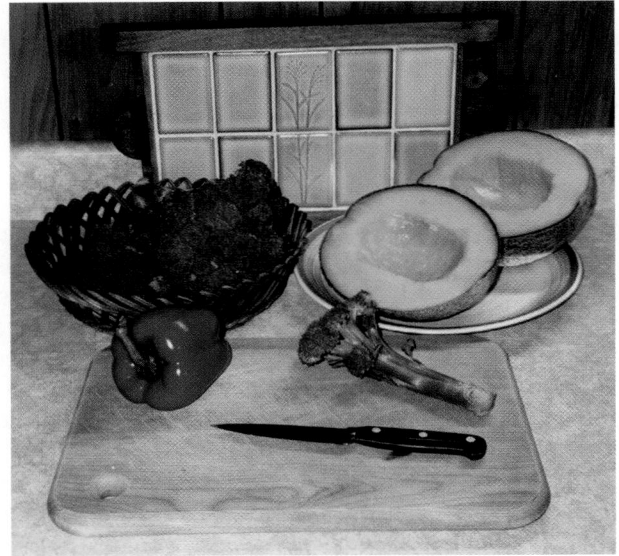

FIGURE 7-4 Broccoli, cantaloupe, and red pepper are excellent sources of both vitamins A and C.

Easily implemented food preparation procedures can minimize loss of vitamin C:

- Store orange juice in an opaque container that holds no more than an amount that can be consumed in a short time.
- Buy ready-to-drink orange juice 3 to 4 weeks before expiration and use within 1 week (Johnston and Bowling, 2002).
- Eat vegetables raw when possible or cook them as quickly as possible; crisp-cooked is better than limp-cooked for retaining the vitamin C content. Boiling the cooking water for 1 minute before adding the food eliminates the dissolved oxygen that would otherwise oxidize the vitamin C. In years past, many food establishments routinely added baking soda to vegetables to enhance their color, but the alkali also destroyed the vitamin C. Fortunately, this practice is now illegal.

Interfering Factors

Individuals who smoke require an additional 35 milligrams of vitamin C, and those exposed to second-hand smoke should obtain the RDA daily. Children exposed to second-hand smoke, even at low levels, had significantly lower plasma ascorbate levels than unexposed children (Preston et al., 2003). After major surgery or extensive burns, a client may need up to 1000 milligrams of vitamin C daily.

Vitamin C is used to mitigate undesirable reactions in food. For example, *nitrates* are chemicals added to smoked and cured meats to preserve them and enhance their flavor. In the small intestine, however, nitrates combine with amino acids to form nitrosamines, which have been linked to some cancers. Because vitamin C blocks the formation of nitrosamines from nitrates, some meat packers add vitamin C to their products to protect against nitrosamine formation.

Toxicity

A dose 10 times the RDA is called a **megadose.** Vitamin C in amounts of 1000 to 2000 milligrams per day has produced nausea, abdominal cramps, and diarrhea. Because vitamin C increases the amount of iron absorbed, persons with diseases characterized by iron overload such as hemochromatosis (see Chapter 8) should avoid ascorbic acid supplementation (Li and Schellhorn, 2008).

Individuals prone to kidney stones are sometimes advised not to take megadoses of vitamin C because it is metabolized to oxalate, and kidney stones are often composed of calcium oxalate. By a different mechanism competing with uric acid for reabsorption by the kidney, megadoses of vitamin C theoretically could increase the risk of urate stones (Gropper, Smith, and Groff, 2009), but the actual risk of kidney stones associated with vitamin C intake has not been established (Li and Schellhorn, 2008).

Excessive vitamin C causes false readings in two common laboratory tests. Some urine glucose tests will read falsely positive. Stool tests for occult blood will read falsely negative.

An occasionally reported consequence of taking megadoses of vitamin C and then abruptly discontinuing them is **rebound scurvy.** The body cannot adjust quickly enough and continues to absorb a meager proportion of the now smaller dose (DePaola et al., 2006). Even without megadose supplements, however, plasma vitamin C levels fall to deficiency levels within 4 weeks of removal of vitamin C from the diet (Levine, Katz, and Padayatty, 2006).

B-Complex Vitamins

The B-complex group encompasses six traditionally recognized vitamins: thiamin, riboflavin, niacin, vitamin B_6, folate, and vitamin B_{12}. Recently added vitamins are pantothenic acid, biotin and choline. Some diseases, including beriberi and pellagra, are associated with deficiencies of a single B vitamin.

Thiamin

For DRIs, see Appendix A. For food and other sources, see Table 7-4. To investigate the vitamin content of a particular item, see "Caffeine and Nutritive Values of Foods" on DavisPlus. For stability, see Table 7-3.

Discovered in the late 19th century when poultry fed polished rice became ill, thiamin was originally named vitamin B_1. It was first isolated from rice bran in 1912.

ABSORPTION, METABOLISM, AND EXCRETION

The human body contains about 30 milligrams of thiamin, about one-half of it located in the skeletal muscles, but the liver, heart, kidneys, and brain also have relatively high concentrations. Thiamin is absorbed in the small intestine, primarily in the jejunum. As a person's energy expenditure increases, the need for thiamin increases. Excess thiamin is mainly excreted in the urine.

FUNCTIONS

Thiamin is a coenzyme in the metabolism of carbohydrate and branched-chain amino acids. It also may play a role in nerve conduction (Gropper, Smith, and Groff, 2009).

DEFICIENCY

Beriberi is the deficiency disease due to a lack of **thiamin.** The enrichment of food products has almost eliminated this disease, but it is still seen even in developed countries. The need for thiamin increases as kilocaloric consumption increases. Individuals whose thiamin status is marginal may become deficient when an increased need for energy is caused by strenuous activity, pregnancy, a growth spurt, or fever.

Cases have been reported of cardiovascular disease (wet beriberi) 20 years after a gastrojejunostomy (Astudillo et al., 2003) and of peripheral neuropathy (dry beriberi) in three adolescents 4 to 6 months after gastric bypass surgery for morbid obesity. In the latter cases, possible poor thiamin status preoperatively and questionable compliance with the postoperative supplementation regimen may have contributed to the disease (Towbin et al., 2004). Despite what is known about the functions of thiamin on a cellular level, that knowledge does not explain all the manifestations of the deficiency disease. *Dry beriberi* is characterized by anorexia, weight loss, muscle weakness and wasting, and peripheral neuropathy. Progression to *wet beriberi* involves the cardiovascular system culminating in right-sided heart failure (Gropper, Smith, and Groff, 2009). In *infantile beriberi,* often presenting between the ages of 2 and 6 months, death may occur within a few hours if no thiamin is administered (Butterworth, 2006).

About 10% to 12% of alcoholic clients develop **Wernicke's encephalopathy,** a neurological disorder caused by thiamin deficiency (Butterworth, 2006). Clients with this syndrome display many motor and sensory deficits often involving eye muscles, balance, and memory. Some clients develop **Korsakoff's psychosis** characterized by amnesia and impaired conceptual functions (Butterworth, 2006). Consequently, clients with alcoholism are often prescribed thiamin by injection. These disorders have also been reported in pregnant women with hyperemesis. See Chapters 10 and 20.

STABILITY AND INTERFERING FACTORS

Air and heat destroy thiamin levels, especially in the presence of alkalis. For this reason, adding baking soda to green vegetables to retain their color or to dried beans to soften them inactivates the thiamin in the vegetables. Also, an enzyme in raw fish, **thiaminase,** destroys up to 50% of thiamin but cooking inactivates the enzyme. Tannic and caffeic acids found in coffee, tea, blueberries, black currants, Brussels sprouts, and red cabbage are also thiamin **antagonists,** but their actions may be prevented by vitamin C and citric acid (Gropper, Smith, and Groff, 2009).

TOXICITY

No adverse effects of thiamin from food or oral supplements have been recorded. Excessive thiamin by injection, however, has been associated with adverse effects, including convulsions, cardiac arrhythmias, and anaphylactic shock (Gropper, Smith, and Groff, 2009).

Riboflavin

For DRIs, see Appendix A. For food and other sources, see Table 7-4. To investigate the vitamin content of a particular item, see "Caffeine and Nutritive Values of Foods" on DavisPlus. For stability, see Table 7-3.

Riboflavin was encountered late in the 19th century when laboratory workers observed a yellow-green fluorescent pigment that formed crystals. Not until the 1930s was riboflavin isolated and eventually named for a sugar it contains (ribose) and the color yellow (flavin).

ABSORPTION, METABOLISM, AND EXCRETION

Most absorption of riboflavin occurs in the proximal small intestine. Small amounts of the vitamin are found in many tissues, the greatest concentrations in the liver, kidneys, and heart. Diet must supply daily needs. The kidneys excrete excess riboflavin so that even an intake of 1.7 milligrams of riboflavin (the amount in a multivitamin tablet) imparts a bright orange-yellow color to urine. Excretion is enhanced by diabetes mellitus, stress, and trauma (Gropper, Smith, and Groff, 2009).

FUNCTIONS AND PHARMACEUTICAL POTENTIAL

Riboflavin is a coenzyme in the metabolism of protein and of other vitamins. Thyroid and adrenal hormones control the conversion of riboflavin to its active coenzymes, which are involved in many oxidative enzyme systems. Riboflavin needs increase as protein needs increase. Clients undergoing major healing processes, such as those with extensive burns, require more riboflavin than the average person.

A proposed use for riboflavin is the inactivation of pathogens in blood products. Riboflavin when exposed to light can inactivate bacteria and viruses and is the basis for a pathogen reduction process for platelets and plasma products (Goodrich et al., 2006). Research is continuing because riboflavin is likely to be safe for this use.

DEFICIENCY

Riboflavin deficiency commonly occurs with thiamin and niacin deficiencies. A person who avoids all dairy products, however, may be deficient in riboflavin alone, a condition called **ariboflavinosis.** Signs of this deficiency that may appear after 4 months of inadequate intake include lesions on the lips and in the mouth, seborrheic dermatitis, and normochromic, normocytic anemia (McCormick, 2006). Other individuals at risk beside milk-avoiders are those with congenital heart disease, with some cancers, with excessive alcohol intake, and women taking oral contraceptives (Gropper, Smith, and Groff, 2009).

STABILITY AND INTERFERING FACTORS

Riboflavin is relatively stable to heat but is sensitive to ultraviolet light. Thus, cardboard milk cartons or opaque plastic bottles are more protective of the vitamin than clear glass bottles.

Iron, zinc, copper, and manganese have been shown to inhibit riboflavin absorption. Drinking alcohol impairs digestion and absorption of riboflavin (Gropper, Smith, and Groff, 2009).

TOXICITY

Large oral doses have not yielded reports of toxicity. High doses have been used in clinical trials as migraine prophylaxis without adverse effects (Gropper, Smith, and Groff, 2009) but the potential for unfavorable events still exists.

Niacin

For DRIs, see Appendix A. For food and other sources, see Table 7-4. To investigate the vitamin content of a particular item, see "Caffeine and Nutritive Values of Foods" on DavisPlus. For stability, see Table 7-3.

Niacin includes nicotinic acid and nicotinamide, both of which provide the vitamin's actions (Gropper, Smith, and Groff, 2009). Niacin deficiency causes a specific disease, pellagra.

ABSORPTION, METABOLISM, AND EXCRETION

Preformed niacin can be absorbed in the stomach but is more easily absorbed in the small intestine (Gropper, Smith, and Groff, 2009). Metabolism by the liver and excretion of excess in the urine is the usual pathway.

Not all of the body's niacin has to come from preformed niacin in food. The liver can convert the amino acid tryptophan to niacin; however, protein synthesis is given a higher priority than niacin formation (Bourgeois, Cervantes-Laurean, and Moss, 2006).

Similarly, not all nutrients present in a food are available to the body. Niacin is found in corn but mostly in a bound form that cannot be absorbed. Treating the corn with lye, as is done in some Latin American cultures, frees the niacin for the body's use.

FUNCTIONS

Requisite for more than 200 enzymes, niacin is a coenzyme required for energy metabolism. Niacin also participates in the synthesis of steroid hormones and fatty acids. Persons with schizophrenia display a diminished flushing response to topical niacin, which may indicate abnormalities in phospholipid metabolism that has been shown in schizophrenia (Cyhlarova et al., 2007; Messamore, Hoffman, and Janowsky, 2003).

DEFICIENCY

Pellagra is the deficiency disease caused by the lack of niacin. In the southeastern United States from 1910 to 1935, the incidence was 170,000 cases per year (Roman, 2006). Contributing factors were poverty and corn-based diets. Currently, pellagra occurs most frequently in alcoholics, the homeless, and persons with malabsorption problems (Delgado-Sanchez, Godkar, and Niranjan, 2008) but has occurred in clients with **anorexia nervosa** (MacDonald and Forsyth, 2005). See Box 7-4 for the clinical signs and symptoms.

To have a deficiency, a person must have a diet lacking in both niacin and tryptophan. Adults can obtain up to 67% of their niacin from complete protein foods. Pellagra has serious effects and is fatal if untreated. One case of pellagra-like dermatitis occurred in a 32-year-old woman 3 months after bariatric surgery (Ashourian and Mousdicas, 2006).

DIETARY REFERENCE INTAKES

Niacin allowances are related to energy intake and are measured in **niacin equivalents (NEs).** One milligram of niacin equivalent is the same as 1 milligram of preformed niacin or 60 milligrams of tryptophan.

Although food composition tables report only preformed niacin, the average American diet contains approximately 900 milligrams of tryptophan equal to 15 milligrams NE (Gropper, Smith, and Groff, 2009).

Box 7-4 ■ *Pellagra*

The "three Ds" are pellagra's major symptoms: dermatitis, diarrhea, and dementia; however, the full triad of symptoms occurs in just 22% of clients, and seldom do all of them appear in children (Ozturk et al., 2001). The dermatitis is a red rash on exposed skin: the face, neck, arms, hands, and feet. The rash is bilaterally symmetrical with a definite border marking its beginning; on the hands and arms, the rash sometimes resembles gloves.

SOURCES AND STABILITY

Coffee and tea contain niacin (Gropper, Smith, and Groff, 2009) and can prevent pellagra in cultures with low protein diets but high intakes of these beverages.

Niacin is a water-soluble vitamin but only small amounts are lost in cooking water. It is the most environmentally stable vitamin.

TOXICITY

Pharmacological doses of niacin, given to lower blood cholesterol, cause flushing and over the long term can cause liver damage. Even reformulation of breakfast cereal to 100% of the RDA of vitamins, including niacin, has caused flushing and a rash in a person who consumed six cupfuls for breakfast that contained almost 3.5 times the UL (Morse, Morse, and Patterson, 1999). A case of niacin toxicity from food is reported in Clinical Application 7-6. It explains how food poisoning outbreaks are investigated and how to preserve evidence.

Vitamin B_6

For DRIs, see Appendix A. For food and other sources, see Table 7-4. To investigate the vitamin content of a particular item, see the Internet site of the United States Department of Agriculture at http://www.nal.usda.gov/fnic/foodcomp/search/. To search for foods highest in the vitamin, see the Internet source Nutrition Data (2008b). For stability, see Table 7-3.

7-6

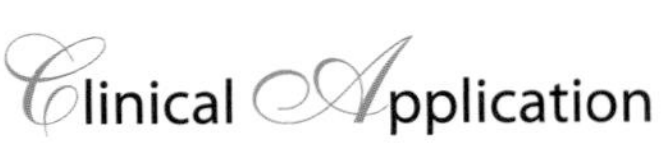

Niacin Toxicity

In late 1980, almost half the residents of a small nursing home became flushed or developed a rash 15–30 minutes after breakfast. To diagnose the problem, the foods consumed were compared. Which food was eaten by all those who became ill but by none of those who did not become ill? The answer was cornmeal mush.

Careful observation and documentation of the sequence of signs and symptoms, which commonly disappear before the physician arrives, may steer the investigators in the right direction. In this nursing home, the signs and symptoms lasted only an average of 50 minutes.

If food poisoning is suspected, none of the food should be discarded before health authorities take samples to examine in the laboratory. The Food and Drug Administration tested the cornmeal from the nursing home's kitchen. It contained more than 1000 milligrams of niacin per pound compared to the recommended amount of 16–24 milligrams per pound. In this case, the offending food was identified but the method of contamination was never positively determined (Bartlett, Morris, and Spengler, 1982).

Vitamin B_6 serves in many roles, but no deficiency disease is associated with it. The name for the pharmaceutical preparation of vitamin B_6 is **pyridoxine.**

ABSORPTION, METABOLISM, AND EXCRETION

The body contains about 165 milligrams of Vitamin B_6, 75% to 88% of it in the muscles. The vitamin is absorbed in the small intestine, mainly in the jejunum, with an overall absorption rate from the average United States diet of 75% (Gropper, Smith, and Groff, 2009). Most excess is excreted in the urine, with very little eliminated via the feces.

FUNCTIONS

Vitamin B_6 is a coenzyme in the metabolism of amino acids. It is involved in the metabolism of more than 100 enzymes, including those that synthesize niacin from tryptophan and heme for hemoglobin.

DEFICIENCY

A deficiency of B_6 is unlikely because large amounts are present in the general diet. Nonetheless, factors such as drug interactions or errors in food processing may cause a deficiency. In the 1950s, severe heat treatment of commercial infant formula produced vitamin B_6 deficiencies (Gropper, Smith, and Groff, 2009).

Clinically, a person with a vitamin B_6 deficiency may present with these signs and symptoms:

- Mouth lesions
- Sleepiness
- Fatigue

Interference with heme production may lead to a hypochromic, microcytic anemia. Infants usually display abnormal electroencephalograms or convulsions (Gropper, Smith, and Groff, 2009).

TOXICITY

No adverse effects of vitamin B_6 from foods have been reported. Sensory neuropathy and severe **ataxia** without weakness have been associated with pyridoxine megadoses greater than 200 milligrams per day but the mechanism of action is not clear (Roman, 2006).

Folate

For DRIs, see Appendix A. For food and other sources, see Table 7-4. To investigate the vitamin content of a particular item, see the Internet site of the United States Department of Agriculture at http://www.nal.usda.gov/fnic/foodcomp/search/. To search for foods highest in the vitamin, see the Internet source Nutrition Data (2008a). For stability, see Table 7-3.

The term for this nutrient as it occurs in foods and body tissues is **folate.** The oxidized and more stable form used to fortify foods and in supplements is **folic acid.** Total body folate levels are estimated to range from 11 to 28 milligrams, about half of which is stored in the liver (Gropper, Smith, and Groff, 2009).

ABSORPTION, METABOLISM, AND EXCRETION

The **bioavailability** of folate from a mixed diet is approximately 50% but rises to about 85% when fortified foods are included (Gropper, Smith, and Groff, 2009). Enzymes in the jejunal and pancreatic secretions and bile convert the folate in foods to the absorbable form used in fortified foods and supplements, which is then absorbed throughout the small intestine, most efficiently in the jejunum, and transported to the liver. In the liver, some of the folate is processed for storage in the tissues or the liver and some is secreted into bile.

When the gallbladder releases bile into the duodenum, folate may again be split off and absorbed. This recycling process, which may account for 100 micrograms of reabsorbed folate daily (Carmel, 2006b), is important in allowing folate stores to be adequate for 2 to 4 months, compared with 1 to 4 weeks for thiamin stores. Excretion of folate occurs via the urine and a minimal amount through the bile into feces. Most of the folate found in feces is of bacterial origin (Gropper, Smith, and Groff, 2009).

FUNCTIONS

Folate is involved in protein synthesis, including that of DNA, RNA, and heme. Thus, folate participates in the reproduction of every cell and is particularly necessary for rapidly growing cells, including those in the gastrointestinal tract, blood, and fetal tissue where absence of adequate amounts soon become clinically apparent.

DEFICIENCY

Poor dietary intake is the most common cause of folate deficiency especially when coupled with abuse of alcohol that affects the enterohepatic recycling of folate, interferes with folate metabolism, and accelerates folate catabolism (Carmel, 2006b). Other clients at risk are those with gastrointestinal diseases marked by malabsorption, with increased losses due to hemodialysis, and rare genetic errors of folate metabolism. The link between folate and neural tube defects in the developing fetus is explained in Chapter 10.

Folate deficiency results in impaired cell division and protein synthesis, including the faulty synthesis of red blood cells. Concentrations in the red blood cells are diminished after about 4 months of low folate intake, and in about 5 months, **megaloblastic anemia** occurs (Gropper, Smith, and Groff, 2009). In addition to laboratory blood changes, a client may have these signs and symptoms:

- Fatigue
- Weakness
- Shortness of breath
- Palpitations

DIETARY REFERENCE INTAKES

Folate RDAs and AIs are given in Dietary Folate Equivalents (DFEs).

One DFE equals

- 1 microgram of food folate
- 0.6 microgram of folic acid from fortified food or as a supplement consumed with food
- 0.5 microgram of a supplement taken on an empty stomach

SOURCES AND STABILITY

Green, leafy vegetables, for which the nutrient is named (Italian for foliage) are good sources but meats and legumes are among the best food sources. (See Table 7-4.)

Folic acid was recently added to the U.S. fortification protocol for grains to reduce the occurrence of neural tube defects (see Chapter 10). Consequently, grain products are now major sources of folic acid.

Folate is easily oxidized by light and acids and some forms are easily destroyed by heat. To minimize losses, vegetables should be cooked quickly.

INTERFERING FACTORS

Zinc deficiency and chronic alcohol intake diminish absorption of folate. Substances in legumes, lentils, cabbage, and oranges impair digestion and absorption of folate (Gropper, Smith, and Groff, 2009).

Methotrexate, an anticancer drug, is a folate antagonist. Its purpose is to interfere with DNA in cancer cells, but it simultaneously affects normal cells. A more commonly used drug, aspirin, displaces folate from its carrier protein after which the displaced folate is excreted. See Chapter 15 for details on the interaction of folic acid and medications.

TOXICITY

No adverse effects of folate from food or folic acid from supplements have been reported. The UL has been set to avoid masking signs of pernicious anemia. See vitamin B_{12} discussion.

Vitamin B_{12}

For DRIs, see Appendix A. For food and other sources, see Table 7-4. To investigate the vitamin content of a particular item, see the Internet site of the United States Department of Agriculture at http://www.nal.usda.gov/fnic/foodcomp/search/. For stability, see Table 7-3.

Vitamin B_{12} is an essential coenzyme in the synthesis of DNA, RNA, and **myelin** and is necessary for normal red blood cell formation. Vitamin B_{12} is stored to a greater extent than the other B vitamins, but diverse causes can precipitate vitamin B_{12} deficiency.

ABSORPTION, METABOLISM, AND EXCRETION

Efficient absorption of vitamin B_{12} requires an explicit protein-binding factor called **intrinsic factor,** secreted by the gastric mucosal cells in the stomach. Vitamin B_{12}, also called **extrinsic factor,** combines with intrinsic factor in the proximal small intestine to protect vitamin B_{12} from digestive enzymes and intestinal bacteria until the complex reaches the ileum, where the vitamin is absorbed about 4 hours after ingestion. About 1% to 2% of large pharmacological doses of vitamin B_{12} circumvents this process and is absorbed passively in the intestine (Carmel, 2006a).

Vitamin B_{12} is not freely absorbed. The amount absorbed depends on the body's storage levels and the amount ingested. At low levels of intake, a large amount of the vitamin is absorbed and vice versa. In addition, in healthy persons, the vitamin can be recycled from bile and intestinal secretions before the remainder is excreted in feces. Thus, a person's stores of vitamin B_{12} last from 3 to 5 years. The principal storage site is the liver, which contains 50% of the body's estimated 2500 microgram supply (Carmel, 2006a).

FUNCTIONS

Vitamin B_{12} is a coenzyme in the synthesis of DNA and RNA and the metabolism of amino acids and fatty acids. Vitamin B_{12} is also essential for the synthesis and maintenance of myelin, the fatty insulation that permits speedy transmission of impulses along the nerves.

DEFICIENCY

As many as 15% of elderly individuals have a deficiency of vitamin B_{12} (Gropper, Smith, and Groff, 2009). Persons may be at increased risk of vitamin B_{12} deficiency because of stomach pathology, intestinal disease, or diet.

Stomach Causes

When a person lacks intrinsic factor, the result is a condition called **pernicious anemia.** The prevalence of this **autoimmune disease** increases with age and is attributed to antibodies against gastric parietal cells and intrinsic factor.

Pernicious anemia can also occur after the surgical removal of the stomach or a large portion of the stomach. In those cases, vitamin B_{12} is not absorbed because intrinsic factor is missing.

Because gastric acid facilitates separation of vitamin B_{12} from the foods containing it, vitamin B_{12} deficiency can be caused by atrophic gastritis. That condition, because it occurs in 10% to 30% of older adults, is a major cause of vitamin B_{12} deficiency (Johnson, 2007). Similarly, prolonged use of medications that block or neutralize gastric acid can impair vitamin B_{12} status.

Intestinal Causes

People with **Crohn's disease** involving the ileum and those whose ileum has been removed do not absorb vitamin B_{12} efficiently. Other intestinal causes of deficiency include conditions causing bacterial overgrowth and parasites.

Dietary Causes

Vitamin B_{12} deficiency can be caused by a diet devoid of animal products. People particularly at risk are the elderly who choose tea and toast for meals, persons with alcoholism who eat poorly, and strict vegetarians. Of particular concern are vegan mothers with subclinical vitamin B_{12} deficiencies whose breastfed babies have developed severe neurological problems (Carmel, 2006a). In another case, a 33-year-old man who had been a strict vegetarian for many years without taking vitamin supplements became irreversibly blind as a result of severe bilateral optic neuropathy. The condition was attributed to deficiencies of vitamin B_{12} and thiamin (Milea, Cassoux, and LeHoang, 2000).

Signs and Symptoms

Symptoms of vitamin B_{12} deficiency can be seen in the circulatory and nervous systems; however, some clients display only neurological symptoms (Carmel, 2006a). Circulatory symptoms include megaloblastic anemia and result in these signs and symptoms:

- Fatigue
- Pallor
- Shortness of breath
- Palpitations.

Neurological manifestations include these signs and symptoms:

- Numbness and tingling in the extremities
- Abnormal gait
- Memory loss
- Possible dementia (Gropper, Smith, and Groff, 2009) that may be irreversible.

Moreover, the mechanism for many of the neurologic changes is unknown (Carmel, 2006a). A case of acute dementia in a 52-year-old client caused by vitamin B_{12} deficiency without other symptoms led the researchers to recommend screening psychiatric clients for vitamin B_{12} and folate deficiencies regardless of age or previous health status (Lerner and Kanevsky, 2002).

Diagnosing vitamin B_{12} deficiency by examining red blood cells is difficult in persons consuming ample folate because folate enables the continued manufacturing of red blood cells in the correct size and number. But folic acid cannot maintain myelin. As a result of the inability to diagnose the deficiency quickly, the neurological deterioration of pernicious anemia continues unabated.

Despite some concerns about missed cases, research indicates that food fortification with folic acid has not caused a major increase in masked vitamin B_{12} deficiency (Mills et al., 2003). Folic acid supplementation in a person with sickle cell anemia, however, did result in a delayed diagnosis of pernicious anemia that had progressed to neuropsychiatric symptoms before it was identified (Dhar, Bellevue, and Carmel, 2003).

Treatment

Traditional treatment of pernicious anemia involves periodic intramuscular injections of vitamin B_{12}. The pharmaceutical names for vitamin B_{12} are **cyanocobalamin** and **hydroxocobalamin.** Oral medication for pernicious anemia requires caution. Neither oral administration nor delivery by sublingual or intranasal modalities has been proven effective for clients with severe neurological involvement (Carmel, 2006a). When the cause is dietary and absorption is normal, oral supplementation with vitamin B_{12} is indicated. However, reliable data on dosage required for food-cobalamin malabsorption due to gastritis are not available (Carmel, 2006a).

SOURCES

Vitamin B_{12} is synonymous with animal products that have derived their cobalamins from microorganisms. Healthy young adults who regularly consume meat, fish, poultry, milk, cheese, or eggs are not at risk of vitamin B_{12} deficiency. Some plant foods may contain vitamin B_{12} from bacterial contamination or, in the case of legumes, from the nitrogen-fixing bacteria on their roots. For strict vegetarians, nutritional yeast and vitamin B_{12}-fortified products (soymilk or tofu) are more appropriate food sources than reliance on bacterial contamination. Products that list vitamin B_{12} rather than cobalamin as an ingredient may include nonbioavailable sources (CDC, 2003).

INTERFERING FACTORS

Megadoses of vitamin C interfere with vitamin B_{12} absorption and utilization. The body's use of vitamin B_{12} is also impaired by a deficiency of vitamin B_6 and by antacids.

TOXICITY

No toxicity from vitamin B_{12} has been recorded from food or supplements or from parenteral doses to clients with pernicious anemia.

Table 7-3 lists factors affecting the stability of the 13 vitamins described thus far. Table 7-4 summarizes the information on the 9 water soluble vitamins.

Other Vitamins

Three additional vitamins are so widely distributed in foods that only special circumstances have produced deficiencies. Long-term **total parenteral nutrition (TPN)** is one such situation. That therapy is detailed in Chapter 14.

PANTOTHENIC ACID

The vitamin **pantothenic acid** serves as a coenzyme in fatty acid metabolism. No cases of deficiency of pantothenic acid have been documented in people who eat a variety of foods, but deficiencies have occurred in prisoner-of-war camps and have been produced experimentally (Trumbo, 2006).

Most adults in the United States consume 4 to 7 milligrams (Gropper, Smith, and Groff, 2009). People with alcoholism or diabetes mellitus may have an increased need for pantothenic acid. Rich food sources include meats, eggs, potatoes, and broccoli. No toxicities have been reported.

BIOTIN

As a coenzyme is the synthesis of fat, glycogen, and amino acids, **biotin** is an essential nutrient because bacterial synthesis in the large intestine is insufficient to meet a person's needs. Dietary biotin is absorbed primarily in the jejunum and small amounts are stored in the muscle, liver, and brain. Food sources include liver, soybeans, egg yolk, legumes, nuts, and cereals.

Deficiencies have been caused by total parenteral nutrition that omitted biotin but also developed in persons with alcoholism or gastrointestinal diseases, those on long-term anticonvulsant therapy, and children with an inborn error of biotin metabolism. Symptoms include a scaly, red rash, alopecia, **paresthesias** of the extremities, depression, and hallucinations (Gropper, Smith, and Groff, 2009).

Toxicity has not been reported.

Avidin, a protein in raw egg white, interferes with absorption by irreversibly binding with biotin. Excessive consumption of raw egg whites has caused biotin deficiency. Cooking the egg white inactivates avidin and thus eliminates the risk.

CHOLINE

The organic compound choline is a precursor for the neurotransmitter **acetylcholine** and for two **phospholipids** that are structural components of all human cell membranes (Linus Pauling Institute, 2008). Deficiency of choline in clients receiving long-term **total parenteral nutrition (TPN),** resulting in fatty liver and hepatocellular damage, helped to establish the essentiality of this nutrient (Zeisel, 2006).

Although not a vitamin by strict definition, choline has been given an Adequate Intake. Choline is widely distributed in foods with the best sources being milk, eggs, liver, and peanuts (Linus Pauling Institute, 2008).

Effects of excessive intake include sweating, salivation, hypotension, hepatotoxicity, and a fishy body odor. The last is due to excessive production and excretion of trimethylamine, a metabolite of choline (Linus Pauling Institute, 2008).

Table 7-5 lists the sources of vitamins by food groups to clarify the potential for inadequate intake if a person should exclude an entire food group.

Vitamin Supplements

Vitamin supplements are not intended as substitutes for a healthy diet because knowledge of vitamins is not complete, and new functions and relationships are

TABLE 7-5 ■ Good Sources of Vitamins by Food Groups

VITAMIN	SYNTHESIS/MISCELLANEOUS	MEATS	MILK	FRUITS/VEGETABLES	GRAINS
A		Liver	Fortified	Deep yellow, dark green leafy	
D	In skin	Salt water fish	Fortified		Fortified cereals
E				Vegetable oil Nuts Leafy vegetables	Wheat germ Whole grains Fortified cereals
K	In intestine			Green leafy Canola, soybean oils	
C				Fresh fruit, especially citrus Vegetables	
Thiamin		Pork		Black beans Black-eyed peas	Wheat germ Fortified cereals
Riboflavin		Meats, esp liver Eggs	Milk	Legumes	Fortified cereals
Niacin	Coffee Tea	Meat Fish Poultry			Whole or enriched grains Fortified cereals
B_6	Orange breakfast drinks	Sirloin steak Salmon Chicken breast		Bananas Nuts Vegetables	Whole grains Fortified cereals
Folate Folic Acid		Liver		Dried peas, beans, lentils Dark green leafy Peanuts	Fortified grain products Whole grains Wheat germ
B_{12}	Nutritional yeast	Meat Fish Poultry Eggs	Milk Cheese	Fortified soymilk, tofu	
Pantothenic Acid	In intestine	Meat Egg yolk		Broccoli Potatoes	Whole grain cereals
Biotin	In intestine	Liver Egg yolk		Legumes Nuts Soybeans	Cereals
Choline		Eggs Liver	Milk	Peanuts	

discovered every year. The single piece of advice given most frequently in the conclusions of researchers, however, is the admonition to eat five servings of fruits and vegetables every day. Fruit eaten out-of-hand is the original fast food. (See Fig. 7-5.)

Individuals wishing to take supplements should consider taking a multivitamin instead of a medley of single vitamins and should not exceed 150% of the RDAIs. This amount will prevent deficiency in healthy individuals, and toxicity is unlikely. Even so, vitamin-taking should be reported to health-care providers along with medications. Although not a major expense for individuals, sales of multivitamins amounted to $4.5 billion in 2007. Users seem to have healthier diets and lifestyles than nonusers (Marra and Boyar, 2009). Multivitamins are sold in many formulations. Dollars and Sense 7-1 suggests ways to economize without sacrificing quality.

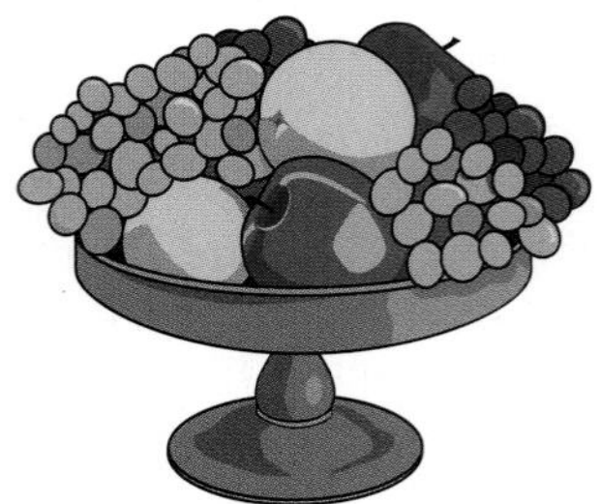

The Original Fast Food

FIGURE 7-5 Fruits eaten out-of-hand are the ORIGINAL fast foods as well as healthy choices.

Dollars & Sense 7-1

Brand-Name versus Generic Multivitamins

Major brand-name and store-brand multivitamins have been found reliable but those sold in discount stores have not passed quality tests. The cut-rate products offered $3 to $21 savings per year over brand-name multivitamins and even less over major store brands (Multivitamins, 2006).

For instance, Centrum A to Zinc®, recommended for premenopausal women, sold for $13 for 180 tablets on the same day that Walgreens Advanced Formula A Thru Z® sold for $10 for 400 tablets. The difference for a year's supply would be $17.23.

See Chapter 15 for quality assurances.

Keystones

- Vitamins are organic substances required in minute quantities and that do not become part of the structure of the body.
- Vitamins A, D, E, and K are fat soluble and require sufficient dietary fat intake and adequate fat digestion for proper utilization.
- Deficiency of vitamin A results in xerophthalmia and night blindness, and deficiency of vitamin D causes rickets and osteomalacia.
- The water-soluble vitamins, C and the B-complex vitamins, are not stored in the body in appreciable amounts, requiring regular intake.
- Vitamins C, B_{12}, thiamin, and niacin have specific diseases associated with deficiency: scurvy, pernicious anemia, beriberi, and pellagra, respectively.
- People who take vitamins should limit their intake to 150% of the RDA in a multivitamin product, except individuals with special needs.
- Two large groups of people for whom synthetic vitamins in fortified food or supplements are recommended are women capable of becoming pregnant (folic acid) and individuals older than 50 years (vitamin B_{12}).

CASE STUDY 7–1

Mr. J, a 79-year-old widowed man, prides himself on caring for himself during the past year since his wife died. His typical meal pattern is:

- Breakfast—egg, toast, jam, coffee
- Lunch—cheese or lunchmeat sandwich, tea
- Dinner—canned stew or hash

Although Mr. J has a refrigerator, he avoids buying fresh fruits or vegetables. He says he has difficulty consuming produce before it spoils. He seldom goes out to eat.

For the past few months, Mr. J has noticed that his gums are tender. He stopped wearing his dentures when his gums began to bleed.

The visiting nurse confirmed inflammation of the gums. When the nurse took Mr. J's blood pressure, she noted a red, flat rash on Mr. J's forearm.

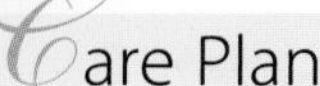

Care Plan

Subjective Data

Sore gums ■ Diet lacks fresh fruits and vegetables

Objective Data

Inflamed gums ■ Erythematous **petechiae** related to blood pressure measurement

Analysis

Possible vitamin C deficiency related to lack of fresh fruit and vegetables as evidenced by sore bleeding gums and petechiae after sphygmomanometer use.

Plan

DESIRED OUTCOMES EVALUATION CRITERIA	ACTIONS/INTERVENTIONS	RATIONALE
Will consume foods containing 90 mg of vitamin C every day within 3 days	Teach the importance of daily vitamin C.	Little vitamin C is stored in the body; should be consumed nearly every day.
	Explore the acceptability of good sources of vitamin C; list amounts necessary to obtain 90 mg; recommend purchasing small quantities.	Foods would be better sources than vitamin supplements because food also supplies other nutrients.
	If the client selects frozen vegetables, teach to boil water 1 minute before adding vegetables and to cook quickly until crisp-tender.	Heat and oxygen destroy vitamin C
	Follow up in 3 days. Report to primary care provider if unimproved.	

Three days later, the nurse determined that Mr. J had not been grocery shopping and his bleeding gums and petechiae persisted. After telephone consultation with his physician, she instructed Mr. J to have the vitamin C blood test the physician ordered and to visit the doctor the following week.

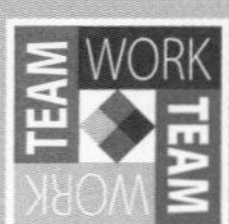

7-1

Physician's Notes

The following Physician's Notes are representative of the documentation found in a client's medical record.

When the doctor saw Mr. J, he wrote the following:

Chief complaint: referred by home health regarding possible vitamin C deficiency

Subjective: Unsure of reason for visit. "Sent by nurse."

Objective: Gingival hypertrophy and inflammation, recent bruising on extremities

Serum ascorbic acid level 0.15 milligrams per 100 milliliters

Analysis: Scurvy

Plan: Replete vitamin C levels with ascorbic acid: 1 gram per day for 5 days, then 500 milligrams per day until normal levels achieved.

Follow up in 2 weeks

Critical Thinking Questions

1. Is this the end of Mr. J's nutritional problems? What additional assessment data would be helpful as you continue to work with Mr. J?
2. Why do you think Mr. J did not follow the nurse's initial advice?
3. Even after the physician prescribes vitamin C, why is it important to improve Mr. J's food intake?

Chapter Review

1. Which of the following vitamins are water-soluble?
   a. A and C
   b. A, D, E, and K
   c. B and C
   d. B, D, E, and K
2. The vitamin that is essential to the synthesis of several blood clotting factors is:
   a. Vitamin A
   b. Vitamin B_6
   c. Vitamin C
   d. Vitamin K
3. Which of the following groups of foods would be the best sources of carotene?
   a. Apricots, cantaloupe, and squash
   b. Asparagus, beets, and sweet potatoes
   c. Broccoli, lettuce, and lima beans
   d. Lemons, oranges, and strawberries
4. Deficiency of vitamin D causes:
   a. Rickets
   b. Pellagra
   c. Night blindness
   d. Beriberi
5. In general, individuals who elect to take a vitamin supplement should:
   a. Buy the most economical product
   b. Limit the amounts to 150% of RDA levels
   c. Obtain a physician's prescription
   d. Select the most advertised product

Clinical Analysis

1. Ms. C is bringing her 3-month-old baby girl to the well-baby clinic. Ms. C states that the baby is taking 6 ounces of a commercial baby formula every 4 hours. Ms. C has not added solid foods to the baby's diet. She was told to wait until the baby is 4 to 6 months old before adding cereal. Ms. C is giving the baby the multivitamin preparation prescribed. She also has added cod liver oil to the infant's diet. "It's only a teaspoonful," she said. Ms. C's grandmother gave Ms. C cod liver oil as a child. Ms. C credits her grandmother's care during her own childhood for her strong bones and teeth. She admires her grandmother, who at age 75 still stands straight and tall. Which of the following pieces of information should the nurse gather first to focus on the situation presented?
   a. The amount of vitamin C in the multivitamin supplement
   b. The conditions under which the vitamins are stored
   c. Ms. C's technique for measuring the vitamins
   d. The total amount of vitamin D the infant receives each day

2. Mr. S has expressed interest in improving his diet. The nurse assessed Mr. S's usual intake, noting the absence of citrus fruit. He stated the acids upset his stomach. Which of the following suggestions to maximize vitamin C content in vegetables is appropriate?
   a. Adding baking soda to the cooking water
   b. Cooking thoroughly to kill any bacteria
   c. Eating good sources raw when possible
   d. Keeping food in a mesh bag to allow air to circulate

3. Ms. M is a Seventh-Day Adventist who has elected a vegan lifestyle and who lives an indoor life. For which of the following vitamin deficiencies would she be at greatest risk without professional dietary advice?
   a. Vitamins A, C, and E
   b. Vitamins B_{12}, D, and niacin
   c. Vitamins B_6, folate, and thiamin
   d. Vitamin K, riboflavin, and biotin

8

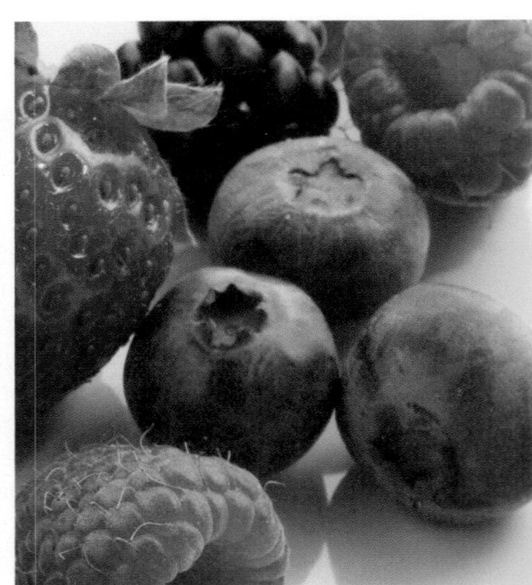

Minerals and Water

LEARNING OBJECTIVES

After completing this chapter, the student should be able to:

- Describe one or more functions of the main nutritive minerals.
- List at least two food sources for each mineral and identify nonfood sources.
- Identify individuals at increased risk for mineral deficiencies.
- Develop strategies to increase clients' calcium intakes from food.
- Devise a plan to increase clients' iron intake from food.
- Describe the locations and functions of water in the body.
- Discuss the body's control mechanisms for maintaining fluid and electrolyte balance.
- Identify methods of assessing water balance in the body.
- Distinguish between heat exhaustion and heat stroke as to signs and symptoms and first-aid treatment.

In a broad sense, minerals are obtained from the Earth's crust. Through the effects of the weather, rocks that contain minerals are ground into smaller particles, which then become part of the soil. Growing plants absorb the minerals from the soil with the water they need. Animals eat the plants, and humans eat both the plants and the animals.

Water is the medium of absorption of nutrients for plants and the basis of the body's nutrient delivery system. In addition, certain forms of minerals are intricately bound to the distribution and movement of water in the body.

Minerals make vital contributions to growth and maintenance of the body's health. This chapter covers minerals important in human nutrition and the role each plays in the body. It describes some general functions of minerals and explains how minerals are classified in nutrition. It details the nutritional implications of the 7 major and 10 trace minerals. Information on minerals appears first and then information on water and its functions.

Functions of Minerals

Minerals represent 4% of total body weight. Like vitamins, minerals help to regulate bodily functions without providing energy and are essential to good health. Unlike vitamins, minerals:

1. Are inorganic substances.
2. Become part of the body's composition.

For instance, calcium and phosphorus combine to give bones and teeth their hardness. Iron attaches to the protein globin to form hemoglobin. Iodine becomes part of the thyroid hormones.

Most minerals serve a variety of functions in the body's regulatory and metabolic processes. Sodium is essential for maintaining fluid balance. Sodium, potassium, and calcium have critical functions in nerve and muscle activity. Potassium and phosphorus play significant roles in acid–base balance. A disruption of the body's balance of any one of these minerals, albeit not necessarily caused by diet, can be life threatening.

Classification of Minerals

Three groups of minerals are considered in nutrition: major, trace, and ultratrace.

Major minerals (macrominerals) and **trace minerals** (microminerals) are differentiated by:

- Amounts present in the body: more or less than 5 grams (approximately 1 teaspoonful)
- Intake requirements: 100 milligrams (approximately 1⁄50 teaspoonful) or less daily.

Despite their small amounts, trace minerals make vital and often unique contributions to the body's functioning.

Ultratrace minerals appear in the DRI tables (see Appendix A). Values have been set only for ULs for three of the five minerals in this category.

Major Minerals

The seven major minerals include calcium, sodium, and potassium, which are familiar to many people in a dietary context. The other four are phosphorus, magnesium, sulfur, and chloride.

Calcium

The body of a 150-pound adult contains approximately 3 pounds of calcium, 90% in the bones and teeth. The remaining 1% of the calcium circulates in the body fluids.

Functions

Calcium, with phosphorus, forms the hard substance of bones and teeth. Ample calcium and phosphorus alone will not guarantee strong bones and teeth, however. Vitamin D is necessary for calcium absorption and protein serves as the matrix that determines the structure of the bone. Exercise, particularly weight-bearing exercise, is also essential for strong bones. Except for slightly demineralized areas, teeth cannot repair themselves so that dental restoration is needed.

Calcium also performs several vital metabolic functions in the nervous, muscular, and cardiovascular systems, for instance:

1. Calcium assists in manufacturing **acetylcholine,** a neurotransmitter (a chemical that enhances transmission of nerve impulses).
2. Calcium acts as a catalyst in initiating and controlling muscle contraction and relaxation. At the beginning of a muscle contraction, calcium is released from its storage area inside the muscle cell. At the end of a contraction, the calcium is gathered into its storage area.
3. Calcium is a catalyst in the clotting process: it aids in the conversion of platelets to thromboplastin and in the conversion of **fibrinogen** to **fibrin.**

Control Mechanisms

Remodeling of bone continues throughout life, such that the bone calcium pool turns over every 8 to 12 years on average in adults, but this turnover does not occur in the teeth (Weaver and Heaney, 2006). One reason for the changes in bone composition is to maintain the adult serum calcium concentration within the normal limits of 8.2 to 10.2 milligrams per 100 milliliters of serum.

Another reason for the movement of calcium in and out of the bones is to renew the bone tissue. In this process, bone cells called **osteoclasts** produce enzymes to destroy the protein matrix that holds the calcium phosphate in place. Other bone cells, called **osteoblasts** produce new matrix protein, which chemically attracts calcium and other nutrients to rebuild the bone.

Several hormones work together to accomplish these activities. Vitamin D (see Chapter 7) is one of these hormones. **Parathyroid hormone** and calcitonin are the other two. Tiny glands behind the thyroid gland in the neck secrete **parathyroid hormone** when the serum calcium level is too low. The thyroid gland secretes **calcitonin** when the serum calcium level is too high.

Figure 8-1 illustrates the complementary actions of parathyroid hormone and calcitonin.

Other hormones affect the body's use of calcium. One prominent one is estrogen.

Dietary Reference Intakes

For DRIs see Appendix A. For food and other sources, see Table 8-1. To investigate the mineral content of a particular item, see "Nutritive Values of Foods" on DavisPlus.

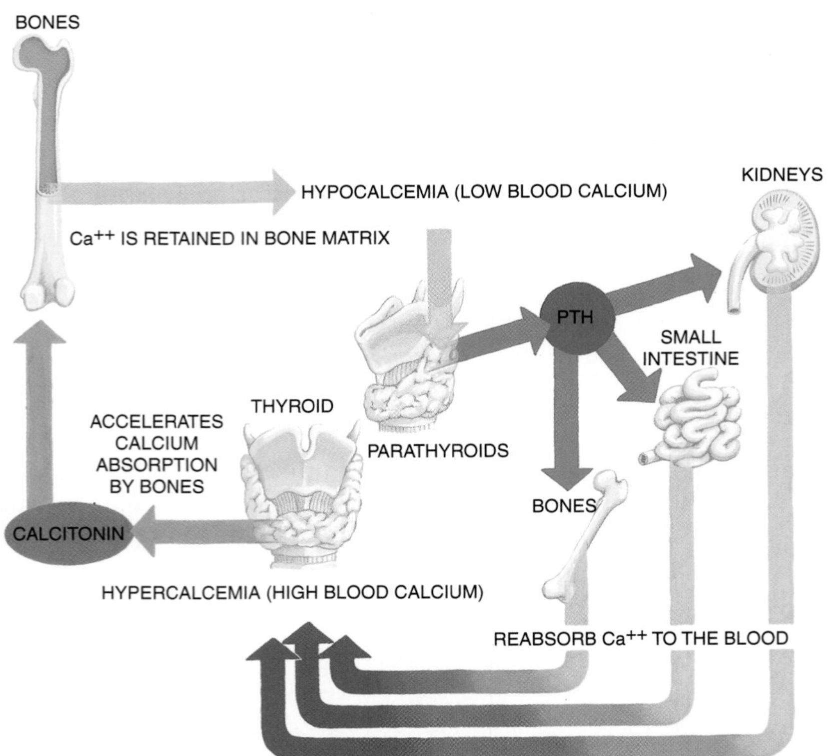

FIGURE 8-1 Parathyroid hormone raises serum calcium levels when they are too low. Calcitonin from the thyroid gland lowers serum calcium levels when they are too high. (Reprinted from Venes, D [Ed.]: *Taber's cylcopedic medical dictionary*, ed 21. FA Davis, Philadelphia, 2010, p 338, with permission.)

TABLE 8-1 ■ Major Minerals

MINERAL	ADULT RDA/AI AND FOOD PORTION*	FUNCTIONS	SIGNS AND SYMPTOMS OF DEFICIENCY	SIGNS AND SYMPTOMS OF EXCESS	BEST SOURCES
Calcium	1000–1200 mg 3.3–4 cups milk	Structure of bones and teeth Nerve conduction Muscle contraction Blood clotting	Tetany Osteoporosis Rickets (premature infants)	Calcification of soft tissue	Milk products Salmon Sardines, Clams Oysters
Phosphorus	700 mg 2.2 cups chili with beans	Structure of bones and teeth Component of DNA and RNA Component of buffers and almost all enzymes Component of ADP and ATP	Increased calcium excretion Bone loss Muscle weakness	Tetany Convulsions Renal insufficiency	Lean meat Fish Poultry Milk Nuts Legumes
Sodium	1.2 to 1.5 grams 0.6 to 0.75 tsp salt	Fluid balance Transmission of electrochemical impulses along nerve and muscle membranes	Hyponatremia	Hypernatremia	Table salt Processed foods Milk and milk products
Potassium	4.7 grams 4 cups white baked beans	Conduction of nerve impulses Muscle contraction	Hypokalemia (not usually dietary)	Hyperkalemia (not usually dietary)	Banana Cantaloupe Winter squash Green leafy vegetables Legumes Salt substitutes
Magnesium	310–420 mg 2.1–2.8 cups spinach	Associated with ADP and ATP Involved in DNA and protein synthesis Influences cardiac and smooth muscle contractility	Impaired CNS function Tetany	Weakness Depressed respirations Cardiac arrest	Green leafy vegetables Seafood Peanut butter Legumes Coffee, tea, and cocoa

TABLE 8-1 ■ Major Minerals (Continued)

MINERAL	ADULT RDA/AI AND FOOD PORTION*	FUNCTIONS	SIGNS AND SYMPTOMS OF DEFICIENCY	SIGNS AND SYMPTOMS OF EXCESS	BEST SOURCES
Sulfur	None	Component of amino acids methionine and cysteine Gives shape to hair, skin, and nails	None known due solely to sulfur	None known due solely to sulfur	Complete protein foods
Chloride	1.8–2.3 grams 0.6–0.75 tsp salt	Component of hydrochloric acid Helps maintain fluid and acid base balance	In infants: neurological impairments	None known	Table salt Salty snacks Processed foods Eggs Meat Seafood

*Examples only; not suggested to be sole source of a day's intake.

Sources

Calcium can be obtained from animal or vegetable sources, but calcium from animal sources is more readily absorbed.

ANIMAL SOURCES

Milk and milk products are the best animal sources of calcium. Even so, only 32% of the available calcium in milk is absorbed (Weaver and Heaney, 2006). In milk, calcium is accompanied by lactose, which increases absorption in infants but not in adults.

Another advantageous component of milk is the protein the osteoblasts need to rebuild the bone matrix. In sum, milk is such an important source of calcium that it is virtually impossible to obtain adequate dietary calcium without dairy products. Figure 8-2 shows a child drinking milk with a "fast food" meal.

See Table 8-2 to evaluate alternate sources of calcium compared to fluid milk. Note the cost in kilocalories.

Milk products supply other nutrients, such as vitamins A and D and are also a major source of riboflavin and protein. See Figure 8-3. Supplements should not substitute for food but sometimes are necessary adjuncts. Clinical Application 8-1 describes some of the contaminants in "natural" calcium supplements and suggestions for choosing a supplement when necessary.

Calcium supplements should be taken:

- In doses of 500 milligrams or less for optimal absorption
- With meals if calcium carbonate (stomach acid enhances absorption)
- Without regard to meals if calcium citrate

PLANT SOURCES

Good plant sources of calcium include turnip and mustard greens, broccoli, cauliflower, kale, legumes, and dried fruits (Gropper, Smith, and Groff, 2009). Some experts question how much calcium the body is actually able to absorb from plant sources because of multiple interfering factors.

Another good plant source that is readily available is calcium-fortified orange juice. A source of calcium for Navajo Americans is the ash derived from the

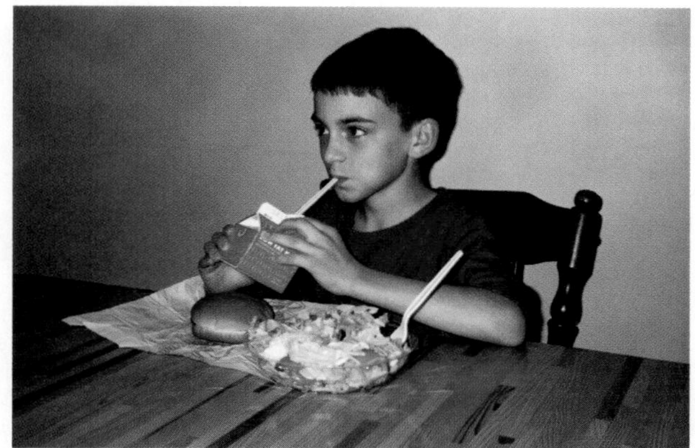

FIGURE 8-2 This child has a balanced meal from a fast food restaurant: a small hamburger, a salad, and milk. Growing bones and teeth need calcium from milk products.

TABLE 8-2 ■ Food Containing Approximately 300 Milligrams of Calcium, Equal to One Cup of Milk

FOOD	AMOUNT	KILOCALORIES
Skim milk	1.0 cup	86
Plain low-fat yogurt	0.7 cup	101
Swiss cheese	1.1 oz	118
Whole milk	1.0 cup	150
Cheddar cheese	1.5 oz	171
Low-fat yogurt with fruit	0.9 cup	199
Cottage cheese, 2% low-fat	2.0 cups	410
Soft ice cream	1.3 cups	479
Cottage cheese, creamed, large curd	2.25 cups	529
Sherbet	2.9 cups	786

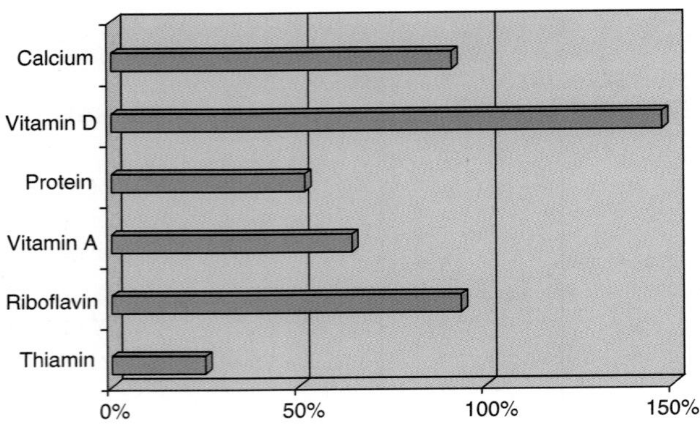

FIGURE 8-3 Milk supplies many nutrients in addition to calcium. Three cups of skim milk provide a woman between 25 and 50 years of age with 91% of her AI for calcium, 147% of her AI for vitamin D, 52% of her RDA for protein, 64% of her RDA for vitamin A, 93% of her RDA for riboflavin, and 25% of her RDA for thiamin. The kilocaloric cost for all of these nutrients is a minuscule 258 kilocalories.

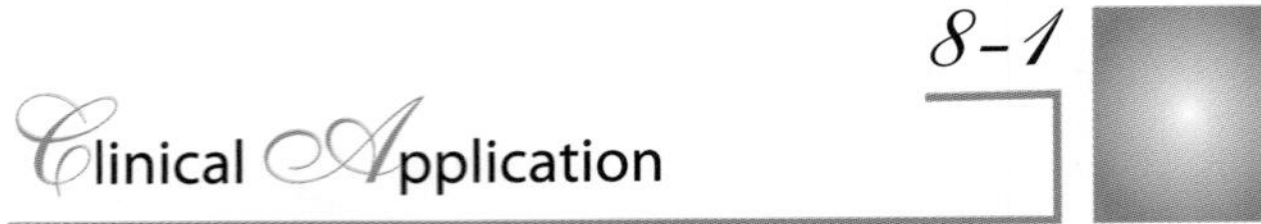

Contents of Natural Calcium Supplements

Shells, dolomite, and bones are natural sources of calcium that are used as dietary supplements. Much of the calcium found in shells and bones is in the form of calcium phosphate, one of the most difficult calcium compounds to absorb. More importantly, shells and dolomite, a limestone product, may be contaminated with aluminum and lead and the latter often contaminates bone meal preparations (Gropper, Smith, and Groff, 2009).

Supplements labeled "USP" or "CL" (see Chapter 15) meet voluntary industry standards for quality, purity, and tablet disintegration or dissolution. To test the dissolvability of a product, place a tablet in one-half cup of vinegar. Stir occasionally over one-half hour after which no particles should be visible.

branches and needles of the juniper tree. The ash is used to flavor various foods, such as cornmeal mush and pancakes and Navajo tea. One teaspoon of the ash supplies roughly the calcium in one glass of milk (Christensen et al., 1998), illustrating the wisdom of traditional ways.

Absorption and Excretion

Calcium is absorbed throughout the small intestine through two distinct processes. In the **duodenum** and proximal **jejunum,** the process is active, through the intestinal cells, and involves a calcium-binding transport protein stimulated by calcitriol. In the distal jejunum and ileum, the process is passive, between the intestinal cells. Lastly, bacteria in the large intestine appear to release calcium from some food fiber, permitting absorption of calcium through that site. Growing children absorb up to 75% of dietary calcium, compared to 30% absorbed by adults.

Excretion takes place in urine (average daily loss of about 170 milligrams) and feces, but also through the skin with an average daily loss of 60 milligrams (Gropper, Smith, and Groff, 2009).

Interfering Factors

In general, the percentage of available calcium absorbed from vegetables is considerably less than that absorbed from milk. The exceptions from which calcium is as easily absorbed as that in milk include:

- Broccoli
- Cabbage
- Bok choy (Chinese cabbage)
- Kale
- Mustard and turnip greens

The difficulty becomes the volume of food necessary to provide the quantity of calcium equal to that in a glass of milk: 2.3 servings of bok choy or 4.5 servings of broccoli (Weaver and Heaney, 2006).

Several factors can interfere with the absorption and retention of calcium. See Table 8-3.

OXALATES

Some plants contain salts of oxalic acid called **oxalates** that bind with the calcium present in some vegetables to produce calcium oxalate, an insoluble substance excreted in the feces. These potent inhibitors are found in high concentrations in spinach and rhubarb (Weaver and Heaney, 2006). Unusually high intake of these and other foods may cause oxalic acid poisoning (see Clinical Application 8-2).

PHYTATES

Cereals contain **phytic acid,** which forms an insoluble complex with calcium. Phytates are the storage form of phosphorus in seeds; however, only foods with heavy concentrations of phytate, such as wheat bran and dried beans, substantially reduce calcium absorption (Weaver and Heaney, 2006).

The overall effect of oxalic and phytic acids on calcium availability in most balanced diets usually is not

TABLE 8-3 ■ Factors Affecting Calcium Absorption and Excretion

INCREASE ABSORPTION	DECREASE ABSORPTION	INCREASE EXCRETION
Lactose (infants)	Oxalic acid	Excessive protein
Vitamin D	Phytic acid	Excessive sodium
	Vitamin D deficiency	Caffeine

8-2

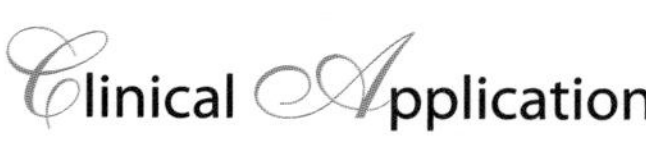

Oxalic Acid Poisoning

Poisoning is possible by ingesting too much of the foods containing oxalic acid, such as:

- Spinach
- Rhubarb
- Gooseberries
- Chard
- Beet leaves

For example, one normal serving of rhubarb contains one-fifth the toxic dose. Rhubarb leaves contain three or four times as much as the stalks so a fairly small amount of leaf can poison a child.

One way to minimize the chance of oxalic acid poisoning is to consume foods that contain calcium with foods high in oxalic acid. The calcium combines with the oxalate, which then passes through the intestine harmlessly but also of necessity decreasing calcium absorption.

significant. People who avoid dairy products, however, need careful attention to meal planning. Ovovegetarian and vegan clients should seek calcium-fortified products, such as orange juice and calcium-set tofu, to bolster their intake of the mineral.

PROTEIN

The impact of dietary protein on calcium absorption is a subject of debate. Over a wide range of protein intakes, however, a one-gram increase in protein intake results in a loss of 1 milligram of calcium in the urine. Such losses resulting from the acid load of the protein may be counterbalanced by high intakes of fruits and vegetables that contribute alkalinity to the equation (Dawson-Hughes, 2006). See the section on potassium and on acid–base balance later in the chapter.

OTHER MINERALS

Magnesium and zinc can impair the absorption of calcium, especially in situations where calcium intake is low. Calcium, magnesium, and zinc use the same absorption mechanism (Gropper, Smith, and Groff, 2009).

Sodium intake can also have a detrimental effect on calcium balance. For every 500-milligram increase in sodium intake, an additional 10 milligrams of calcium is spilled in the urine (Dawson-Hughes, 2006)—a small amount compared to the RDA but the amount could be important in young women consuming high-salt, low-dairy diets. In adolescent girls, sodium intake correlates more strongly with excreted urinary calcium than does calcium intake (Weaver and Heaney, 2006).

CAFFEINE

Caffeine stimulates urinary excretion of calcium (Gropper, Smith, and Groff, 2009), which may become important when caffeinated beverages replace milk in the diet. Caffeine equal to 2 to 3 cups of coffee accelerated bone loss from the spine and total body in postmenopausal women who consumed less than 744 milligrams of calcium per day (Weaver and Heaney, 2006). Therefore, if a person's calcium intake is low or marginal, drinking many caffeinated beverages could adversely affect bone health.

Deficiencies

Calcium deficiency in children can contribute to poor bone and tooth development. Rickets is typically more directly related to vitamin D deficiency than to calcium deficiency except in premature infants, whose skeletons still need much added minerals. Two other conditions related to calcium balance are osteoporosis and tetany.

OSTEOPOROSIS

According to the World Health Organization, **osteopenia** is bone mineral density 1 to 2.5 standard deviations below the mean of healthy young adults, whereas **osteoporosis** is bone mineral density greater than 2.5 standard deviations below the mean. Osteoporosis permits minimal trauma to cause fractures commonly affecting the hip, wrist, or vertebrae.

Two major factors in the development of osteoporosis are:

1. The bone mass developed from birth to age 30
2. The rate at which bone mass is lost in later life

In girls and women, 99% of total bone body mineral content is achieved by age 22. Total body bone mass remains fairly constant through the reproductive years, but decreases in the aging adult, most markedly in postmenopausal women but also in men (Weaver and Heaney, 2006). The most rapid loss of bone occurs in the first 5 years after menopause. Intuitively, then, estrogen treatment might help prevent osteoporosis but is not first-line therapy because of increased risks of heart disease, stroke, breast cancer, pulmonary emboli, and deep vein phlebitis (Dawson-Hughes, 2006).

Selective estrogen receptor modulators (SERMs) are currently under clinical development to prevent and treat postmenopausal osteoporosis. The new drugs are expected to preserve bone without stimulating breast or endometrial tissues (de Villiers, 2010).

Osteoporosis is most common in postmenopausal, fair-complexioned white women; however, all are not equally affected. See Genomic Gem 8-1. Men and black women lose bone mass also, but because their skeletons are generally heavier, they are at lower risk. Blacks have higher bone mineral density than whites and Asians, a difference that is noted beginning in early childhood (Dawson-Hughes, 2006).

Figure 8-4 shows normal and osteoporotic cancellous bone. Figure 8-5 displays x-ray films of normal and osteoporotic bones. Clinical Application 8-3 details prevalence, major risk factors, diagnostic aids, and treatment approaches for osteoporosis.

Two lifestyle factors impacting bone include:

1. Smoking
2. Alcohol consumption

Women who smoke have lower bone density and faster rates of bone loss than women who do not smoke. Men who smoke have lower bone mineral density, faster rates of bone loss, and higher fracture risk than men who do not smoke (Dawson-Hughes, 2006).

Genomic Gem 8-1
Osteoporosis Is Familial

About 80% of the variance in peak bone mass is an inherited trait. Likewise, the propensity for rapid or slow bone loss in later life has a less prominent genetic link that is not well defined. Alleles for vitamin D receptors are known to interact with calcium intake. Women with a low bone density genotype not only lose bone more rapidly when calcium intake is very low but also do not compensate by increasing the rate of calcium absorption when intake is reduced. Research in this area is ongoing. (Dawson-Hughes, 2006).

Alcohol consumption has been reported to have varying effects on bone health. Ethanol directly impacts bone tissue by suppressing bone formation. Chronic alcohol abuse and osteoporosis commonly occur together in men.

Relatively minor risk factors for decreased calcium metabolism (alcohol, caffeine, high-protein intake unopposed by adequate fruits and vegetables, phytic acid-containing and oxalic acid-containing foods, sodium, and smoking), when combined, and especially when coupled with low-calcium and vitamin D

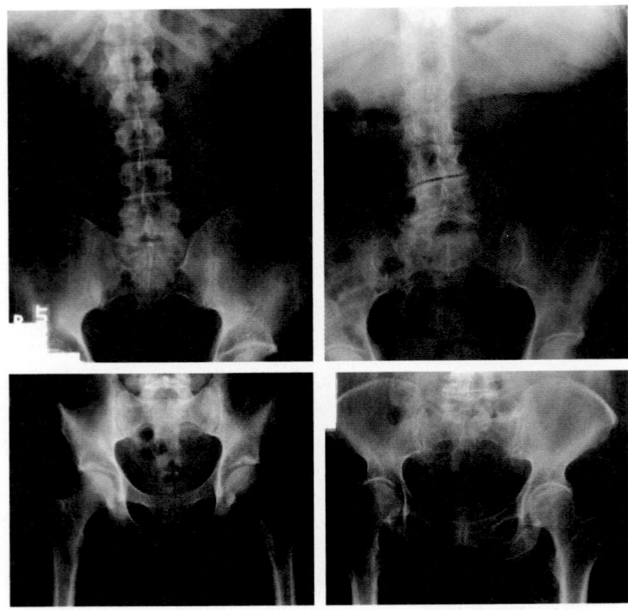

FIGURE 8-5 X-ray films of a normal bone on the left and an osteoporotic bone on the right. (Courtesy of Dr. Russell Tobe.)

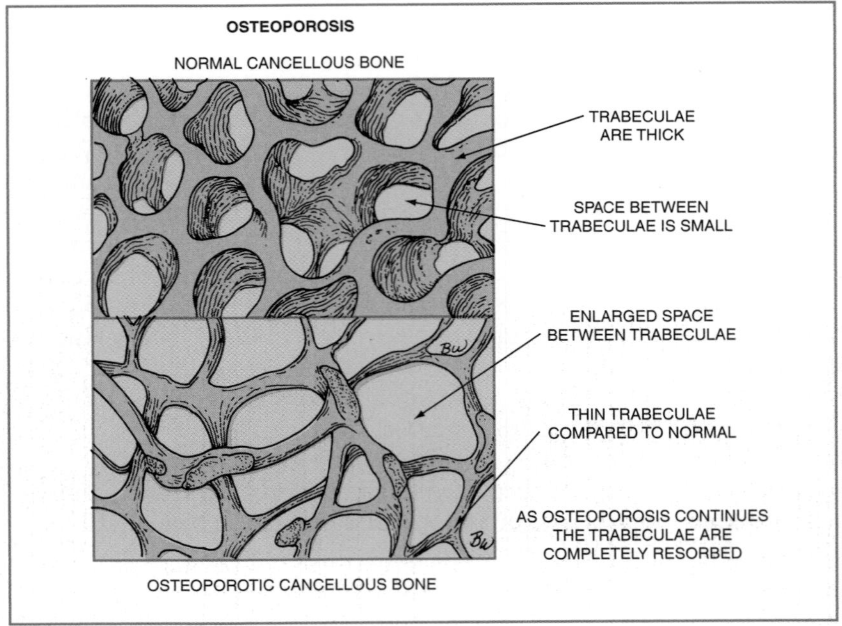

FIGURE 8-4 Sketch of normal and osteoporotic cancellous bone showing enlarged spaces and thinner bony structure in the latter. (Reprinted from Venes, D [Ed.]: *Taber's cylcopedic medical dictionary*, ed 21. FA Davis, Philadelphia, 2010, p 1659, with permission.)

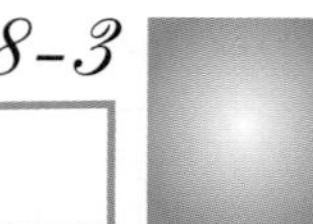

Clinical Application 8-3

Osteoporosis Prevalence, Risk Factors, Diagnosis, and Treatment

PREVALENCE

- An estimated 10 million people in the United States, 80% of them women, have osteoporosis, the major factor in fractures in the elderly.
- Annually in the United States, osteoporotic fractures occur at the hip (300,000), at the spine (700,000), or at the forearm (250,000), totaling approximately $18 billion in direct costs (Lanham-New, 2006).

MAJOR RISK FACTORS IN WHITE POSTMENOPAUSAL WOMEN

- Personal history of fracture as an adult. Forearm fractures are "sentinel events" that should trigger assessment for osteoporosis but frequently do not (Cuddihy et al., 2002).
- History of fragility fracture in a **first-degree relative.**
- Low body weight (less than 127 pounds)
- Current smoking
- Use of corticosteroid therapy (equal to 5 milligrams prednisone daily) for more than 3 months (Khosia and Melton, 2007)

DIAGNOSIS

- History and physical examination including assessment for height loss and posture changes
- Measurement of bone mineral density (BMD) if postmenopause. Until 30% to 40% of bone mass is lost, it is not detectable on x-ray film (see Fig. 8-5), but dual-energy x-ray absorptiometry (DEXA) permits earlier diagnosis.

TREATMENT

- Optimize nutrition, including protein, vitamin D, and calcium. Supplements when indicated. High intakes of calcium reduce bone resorption by reducing parathyroid hormone secretion (Heaney, 2006).
- Exercise to the extent fragility permits.
- May consider medications to affect bone metabolism in conjunction with, not instead of, nutrition and exercise. More than half the women on pharmacotherapy to prevent or treat osteoporosis had inadequate serum vitamin D levels (Holick et al., 2005).

intake, might make a decided difference in an individual's bone health. Diet and lifestyle interventions are not sufficient treatment for established osteoporosis; however, they are part of the therapeutic plan (Dawson-Hughes, 2006).

TETANY

Despite the hormonal control of serum calcium and the large reservoir in the bones, serum calcium levels sometimes fall below normal. An actual lack of calcium or a lack of ionized calcium may cause tetany. A serum calcium level that is too low is called **hypocalcemia.** If the signs and symptoms described here appear, the condition is called **tetany.** Causes include parathyroid deficiency, **alkalosis**, and (in infants) vitamin D deficiency (see Chapter 7).

Parathyroid deficiency has been caused by accidental removal of the parathyroid glands during thyroidectomy but more commonly is caused by edema following thyroid surgery or by thyroid disease. Of 170 clients undergoing total thyroidectomy, 41 developed transient and 2 developed permanent hypoparathyroidism. Measuring intact parathyroid hormone levels 24 hours after surgery plus serum calcium levels on the second postoperative day were found to be the best predictors of postoperative hypoparathyroidism (Asari et al., 2008).

In **alkalosis,** because of the excessive alkalinity of body fluids, a greater number of calcium ions than usual are bound to serum proteins, effectively inactivating calcium and impairing nerve and muscle function. (See Acid–Base Balance later in this chapter.) Alkalosis may be caused by:

- Losing acid (due to vomiting or gastric suction)
- Ingesting alkalis (e.g., sodium bicarbonate)
- Breathing too rapidly, either in response to fear or through mechanical ventilation

The result of rapid breathing is excessive loss of carbon dioxide. In the blood, carbon dioxide is transported as carbonic acid. Thus, when too much carbon dioxide is exhaled, the alkalinity of the blood increases and produces tetany.

Early symptoms of tetany are:

- Nervousness
- Irritability
- Numbness
- Tingling of the extremities and around the mouth
- Muscle cramps

Diagnostic signs of tetany are Trousseau's sign and Chvostek's sign.

In **Trousseau's sign,** inflation of the blood pressure cuff above systolic pressure for 3 minutes causes ischemia of the peripheral nerves, increasing their excitability.

In **Chvostek's sign,** a tap over the facial nerve in front of the ear causes a twitch of the facial muscles on that side. Figure 8-6 depicts these diagnostic signs.

Because of the many functions of calcium, tetany is a medical emergency. Untreated, tetany can progress to:

- blood clotting irregularities,
- heart dilatation,
- respiratory paralysis,
- seizures, or
- coma.

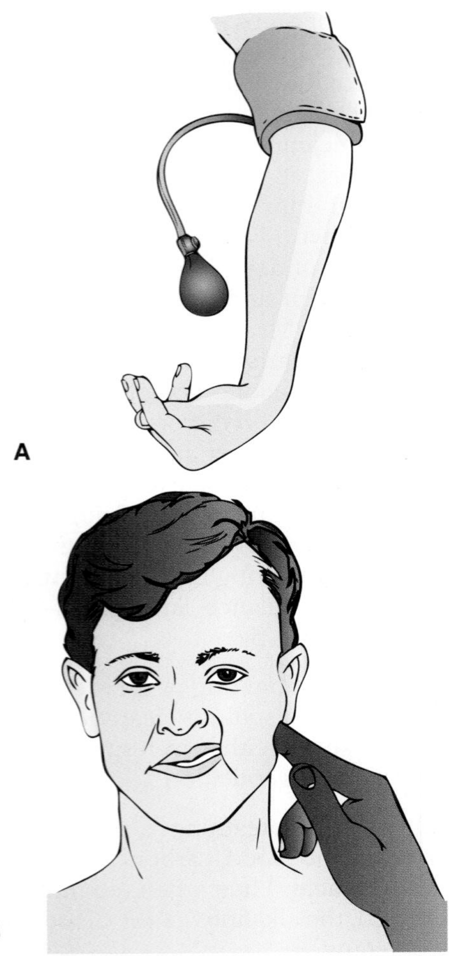

FIGURE 8-6 Indications of hypocalcemia. *A*, Positive Trousseau's sign. *B*, Positive Chvostek's sign. (Reprinted from Phillips, L: *Manual of I.V. therapeutics*, ed 4. FA Davis, Philadelphia, 2005, pp 128, 129, with permission.)

Toxicity

For basic information on mineral toxicity, see Table 8-4. A serum calcium level that is too high, above 11 milligrams per 100 milliliters of serum in adults, is called **hypercalcemia.** Kidney stones are not usually caused by dietary calcium but by malfunctioning kidneys that permit too much calcium to be spilled into the urine (Weaver and Heaney, 2006).

Milk-alkali syndrome, currently the third most common cause of hypercalcemia (Ulett, Wells, and Centor, 2010), was associated with the milk and cream antacid treatment of peptic ulcers common years ago. A recent resurgence in cases involved heart–lung transplant clients who received glucocorticoid immunosuppressive therapy and were given calcium carbonate to prevent peptic ulcer disease and osteoporosis. Other individuals with the syndrome include those taking glucocorticoids, postmenopausal women taking calcium carbonate to prevent osteoporosis, and a pregnant woman self-medicating with antacid tablets for dyspepsia (Bailey et al., 2008).

These cases emphasize the importance of carefully taking a client's dietary and medication history as well as teaching a client about over-the-counter and prescription medications. Early diagnosis of milk-alkali syndrome could limit permanent kidney dysfunction (Beall et al., 2006).

Phosphorus

Phosphorus occurs in bones and teeth as calcium phosphate. The body of a 154-pound man contains about 700 grams of phosphorus—85% in bone,

TABLE 8-4 ■ Mineral Toxicities

	SIGNS AND SYMPTOMS	NUTRITIONAL CAUSES	ASSOCIATED CONDITIONS
Calcium	Calcium deposits in the soft tissues of the body	Almost never	Hyperparathyroidism Vitamin D poisoning (most frequent in infants) Antacids Milk alkali syndrome
Phosphorus	Calcifications in soft tissue	Dietary overload unusual Occurred in infants during the first few weeks of life from diet consisting solely of cow's milk	Overmedication with vitamin D Phospholipids in TPN (Knochel, 2006).
Sodium	Sodium balance important for people with hypertension, heart disease, or kidney disease (Chapters 18, 19)	Healthy people excrete excess sodium without immediate adverse effects except in salt-sensitive individuals.	Long-range adverse effects due to calcium loss
Potassium	Hyperkalemia (Table 8-7)	Rarely caused by excessive dietary intake Intravenous potassium should be given only to clients excreting urine.	Diabetic acidosis Kidney failure Adrenal insufficiency Severe dehydration Transfusion with old blood (Clinical Application 8-5)

TABLE 8-4 ■ Mineral Toxicities (Continued)

	SIGNS AND SYMPTOMS	NUTRITIONAL CAUSES	ASSOCIATED CONDITIONS
Magnesium	Hypotension Nausea Vomiting Lethargy Confusion Slow pulse Depressed respirations Loss of patellar reflex	Not ordinarily seen	Kidney disease
Sulfur			Environmental causes such as air pollution with sulfur dioxide (Komarnisky, Christopherson, and Basu, 2003).
Iron	Accumulated mineral damages tissues	Most people at little risk of iron toxicity from diet	Iron metabolism disorders Chronic alcoholism Iron poisoning can be fatal.
Iodine	Burning of mouth, throat, and stomach Nausea Vomiting Diarrhea Fever Hypothyroidism, Hyperthyroidism, Thyroiditis.	Japanese infants: Congenital hypothyroidism due to large amounts of seaweed consumed by their mothers during pregnancy (Nishiyama et al., 2004)	
Fluoride	Mottled, discolored but sound teeth	Drinking water with a fluoride concentration of 2 parts per million Overuse, swallowing of fluoridated dental products	Fluorosis in children up to 8 years of age
	Bone and kidney dysfunction	Drinking water with a fluoride concentration of 4 parts per million	Increased dental caries
Zinc	Gastric problems Suppression of immune response Decrease in high-density lipoprotein (HDL) cholesterol (King and Cousins, 2006).	Supplemental doses three times the RDA can interfere with copper absorption leading to copper deficiency (Gropper, Smith, and Groff, 2009).	
Copper	Accumulation of copper in the liver, kidneys, brain, and cornea of the eye.	Consuming acidic foods stored in copper vessels Infants fed water high in copper	Clients treated with an artificial kidney that used copper tubing Wilson's disease
Selenium	Fatigue Nausea Vomiting Diarrhea Nail and hair brittleness and loss (Gropper, Smith, and Groff, 2009).	Persons overdosing with supplements	Miners
Chromium	Disagreeable metallic taste	Contaminated foods	Inhalation of chromium in an industrial setting. Stainless steel welding may be the most common source of this contamination (Stoecker, 2006).
Manganese	Signs/symptoms similar to Parkinson's disease Monotone voice Neurological abnormalities.	Parenteral nutrition, especially in neonates	Decreased liver function Cholestasis Miners exposed to manganese dust Welders exposed to manganese fumes
Molybdenum	Gout-like symptoms (Gropper, Smith, and Groff, 2009).	Eating food from regions with high levels in the soil	

14% in soft tissue, and 1% in body fluids (Gropper, Smith, and Groff, 2009). Phosphorus is closely associated with calcium in both foods and interrelated metabolic body functions. See Clinical Application 8-4 for information on phosphorus intake and calcium balance.

Phosphorus is a component of DNA and RNA. The storage forms of energy, **adenosine diphosphate (ADP)** and **adenosine triphosphate (ATP),** contain phosphorus. Phosphorus is an essential mineral in **phospholipids,** which are structural components of cells. Lecithin, a part of cell membranes, and myelin, the insulating covering of many nerves, are phospholipids. Phosphorus is contained in almost all enzymes, and phosphorus compounds function as buffers to maintain the blood's pH as slightly alkaline.

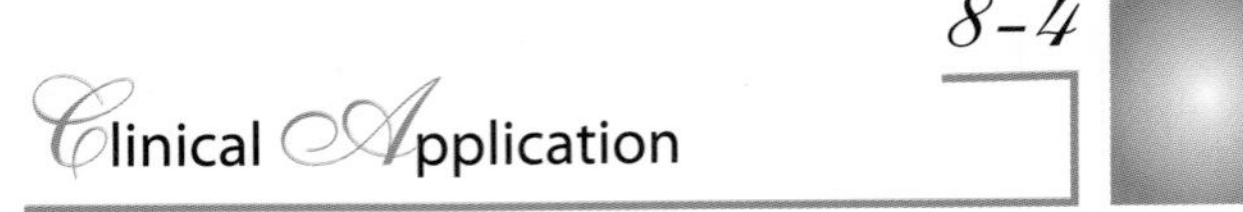

8-4

Clinical Application

Phosphorus Intake and Calcium Balance

In the past, the ratio of calcium to phosphorus was considered crucial to proper calcium balance. Now authorities think that the calcium-to-phosphorus ratio is less important than an adequate calcium intake for adults; however, authorities still think infants and children need correctly balanced intakes. Calcium to phosphorus ratios no less than 1.1 nor more than 2.0 are recommended for infant formulas. On the other hand, athletes and others with high energy expenditure often consume amounts of phosphorus greater than the UL with no apparent ill effects (Institute of Medicine, 2001).

Health authorities have expressed concern about cola beverages supplanting milk in the diets of young people. Unlike milk, in which the phosphate is balanced by calcium and vitamin D content, cola beverages contain phosphoric acid and no calcium. If insufficient calcium is available to neutralize phosphoric acid, the body will take calcium from the bones.

Control Mechanism

Between 50% and 70% of dietary phosphorus is absorbed primarily from the duodenum and jejunum. Vitamin D enhances absorption. Excessive intakes of aluminum, calcium, and magnesium inhibit it (Gropper, Smith, and Groff, 2009). Unabsorbed phosphorus is eliminated in the feces.

Low levels of serum phosphorus stimulate the kidney to produce more active vitamin D (calcitriol). Vitamin D increases the absorption of phosphorus from the intestinal tract and enhances phosphate resorption from the bones. In response to parathyroid hormone, the kidneys excrete excess phosphorus.

Dietary Reference Intakes and Sources

For DRIs see Appendix A. For food and other sources, see Table 8-1. To investigate the mineral content of a particular item, see the Internet site of the United States Department of Agriculture at http://www.nal.usda.gov/fnic/foodcomp/search/.

In many plants, much of the phosphorus is found as phytate which limits its bioavailability to 50%. Depending on a person's habits, cola beverages (that contain 25 to 40 milligrams of phosphorus in phosphoric acid) can contribute significantly to intake (Gropper, Smith, and Groff, 2009).

Deficiency

Although calcium and magnesium impair phosphorus absorption, deficiency is unlikely in healthy persons consuming a normal diet. Deficiency, however, has occurred in clients receiving total parenteral nutrition (TPN) with insufficient phosphorus.

In addition, certain medications or diseases can produce **hypophosphatemia.** For example, persons ingesting a diet low in phosphorus while also taking a phosphate-binding drug, such as the antacid aluminum hydroxide have experienced hypophosphatemia. These conditions have precipitated hypophosphatemia:

- Malabsorption disorders
- Severe burns
- Uncontrolled diabetes mellitus

Also, **refeeding syndrome,** a condition related to imbalances in phosphorus, occurs when wasted or starved clients are given nutrients in excess of what their bodies can handle (see Chapter 22).

In the client with alcoholism, the clinical picture of severe hypophosphatemia could be mistaken for Wernicke's encephalopathy or delirium tremens because the client may suffer from hallucinations (Knochel, 2006).

Hyperparathyroidism is a disease causing excess excretion of phosphorus. In this disease, parathyroid hormone causes withdrawal of calcium from the bones. Because the two minerals, calcium and phosphorus, are combined in the bones, phosphorus is lost along with calcium. Chronic kidney disease often produces the same result.

Reflecting the wide distribution and functions of phosphorus in the body, deficiency affects many organs and systems. Signs and symptoms of hypophosphatemia include:

- Impaired growth
- Osteomalacia
- Proximal muscle atrophy and weakness
- Cardiac arrhythmias
- Respiratory insufficiency
- Nervous system disorders (Knochel, 2006).

Toxicity

For basic information on mineral toxicity, see Table 8-4. Decreased renal excretion of phosphorus is the most common cause of **hyperphosphatemia**.

The Food and Drug Administration has posted a warning regarding oral sodium phosphate bowel cleansing products that caused acute renal failure in 22 clients who used these products. Increased risk of this acute phosphate nephropathy occurs in individuals:

- Of advanced age
- With kidney disease or decreased intravascular volume
- Using medicines that affect renal perfusion or function

- Possibly those medicated with nonsteroidal anti-inflammatory drugs (U.S. Food and Drug Administration [FDA], 2006b).

Previous cases of hyperphosphatemia causing serious neurological damage were attributed to sodium phosphate bowel cleansing products administered rectally to individuals with bowel diseases. Clients with conditions that increase the permeability of the intestine are at special risk when using these ordinarily harmless products.

Sodium

The body of a 154-pound adult contains about 105 grams (3.5 ounces) of sodium. Approximately 70% of the sodium in the body is in the blood and other extracellular fluids and in nerve and muscle tissue. The other 30% is on the surface of the bone crystals where it is available for release to counteract a low serum sodium level (Gropper, Smith, and Groff, 2009).

Sodium, which has a major role in maintaining fluid balance in the body, is also necessary for the transmission of electrochemical impulses along nerve and muscle membranes and is a component of two phosphate buffers.

The intestine readily absorbs sodium. At most, 5% of dietary sodium travels within the intestine to remain in the feces. All the remaining 95% of ingested sodium is absorbed into the bloodstream. To maintain a normal level of sodium in the blood, the kidney either reabsorbs sodium and returns it to the bloodstream or allows it to be spilled in the urine. A hormone from the adrenal cortex, **aldosterone,** stimulates the kidney to return sodium to the bloodstream. (See the section on Water Balance.)

Dietary Reference Intakes and Sources

For DRIs see Table 8-5. For food and other sources, see Table 8-1. To investigate the mineral content of a particular item, see "Nutritive Values of Foods" on DavisPlus.

Table salt, the major dietary source of sodium, is 40% sodium and 60% chloride. One teaspoonful (5 grams) of salt contains about 2 grams of sodium, nearly the UL. Many foods, such as milk, milk products, and several vegetables, are naturally high in sodium.

Most dietary sodium is derived from the salt or sodium-containing additives in processed foods, despite the fact that salt is not so crucial to maintaining year-round food stocks as it was years ago, when, for instance, meat was salted to preserve it. Table 8-6 compares the sodium content of relatively unprocessed foods with processed versions.

Deficiency

Sodium deficiency is typically caused by increased sodium loss from:

- Diarrhea
- Vomiting
- Heavy sweating
- Kidney disease

TABLE 8-5 ■ DRIs for Sodium, Potassium, Chloride, and Water

	SODIUM	POTASSIUM	CHLORIDE	WATER, TEMPERATE CLIMATES
AI Younger Adults	1.5 grams*	4.7 grams	2.3 grams	3.7 liters, men 19–30 years 2.7 liters, women 19–30 years
AI Ages 50–70 Years	1.3 grams	4.7 grams	2.0 grams	
AI Ages 71 and Older	1.2 grams	4.7 grams	1.8 grams	
UL	2.3 grams, adults†	Not established		

*Does not apply to highly active such as endurance athletes.
†May be lower for salt-sensitive individuals and higher for unacclimatized individuals exercising in a hot environment (Institute of Medicine, 2004a).

TABLE 8-6 ■ Comparison of Sodium Content in Fresh and Processed Foods

FRESH FOOD	SODIUM (MG)	PROCESSED FOOD	SODIUM (MG)
Natural Swiss cheese, 1 oz	74	Pasteurized, processed Swiss cheese, 1 oz	388
Lean roast pork, 3 oz	65	Lean ham, 3 oz	930
Whole raw carrot, 1	25	Canned carrots, ½ cup	176
Tomato juice, canned without salt, 1 cup	24	Tomato juice, canned with salt, 1 cup	881

Hyponatremia is the technical name for low serum sodium, less than 135 **milliequivalents** per liter in adults. Low serum sodium because of excess retained water, is called **dilutional hyponatremia.**

To convert milligrams to milliequivalents, see Clinical Calculation 8-1.

The organ most sensitive to hyponatremia is the brain (Yool, 2007), the impairment of which is evident in the signs and symptoms listed in Table 8-7. Too rapid correction of hyponatremia presents a risk of *osmotic demyelinating disease* causing motor nerve dysfunction including quadriplegia (Oh and Uribarri, 2006).

Toxicity

For basic information on mineral toxicity, see Table 8-4. The reported 4 to 6 grams of sodium in the average American diet is probably an underestimate. Frequently such surveys do not account for all sources of sodium.

An excess of sodium in the blood, greater than 145 milliequivalents per liter in adults, is called **hypernatremia.** Its signs and symptoms appear in Table 8-7.

Electrolyte Imbalances

Table 8-7 lists the normal values for serum sodium and serum potassium, along with the technical names and some of the signs and symptoms for deviations from normal. Many other signs, including the direct measurement of serum electrolytes and the results of electrocardiograms, assist in diagnosis. Dire consequences can result from any of these four imbalances. If the nurse recognizes and reports early signs and symptoms, the need for drastic treatment measures may be averted.

Potassium

The body of a 154-pound adult contains about 245 grams of potassium, approximately 8 ounces. Over 85% of ingested potassium is absorbed from the small intestine and possibly the colon (Gropper, Smith, and Groff, 2009). From 95 to 98% of the body's potassium is inside the cells, where it helps to control fluid balance.

In addition to fluid balance, potassium is essential for the conduction of nerve impulses and the contraction of muscles, including the heart. Potassium also helps maintain the body's **electrolyte** and acid–base balance. The potassium in fruits and vegetables, but not in supplements or food additives, acts to neutralize diet-derived acids in high-protein foods and thus prevents bone demineralization. Increased bone turnover and kidney stones are adverse consequences of bone titration of excess diet-derived acids (Institute of Medicine, 2004b).

The kidney responds to systemic alkalosis by excreting potassium to conserve hydrogen. Retaining the hydrogen will make the blood more acidic and help to correct the alkalosis. Conversely, in **acidosis**, the body responds by excreting hydrogen and retaining potassium. Similarly, when aldosterone stimulates the kidney to retain sodium, potassium is excreted to maintain electrolyte balance.

Dietary Reference Intakes

For DRIs see Table 8-5. For food and other sources, see Table 8-1. To investigate the mineral content of a particular item, see "Nutritive Values of Foods" on DavisPlus.

Clinical Calculation 8-1

Converting Milligrams to Milliequivalents

Milligram is a measure of weight. Milliequivalent is a measure of the concentration of electrolytes (number of particles) per volume of solution. The concentration of electrolytes in any given solution determines its chemical activity.

Electrolytes are expressed as milliequivalents per liter of solution whether referring to blood values or intravenous solutions.

To convert milligrams to milliequivalents, it is necessary to know the number of milligrams per liter, the molecular weight of the substance, and its valence. Valence, a number indicating the combining power of an atom, is found in many dictionaries.

A teaspoonful of table salt in 1 L of water will produce a 0.5% solution. A teaspoonful is roughly 5 g. Since table salt is 40% sodium and 60% chloride, the liter of 0.5% salt water would contain 2 g (2000 mg) of sodium and 3 g (3000 mg) of chloride.

Two other values are needed: atomic or molecular weights, and valences. The atomic weight for sodium is 22.9898. Sodium has a valence of 1. The formula for converting milligrams to milliequivalents is:

$$\text{mEq/L} = \frac{(\text{mg/L}) \times \text{valence}}{\text{molecular weight}} = \frac{2000 \times 1}{22.9898} = 87 \text{ mEq/L of sodium}$$

Continuing, we can use the same formula with different values to calculate the milliequivalents of chloride. The atomic weight for chlorine is 35.453. Chlorine has a valence of 1.

Filling in the values for chloride, we have:

$$\text{mEq/L} = \frac{(\text{mg/L}) \times \text{valence}}{\text{molecular weight}} = \frac{3000 \times 1}{35.453} = 85 \text{ mEq/L of chloride}$$

Then, adding the sodium and chloride, we have:

$$87 + 85 = 172 \text{ mEq/L in the 0.5-percent solution.}$$

TABLE 8-7 ■ Signs and Symptoms of Abnormal Serum Sodium and Potassium Levels

	LOW	NORMAL	HIGH
Sodium			
Lab value	Less than 135 mEq/L	135–148 mEq/L	Greater than 148 mEq/L
Condition	Hyponatremia		Hypernatremia
Symptoms	Irritability Anxiety		Thirst Fatigue
Signs	Muscle twitching Fingerprinting over the sternum Seizures Coma Permanent neurological damage Respiratory arrest		Flushed skin Sticky mucous membranes Agitation Coma
Potassium			
Lab value	Less than 3.5 mEq/L	3.5–5.0 mEq/L	Greater than 5.0 mEq/L
Condition	Hypokalemia		Hyperkalemia
Symptoms	Nausea and/or vomiting Paresthesias, especially lower extremities Disorientation		Irritability Abdominal cramps
Signs	Decreased bowel sounds Diminished reflexes Muscle weakness Weak, irregular pulse Coma		Weakness, especially lower extremities Irregular pulse Characteristic electrocardiograph changes Cardiac arrest

Sources of Potassium

Potassium is present in all plant and animal cells but the best sources are unprocessed foods. Only fats, oils, and white sugar have negligible amounts of potassium. (See Table 8-1.) Dietary instructions may focus on fruit sources because the client might also need to limit sodium which occurs in greater amounts in vegetables and dairy products than in fruits. Potassium might also be obtained from salt substitutes that often replace the sodium with potassium.

Deficiency

A potassium deficiency is related to diet only in cases of severe protein-energy malnutrition. **Hypokalemia,** a serum potassium less than 3.5 milliequivalents per liter, can be fatal if prolonged or severe. Hypokalemia may be caused by:

- Increased losses in urine, stool, or sweat (cystic fibrosis, see Chapter 20)
- Alkalosis
- Overhydration with plain water by perspiring athletes

For signs and symptoms, see Table 8-7.

Toxicity

For basic information on mineral toxicity, see Table 8-4. A potassium level greater than 5.0 milliequivalents per liter is hyperkalemia. Signs and symptoms of hyperkalemia appear in Table 8-7.

Hyperkalemia may also be caused by excessive destruction of cells in burns, crushing injuries, or severe infections. No symptoms may be apparent until blood levels of potassium are very high and skeletal muscle weakness is seen. One adverse effect of blood transfusion with old blood is elevated serum potassium or hyperkalemia. Clinical Application 8-5 covers that possibility.

Magnesium

The body of a 154-pound adult contains about 35 grams (1.2 ounces) of magnesium. About 55 to 60% of the magnesium is in bone, 20 to 25% in soft tissue, and 1% in body fluids (Gropper, Smith, and Groff, 2009).

Absorption, Elimination, and Functions

Magnesium is absorbed throughout the small intestine, mostly in the distal jejunum and ileum and may be absorbed from the colon if disease has impaired small intestine absorption. Of usual intakes, from 40% to 60% is absorbed, but a smaller percentage is absorbed at high intakes and a larger percentage at low intakes.

Excess magnesium is eliminated by the kidneys. Such excretion can be increased by protein, alcohol,

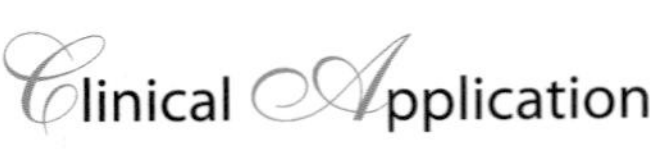
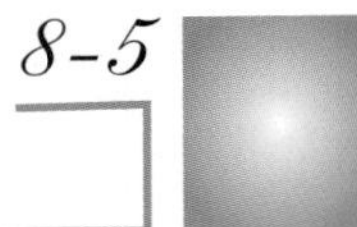

8-5 Clinical Application

Hyperkalemia After Blood Transfusion

Red blood cells do not live as long in the blood bank as they do in the human body. Potassium is the major cation in red blood cells (intracellular). When the red blood cells die and their cell walls rupture, potassium is spilled into the serum.

Blood that has been stored for a prolonged period may contain up to 30 mEq per liter of potassium due to the destruction of the red blood cells. This may not sound like a large amount, but potassium is usually administered intravenously at a concentration of 40 mEq per liter to a person who is potassium depleted. The person receiving a blood transfusion may have a serum potassium level that is nearly normal, and the old blood containing a higher concentration of potassium may push him or her into hyperkalemia. The nurse should be aware of the age of blood products and identify clients at risk of hyperkalemia.

and caffeine consumption (Gropper, Smith, and Groff, 2009).

Magnesium is involved in more than 300 essential metabolic reactions. It is associated with ADP and ATP in energy metabolism. Magnesium is involved in DNA synthesis and degradation, in protein synthesis, and insulin action. It influences cardiac and smooth muscle contractility directly and through calcium utilization (Gropper, Smith, and Groff, 2009).

Dietary Reference Intakes and Sources

For DRIs see Appendix A. For food and other sources, see Table 8-1. To investigate the mineral content of a particular item, see the Internet site of the United States Department of Agriculture at http://www.nal.usda.gov/fnic/foodcomp/search/.

Magnesium is widely distributed in foods, especially plant foods, because it is part of the chlorophyll molecule. Removing the germ and outer layers of the wheat kernel can remove 80% of its magnesium content. Beverages such as coffee, tea, and cocoa are also rich in magnesium (Gropper, Smith, and Groff, 2009).

Interfering Factors and Deficiency

Calcium and phosphorus can inhibit magnesium absorption especially when magnesium intake is low and that of the other minerals is high. Pure magnesium deficiency from inadequate dietary intake has not been reported.

Diabetes mellitus is commonly associated with magnesium deficiency, presumably due to renal losses, and several studies have identified deficiencies in acutely or chronically ill clients (Rude and Shils, 2006). Deficiency may also result from:

- Excessive vomiting or diarrhea
- Protein malnutrition
- Diuretic therapy (Gropper, Smith, and Groff, 2009)

Insufficient magnesium impairs central nervous system activity and increases muscular excitability. Magnesium deficiency may exacerbate the increased neuroirritability in cases of acute alcohol withdrawal. Although the value of magnesium in preventing migraine headaches is low, its lack of severe adverse effects makes it a good treatment option particularly during pregnancy (Schurks, Diener, and Goadsby, 2008). Chapter 10 has more information on magnesium and eclampsia.

Because magnesium metabolism is intricately linked to calcium metabolism, magnesium-deficient clients display the signs of tetany. Other signs include:

- Personality changes
- Anorexia
- Nausea
- Vomiting (Heimburger, McLaren, and Shils, 2006).

Toxicity

For basic information on mineral toxicity, see Table 8-4. Ordinarily, magnesium levels do not build up in the blood except as a result of kidney disease. In fact, oral magnesium can cause diarrhea—Epsom salt is magnesium sulfate.

Because of magnesium's close link to calcium, the effects of magnesium toxicity can be blocked by administering calcium.

Sulfur

The adult body contains approximately 175 grams of sulfur, a component of the cytoplasm of every cell. Sulfur is especially notable in hair, skin, and nails where it contributes to their shape. Sulfur is a component of thiamin, biotin, insulin, and heparin and of the amino acids methionine and cysteine. A protective function of sulfur is that of combining with toxins to neutralize them.

The major source of sulfate for humans is provided through the amino acid pool (see Fig. 5–2) by catabolism of the sulfur-containing amino acids methionine and cysteine. Dietary intake of foods containing these amino acids helps to replenish the supply. See Table 8-1. Cases of deficiency of sulfur alone are unknown. Only people with a severe protein deficiency lack this mineral. *For basic information on mineral toxicity, see Table 8-4.*

Chloride

Chloride plays a major role in maintaining fluid balance and acid–base balance. The body of a 154-pound adult contains approximately 105 grams of chloride. Of the body's chloride, 88% is found in extracellular fluids such as the hydro*chloric* acid in the stomach and 12% is found in intracellular fluids. Chloride also is released by white blood cells as they fight substances foreign to the body. Chloride is almost completely absorbed through the small intestine and is excreted primarily by the kidney as a result of sodium regulation (Gropper, Smith, and Groff, 2009).

For DRIs see Table 8-5. For food and other sources, see Table 8-1.

The DRI levels were established proportionate to the AI for sodium because nearly all dietary chloride is derived from salt. Table salt, which is 60% chloride, contains about 3 grams of chloride per teaspoon (5 grams).

Normally, most chloride is excreted by the kidney; however, loss of gastrointestinal fluids through severe vomiting, nasogastric suctioning, or diarrhea is a common cause of chloride deficiency. Chloride deficiency has occurred in infants because chloride was omitted from their formulas. Long-term sequelae in some of these children included cognitive impairments, visual–motor difficulties, and attention deficit disorder (Kaleita, Kinsbourne, and Menkes, 1991).

Sodium and chlorine are so chemically active that in nature they are always found bound to each other or to other elements. Table salt is a compound of sodium (an unstable, silvery white, waxy, soft metal) and chlorine (a greenish yellow poisonous gas). See Box 8-1.

Trace Minerals

Many trace minerals occur in such small amounts that they are difficult to measure and analyze; thus, their physiological functions and possible roles in nutrition are not completely understood.

Ten trace minerals have well-known bodily functions, and nine of them have been assigned RDAs or AIs. Four of them are commonly recognized for their relationship to health:

1. Iron
2. Iodine
3. Fluoride
4. Zinc

Box 8-1 ■ *Elementary Chemistry*

An element is a primary, simple substance that cannot be broken down by ordinary chemical methods into any other substance. Oxygen is an element, as are sodium, chlorine, and the other minerals considered earlier.

Atoms

Elements are composed of smaller parts called atoms. In the center of an atom is the nucleus, which contains protons and neutrons and gives an atom its weight and mass. Circling around the nucleus like satellites are electrons. These electrons are arranged in a consistent manner: a maximum of two in the orbit or shell closest to the nucleus, and a maximum of eight in each of the outer shells. The ability of an atom to react chemically depends on the number of "empty slots" in the outermost electron shell.

Chemical Bonding

A compound is a substance created by the chemical bonding (joining) of two or more different kinds of atoms (elements). A chemical bond is the force that binds atoms together. A compound is formed when atoms share electrons or when one atom donates one or more electrons to another atom. For example, water (a liquid) is formed when two atoms of hydrogen (a colorless, odorless gas) are joined with one atom of oxygen (another colorless, odorless gas), hence the abbreviation H_2O.

A sodium atom has only one electron in its outer shell; a chlorine atom has seven. In close proximity, the sodium atom donates the electron in its outer shell to the outer shell of the chlorine atom. With the loss of its electron, the sodium now has an electrical charge of +1 and is called a sodium ion (Na^+). Ions with positive charges are referred to as cations. The chlorine atom, which gained an electron, now has a charge of −1 and is called a chloride ion (Cl^-). Ions with negative charges are referred to as anions.

Because these ions have opposite charges (+ and −), they are attracted to one another and unite, forming sodium chloride (NaCl). The chemical bond that holds the sodium and chloride ions together is called an **ionic bond.** Sodium can donate its single electron to other elements beside chlorine, and other elements can form ionic bonds as well. (See Fig. 8-7.)

Electrolytes

An **electrolyte** is an element or compound that, when dissolved in water, separates (dissociates) into ions capable of conducting an electrical current. These electrically charged particles are then available to take part in other chemical reactions. Clinical Application 8-6 gives examples of uses and hazards related to electrolytes in the body.

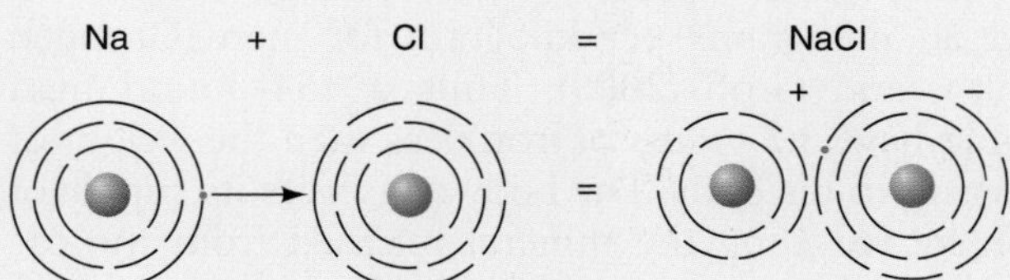

FIGURE 8-7 Formation of an ionic bond. An atom of sodium loses an electron to an atom of chlorine. The two ions formed have unlike charges, are attracted to one another, and form a molecule of sodium chloride. (Reprinted from Scanlon, VC, and Sanders, T: *Essentials of anatomy and physiology*, ed 5. FA Davis, Philadelphia, 2007, p 26, with permission.)

8-6

Clinical Application

Diagnostic Uses and Potential Hazards of Electrolytes

Skin sensors attached to an electrocardiograph can trace the electrical activity of the heart. The resulting graphic record is called an **electrocardiogram (ECG)**. The machine's sensors on the skin can detect the electric current because blood is an electrolyte solution and thus capable of conducting electricity. The same principle applies to the use of an electroencephalograph, a device that traces brain-wave activity. The record obtained from this machine is called an **electroencephalogram (EEG)**.

The characteristics of electrolyte solutions that allow these machines to sense electrical activity can also be hazardous. A fluid-filled tube, such as a nasogastric tube or catheter, can conduct stray electricity from faulty electrical devices to the client's heart and could result in dysrhythmias. The electricity in the shock may be minuscule but enough to be fatal if it happens at the wrong time in the cardiac cycle. The health-care worker should be vigilant for defective electrical equipment, tagging it for repair and replacing it immediately.

The other six are:

1. Selenium
2. Chromium
3. Copper
4. Manganese
5. Cobalt
6. Molybdenum

Five additional trace minerals, termed ultratrace minerals, arsenic, boron, nickel, silicon, and vanadium, appear in the DRI tables, but RDAs or AIs are not determinable.

Iron

For a nutrient with functions as vital as those of iron, the amount in the body is very slight—approximately 38 milligrams per kilogram of body weight for women and 50 milligrams per kilogram for men (Gropper, Smith, and Groff, 2009). Thus a 154-pound man would have 3.5 grams of iron, less than the weight of a penny, in his body. The body conserves its supply of iron by recycling the mineral released from the catabolism of worn-out red blood cells.

Functions

Iron is essential to the formation of hemoglobin, the component of the red blood cell that transports approximately 98.5% of the oxygen in the blood. **Hemoglobin** is composed of **heme,** the nonprotein portion that contains iron, and globin, a simple protein.

Iron is also a component of **myoglobin,** a protein located in muscle tissue. Myoglobin stores oxygen within the muscle cells. When the body needs an immediate supply of oxygen, such as during strenuous exercise, myoglobin releases its stored oxygen.

Iron is also present in enzymes that support energy metabolism and the synthesis and catabolism of neurotransmitters. The iron content of parts of the brain is comparable to that in the liver and continues to increase until the third decade of life (Chitambar and Asok, 2006).

About 80% of the iron in a healthy body is available for carrying oxygen: hemoglobin contains 65%, myoglobin 10%, and iron-containing enzymes 3%. The remainder is stored. The main storage form of iron in the body is a protein–iron compound called **ferritin.** It is kept in the liver, spleen, and bone marrow for future use.

Absorption

The body tightly conserves its supply of iron. Dietary iron is absorbed throughout the small intestine, most efficiently in the duodenum. When red blood cells are destroyed after their usual life span of 120 days, their iron is stored for reuse. Once iron is absorbed, there is no effective mechanism for excreting the excess. Fortunately, under normal conditions, the body is selective about absorbing iron.

FACTORS AFFECTING AMOUNTS

As the body's need for iron increases, so does the proportion absorbed. In a healthy person, up to 15% of the iron in foods is absorbed whereas a person who is iron deficient may absorb as much as 35% (Gropper, Smith, and Groff, 2009).

The amount of dietary iron that is absorbed is determined by the amount of ferritin present in the intestinal mucosa. The iron obtained from ingested food is bound to a protein called **apoferritin** in the intestinal mucosa to form ferritin. When the total supply of apoferritin has been bound to iron, any additional iron in the gut is rejected and eliminated in the feces. Similarly, iron within the apoferritin that is not needed remains in the intestinal cell to be sloughed off and excreted in the feces (Gropper, Smith, and Groff, 2009).

Absorbed iron combines with a protein in the blood, **transferrin,** which transports iron to the bone marrow for hemoglobin synthesis, to the liver or spleen for storage, or to the body cells for use. Hemoglobin synthesis requires many other substances, including adequate protein and traces of copper, in addition to iron but the shortages most likely to impair synthesis of red blood cells are:

- Iron
- Cobalamin
- Folate (Chitambar and Asok, 2006)

FACTORS AFFECTING ABSORPTION RATES

Two types of iron are found naturally in food:

1. Heme iron
2. Nonheme iron

Heme iron is bound to the hemoglobin and myoglobin in meat, fish, and poultry. From 50% to 60% of the total iron in these animal sources is heme iron. Because heme iron is composed of **ferrous iron** (Fe^{2+}), it is rapidly transported and absorbed intact.

Nonheme iron is the other 40 to 50% of the total iron in meat, fish, and poultry, and all the iron in plant sources (Gropper, Smith, and Groff, 2009).

The absorption of nonheme iron is slow because it is closely bound to organic molecules in foods as **ferric iron** (Fe^{3+}). In the acidic medium of the stomach, oxygen is removed from ferric iron during a chemical reaction called reduction. The end product is ferrous iron, which is more soluble and bioavailable. See Figure 8-8 for an overview of the steps involved in the process of iron absorption.

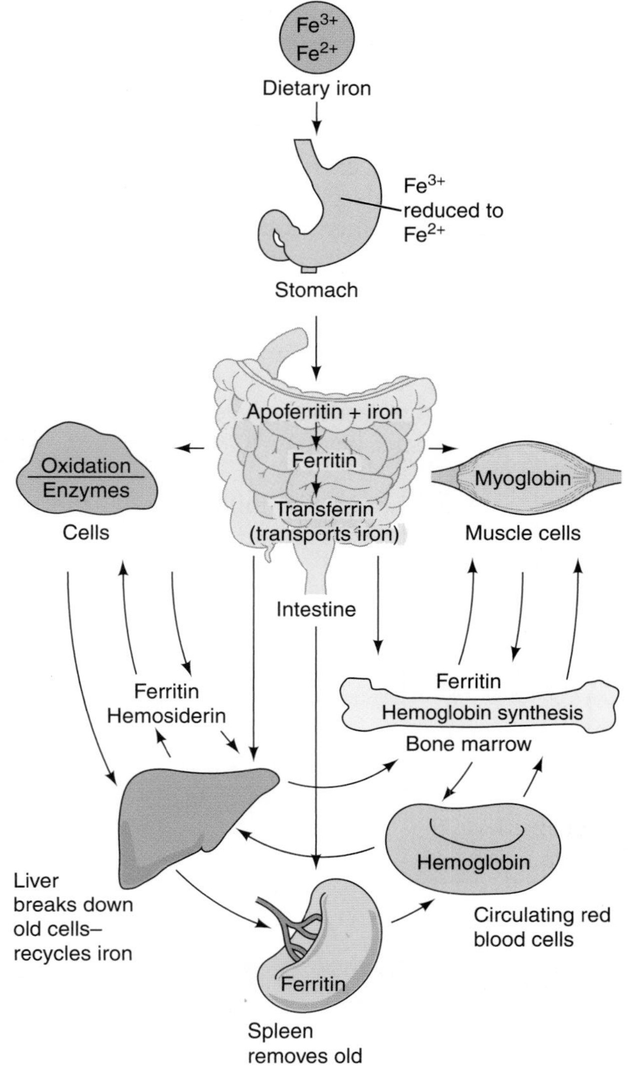

FIGURE 8-8 In the process of dietary iron absorption, iron is absorbed primarily in the small intestine and may be transported or stored to meet the body's needs.

FACTORS ENHANCING ABSORPTION

Several factors increase the absorption of iron through different mechanisms.

- Alcohol in large amounts damages the intestine, which then permits absorption of increased amounts of iron.
- Acids, such as ascorbic and citric, increase absorption by combining with the iron in a soluble compound, thus preventing formation of insoluble iron complexes.
- MFP Factor (meat, fish, poultry) increases the absorption of nonheme iron when meat, fish, or poultry is consumed at the same time.

FACTORS INTERFERING WITH ABSORPTION

Other minerals compete with iron for absorption.

- Calcium, in foods or in supplements, decreases iron absorption by up to 70% and excesses of zinc or manganese may also decrease iron absorption (Gropper, Smith, and Groff, 2009).
- Phytic acid from cereals (whole grains, legumes, and maize) forms insoluble complexes with iron.
- Oxalic acid from certain berries and vegetables (see the calcium section) combines with iron, reducing its availability.
- Decreased gastric acid, whether because of antacid medications or gastric resection, lessens the iron that is absorbed.
- Polyphenols found in coffee, tea, and cocoa and also in spinach can lock out nonheme from the absorption process (Chitambar and Asok, 2006), thus reducing iron absorption by over 60%. Coffee, taken with or just after a meal, may reduce iron absorption by 40% (Gropper, Smith, and Groff, 2009).

Table 8-8 summarizes the factors that affect iron absorption. People who consume vegetarian diets should be especially careful to construct optimal menus. Practical suggestions to enhance iron and zinc nutrition in vegetarian diets are given in Table 8-9.

Excretion

No known mechanism exists to regulate the excretion of iron. Small amounts of iron are lost daily via the gastrointestinal tract, shed skin cells, and urine even in healthy people. Certain medications and diseases increase the losses.

Physiologic status also influences iron loss. Postmenopausal women lose an average of 0.8 milligrams of iron per day, men about 1 milligram per day, whereas women of reproductive age lose an average of 1.3 to 1.4 milligrams per day (Gropper, Smith, and Groff, 2009).

Blood contains about 0.5 milligram of iron per milliliter, so a blood donor would lose 250 milligrams per unit donated (Wood and Ronnenberg, 2006). Someone who donates every 2 months, then, would have to replace iron at the rate of 4 milligrams per day over and above the RDA all year long.

TABLE 8-8 ■ Factors Affecting Iron Absorption

INCREASE	DECREASE
Large alcohol intake	Phytic or oxalic acids
Meat, fish, or poultry	Coffee or tea (tannins)
Vitamin C	Less gastric acid, antacids Calcium and zinc

Dietary Reference Intakes

For DRIs see Appendix A. For food and other sources, see Table 8-10. To investigate the mineral content of a particular item, see "Nutritive Values of Foods" on DavisPlus.

Two groups need increased amounts of iron: people participating in intense physical exercise and vegetarians. Those who exercise strenuously on a regular basis require an estimated 30% to 70% more iron than baseline (Wood and Ronnenberg, 2006). Because the authors of the RDAs assume that 75% of iron intake is derived from heme iron sources, they suggest that vegetarians double the RDA amounts (Institute of Medicine, 2001).

Sources

The Western diet contains an estimated 5 to 7 milligrams of iron per 1000 kilocalories. In the United States, one-third of dietary iron is supplied by grains, one-third by meats, and one-third by other sources. Absorption also varies among the sources of iron. Ten to 30% of iron is absorbed from liver and other meats; less than 10% is absorbed from eggs; and less than 5% is absorbed from grains and most vegetables.

TABLE 8-9 ■ Improving Iron and Zinc Nutrition In Vegetarian Diets

GOAL	STRATEGY	RATIONALE
Increase the total amount of iron and zinc consumed.	Select foods rich in iron and zinc at all meals. Consume cereals and pasta fortified with these nutrients.	Obtaining sufficient iron and zinc without animal products requires careful planning.
Make use of contamination iron.	Use cast iron cookware or steel woks for vegetable casseroles or curries, spaghetti sauces, or stewed fruits.	Moist, acidic foods have increased iron content when thus cooked for a long period. Even 20 minutes has shown an effect (Fairweather-Tait, Fox, and Mallilin, 1995).
Expand the intake of absorption enhancers.	Consume fermented foods such as yogurt and oriental soy products (tempeh, miso, natto, and soy sauce). Include a good source of vitamin C at every meal.	Certain organic acids (citric, lactic, malic, and tartaric) prevent the formation of insoluble iron and zinc phytates. Ascorbic acid is the most effective enhancer of nonheme iron absorption when consumed with the nonheme iron. It reduces ferric to ferrous iron that is more soluble at the pH of the duodenum and small intestine.
Reduce the intake of absorption antagonists.	Consumption of both sprouted whole-grain cereals and legumes and yeast-leavened baked products can potentially reduce the phytic acid content of a meal. Soak legumes before cooking. Delay drinking coffee and tea until at least 2 hours after meals.	Microbial fermentation can enhance bioavailability of iron and zinc via hydrolysis induced by microbial phytase enzymes derived from microflora on the surface of cereal grains or from yeast. Since phytic acid is relatively water soluble, soaking reduces the phytic acid of most legumes These beverages reduce nonheme iron absorption 40%–60%.
Avoid taking high doses of mineral supplements.	Dietary sources alone are unlikely to compromise iron and zinc status.	Antagonistic interactions between copper and zinc and between nonheme iron and zinc are most likely when high doses of supplemental zinc and nonheme iron are ingested without food.

SOURCE: Adapted primarily from Gibson, Donovan, and Heath (1997).

TABLE 8-10 ■ Trace Minerals

MINERAL	ADULT RDA/AI AND FOOD PORTION CONTAINING IT*	FUNCTIONS	SIGNS AND SYMPTOMS OF DEFICIENCY	SIGNS AND SYMPTOMS OF EXCESS	BEST SOURCES
Iron	8–18 mg (female) 8 mg (male) 3–6.8 oz Braunschweiger	Component of hemoglobin	Fatigue, lightheadedness Shortness of breath Hypochromic, microcytic anemia	Hemosiderosis Hemochromatosis	Liver, other red meats Clams Oysters Lima and navy beans Green leafy vegetables Dried fruit
Iodine	150 µg 0.3 tsp iodized salt	Component of thyroid hormones	Goiter Cretinism Myxedema	Acne-like lesions Goiter	Iodized salt Saltwater seafood
Fluoride	3–4 mg 3–4 L fluoridated water	Hardens teeth	Dental caries	Mottled teeth Increased caries	Fluoridated water Seafood Brewed tea
Zinc	8–11 mg 2.6–3.5 oz beef chuck roast, lean only	Component of 70 enzymes Involved in DNA and RNA synthesis Necessary for collagen formation Serves role in immunity	Growth failure Hypogonadism Delayed wound healing Impaired night vision Impaired taste Delayed sexual maturation	Copper deficiency Decreased HDL cholesterol Suppressed immune response	Red meat, especially organ meat Seafood, especially oysters Poultry Pork Dairy products
Copper	900 µg 1.5 oz lobster	Cofactor for enzymes involved in hemoglobin synthesis and cell respiration Necessary for melanin formation	Anemia Demineralization of skeleton Depigmentation of skin and hair Impaired immune function Menkes' disease	Copper deposits in liver, kidneys, brain, spleen, and cornea Wilson's disease	Organ meats Shellfish Nuts Seeds Dried fruit
Selenium	55 µg 0.5 oz oil-roasted mixed nuts	Part of many enzymes Necessary for iodine metabolism Reciprocal sparing relationship with vitamin E Protects against the toxicity from mercury, cadmium, and silver	Keshan cardiomyopathy	Sour milk or garlic breath odor Fatigue Nail and hair loss	Brazil nuts Organ meats Seafood Dairy products
Chromium	20–35 µg 0.6–1.1 egg yolks	Potentiates action of insulin	Weight loss Impaired glucose utilization Elevated blood lipids Peripheral neuropathy	Rarely related to food Metallic taste	Meats, especially organ meats Fish Poultry Whole grains
Manganese	1.8–2.3 mg 3–4 tsp blanched hazelnuts or filberts	Involved in amino acid and CHO metabolism Required for bone formation	Dermatitis Decreased growth of hair and nails Skeletal defects Changes in hair and beard color	Accumulated mineral in brain In miners: liver damage and Parkinson-like syndrome—monotone voice, CNS impairment	Whole grains Dried fruits Nuts Green, leafy vegetables
Cobalt	Not established	Component of vitamin B_{12}	Not reported		Meat Poultry Fish Shellfish Milk
Molybdenum	45 µg ¼ cup navy beans, cooked†	Cofactor for enzymes involved in catabolism of sulfur-containing amino acids and purines	TPN clients only: tachycardia, headache, mental disturbances, coma	Hyperuricemia Gout	Legumes Nuts Yogurt†

*Examples only; not suggested to be sole source of a day's intake.
†Nutrition Fact Sheet: Molybdenum.

Many foods are fortified with iron, but its bioavailability depends on the compounds used. If the added iron is elemental iron, very little can be absorbed (Wood and Ronnenberg, 2006). Iron from spinach, iron supplements, and contamination iron are absorbed at a 2% rate. Clinical Application 8-7 describes one way iron becomes available from nonfood sources.

Deficiency

Iron deficiency can be determined by laboratory tests such as plasma ferritin and transferrin saturation before a person's hemoglobin value drops sufficiently to diagnose anemia, in which iron stores are severely depleted (Gropper, Smith, and Groff, 2009). The anemic client often complains of lightheadedness, shortness of breath on exertion, and possibly soreness of mouth and tongue, and physical examination reveals pallor and probably an increased pulse rate. Iron-deficient children show reduced attention spans and poor learning that improves with iron therapy (Chitambar and Asok, 2006).

A person who is anemic has insufficient hemoglobin to provide oxygen to the cells of the body. The features of the red blood cells are characteristic of various anemias. In iron-deficiency anemia, the red blood cells are microcytic (smaller than normal) and hypochromic (contain less hemoglobin, giving the cell less color than normal).

RISK OF DEFICIENCY

In the United States, individuals at greatest risk of iron deficiency are 1- to 2-year old children and women of childbearing age (Wood and Ronnenberg, 2006) but **bariatric** surgical procedures that bypass the duodenum may lead to deficiency if supplements are not given (Heimburger, McLaren, and Shils, 2006). Other illnesses or treatments that increase gastrointestinal blood loss such as long-term use of nonsteroidal anti-inflammatory medications should be considered when assessing iron nutriture. More information on iron deficiency in pregnant women is included in Chapter 10. Iron deficiency in children appears in Chapter 11.

ASSESSMENT DATA

Although no single test is diagnostic for iron deficiency, a common test to determine the hemoglobin level of the blood delivers valuable assessment data. The normal level for men is 14 to 18 grams per 100 milliliters of blood; for women it is 12 to 16 grams. Another common laboratory test is the **hematocrit,** which measures the percentage of red blood cells in a volume of blood. Normal hematocrit levels are 40% to 54% for men and 36% to 46% for women. Persons living above 4000 feet in altitude will have higher normal values. Unfortunately, low hemoglobin and hematocrit levels are late indicators of iron deficiency.

In early iron deficiency, before hemoglobin and hematocrit readings drop, **serum transferrin** levels rise. The person with early iron deficiency will, providing the body is attempting to compensate, manufacture more transferrin to increase iron-carrying capacity. Similarly, serum ferritin is a good indicator of iron stores under most conditions but can be falsely high due to infection and inflammation (Wood and Ronnenberg, 2006).

TREATMENT

Iron is absorbed best when taken on an empty stomach, but gastrointestinal side effects often provoke noncompliance. Even taking the supplement with food or close to mealtime is better than not taking it at all. Accompanying the supplement with meat or vitamin C-rich foods and avoiding tea, milk, and cereals should increase absorption. Also, beginning at a lower dosage and then increasing it as tolerance develops is sometimes a useful strategy. Enteric coated preparations are available but may not dissolve until beyond the duodenum, where absorption is most effective. An increase in hemoglobin level of 1 gram per week would indicate successful treatment (Chitambar and Asok, 2006).

After a person has been treated for iron deficiency, iron therapy should be continued for several months after hemoglobin and hematocrit levels return to normal. This prolonged therapy will enable the body to rebuild iron stores.

In developing countries with high levels of infectious diseases, iron administration for anemia has been followed by increased morbidity from infections.

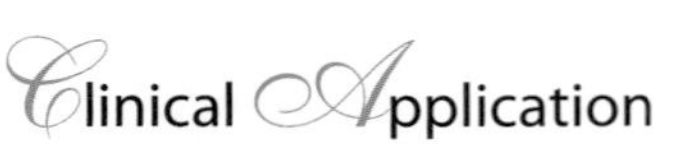

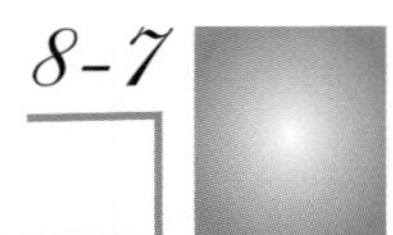

Contamination Iron

Cooking in iron pots can increase the iron content of foods. This source of dietary iron is called **contamination iron**. Significant transfer occurs during simmering of acidic foods, especially tomatoes. For instance, 3½ oz of spaghetti sauce cooked for 3 hours in a cast iron pot contains almost 90 mg of iron, compared to less than 5 mg of iron when cooked in a glass container (Zhou and Brittin, 1994). The East Indian practice of cooking curries in cast iron woks also was shown to increase iron content 4- to 12-fold (Fairweather-Tait, Fox, and Mallillin, 1995). The absorption rate of contamination iron is the same as that of supplements, 2%.

Bacteria also require iron, and when the body's supply increases, they thrive.

Toxicity

For basic information on mineral toxicity, see Table 8-4. Iron absorption is effectively controlled in healthy people even when meat intake is high and foods are fortified.

Surplus iron is stored in the liver as **hemosiderin**. When large amounts of hemosiderin are deposited in the liver and spleen, a condition called **hemosiderosis** results. If prolonged, it can lead to **hemochromatosis,** a disease of iron metabolism in which iron accumulates in and damages tissues. (See Genomic Gem 8-2.)

Genomic Gem 8-2
Hereditary Hemochromatosis

Although 5 of every 1000 persons of northern European descent are **homozygous** for this mutation, the phenotypic expression varies greatly. This autosomal recessive disease is associated with mutations in genes on chromosome 6 with resultant decreased cellular uptake of iron. As in sickle cell disease, substitutions of single incorrect amino acids are responsible for hereditary hemochromatosis. Depending upon the location of the substitution, the client may have a severe or not-so-severe illness, but once identified, his first degree relatives should be screened.

Classic symptoms include hepatomegaly, diabetes, and hyperpigmentation. Treatment involves regular removal of blood (200 to 250 milligrams of iron per unit) through phlebotomy until a satisfactory serum ferritin level is achieved. Dietary interventions can also be therapeutic:

- Avoid iron and vitamin C supplements, including multivitamin–multimineral preparations.
- Consume red or organ meats in moderation.
- Avoid alcohol.
- Do not consume raw shellfish lest it contain an organism *(Vibrio vulnificus)* that can cause fatal infections in persons with iron overload and cirrhosis (Chung, Misdraji, and Sahani, 2006).

Eventually organ failure may lead to cardiac failure and death. The disease is most common in males and typically becomes symptomatic around the age of 20 (Gropper, Smith, and Groff, 2009).

Clients with alcoholism, although often lacking many other nutrients, sometimes suffer from iron overload. Some alcoholic beverages themselves contain a significant amount of iron. For example, inexpensive red wines contain 10 to 350 milligrams of iron per liter.

Dietary iron overload is common in parts of sub-Saharan Africa. It results from the consumption of large volumes of beer home-brewed in iron pots or ungalvanized steel drums from which it acquired a high iron content. Such Zimbabwean beer contained 52 milligrams of iron per liter (Wood and Ronnenberg, 2006).

Toxicity from supplemental iron tablets is a major threat to children. The body's absorptive controls for dietary iron are circumvented by the large amounts of soluble iron in pharmaceutical preparations. In the United States, iron is the most common cause of accidental pediatric poisoning deaths in children younger than the age of 6 years. See Box 8-2.

Symptoms of acute iron poisoning can occur with doses of 20 to 60 milligrams per kilogram of body weight (Wood and Ronnenberg, 2006). Ferrous sulfate, the most commonly prescribed iron supplement, consists of 30% elemental iron so that minimal toxic dose could result from three and one-half 195-milligram tablets taken by a 22-pound child. Signs and symptoms begin with acute gastroenteritis within 6 hours of iron ingestion, followed by a latent period of up to 24 hours, then shock, seizures, and liver failure (*Merck Manual,* 2005).

The Consumer Product Safety Commission requires child-resistant packaging for iron preparations in certain forms and specified strengths, and the Food and Drug Administration requires a warning label on solid dosage forms of iron (FDA, 2003).

Iodine

In the human body, iodine usually is found and functions in its ionic form, iodide. The body of the average adult contains about 15 to 20 milligrams of iodide. The thyroid gland in the neck contains 70% to 80% of the total body iodide and takes up approximately

Box 8-2 ■ *Precautions to Prevent Medication Poisoning in Children*

Health-care providers should impress upon parents the enormous threat medications and supplements pose for small children. The products should be stored:

- Out of reach
- Out of sight
- With child-resistant caps intact

Adults should take medicines out of the child's view to avoid modeling a behavior that could harm the child.

If a child ingests any medication or supplement, a poison control center should be consulted ***immediately*** without waiting for signs and symptoms to appear.

120 micrograms of iodide per day (Gropper, Smith, and Groff, 2009).

Function and Control of the Thyroid Gland

The only known function of iodine is its participation in the synthesis of thyroid hormones, which are essential for proper maturation of the nervous system, particularly in utero and for the first few years after birth. Devastating consequences result from deficiency of iodine during those years. See Deficiency.

The thyroid gland secretes **thyroxine (T_4)** and **triiodothyronine (T_3)** in response to the **thyroid-stimulating hormone (TSH)** from the anterior pituitary gland. Both T_3 and T_4 increase the rate of oxidation in cells, thereby increasing the rate of metabolism. When serum levels of T_3 and T_4 are adequate, secretion of TSH ceases. This is called a **negative feedback cycle:** TSH stimulates T_4 and T_3 production until a sufficient level of those hormones stops the secretion of TSH; when T_4 and T_3 levels drop, more TSH is secreted.

Absorption and Excretion

Iodine is easily absorbed from all portions of the intestinal tract, including the stomach, and excreted by the kidneys, which have no mechanism to conserve iodine. After performing their functions, T_4 and T_3 are degraded by the liver, and the iodine content is excreted in bile. Some iodine is lost in sweat, which may be important in hot climates if intake is low (Gropper, Smith, and Groff, 2009).

Dietary Reference Intakes and Sources

For DRIs see Appendix A. For food and other sources, see Table 8-10.

Iodine can come from foods, either naturally present or fortified, or from incidental sources.

IN FOODS AND WATER

Foods that are naturally high in iodine include saltwater fish, shellfish, and seaweed. The iodine content in plants varies with the mineral content of the soil in which they are grown. Table salt fortified with iodine (100 micrograms of iodine in ¼ teaspoon of salt) has been available in the United States since 1924.

Iodine has antibacterial properties and is sometimes used to purify drinking water. If the region is also iodine deficient, the mineral in the water can serve both purposes (Dunn, 2006).

INCIDENTAL

Sometimes iodine is present as a side effect of processing. For example, iodine solutions can be used to sterilize milk pasteurization vats; some iodine may remain on the vat and be mixed into the next batch of milk to be processed. Iodine is also used to improve the texture of bread dough.

Deficiency

Because almost every country in the world has iodine deficient areas, an estimated 50% of the world's population is iodine deficient. Since the introduction of iodized salt, overt deficiency has been rarely encountered in North America even though most processed foods do not contain iodized salt (Dunn, 2006). At particular risk of deficiency are vegans who consume sea salt, which contains virtually no iodine because of processing methods.

An infant of a vegan mother was diagnosed with hypothyroidism soon after birth (Borak, 2005). Two lifelong residents of the United States developed iodine deficiency because they avoided iodized salt and seafood (Nyenwe and Dagogo-Jack, 2007). Diagnosis of thyroid malfunction can be readily evaluated by measuring protein-bound iodine and the serum levels of T_4 and T_3.

LOCAL EFFECTS

When the thyroid gland does not receive sufficient iodine, it increases in size, attempting to increase production. The gland may reach 1 to 1.5 pounds (about 500–700 grams). This enlargement of the thyroid is called **goiter** (see Fig. 8-9). Sometimes the gland may attain sufficient size to impede breathing or swallowing. Unfortunately, in rare cases, replacement of iodine does not reduce the goiter, especially after long-standing deficiency, so that surgery or radiotherapy may be needed.

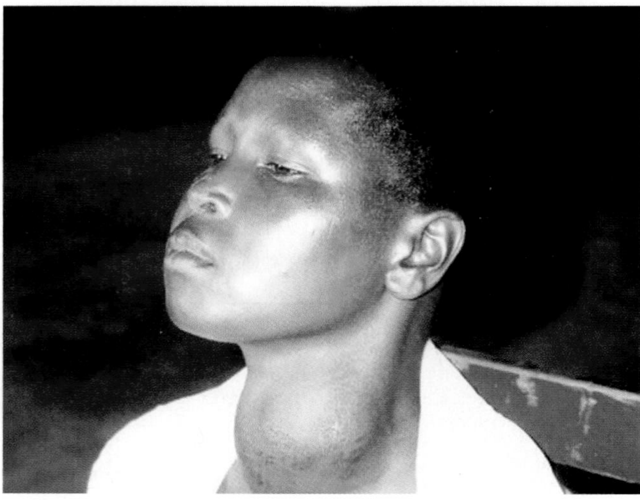

FIGURE 8-9 Woman with a goiter. (Reprinted from Kenya Medical Mission Web site, with permission.)

In some cases, prolonged iodine deficiency can short-circuit the negative feedback control system, resulting in thyroid nodules that produce T_3 and T_4 in response to dietary iodine rather than to TSH. Iodine given to these people may cause **hyperthyroidism** (Dunn, 2006).

Because of iodine-poor soil, the Great Lakes States and the Rocky Mountain States once were considered the "goiter belt." Now that food is distributed nationally and internationally and iodized salt is readily available, goiter is less common in this country. One case of goiter in a vegan woman and her newborn infant was reported in the United Kingdom (Shaikh et al., 2003).

In contrast, worldwide, 211 million people have goiter, and 1.6 billion people are at risk for iodine deficiency, particularly in mountainous areas or those with eroded soil. When a population's prevalence of goiter is 10% or more, it is termed **endemic** goiter (Gropper, Smith, and Groff, 2009).

SYSTEMIC EFFECTS

Severe **hypothyroidism** during pregnancy results in **cretinism** in the newborn. As a consequence of the mother's thyroid deficiency, the infant exhibits mental and physical retardation. Cretinism is a congenital condition (present at birth). Prevention focuses on diagnosing and treating iodine deficiency in pregnant women.

Hypothyroidism due to iodine deficiency occurring in older children and adults is called **myxedema.** In areas where salt fortification is difficult to implement, treatment may consist of iodized oil. If administered orally, it could suffice for a year, by injection for 3 or more years (Dunn, 2006).

Interfering Factors

Substances called **goitrogens** may block the body's utilization of iodine. Goitrogens found in vegetables belonging to the cabbage family, including cauliflower, broccoli, Brussels sprouts, rutabaga, and turnips, are unlikely to cause goiter because of the relatively small amounts consumed. The only food linked to goiter is cassava, a starchy root eaten in developing countries (recall konzo in Chapter 5). A metabolite of cassava prevents uptake of iodine by the thyroid.

Toxicity

For basic information on mineral toxicity, see Table 8-4. The lowest iodide intake level producing observable adverse effects is about 1700 micrograms per day.

Fluoride

In body fluids, fluorine exists as fluoride, a salt of hydrofluoric acid, or as an ion. About 99% of the body's fluoride accumulates as fluorapatite in bones and teeth. Fluoride seems to make bone mineral less soluble and hence less likely to be reabsorbed.

Nearly 100% of soluble fluoride found in fluoridated water and toothpaste is rapidly absorbed from the stomach and small intestine, but absorption diminishes to 50% to 80% when fluoride is consumed with solid foods or with calcium-containing beverages. Increased gastric secretion increases its rate of absorption, and aluminum hydroxide (an antacid) inhibits absorption. Approximately 90% of excess fluoride is rapidly excreted in urine, most of the remainder in feces, and only minor amounts in sweat (Gropper, Smith, and Groff, 2009).

Functions

In addition to its function in bone, fluoride in plaque and saliva inhibits demineralization and enhances remineralization of early carious lesions. Drinking fluoridated water and using fluoride toothpaste and other dental products can raise the concentration of fluoride in saliva 100- to 1000-fold for 1 to 2 hours (Centers for Disease Control and Prevention [CDC], 2001b). Adults as well as children can benefit from these interventions.

Dietary Reference Intakes and Sources

For DRIs see Appendix A. For food and other sources, see Table 8-10.

Food and beverages prepared with fluoridated water contain increased fluoride. Tea accumulates fluoride in the leaves so that brewed tea contains 1 to 6 milligrams per liter; decaffeinated varieties contain the larger quantities (Gropper, Smith, and Groff, 2009).

For children, recommendations for dietary supplements are based on the child's age and the concentration of fluoride in the child's drinking water (CDC, 2001b). See Chapter 11.

Water fluoridation is one of the 10 great public health achievements of the 20th century (CDC, 2008c). Nationally, the prevalence of any dental caries among children 12 to 17 years of age declined from 90% in 1971 to 1974 to 67% in 1988 to 1991, and the mean number of missing, decayed, or filled teeth fell from 6.2 to 2.8 (CDC, 2001b).

Fluoridated drinking water costs less than a dollar per person per year (DePaola et al., 2006). Recommended concentrations are 0.7 to 1.2 parts per million (ppm), depending on the average maximum daily air temperature of the area.

The U.S. Environmental Protection Agency (EPA), which is responsible for the safety and quality of drinking water in the United States, sets a maximum allowable limit for fluoride in community drinking water at 4 ppm (CDC, 2001b). A concentration of one part per million provides 1 milligram of fluoride per liter.

The goal for *Healthy People 2010* is to give 75% of people served by community water supplies access to optimally fluoridated water, a level that had been achieved by 25 states and the District of Columbia in 2006 (Fig. 8-10). Nationwide, in the same year, 69% of people served by community water systems received optimally fluoridated water (CDC, 2008c). Information on county and community water systems can be obtained at http://apps.nccd.cdc.gov/mwf/index.asp.

Concern has been raised that children consuming conditioned water or bottled water instead of fluoridated tap water would receive suboptimal amounts of fluoride. Steam distillation removes all the fluoride and reverse osmosis units remove 65 to 95%, but water softeners and charcoal/carbon filters generally do not remove significant fluoride from water (American Dental Association, 2003).

After the FDA approved a health claim for fluoridated bottled water containing 0.6 to 1.0 milligrams of fluoride per liter to read "Drinking fluoridated water may reduce the risk of dental caries or tooth decay," another concern regarding possible excessive intake arose. The FDA specifically states that the health claim is not intended for use on bottled water products specifically marketed for use by infants for whom lesser amounts of fluoride are appropriate (FDA, 2006a). The FDA health claim ruling was followed by new guidelines from the American Dental Association regarding the use of fluoridated water to reconstitute infant formulas (see Toxicity).

Toxicity

For basic information on mineral toxicity, see Table 8-4. Death may occur with intake as low as 5 milligrams of fluoride per kilogram of body weight (Gropper, Smith, and Groff, 2009).

The American Dental Association specifically recommends the following actions to avoid excessive fluoride in infants from birth to 1 year:

- Breastfeeding (Babies who are breastfed do not appear to exceed the optimal amount of fluoride).
- Using ready-to-feed formula with known quantities of fluoride.
- Consulting the physician or dentist, when using powdered or liquid concentrate infant formula, about the correct source of water to dilute the formula and whether the water should be sterilized to meet the infant's special medical needs (American Dental Association, 2006).

Because young children tend to swallow toothpaste, children who begin using fluoride toothpaste when younger than 2 years of age are at higher risk of enamel fluorosis than children who begin later or do not use fluoridated toothpaste (CDC, 2001b).

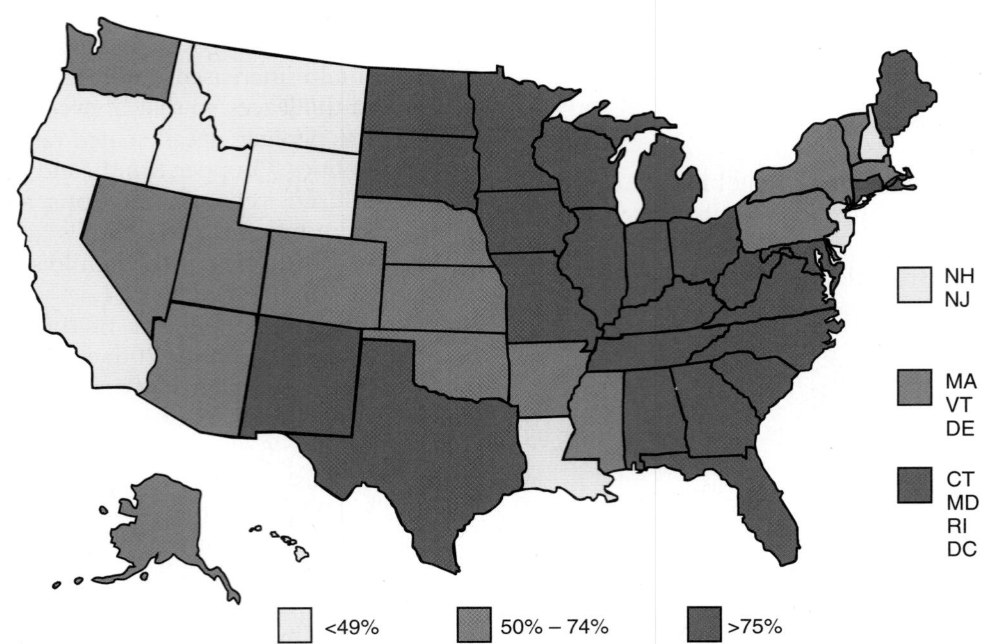

FIGURE 8-10 Percentage of state populations with access to fluoridated water through public water systems in the year 2006. (SOURCE: CDC, 2008b.)

Package labeling directs caregivers to limit the amount of fluoridated toothpaste for children younger than 6 years of age to "a pea-sized amount" and to consult a dentist or physician before using such toothpaste for a child younger than 2 years of age.

Zinc

Zinc in adult humans, 1.5 grams in women and 2.5 grams in men, is found in all body organs, primarily the liver, kidneys, muscle, skin, and bones. Zinc is incorporated into the structure of at least 70 and perhaps more than 200 enzymes.

One essential respiratory enzyme, *carbonic anhydrase*, catalyzes carbon dioxide and water into carbonic acid to allow rapid disposal of carbon dioxide (Gropper, Smith, and Groff, 2009). Zinc is essential for the growth and repair of tissues because it is involved in the synthesis of DNA and RNA. Zinc is associated with insulin and is a component of a protein, *gustin*, involved in taste acuity. The production of active vitamin A for the visual pigment rhodopsin requires zinc. It is integral to collagen formation for wound healing and plays a role in providing immunity.

Whether zinc is effective in warding off or minimizing symptoms of the common cold is unproved (Caruso, Prober, and Gwaltney, 2007; Gropper, Smith, and Groff, 2009; Marshall, 2006). Moreover, taking zinc lozenges every 2 to 3 hours while awake would deliver zinc in excess of the UL. Some individuals have suffered gastrointestinal symptoms and mouth irritation attributed to the lozenges (King and Cousins, 2006).

Absorption, Control, and Excretion

Zinc is released from foods in the acid environment of the stomach and absorbed from the small intestine through the same absorption sites as iron. Control of zinc levels is achieved through limitations on absorption that varies from 10% to 59%.

Most zinc is excreted in feces. Small amounts are lost in urine, in exfoliated skin cells, in sweat, in semen, and in menstrual flow. Because hair contains about 0.1 to 0.2 milligrams of zinc per gram, hair loss is also a route for zinc depletion (Gropper, Smith, and Groff, 2009).

Dietary Reference Intakes and Sources

For DRIs see Appendix A. For food and other sources, see Table 8-10. To investigate the mineral content of a particular item, see the Internet site of the United States Department of Agriculture at http://www.nal.usda.gov/fnic/foodcomp/search/.

Vegetarians are advised to consume twice as much zinc as persons consuming a mixed diet (Institute of Medicine, 2001).

In the body, zinc is recovered from pancreatic and biliary secretions in the gastrointestinal tract for reuse (Gropper, Smith, and Groff, 2009).

Interfering Factors

Conditions or medications that decrease gastric acidity impede zinc absorption. Iron and zinc compete for the same absorption sites. Zinc and nonheme iron interact when ingested together in solution but not when taken with a meal; however, mineral supplements with an iron to zinc ratio of 2:1 or greater inhibit zinc absorption (Gropper, Smith, and Groff, 2009).

In a similar reaction, zinc and calcium or copper may interact. In addition, phytates, oxalates, tannins, and **chelating agents** all reduce the absorption of zinc.

Deficiency

Zinc intake correlates directly with protein consumption. Groups at risk because of limited meat intake include the poor, the elderly, and vegetarians. Zinc deficiency in adults can also occur as a result of diseases that either hinder zinc absorption or cause excessive amounts of zinc to be excreted in urine. Some of the clinical conditions that may precipitate zinc deficiency include:

- Alcoholism
- Chronic illness
- Stress
- Trauma
- Surgery
- Diseases causing malabsorption (Gropper, Smith, and Groff, 2009).

Zinc deficiency causes:

- Growth retardation and delayed sexual maturation in children
- Alopecia
- Loss of taste sensation
- Poor wound healing
- Impaired immunity (Gropper, Smith, and Groff, 2009)

In developing countries, zinc supplementation has been effective in decreasing mortality and morbidity from acute and chronic diarrhea. The World Health Organization and UNICEF recommend that treatment for acute diarrhea include zinc supplementation.

A rare autosomal recessive disease, **acrodermatitis enteropathica,** causes zinc deficiency that is fatal if untreated. A mutation in a zinc transport protein causes poor absorption (Griffin, 2007). Oral zinc sulfate rapidly alleviates the symptoms.

Toxicity

For basic information on mineral toxicity, see Table 8-4. Because zinc can be toxic if consumed in excessive amounts, it should be obtained from foods, not from routine or long-term supplementation.

Copper

The healthy adult body contains less than 150 milligrams of copper, most located in the liver (the main storage site), brain, and kidneys (Gropper, Smith, and Groff, 2009). Copper is a cofactor for enzymes involved in hemoglobin synthesis and cell respiration, and is required for melanin pigment formation.

Gastric secretions aid in the release of bound copper in foods. Although some absorption is possible in the stomach, most copper is absorbed from the small intestine, chiefly the duodenum. Typically, 50% of ingested copper is absorbed but increases with low intake and decreases with high intake. The major route of excretion is via biliary tract into the feces, which serves to control copper balance (Gropper, Smith, and Groff, 2009).

Dietary Reference Intakes and Sources

For DRIs see Appendix A. For food and other sources, see Table 8-10. To investigate the mineral content of a particular item, see the Internet site of the United States Department of Agriculture at http://www.nal.usda.gov/fnic/foodcomp/search/.

In the United States, adult intake averages 1 to 2 milligrams. The body may also recycle copper from digestive secretions (Gropper, Smith, and Groff, 2009).

Interfering Factors and Deficiency

High intakes of zinc, iron, calcium, phosphorus, and phytate interfere with copper absorption. Phytates hinder absorption by forming more stable complexes with copper than with calcium or iron. Vitamin C reduces copper to a less absorbable form.

Individuals at increased risk of copper deficiency are those:

- Taking large amounts of antacids or zinc supplements (40 milligrams per day)
- With gastrointestinal diseases permitting malabsorption
- With kidney diseases that increase losses

Deficiency also has occurred as a result of the administration of total parenteral nutrition (TPN) solutions deficient in copper (Gropper, Smith, and Groff, 2009). In an unusual case, copper deficiency was caused by swallowed coins that released zinc into the body (Hassan, Netchvolodoff, and Raufman, 2000).

Because of copper's link with iron utilization, copper deficiency produces a hypochromic, microcytic anemia. Other manifestations of copper deficiency are:

- Skeletal demineralization
- Impaired immune function
- Depigmentation of the skin and hair

A hereditary abnormality that blocks the absorption of copper from the gastrointestinal tract causes **Menkes' disease.** The disease is inherited as an X-linked recessive trait. Intravenous administration of copper only partially corrects the vascular and neurological problems (Gropper, Smith, and Groff, 2009).

Toxicity

For basic information on mineral toxicity, see Table 8-4.

A genetic mutation causes **Wilson's disease,** which is inherited as an autosomal recessive trait affecting copper metabolism. A dietary prescription to avoid foods high in copper can augment chelation therapy and zinc supplements.

Selenium

The amount of selenium in the body ranges from 13 to 30 milligrams. Most selenium occurs in proteins as a component of amino acids, in which it can substitute for sulfur in methionine and cysteine. Selenium is part of an enzyme that works with vitamin E to protect cellular compounds from oxidation. In this role, selenium functions as an antioxidant. Selenium and vitamin E have a reciprocal sparing relationship (each spares the other).

Selenium is part of many enzymes in the body and is necessary for iodine metabolism. It also protects against the toxicity of mercury, cadmium, and silver (Burk and Levander, 2006).

The highest concentrations of this mineral occur in the thyroid gland, kidneys, liver, heart, pancreas, and muscle. An estimated 80% of selenium is absorbed through the small intestine, primarily the duodenum. Excretion into urine and feces is thought to be the mechanism to maintain homeostasis of the nutrient, but some is also lost through the lungs and skin (Gropper, Smith, and Groff, 2009).

Dietary Reference Intakes and Sources

For DRIs see Appendix A. For food and other sources, see Table 8-10. To investigate the mineral content of a particular item, see the Internet site of the United States Department of Agriculture at http://www.nal.usda.gov/fnic/foodcomp/search/.

Selenium can unspecifically substitute for methionine in some proteins (Alexander, 2007). Adolescence, pregnancy, and lactation increase the need for selenium, whereas a high intake of vitamin E reduces it. The amount of selenium present in plant foods depends on the selenium content of the soil and water where the foods are grown.

Selenium in fish, especially if contaminated with mercury (see Chapter 10), may have low bioavailability because of unabsorbable mercury–selenium complexes (Gropper, Smith, and Groff, 2009).

Deficiency and Toxicity

Selenium deficiencies have been produced in animals but are unlikely in humans who eat meat on a regular basis. Nevertheless, some exceptions exist, notably clients receiving long-term special formulas such as those for:

- Phenylketonuria
- TPN

Several TPN clients developed heart disease that responded to selenium treatment.

A deterioration of the heart due to selenium deficiency has occurred in residents of China's Keshan province. The fatality rate of **Keshan disease** is as high as 80%, and once heart failure occurs, supplementation does not reverse it. Coxsackie virus appears to be a cofactor in the development of Keshan disease. Without adequate selenium, benign strains of the virus mutate into virulent strains to which some of the symptoms of Keshan disease are attributed.

Signs and symptoms of selenium deficiency include:

- Poor growth
- Muscle pain and weakness
- Depigmentation of hair and skin
- Whitening of nail beds (Gropper, Smith, and Groff, 2009).

For basic information on mineral toxicity, see Table 8-4. Selenosis, toxicity from selenium, has occurred in miners and people overdosing with supplements.

Chromium

The adult body contains approximately 4 to 6 milligrams of chromium. High concentrations are found in the kidney, liver, muscle, spleen, heart, pancreas, and bone. Only about 0.4% to 2.5% of dietary chromium is absorbed probably throughout the small intestine. Ninety-five percent of excretion is via the urine, the content of which reflects current intake, not chromium status.

Chromium potentiates the action of insulin but the mechanism of action is uncertain. Supplementation has improved blood glucose in individuals with low chromium status, but not those with normal stores. No support has been found for chromium supplementation to increase strength or muscle or to decrease fat tissue (Gropper, Smith, and Groff, 2009).

For DRIs see Appendix A. For food and other sources, see Table 8-10.

Severe trauma and stress, through related elevated secretion of glucagon and cortisol, may increase the need for chromium. Vitamin C may enhance absorption, but antacids and phytates decrease absorption.

Individuals receiving TPN without chromium have shown these signs of deficiency:

- Weight loss
- Peripheral neuropathy
- Impaired glucose utilization
- High plasma levels of free fatty acids

Mild chromium deficiency is a risk factor for metabolic syndrome (see Chapter 18) (Gropper, Smith, and Groff, 2009).

For basic information on mineral toxicity, see Table 8-4. Chromium toxicity occurs rarely and under unusual circumstances. A 33-year-old white woman ingested chromium picolinate, 1200–2400 micrograms per day, to enhance weight loss. After 4 to 5 months, she achieved weight loss, but also acquired anemia, liver dysfunction, and kidney failure (Cerulli et al., 1998).

Manganese

The body contains only 10 to 20 milligrams of manganese, which is found in highest concentrations in the bones, liver, pancreas, and kidneys. Manganese is involved in the formation of bone and in amino acid, cholesterol, and carbohydrate metabolism.

Absorption throughout the small intestine varies from 1% to 14% and is inhibited by nonheme iron, copper, oxalates, phytates, and fiber (Gropper, Smith, and Groff, 2009). Excretion is primarily via the bile, with small losses through sweat and skin desquamation.

For DRIs see Appendix A. For food and other sources, see Table 8-10. To investigate the mineral content of a particular item, see the Internet site of the United States Department of Agriculture at http://www.nal.usda.gov/fnic/foodcomp/search/.

Deficiency is unlikely except when manganese is deliberately eliminated from the diet. Among other signs and symptoms, the client displays:

- Dermatitis
- Decreased growth of hair and nails
- Changes in hair color

For basic information on mineral toxicity, see Table 8-4. Whole-blood manganese levels do not necessarily correlate with the accumulated mineral in the brain (Iinuma et al., 2003).

Industrial toxicity may be related to transport of fumes to the brain via the olfactory nerve which bypasses the blood-brain barrier (Flynn and Susi, 2009). Parenteral administration of manganese, which bypasses the regulatory mechanism of the gut, has caused hypermanganesemia with seizures in one child (Hsieh et al., 2007) and magnetic resonance imaging (MRI) changes in two others.

Cobalt

For food and other sources of cobalt, see Table 8-10. DRIs for cobalt have not been established.

As an essential component of the vitamin B_{12} molecule, cobalt is necessary for red blood cell formation, but a role for the ionic form of cobalt has not been demonstrated (Gropper, Smith, and Groff, 2009). Cobalt deficiency has not been reported in humans or animals.

Molybdenum

Molybdenum, a cofactor for enzymes involved in catabolism of sulfur-containing amino acids and **purines**, is found primarily in the liver, kidneys, and bone. About 50% to 90% of ingested molybdenum is absorbed although little is known about the mechanism of absorption. Molybdenum is mainly excreted in urine, but small amounts are lost via bile in feces and in sweat and hair (Gropper, Smith, and Groff, 2009).

For DRIs see Appendix A. For food and other sources, see Table 8-10.

Molybdenum deficiency is rarely found except if the diet is especially rich in sulfate, copper, or tungstate (Gropper, Smith, and Groff, 2009). Deficiency has been reported in a client receiving prolonged TPN who displayed tachycardia, headache, mental disturbances, and coma (Sardesai, 1993).

For basic information on mineral toxicity, see Table 8-4. At intakes of up to 1500 micrograms per day, molybdenum seems to be relatively nontoxic.

Figure 8-11 illustrates the food groups contributing to the intake of major and trace minerals.

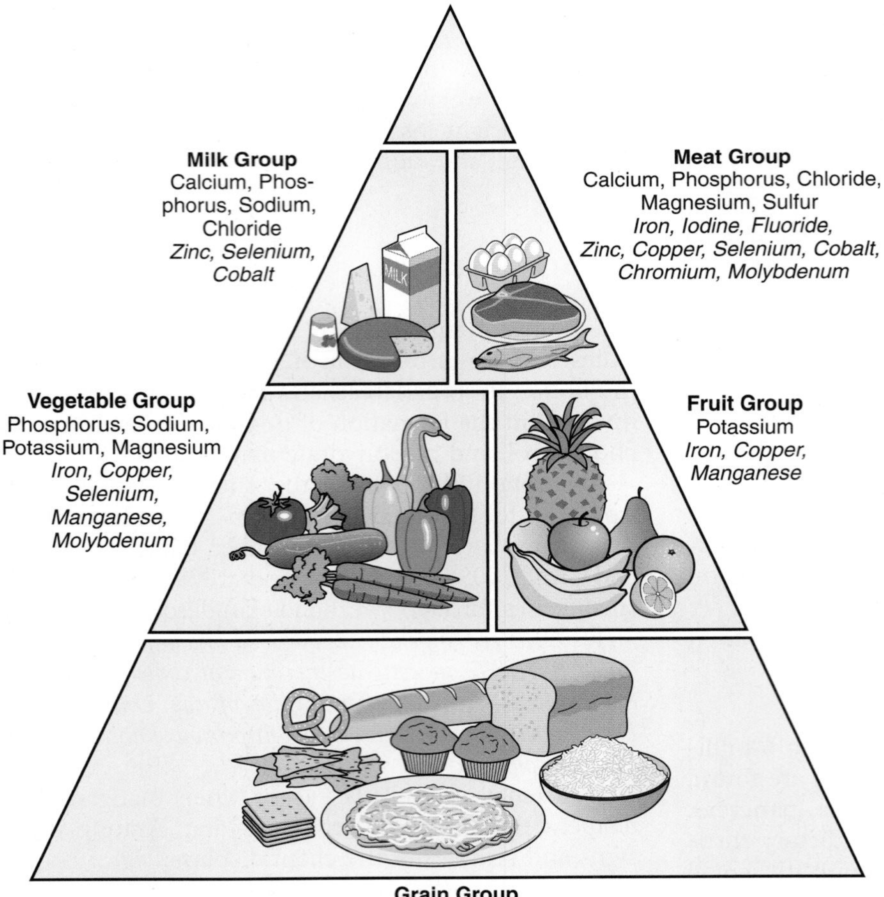

FIGURE 8-11 This pyramid illustrates the food groups supplying the various minerals. Italics indicate trace minerals.

Ultratrace Minerals

For DRIs see ULs in Appendix A. Clear biological functions in humans have not been identified.

Arsenic is found mostly in skin, hair, and nails. Environmental sources of arsenic are pesticides and fallout from smelters and coal-fired power plants (Gropper, Smith, and Groff, 2009).

Most people acquire arsenic from food, in an organic form, but individuals most severely affected with overdoses receive it from drinking water, in a more toxic inorganic form and in higher amounts. Arsenic in drinking water is associated with gastroenteritis, neurological manifestations, vascular changes, diabetes, and cancers. The U.S. Environmental Protection Agency has set a maximum contaminant level for arsenic in drinking water of 10 micrograms per liter (Abernathy, Thomas, and Calderon, 2003).

Boron is found mainly in bone, teeth, nails, and hair. The body contains between 3 and 20 milligrams of boron, which is thought to influence embryogenesis, bone development, cell membrane function, and the immune response. Plant foods are particularly rich in boron (Gropper, Smith, and Groff, 2009).

Nickel is found in highest concentrations in the thyroid and adrenal glands. It is also found in hair, bone, and other soft tissues. Nickel is released into the environment with the combustion of nickel-containing products and is found in higher levels in foods of plant rather than animal origin. Most absorbed nickel is excreted in urine (Gropper, Smith, and Groff, 2009).

Silicon is found in greatest concentrations in bone, skin, blood vessels, and tendons. Intake comes from plant foods with cereal grains and root vegetables especially rich sources. The kidney is the major organ of excretion (Gropper, Smith, and Groff, 2009).

Vanadium is found mainly in bone, teeth, lung, and thyroid gland. Rich food sources include shellfish, black pepper, parsley, and dill seed. Vanadium toxicity produces:

- A green tongue (due to vanadium deposits)
- Gastrointestinal disturbances
- Mental dysfunction
- Hypertension
- Renal toxicity (Gropper, Smith, and Groff, 2009)

Other Minerals Impacting Health

Aluminum, lead, and mercury are found in the body, not because of nutritional needs but as the result of environmental contamination. See Clinical Application 8-8 and Chapter 10.

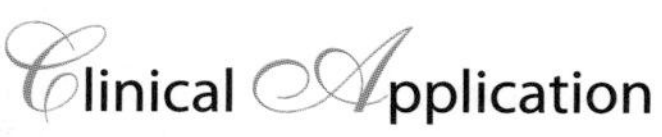

8-8

Lead Poisoning (Plumbism)

Lead is a contaminant in the human body. The effects of lead toxicity, such as neurological damage and retardation, can be devastating and permanent. Black and Hispanic children are at greater risk of lead poisoning than white children, as are all low-income children. No blood lead level (BLL) has been declared safe and one of 70 micrograms or higher is a medical emergency (Meyer et al., 2003).

Not food, but lead-based paint in older homes is the primary source of poisoning in inner-city children, as was the case of a 2-year-old child who died from acute lead poisoning (CDC, 2001a). Children may eat paint chips that have an appealing sweet taste but a principal mode of ingestion is lead dust on hands, toys, and household objects. Lead paint in homes built before 1950 pose a particular risk for children.

Other sources of lead are solder in metal food and beverage cans and lead that leaches out of glazes on serving utensils and containers, especially those containing acidic juices and wine (Hackley and Katz-Jacobson, 2003). However, in the 1980s, lead was eliminated from solder in cans packaged in the United States. Reports of ingestion of lead from dishware or foreign packaging materials still appear sporadically and imported toys have recently been implicated. These cases of lead poisoning in children had been discovered by astute clinicians:

- Candy packaged in lead-containing wrappers from Mexico (CDC, 2002a).
- Candy in ceramic jars from Mexico and a spice purchased in Iraq (CDC, 1998).
- A product called Sindoor used for food coloring and consumed by a breastfeeding mother thus poisoning a 13-month-old boy and his parents (Vassilev et al., 2005).

Other nonfood products causing lead poisoning after ingestion include toy jewelry, pool cue chalk, curtain weights, and fishing sinkers (CDC, 2004 and 2006a; Miller et al., 1996; Mowad, Haddad, and Gemmel, 1998).

Although fetuses and children are the most susceptible to damage from lead poisoning, adults can be affected also. About 9% of total body lead in adults is accumulated in the bones, where it remains for decades. Of special concern are pregnant and lactating women whose bone turnover releases sequestered lead into the bloodstream that readily crosses the placenta. Blood lead levels reflect only recent or continued lead exposure, not accumulated bone lead levels (Cleveland et al., 2008), which complicates case finding.

In addition to lead-based paint, older homes also may have plumbing that could contaminate drinking water. Ten infants were poisoned from formula reconstituted with lead-contaminated water (Shannon and Graef, 1992). Since boiling increases the concentration of lead in water, the need to boil water for infant formula needs individual evaluation. To decrease the chance of lead leaching into drinking or cooking water:

1. Run water for 2 minutes in the morning before drawing water to drink
2. Use cold water for cooking and drinking.

Local health departments are able to direct people to appropriate laboratories if they wish to have their water tested.

Continued

Clinical Application—cont'd 8-8

Early diagnosis and treatment of lead poisoning are essential. Even children successfully treated and kept away from further intake showed lasting brain damage in 25% of cases. Foremost is the avoidance of further exposure through environmental control. Nutritional tactics can be used in addition:

- Iron and calcium supplementation can be started so these minerals will compete with lead for absorption.
- A reduced-fat diet and frequent meals decrease gastrointestinal absorption of lead.

Use of chelating agents that will bind with lead are recommended if the blood lead level is greater than 45 micrograms per 100 milliliters; however, experts should be consulted because fatal hypocalcemia has occurred following inappropriate prescribing (CDC, 2006b).

Aluminum, a metal frequently found in the environment, puts clients especially at risk when it contaminates pharmaceutical products used for hemodialysis or parenteral nutrition (see Chapter 14) because such intake bypasses any possible defense by the gastrointestinal system. Aluminum toxicity can cause serious central nervous system and bone effects.

In 2004, the U.S. Food and Drug Administration mandated labeling requirements for aluminum content in all parenteral solution components and set maximum exposure values. Some concerns remain:

- One study determined that meeting the FDA exposure regulation was possible only in clients weighing more than 50 kilograms (110 pounds), whereas almost half the exposure to aluminum occurred in babies weighing less than 3 kilograms or 6.6 pounds (Poole et al., 2008).
- Another study measured the concentration of aluminum in parenteral nutrition solutions. In the pediatric and neonatal solutions tested, the amount of aluminum met or exceeded maximum permissible concentrations (Speerhas and Seidner, 2007).

On a positive note, routine testing of hemodialysis clients' serum aluminum levels led to elimination of pumps that presumably contaminated the dialysate. The clients displayed no symptoms and their blood levels of aluminum decreased after the pumps were removed from service (CDC, 2008a).

Mineral Supplementation

Excessive intake of nutrients can be as harmful as insufficient intake. For most healthy people, foods are the preferred source of minerals. Notable exceptions are women who are capable of becoming pregnant, the elderly, and persons with restricted diets such as vegetarians.

People who take supplements are advised to not take more than the RDAs or AIs for each mineral without consulting their health-care providers. Healthy postmenopausal women and adult men should not take iron supplements (Marra and Boyar, 2009). In the case of some minerals, toxicity is possible at levels slightly above the recommended intake amounts. In addition, an excess of one mineral may cause a deficiency of another.

Water in Human Nutrition

Water is the largest single constituent of the human body, and the need for water is more urgent than the need for any other nutrient. Humans can live a month without food but only 6 days without water.

More than half of body weight is water, which is found in and around the cells, within the blood and lymph vessels, and in various body cavities. Some tissues have significantly more water than others:

- Muscle tissue is 70% water.
- Fat tissue is 30% water.
- Bone tissue is 10% water.

A man's body is 60% to 65% water, whereas a woman's body is just 50% to 54% water. Men have higher water content than women because of their greater muscle mass. The body of a 70-kg (154-lb) man would contain about 42 liters of water.

Age also affects the proportion of water in a body. Compared with the 50% to 65% for women and men, an infant's body is 75% water. Premature infants may be 80% water by weight. Infants, especially premature infants, are at high risk of fluid imbalances because of the proportion and distribution of water in their bodies. The adult proportion of water to body weight is reached at about 3 years of age (Gropper, Smith, and Groff, 2009).

Fluid Compartments

Body fluids are contained in intracellular and extracellular compartments (see Fig. 8-12). These compartments are separated by semipermeable membranes, which allow some substances to pass through and prevent the passage of other substances. Water passes freely through the membranes.

Thirteen water transport proteins, called **aquaporins**, have been identified in humans, each with a distinct distribution throughout the body (Hibuse et al., 2006). Thirteen is the final number because the human

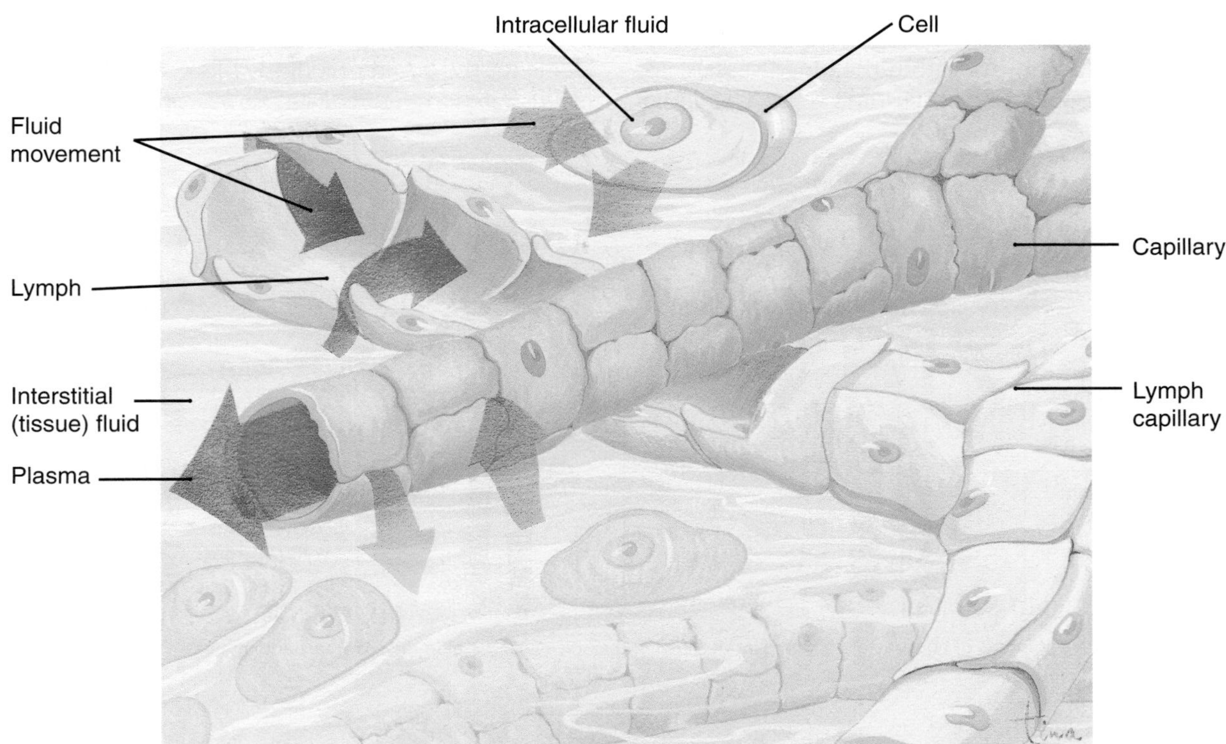

FIGURE 8-12 Water compartments, showing the names water is given in its different locations and the ways in which water moves between compartments. (Reprinted from Scanlon, VC, and Sanders, T: *Essentials of anatomy and physiology*, ed 5. FA Davis, Philadelphia, 2007, p 29, with permission.)

genome project is complete (Ishibashi, Hara, and Kondo, 2009). Aquaporins are membrane proteins that function as water-selective channels in the plasma membranes of many cells and help to explain the speed at which water moves across cell membranes, including the selective absorption found in different areas of the kidney.

To illustrate the enhanced transport for instance, water flows through aquaporin 1 at a rate of three billion water molecules per second per aquaporin channel (Gade and Robinson, 2006). Aquaporins 1 and 4 play important roles in homeostasis of fluids in the brain, a critical function given the rigid skull that restrains expansion of its contents. For example, approximately 500 to 600 milliliters of cerebrospinal fluid is synthesized daily, three or four times the entire volume of the cerebrospinal fluid in the body (Yool, 2007).

Clinically, researchers have found aquaporin 4 levels increased in human brains after traumatic brain injury, within brain-derived tumors, and around brain tumors (Hu et al., 2005). At least five aquaporins have been found in the eye and that discovery may lead to new treatments for glaucoma, corneal edema, and other diseases of the eye involving abnormalities in intraocular pressure or tissue hydration (Verkman, 2003).

The inner ear is also rich in diverse aquaporins (Yool, 2007). As more is learned about aquaporins in health, it may be possible to develop new drug treatments to target specific areas of malfunction in disease, for instance, in hydrocephalus.

Intracellular Fluid

The fluid inside the cells is called intracellular. In adults, intracellular water constitutes 65% of body water. In infants, 46% of the body water is intracellular.

Extracellular Fluid

All fluid outside cells is extracellular. In adults, 35% of the body's water is extracellular; in infants, 54% is extracellular. Figure 8-13 illustrates the proportions of intracellular to extracellular fluid in men, women, and infants. The difference is important because extracellular fluid is more easily and rapidly excreted than is intracellular fluid. **Extracellular fluid** includes interstitial, intravascular, lymph, and transcellular fluids.

INTERSTITIAL FLUID

Located between the cells or surrounding the cells, interstitial fluid assists in transporting substances between the cells and the blood and lymph vessels.

INTRAVASCULAR FLUID

Intravascular fluid is found within the blood vessels, arteries, arterioles, capillaries, venules, and veins. The liquid part of the blood is called plasma; minus the clotting elements, the liquid part of the blood is called serum. As is illustrated in Figure 8-14, 91.5% of plasma is water.

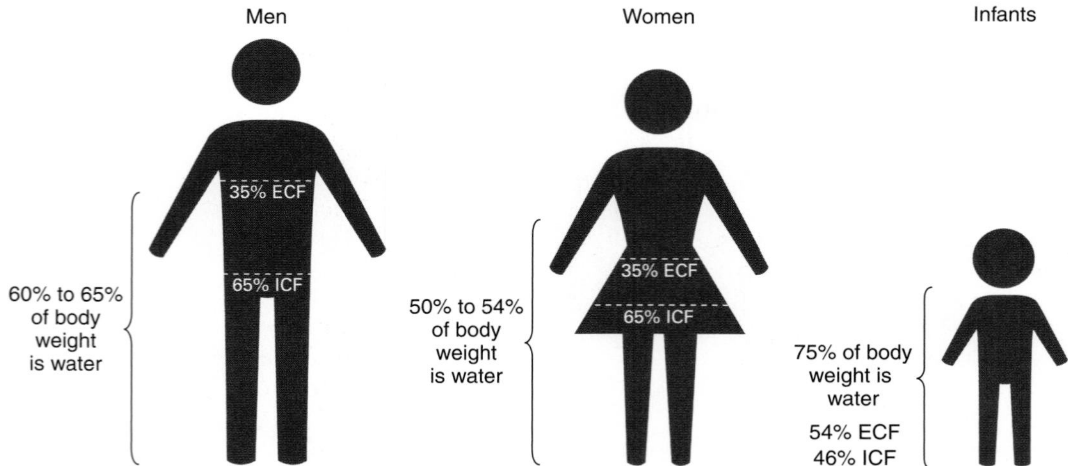

FIGURE 8-13 The relative amounts of body weight that are intracellular and extracellular water in men, women, and infants.

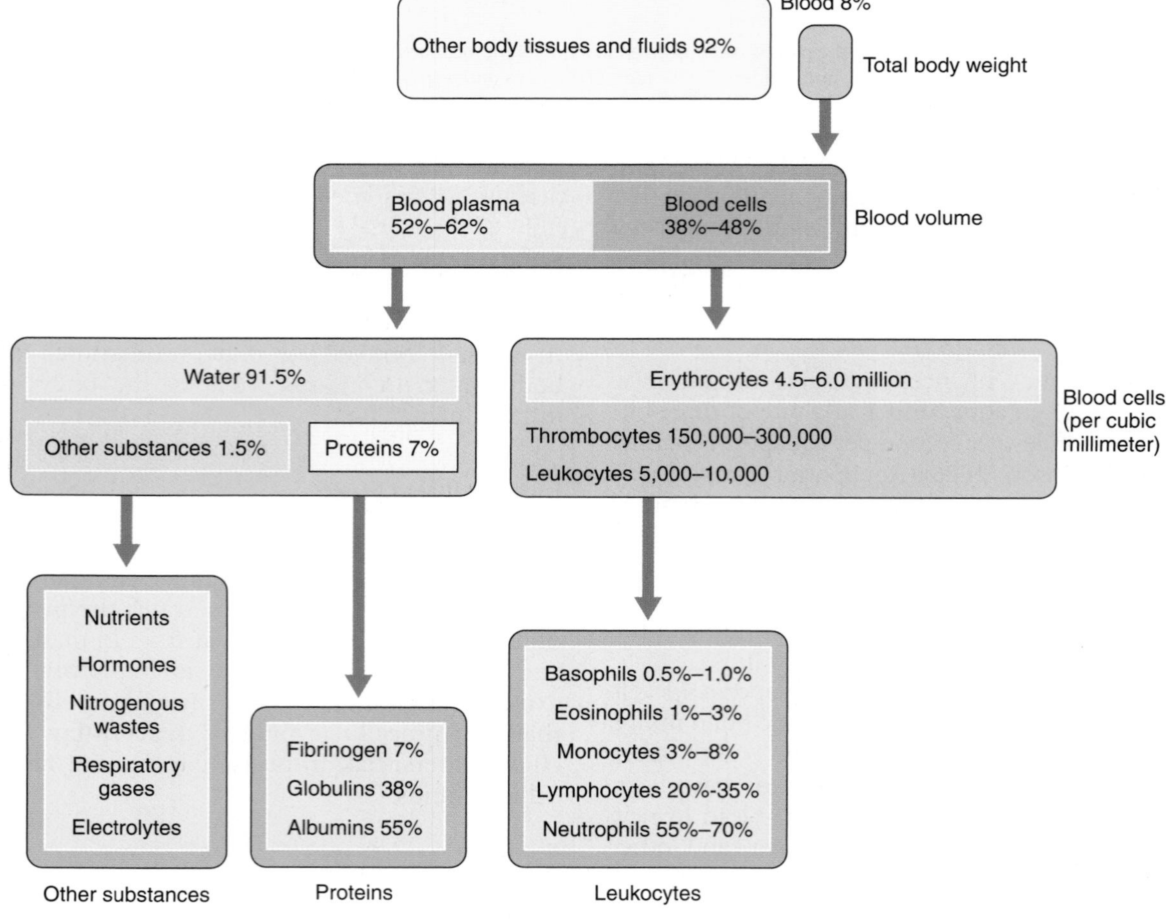

FIGURE 8-14 Blood constitutes 8% of body weight. The largest single component of the blood is water. (Reprinted from Venes, D [Ed.]: *Taber's cylcopedic medical dictionary*, ed 21. FA Davis, Philadelphia, 2010, p 283, with permission.)

LYMPHATIC FLUID

The venous system cannot collect and return all the fluid from the tissues to the heart. Lymph, via the lymphatic vessels, assists in returning the fluid part of blood to the heart.

TRANSCELLULAR FLUID

Transcellular fluids include cerebrospinal fluid, pericardial fluid, pleural fluid, synovial fluid, intraocular fluids, and gastrointestinal secretions. Transcellular fluids are constantly being secreted into their spaces and reabsorbed into the vascular system. Figure 8-15 shows the approximate distribution of water in the four compartments.

Usage

No storage tanks for water exist in the body; water continually moves from one body compartment to another and is often reused by the body to perform different tasks.

Functions

As a component of cells, water helps give the body shape and form, and as the major constituent of blood, it helps to maintain blood volume and blood pressure. It is part of the structure of many of the body's large molecules, such as protein and glycogen.

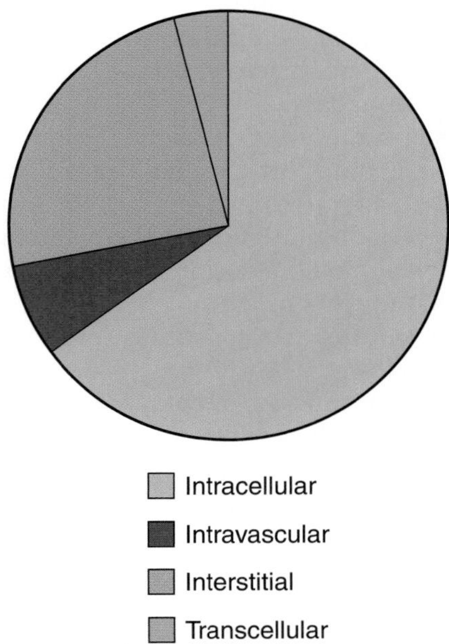

FIGURE 8-15 Proportionate amounts of water in the four fluid compartments in the body. (Reprinted from Williams, L, and Hopper, P: *Understanding medical surgical nursing,* ed 3. FA Davis, Philadelphia, 2007, p 59, with permission.)

Some body water also serves as a lubricant, as in mucus secretions and joint fluid.

Water helps to regulate body temperature by absorbing the heat produced by fever and the heat resulting from metabolic processes. On average, tissue metabolism generates 100 kilocalories per hour. The blood carries excess heat to the skin, where it is dissipated by sweating or radiation.

Water is a **solvent** for minerals, vitamins, glucose, and other small molecules. (The substance that is dissolved in a solvent is called a **solute.**) See Box 8-3 for a list of the functions of water in the body.

Absorption

A small amount of water can be absorbed into the bloodstream from the stomach but a liter of water can be absorbed from the small intestine in an hour.

Under conditions that disrupt an individual's automatic adaptive mechanisms, water may be retained. The accumulation of excessive amounts of fluid between the cells (in the interstitial compartments) is called **edema.** Conditions that may cause such water retention include:

- Hypothyroidism
- Heart failure
- Severe protein deficiency
- Some kidney conditions

When finger pressure displaces excess fluid over a bony area the sign is termed **pitting edema**. Although the fluid remains inside the body, it is lost to circulation. (See Figure 8-16.)

As a result of injury or trauma, capillary permeability increases so that more fluid and cells can travel to the site of the injury to begin repairs, or healing. This process also causes swelling, or edema, at the site of an injury—blisters at the site of burns, for example. Fluid leaves the vessels and accumulates in the skin. As noted in Chapter 22, correct fluid replacement is a high priority for severely burned clients.

In most cases, localized edema is not life-threatening. The accumulation of fluid in the brain (cerebral edema) or in lung tissue (pulmonary edema), however, is life-threatening. Cerebral edema may result from

Box 8-3 ■ *Functions of Water*

- Gives shape and form to cells.
- Maintains blood volume and blood pressure.
- Helps form the structure of large molecules.
- Serves as a lubricant and a solvent.
- Helps regulate body temperature.
- Transports nutrients to and waste away from cells.
- Is a medium for and participant in chemical reactions.

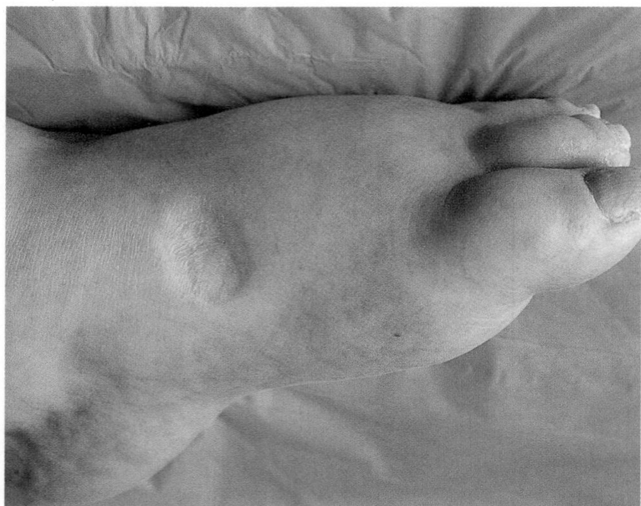

FIGURE 8-16 Finger or thumb pressure over a bony area displaces edematous fluid; shown here as pitting edema of the foot. (Reprinted from Williams, L, and Hopper, P: *Understanding medical surgical nursing*, ed 3. FA Davis, Philadelphia, 2007, p 357, with permission.)

tumors, toxic chemicals, or infection. Pulmonary edema can be a consequence of a failing heart or irritation of the lung, as seen in a client who inhales toxic gases.

Excessive water also can be dispersed throughout the body. This condition is called **water intoxication,** which can be caused by excessive water intake (either by the intravenous or gastrointestinal route), cerebral concussion, or hormonal disorders. Many of the symptoms are caused by diluting the concentration of the electrolytes in the body's fluid compartments.

Dietary Reference Intakes

For DRIs see Table 8-5.

Approximately 80% of water needs are expected to come from fluids and 20% from foods. Larger intakes are required by physically active people or those in a hot environment.

The previously publicized negative effects of caffeine and alcohol on water balance have been refuted by evidence showing the diuretic effects of those substances to be transient. Thirst and mealtime beverages are usually adequate to maintain hydration. Acute water toxicity is a hazard in individuals rapidly consuming much more than the kidneys' maximal excretion rate of 0.7 to 1.0 liter per hour (Institute of Medicine, 2004b).

Ordinarily, breast milk alone can supply an infant's needed water even in a desert. At the opposite end of the age spectrum, older adults often have a blunted sense of thirst and may have their water needs impacted by disease and medication.

Physiology of Body Fluids

To help with understanding the information in this section, see Box 8-1.

The Effect of Electrolytes on Water Balance

Each fluid compartment has an electrolyte composition that serves its needs and has automatic mechanisms designed to keep it electrically neutral, or balanced. The positive ions within a compartment must equal the negative ones. When shifts and losses occur, compensating shifts and gains reestablish electroneutrality.

Important Body Electrolytes

Mineral ions strongly influence not only water balance but also osmotic pressure, blood pressure, and acid–base balance.

See Table 8-11 for a summary of the major body electrolytes.

Osmotic Pressure

Osmosis is the movement of water (or another solvent) across a semipermeable membrane from an area with fewer particles to one with more particles. The result, as long as the difference is reasonable, is an equalization of concentration on either side of the membrane. Clinical Application 8-9 describes an experiment to demonstrate osmosis.

Osmosis is a passive process. The movement of some substances, however, is active. Some substances require active transport mechanisms to push them through a membrane. Two such transport mechanisms are the sodium pump and the potassium pump. Located in cell membranes, these pumps are actually proteins that move ions.

Sodium pumps move sodium ions out of cells (and water follows).

Potassium pumps move potassium ions into cells.

In this manner, the body maintains electrolyte concentrations of the intracellular and extracellular fluid compartments. Active transport requires energy to operate.

DETERMINATION OF OSMOTIC PRESSURE

When two solutions on either side of a semipermeable membrane have different concentrations, pressure develops. This pressure, which is exerted on the semipermeable membrane, is called **osmotic pressure.**

TABLE 8-11 ■ Major Body Electrolytes

ELECTROLYTE	FLUID COMPARTMENT*	FUNCTIONS
Cations		
Sodium (Na^+)	Extracellular	Major cation in ECF. Na^+ concentration in fluids determines the distribution of H_2O by osmosis. With Cl^- and HCO_3^-, Na^+ regulates acid-base balance.
Potassium (K^+)	Intracellular	Major cation in ICF. K^+ with Na^+ maintains water balance. With Na^+ and H^+, K^+ regulates acid-base balance.
Calcium	Extracellular†	Participates in permeability of cell membranes, transmission of nerve impulses, muscle action.
Magnesium (Mg^{2+})	Intracellular	Regulates nerve stimulation and normal muscle action.
Anions		
Chloride (Cl^-)	Extracellular	Major anion in ECF. Helps maintain water balance and acid–base balance.
Bicarbonate (HCO_3^-)	Extracellular	Most important ECF buffer.
Phosphate (HPO_4^{2-})	Intracellular	Within the ICF, phosphates and proteins buffer 95% of the body's carbonic acid and 50% of other acids.

*ECP and ICF both contain all the cations and anions listed in this table but are labeled as either ECP or ICF according to the concentration. For example, sodium ions make up 142 of the total 155 milliequivalents per liter (of the cations) in the ECF.

†Of the cations, 3% in ECF and 1% in ICF.

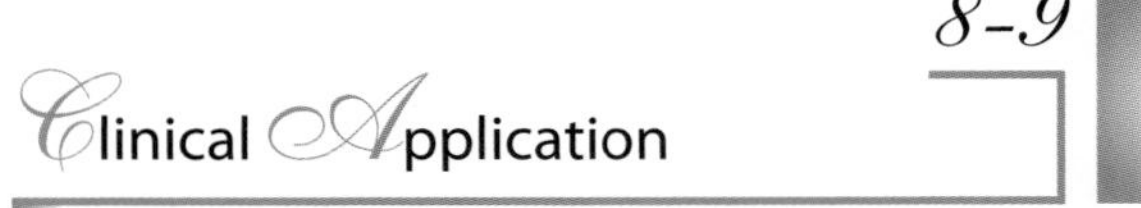

Osmosis in the Kitchen

To make sauerkraut, cabbage is sliced very finely and placed in the bottom of a crock. Salt is added to the dry cabbage in layers that are tamped down until the crock is full. At this point, liquid will have gathered, pulled from the cabbage pieces by the concentrated salt. A heavy plate topped with bags of water is placed atop the cabbage to continue squeezing the water from the cabbage as it ferments. The crock is covered with a cloth. After 5 or 6 weeks, the crock is full of juice and the cabbage has become sauerkraut.

To make a small batch of sauerkraut, use 2 teaspoons of canning salt per pound of cabbage.

Osmotic pressure causes a solvent such as water to cross the membrane, while the solutes (particles) that are outside the membrane cannot go through.

The size of the molecule and its ability to ionize determines the number of particles in a given concentration. Electrolytes readily ionize in solution. Disaccharides and monosaccharides do not ionize.

OSMOLALITY AND NUTRITION

The measure of the osmotic pressure exerted by the number of particles per volume of liquid is referred to as its **osmolarity.** The unit of measure for osmotic activity is the **milliosmole.** Clinically, osmolarity is usually reported in milliosmoles per liter. **Osmolality,** in contrast, is the measure of the osmotic pressure exerted by the number of particles per weight of solvent, usually reported in milliosmoles per kilogram. The normal value for osmolality of human blood serum is about 275 to 295 milliosmoles per kilogram.

In dilute aqueous solutions as in the body, only a small numerical difference is found between osmolarity and osmolality (Gropper, Smith, and Groff, 2009). The primary determinant of osmolality in the extracellular fluid is sodium.

Fluids are designated **isotonic** if they approximate the osmolality of blood plasma, Two commonly administered isotonic intravenous fluids are 5% glucose in water and 0.9% sodium chloride. Fluids exerting less osmotic pressure than plasma are labeled **hypotonic.** Those exerting greater osmotic pressure than plasma are called **hypertonic**.

Achieving the correct osmolality of fluids administered intravenously (by needle or tube into the vein) is very important. A solution that is too concentrated pulls water out of the red blood cells, and the cells shrivel and die. A solution that is too weak allows water to be pulled into the red blood cells until the cells burst. For these reasons, isotonic solutions are given with red blood cell products.

Intravenous solutions containing sufficient nutrients to provide all a person's known needs are so hypertonic that they must be infused into a very large vein so that they are diluted quickly by the large volume of blood flowing past the infusion port or catheter. This procedure is described in Chapter 14.

Oral fluids also can be categorized by osmotic pressure. Plain water is hypotonic. Whole milk at 275 milliosmoles per liter is close to isotonic but is not recommended for infants for another reason (see Chapter 11). Ginger ale, with 510 milliosmoles per liter, and 7-Up®, with 640, are both hypertonic. The significance of these differences will become apparent in the section on treatment of fluid volume abnormalities.

SERUM ELECTROLYTES

The electrolyte content of blood can also be reported in milliequivalents per liter. The normal serum sodium level is 135 to 145 milliequivalents per liter. In most cases, because sodium is the most influential extracellular ion, osmolarity of the extracellular fluid can be estimated clinically by doubling the serum sodium value. Normal serum sodium doubled would be 270 to 296 milliosmoles per liter. Normal osmolality of the serum is about 300 milliosmoles per kilogram. This simple method gives a close approximation.

The other ion that health-care providers monitor carefully in clients with potential fluid and electrolyte imbalances is potassium. Most of the potassium in the body is inside the cells, at a concentration of 150 milliequivalents per liter. By contrast, potassium concentration in the blood is only 3.5 to 5.0 milliequivalents per liter. Even slight variations above or below these values can produce severe consequences. The heart muscle is particularly sensitive to high or low levels of potassium; abnormal levels can produce cardiac arrest.

The Effect of Plasma Proteins on Water Balance

The body has highly developed mechanisms that maintain a constant flow of water and:

- Nutrients to cells
- Waste materials from cells

Adequate blood pressure is necessary for this transport system to function. Blood pressure is the force exerted against the walls of the arteries by the beating heart. It is reported in two numbers, for example, 120/80 (measured in millimeters of mercury). The top number is the pressure when the heart beats, called **systolic pressure.** The bottom number is the pressure between beats, called the **diastolic pressure.** One of the factors necessary to maintain blood pressure is a sufficient volume of blood in the arteries and veins.

Water and nutrients in the blood are pushed out through the thin walls of the capillaries into the interstitial fluid by **hydrostatic pressure** (blood pressure) supplied by the heart. From the interstitial compartment, the water and nutrients cross cell membranes to bathe and nourish the cell. Plasma proteins, including **albumin,** remain in the capillaries because they are too large to squeeze through the capillary wall.

Inside the blood vessels, the plasma proteins exert **colloidal osmotic pressure** (COP). The COP, now greater than the hydrostatic pressure, pulls water and waste materials from the interstitial fluid into the capillaries to maintain blood volume. Clinical Application 8-10 describes a condition in which a low serum protein is the cause of water imbalance.

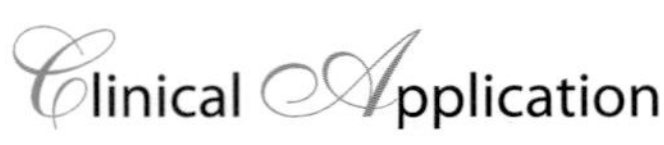

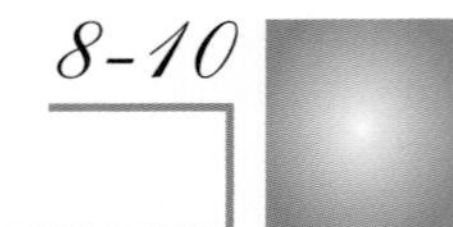

8-10

Clinical Application

Protein–Energy Malnutrition and Water Balance

Starving children often look plump (see Fig. 5-3), because they are edematous. Such children are victims of **kwashiorkor,** a disease of protein-energy malnutrition, which commonly occurs in children just after weaning when their diets do not have as much protein as found in their mothers' milk.

Protein plays a crucial role in maintaining fluid volume in blood vessels. Children with kwashiorkor develop edema because they do not have enough plasma proteins remaining in the capillaries to pull water back into the circulatory system. Thus, water accumulates in the interstitial spaces. After treatment begins, plasma proteins will pull the retained water into the blood and the children will appear emaciated.

Regulation of Water Intake and Excretion

The body has mechanisms regulating both the intake and the excretion of water. Normally, thirst governs water intake. Excretion is controlled mainly by two hormones:

1. Antidiuretic hormone causes the body to reabsorb (retain) water.
2. Aldosterone causes the body to retain sodium.

Thirst Mechanism

Thirst is the desire for fluids, especially water. Thirst normally occurs when 10% of the intravascular volume is lost or when cellular volume is reduced by 1 to 2%. When blood has too little water, the blood's osmotic pressure increases. Special sensors in the **hypothalamus** monitor the osmotic pressure as the blood circulates in the brain. When the hypothalamus detects an increase in osmotic pressure, the gland triggers a desire to drink.

Antidiuretic Hormone

If thirst is not alleviated, the sensors in the hypothalamus increase the secretion of **antidiuretic hormone (ADH)** from the posterior pituitary gland. ADH, also named **vasopressin,** causes the kidneys to return more water to the bloodstream rather than spill it into the urine.

ADH also constricts arteries to increase blood pressure similar to putting a finger over the end of a garden hose, narrowing its diameter, thus increasing the water pressure.

In **diabetes insipidus,** the hypothalamus does not secrete ADH or the kidneys do not respond appropriately. If the hypothalamus is not secreting ADH, a pharmaceutical preparation can be given. Clinical Application 8-11 provides information about a condition called syndrome of inappropriate secretion of antidiuretic hormone (SIADH).

Aldosterone

The release of **aldosterone,** a hormone secreted by the adrenal glands, is another water-balancing mechanism in the body. Aldosterone causes sodium ions to be returned to the bloodstream by the kidneys rather than to be spilled into urine. Sodium, the most influential extracellular ion, pulls water along with it.

The stimulus for the release of aldosterone is decreased pressure of the blood supplying kidney tissue. In response, the kidneys produce **renin** that acts with secretions from the liver and the lungs to produce **angiotensin II.** The cascade continues as shown in Figure 8-17.

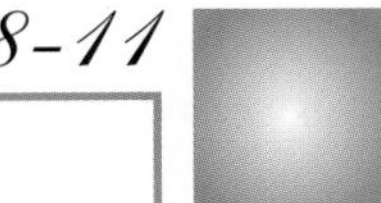

Clinical Application 8-11

Syndrome of Inappropriate Secretion of Antidiuretic Hormone (SIADH)

Normally, increased blood osmolality stimulates the posterior pituitary gland to release ADH. When enough water is returned to the bloodstream by the kidney, ADH secretion stops. Several diverse situations cause ADH to be released inappropriately including:

- Central nervous system disorders
- Lung disease
- Some tumors
- Certain drugs
- Surgery
- Emotional stress

The signs and symptoms of SIADH are those of hyponatremia (see Table 8-7). In this case, it is dilutional hyponatremia. The client has enough sodium, but it is diluted in too much retained water dispersed throughout the body so that symptoms of volume overload are seldom apparent. Neurological signs are attributed to cerebral edema.

Effective treatment of SIADH depends on discovering and removing the cause. In milder cases, fluid restriction—wherein the client is given precisely prescribed amounts of fluids throughout the day—may suffice. Over a period of several days, the client's body will excrete the extra water. Beyond that, treatment may involve diuretic therapy and sometimes saline infusions with careful monitoring of the effects on blood values to avoid complications associated with too rapid correction of the hyponatremia.

Another side of sodium retention is potassium loss. Within fluid compartments, positively charged particles must equal negatively charged ones. When sodium is retained, to maintain electroneutrality, the kidney excretes more potassium, under the influence of aldosterone.

Acid–Base Balance

The body is well equipped to digest and metabolize acidic and basic foods without jeopardizing its acid–base balance. The use of substances such as baking soda to treat an upset stomach should be discouraged, however, because the baking soda can be absorbed into the blood, thereby affecting the total body systems. Antacids designed to treat stomach upsets and used according to directions, are a better choice than baking soda.

Electrolytes play an important role in maintaining the correct acidity or alkalinity of various body fluids. Acids are compounds that yield hydrogen ions when dissociated in solution. The more hydrogen ions a solution contains, the more concentrated the acid. Bases, or alkalis, are substances that accept hydrogen ions. Acidity or alkalinity is measured by a scale called **pH** for *potential of hydrogen*.

The pH scale ranges from 0 to 14: acids are rated 0 to 6.999; 7.0 is neutral; bases (alkalis) are greater than 7. One on the scale would indicate a strong acid, and 14 a strong base. Figure 8-18 illustrates the pH scale, showing placement of acid, neutral, and alkaline fluids. The difference between units is 10-fold. Thus, lemon juice at a pH of 2 is 10 times as acidic as orange juice with a pH of 3.

The action of the lungs, kidneys, and buffer systems of the body maintains the balance between too much and too little acid in body fluids. These buffer systems minimize significant changes in the pH of body fluids by controlling the hydrogen ion (H^+) concentration. **Buffers** are substances that can neutralize both acids and bases. **Bicarbonate** (HCO_3^-) is the most important buffer in the extracellular fluid. Phosphate (HPO_4^{2-}) and proteins are two important buffers in the intracellular fluid.

Extracellular Fluid

The normal pH of the extracellular fluid is 7.35 to 7.45. It is slightly alkaline despite the acidity of the waste products of metabolism. A blood pH below 6.8 or above 7.8 is usually fatal (Fournier, 2009). The body is continually working to maintain the pH within this narrow range. Extracellular fluid contains both positive sodium ions (Na^+) and negative bicarbonate ions (HCO_3^-).

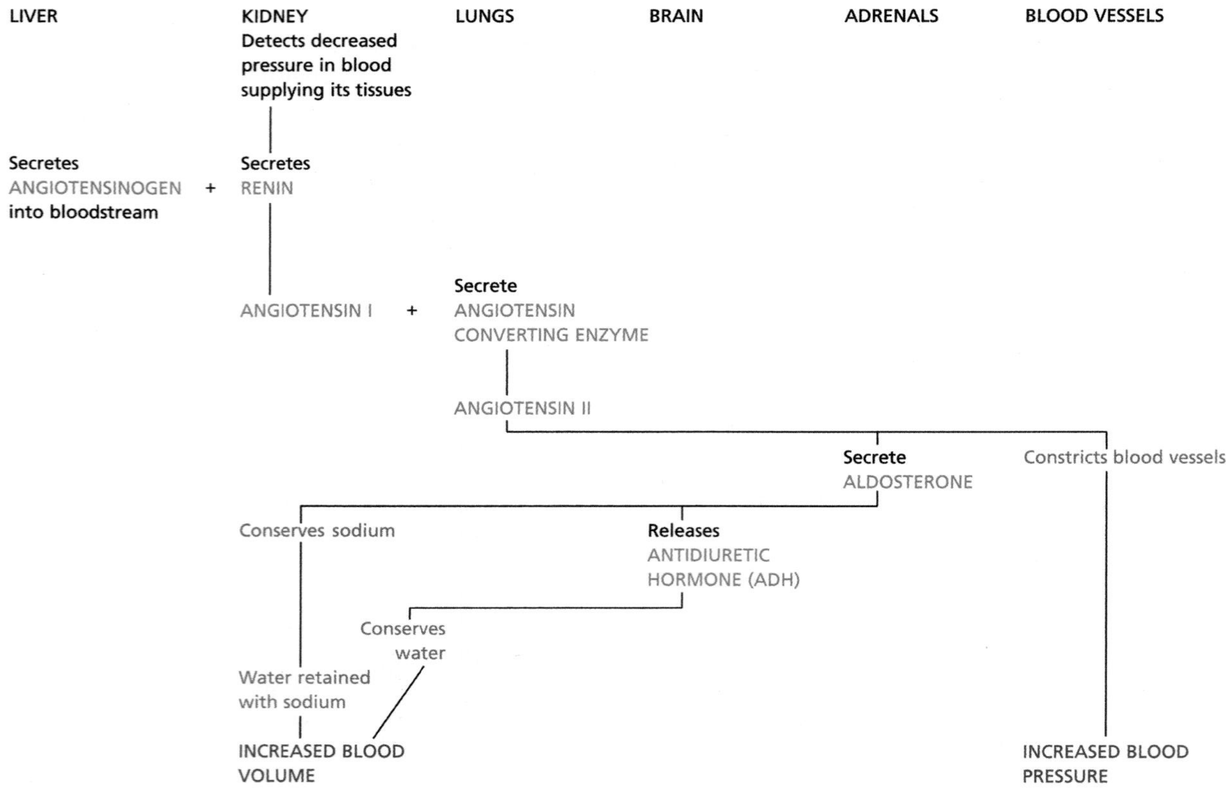

FIGURE 8-17 Hormonal control of water balance. Although the kidneys do most of the work, the complex process also involves the liver, lungs, brain, adrenal glands, and blood vessels.

When a strong acid is introduced into the fluid, a chemical reaction takes place yielding sodium chloride (a salt), which is neutral, and carbonic acid (a weak acid). **Carbonic acid** breaks down to carbon dioxide and water, which are excreted by the lungs (exhaled) and kidneys respectively.

When a strong base (alkali) enters the system, carbon dioxide and water (the two main waste products of cellular metabolism) react to form carbonic acid to counteract the alkaline effect of the base. The end products of this reaction are water and a weak base that does not drastically affect the pH.

RESPIRATORY SYSTEM

The lungs help maintain pH by varying the amount of carbon dioxide (CO_2) exhaled. Retained carbon dioxide makes the body fluids more acidic because it reacts to form carbonic acid, a source of hydrogen ions. Too much carbonic acid, or too much of any acid, results in acidosis, a condition that causes the lungs to automatically increase the rate and depth of breathing, eliminating more carbon dioxide and water.

This respiratory response to acidosis begins within minutes of an increase in acidity. Respiratory compensation for acidosis is 50% to 75% effective and is an extremely important component in the regulation of pH.

RENAL SYSTEM

The respiratory system acts quickly but can eliminate only carbonic acid. Other acids, as well as excess carbonic acid, must be eliminated in urine. The kidney spills or retains hydrogen, sodium, and bicarbonate ions as necessary to maintain an acceptable pH in blood. For example, in response to acidosis, the kidneys excrete hydrogen ions and reabsorb sodium and bicarbonate ions. Conversely, in response to alkalosis, the kidneys conserve hydrogen ions and excrete sodium and bicarbonate ions. The kidneys initiate these actions within 24 hours but require 3 to 4 days to compensate for changes in blood pH.

Neither the respiratory nor the renal systems will overcompensate to send the client into the opposite state (Fournier, 2009).

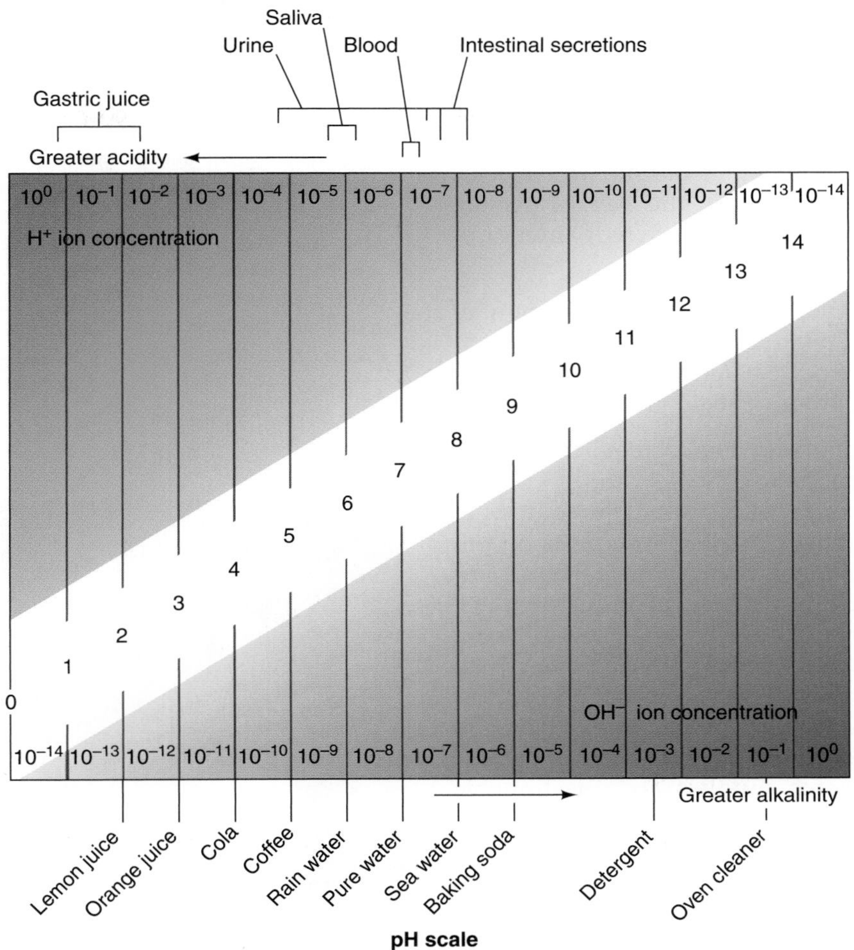

FIGURE 8-18 Representation of the pH scale with usual readings for body fluids, beverages, and household products. (Reprinted from Venes, D [Ed.]: *Taber's cylcopedic medical dictionary*, ed 21. FA Davis, Philadelphia, 2010, p 1764, with permission.)

Intracellular Fluid

The normal pH of the intracellular fluid is 6.8 to 7.0, slightly acid to neutral. Within the intracellular fluid, organic phosphates and proteins are the most important buffers. These substances buffer 95% of the body's carbonic acid and 50% of other acids. Protein is the most powerful and plentiful buffer system in the body.

Of the body's proteins, hemoglobin has the largest buffering capacity. Thus, red blood cells have 70% of the buffering power of the blood. This buffering capacity allows large quantities of carbon dioxide to be transported from the tissues to the lungs, with only a small change in venous pH compared with arterial pH.

When blood contains excessive hydrogen ions, they move into the cells to be buffered. Then, to maintain electroneutrality, potassium moves from the intracellular to the intravascular compartment, raising serum potassium levels.

Water Balance and Imbalances

For optimum health, water intake must equal water output. The body has automatic monitoring and regulating mechanisms to achieve this homeostasis.

Sources of Water

Much of our water is consumed in other beverages. Skim milk is 91% water, and whole milk is 88% water. Water itself may contain other nutrients. Hard water has calcium, magnesium, and often iron. Water conditioners used to soften water replace those minerals with sodium. Drinking softened water increases some people's sodium intake excessively. For this reason, most experts recommend that the cold water in the kitchen be unsoftened.

We obtain about 4 cups of water per day in foods. Some foods that are solids also have a high water content: head lettuce is 96% water, celery is 95% water, and raw carrots are 88% water. See "Nutritive Values of Foods" on DavisPlus for other examples.

Water is also a product of metabolism, which yields about 1 cup of water per day in the average person. Each energy nutrient produces a different amount of metabolic water:

- 1 gram of carbohydrate produces 0.60 gram of water.
- 1 gram of fat produces 1.07 grams of water.
- 1 gram of protein produces 0.41 gram of water.

In contrast, 1 ounce of pure alcohol requires 8 ounces of water for its metabolism.

Consumers can choose from multiple sources of drinking water. An estimated 6 billion gallons of bottled water are consumed annually in the United States compared to the estimated 22.8 billion gallons of tap water. Ironically, bottled water not only is not necessarily safer than tap water, but 25% or more of bottled water *is* tap water. See Table 8-12 for a brief comparison of these two main sources of drinking water and Dollars and Sense 8-1 for choices influenced by culture.

Yet, many city water supplies are questionable because of aging distribution systems and a deteriorating regulatory climate. The National Resources Defense Council graded water quality in 19 cities, concluding that drinking water purity has improved slightly during the past 15 years in most cities but that overall tap water quality varies widely from city to city. Only six cities received a grade of good or excellent (2003).

Losses of Water

We lose water in obvious ways, called **sensible water losses,** as in perspiration and urine. We also lose water in less obvious ways, called **insensible water losses,** as through breathing.

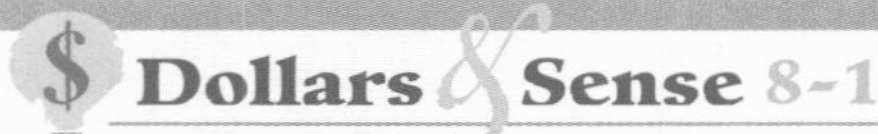

Dollars & Sense 8-1

Culture Influences Water Choices

Economic and health issues regarding choices of drinking water concern immigrant families. One survey showed that 34% of Latino parents never drank tap water, and 44% never gave it to their children, typically because they thought it caused illness which may have been true in their native countries.

Not only is bottled water as much at 10,000 times more expensive than tap water (see Fig. 8-19), the quantity of fluoride in bottled water is uncertain. Lack of fluoride may increase the risk for dental caries (Hobson et al., 2007).

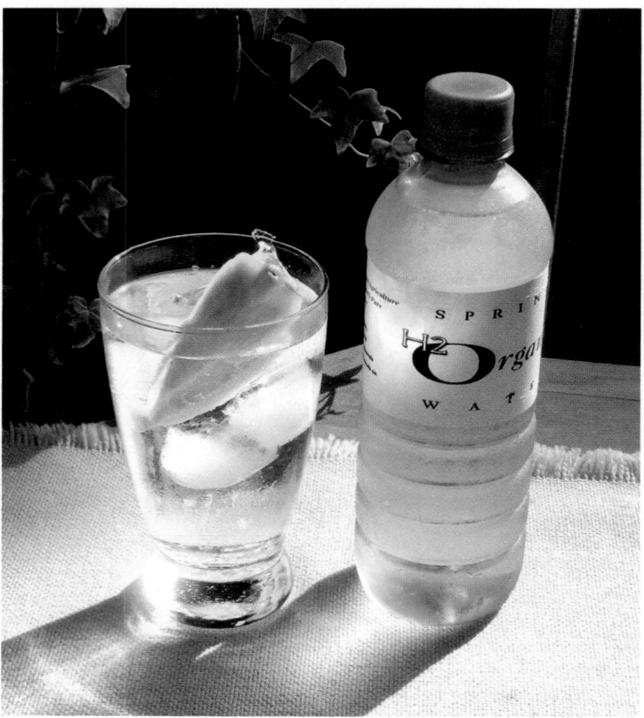

FIGURE 8-19 If a person consumes 8 glasses of water daily, tap water would cost approximately 33 cents per year; bottled water, approximately $200 (Hobson, 2007).

TABLE 8-12 ■ Comparison of Bottled Water and Municipal Water Regulations

	BOTTLED WATER	MUNICIPAL WATER
Regulatory Agency	Food and Drug Administration (FDA)	Environmental Protection Agency (EPA)
Subject to Regulation	Only that sold state-to-state, = 30%–40% of bottled water	All systems serving >24 people
Number of States Regulating Intrastate Bottlers	40	
Coliform Testing	Once a week	100+ times a month
Chemical Testing	Annually	Quarterly
Certified Labs to Test	No	Yes
Reporting to State or Federal Governments	Not mandatory	Yes

SOURCES: Chalupka (2005); National Resources Defense Council (1999).

Sensible Water Losses

Sensible water losses include losses of the major extracellular ions, sodium and chloride. Three important routes commonly account for sensible water losses:

1. Through the skin as perspiration
2. Through the kidney as urine
3. Through the gastrointestinal tract in the feces

PERSPIRATION

Evaporation of sweat is the main means of dissipating the body's heat produced by exercise. In extreme cases, a person may perspire at the rate of 2 liters per hour. For example, during a marathon race, runners may lose 6% to 8% of their body weight, primarily as perspiration. A 150-pound person could then lose 9 to 10½ pounds, or 4.3 to 5 liters, of fluid.

Sweat is not pure water. It is salty to the taste, hypotonic, and its composition varies from person to person. On average, one liter of perspiration contains, with wide ranges for each, approximately:

- 35 milliequivalents of sodium
- 5 milliequivalents of potassium
- 1 milliequivalent of calcium
- 0.8 milliequivalent of magnesium
- 30 milliequivalents of chloride (Sawka et al., 2007)

Consequently, even a sweat loss of 5 or 6 liters entails small amounts of electrolytes so that rehydration with water should suffice (Gropper, Smith, and Groff, 2009).

Exposure to extreme heat can be life-threatening. From 1999 to 2003, 3442 deaths resulted from exposure to extreme heat, either alone (65%) or by complicating other illnesses leading to death (35%) (CDC, 2006c). Even with prompt medical care, 15% of heatstroke cases are fatal (CDC, 2002b), and 20 to 33% of survivors sustain irreversible brain injury (Lewis, 2007). Persons at greatest risk of heat-related illness are:

- Young children
- Older adults
- Individuals with chronic medical (especially cardiovascular) conditions (CDC, 2006c)

See Table 8-13 for a capsule comparison of the most serious conditions resulting from exposure to extreme heat.

URINE

In the normal, healthy person with average exertion throughout the day, urine output is roughly equal to liquid intake. A well-hydrated individual produces light yellow or straw-colored urine. A minimum amount of urine must be excreted each day to carry away the waste products resulting from metabolic processes. This function, called obligatory excretion, eliminates 400 to 600 milliliters per day.

The hourly urine output of seriously ill clients is monitored but the amounts must be interpreted in relation to the client's situation. Even if a person is losing massive amounts of fluid through the gastrointestinal

TABLE 8-13 ■ Serious Heat-Related Illnesses

		HEAT EXHAUSTION	HEAT STROKE-MEDICAL EMERGENCY
Pathophysiology		Loss of water and salt in sweat	Loss of body temperature regulation Progresses to multiple organ dysfunctions
Symptoms		Headache Weakness, fatigue Dizziness, fainting Muscle cramps	Lethargy Throbbing headache Disorientation
Signs		Coherent	Delirium Convulsions Coma
	Temperature	Usually <102.2°F	>103°F
	Pulse	Weak, thready, rapid	Full, bounding, rapid
	Respirations	Shallow, rapid, quiet	Difficult, loud
	Skin	Cool, clammy, sweaty	Flushed, hot, dry (unless just progressed from heat exhaustion)
Treatment		Move to cool location Lie down Elevate feet Loosen clothing Monitor temperature If able to drink: ½ tsp salt in ½ glass of water orally every 15 min until medical help arrives	Move to cool location Lie down Elevate head Remove clothing Ice bags to neck, axillae, groin Spray with water while fanning Monitor airway, breathing, circulation until medical help arrives

tract, such losses do not rid the body of metabolic wastes as efficiently as the kidney does. Adults should excrete 40 to 80 milliliters per hour—although the amount varies throughout the day and night. Clinical Calculation 8-2 shows a method of determining a desirable hourly urine output for children.

GASTROINTESTINAL SECRETIONS

Abnormal gastrointestinal function can cause extensive fluid loss. Location of the loss determines signs and symptoms. Gastric juice is acid, whereas intestinal juices are alkaline. Therefore, conceptually, gastrointestinal losses are divided into those lost above the outlet of the stomach, the pylorus, and those lost below it.

Above The Pylorus

The common causes of losses above the pylorus are vomiting or stomach suctioning. Two organs secrete digestive juices above the pylorus: the salivary glands in the mouth and the gastric glands in the stomach. The ions lost in secretions above the pylorus are:

- Sodium
- Potassium
- Chloride
- Hydrogen

About 1 liter of saliva per day is mixed with food or just swallowed. The stomach secretes about 1.5 to 2.5 liters of gastric juice per day. If gastric juices are lost, hydrogen ions in the hydrochloric acid are also lost, putting the person at risk for alkalosis.

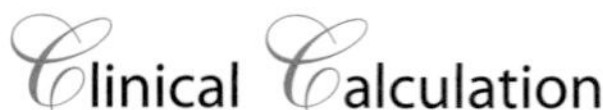
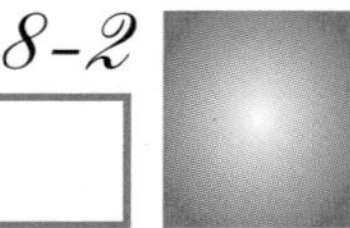

8-2 Clinical Calculation

Hourly Urine Output in Children

Children should excrete between 0.5 and 2 milliliters of urine per kilogram of body weight per hour. What would be a normal hourly urine output for a child who weighs 50 pounds?

First, convert pounds to kilograms. There are 2.2 pounds per kilogram.

$$\frac{50 \text{ lb}}{2.2 \text{ lb/kg}} = 22.7 \text{ kg}$$

To find the desirable range of output, multiply the child's weight in kilograms by the desired factors of 0.5 to 2 mL per kilogram.

$$22.7 \times 0.5 = 11.4 \text{ mL/h}$$
$$22.7 \times 2 = 45.4 \text{ mL/h}$$

Thus, a 50-lb child normally should excrete between 11 and 45 mL/h of urine.

Below the Pylorus

The usual causes of losses below the pylorus are diarrhea and intestinal suctioning. Gastrointestinal secretions below the pylorus contain:

- Sodium
- Potassium
- Bicarbonate

Two to 3 liters of intestinal secretions per day flow into the bowel to digest food. Normally, bile is released from the gallbladder into the small intestine at the rate of 1 liter per day. The total gastrointestinal secretions amount to 6.5 to 8.5 liters per day. Yet, because water is absorbed back into the blood from the large intestine, normal feces from an adult contain only 100 to 200 milliliters of water.

Insensible Water Losses

An invisible amount of water is lost through the lungs and the skin. These are insensible losses. Between 800 and 1000 milliliters of water is lost each day via the lungs and skin. Breath is visible only in very cold weather. Even in warmer weather and indoors, people lose 400 milliliters of water per day in exhaled air. Deep respirations or a dry climate increase the amount of water lost.

The insensible loss of water through the skin is evaporative. It is almost pure water and nearly electrolyte-free. This insensible water loss amounts to 6 milliliters per kilogram of body weight in 24 hours, which is a baseline amount.

Environmental conditions influence the amount of water lost. Greater losses occur:

- At high temperatures
- At high altitudes
- In low humidity

Clinical Calculation 8-3 shows how to estimate insensible water loss. Burns, phototherapy, radiant warmers, or fever will increase the amount of insensible water loss. Fever increases evaporative losses by about 12% per Celsius degree of temperature elevation.

Clinical Calculation 8-4 shows how **evaporative water losses** are calculated. Table 8-14 lists average fluid gains and losses for 24 hours.

Assessment of Water Balance

Gathering data on water losses is quite straightforward: daily weight or documenting intake and output.

Weight

Daily weight is the single most important indicator of fluid status. An easy way to relate volume to weight is

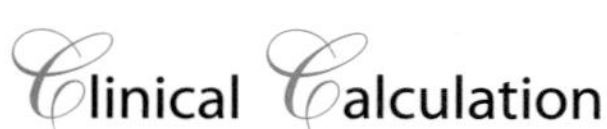
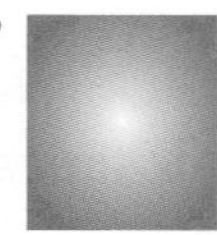

8-3

Clinical Calculation

Insensible Water Loss Through the Skin

The rule of thumb for insensible water loss through the skin is 6 mL/kg per 24 hours. How much insensible water loss would be expected for a 154-lb client?

First, convert pounds to kilograms:

$$\frac{154 \text{ lb}}{2.2 \text{ lb/kg}} = 70 \text{ kg}$$

Then multiply the client's weight in kilograms by the estimated standard:

$$70 \text{ kg} \times 6 \text{ mL/kg} = 420 \text{ mL}$$

Thus, this client's insensible water loss in a 24-hour period is expected to be 420 mL.

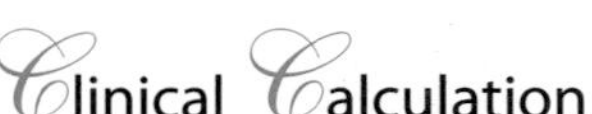
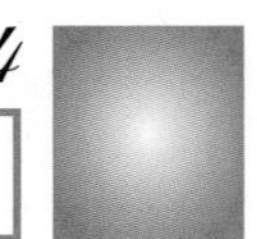

8-4

Clinical Calculation

Evaporative Water Loss in Fever

Fever increases the amount of evaporative loss by 12% for every degree Celsius of fever. If the 154-lb client in Clinical Calculation 8-3 had a fever of 102.2ºF, how much additional evaporative loss would he or she sustain?

Temperatures can be reported in Fahrenheit or Celsius degrees, and the conversion formulas account for the fact that the Celsius scale sets freezing at zero and the Fahrenheit sets it at 32 degrees.

To convert Fahrenheit to Celsius, subtract 32 and multiply by 5/9.

$$102.2 - 32 = 70.2 \times 5/9 = 39^{\circ}\text{C}$$

Normal body temperature on the Celsius scale is 37 degrees.

To convert Celsius to Fahrenheit, multiply by 9/5 and add 32.

$$37 \times 9/5 = 66.6 + 32 = 98.6^{\circ}\text{F}$$

The client had insensible losses of 420 mL.

The client has an elevation of 2ºC, which would increase evaporative loss by 24%.

420 mL × 0.24 = 100.8 mL additional evaporative water loss.

420 mL + 100.8 mL = 520.8 total insensible water loss through the skin

to remember "a pint is a pound the world around." One liter is 1 kilogram or 2.2 pounds.

Acute weight loss in adults is rated as follows:

Mild volume deficit, 2% to 5% loss;
Moderate volume deficit, 5% to 10% loss;
Severe volume deficit, >10% loss.

Fluid balance in an infant is much more precarious than in an adult. Because a greater proportion of the

TABLE 8-14 ■ Average Fluid Gains and Losses in Adults in 24 Hours

FLUID GAINS		FLUID LOSSES*	
Energy metabolism	300 mL	Kidneys	1200–1500 mL
		Skin	500–600 mL
Oral fluids	1100–1400 mL	Lungs	400 mL
Solid foods	800–1000 mL	Intestines	100–200 mL
Total Gains	2200–2700 mL	**Total Losses**	2200–2700 mL

*Includes sensible and insensible losses.

Box 8-4 ■ *Third-Space Losses*

Large amounts of fluid can accumulate in several places in the body outside the normal circulation. These losses are called **third-space losses.** Certain diseases cause **ascites,** the accumulation of fluid (often amounting to several liters), not within the bowel but around it in the abdominal cavity. Other third-space losses involve internal bleeding or the collection of fluid in the chest cavity. An alert nurse can spot an early clue to third-space losses: decreasing urine output despite seemingly adequate fluid intake.

infant's body water is in the extracellular space, infants can lose water more rapidly than adults. Therefore, a loss of 5% of body weight in an infant merits medical attention.

Weight changes can be caused by metabolic events as well as by fluid shifts. If a client receives no oral, enteral, or parenteral nutrition, the loss of body tissue may amount to 0.3 to 0.5 kilogram per day.

Similarly, the loss of effective circulatory volume is not always an external loss. Weight gain may mean circulatory loss. See Box 8-4 for insight into fluid losses within the body.

Intake and Output

In a healthy person, liquid intake and output should be approximately equal. Measuring intake is easier than measuring output, but it still is frequently inaccurate. Most institutions post the amounts that food and beverage containers hold. Amounts remaining should be measured and subtracted from the total liquid served.

Rather than assume that clients have consumed everything missing from the pitcher or tray, the nurse should ask if they drank the fluid (as opposed to, for instance, giving it to a visitor). Updating the intake form throughout the day rather than at the end of a shift is likely to produce a more complete record. Record the amount of water from ice chips as one-half of their volume. One cup of ice chips yields only ½ cup of water.

Fluid lost into a dressing or a diaper can be estimated by weighing it. Subtract the dry material's weight from the total. One gram of weight equals 1 milliliter of water. **Specific gravity** is the weight of a substance compared with that of distilled water. Normal specific gravity of urine is 1.010 to 1.025, but a lower value is common in newborns. So, although the weight of a diaper wet with urine is not exactly the same as if it were wet with water, this method of recording incontinent urine is adequate in most situations.

In a sick person, intake and output totals may not balance every day. The client's intake and output should be assessed over a period of several days, because a single-day evaluation can lead to missing the big picture. See Clinical Application 8-12 for teaching and documentation tips regarding fluid intake and Box 8-5 for practical assessment tips regarding output.

Water Imbalances

Fluid volume is unbalanced if it is insufficient or excessive. Signs and symptoms of both are shown in Table 8-15. To assess fluid volume through observation of hand veins, raise the client's hand above the heart. Normally, the veins will collapse in 3 to 5 seconds. Then lower the hand below the heart. The veins should refill in 3 to 5 seconds. The veins of a person with insufficient fluid volume require more than 5 seconds to refill. Reverse the procedure to assess excessive fluid volume in which the veins will take more than 5 seconds to empty.

Fluid compartments do not operate in isolation: if one is out of balance, the other compartments eventually will be affected as the body attempts to equalize osmotic pressure across the compartments.

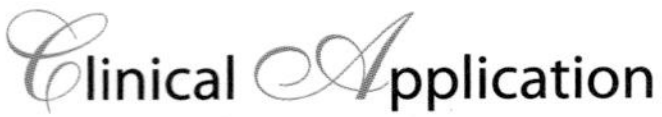
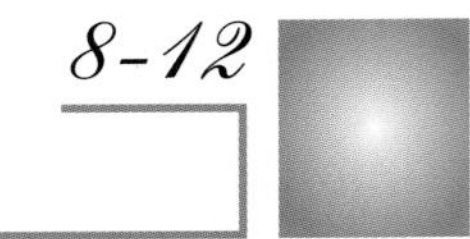

8-12 Clinical Application

Avoiding Misinterpretation

One client was told to "drink a lot of fluid" when he was discharged from the hospital. He interpreted this to be 3 to 4 gallons per day! His kidneys did their best, but kidneys cannot excrete plain water. In a few days, the client was back in the hospital for correction of electrolyte imbalance.

- Be specific when teaching clients.
- Document both the teaching content and the client's response to the information.

Box 8-5 ■ *Visual Assessment of Fluid Balance*

In persons with normal organ function, a good day-to-day measure of hydration status is the color of urine. Urine of light yellow color usually reflects normal fluid balance whereas concentrated urine of a deeper color may indicate dehydration.

TABLE 8-15 ■ Signs and Symptoms of Abnormal Fluid Volume

	INSUFFICIENT FLUID VOLUME	EXCESSIVE FLUID VOLUME
Symptoms		
Gastrointestinal	Thirst Loss of appetite (decreased blood to intestines)	Nausea Loss of appetite (edema of the bowel)
Signs		
General	Weight loss Depressed fontanel (infant) Sunken eyes (infant) Lack of tears when crying (infant)	Weight gain Edema
Skin and mucous membranes	Dry mucous membranes Decreased skin **turgor** (not reliable in elderly)	Skin stretched and shiny
Cardiovascular system	**Orthostatic hypotension** (pressure decrease of 15 mm Hg in systolic or diastolic) Increased pulse rate upon standing Increased hematocrit values (unless red blood cells also lost) Narrowing **pulse pressure** Filling of dependent hand veins takes longer than 5 seconds	Decreased hematocrit values Increasing pulse pressure Emptying of elevated hand veins takes longer than 5 seconds.
Urinary	Decreased urine output Concentrated urine	**Polyuria** Dilute urine
Gastrointestinal	Vomiting (decreased blood to intestines) Longitudinal furrows on tongue	Vomiting (edema of intestines)
Central nervous system	Confusion, disorientation	Deteriorating consciousness

Insufficient Fluid Volume Treatment

Treating insufficient fluid volume with appropriate fluids is essential, as is correcting the cause. Hypotonic fluids are given to replace fluid volume and correct electrolyte imbalances intravenously if necessary but orally if possible (Clinical Application 8-13).

Oral electrolyte solutions, although clearly lifesaving and effective in maintaining hydration, do not necessarily reduce stool volume or the duration of diarrhea. Although hypotonic, plain water orally is not advised for treating insufficient fluid volume because it is likely to inhibit thirst and to increase urine output.

Thickened hydration solutions are also available for clients who have difficulty swallowing thin liquids. A dietitian should be consulted before using food thickeners, inasmuch as some of them bind with water, making water less available for absorption.

An alternative to intravenous rehydration in selected clients is the use of hypodermoclysis. In this technique, fluid is introduced into the subcutaneous tissue, in the thighs or abdomen, for instance, usually by means of a pair of long needles. A drug may be used to aid in dispersal of the solution.

If hypertonic solutions are given orally to correct fluid loss, the concentrated solution would remain in the stomach longer than water, providing satiety and restraining water intake. In addition, as hypertonic solutions draw fluid from the bowel wall into the lumen, the result is osmotic diarrhea. Some commercial laxatives and enemas are hypertonic solutions.

Maximal sodium and water absorption is thought to occur with a glucose concentration of 10 to 25 grams per liter. Higher concentrations allow less sodium and water to be absorbed in addition to causing osmotic diarrhea. Cola beverages (750 milliosmoles per liter) and apple juice (730 mmol/L) are poor choices for rehydration in prolonged diarrhea, owing to their high glucose and low electrolyte concentrations (Oral Therapy, 2004).

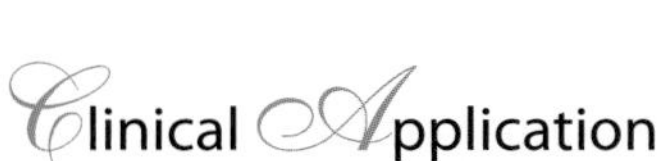

8-13

Oral Electrolyte Solutions

Originally, oral electrolyte solutions were designed to combat diarrheal diseases in developing countries. They proved so useful that they have since been modified for use in Western nations. One commonly used oral electrolyte solution is Pedialyte®. It is available over the counter without a prescription. One liter of Pedialyte contains sodium chloride and potassium citrate yielding the following electrolytes:

Cations	Anions
45 mEq sodium (Na^+)	35 mEq chloride (Cl^-)
20 mEq potassium (K^+)	30 mEq citrate, a base ($^-$)
65 mEq cations	65 mEq anions

Pedialyte is mildly hypotonic, about 250 milliosmoles per liter, and also contains a concentration of glucose that promotes sodium and water absorption, 25 g/L.

Pedialyte is designed for maintenance of an infant or child experiencing vomiting or diarrhea. If the client becomes dehydrated, as evidenced by loss of 5% of body weight, medical attention is needed. Intravenous fluids or an oral rehydration solution of different composition from Pedialyte may be prescribed for the dehydrated client.

Excessive Fluid Volume Treatment

When a person becomes ill and the control mechanisms stop working, the individual can retain fluid intracellularly or extracellularly. In addition, a person can overwhelm his or her own homeostatic mechanisms with voluntary water consumption. Such cases were reported in 17 military trainees who were hospitalized to treat overhydration (O'Brien et al., 2001) and in hyponatremic Boston Marathon runners (Almond et al., 2005).

As with insufficient fluid volume, the remedy for excessive fluid volume is to treat the cause. Osmotic diuretic drugs such as mannitol remain in plasma. By increasing the osmotic pressure there, these drugs pull excess fluid from the cells to be excreted by the kidney.

Nutritionally, the client may be on a restricted fluid regimen. The physician may prescribe an intake of no more than 1000 milliliters in 24 hours. This amount compensates for insensible losses through the skin and lungs. It is essential to supply fluid as prescribed and to teach the client the reason for the restriction. Over a period of several days, the obligatory urine output and any diuretic therapy will help the client's body excrete the excess fluid.

Keystones

- Minerals are inorganic substances that help regulate body functions without providing energy, but unlike vitamins, minerals become part of the body's structure and enzymes.
- Major minerals are present in the body in amounts of 5 grams (1 teaspoonful) or more; the daily recommended intake is 100 milligrams or more.
- Trace minerals are those present in small amounts with daily intakes less than the major minerals; however, even small amounts support essential functions.
- Either insufficient or excessive mineral intake can cause illness, so persons fed artificially, in particular, should be carefully monitored.
- In the United States, increasing the intake of iron and calcium has the potential to improve the health of millions of people.
- Unless medically indicated, people who take mineral supplements should limit intake to RDA or AI levels and select pharmaceutical preparations rather than natural supplements, that may have uncertain strengths and unwelcome contaminants.
- Water is our most essential nutrient. It constitutes at least half of everyone's body weight so that the single most important measure of fluid balance is daily weight.
- The movement, distribution, and composition of body fluids are influenced and controlled by electrolyte and plasma protein concentrations. The major cations are sodium in the extracellular fluid and potassium in the intracellular fluid.
- Acid–base balance is maintained in the body by the action of the lungs, kidneys, and chemical buffers.
- The body's sources of water include beverages, foods, and water from the metabolism of the energy nutrients. Water can be lost through the skin, lungs, kidneys, and intestinal tract.

CASE STUDY 8–1

Mrs. B is a 34-year-old woman who has related her fear of osteoporosis to the nurse. A recent visit to a 75-year-old aunt crystallized this fear. The aunt has become stooped and recently broke her hip. Mrs. B is especially concerned because she has often been told she resembles this aunt. Mrs. B asks, "Is there anything I can do to prevent this from happening to me?"

A 24-hour recall of dietary intake revealed a total of 1 cup of milk and no other dairy products. Mrs. B did consume two 3-oz servings of meat. Mrs. B has three small children and stated that they are exercise enough for her. She sits outside and watches them play on every nice day.

Mrs. B is 5 ft 3 in. tall and weighs 110 lb. She is white with fair skin.

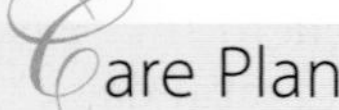

Care Plan

Subjective Data

Fear of osteoporosis ■ Family history positive for osteoporosis ■ Less than AI for calcium previous 24 hours ■ Met MyPyramid guideline for meat group previous 24 hours ■ No planned exercise program

Objective Data

Height: 5 ft 3 in. ■ Weight: 110 lb ■ White, fair, slight build

Analysis

Self-identified need regarding prevention of osteoporosis related to aunt's history of disease.

CASE STUDY *(Continued)*

Plan

DESIRED OUTCOMES EVALUATION CRITERIA	ACTIONS/INTERVENTIONS	RATIONALE
Client will list appropriate actions to maintain a strong skeleton after teaching session.	Teach client how to consume 1000 mg of calcium daily: 3 cups of milk or equivalent.	One cup of milk contains approximately 300 mg of calcium + 100 mg from other sources.
	Teach client factors favoring calcium absorption: vitamin D.	If client chooses unfortified dairy products for calcium content, vitamin D may become insufficient depending on available sun exposure.
	Teach client role of exercise in strengthening bones.	Weight-bearing exercise stimulates the osteoblasts to build bone.

At a follow-up visit, Mrs. B indicated she had increased her consumption of dairy products but had not begun a planned exercise program. The nurse referred Mrs. B to a local Women's Health Center.

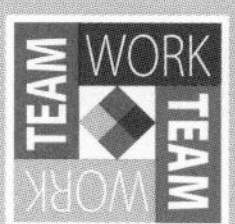

8-1

Director of Women's Health Center's Notes

The following Director of Women's Health Center's Notes are representative of teamwork documentation.

Subjective

Interested in strengthening bones due to fear of familial osteoporosis

States no activity impediments

Objective

BMI = 19.5

Passed Intake Activity Screen

Analysis

Increased risk of osteoporosis based on family history and physical characteristics.

Plan

Suggest ultrasound heel BMD for baseline value

Beginning level walking program with group 3 times weekly, solo 3 times weekly.

Critical Thinking Questions

1. What additional dietary information would you need before recommending good sources of calcium for Mrs. B?
2. What other assessment data would be helpful to broaden the scope of preventing osteoporosis?
3. Is the problem described in the Case Study a significant one for a 34-year-old woman? Why or why not?

CASE STUDY 8-2

Mr. N, a 75-year-old retired office worker, recently arrived from his summer home in the North to his winter home in Florida. He had anticipated enjoying the 85°F weather. He left temperatures in the 40s. Although Mr. N had hired someone to care for his small yard while he was away from Florida, he still had to do a number of chores, which he tackled with a vengeance.

After 1½ hours, Mr. N began to get a headache. He felt a bit weak and dizzy but continued his work. He was nearly finished with the outside tasks.

Half an hour later, Ms. N found her husband lying on the ground and called to their neighbor, a retired nurse.

The nurse noted that Mr. N's skin was pale and cool but that he was perspiring profusely. He was conscious and coherent but said he felt weak. The nurse took Mr. N's pulse. It was 90 beats per minute, regular but weak. His respirations were 12 per minute and shallow.

The nurse provided the emergency care described in the following care plan. (Of course, she did not write it all out before helping Mr. N.)

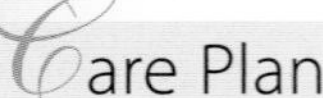

Care Plan

Subjective Data

Had worked outside in 85°F heat 2 hours ■ Headache, weakness, dizziness ■ Recently arrived from colder climate

Objective Data

Conscious, coherent ■ Skin pale, cool, wet with perspiration ■ Pulse 90, regular and weak ■ Respirations 24 and shallow

Analysis

Heat stress related to excessive loss of hypotonic fluid (sweat) as evidenced by wet, pale skin and weak, rapid pulse.

Plan

DESIRED OUTCOMES EVALUATION CRITERIA	ACTIONS/INTERVENTIONS	RATIONALE
Client will remain conscious and oriented, with a pulse rate no greater than 90 beats/min, until the emergency team arrives.	Instruct Ms. N to call emergency medical services and return to help.	In an emergency situation, the nurse stays with the client. Potential electrolyte imbalance requires medical care.
	Loosen Mr. N's clothing.	Loosening the clothing will allow maximum air exchange and permit relaxation.
	With Ms. N, move client to shade or provide shade where he lies.	Mr. N must get out of the sun. Depending on the situation, he might be moved indoors, but perhaps the two women could not manage to move him.
	Keep client lying down with legs elevated slightly.	Lying down permits maximum blood circulation to the brain. Raising the legs increases the return of blood to the heart. The head should not be lowered because this causes venous congestion in the brain.
	Ask Ms. N to prepare a ½ glass water with ½ teaspoonful of salt in it. Administer salty water to Mr. N.	Although this is a hypertonic solution, sodium is readily absorbed by the intestine, so it is unlikely to cause osmotic diarrhea. Only 5% of consumed sodium remains in the feces. The kidneys control sodium levels in the blood. This client has lost water and sodium chloride in perspiration.

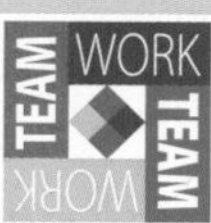

8-2

Emergency Medical Technition's Notes

The following Emergency Medical Technition's notes are representative of teamwork documentation.

Chief Complaint

Collapsed while performing yard work

Subjective

Oriented to person, place, time

Hesitant in answers

Wife reports 75 years old, no chronic illnesses, no daily medications

Objective

Temperature 101.0°F axillary

Pulse 108, weak, thready

Respirations 22, shallow

B/P 105/70

Skin cool, clammy

Analysis

Heat exhaustion

Plan

Rehydrate with 0.9% sodium chloride at 250 mL/hour

Monitor vital signs every 5 minutes

Transport to Emergency Department

Critical Thinking Questions

1. Reread the narrative. At what points in the narrative or in your expansion of the story could you envision Mr. N avoiding this incident?
2. The case study narrative does not discuss Mr. N's usual dietary intake. What dietary modifications can you think of that would make Mr. N's situation of overworking in the heat more critical?
3. What would you include in a presentation on preventing heat-related illnesses for an audience of elderly residents such as Mr. N, who follow the sun for the winter?

Chapter Review

1. Like vitamins, minerals give no energy to the body. Unlike vitamins, minerals:
   a. Are completely absorbed from the intestinal tract
   b. Become part of the structure of the body
   c. Cause few clinical problems because of their great abundance in foods
   d. Cannot accumulate to the extent that they cause problems
2. From which of the following sources of iron is the greatest percentage of iron absorbed by the average person?
   a. Eggs
   b. Ferrous sulfate tablets
   c. Meat
   d. Vegetables
3. Which of the following individuals would be at greatest risk for a mineral deficiency?
   a. Someone who consumes no dairy products
   b. Someone who consumes no shellfish
   c. Someone who consumes no red meat
   d. Someone who drinks tea or coffee with every meal
4. Which of the following people has the greatest percentage of body weight as water?
   a. A 154-pound man
   b. A 120-pound woman
   c. An 18-pound boy, 14 months old
   d. An 8-pound girl, 4 days old
5. Heat exhaustion is caused by:
   a. Insufficient secretion of ADH
   b. Loss of water and salt in sweat
   c. Inability to perspire
   d. Retention of excessive water

Clinical Analysis

Mrs. H is a 30-year-old mother of three children, all younger than 5 years of age. On her 6-week postpartum visit, her hemoglobin level was 10 grams per 100 milliliters of blood. She is given a prescription for ferrous sulfate and referred to the office nurse for nutrition counseling regarding her iron intake.

Mrs. H tells the nurse that she eats what the children eat: cold cereal and milk for breakfast, peanut butter and jelly sandwiches and maybe a banana for lunch, and casseroles of tuna or hamburger for dinner. Mrs. H is a heavy coffee drinker, consuming 10 cups per day, two with each meal and a total of four others during "coffee breaks."

The H family is lower-middle class. Mr. H is a long-distance truck driver and is away from home for long intervals. Mrs. H has some knowledge of iron needs and sources because of her three pregnancies. She is reluctant to continue the ferrous sulfate she has been taking throughout her pregnancy. "It binds me up," she tells the nurse. Also, Mrs. H maintains she cannot eat liver: "It gags me."

1. Which of the following statements by Mrs. H would indicate she understood the nurse's instructions correctly?
   a. "I should eat a little meat, fish, or poultry with every meal containing grain, fruit and vegetable sources of iron."
   b. "I should increase the fiber in my diet because it will increase the absorption of iron."
   c. "If I want an alcoholic beverage, beer contains the most iron in a readily absorbable form."
   d. "Since I am taking an iron supplement, it is not important how I eat."
2. To meet the safety needs of the H children, the nurse instructs Mrs. H to keep her ferrous sulfate in a locked cupboard. The reason for this is:
   a. Interactions of iron tablets with vitamin supplements intended for children can cause deficiencies of water-soluble vitamins.
   b. The human body has no effective means of excreting an overload of iron.
   c. Iron poisoning, although rare, can occur if a child ingests more than 30 tablets of ferrous sulfate.
   d. Because iron binds with calcium, an overdose of iron would cause rickets.

Baby I, a 4-month-old boy, has developed diarrheal stools within the past 2 days. At birth he weighed 7 pounds 8 ounces. Since then he has gained steadily. Three days ago he weighed 12 pounds 8 ounces. Baby I's present weight is 12 pounds 2 ounces.

Mrs. I has been feeding the baby his usual formula. He drinks eagerly but then has an explosive bowel movement with loud crying. Baby I has had six bowel movements per day instead of his usual two.

3. With this history, what physical assessment measures would the nurse include initially?
   a. Condition of hair, strength of grasp, presence of sucking reflex
   b. Heart sounds, lung sounds, blood pressure
   c. Skin turgor, fontanel fullness, moisture of mucous membranes
   d. Urine specific gravity, observation of diaper rash
4. Which of the following recommendations by the nurse would show understanding of supportive care of this client?
   a. Give Baby I whole milk to maintain nutrition.
   b. Continue, as Mrs. I has been doing, to allow the bowel to empty itself.
   c. Substitute orange juice for the formula for 3 days.
   d. Start Baby I on an oral electrolyte solution.

9

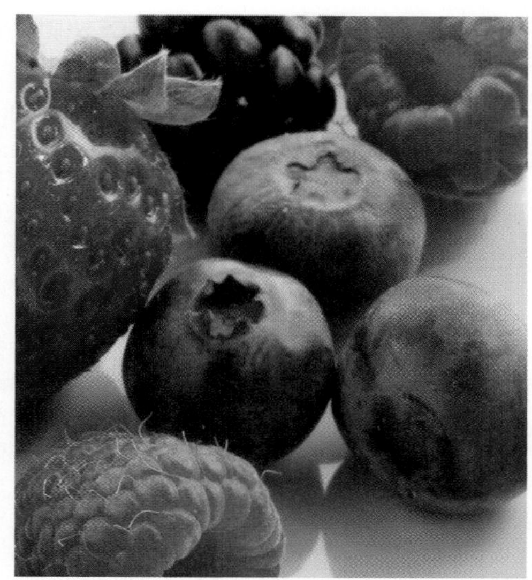

Digestion, Absorption, Metabolism, and Excretion

LEARNING OBJECTIVES

After completing this chapter, the student should be able to:

- List the anatomic structures that make up the gastrointestinal tract.
- Describe the processes of digestion, absorption, metabolism, and excretion.
- Discuss how cells use nutrients.
- Describe appropriate dietary treatments for lactose intolerance, lipid malabsorption, food allergies, and gluten-sensitive enteropathy.
- List the ways the body eliminates waste.

Every part of the human body requires nutrients from food for energy, maintenance, and growth. Food is composed of complex substances that must be broken down to simpler forms for cell use.

The **cell** is the ultimate destination for food's nutrients. Digestion, absorption, and metabolism are the three interrelated processes that act on food to prepare it for use. A fourth process, excretion, is the elimination of undigestible or unusable substances. This chapter discusses all the bodily activities, organs, and systems involved in these major processes.

Overview of the Major Processes

The first step in preparing food for use is digestion. During **digestion,** food is broken down mechanically and chemically in the gastrointestinal tract into forms small enough for **absorption** into the blood or lymphatic system.

After absorption, the nutrients usually are transported to the liver, where they may be adjusted to suit the body's needs. **Metabolism,** the sum of all physical and chemical changes that take place in the body, determines the final use of individual nutrients as well as medications. What the cells cannot use becomes waste that is eliminated through **excretion.**

Digestion

Digestion takes place in the alimentary canal with the aid of its accessory organs.

Alimentary Canal

The **alimentary canal** is a long, muscular tube that extends through the body from the mouth to the anus. It includes:

- The oral cavity
- Pharynx
- Esophagus
- Stomach
- Small intestine
- Large intestine

Muscle rings, called **sphincters,** separate segments of the alimentary canal. The sphincters act as valves to control the passage of food. When the muscles contract, the passageway closes; when the muscles relax, the passageway opens.

The **mucosa** lines the alimentary canal and secretes **mucus,** which lubricates the canal and helps facilitate the smooth passage of food. The mucosa secretes the digestive enzymes of the stomach and small intestine.

Accessory Organs

Three **organs** located outside of the alimentary canal are considered part of the digestive system—the liver, gallbladder, and pancreas. They make important contributions to the digestive process.

LIVER

The **liver** is the second largest single organ in the body (skin is the largest). The liver performs many functions, but its primary digestive function is the production of **bile,** which breaks down dietary fats. Bile exits the liver via the hepatic **duct** (a narrow tube that permits the movement of fluid from one organ to another).

GALLBLADDER

The **gallbladder** is a 3- to 4-inch sac that concentrates and stores bile until it is needed in the small intestine. Bile is delivered to the small intestine through the common bile duct. About 2 to 3 cups of bile are secreted each day into the alimentary canal.

PANCREAS

The **pancreas** secretes enzymes that are involved in the digestion of all the energy nutrients. These secretions are collectively known as pancreatic juice. Pancreatic juice is carried to the small intestine via the pancreatic and common bile ducts.

Digestive Action

Mechanical and chemical digestion occur simultaneously throughout the alimentary canal. **Mechanical digestion** is the physical breaking down of food into smaller pieces. **Chemical digestion** involves the splitting of complex molecules into simpler forms.

Mechanical Digestion

Examples of mechanical digestion include chewing, or **mastication,** and swallowing, peristalsis, and emulsification. **Peristalsis** is a wavelike movement that propels food through the entire length of the alimentary canal. This one-way movement is caused by the alternate contraction and relaxation of the circular and longitudinal muscles that make up the external muscle layer of the alimentary canal. Other muscular activity churns the food, reducing it to successively smaller particles and mixing it with digestive secretions. All of these muscular actions are regulated by a network of nerves within the wall of the alimentary canal.

Chemical Digestion

Many **chemical reactions** are involved in digestion. **Hydrolysis** is a chemical reaction in which a substance is split into two smaller and simpler substances by the addition or the taking up of the elements of water. When the substance is split one hydrogen (H) attaches to one of the products and the hydroxyl (OH) attaches to the other product. For example, the conversion of starch to maltose, of fat to glycerol and fatty acids, and of protein to amino acids all involve hydrolysis. The hydrolysis of nutrients is achieved mostly through the action of digestive enzymes, which are present in:

- Saliva
- Gastric juice
- Pancreatic juice
- Intestinal juice.

Each enzyme is specific in its action, and it acts only upon a particular substance. Enzymes sometimes require the presence of additional substances, such as activators, coenzymes, or hormones, for activation. More than 500 enzymes are involved in the digestive process; this chapter discusses a few of the major ones.

In addition to enzymes, other secretions and chemicals are used in digestion. For example, mucus lubricates passages and facilitates the movement of food. It also protects the inside walls of the alimentary canal from acidic solutions. Another example is **electrolytes,** which are substances that conduct an electric current in solution. **Hydrochloric acid (HCl)** is an electrolyte and performs many functions necessary to the digestive process. A third example is bicarbonate, which is a basic solution, and enters the small intestine and assists in digestion. Bicarbonate is discussed in more detail in Chapter 8.

SECRETIONS

The quantity of mucus, electrolytes, water, and enzymes released during the digestive process depends on several factors:

Hormones frequently initiate a given secretion. For example, the presence of food in the stomach stimulates the cells to release a hormone called gastrin. Gastrin stimulates the release of hydrochloric acid. When the stomach's content is sufficiently acidic, it turns off further release of gastrin. When gastrin is no longer being released, hydrochloric acid is no longer released.

Emotions and conditioned responses can affect the amount of a secretion released. For example, the smell of a roasting turkey on Thanksgiving causes the release of hydrochloric acid in the stomach. Stress and tension can also produce this effect, sometimes with deleterious results.

The food in the gastrointestinal tract can influence the release of alimentary canal secretions. Drinking coffee, for instance, causes a hormone to be released into the stomach that in turn causes the secretion of hydrochloric acid. Another trigger, for the release of bile from the gallbladder, is the presence of fat in the small intestine. A chain of reactions whereby one event causes another and then another is very common in all biological **systems.**

END PRODUCTS

Four to 6 hours after a meal, the body has broken down the food into some trillion molecules. Each of the energy nutrients is broken down into simpler molecules.

- Carbohydrates are digested into monosaccharides.
- Fats are broken down into molecules of glycerol, fatty acids, and monoglycerides.
- The end products of protein digestion are amino acids and small peptides.

Researchers think that as much as one-third of dietary protein is absorbed into mucosal cells as dipeptides and tripeptides. Vitamins, minerals, and water are also released during digestion.

The Food Pathway

Food passes through the mouth into the oral cavity, where it is chewed and exposed to chemicals in the saliva. The tongue voluntarily forces the mass of food, called a **bolus,** into the pharynx, which is responsible for the reflex action of swallowing. The bolus then enters the esophagus, a muscular, mucus-lined tube, and is propelled downward by peristalsis to the stomach.

Both mechanical and chemical digestion occur in the stomach, reducing the food to a semifluid mass that is released into the small intestine. Further digestion takes place in the small intestine, and most of the absorption of nutrients occurs there as well. Any food remaining after digestion and absorption passes into the large intestine and is excreted as fecal matter.

Oral Cavity

The **oral cavity,** the hollow space in the skull directly behind the mouth, includes the roof of the mouth, the cheeks, and the floor of the mouth. Within the oral cavity are the teeth, tongue, and openings of the ducts of the salivary glands.

DIGESTIVE ACTION

Food entering the oral cavity is chewed and, thus, broken into smaller particles. This mechanical action increases the surface area of the food for exposure to saliva, a digestive secretion produced by the **salivary glands.** Saliva moistens and softens the food for swallowing and contains the digestive enzyme known as **salivary amylase,** which converts starch to maltose (a disaccharide) or to the shorter chains of glucose. Because simple sugars (monosaccharides) require no digestion, some absorption may occur in the mouth. The chemical digestion of more complex carbohydrates (starch) continues until the hydrochloric acid in the stomach halts the action of the salivary amylase. Box 9-1 discusses the dietary treatment of dysphagia.

Pharynx

The **pharynx** is a muscular passage between the oral cavity and the esophagus. No digestive action occurs there. The pharynx continues the movement of the bolus by the reflexive action of swallowing. The bolus then enters the esophagus.

Esophagus

The **esophagus** is a muscular tube about 10 inches long that takes food from the pharynx to the stomach. No digestive action occurs there. Peristalsis forces the bolus into the stomach with the help of mucous secretions. Between the esophagus and the stomach is the **cardiac sphincter** (the first portion of the stomach is called the cardia), which opens to permit passage of food. The sphincter then closes to prevent the backup of stomach contents.

Stomach

The **stomach** is a J-shaped sac that extends from the esophagus to the small intestine. Folds in the mucous membrane, called **rugae,** allow the stomach to expand and to smooth out when full. There is no need to eat constantly, partly because the stomach serves as a reservoir for food—it takes 4 to 6 hours for food to pass completely through to the small intestine. The stomach influences appetite, by signaling to decrease intake when distended and to increase intake when empty and contracting (Colaizzo-Anas, 2007). Stomach size also influences the amount of food eaten, and its size is related to the amount of food habitually eaten.

Gastric juice, the collective secretions of the stomach, consists of hydrochloric acid, mucus, and the enzymes pepsin, **rennin,** and **gastric lipase.** Many factors influence the rate of gastric emptying, including the amount of gastric juice, meal composition (percent of fat, carbohydrate [CHO], or protein), meal

Box 9-1 ■ *Dietary Treatment for Dysphagia*

One in 17 people, including 6.2 million Americans older than age 60, have a swallowing disorder called dysphagia, literally meaning difficulty in swallowing (Galvan, 2001). A swallowing disorder may cause coughing, but not always. As a result, food particles may pass into the lungs (aspiration), allowing bacteria to multiply. Studies show that aspiration occurs in 43%–54% of patients who have had strokes. Of these patients, 37% develop pneumonia and 3.8% die of it (Galvan, 2001). Diets for dysphagia that safely meet nutrient needs range from nothing by mouth (NPO) to total oral feedings. Candidates for oral feedings should demonstrate the ability to perform a safe swallow by a bedside evaluation or a modified **barium swallow,** be alert and able to follow directions, and be oriented to self and the task of eating.

Dysphagia diets provide graduated steps from the most easily managed food to the ones most difficult to manage:

- Liquids range from thick to thin.
- Solids range from pureed to regular.
- The most conservative starting point is thickened liquids and pureed textures.
- Liquids and solids may be progressed independently.
- High-protein, high-calorie between-meal feedings as necessary.

Precise diet orders specify both the texture of solid foods and the consistency of liquids as well as other therapeutic modifications. To address the multiplicity of dysphagia diet terminology and practices, a multidisciplinary task force developed The National Dysphagia Diet (NDD) based on existing scientific evidence (McCallum, 2003). The NDD has four levels:

Level 1: Dysphagia Pureed

- Homogenous, cohesive, pudding like
- Requires minimum chewing

Level 2: Dysphagia Mechanically Altered

- Cohesive, moist, semisolid
- Requires some chewing ability.

Level 3: Dysphagia Advanced

- Semisolid, easy-to-cut meats, vegetables, and fruits
- Requires some chewing ability.

Level 4: Regular

- Any solid texture

Hydration is also a challenge for clients with dysphagia; as a result, thickening agents are commonly used to increase a client's fluid intake. Using thickening agents to modify beverages, soups, and pureed foods is both an art and a science. Commercial thickening agents, instant potato flakes, unflavored gelatin, and dehydrated baby foods and cereals can all be used. The nurse should recognize that thickeners may:

- Become thicker with time.
- Add significant carbohydrate kilocalories to clients' diets.
- React differently in various foods.
- Affect palatability of the thickened item.

In addition, being aware that some foods—such as ice cream and gelatin—change their consistency at body temperature is important, and so is following recipes and mixing complementary flavors. For example, tomato juice can be used to thin spaghetti sauce. Another important thing to note is that each patient needs his or her diet highly individualized. For instance, foods with mixed consistency such as vegetable soups with chunks and cereal with milk may not be appropriate for an individual who cannot swallow such foods. For individuals who have problems forming a food bolus, foods such as rice, scrambled eggs, corn, peas, and legumes may cause problems because these foods do not form a cohesive bolus. For other patients, foods that crumble, such as crackers, cornbread, and unmoistened ground meats, may not be appropriate.

A preprinted sheet of dos and don'ts is of limited usefulness for many clients. A nurse, speech therapist, occupational therapist, and registered dietitian may collectively devote many sessions to the developing individualized diet plans and determining the best positions for clients during feeding times. Usually the client should sit upright with hips at a 90-degree angle, shoulders slightly forward, and feet flat on the floor or firmly supported (American Dietetic Association, 2000).

The nurse can do much to help these clients by referring them to other health-care providers who can spend time working with them.

Signs and symptoms of dysphagia include:

- "Gurgly" voice
- Coughing or choking with food and fluid intake
- Nasal regurgitation
- Pocketing of food in cheeks
- Drooling
- Difficulty in initiating a swallow
- Excessive chewing
- Poor tongue control
- Poor lip closure
- Lack of body position control
- Slurred speech
- Refusal to eat
- Absence of gag reflux
- Excessive time spent eating
- Multiple swallows required to clear a single bolus of food
- Pain on swallowing
- Verbal complaints of food stuck in the throat
- Lack of attention to eating

On observation, these clients may have a documented weight loss, edema, poor skin turgor, and open wounds. These are all signs of poor nutrition.

For the client, safe swallowing includes the following tips:

- Eat slowly.
- Avoid distractions while eating.
- Do not talk while eating.
- Remove loose dentures.
- Sit up while eating.
- Position head correctly.
- Use a teaspoon and take only one-half teaspoon of food or liquids at a time.
- Swallow completely between bites or sips.
- Select foods and fluids of appropriate consistency

particle size, and some hormones. Liquids empty in less time than solids do. The primary hormone that influences gastric emptying is **cholecystokinin** (CCK), which inhibits gastric emptying. Another hormone, leptin, which is secreted in the gastric mucosa in addition to fat cells, enhances the action of CCK (Colaizzo-Anas, 2007).

DIGESTIVE ACTION

In the stomach, the chemical digestion of protein begins and further mechanical digestion takes place. Some water and minerals, certain drugs, and alcohol are absorbed in the stomach. Even before food enters the mouth, the sight or smell of food can cause the gastric mucosa to excrete the hormone **gastrin.** This hormone stimulates the secretion of gastric juice so that there is some present in the stomach when the food arrives. Mucus partially protects the stomach's lining from the corrosive effects of gastric juice.

The hydrolysis of protein begins when hydrochloric acid activates and then converts **pepsinogen** to its active form, **pepsin.** A protein molecule consists of hundreds of amino acids joined by **peptide bonds.** Such chains of amino acids linked by peptide bonds are called **polypeptides.** Pepsin breaks down large polypeptides into smaller ones. In infants, the milk protein casein is broken down by the enzyme rennin, which coagulates (curdles) the milk. In addition to activating pepsin, hydrochloric acid destroys harmful bacteria, makes certain minerals such as iron and calcium more absorbable, and maintains the pH (1–2) of the gastric juice.

Another enzyme, gastric lipase, breaks down some milk butterfat molecules into smaller ones. This enzyme is most active in infants; the more alkaline environment of an infant's stomach enables gastric lipase to work more effectively than it does in adults.

The mechanical digestion occurring in the stomach comes from the churning action of the stomach's muscular walls. This activity agitates the contents of the stomach, thoroughly mixing the food with gastric juice. In this way, the food is reduced to a semifluid mass of partially digested material called **chyme.** Peristaltic waves push the chyme toward the **pyloric sphincter,** the valve separating the stomach from the small intestine. With each peristaltic wave, a small amount of **chyme** is forced through the pyloric sphincter into the small intestine.

Gastroparesis, delayed gastric emptying, can be caused by a variety of pathologies including diabetes mellitus, neuropathic disorders, connective tissue diseases, infiltrating diseases, and postsurgical complications. Symptoms of gastroparesis include:

- Nausea
- Vomiting
- Early satiety
- Bloating or fullness
- Abdominal discomfort

Many clients are asymptomatic (no symptoms). Complications of gastroparesis include:

- Fluid and electrolyte abnormalities
- Inadequate nutritional intake
- Weight loss
- Difficult blood glucose control

Dietary treatment includes small feedings, low-fat foods, low-residue foods, and frequent feedings. Gastric motor and sensory function is complex and the care of clients with gastroparesis is a challenge.

Ileus, a temporary loss of peristalsis, is another common pathology of gastrointestinal motility. Dietary treatment for ileus is nothing by mouth, or NPO, until the problem is resolved medically.

Small Intestine

The **small intestine** is the longest portion of the alimentary canal, approximately 20 feet (610 cm) in length. It extends from the pyloric sphincter of the stomach to the large intestine. The small intestine is looped and coiled in the central part of the abdominal cavity, surrounded by the large intestine. It consists of three parts: the **duodenum** is the first 10 inches, the **jejunum** is the middle 8 feet, and the **ileum** is the last 11 feet. Ninety percent of the digestive action in the alimentary canal and nearly all end-product absorption of digestion occur in the small intestine.

The entry of chyme into the duodenum stimulates the secretion of two hormones, secretin and CCK. Collectively, these hormones are responsible for the secretion and release of bile and the secretion of pancreatic juice.

Secretin stimulates the production of bile by the liver and the secretion of sodium bicarbonate juice by the pancreas. The bile salts in bile emulsify fats, and sodium bicarbonate juice (which is alkaline) neutralizes the gastric juice that enters the duodenum. This neutralization is necessary to prevent damage to the lining of the duodenum. Mucus secreted by intestinal glands also provides some measure of protection against such damage.

CCK stimulates the contraction of the gallbladder, an action that forces stored bile into the duodenum. It also stimulates the secretion of pancreatic enzymes, which are essential for the breakdown of carbohydrates, fats, and proteins.

Intestinal juice is also secreted in response to the presence of chyme in the duodenum. The peristaltic action of the small intestine mixes the bile, the pancreatic juice, and the intestinal juice with the chyme as it moves toward the colon. The collective action of these juices yields the final products of digestion.

DIGESTION OF CARBOHYDRATES

The action of pancreatic and intestinal enzymes completes carbohydrate digestion. Pancreatic **amylase** breaks down any remaining starch into maltose. And the action of three enzymes (maltase, sucrose, and lactase) located in the walls of the small intestine reduces the disaccharides maltose, sucrose, and lactose to monosaccharides. Each of these enzymes is specific for a given disaccharide:

Maltase breaks down maltose to glucose and glucose.
Sucrase breaks down sucrose to glucose and fructose.
Lactase breaks down lactose to glucose and galactose.

Often, low levels of these intestinal enzymes leads to intolerances for the respective disaccharides.

In fact, approximately 70% of the world's population has some degree of lactose intolerance from a lack of the intestinal enzyme lactase. Clinical Application 9-1 discusses carbohydrate intolerances, including lactose intolerance. Table 9-1 lists food items that are lactose-free, low in lactose, and high in lactose. Table 9-2 contains a lactose-restricted diet with a sample menu.

DIGESTION OF FATS

Fats are emulsified by bile salts in the small intestine before they are digested further. **Emulsification** is the physical breaking up of fats into tiny droplets. In this

Clinical Application 9-1

Intolerances

Some individuals are deficient in the enzyme lactase and are unable to digest lactose into glucose + galactose. The resulting condition is called lactose intolerance.

Lactose intolerance, the most common of these conditions, may occur in 60%–100% of Hispanics, Blacks, and Southeast Asians. The condition can be hereditary or can be secondary to other disease processes involving the small intestine. After eating or drinking milk products, the client commonly experiences these symptoms of lactose intolerance:

- Abdominal cramping and pain
- Loose stools
- Flatulence (gas)

Dietary treatment of lactose intolerance involves three steps:

1. Identifying food items that contain lactose
2. Eliminating all sources of lactose from the diet
3. Establishing an individual tolerance level on a trial-and-error basis. The tolerance levels for lactose vary widely.

LACTOSE IN CHEESES

The lactose content of cheeses varies. One gallon of milk is required to produce 1 lb of cheese. During cheese making, liquid **whey** is separated from the solid curd (similar to the curd in cottage cheese). Most of the lactose in cheese is contained in the whey. In ripened cheese, the small amount of lactose entrapped in the curd is transformed into lactic acid, which does not require lactase for absorption.

Generally, cheese must age for more than 90 days to be lactose free. These cheeses are considered hard-ripened (low in lactose):

- Blue
- Brick
- Brie
- Camembert
- Cheddar
- Colby
- Edam
- Gouda
- Monterey
- Muenster
- Parmesan
- Provolone
- Swiss.

These cheeses are considered soft cheeses and thus contain more lactose:

- Cream cheese
- Neufchatel
- Ricotta
- Mozzarella
- Cottage cheese.

PRODUCTS

Clients on a lactose-free diet should read all labels carefully to see if milk or milk solids, lactose, or whey have been added to the products. Many toothpastes and over-the-counter medications contain a small amount of lactose. Generally, the amount is very small and is tolerated well.

Lactaid is an over-the-counter product specially designed for individuals with lactose intolerance. Lactaid is a natural enzyme that is available in a tablet form. Some grocery stores also sell milk that has been pretreated with the lactase enzyme. This product will digest 70% of the lactose in milk into glucose and galactose. As a result, most lactose-intolerant persons can drink Lactaid-treated milk or, after consuming the tablets, eat foods that contain lactose and digest the lactose comfortably. Milk treated with Lactaid is slightly sweeter than regular milk. The sweeter taste results naturally when lactose is broken into glucose and galactose.

A lactose-restricted diet may be low in calcium, riboflavin, and vitamin D. Clients should be instructed in alternative sources of these nutrients or advised to take supplements.

TABLE 9-1 ■ Lactose in Foods
Lactose-Free Foods
Broth-based soups unless made with added whey
Plain meat, fish, poultry, peanut butter
Breads that do not contain milk, dry milk solids, or whey
Cereal, crackers
Fruit, plain vegetables
Desserts made without milk, dry milk solids, or whey
Tofu and tofu products, such as tofu-based ice cream substitute
Nondairy creamers
Low-Lactose Foods (0–2 grams/serving)
Milk treated with lactase enzyme, ½ cup
Sherbet, ½ cup
Aged cheese, 1–2 oz
Processed cheese, 1 oz
Butter or margarine
Commercially prepared foods containing dry milk solids or whey
Some medications and vitamin preparations may contain a small amount of lactose. Generally, the amount is very small and is tolerated well.
High-Lactose Foods (5–8 grams/serving)
Milk (whole, skim, 1%, 2%, buttermilk, sweet acidophilus), ½ cup
Powdered dry milk (whole, nonfat, buttermilk—before reconstituting), ⅛ cup
Evaporated milk, ¼ cup
Sweetened condensed milk, 3 tbsp
Party chip dip or potato topping, ½ cup
White sauce, ½ cup
Creamed or low-fat cottage cheese, ¾ cup
Dry cottage cheese, 1 cup
Ricotta cheese, ¾ cup
Cheese food or cheese spread, 2 oz*
Sour cream, ½ cup
Heavy cream, ¾ cup
Ice cream or ice milk, ¾ cup
Half and half, ½ cup
Yogurt, ½ cup†

*Lactose content is higher than that of aged cheese and of processed cheese because of the addition of whey powder and dry milk solids.
†Yogurt may be tolerated better than foods with similar lactose content because of hydrolysis of lactose by bacterial lactase found in the culture. Tolerance may vary with the brand and processing method.

way, more surface area of the fat is exposed to the chemical action of the enzyme pancreatic lipase. Pancreatic lipase completes the digestion of fats by reducing triglycerides to diglycerides and monoglycerides, fatty acids, and glycerol.

Lingual lipase is an important enzyme in infants, although not in adults.

DIGESTION OF PROTEIN

Although hundreds of enzymes are involved in protein digestion, this text reviews only a few of the major ones. The shorter polypeptides, resulting from the stomach's digestive action, are broken down further by pancreatic and intestinal enzymes. Two of the major pancreatic enzymes are **trypsin** and **chymotrypsin,** which have inactive precursors that are activated by other enzymes.

The intestinal wall also secretes a group of enzymes known as **peptidases,** which act on the smaller molecules produced by the pancreatic enzymes, reducing them to single amino acids and small peptides, the final products of protein digestion.

Table 9-3 summarizes the digestion of carbohydrates, fats, and proteins by body organ (mouth, stomach, and small intestine) and identifies action as mechanical or chemical.

Absorption

The end products of digestion move from the gastrointestinal tract into the blood or lymphatic system in a process called **absorption.** The **lymphatic system** transports **lymph** from the tissues to the bloodstream, which is technically part of the circulatory or cardiovascular system. All fluid in the lymphatic system enters the blood after it collects in the thoracic duct, which opens into the subclavian vein. Lymph enters the bloodstream through the subclavian vein. Only after nutrients have been absorbed into either the blood or lymphatic system can the body's cells use them.

The end products of digestion include monosaccharides from carbohydrate digestion, fatty acids and glycerol (and often monoglycerides) from fats, and small peptides and amino acids from protein digestion. Absorption occurs primarily in the small intestine.

Small Intestine

The inner surface of the small intestine has mucosal folds, villi, and microvilli to increase the surface area for maximum absorption (Fig. 9-1). The mucosal folds are like pleats in fabric. On each fold (pleat) are millions of finger-like projections, called **villi.** Each villus has hundreds of microscopic, hair-like projections (resembling bristles on a brush), called **microvilli,** on its surface. The large surface area resulting from this arrangement fosters the movement of nutrients into the blood or lymphatic system. The structure of the mucosa serves as a unit that accomplishes the absorption of nutrients.

Within each villus is a network of blood capillaries and a central lymph vessel called a **lacteal.** The villi absorb nutrients from the chyme by way of these blood and lymph vessels. Monosaccharides, amino acids, glycerol (which is water soluble), minerals, and water-soluble vitamins are absorbed into the blood in the **capillary** network. Because short- and medium-chain

TABLE 9-2 ■ Lactose-Restricted Diet

Description
This diet restricts foods that contain lactose. Soy milk substitutes are used as a milk replacement. Individual tolerances should be taken into consideration, because some clients may tolerate foods low in lactose (see Table 10-1).
Note: All labels should be read carefully for the addition of milk, lactose, or whey.

Indications
This diet is used for the management of patients exhibiting the signs and symptoms of lactose intolerance, Crohn's disease, short bowel syndrome, or colitis. Persistent diarrhea and excessive amounts of gas may be lessened by decreasing lactose intake.

Nutritional Adequacy
This diet is low in calcium, riboflavin, and vitamin D. Supplementation is recommended.

FOOD GROUP	ALLOWED	AVOIDED
Milk	Hard, ripened cheese Ensure® Sustacal® Ensure Plus® Soy milk Lactaid-treated milk Coffee Rich®	Unripened cheese Fluid milk Powdered milk Milk chocolate Cream Most chocolate drink mixes Most coffee creamers
Breads and Cereals	Most water-based bread (French, Italian, Jewish, Graham crackers) Ritz crackers without cheese	Bread to which milk or lactose has been added (check label)
Fruits	Any	None
Vegetables	Fresh, frozen or canned without milk	Creamed, buttered, or breaded vegetables
Meat	Those not listed under "Avoided" Kosher prepared meat and/or milk products	Breaded or creamed meats, fish, or poultry Most luncheon meats Sausage Frankfurters
Desserts and Miscellaneous Items	Angel food cake Gelatin desserts Milk-free cookies Popcorn made with milk-free margarine Pretzels Mustard, catsup, pickles	Most commercially made desserts Sherbet Ice Cream Toffee Cream candies Most chewing gums

SAMPLE MENU

Breakfast	Lunch/Dinner
½ cup orange juice ½ cup cream of wheat 2 slices whole grain milk-free bread 2 tsp milk-free margarine Jelly Coffee ½ cup nondairy "creamer"	3 oz baked chicken Baked potato ½ cup carrots Sliced tomato 1 slice milk-free bread 2 tsp milk-free margarine Angel food cake with fresh fruit topping Coffee

fatty acids have fewer carbons in their chain length, they are more water soluble than long-chain fatty acids. Thus, they are absorbed directly into the blood as well.

These water-soluble nutrients, including short- and medium-chain fatty acids, eventually enter into hepatic portal circulation (via the portal vein) and travel to the liver. **Hepatic portal circulation** is a subdivision of the vascular system by which blood from the digestive organs and spleen circulates through the liver before returning to the heart. In the liver, the nutrients are modified according to the body's needs.

Because long-chain fats are not soluble in water and blood is chiefly water, fat-soluble nutrients cannot be absorbed directly into the blood. Instead, fat-soluble nutrients—including long-chain fatty acids, any monoglycerides remaining from fat digestion, and fat-soluble vitamins—are first combined with bile salts as a carrier. Then, this complex of fat-soluble materials is absorbed into the cells lining the intestinal wall.

Once the fat is absorbed, the bile separates from it and returns to recirculate. Within the intestinal cells, an enzyme reduces any remaining monoglycerides to

TABLE 9-3 ■ Summary of Digestion

NUTRIENT	MOUTH AND ESOPHAGUS	STOMACH	SMALL INTESTINE
Carbohydrates Yield ↓	Mechanical Mastication Swallowing Peristalsis Mucus Chemical Salivary amylase	Mechanical Peristalsis Mucus Chemical None	Mechanical Peristalsis Mucus Chemical Pancreatic enzymes: Pancreatic amylase Intestine enzymes: Maltase Sucrase Lactase
Monosaccharides			
Fats Yield ↓	Mechanical Mastication Swallowing Peristalsis Mucus Chemical None Lingual lipase in infants	Mechanical Peristalsis Mucus Chemical Gastric lipase†	Mechanical Peristalsis Mucus Gallbladder: Bile* Chemical Pancreatic enzymes: Pancreatic lipase
Glycerol, fatty acids, and monoglycerides			
Proteins Yield ↓	Mechanical Mastication Swallowing Peristalsis Mucus Chemical None	Mechanical Peristalsis Mucus Chemical Rennin Pepsin Hydrochloric acid	Mechanical Peristalsis Mucus Chemical Pancreatic enzymes: Trypsin, Chymotrypsin Intestinal enzymes: Peptidases
Amino acids and small peptides			

*Emulsifies fat.
†Digests butterfat only.

fatty acids and glycerol. In a process called triglyceride synthesis, the fatty acids, glycerol, and absorbed long-chain fatty acids recombine (within the intestinal cells) to form human triglycerides.

Next, special proteins cover the newly formed triglycerides and any other fat present (such as cholesterol) to form lipoproteins called **chylomicrons,** which are released into the lymphatic system via the lacteals. Remember that the lymphatic system is connected to the blood system. The protein wrapping these packages of fat enables the chylomicrons to move into the blood via the **thoracic** lymphatic duct (and hence into portal blood). In the liver, lipids are also modified to suit the needs of the body before distribution to body cells. Table 9-4 describes some of the nutrient modifications made in the liver.

The **ileocecal valve,** which relaxes and closes with each peristaltic wave controls further passage of undigested food. This valve prevents backflow and ensures that chyme remains in the small intestine long enough for sufficient digestion and absorption.

The small intestine's structure decreases in size, or wastes away, during starvation, stress, medically indicated bowel rest, and whenever the small bowel is not used. After 1 week of a protein-deficient diet, the microvilli shorten (Colaizzo-Anas, 2007). Even an individual who is ill with a flulike virus and does not eat for several days may need several additional days to regain his appetite after recovery from the illness. Eating six small low-fat meals daily assists in appetite recovery. See Dollars and Sense 9-1.

Large Intestine

The **large intestine,** also called the **colon,** extends from the ileum (last part of the small intestine) to the anus. When chyme leaves the small intestine, it enters the first portion of the large intestine, the **cecum** (the appendix, an organ with no known function, is attached to the cecum). It then travels slowly through the remaining parts of the large intestine: the ascending colon, the transverse colon, the descending

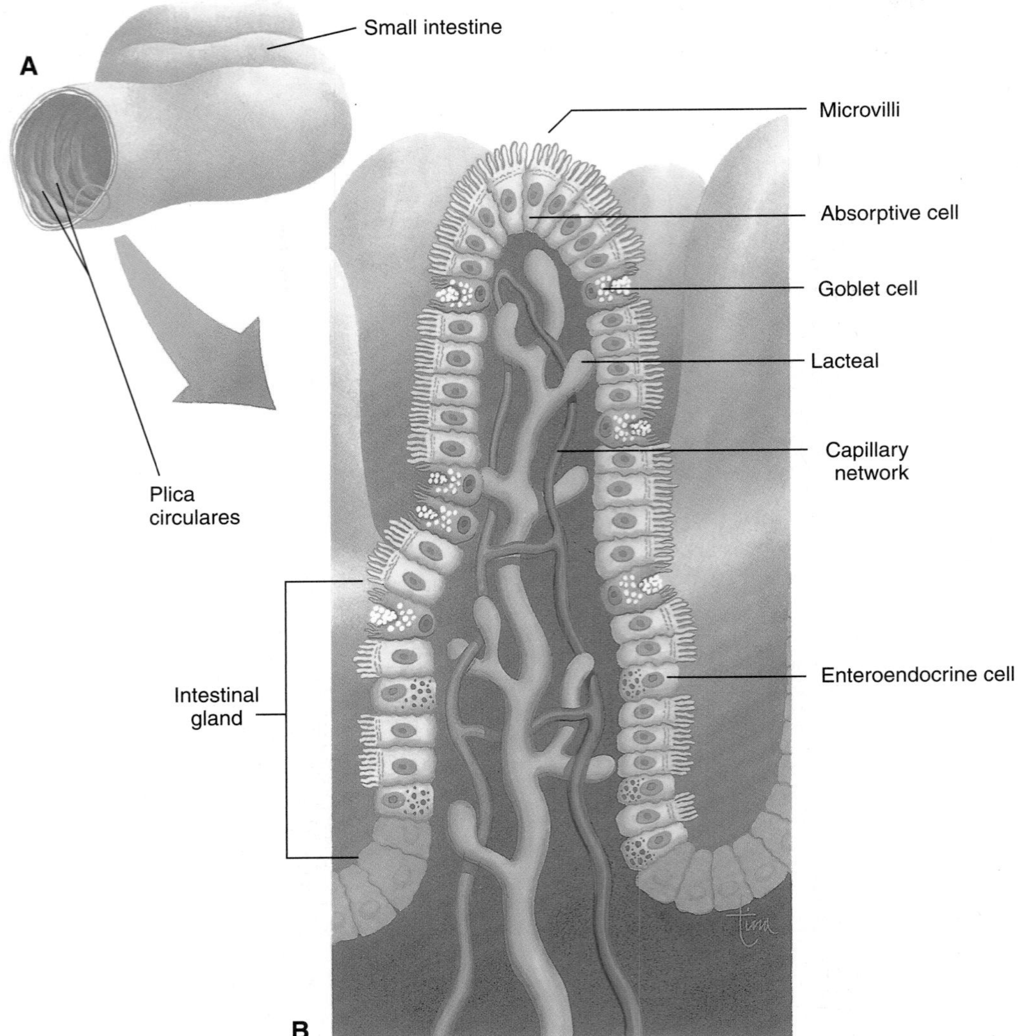

FIGURE 9-1 Cross-section of the small intestine. The multiple folds greatly increase the surface area of the small intestine. (Reprinted from Scanlon, VC, and Sanders, T: *Essentials of anatomy and physiology*. FA Davis, Philadelphia, 2003, with permission.)

TABLE 9-4 ■ Metabolic Modifications in the Liver

ENERGY NUTRIENT	MODIFICATION
Carbohydrates	Fructose and galactose changed to glucose, excess glucose converted to glycogen
Lipids	Lipoproteins formed, cholesterol synthesized, triglycerides broken down and built
Amino Acids	Nonessential amino acids manufactured, excess amino acids deaminated and then changed to carbohydrates or fats, ammonia removed from the blood, plasma proteins made
Other	Alcohol, drugs, and poisons detoxified

colon, the sigmoid colon, the **rectum,** and the anal canal.

Water is the main substance absorbed by the large intestine. However, the absorption of some minerals and vitamins also occurs in the colon. Up to 80% of the water is extracted in the cecum and the ascending colon and returned to the bloodstream. Vitamins synthesized by intestinal bacteria, including vitamin K and some of the B-complexes, are absorbed from the colon. After absorption and digestion have taken place, the remaining waste products are eliminated in the feces through the rectum.

Elimination

Absorption of water into the bloodstream slowly reduces the water content of the material left inside the large intestine, and the waste product (feces) has a solid consistency. Mucus, the only secretion of the large intestine, provides lubrication for the smooth passage of the feces. By the time feces reach the rectum, it consists

Dollars & Sense 9-1

Reintroducing Food After an Illness

Dehydration can be costly because the cells of the gastrointestinal tract turn over every few days. Therefore, if one cannot or will not eat for just a few days, gastrointestinal cell replacement ceases. Among the reasons for not eating are the stomach flu, common cold, a major dental procedure, or childhood illnesses such as measles.

In all these situations, the client will experience some discomfort when food is reintroduced. Symptoms may include abdominal cramping and diarrhea. To prevent a costly trip to the emergency room because of dehydration, everyone should consume liquids if at all possible when ill. If emeses (vomiting) prevent intake, introduce liquids first during recovery, not spicy or solid foods. Good liquid choices include:

- Popsicles
- Apple juice
- Grape juice
- Cranberry juice
- Broth
- Tea
- Gelatin

Mothers should keep these items on hand in the event their children become ill.

TABLE 9-5 ■ Factors Decreasing Absorption

Medications	Antacids Laxatives Birth control pills Anticonvulsants Antibiotics
Parasites	Tapeworm Hookworm
Surgical Procedures	Gastric resections Any surgery on the small intestine Some surgical procedures on the large intestine
Disease States	Infection Tropical sprue Gluten-sensitive enteropathy Hepatic disease Pancreatic insufficiency Lactase deficiency Sucrase deficiency Maltase deficiency Circulatory disorders Cancers involving the alimentary canal
Medical Complications	Effects of radiation therapy Chemotherapy

Note: Most of these conditions are discussed in later chapters.

of 75% water and 25% solids. The solids include cellular wastes, undigested dietary fiber, undigested food, bile salts, cholesterol, mucus, and bacteria.

Indigestible Carbohydrates

The body cannot digest some forms of carbohydrates because it lacks the necessary enzyme to split the appropriate molecule. Some vegetables and legumes contain these indigestible sugars and fibers. Intestinal gas is formed partly in the colon by the decomposition of undigested materials. Foods that may cause intestinal gas in one person may not in another because each person has slightly different bacterial colonies in the colon.

Factors Interfering with Absorption

Malabsorption is the inadequate movement of digested food from the small intestine into the blood or lymphatic system. Malabsorption can cause malnutrition. Table 9-5 lists factors that interfere with the absorption of nutrients. Note in the table that many diseases, medications, and some medical treatments have a negative impact on the absorption of nutrients. Clinical Application 9-2 discusses surgical removal of all or part of the alimentary canal and the effect on absorption. Clinical Application 9-3 discusses inadequate absorption.

The cells lining the inside layer of the small intestine have a very short life. The smallest structures are replaced every 2 to 3 days. Although this rapid cell

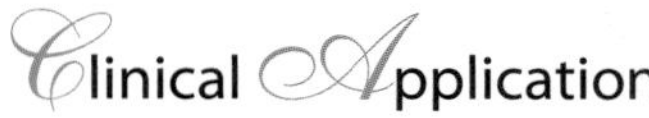

Clinical Application 9-2

Surgical Removal of All or Part of the Alimentary Canal

Clients may need to have a portion of the small intestine surgically removed for a variety of reasons. These clients are frequently at a nutritional risk because they are either permanently or temporarily unable to absorb essential nutrients. In such cases, a nutritional assessment is indicated. In the past, some clients elected to have a portion of the alimentary canal removed to lose weight. This procedure is discussed in Chapter 16.

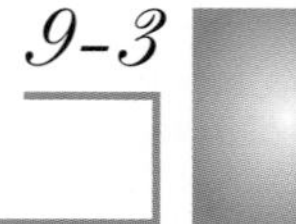

Clinical Application 9-3

Inadequate Absorption

Visually inspecting a client's feces can confirm a suspicion of poor digestion or absorption. Large chunks of food indicate a problem with digestion. A large amount of liquid or near-liquid stools suggests poor absorption. A simple question directed to the client, such as "Are your stools formed?" can provide some information. Sometimes, however, a client's concept of normal may be different from the health-care provider's.

turnover helps to promote healing after injury, it also allows vulnerability to any nutritional deficiency or process that might interfere with cell reproduction. Genomic Gem 9-1 describes celiac disease, in which ingestion of gluten causes an autoimmune response that damages the lining of the small intestine.

Gut failure describes a situation in which the small intestine fails to absorb nutrients properly. Symptoms of gut failure include:

- Diarrhea
- Malabsorption
- Poor response to oral feedings

A vicious cycle starts when the cells lining the small intestine fail to reproduce because they do not have the necessary nutrients for cell replacement. The result is chronic diarrhea caused by malabsorption. In turn, the malabsorption leads to malnutrition, which prevents cell reproduction. See Figure 9-2.

STEATORRHEA

Some diseases and medications result in the malabsorption of fat. In these conditions, clients have **steatorrhea,** or fat in the stools. In many cases, the inhibition of pancreatic lipase, an enzyme necessary for the digestion of fats, causes the condition. Treatment typically involves using medications and decreasing dietary fat.

Food Allergies

A food **allergy** is sensitivity to a food that does not cause a negative reaction in most people. Clients commonly use the term **food allergy** as a generic term that encompasses a broad range of symptoms triggered by certain foods. The medical community reserves the term to immunologically mediated abnormal reactions to foods that are life-threatening.

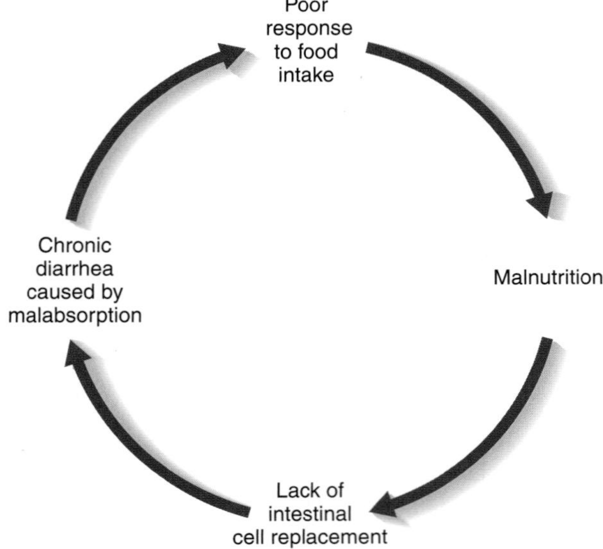

FIGURE 9-2 "Gut failure." Gut failure is a self-perpetuating cycle. Poor response to food intake leads to poor intestinal cell regeneration, which leads to chronic diarrhea caused by malabsorption.

Genomic Gem 9-1
Nontropical Sprue

Nontropical **sprue** is a disorder of the small intestine. This disease is commonly referred to as **celiac disease** or **gluten-sensitive enteropathy.** Celiac disease is a genetically determined condition in which certain grain proteins cause an autoimmune response that damages the lining of the small intestine, causing blunting of the villi and malabsorption of nutrients (Raymond, Heap, and Case, 2006). Approximately 1 of every 133 Americans and one in 266 people worldwide have this genetic defect (Raymond, Heap, and Case, 2006). Gluten-sensitive enteropathy results from the toxic effects that occur from the ingestion of **gluten,** a protein present in wheat, rye, and barley. Oats may be problematic if they were grown in soil previously planted with wheat, rye, or barley. In the United States, such crop rotation is a common practice. Individuals with celiac disease suffer from a wide variety of nutritional problems.

The toxic effect of gluten results in the destruction of intestinal cells. This effect may be related to an allergic reaction and can be either severe or mild. In the severe form, the loss of intestinal mucosa causes malnutrition by impairing the intestine's ability to absorb nutrients, including carbohydrates, proteins, fats, and fat-soluble vitamins.

Lactose intolerance is common in clients with the severe form. The potential risks extend even further: premature osteoporosis, colon cancer, autoimmune disorders (including thyroid disease and type 1 diabetes), arthritis, miscarriage, and birth defects (Duyff, 2008).

Treatment of celiac plus lactose intolerance involves using a high-kcalorie lactose-free, gluten-free diet. This is a complex diet for a dietitian to plan and for the client to follow. These clients are often malnourished. As such, the client benefits from being kept on the lactose-free restriction only until intestinal cell regeneration occurs. Unfortunately, in some clients, the cells of the villi never regenerate because the condition went undiagnosed or untreated for years or treatment was never sought.

In milder forms, only a gluten-restricted diet is indicated for treatment. Removal of all forms of wheat, rye, and barley from the client's diet frequently results in remission or improvement within weeks. See Table 9-6 for lists of foods containing gluten, including several prepared foods containing thickened sauces. For a positive outcome, the client on a gluten-restricted diet must have extensive teaching. Table 9-7 lists products that can be substituted for flour in many recipes.

A true allergy requires meticulous avoidance of the implicated food to minimize the risk of potentially life-threatening reactions. Avoidance includes:

- No eating
- No touching
- No smelling

Individuals may be genetically predisposed to a food allergy.

TABLE 9-6 ■ Gluten-Restricted Diet

Description
This diet is free of cereals that contain gluten: wheat, oats, rye, and barley. Oats may be included in the diet if the oats are guaranteed to be gluten free.

Indications
This diet is used to treat the primary intestinal malabsorption found in celiac disease.

Adequacy
Kilocalorie (energy) intake may be inadequate to replace previous weight loss. This diet may not meet the RDA for B-complex vitamins, especially thiamin. Iron intake may be inadequate for the premenopausal woman.

FOOD GROUPS	FOODS THAT CONTAIN GLUTEN	FOODS THAT MAY CONTAIN GLUTEN	FOODS THAT DO NOT CONTAIN GLUTEN
Beverage	Cereal beverages (e.g., Postum®), malt, Ovaltine®, beer and ale	Commercial* chocolate milk, cocoa mixes, other beverage mixes, dietary supplements	Coffee, tea, decaffeinated coffee, carbonated beverages, chocolate drinks made with pure cocoa powder, wine, distilled liquor
Meat and Meat Substitutes		Meat loaf and patties, cold cuts and prepared meats, stuffing, breaded meats, cheese foods and spreads; commercial souffles, omelets, and fondue; soy protein meat substitutes	Pure meat, fish, fowl, egg, cottage cheese, peanut butter
Fat and Oils		Commercial salad dressing and mayo, gravy, white and cream sauces, nondairy creamer	Butter, margarine, vegetable oil
Milk	Milk beverages that contain malt	Commercial chocolate milk	Whole, low-fat, and skim milk; buttermilk
Grains and Grain Products	Bread, crackers, cereal, and pasta that contain wheat, oats (if not gluten free), rye, malt, malt flavoring, graham flour, Durham flour, pastry flour, bran, or wheat germ; barley; millet; pretzels; communion wafers	Commercial seasoned rice and potato mixes	Specially prepared breads made with wheat starch,† rice, potato, or soybean flour or cornmeal; pure corn or rice cereals; hominy grits; white, brown, and wild rice; popcorn; low-protein pasta made from wheat starch
Vegetables		Commercially seasoned vegetable mixes; commercial vegetables with cream or cheese sauce; canned baked beans	All fresh vegetables; plain commercially frozen or canned vegetables
Fruits		Commercial pie fillings	All plain or sweetened fruits; fruit thickened with tapioca or cornstarch
Soup	Soup that contains wheat pasta; soup thickened with wheat flour or other gluten-containing grains	Commercial soup, broth, and soup mixes	Soup thickened with cornstarch, potato rice or soybean flour; pure broth
Desserts	Commercial cakes, cookies, and pastries	Commercial ice cream and sherbet	Gelatin; custard; fruit ice; specially prepared cakes, cookies, and pastries made with gluten-free flour or starch; pudding and fruit filling thickened with tapioca, cornstarch, or arrowroot flour
Sweets		Commercial candies, especially chocolates	
Miscellaneous		Ketchup, prepared mustard, soy sauce, commercially prepared meat sauces and pickles, vinegar, flavoring syrups (syrups for pancakes or ice cream)	Monosodium glutamate, salt, pepper, pure spices and herbs, yeast, pure baking chocolate or cocoa powder, carob, flavoring extracts, artificial flavoring

SAMPLE MENU

Breakfast	Lunch/Dinner
½ cup orange juice	Chicken breast
Cocoa Puffs®, Sugar Pops®, Puffed Rice®	Baked potato
2 slices gluten-free bread	½ cup broccoli
1 poached egg	Lettuce/tomato salad
1 cup milk	French dressing
2 tsp margarine	Sour cream
Jelly	½ cup milk
	Cornstarch pudding

*The terms *commercially prepared* and *commercial* are used to refer to partially prepared foods purchased from a grocery or food market and to prepared foods purchased from a restaurant.
†Wheat starch may contain trace amounts of gluten. Avoid if not tolerated.
Note: Medications may contain trace amounts of gluten. A pharmacist may be able to provide information on the gluten content of medications.

TABLE 9-7 ■ Gluten-Free Substitutions for 2 Tablespoons of Wheat Flour
3 tsp cornstarch
3 tsp potato starch
3 tsp arrowroot starch
3 tsp quick-cooking tapioca
3 tbsp white or brown rice flour

Some food allergies may be due to an alteration in absorption. The susceptible person absorbs a part of a food before it has been completely digested. The incomplete digestion of protein in particular is responsible for many allergic reactions. Box 9-2 provides a list of food allergy triggers.

Box 9-2 ■ *Food Allergy Triggers*

Common triggers for food allergies include:

- Eggs
- Milk
- Peanuts
- Fish

Less common triggers include:

- Fruits
- Vegetables
- Tree nuts
- Wheat

Metabolism

After digestion and absorption, nutrients are carried by the blood (usually after being modified in the liver cells) to all cells of the body. After entry into the cells, the nutrients from food undergo many chemical changes, which result in either the release of energy or the use of energy.

Metabolism is the sum of all chemical and physical processes continuously going on in living organisms, comprising both anabolism and catabolism. Catabolic reactions usually result in the release of energy. Anabolic reactions require energy.

Catabolic Reactions

In the cells, glucose, glycerol, fatty acids, and amino acids can be broken down even further. These nutrients are held together by bonds that require energy to form and that, when broken, release energy. The breakdown of the fuel-producing nutrients yields carbon dioxide, water, heat, and other forms of energy. Eventually, the carbon dioxide is exhaled, and the water becomes part of the body fluids or is eliminated in urine. Fifty percent or more of the total potential energy usually is lost as heat. The remaining available energy is temporarily stored in the cells as adenosine triphosphate (ATP).

ATP, a high-energy compound that has three phosphate groups in its structure, is thus available in all cells. Practically speaking, ATP is the storage form of energy for the cells because each cell has enzymes that can initiate the hydrolysis (breakdown through the addition of water) of ATP. In this reaction, one or more phosphate groups split off and subsequently release energy. If one phosphate group is removed, the result is ADP (adenosine diphosphate) plus phosphate.

Many steps are involved in the catabolic process responsible for the release of this energy. These steps require one or more of the following agents: enzymes, coenzymes, or hormones. Some vitamins and minerals act as coenzymes. Oxygen is also necessary for the full release of any potential energy. The addition of oxygen to the reaction is called **oxidation.** During the many steps that occur, energy is released little by little and stored as ATP.

The breakdown process includes the formation of intermediate chemical compounds such as **pyruvate** (pyruvic acid) and **acetyl CoA.** Acetyl CoA can be broken down further by entering a series of chemical reactions known as the **Krebs cycle** or the TCA (tricarboxylic acid) cycle. Figure 9-3 is a simplified schematic of the steps involved in the release of energy by the cells. The Krebs cycle is discussed in more detail in Chapter 22.

STORAGE OF EXCESS NUTRIENTS

If the cells do not have immediate energy needs, the excess nutrients are stored. Glucose is stored as glycogen in liver and muscle tissue; surplus amounts are converted to fat. Glycerol and fatty acids are reassembled into triglycerides and stored in adipose tissue. Amino acids are used to make body proteins; any excess is deaminated (stripped of nitrogen) and ultimately used for glucose formation or stored as fat. If energy is not available from food, the cells will seek energy in those body stores. Fat cannot be used to meet the body's need for glucose; however, protein can be converted into glucose. If CHO intake is inadequate, the body will break down lean body mass (protein stores) to meet its glucose need.

Anabolic Reactions

Once immediate energy needs have been met, cells utilize nutrients as needed for growth and repair of body tissue. The cellular supply of ATP is used first. When this instant energy source is exhausted, glycogen and fat stores are used. In addition to building up body protein, other anabolic reactions include the recombination of

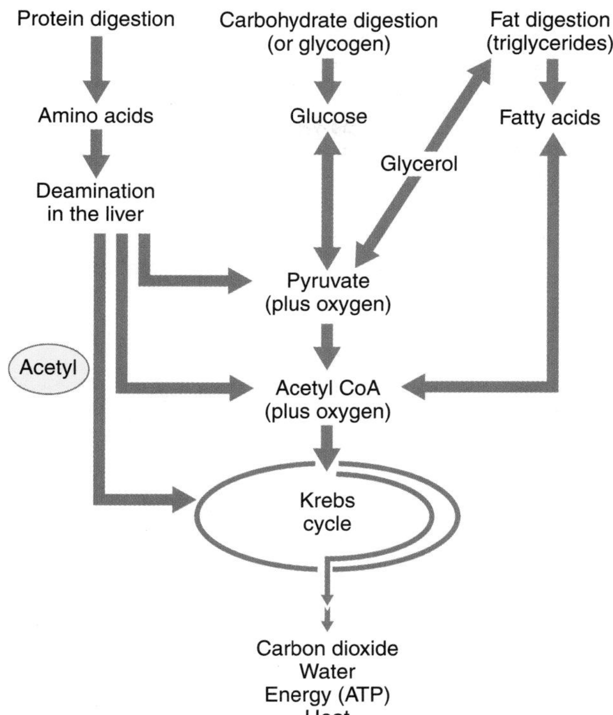

FIGURE 9-3 Energy production in the cells. Energy is released bit by bit during the further breakdown of amino acids, glucose, glycerol, and fatty acids.

glycerol and fatty acids to form triglycerides and the formation of glycogen from glucose.

Excretion of Waste

Materials of no use to the cells become waste that is eliminated through excretion. Solid waste and some liquid is disposed of in the feces. The digestive system needs assistance from other body systems in the disposal of nonsolid waste. The lungs dispose of gaseous waste. Most liquid waste is sent first to the kidneys and then to the **bladder** to be eliminated in the urine. Some liquid waste is disposed of by the skin through perspiration.

Carbon dioxide (CO_2) is a gas that is eliminated through the lungs each time one exhales. The amount of carbon dioxide exhaled depends on the type of fuel (lipid, protein, or carbohydrate) or the source of fuel that the body is currently burning for energy. For example, more CO_2 is produced when carbohydrates are utilized than when protein or fat are used.

The skin removes some of the liquid waste in the form of perspiration or water, and some is excreted in the feces. The kidneys eliminate most of the excess water, sodium, hydrogen, and urea. **Urea** is synthesized in the liver from the nitrogen resulting from the breakdown of amino acids. Some water is also removed from the body each time one exhales.

Keystones

- The cell is the ultimate destination for the nutrients in food.
- Digestion is the process whereby food is broken down for use by cells: carbohydrates are broken down to monosaccharides; fats are reduced to glycerol and fatty acids; and proteins are split to yield amino acids.
- Secretions from the salivary glands, stomach, small intestine, liver, and pancreas assist in chemical digestion.
- Absorption refers to the movement of food from the gastrointestinal tract into the blood and lymphatic systems.
- Metabolism involves anabolism and catabolism. The liver plays a major role in metabolism.
- Energy is released little by little from the end products of digestion in a series of chemical reactions.
- Energy nutrients not needed immediately by the cells are stored as glycogen and adipose tissue.
- The human body cannot convert fat into glucose but it can convert protein into glucose.
- The metabolism of food produces waste. Waste products are released from the body in feces, urine, perspiration, and exhaled air.
- Many ailments and diseases, including malaborption, disaccharide intolerances, allergies, and gluten-sensitive enteropathy, are related to the structure and function of the gastrointestinal system.

CASE STUDY 9–1

Mr. H is 25 years old, 6 ft tall and weighs 170 lb (dressed without shoes). He has a medium frame, as determined by measuring his wrist circumference. Mr. H has been admitted to the hospital for an elective arthroscopic (surgical procedure) on his right knee. During the nursing admission process, Mr. H complained of gas pains and frequent loose stools. He stated that he does not avoid any particular foods and has a healthy appetite. He claims to drink about 3 cups of milk each day. The client complains of losing 5 lb during the previous month. Mr. H uses the restroom twice during the interview to "move his bowels." The second time you inspect the stool. The client's stool is loose and unformed.

The next day you note that a diagnosis of lactose intolerance has been made. A lactose-restricted diet is ordered.

The following nursing care plan originates on the day the client is admitted. The physician uses the information collected from the nurse in making his or her diagnosis. Please note that the client has already met the first desired outcome and part of the second; the outcomes have been charted. The client has not met the third desired outcome.

Care Plan

Subjective Data

Client complains of gas pains and loose stools. Client states that he does not avoid any particular foods. He drinks milk.

Objective Data

Client observed to use the restroom twice in 9 minutes to defecate. Visual inspection shows loose and unformed stool.

Analysis

Diarrhea related to client's complaints of loose unformed stools as evidenced by the client's need to use the restroom twice in a 9-minute period and by direct observation of one loose and unformed stool.

Plan

DESIRED OUTCOMES EVALUATION CRITERIA	ACTIONS/INTERVENTIONS	RATIONALE
The client will assist in ruling out causes for his loose stools and report his signs and symptoms to the nurse.	Teach the client to observe and record the pattern, onset, frequency, characteristics, amount, time of day, and precipitating events related to occurrence of diarrhea. Refer client to the dietitian to determine usual food intake and nutritional status.	Observation and documentation of the client's response to these factors will assist in determining the cause of his loose stools.
	Determine exposure to recent environmental contaminants, such as drinking water, food-handling practices, and proximity to others who are ill.	
	Review drug intake for medications affecting absorption (see Table 9-5).	
The client will eliminate causative factors at once after these factors have been determined.	Follow through with the elimination of causative factors, restrict intake if necessary, note change in drug therapy, if any.	Elimination of the causative factors should decrease the frequency of loose, unformed stools. The client needs to be instructed on the relationship of his diarrhea to causative factors.
The client will have formed stools within 24 hours after the causative factors have been eliminated.	Document stool consistency.	Whenever possible, an objective measure should be used to evaluate the success of any client intervention. Stool consistency is an objective measure for treatment response to diarrhea and malabsorption.
If he or she is willing, refer the client to the registered dietitian.		

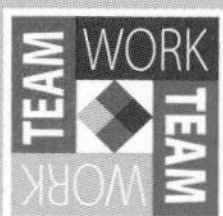

9-1

Dietitian's Note

The following Dietitian's Notes are representative of the documentation found in a client's medical record. The SOAP acronym refers to subjective and objective information, assessment, and plan. Subjective is what the client reports. Objective is what has been previously documented, such as doctor's diagnosis, laboratory information, results of diagnostic procedures and measurements. Assessment is the interviewer's interpretation of the subjective and objective information combined. Dietitians may chart the nutrition diagnosis here. Plan is action or actions the provider intends to do as a result of the assessment.

SOAP: Client states he has no prior knowledge of food- and nutrition-related recommendations. States he feels much better after milk restriction. Client expressed interest in learning more about diet. Formerly client drank 3 glasses of milk per day. He is concerned about calcium and vitamin D deficiencies. He misses eating soft and fresh cheese. Client claims a recent 5-pound weight loss that he attributes to frequent loose stools.

Objective: Prescribed diet (Rx) = lactose restricted diet; Medical Diagnosis (Dx) = lactose intolerance

Assessment: Food- and nutrition-related knowledge deficit related to weight loss and loose stools as evidenced by client statements that he has no prior exposure to lactose-restricted diet and cessation of loose stools 24 hours after the diet was started. Oral and written instructions were provided. Special emphasis was placed on food sources of calcium and vitamin D that are low in lactose. Patient demonstrated an understanding of the diet by verbally planning a lactose-free menu for one diet without error.

Plan: Recommend a calcium and vitamin D supplement. Client instructed to call the outpatient dietitian with questions. The phone number was provided. Follow-up visit in 1 week.

Critical Thinking Questions

1. The client asks you how long he will need to follow this diet and whether he will ever be able to reintroduce milk to his diet. What do you tell him?
2. What would you tell the client if the diet were only partially effective in controlling the diarrhea?

Chapter Review

1. An appropriate snack for a child on a gluten-free diet would be:
   a. Crackers and peanut butter
   b. Half of a cheese sandwich
   c. Potato chips and an oatmeal cookie
   d. Rice cakes and a banana
2. Solid body waste is stored in the:
   a. Large intestine
   b. Gallbladder
   c. Small intestine
   d. Stomach
3. Gaseous waste is expelled:
   a. In the urine
   b. In the feces
   c. Through the lungs
   d. Through the skin
4. The end products of protein digestion are:
   a. Glycerol and fatty acids
   b. Amino acids
   c. Fatty acids
   d. Monosaccharides
5. A food commonly responsible for an allergic reaction is:
   a. Chicken
   b. Peanuts
   c. Rice
   d. Carrots

Clinical Analysis

1. The nurse is visiting Mr. D, who is receiving home health care. His caregiver is concerned that Mr. D chokes on liquids but swallows semisolid food well. Which of the following actions by the nurse would be the most appropriate?
   a. Recommend a soft diet.
   b. Recommend a fluid restriction.
   c. Refer Mr. D to a speech therapist.
   d. First, advise client to drink thickened liquids and then refer to both a speech therapist and then a registered dietitian.

2. Brenda, a 3-year-old, has been admitted to the pediatric unit with a diagnosis of celiac disease. The doctor ordered a gluten-free diet. Which of the following meals would be compatible with the diet order?
   a. Goulash, green beans, and milk
   b. Hamburger on bun, French fries, and a chocolate shake
   c. Tomato soup, grilled cheese, applesauce, and a cookie
   d. Baked chicken, baked potato, sour cream, green beans, peaches, and milk

3. Mr. P is on a low-fat diet (20 grams) to control his steatorrhea. An appropriate snack would be:
   a. Fruit
   b. Nuts
   c. Cheese
   d. Cookies

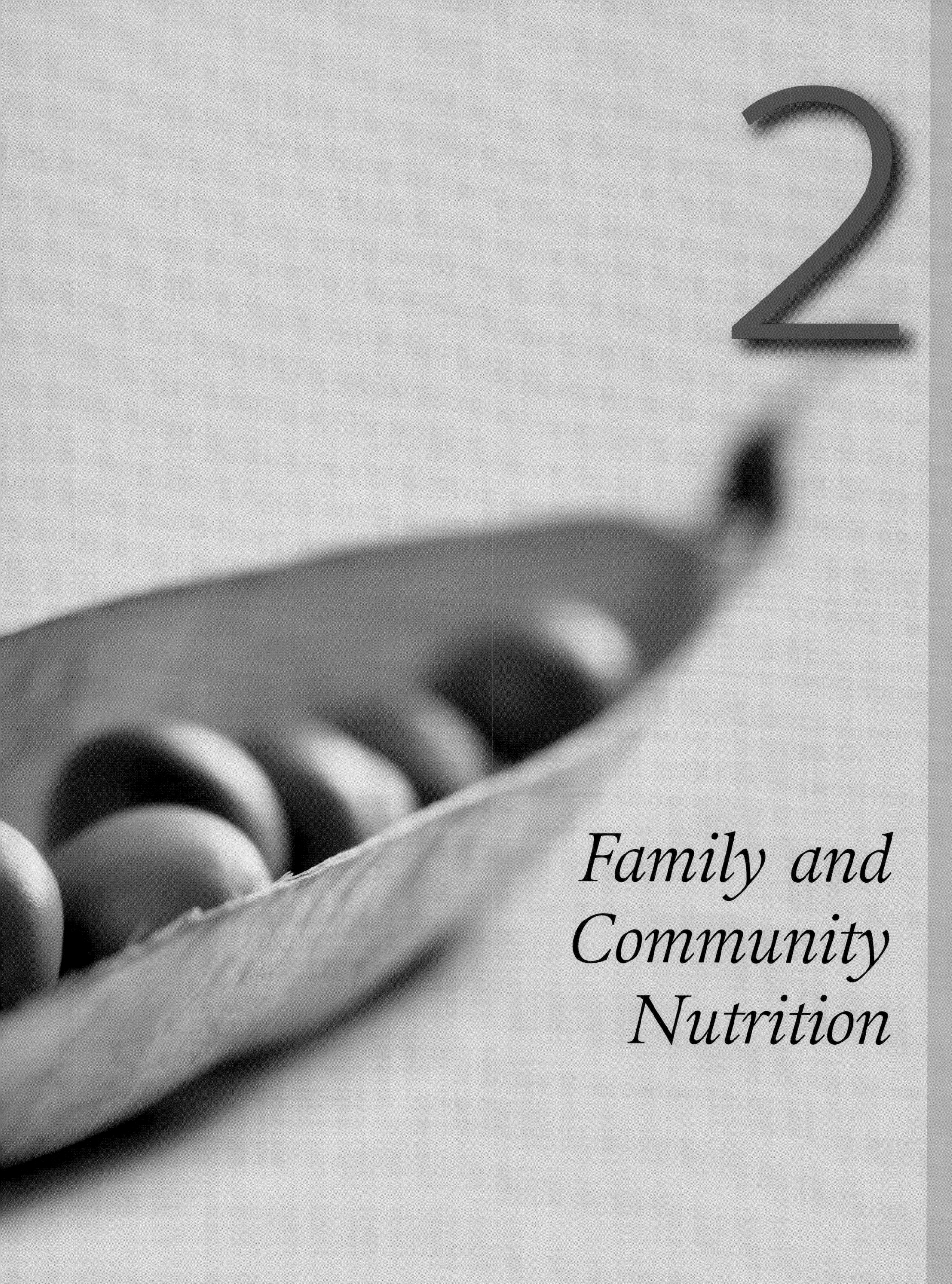

2

Family and Community Nutrition

10

Life Cycle Nutrition: Pregnancy and Lactation

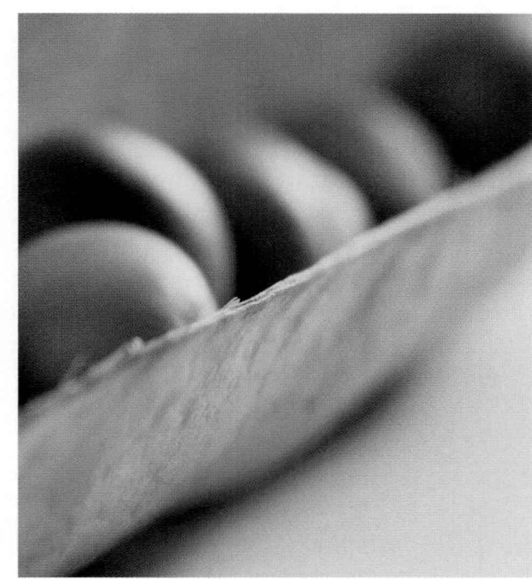

LEARNING OBJECTIVES

After completing this chapter, the student should be able to:

- Compare the nutritional needs of a pregnant woman with those of a nonpregnant woman of the same age.
- Contrast the nutritional needs of a pregnant adolescent with those of a pregnant adult.
- Explain why folic acid intake is critical for women of childbearing age.
- Identify substances to be avoided by pregnant and breastfeeding women.
- Discuss the dietary treatment of common problems of pregnancy.
- List three advantages that breastfeeding confers on the mother.

The needs for many nutrients change at different stages of life. Human beings are most vulnerable to the impact of poor nutrition during periods of rapid growth. This chapter focuses on the period of most rapid growth, that of the unborn child. If the essential nutrients are not present to support growth during that critical time, permanent damage to tissues and organs can occur.

Nutrition During Pregnancy

An expectant mother's nutritional status can affect the outcome of pregnancy. For example, during the first month of **gestation**, the mother must be well nourished so that the **placenta** that forms will be healthy. Because all the **embryo** and **fetus's** major body organs form within 2 to 3 months of conception, nutrition during this time is critical to the health of the child. Required nutrients come from the mother's diet or body stores.

The placenta is not just a passive conduit for nutrients, however. It regulates fetal growth and development. It can selectively extract nutrients of the appropriate form from the maternal blood, certain fatty acids for instance, and transfer them to the fetus (Pardi and Cetin, 2006). The placenta also provides a barrier to the transfer of some substances such as maternal red blood cells and bacteria. Large molecules, including insulin and enzymes, are not transferred (Brown, 2008).

After the birth and weaning of a child, the mother needs time to rebuild her nutrient stores. Birth to conception intervals shorter than 18 months and longer than 59 months are significantly associated with increased risk of preterm birth, **low-birth-weight (LBW) infant,** and **small-for-gestational age (SGA) infant** (Conde-Agudelo, Rosas-Bermudez, and Kafury-Goeta, 2006). Whether related to birth spacing or not, these complications are not evenly distributed throughout the population. Black women are almost twice as likely as white women to give birth to a LBW infant (Centers for Disease Control and Prevention [CDC], 2007a).

The best action an expectant mother can take for her unborn child is to enter the pregnancy with good nutrient stores and to consume a well-balanced diet while pregnant. She must also avoid harmful substances, such as alcohol and contraindicated drugs, including over-the-counter and prescription preparations.

From **implantation** to birth, the fertilized **ovum** (which weighs less than 100 micrograms) develops into an infant who weighs about 3.4 kilograms (7.5 pounds) on average. During this period of rapid growth and development, the mother needs additional nutrients, including kilocalories, protein, and certain vitamins and minerals.

Energy Needs

For DRIs for macronutrients, see Appendix A. For digestible carbohydrate and protein DRIs, see Table 10-1.

Increased energy is needed to sustain the mother and for the development of the fetus and the placenta. From the fourth through the sixth month, the second trimester, much of this energy supports the growth of the uterus (womb) and other maternal tissues. During the seventh through ninth months, the third trimester, much of the energy supports the fetus and the placenta. To meet this increased metabolic workload and to spare protein for tissue building, a pregnant woman needs an extra:

- 340 kilocalories per day in the second trimester
- 452 kilocalories per day in the third trimester.

Energy intake should be distributed throughout the day to maintain maternal blood glucose levels because glucose is the fetus's major and preferred fuel (Brown, 2008; Turner, 2006).

Fat Needs

For DRIs for fat, see Appendix A.

Because the rapidly developing fetal organs incorporate long-chain *n*-3 and *n*-6 essential fatty acids into their cell walls, the accumulated need of essential fatty acids for pregnancy is approximately 620 grams (Jones and Kubow, 2006). One member of the *n*-3 family is docosahexaenoic acid (DHA), a critical component of cell membranes in the brain and the retina. So important is DHA to fetal growth that the placenta actively transfers it to the fetus in preference to other fatty acids (Koletzko et al., 2008). The body is able to convert alpha-linolenic acid to DHA but only in limited amounts (Brown, 2008). See Chapter 18 for more information on omega-3 fatty acids.

The AIs for *n*-6 fatty acids (linoleic acid) and *n*-3 fatty acids (alpha-linolenic acid) are increased during pregnancy and lactation compared to amounts designated for other women.

Food sources of linoleic acid are the following oils:

- Corn
- Safflower
- Sunflower

Alpha-linolenic acid is found in these oils:

- Canola
- Flaxseed
- Soybean
- Walnut (see Chapter 18)

Important sources of DHA are fish and shellfish, because conversion by the body is not required. Consequently, a pregnant woman's diet should contain oils as well as seafood within the limits described under Certain Species and Amounts of Fish.

Protein Needs

For DRIs for protein, see Appendix A and Table 10-1.

Protein is required to build fetal **tissue**. The mother also needs adequate protein for growth of her tissues. Her blood volume increases in anticipation of blood loss at delivery. Her breasts develop in preparation for lactation. Her uterus enlarges and contains a sac filled

TABLE 10-1 ■ RDAs and AIs for Selected Minerals and Energy Nutrients

LIFE STAGE GROUP	CALCIUM* (MG/DAY)	FLUORIDE* (MG/DAY)	IODINE (μg/D)	IRON (MG/DAY)	ZINC (MG/DAY)	DIGESTIBLE CARBOHYDRATE (G/DAY)†	PROTEIN (GRAMS/DAY)
Pregnancy							
<19 years	1300	3	220	27	12	175	71
19–50 years	1000	3	220	27	11	175	71
Lactation							
<19 years	1300	3	290	10	13	210	71
19–50 years	1000	3	290	9	12	210	71

*AI.

†Based on its role as primary energy source for the brain.

Values in boldface indicate RDA; AIs are in light face.

SOURCE: Adapted from http://www.iom.edu/Object.File/Master/21/372/0.pdf.

with **amniotic fluid**. For those reasons, the RDA for protein for pregnant women is 54% more than for nonpregnant women. Translating this need to the exchange system, 2 extra cups of milk (16 grams of protein) and 1.5 additional ounces of meat (10.5 grams of protein) would more than meet the increased protein requirement.

Protein intake becomes a hazard to the fetus when the mother has phenylketonuria and is eating inappropriately. Because approximately 3000 to 4000 women of childbearing age in the United States have phenylketonuria without severe mental retardation (Turner, 2006), all women should be asked directly if they have ever had a special diet prescription. The health-care provider should investigate further when a woman cites a history of troubled pregnancies, congenital abnormalities, a mentally retarded infant, spontaneous abortion, or stillbirth. See Clinical Application 5–2 and Genomic Gem 5-1.

Vitamin Needs

Pregnant women have an increased need for some vitamins. They must avoid taking excessive amounts of others because of potential hazard to the fetus.

Water-Soluble Vitamins

For DRIs for vitamins during pregnancy and lactation, see Appendix A. For selected vitamins during pregnancy and lactation, see Table 10-2.

A pregnant woman's RDA for vitamin C is 13% higher than that of a nonpregnant woman. Vitamin C is necessary for collagen formation and tissue building.

The RDAs for all the B vitamins except biotin are modestly increased for pregnancy. The increased requirements are understandable—particularly for thiamin, niacin, and vitamin B_6, which are coenzymes involved in energy metabolism. See the section on hyperemesis gravidarum for information specific to thiamin deficiency. Two other B vitamins are of special concern in pregnancy: vitamin B_{12} and folic acid.

VITAMIN B_{12}

For DRIs for vitamins during pregnancy and lactation, see Appendix A. For selected vitamins during pregnancy and lactation, see Table 10-2.

The vitamin B_{12} RDA is only slightly increased for pregnant and lactating women. The placenta appears to concentrate vitamin B_{12} because serum levels in the newborn are about twice the maternal levels. Because only newly absorbed vitamin B_{12} is readily transported across the placenta, pregnant vegans will need a supplemental source (Turner, 2006).

In addition, vegetarians should be knowledgeable about the cobalamin content of their food or seek nutritional advice, because neurological impairment has occurred in their infants (CDC, 2003). Fortified food and supplements made from cobalamin provide a physiologically active form of the vitamin, whereas products that list only vitamin B_{12} might include non-bioavailable sources.

FOLIC ACID

For DRIs for vitamins during pregnancy and lactation, see Appendix A. For selected vitamins during pregnancy and lactation, see Table 10-2.

The RDA for folic acid for all women of childbearing potential specifies synthetic folic acid from fortified foods or supplements. In addition, food folate from a varied diet is expected to be consumed.

These recommendations are based on clinical studies that showed that 4 milligrams of folic acid daily prevented 72% of neural tube defects (NTDs) in infants of women who had already borne an afflicted child (MRC Vitamin Study Research Group, 1991). See Box 10-1. The CDC quickly recommended the treatment for such high-risk women (CDC, 1992). A later trial demonstrated that

TABLE 10-2 ■ RDAs and AIs for Selected Vitamins for Pregnancy and Lactation

LIFE STAGE GROUP	VITAMIN A (μg/DAY)	VITAMIN C* (MG/DAY)	VITAMIN D† (μg/DAY)	VITAMIN E (MG/DAY)	THIAMIN (MG/DAY)	NIACIN (MG/DAY)	VITAMIN B_6 (MG/DAY)	FOLATE‡ (μg/DAY)	VITAMIN B_{12} (μg/DAY)
Pregnancy									
<19 years	750	80	5	15	1.4	18	1.9	600	2.6
19–50 years	770	85	5	15	1.4	18	1.9	600	2.6
Lactation									
<19 years	1200	115	5	19	1.4	17	2.0	500	2.8
19–50 years	1300	120	5	19	1.4	17	2.0	500	2.8

*Smokers require an additional 35 mg/day of vitamin C.
†AI.
‡Women able to become pregnant should consume 400 micrograms of synthetic folic acid from fortified foods/supplements besides food folate.
Values in boldface indicate RDA; AIs are in light face.
SOURCE: Adapted from http://www.iom.edu/?id=7296&redirect=0.

Box 10-1 ■ *Neural Tube Defects: Occurrence, Pathophysiology, and Side Effects of Supplementation*

Neural tube defects (NTDs) are the most common preventable type of birth defect in the world, and affect approximately 1 in 3000 pregnancies in the United States annually (CDC, 2008e).

The neural tube is embryonic tissue that develops into the brain and spinal cord. A critical time in the development of this structure is from conception through the fourth week of pregnancy. Interference with normal development at that time produces major congenital defects, including **anencephaly, meningoencephalocele, spina bifida,** and **meningocele.** Unfortunately, the neural tube develops before many women are aware they are pregnant.

As a multifactorial condition, the exact connection of NTDs to folic acid is unclear but folate is directly or indirectly essential for cell function, division, and differentiation. Pinpointing the mechanism by which folic acid aids normal closure of the neural tube is difficult because more than 25 proteins are involved in folate pathways (De Marco et al., 2006).

In addition to preventing NTDs, folic acid seems to reduce the risk of other birth defects, especially cardiac anomalies and orofacial clefts and its relationship to other conditions is under investigation (Johnston, 2007).

0.8 milligrams of folic acid given 1 month before and continuing into the first trimester prevented NTDs in women without a history of the disorder (Czeizel and Dudas, 1992).

Despite recommendations for women of childbearing age to increase folic acid intake, most women did not follow the recommendation. Consequently, folic acid has been added to the enrichment protocol for cereal-grain products in the United States. Forty-one other countries fortify foods with folate. Thus 140 micrograms of folic acid has been incorporated into each 100 grams of enriched flour since 1998 (Johnston, 2007) at a cost of pennies per person per year (CDC, 2008d).

Following the initiation of folate fortification, the prevalence of spina bifida decreased 31% and of anencephaly 26% (Blom et al., 2006) primarily in infants born to non-Hispanic white and Hispanic women. No significant change in prevalence has been seen in babies born to non-Hispanic black women (CDC, 2007b). See Genomic Gem 10-1 for more information on risk factors for NTDs.

By 2007, 60% of women of childbearing age surveyed still were not taking a daily supplement containing folic acid. Moreover, women ages 18 to 24 years, who have the highest rate of unintended pregnancies, are the least knowledgeable about folic acid and the least likely to consume a folic acid supplement (CDC, 2008e). Health-care providers need to increase their efforts to promote adequate folic acid intake among fertile women. Specific target populations include:

- Young women
- Hispanic and black women
- Women with low incomes
- Women with less than a high school education (American Dietetic Association [ADA], 2008)

Genomic Gem 10-1

The Genesis of Neural Tube Defects

Most cases of NTD occur in women without a history of the disorder (Pitkin, 2007) but there is evidence of a genetic component to this multifactorial condition. Heritability is estimated to be 60% with multiple genes involved but their identity and specific contributions to producing the defect remain to be discovered (Kibar, Capra, and Gros, 2007). Because folic acid is so clearly protective, much research has focused on its metabolic pathways. Variants of several folate-related genes have been significantly associated with risk for NTDs.

Among other findings suggesting a genetic component are:

- Three- to fivefold increased risk of a second affected child for couples with one child with a NTD (Kibar, Capra, and Gros, 2007)
- Ethnic and racial differences in NTD prevalence—highest in Hispanics, lowest in blacks and Asians (Mitchell, 2005)
- Evidence that factors related to NTDs may be transmitted preferentially from the mother's side of the family (Byrne and Carolan, 2006).

Among the environmental factors associated with NTDs, the estimated "other 40% causality," are maternal diabetes, maternal obesity, and maternal hyperthermia along with antiepileptic medications (De Marco et al., 2006). While awaiting clear understanding of causality, the ability to prevent approximately 70% of NTDs through the administration of folic acid is a remarkable advance.

Fat-Soluble Vitamins

For DRIs for vitamins during pregnancy and lactation, see Appendix A. For selected vitamins during pregnancy and lactation, see Table 10-2.

The RDA for vitamin E and the AI for vitamin K are the same for pregnant women as for mature nonpregnant women. Interfering with normal physiology can create problems, however. During normal pregnancy, the placenta transfers limited amounts of vitamin K to the fetus. A greater risk of vitamin K deficiency may ensue after maternal bariatric surgery. Five cases of severe intracranial bleeding possibly related to vitamin K deficiency resulted in two severely disabled children and three neonatal deaths, including one infant with generalized bone malformation (Eerdekens et al., 2010).

Vitamins D and A merit special mention even for normal pregnancies.

VITAMIN D

The same controversy about the adequacy of the AI for vitamin D (see Chapter 7) spills into discussions regarding the needs of pregnant women (Hollis, 2007). In fact, the AI of 5 micrograms is half of the RDA that was promulgated in 1989 (Turner, 2006) and half of what is recommended in Britain (Camadoo, Tibbott, and Isaza, 2007).

The chief function of vitamin D during pregnancy is to maintain healthful serum levels of calcium and phosphorus (Turner, 2006). Despite the placenta's capability to produce active vitamin D (Holick, 2006), maternal vitamin D deficiency may limit fetal bone mineral accumulation and may affect long-term childhood bone status (Abrams, 2007).

Even short term, maternal vitamin D deficiency during pregnancy and lactation produced hypocalcemic seizures in a 1-week-old infant. Both parents were Asian vegetarians and the mother, dressed in whole-body coverings, took no supplements during pregnancy. Treatment with vitamin D and calcium stopped the infant's seizures within 3 days and returned his blood calcium levels to normal (Camadoo, Tibbott, and Isaza, 2007).

VITAMIN A

Large intakes of vitamin A consumed by pregnant women have been related to birth defects. Vitamin A as retinol or retinoic acid in excess of 10,000 IU per day or treatment with **isotretinoin** during the first trimester increase the risk of **retinoic acid syndrome**. The characteristic fetal deformities include:

- Small ears or no ears
- Abnormal or missing ear canals
- Brain malformation
- Heart defects

Three ounces of beef liver may contain 27,000 IU and 3 oz of chicken liver, 12,000 IU. A pregnant woman who eats liver regularly may consume enough vitamin A to pose a risk to her baby. She also should be sure that her multivitamin or prenatal supplement contains no more than 5000 IU of preformed vitamin A, and she should not take any vitamin A supplements beyond that amount (March of Dimes, 2006).

Some prenatal vitamins substitute beta-carotene, which is not associated with birth defects, for preformed vitamin A or omit vitamin A entirely. Table 10-3 lists the RDAs and ULs in micrograms and International Units for vitamin A for pregnancy and lactation. Remember the conversion to IUs depends on the source. (See Clinical Calculation 7-1.)

Isotretinoin, a vitamin A metabolite used to treat severe acne, is hazardous to the fetus with almost a 30% risk of malformations if a woman is exposed to isotretinoin during the first trimester (Malvasi et al., 2009). Despite a pregnancy prevention program started by the manufacturer of isotretinoin in 1988 and subsequent upgrades (one called iPLEDGE), women are still becoming pregnant while taking the drug. Requiring client registration and negative pregnancy tests before each prescription is dispensed have not eliminated the danger to fetuses.

Women of childbearing age taking isotretinoin should adhere to strict contraceptive protocols, including simultaneous use of two reliable methods. A woman who ceased taking isotretinoin three months before becoming pregnant still manifested teratogenic effects: conjoined twins (Malvasi et al., 2009). Furthermore, no one should donate blood during or for 30 days after cessation of therapy with isotretinoin (U.S. Food and Drug Administration [FDA], 2005).

Follow-up of the iPLEDGE program indicated 148 pregnancies occurred in the first 16 months of the program (U.S. Food and Drug Administration, September 2007). Similarly, an analysis of Kaiser Permanente's program to improve pregnancy testing rates and reduce fetal exposure did not change the rate of fetal exposure to the drug. The client's failure to use two contraceptive methods was the most common reason for fetal exposure (Cheetham et al., 2006).

In contrast, vitamin A deficiency is a greater problem than toxicity in developing countries. Gestational nightblindness relating to low levels of serum retinol was diagnosed in 17.9% of postpartum women at one hospital in Brazil (Saunders et al., 2004) and

TABLE 10-3 ■ DRIs for Vitamin A During Pregnancy and Lactation

	RDA		UL	
	Micrograms as RAEs (Retinol Activity Equivalents)	International Units	Micrograms as pre-formed only	International Units
Pregnancy				
<19 years	750	2475	2800	9240
19–50 years	770	2541	3000	9900
Lactation				
<19 years	1200	3960	2800	9240
19–50 years	1300	4290	3000	9900

maternal night blindness was associated with an increased risk of low birthweight infants in South India (Tielsch et al., 2008).

Mineral Needs

For DRIs for minerals during pregnancy and lactation, see Appendix A. For selected minerals during pregnancy and lactation, see Table 10-1.

The trace mineral iron plays a major role in the health of the mother and fetus and therefore appears first in the discussion. Other minerals of special concern in pregnancy are calcium, iodine, fluoride, and zinc.

Iron

For DRIs for minerals during pregnancy and lactation, see Appendix A. For selected minerals during pregnancy and lactation, see Table 10-1.

During pregnancy, the mother's plasma volume increases about 45 to 50% by the 34th week of gestation and her red cell mass increases about 33%. Besides supporting the mother's increased blood volume, iron supports the red blood cells in the fetus, placenta, and umbilical cord. As a result, the net iron cost of a singleton (one fetus) pregnancy is estimated at 1 gram. Even moderate iron deficiency anemia is associated with twice the risk of maternal death.

The fetus receives sufficient iron from the mother's stores unless the mother is severely anemic (Turner, 2006), but maternal anemia at the beginning of pregnancy increases the risk of preterm delivery and low birth weight infants by two or three times. Long-term, iron deficiency during pregnancy is related to lower scores on intelligence, language, gross motor, and attention tests when the child is 5 years old (Brown, 2008).

Fortunately, the body adjusts to limited or abundant iron sources, and iron absorption is enhanced in the second and third trimesters of pregnancy. Rates of iron absorption vary so that women who begin pregnancy:

- With adequate iron stores absorb about 10% of ingested iron
- With low iron stores absorb about 20%
- Anemic absorb about 40%

The RDA for iron for pregnancy assumes an absorption rate of 20%. Supplementation with 30 milligrams of iron daily is generally recommended after the first trimester, usually prescribed as a stand-alone tablet since just 5% of the iron in multimineral supplements is absorbed compared with 10% in an iron-only supplement (Brown, 2008). Even when she takes supplements, a woman's hemoglobin and hematocrit should be monitored regularly. Lower values are expected during the first and second trimesters because expanding blood volume dilutes the concentration of red blood cells.

Prescribed iron supplements may not be taken. Economic factors or side effects, such as nausea, cramps, gas, and constipation, may influence intake. Although oral iron preparations are best absorbed if taken 1 hour before or 2 hours after meals, individualizing the schedule is better than the client choosing to eliminate the supplement altogether. Clinical Application 10-1 illustrates the principle of knowing the client as well as the subject matter.

Calcium

For DRIs for minerals during pregnancy and lactation, see Appendix A. For selected minerals during pregnancy and lactation, see Table 10-1.

Throughout pregnancy, approximately 25 to 30 grams of calcium are transferred to the fetus, most of it in the third trimester. Typically, at 28 weeks, 100 milligrams per day is deposited in the fetal skeleton; at 35 weeks, 350 milligrams per day (Holick, 2006). More calcium is absorbed by the intestine during pregnancy because of increased maternal vitamin D to meet the fetus's needs (Turner, 2006).

Some evidence suggests that both pregnancy and lactation are associated with a loss of bone mineral

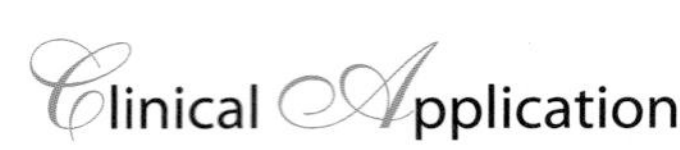

Clinical Application 10-1

Effective Teaching

Often the facts presented by a health-care provider are misunderstood by the client or perceived as counter to the client's goals. The following incidents illustrate the point (Galloway and McGuire, 1996).

1. When anemic pregnant women were given iron tablets, they took the supplement until they felt better and then stopped, thinking they were cured. Prevention is a new concept to people in many countries.
2. Anemic pregnant women accepted the notion of iron supplements to correct "too little blood" but were fearful that too much iron would give them too much blood so that they would bleed more extensively at delivery.
3. Presenting the idea that iron would produce bigger babies was a disincentive for anemic pregnant women who thought they then would face a more difficult labor.

Teaching is more than presenting facts, especially when the goal is changed behavior. Local knowledge and cultural perspective are essential to the health-care provider promoting a new health practice. For instance, it would help to know that some Puerto Rican women are likely to avoid iron as a "hot" food during pregnancy (Purnell and Paulanka, 2008).

density, as much as 5%, which is replaced after weaning (Karlsson, Ahlborg, and Karlsson, 2005). Chapters 7 and 8 describe the effects and interactions of calcium and vitamin D.

Transient osteoporosis is a rare, self-limiting syndrome typically characterized by hip pain in the third trimester of pregnancy accompanied by radiologic osteopenia; other joints may be affected as well. Etiology is unclear, with the left hip more often involved than the right and bilateral hips affected in 25% to 30% of pregnant women. Usual treatment is supportive during the mean duration of 6 to 8 months. Spontaneous resolution is the usual outcome (Ma and Falkenberg, 2006).

Follow-up of five women with pregnancy osteoporosis, most of whom suffered vertebral fractures in their first pregnancy, found osteoporosis in 53% of their **first-degree relatives** versus 15% of the controls. Some women who develop pregnancy osteoporosis may have genetically determined low peak bone mass that increases their risk for bone loss (Peris et al., 2002).

Iodine, Fluoride, and Zinc

For DRIs for minerals during pregnancy and lactation, see Appendix A. For selected minerals during pregnancy and lactation, see Table 10-1.

As part of thyroid hormones, iodine is essential to the control of metabolism. During the second half of pregnancy, resting energy expenditure increases by as much as 23%. The RDAs for iodine are increased 46 and 93% for pregnant and lactating women over those of other women. In the United States, a pregnant woman's usual need for iodine is met by the use of iodized salt. Severe maternal deficiency can cause cretinism in the newborn. See Chapter 8.

The fetus begins to develop teeth at the tenth to twelfth week of pregnancy. Fluoride crosses the placenta so that the concentration in fetal circulation is one-fourth that of the mother; fluoride is found in fetal bones and teeth. Supplements taken during pregnancy, however, have not been shown to prevent caries in preschool children (DePaola et al., 2006). The AI for pregnancy and lactation is the same as for nonpregnant women.

Zinc is not mobilized from the mother's tissues. To provide for the fetus, the mother needs regular intake. Marginal zinc deficiency has been associated with preterm delivery and labor complications, but serum zinc measurement lacks a well-established standard (King and Cousins, 2006). The RDAs for pregnant and lactating women are about 50% higher than those for other women. Lean meat from beef chuck roast, 3.5 to 4 ounces, would provide these RDAs.

Water and Weight Gain

Plasma volume during pregnancy expands by about 50%, necessitating a fluid intake of about 9 cups daily (Brown, 2008). See Box 8-5.

The recommended weight gain during pregnancy has varied over the years. Clinical Calculation 10-1 shows how to determine a goal for weight gain in pregnancy based on prepregnancy weight. On average, a woman of normal weight should gain 2 to 4 pounds during the first trimester, followed by 1 pound per week for the remainder of the pregnancy. Regardless of prepregnancy height and weight, a woman should gain at least 15 pounds during pregnancy (CDC, 2008b). Figure 10-1 is a graph for plotting weight gain; Table 10-4 shows the typical distribution of pounds between the baby and the mother's tissues.

Approximately 40% of U.S. women gain within the recommended ranges (Brown, 2008) even though about half of pregnant women are given no advice or inappropriate advice regarding desirable weight (Turner, 2006). Gaining less than recommended is associated with fetal growth retardation, low birth weight, and increased **perinatal mortality**. In 2005, 10% of women carrying single fetuses gained less than 15 pounds, events more likely in older women and in non-Hispanic black women (CDC, 2008b).

At the upper end of the spectrum, gaining more than recommended is associated with large babies, Caesarean deliveries, and postpartum weight retention (Brown, 2008) as well as gestational diabetes and preeclampsia (see following sections). In 2005, 20% of women gained more than 40 pounds, most common among non-Hispanic white women (CDC, 2008c).

Meal Pattern

Mature women who become pregnant require relatively few modifications in MyPyramid recommendations for adults. An example for a 22-year-old, 125-pound woman who is physically active 30 to 60 minutes per day is shown in Table 10-5.

Except for iron, MyPyramid recommendations should suffice for healthy women. Self-selected meal plans should be varied enough to provide all the required nutrients (ADA, 2008).

Pregnant teenagers need nutrients to provide for their own growth as well as that of the fetus. A client, 16 years old, weighing 120 pounds who is physically active 30 to 60 minutes per day would require additional grains, vegetables, and meat/beans in the second and third trimesters as shown in Table 10-5. Clinical Application 10-2 relates the particular hazards of teenage pregnancy.

Women of dissimilar ages, sizes, and lifestyles would require different intakes. Individualized meal

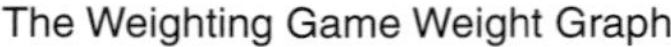

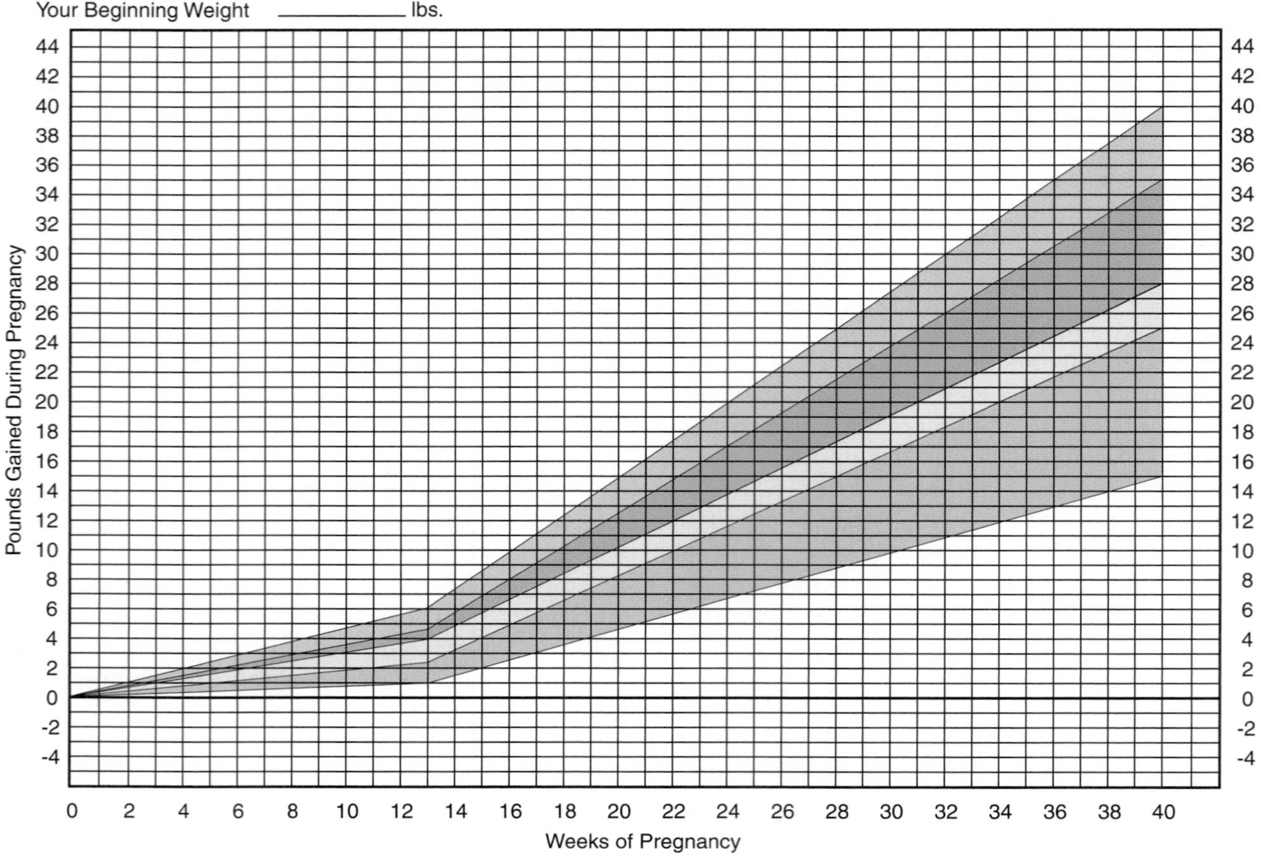

Adapted from the National Academy of Science's Nutrition during Pregnancy, 1990.

FIGURE 10-1 Example of a chart on which a woman can plot her weight gain during pregnancy. Goals are shown in pink/orange for women who begin pregnancy underweight, in orange/yellow for normal weight women, and in blue for overweight women. (Reprinted from GREAT BEGINNINGS: The Weighting Game Weight Graph, 1991. Courtesy of National Dairy Council, with permission.)

TABLE 10-4 ■ Here's How It All Adds Up

Baby	7–8½ pounds
Amniotic fluid	2 pounds
Placenta	2–2½ pounds
Increased blood volume	4–5 pounds
Tissue fluid	3–5 pounds
Increased weight of uterus	2 pounds
Body changes for breastfeeding	1–4 pounds
Mother's stores*	4–6 pounds
Total	25–35 pounds

*Mother's stores are reserves of extra fat and probably a little protein. These serve as a source of energy to support the work of pregnancy. These stores also supply energy for labor and delivery and for milk production after birth.

SOURCE: Reprinted from GREAT BEGINNINGS: The Weighting Game Weight Graph, 1991. Courtesy of National Dairy Council, with permission.

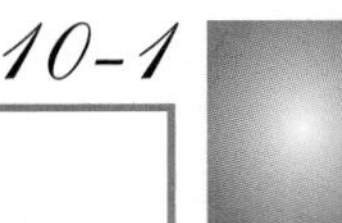

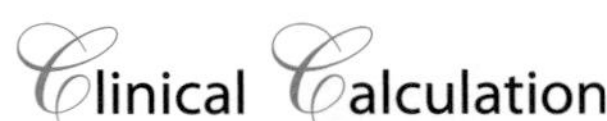

Clinical Calculation 10-1

Determining Recommended Weight Gain During Pregnancy

Body mass index (BMI) = Weight in kilograms/Height in meters^2

Suppose a woman is 5 ft, 4 in. tall and weighs 125 lb.

5 ft, 4 in. = 64 in.

1 m = 39.371 in.

$$\frac{64}{39.371} = 1.6 \text{ m}$$

$$\frac{125 \text{ lb}}{2.2 \text{ lb/kg}} = 56.8 \text{ kg}$$

$$\text{BMI} = \frac{56.8}{(1.6)^2} = \frac{56.8}{2.56} = 22.2$$

Looking at the table below, we see that 22.2 is in the normal category. Recommended weight gain for this woman is 25 to 35 lb.

Recommended Weight Gain for Pregnancy

BMI CATEGORY	KILOGRAMS	POUNDS
<19.8 = Low	12.5–18	28–40
19.8–26 = Normal	11.5–16	25–35
26–29 = High	7–11.5	15–25
>29 = Obese	6.8	15

Young adolescents and black women should strive for gains at the upper end of the recommended range. Women whose height is less than 157 cm (62 in) should strive for gains at the lower end of the range.

Source: Reprinted with permission from Nutrition During Pregnancy. © 1990 by the National Academy of Sciences. Published by National Academy Press, Washington, DC.

planning based on age, height, prepregnancy weight, and activity level is available at http://www.mypyramid.gov/mypyramidmoms/index.html.

Careful food selection is critical for all pregnant women but especially for pregnant teens who may have unbalanced diets and for women who restrict or eliminate whole categories of food such as vegetarians. Thorough nutritional assessment, ideally before pregnancy or at least very early in pregnancy, could yield huge dividends by decreasing complications and improving newborns' health. Dollars and Sense 10-1 describes some food assistance programs available to improve nutrition.

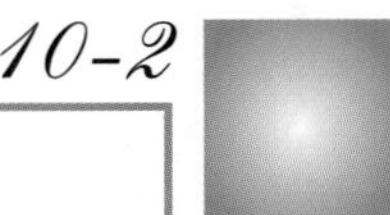

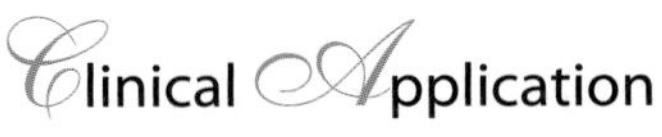

Clinical Application 10-2

Teenage Pregnancy

The average girl does not reach her full height or attain gynecologic maturity until age 17. When pregnant before that age, she herself is still growing and has a fetus to nourish as well. Infants born to still-growing adolescents, weigh an average of 155 grams (0.3 lb) less than those born to adult women. Rates of spontaneous abortion, preterm delivery, and low birth weight are higher in growing than in non-growing adolescents.

Adolescents who were overweight or obese before becoming pregnant have increased risks of Caesarean delivery, hypertension, gestational diabetes, and large infants (Brown, 2008).

Because many pregnant adolescents have low incomes, referral to appropriate sources of assistance is a crucial part of their nutritional care.

TABLE 10-5 ■ MyPyramid for Pregnancy and Lactation

	PREGNANT ADULT, 2ND TRIMESTER*	PREGNANT ADULT, 3RD TRIMESTER	PREGNANT ADOLESCENT, 2ND TRIMESTER†	PREGNANT ADOLESCENT, 3RD TRIMESTER	LACTATION, BIRTH TO 12 MONTHS‡
Grains (½ Whole), Ounces	8	9	8	9	9
Vegetable, Cups (Vary Selections)	3	3.5	3	3.5	3.5
Fruit, Cups	2	2	2	2	2
Milk, Cups	3	3	3	3	3
Meat and Beans, Ounces	6.5	6.5	6.5	6.5	6.5
Oils, Teaspoons	7	8	7	8	8
Extra Fats & Sugars, kilocalories	360	410	360	410	410

*Calculated for a 22-year-old, 5 ft, 4 in. tall, 125 lb before pregnancy, who is physically active 30–60 minutes per day.
†Calculated for a 16-year-old, 5 ft 4 in. tall, 120 lb before pregnancy, who is physically active 30 to 60 minutes per day.
‡Calculated for a 22-year-old, 5 ft 4 in. tall, 130 lb, who is physically active 30 to 60 minutes per day.

Dollars & Sense 10-1
Food Assistance

Supplemental food assistance is available for families in the Food Stamp Program and for women and children in the Supplemental Feeding Program for Women, Infants, and Children **(WIC).** The latter program served 7.9 million people in 2004, including 4 million children and 2 million infants. It provides supplemental foods monthly to low-income pregnant or postpartum women, infants, and children up to age 5. WIC is available in all 50 states plus 40 other territories and jurisdictions (United States Department of Agriculture, 2006).

Substances to Avoid

While pregnant or nursing, women are urged to limit caffeine intake and to eliminate these items from their diets:

- Alcohol
- Soft cheeses and ready-to-eat meats,
- Certain species and amounts of fish
- Undercooked meat and unwashed produce

Serious allergies to nuts and seeds affect less than 1% of the population. See Chapter 11 for information on food allergies. The American Academy of Pediatrics (APA) currently does not recommend dietary restrictions—to protect children from allergies—during pregnancy or lactation (2008).

Alcohol

A pregnant woman who drinks alcoholic beverages is endangering her baby because alcohol readily crosses the placenta, and the fetus has inadequate enzymes to detoxify it. Although the number and severity of negative effects can range from subtle to serious, they are always lifelong (CDC, 2005). Approximately 40% of fetuses born to women who drink heavily early in pregnancy will develop Fetal Alcohol Syndrome (Brown, 2008). The fetus is most vulnerable during the first trimester when basic structural development occurs.

First recognized in 1973, **fetal alcohol syndrome (FAS)** is most easily diagnosed between the ages of 4 and 14. FAS has specific diagnostic criteria:

- Three characteristic facial features: smooth philtrum, thin upper lip, and small palpebral fissures (see Fig. 10-2). These signs may become less distinct or disappear in adolescence and adulthood (Lupton, Burd, and Harwood, 2004).
- Growth problems (height or weight at or below the 10th percentile)
- Central nervous system abnormalities, such as head circumference at or below the 10th percentile, neurological problems, or functional deficits.

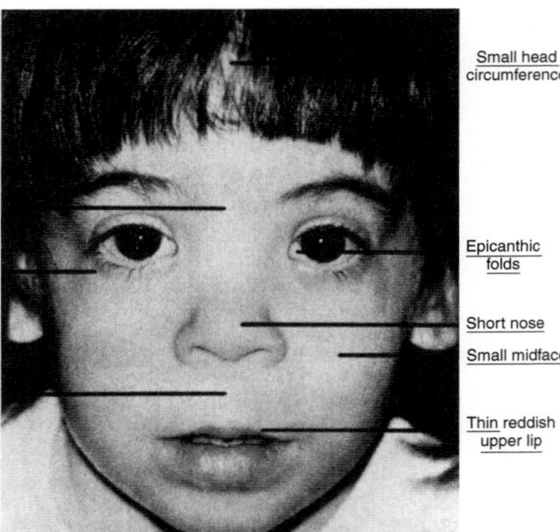

FIGURE 10-2 Specific facial signs of fetal alcohol syndrome include microcephaly, or small head size; small eyes and/or short eye openings; and an underdeveloped upper lip with flat upper lip ridges. (Reprinted from Feldmen, EB: *Essentials of clinical nutrition.* FA Davis, Philadelphia, 1988, p 164, with permission.)

In 1996, the term Fetal Alcohol Spectrum Disorder was introduced to encompass several diagnostic categories covering the wider range of alcohol effects in infants and children that do not meet the criteria for FAS.

Because researchers have not been able to determine safe levels of alcohol during pregnancy, women should be encouraged to abstain. The task of protecting the unborn is formidable. One of the goals of Healthy People 2010 is to increase to 94% the percentage of pregnant women abstaining from alcohol use (CDC, 2002).

Surveys indicate approximately 10% of pregnant women used alcohol, and approximately 2% engaged in binge drinking or frequent use of alcohol. Moreover, more than 55% of the women not using birth control reported alcohol use and 12% reported binge drinking (CDC, 2004a).

For women engaging in risky drinking behaviors and not using effective contraceptive methods, brief interventions by health-care providers have succeeded in reducing such risk (CDC, 2005). Information on prenatal alcohol screening and intervention programs is available at:

http://www.cdc.gov/ncbddd/fas
http://www.fascenter.samhsa.gov

In addition, curricular materials for parents, educators, and juvenile justice workers are available at:

http://www.cdc.gov/ncbddd/fasd/freematerials.html

Soft Cheeses and Ready-to-Eat Meats

Listeriosis is a bacterial infection causing a meningoencephalitis and/or septicemia that is particularly virulent for fetuses. The case-fatality rate is 30% in newborns and almost 50% if the onset occurs in the first 4 days of life (Heymann, 2004). The infection can damage the heart, brain, lungs, and eyes resulting in blindness. The causative organism, *Listeria monocytogenes,* is transmitted from the mother (who may be asymptomatic) to the fetus in utero or through the birth canal.

The organism can grow at refrigeration temperatures, at a pH of 5.0 or higher, and in salt concentrations as high as 12% (Chettle, 2008). Outbreaks of listeriosis have been associated with raw or contaminated milk, soft cheeses, smoked seafood, and ready-to-eat meats. Widespread outbreaks have occurred affecting:

- 50 people in 11 states, with 6 adult deaths and 2 spontaneous abortions, traced to hot dogs from a single packing plant (CDC, 1999)
- 29 people in 10 states, with 4 deaths and 3 spontaneous abortions, probably caused by deli turkey meat (CDC, 2000a)
- 12 people in North Carolina, with 5 stillbirths, 3 premature deliveries, 2 infected newborns, postpartum meningitis, and a brain abscess, that involved a soft Mexican cheese made with raw milk (CDC, 2001a).
- 5 people in Massachusetts, with 3 adult deaths, 1 stillbirth, and 1 premature delivery attributed to post-pasteurization contamination at a small milk bottling plant (CDC, 2008a).

Listeria infections during pregnancy can cause influenza-like symptoms, with fever and chills. The **incubation period** may be 3 to 70 days after a person has eaten the contaminated food (Heymann, 2004). In addition to the general rules for safe food handling, pregnant women should:

- Avoid soft cheeses (feta, Brie, Camembert, blue-veined, and Mexican-style cheese). However, hard cheeses, processed cheeses, cream cheese, cottage cheese, and yogurt may be eaten safely.
- Cook leftover foods or ready-to-eat foods (hot dogs, sausage, deli meats) until steaming hot (165°F).
- Not eat refrigerated meat spreads at all or refrigerated smoked seafood without cooking it.
- Not consume unpasteurized milk or foods made from it.

Certain Species and Amounts of Fish

Nearly all fish and shellfish have traces of mercury from environmental pollution that contaminates bodies of water where bacteria convert it to the more toxic form, methylmercury (March of Dimes, 2006). Because of high levels of mercury in some species of fish (those that grow larger and live longer), the Food and Drug Administration and the Environmental Protection Agency have advised pregnant women and women who may become pregnant, nursing mothers, and young children to avoid eating:

- Shark
- Swordfish
- King mackerel
- Tilefish

If chosen as the week's seafood meals, albacore tuna or tuna steak should be limited to 6 ounces per week, whereas up to 12 ounces per week may be consumed of species of seafood with lower amounts of mercury:

- Shrimp
- Canned light tuna
- Salmon
- Pollock
- Catfish

Fish sticks and fish sandwiches at fast food restaurants generally contain species with lower amounts of mercury. Local advisories should be sought to determine the safety of recreationally caught fish. If no local advice is available, a general rule is to limit local seafood consumption to 6 ounces per week (U.S. Department of Health and Human Services, 2004).

Developing nervous tissue is at particular risk, hence the warning regarding pregnant women and young children. Effects of methylmercury include poor performance on tests of:

- Attention
- Fine-motor function
- Language
- Visual–spatial abilities
- Memory (Hart, 2005)

Over time, the body eliminates mercury, but it can accumulate in the body faster than it can be removed.

Undercooked Meat, Unwashed Produce, and Cat Litter

Health-care providers should reinforce the principles of food hygiene to pregnant women. An infection with *Toxoplasma gondii* causes an estimated 400 to 4000 cases of congenital **toxoplasmosis** annually, producing:

- Mental retardation
- Blindness
- Epilepsy

The wide range of the estimate occurs because the disease is not nationally reportable or widely recognized as a threat by pregnant women. Only 48% of mothers of affected infants recognized risk factors of the disease, a situation that possibly could have been prevented by education.

However, only systematic serologic screening of all pregnant women at prenatal visits or of all newborn infants at birth would prevent or detect a higher proportion of these congenital infections (Boyer et al., 2005). Treatment of acute infection in pregnancy has reduced fetal infection by about 50% (CDC, 2000b). The protozoan is spread via undercooked meat, unwashed fruits and vegetables, contaminated soil, and cat feces. To prevent the infection, the pregnant woman should:

- Cook meat, poultry, and seafood thoroughly.
- Clean items that those raw foods have contacted with hot soapy water.
- Peel or meticulously wash raw fruits and vegetables before eating.
- Keep cats indoors and feed them only cooked food or prepared cat food.
- Avoid changing cat litter or, if not possible, use mask and gloves and wash hands carefully afterwards.

The FDA has compiled an extensive free educational kit on food safety for pregnant women and medical professionals. Available in English and Spanish, topics include methylmercury, Listeria, and Toxoplasma. Health educators can learn how to obtain the materials at http://www.fda.gov/downloads/Food/ResourcesForYou/HealthEducators/UCM094856.pdf.

Caffeine

The effects of caffeine consumption during pregnancy have been studied with inconsistent results, often testing the effects of coffee, which contains hundreds of substances, some of which have actions similar to those of caffeine (Brown, 2008). Neither coffee nor caffeine has been associated with preterm delivery.

Overall, caffeine intake of less than 300 milligrams per day (see "Caffeine" on DavisPlus) is unlikely to delay conception or to increase the risk of spontaneous abortion or birth defects. Neither is that level of intake likely to affect fetal growth in nonsmoking women (Higdon and Frei, 2006). In one study, mean birth weight decreased by 28 grams per 100 milligrams of caffeine consumed daily, but the authors concluded that this small amount is likely to be clinically important only in women consuming 600 milligrams or more of caffeine daily. Decaffeinated coffee did not increase risk for any **perinatal** outcome (Bracken et al., 2003).

Problems and Complications of Pregnancy Affecting Nutrition

The physiological changes that take place in a woman's body during pregnancy may cause a variety of conditions. Some of the common problems, such as morning sickness and leg cramps, are usually annoying but only occasionally require medical intervention. Other conditions, such as hypertensive disorders of pregnancy and gestational diabetes, can be hazardous and demand medical intervention.

Common Problems

Four of the most common problems of pregnancy are:

1. Morning sickness
2. Leg cramps
3. Constipation
4. Heartburn

Pica is a regional practice that is mainly influenced by culture.

MORNING SICKNESS

Hormonal changes, some of which produce relaxed gastrointestinal muscle tone, cause the nausea and vomiting of pregnancy. About 70% to 85% of pregnant women feel nauseated, and about half experience vomiting (Jewell and Young, 2003). Compared to women without morning sickness, women with it consumed significantly less meat and more carbohydrate in the first trimester, differences that were maintained throughout the pregnancies. In addition, the women with morning sickness delivered ½ week earlier than those without it (Latva-Pukkila, Isolauri, and Laitinen, 2010).

The occurrence and duration of these events vary widely, and they are not confined to mornings. Control of the problem without medication is the goal. Eating dry crackers before getting out of bed is the classic preventive. Other suggestions are to:

- Avoid fatty foods.
- Eat fruits and complex carbohydrates in small, frequent meals.
- Consume cold foods rather than hot foods.
- Drink liquids between rather than with meals.
- Eat a high-protein snack at bedtime.

In most cases, morning sickness subsides after the first trimester. With the usual caution regarding herbal products (see Chapter 15), ginger appears to be a fairly low-risk and effective treatment for nausea and vomiting associated with pregnancy (Ozgoli, Goli, and Simbar, 2009). Vitamin B_6 (pyridoxine hydrocholoride) does not appear to adversely affect fetal brain development and can be used to control nausea and vomiting of pregnancy when clinically indicated (Nulman et al., 2009).

LEG CRAMPS

Pregnant women often complain of leg cramps. One cause may be neuromuscular irritability due to low serum calcium, but the evidence that supplemental calcium reduces cramping is weak. Because of its close link to calcium metabolism, magnesium deficiency has been postulated to cause leg cramps. Magnesium supplementation just above the UL, however, produced no significant effect on frequency or intensity of leg cramps in women between 18 and 36 weeks pregnant (Nygaard et al., 2008). Evidence for effective nonpharmacological treatment of leg cramps, even those caused by varicose veins in pregnancy, is sparse (Bamigboye and Smyth, 2007).

Staying well hydrated is of prime importance, followed by maintaining adequate intakes of potassium, sodium, calcium, and magnesium. A noninvasive procedure to prevent muscle cramps is to stretch the muscles before exercise and, for nighttime cramps, before bedtime.

CONSTIPATION

Decreased gastrointestinal muscle tone and the growing uterus pressing on the intestines cause constipation that may affect up to 24% of pregnant women (Bradley et al., 2007). Adequate fluid intake, regular exercise, and a high-fiber diet should relieve this condition. Ideally, the suggested amount of fiber intake, 30 grams per day, should be achieved with food rather than pharmaceutical preparations. Foods high in fiber but relatively low in kilocalories are listed in Table 10-6. If needed, dietary supplements of bran or wheat fiber are likely to help women experiencing constipation in pregnancy (Jewell and Young, 2001).

HEARTBURN

A burning sensation beneath the breastbone is called heartburn. Hormonal changes cause relaxation of the cardiac sphincter, located between the esophagus and the stomach. That and the upward pressure on the diaphragm from the enlarging uterus can cause reflux of gastric contents into the esophagus and the burning sensation.

Avoiding spicy or acidic foods and taking small, frequent meals can control heartburn. Other helpful measures include sitting up for an hour after a meal as well as elevating the head while sleeping. Pregnant women should not self-medicate with sodium bicarbonate or antacids. The bicarbonate can be absorbed, producing alkalosis. Antacids decrease iron absorption by decreasing gastric acids, thus increasing the risk of anemia.

PICA

Pica is the compulsive ingestion of nonfood items, usually dirt, clay, laundry starch, baking soda, or ice. It is an ancient behavior. Most notable in some regions of the southern United States, pica occurs in conjunction with inadequate diets due to poverty, but it also occurs in women at other socioeconomic levels. Many women with pica have it only during pregnancy, believing it cures the annoyances of pregnancy or ensures a beautiful baby. Others contend that the substances they ingest taste good to them.

Health concerns about pica include:

- Inadequate nutrition due to substitution of nonfood items for nutritious foods
- Iron-deficiency anemia
- Constipation
- Lead poisoning

Eating ice or freezer frost, seemingly specific to iron deficiency, ceases within 1 to 2 weeks after beginning iron therapy (Chitambar and Antony, 2006). Consuming laundry starch interferes with iron absorption.

Ingestion of clay may lead to fecal impaction. Sometimes the substance ingested contains lead, as

TABLE 10-6 ■ Nutrient-Dense Foods High in Fiber

FOOD	QUANTITY	GRAMS OF DIETARY FIBER	KILOCALORIES
Grains			
All Bran	½ cup	9	81
Bran buds	⅓ cup	13	75
100% Bran	⅓ cup	8	83
Fruits			
Apple, raw with skin, chopped	1 cup	3	65
Orange sections, raw	1 cup	4	85
Pear, raw with skin	One small	5	86
Prunes, cooked, unsweetened	½ cup	4	133
Vegetables/Legumes			
Baked beans, in tomato sauce with pork	½ cup	5	116
Brussels sprouts, cooked from frozen	1 cup	6	65
Kidney beans, canned	½ cup	7	108
Navy beans, cooked from dry	½ cup	10	128
Green peas, cooked from frozen	½ cup	4	62

occurred in 15 women, 70% of them Hispanic, with lead poisoning caused by pica. Because lead freely crosses the placenta, their infants had higher blood levels than the women (Shannon, 2003).

Ingestion of large amounts of baking soda has caused severe metabolic alkalosis that was initially thought to be an atypical preeclampsia before the pica was discovered (Grotegut et al., 2006).

Women who have migrated to an area where pica is uncommon may continue the custom. A caring, nonjudgmental interviewer may encourage a woman to reveal that she has a craving for and is eating nonfood items. The interview could lead to preventive therapy and a teaching opportunity.

Complications of Pregnancy

Three complications of pregnancy with nutritional ramifications are:

- Hyperemesis gravidarum
- Hypertensive disorders of pregnancy
- Gestational diabetes

HYPEREMESIS GRAVIDARUM

Severe nausea and vomiting persisting after the 14th week of pregnancy is called **hyperemesis gravidarum**. Its incidence is reported to be higher in multiple pregnancies and other conditions associated with increased pregnancy hormone levels. The etiology and pathogenesis are unknown. It develops most often in Western countries and in first pregnancies.

Estimated to occur in 2% of pregnancies, hyperemesis gravidarum can be life-threatening, causing:

- Dehydration
- Electrolyte imbalance
- Weight loss
- Rarely, esophageal rupture (Eroglu et al., 2002; Liang et al., 2002)
- Rarely, renal failure (Hill, Yost, and Wendel, 2002)

Because of the physiological increase in blood volume that occurs in pregnancy, hypovolemia due to hyperemesis gravidarum can become severe without clinical signs. The body's adaptive response causes vasoconstriction of uterine vessels, reducing its blood supply up to 20% without a notable change in the woman's blood pressure (Wagner et al., 2000).

Major vitamin deficiencies have resulted from hyperemesis gravidarum:

- Vitamin K deficiency in a 32-week preterm infant caused severe intracranial hemorrhage. The infant's blood depicted vitamin K deficiency whereas the mother's coagulation status was normal (Eventov-Friedman, Klinger, and Shinwell, 2009).
- Deficiencies of vitamins B_6 and B_{12} can result in peripheral neuropathy.
- Deficiency of thiamine has caused Wernicke's encephalopathy in pregnant clients (Indraccolo et al., 2005; Wagner et al., 2000).

See Chapters 7 and 20 for information on Wernicke's encephalopathy. Sometimes Wernicke's encephalopathy has resulted in fatal outcomes in the mother or the fetus (Chiossi et al., 2006). Prophylactic thiamine supplementation should be considered in the care of hyperemesis (Chiossi et al., 2006; Selitsky, Chandra, and Schiavello, 2006).

Hyperemesis gravidarum requires treatment for the health of the woman and the fetus. Many approaches have been used to treat hyperemesis gravidarum:

- Pyridoxine
- Ginger
- Rehydration
- Enteral and parenteral nutritional support
- Antiemetics (without teratogenic effects)
- Corticosteroid therapy

HYPERTENSIVE DISORDERS OF PREGNANCY

Hypertensive disorders affect 6% to 8% of pregnancies (Brown, 2008) and include:

- Chronic hypertension
- Gestational hypertension
- Preeclampsia
- Eclampsia

Hypertension is blood pressure greater than 140 mm Hg systolic or greater than 90 mm Hg diastolic. Fetal complications include growth restriction, prematurity, and stillbirth. Distinctions among the categories and a summary of risks, pathophysiology, and treatments follow.

- *Chronic hypertension* existed before pregnancy—or is diagnosed in retrospect when gestational hypertension or the hypertension of preeclampsia do not resolve after delivery. Blood pressures higher than 160 mm Hg systolic or 110 mm Hg diastolic are associated with increased risk of preterm delivery, fetal growth retardation, or fetal mortality (Brown, 2008).
- *Gestational hypertension* occurs after 20 weeks of gestation without proteinuria. About 25% of these women will develop preeclampsia (ADA, 2008).
- **Preeclampsia** occurs after 20 weeks of pregnancy with proteinuria. It affects 3% to 5% of pregnant women in the United States (Turner, 2006). Risk factors for preeclampsia include:
  - First pregnancy
  - Multiple fetuses
  - Mother older than 35 years

- African American race
- Obesity
- History of preeclampsia
- Chronic hypertension.

- **Eclampsia** is the occurrence in preeclamptic women of seizures not attributable to another cause. It is an obstetrical emergency. The woman requires intensive care because she is at high risk for cerebral hemorrhage, circulatory collapse, and kidney failure. The fetus, too, is in grave danger.

All forms of hypertension in pregnancy are related to inflammation, **oxidative stress**, and damage to the **endothelium** resulting in impaired blood flow, increased clotting tendencies, and **plaque** formation (Brown, 2008). A review of some genetic factors related to preeclampsia appears as Genomic Gem 10-2.

Chronic hypertension in a pregnant woman requires careful management. Sodium restriction is not recommended for everyone because of the risk of impaired fetal growth. If a woman's salt-sensitive hypertension was managed successfully before pregnancy with a sodium-restricted diet, that approach is usually continued (Brown, 2008).

Definitive treatment of preeclampsia, aside from delivery of the fetus and placenta, awaits elucidation of its cause. Without question, careful monitoring of pregnant women and early intervention is crucial. Better antioxidant status in the blood significantly reduces risk of preeclampsia, and calcium supplements appear to reduce risk of preeclampsia in high-risk women with low calcium intakes (ADA, 2008).

Genomic Gem 10-2
Susceptibility to Preeclampsia

Transmission of genetic risk factors for preeclampsia can occur through the mother or the father. Women who were born after a preeclamptic pregnancy were more than twice as likely to have preeclampsia in their first pregnancy as women without such history, whereas men born after a preeclamptic pregnancy had a 50% increased risk of fathering a preeclamptic pregnancy. These familial associations were stronger in the clinically more severe forms of preeclampsia (Skjaerven et al., 2005).

An exaggerated inflammatory response to pregnancy may occur in genetically susceptible women. Those who were homozygous for a particular allele had the greatest risk for preeclampsia. Black women with preeclampsia were more than three times as likely as normotensive black women to have certain combinations of alleles; white women twice as likely. Other inflammatory factors such as bacterial and viral infections may exaggerate the normal inflammatory response to pregnancy. Many infectious organisms have been associated with preeclampsia, including herpes simplex and streptococcus (Haggerty et al., 2005).

Eclampsia may occur even 12 days after delivery (Brown, 2008). For both prophylaxis against and treatment of eclampsia, magnesium sulfate has been used for decades and contributes to the very low mortality rates in developed countries without harm to the fetus (Rude and Shils, 2006).

Very long-term health effects have emerged after hypertensive disorders of pregnancy. Preeclampsia can continue to affect women 20 to 30 years after the delivery when these women have increased cardiovascular mortality rates. Whether their preeclampsia damaged blood vessels leading to cardiovascular disease or if women at risk for cardiovascular disease develop preeclampsia still must be determined (Fedorka and Heasley, 2008).

GESTATIONAL DIABETES

The emergence of diabetes in pregnancy, **gestational diabetes,** is considered to be a form of type 2 diabetes (see Chapter 17) that usually appears between weeks 24 and 28 of gestation when the body's insulin requirement is greatly increased (Anderson, 2006). It affects 3 to 7% of pregnant women who seem to have a predisposition to insulin resistance and type 2 diabetes. The physiological changes of pregnancy bring out the disease (Brown, 2008).

Among these changes is the production of hormones by the placenta that decrease insulin sensitivity and increase insulin resistance in the mother to ensure a constant, optimum level of glucose for the fetus. When the mother's insulin supply is inadequate or ineffective, her high blood glucose is transferred to the fetus who secretes his own insulin to lower the glucose content of his blood by converting it to fat, hence the hallmark result of diabetes in pregnant women: large newborns.

Risk factors for gestational diabetes are:

- Occurrence of gestational diabetes in a previous pregnancy
- Previous delivery of an infant weighing more than 9 pounds
- Family history of diabetes
- Maternal obesity (greater than 120% of ideal body weight).

Most women return to normal glucose levels after delivery; however, 40% to 60% of them may develop type 2 diabetes in 15 to 20 years. Maintaining a reasonable body weight and a regular exercise program decreases the risk of developing type 2 diabetes (Anderson, 2006).

Treatment of gestational diabetes, requiring an aggressive team approach, is included in Chapter 17. Because insulin does not cross the placenta, insulin is the recommended method of controlling blood glucose during pregnancy (Deglin and Vallerand, 2009). Clinical trials of oral antidiabetic agents during pregnancy have been conducted (Ecker and Greene, 2008).

The Breastfeeding Mother

One of the goals of *Healthy People 2010* is to increase to:

- 75% the proportion of mothers who breastfeed in the early postpartum period
- 50% those who breastfeed until the infant is 6 months old
- 25% those who breastfeed until the infant is 1 year old

In 2005–2006, 77% of infants had received some breast milk, exceeding the *Healthy People 2010* goal. Mexican American and non-Hispanic whites exceeded the goal but just 65% of non-Hispanic black infants were ever breastfed, still a significant increase from 36% in 1993–1994. The longer term breastfeeding goals were not met (McDowell, Wang, and Kennedy-Stephenson, 2008).

Breastfeeding rates varied greatly within the Mexican American community. When *immigrant* is defined as born outside of the United States, 59% of Mexican immigrant mothers breastfed for at least 6 months compared with 24% of Mexican nonimmigrants. For immigrant women, breastfeeding may be the common and expected method of feeding whereas women born in the United States may see breastfeeding as just one of multiple feeding options (Gibson-Davis and Brooks-Gunn, 2006). Figure 10-3 shows the percentage of 6-month-old infants by race/ethnicity being breastfed in the United States from 1993 through 2004. Chapter 11 covers the advantages of breast milk for the infant.

Nutritional Needs

For DRIs during pregnancy and lactation, see Appendix A. For selected energy nutrients and minerals, see Table 10-1.

The MyPyramid recommendations for a breastfeeding mother are the same as those for the third trimester of pregnancy. See Table 10-5.

A common recommendation for the breastfeeding woman is to drink a glass of fluid with meals and whenever she breastfeeds, and to limit caffeinated beverages to two cups per day.

Calcium

The primary source of calcium in human milk is calcium resorbed from the mother's bones, a process that is not prevented by increased calcium intake from foods or supplements. Moreover, the lost skeletal calcium is rapidly replaced after weaning with compete recovery occurring in most women even with closely spaced pregnancies and long periods of lactation. In general, lactation duration does not appear to be associated with increased fracture risk or osteoporosis in later life (Picciano and McDonald, 2006).

Mobilization of calcium from the mother's bones also frees sequestered lead. Some evidence suggests that a higher maternal dietary intake of polyunsaturated fatty acids may limit the transfer of lead from bone to breast milk (Arora et al., 2008).

Energy

The average lactating woman produces 26 ounces of milk daily but the amount varies greatly. Emptying the breast stimulates more milk production. Breast milk contains about 20 kilocalories per ounce, now the standard for term infant formulas. (See Chapter 11.) Some of the energy for the milk comes from the

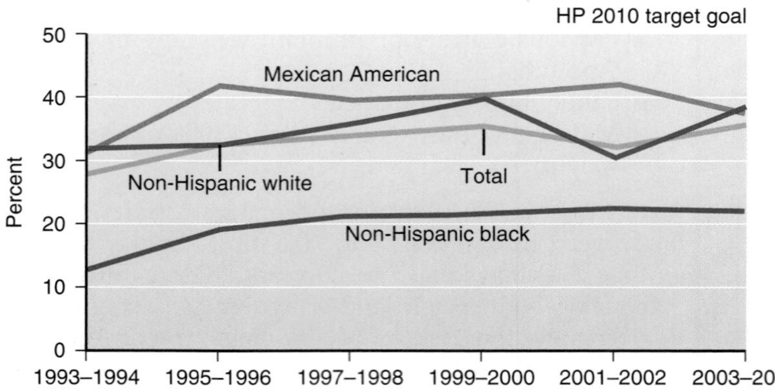

FIGURE 10-3 U.S. breastfeeding rates, 1993–2004: percentage of infants who were still breastfed at 6 months of age by race-ethnicity group. (SOURCE: McDowell, Wang, and Kennedy-Stephenson, 2008.)

mother's dietary intake, some from fat stores accumulated during pregnancy.

Effect of Maternal Deficiencies

The mammary gland can extract most nutrients from the circulation so that breast milk may contain adequate levels of nutrients even when the mother's intake is inadequate. Levels of water-soluble vitamins in human milk depend on maternal intake, and evidence suggests that the mammary gland may take priority in folate use over the mother's own blood-forming needs. Persistent maternal vitamin deficiencies, however, may result in inadequate concentrations in the milk (Picciano and McDonald, 2006). For instance, vitamin B_{12} deficiency in vegetarian mothers has caused growth failure and neurologic impairment in their breastfeeding infants (CDC, 2003; Kanra et al., 2005). Vitamin B_{12} deficiency can cause irreversible neurologic damage in infancy and worse outcomes if deficiency also occurred in utero (Kanra et al., 2005).

In contrast, the concentrations of the major minerals in human milk do not correspond to the mother's blood levels but the trace minerals selenium and iodine do depend upon maternal dietary intake (Picciano and McDonald, 2006). As recounted in Chapter 8, iodine is critical for normal neurological development and is the one mineral, along with vitamins thiamin, riboflavin, vitamins B_6 and B_{12}, and vitamin A categorized as priority nutrients. Because low maternal intake or stores of these nutrients are reflected in human milk, supplementing the lactating mother can restore her milk to adequate levels (Allen, 2005) thus providing a healthier intake for the nursing infant.

Benefits to the Mother

Several advantages to the mother are associated with breastfeeding. Breast milk is less expensive than formula (see Dollars and Sense 10-2) and is always ready at the correct temperature. Contamination during formula making is usually not a concern. Nursing the infant encourages the new mother to sit down several times a day. On the other hand, without pumping her breasts and storing the milk (see Chapter 11), the task of feeding the infant is hers alone.

Breastfeeding has unique advantages:

1. Helps the uterus return to its nonpregnant state more quickly.
2. Assists in birth spacing under certain conditions.
3. May be protective against later breast cancer.

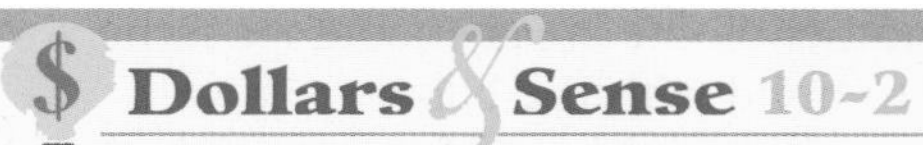

Savings with Breastfeeding

Breastfeeding is less costly than bottle feeding. The additional foods the mother consumes are less expensive than infant formula that may cost a family $700 the first year. In addition to individual benefits, breastfeeding can help the environment by reducing costs and waste associated with formula production, marketing, and distribution (ADA, 2005).

Aids Uterine Involution

During breastfeeding, the sucking of the infant stimulates the release of **oxytocin** from the posterior pituitary gland in the brain. Oxytocin causes the uterine muscles to contract and helps return the uterus to its nonpregnant size while reducing postpartum blood loss.

Assists in Birth Spacing

The effectiveness of full or nearly full breastfeeding as a contraceptive technique has been confirmed in both developing and developed countries (Picciano and McDonald, 2006) but it is not as effective as other methods of contraception. Consequently, breastfeeding is not suggested as the sole means of birth spacing if other methods are available and acceptable to the client. Because estrogen inhibits lactation, means of contraception other than those containing estrogen are advised if the woman continues to breastfeed.

Lessens Risk of Cancer

Over the long term, breastfeeding has been associated with a decreased risk of breast cancer later in life, especially among premenopausal women. The risk reduction is directly related to lifetime duration of breastfeeding (Picciano and McDonald, 2006). Less-convincing evidence suggests an association between breastfeeding and a reduction in the risk of maternal ovarian cancer (Ip et al., 2007). Some of the factors in cancer's complex etiology are described in Chapter 21.

Techniques of Breastfeeding

The medical and nursing staff will assist the mother to start breastfeeding her infant. Even mothers of twins and premature babies can successfully breastfeed with additional education and support. Some general principles to aid in breastfeeding have been established.

The mother and infant should be permitted to spend as much time together as possible during the first 24 hours after birth. This practice permits bonding of infant and mother. Some areas encourage fathers to "room in" also to bond with the baby.

One correct position for breastfeeding is shown in Figure 10-4. It is "tummy-to-tummy." The infant should face the breast squarely. If the breast is very large, the mother must take care to prevent it from blocking the infant's nose lest it impede infant's breathing. When nursing, the infant should grasp the entire areola (the colored portion around the nipple) to prevent the nipples from becoming sore.

Most infants will take 80% to 90% of the milk from each breast in the first 4 minutes of nursing. Because nursing stimulates further milk production, the mother should alternate breasts to start the feeding. This method allows the infant to vigorously stimulate milk production in the first breast offered and to finish feeding on the other breast if it is still hungry or is just enjoying the experience.

Encouraging Breastfeeding

Pediatricians are encouraged to provide information on the benefits and methods of breastfeeding so that the mother can make an informed choice (AAP, 2005). Prenatal encouragement increases breastfeeding rates and identifies potential problem areas.

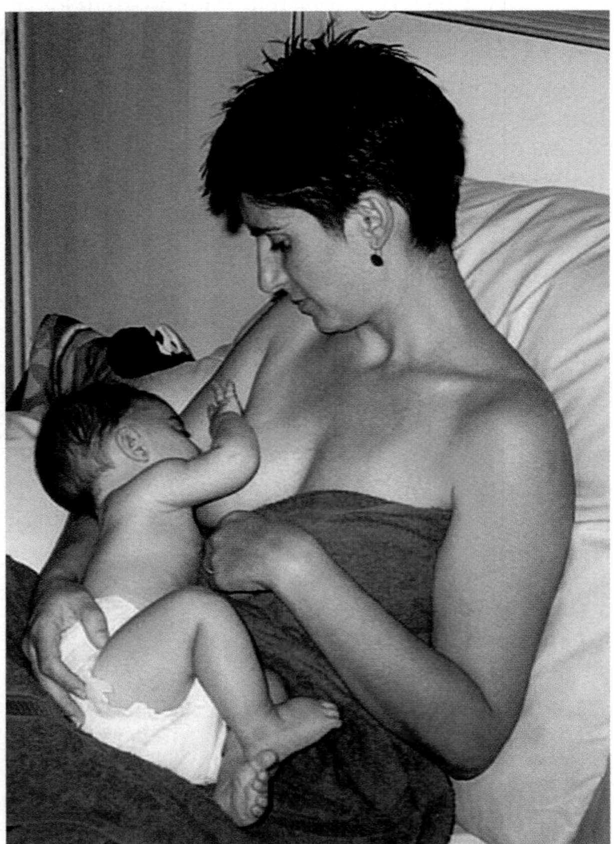

FIGURE 10-4 One correct breastfeeding position, "tummy-to-tummy." The infant takes the entire areola in its mouth. Notice how focused the mother is on the baby.

Hospital and birthing center practices should focus on rooming in, early and frequent breastfeeding, skilled support, and avoidance of artificial nipples, pacifiers, and formula. Infants should be assessed while nursing at 2 to 4 days of age, with liberal use of referral and support groups, including lactation consultants and peer counselors (Brown, 2008). Box 10-2 summarizes a program to increase breastfeeding worldwide.

Knowledge of and respect for a family's cultural traditions will assist the health care provider when promoting breastfeeding. For instance, one group of Native Americans saw breastfeeding as the "natural way" or even as a moral choice calling it the "right way" to feed a baby. Decision-making in this and other traditional societies involves not just the mother but also the family and the community. In such situations, educational efforts should be directed at the

Box 10-2 ■ *The Baby-Friendly Hospital Initiative*

The Baby-Friendly Hospital Initiative (BFHI) is a global UNICEF/WHO-sponsored effort to promote breastfeeding. As of July 2008, 65 of these designated hospitals and birth centers were in the United States (Baby-Friendly, 2006a).

The WHO and UNICEF recommend implementing the following practices in every facility providing maternity services and care for newborn infants:

Ten Steps to Successful Breastfeeding

1. Have a written breastfeeding policy routinely communicated to all health-care staff.
2. Train all health-care staff in skills necessary to implement this policy.
3. Inform all pregnant women about the benefits and management of breastfeeding.
4. Help mothers initiate breastfeeding within a half hour (U.S., 1 hour) of birth.
5. Show mothers how to breastfeed and how to maintain lactation even if they are separated from their infants.
6. Give infants no food or drink other than breast milk unless *medically* indicated.
7. Practice rooming-in: Allow mothers and infants to remain together 24 hours a day.
8. Encourage unrestricted breastfeeding.
9. Give no pacifiers or artificial nipples to breastfeeding infants.
10. Foster the establishment of breastfeeding support groups and refer mothers to them on discharge from the hospital or clinic (Baby-Friendly, 2004, 2006b).

In addition, Baby-Friendly institutions are expected to abide by the WHO International Code of Marketing of Breast Milk Substitutes that forbids accepting free formula or other gifts and grants from formula producers. Distributing sample packs of formula or literature bearing the name of a formula product to breastfeeding mothers is also not permitted (Baby-Friendly, 2006b).

larger group to increase acceptance of and support for breastfeeding (Dodgson et al., 2002).

Adoptive mothers have successfully breastfed their infants by using physical stimulation and breast pumps to establish a milk supply. A breastfeeding supplementer system, the Lact-Aid Nursing Trainer System, is available to provide additional milk while the infant is nursing at the breast. Compelling stories of women who have breastfed adopted infants offer encouragement to others (Adoptive Breastfeeding Resource, 2008).

On the other hand, overselling of the benefits and ease of breastfeeding has resulted in starvation deaths of infants (see Chapter 11). Not only should the mother's choice be respected and supported, but also the infant's condition should be monitored appropriately regardless of the feeding method chosen.

Maternal Contraindications to Breastfeeding

Most women can feed their infants at breast. A few contraindications to breastfeeding include the mother's use of illegal drugs and certain medications, particular illnesses in the mother, and the mother's exposure to toxic chemicals. Galactosemia, an absolute contraindication due to a metabolic defect in the infant, is covered in Chapter 11.

Medication Use

Mothers are sometimes counseled to interrupt breastfeeding or to wean the infant, without a compelling medical reason (Crenshaw, 2005). Although many medications the mother takes are secreted in breast milk, most do not affect the milk supply or the infant when taken in recommended doses. However, compatibility with breastfeeding has not been established for all psychotropic drugs (Fortinguerra, Clavenna, and Bonati, 2009).

Particularly if the medication can be administered directly to infants, the amount received in breast milk is unlikely to be harmful, but the capabilities of the livers and kidneys of premature and young infants as well as the characteristics of the medication should be considered. In rare cases, a mother's metabolism of a drug endangers a breastfeeding infant. See Genomic Gem 10-3.

Diagnostic radioactive compounds require temporary cessation of breastfeeding until the drug has left the mother's system; therapeutic doses are a contraindication. Cytoxic drugs, illegal drugs, psychotropic drugs, some anticonvulsants, salicylates, and ergot derivatives all have had significant effects on nursing infants or raise concerns because the effect on nursing infants is unknown (Breastfeeding, 2004). The physician should be consulted about both prescription and nonprescription drugs the mother takes.

Substances that are commonly not thought of as drugs may also affect the breastfed infant. These include alcohol and caffeine. The American Academy of Pediatrics recommends against the use of alcohol by breastfeeding mothers except for an occasional small drink and then only if a 2-hour delay occurs until the next feeding (AAP, 2005).

A premature infant suffered from acute and chronic prenatal and postnatal exposure to caffeine and related

Genomic Gem 10-3

Ultrarapid Metabolizers of Codeine

The FDA has issued a warning to health care providers about a very rare but potentially lethal side effect that can affect the infants of nursing mothers who are taking codeine-containing analgesics. Some people are ultrarapid metabolizers of codeine with a specific **cytochrome P450 enzyme** (CYP2D6 genotype). See Chapter 15 for a discussion of these isoenzymes.

People with a certain variation in a liver enzyme allows them to convert codeine to its active metabolite, morphine, more rapidly and completely than other people (FDA, 2007a). A breastfeeding mother with this genotype can accumulate unusually high morphine levels in her serum and breast milk, putting her nursing infant at risk for morphine overdose. One healthy, 13-day-old breastfeeding baby died of such a morphine overdose even though his mother was taking codeine at a reduced dose because she, too, had suffered side effects (FDA, 2007b).

The prevalence of the ultra-rapid metabolizers of codeine varies for different populations, less than 10% for most groups. In some groups of North Africans, Ethiopians, and Saudis the prevalence may be as high as 28%. The FDA has cleared a genetic test that can determine a person's CYP2D6 genotype, thus identifying individuals who can rapidly metabolize codeine (FDA, 2007b).

Because codeine has been used for postpartum pain for decades and is generally considered the safest narcotic pain reliever for breastfeeding mothers, absent genotyping of every new mother, careful, informed observation of mothers and infants is critical. Health care providers should teach nursing mothers who may be taking codeine about the signs of morphine overdose in themselves (extreme sleepiness and constipation) and in infants (increased sleepiness, trouble breastfeeding, breathing difficulties, and limpness). The mother should report any of those signs to the doctor or seek other medical attention immediately.

Newborn breastfed babies usually nurse every two to three hours and shouldn't sleep more than four hours at a time. Mothers should also be aware that morphine may remain in the infant's body for up to several days after the last codeine dose (FDA, November 2007).

compounds in a tea-like beverage (mate) the mother consumed. The baby's irritability, due to either the stimulatory effects of the caffeine or to a withdrawal syndrome, gradually improved by 84 hours of age, although intermittent irritability was still present when the infant was discharged at 24 days of age. The mother was strongly advised to initiate a progressive reduction of mate consumption to a maximum of two cups a day for the duration of breastfeeding (Martin et al., 2007).

Altered Physiology or Pathology

In the United States, absolute contraindications to breastfeeding include active untreated tuberculosis and some viral infections. Acute or chronic diseases in the mother such as heart disease, severe anemia, and nephritis also may preclude breastfeeding.

Maternal infection with human immunodeficiency virus (HIV) is a contraindication in the United States. If an uninterrupted supply of safe, nutritionally adequate breast milk substitute is available (as is possible in industrialized countries), HIV-infected women should be counseled not to breastfeed their infants. In developing countries where the risks of malnutrition, diarrhea, and other infectious diseases may be more immediate than the risk of HIV, mothers are encouraged to breastfeed.

Women infected with human T-cell leukemia virus, type 1 (HTLV-1) should not breastfeed (State of New Jersey, 2009). Herpes infections preclude breastfeeding only if the mother has herpetic lesions on the breast.

Exposure to Toxic Chemicals

Certain chemicals, such as DDT and PCB, have been shown to be **teratogenic**, causing congenital defects. Concern has been raised about the transmission of toxic chemicals to the infant through breast milk. Once ingested, if the body has no means of excreting the chemicals, the contaminants are stored in adipose tissue. When the lactating mother's fat stores are mobilized to produce milk, it, too, contains the chemicals.

Some experts think that the risk to the infant is minimal unless the mobilization of the mother's fat is due to inadequate intake. Others say that there is no hazard unless the woman has had occupational exposure to the chemicals or has consumed a large amount of fish from contaminated waters. Women with concerns about the issue should discuss them with their health-care providers.

Keystones

- To support her own and the fetus's growth, a pregnant woman requires increased intake of many nutrients, especially kilocalories, protein, folic acid, and iron. Vitamin B_{12} status should be assessed in vegans.
- All women capable of becoming pregnant should consume 400 micrograms of folic acid from fortified foods or supplements to decrease risk of neural tube defects in the embryo.
- The pregnant woman should avoid ingesting alcohol, soft cheeses, ready-to-eat meats, certain species and amounts of fish, undercooked meats, unwashed produce, and immoderate amounts of preformed vitamin A.
- Nutritional interventions are sometimes helpful for common complaints of pregnancy: morning sickness, leg cramps, constipation, and heartburn. Tact and diplomacy may be required to counsel women who have pica.
- Medical intervention and nutritional support are indicated for clients with hyperemesis gravidarum, hypertensive disorders of pregnancy, or gestational diabetes.
- Some maternal contraindications to breastfeeding are ingestion of certain medications and drugs, some illnesses, including AIDS and untreated tuberculosis, and exposure to toxic chemicals.

CASE STUDY 10-1

Ms. T is a 21-year-old sexually active woman who has been followed in a family planning clinic for 3 years. She has been faithful about keeping appointments and taking her oral contraceptives. She also takes the multivitamin/multimineral supplement containing 400 micrograms of folic acid about four times a week "when she remembers and eats breakfast." She is taking no other medications. She and her immediate family have no known allergies. Now she relates that she is seriously considering becoming pregnant and wonders if they can afford to start a family. Her boyfriend proposed at her 21st birthday celebration. The couple has no pets but they do enjoy outdoor sports. Ms. T denies knowledge of means to minimize fetal risk and states she drinks a beer or a glass of wine on Saturdays and Sundays. She does not smoke. She received the standard measles, mumps, and rubella (MMR) vaccination as a child.

Ms. T is a 5-ft 3-in. woman and weighs 104 lb. She has a small frame. Her hemoglobin was 14 g/dL and hematocrit was 42% last month.

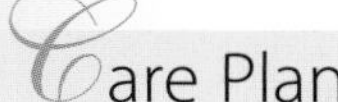

Care Plan

Subjective Data

Expressed interest in becoming pregnant ■ Concerned about the costs of parenthood ■ Regular moderate alcohol intake ■ History of compliance with medical regimen ■ Immunized against measles, mumps, and rubella

Objective Data

89% of healthy body weight ■ Hemoglobin 14 g/dL, within normal limits (WNL) ■ Hematocrit 42%, within normal limits (WNL)

Analysis

Increased risk to potential fetus related to current lifestyle and underweight

Plan

DESIRED OUTCOMES EVALUATION CRITERIA	ACTIONS/INTERVENTIONS	RATIONALE
Will affirm today her intention to abstain from alcohol when attempting to achieve a pregnancy and throughout gestation.	Teach Ms. T about fetal alcohol syndrome.	No amount of alcohol is presumed to be safe in pregnancy.
	Use photographs of affected children.	"A picture is worth 1,000 words." Photographs introduce visual learning and impact feelings.
Will take multivitamin, multimineral supplement every day beginning tomorrow.	Reiterate that vitamin preparation should contain 400 micrograms of folic acid.	This is the RDA for all women capable of becoming pregnant.
	Review the value of a varied diet and good sources of food folate.	The RDA also emphasizes the importance of food folate.
Will eat breakfast or equivalent morning nourishment every day beginning tomorrow.	Review Dietary Guidelines with Ms. T. Explore means to take nourishment in morning.	This is a good habit to acquire. Once Ms. T achieves pregnancy, supplying the embryo/fetus with a steady supply of nutrients is critical.
Will recount the limits to vitamin A intake during pregnancy by next visit.	Inform Ms. T of RDA for vitamin A in pregnancy. Alert Ms. T to the large amounts of preformed vitamin A in liver and liver products. Caution against supplements of vitamin A in addition to the multivitamin, multimineral tablet.	Teratogenic effects usually occur during the first trimester.
	Discuss the safety of beta-carotene (provitamin A) in pregnancy.	Beta-carotene has not been associated with birth defects. Supplements containing provitamin A are considered safe for pregnant women at the RDA level.

(Continued on the following page)

CASE STUDY *(Continued)*

DESIRED OUTCOMES EVALUATION CRITERIA	ACTIONS/INTERVENTIONS	RATIONALE
Will list actions to take to minimize exposure to Listeria infection by 10 weeks before attempted conception.	Provide Ms. T with a list of cheeses to avoid and those that are considered safe. Review rules for safe handling of ready-to-eat meats.	Because the incubation period of Listeria is up to 10 weeks, avoidance of possibly contaminated food should begin well before conception.
	Alert her to report flu-like symptoms promptly to her primary health-care provider.	Antimicrobial therapy may prevent fetal infection and the associated high mortality.
Will monitor own intake of fish to remain within recommended limits by conception.	Emphasize complete abstinence from shark, swordfish, King mackerel, and tilefish. If available, use food models showing the weekly limits of 12 ounces or 6 ounces of fish.	These advisories from the FDA and the EPA to minimize the exposure of the fetus to methylmercury show the seriousness of the threat.
Will discuss discontinuing oral contraceptive therapy and attempting conception with the primary health-care provider before changing her regimen.	Advise Ms. T about the possibility of birth defects with some oral contraceptives.	Progestins may cause birth defects if taken early in pregnancy.
Will continue planning optimal nutrition for herself and her prospective child.	Refer Ms. T to local WIC program.	If eligible, she could begin receiving food assistance when she becomes pregnant.

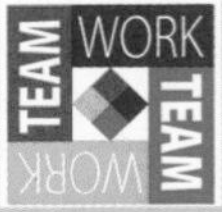

10-1

WIC Program Director's Notes

The following WIC Program Director's Notes are representative of the documentation found in a client's medical record.

Subjective: *Interested in possible food assistance when she achieves pregnancy*

Objective: *Completed WIC application*

Analysis: *Meets eligibility requirements for*

- *Residency in state*
- *Household income*
- *Nutrition risk due to underweight—documented by family planning nurse*

Does not currently meet categorical eligibility requirement:

- *Is not pregnant*
- *Has no dependent children.*

Plan: *Place application in pending file*

Encourage client to activate application when becomes pregnant

Critical Thinking Questions

1. If Ms. T were to achieve a pregnancy, what would her month-by-month recommended weight gain be? If she expresses concern about "gaining too much weight" when within the recommended amounts, how would you counsel her?
2. Are there other issues you believe ought to be raised with Ms. T before she attempts to become pregnant? Are they more or less important than the ones addressed in the Care Plan? Why?
3. Assuming Ms. T becomes pregnant, how would you approach anticipatory guidance regarding complications of pregnancy affected by nutrition?

Chapter Review

1. Throughout pregnancy and lactation, a woman should consume 2 cups of ____ daily.
   a. Vegetables
   b. Fruit
   c. Milk
   d. Meat or beans
2. Which of the following substances are contraindicated during pregnancy?
   a. Alcohol and swordfish
   b. Cocoa and peanut butter
   c. Coffee and well-done beef
   d. Tea and cheddar cheese
3. Which of the following principles is not recommended by the Baby-Friendly Hospital Initiative?
   a. Feeding on demand
   b. Keeping mother and infant together 24 hours a day
   c. Hydrating the infant with sterile water until the mother's milk supply is established
   d. Putting the infant to breast within 1 hour of birth
4. The RDA for folic acid specifies 400 micrograms of synthetic folic acid from fortified foods or supplements for:
   a. All women capable of becoming pregnant
   b. Women taking oral contraceptive medications
   c. Women of northern European descent
   d. Breastfeeding mothers
5. If a pregnant woman complains of heartburn, she should be instructed to:
   a. Increase her intake of milk products
   b. Decrease her overall food intake
   c. Rest in bed after eating
   d. Avoid spicy or acidic foods

Clinical Analysis

Ms. S is a 15-year-old girl who thinks that she is 2 months pregnant. She confides to the school nurse that she is not sure if she should have an abortion. She has not told anyone else of the pregnancy. Her purpose in disclosing the information to the school nurse is to obtain assistance with weight control so she has more time to make up her mind.

1. Based on the above information, which one of the following interventions would be of highest priority at this time?
   a. Designing a weight-control program that is high in calcium
   b. Giving information on the desirability of breastfeeding the infant
   c. Instructing the girl regarding substances that are likely to harm the fetus
   d. Scheduling a visit with a social worker to help the girl decide on a course of action
2. Knowing that adolescents are often lacking in certain nutrients, the nurse would want to assess the girl's intake of:
   a. Cola, coffee, and tea
   b. Fruits, vegetables, milk, and red meat
   c. Fried foods and pastries
   d. Poultry, seafood, and white bread
3. Ms. S complains of morning sickness. The nurse instructs her to:
   a. Eat breakfast later in the morning
   b. Drink at least two glasses of liquid with every meal
   c. Increase her intake of whole-grain breads and cereals to 2 ounces per meal
   d. Drink a large glass of skim milk at bedtime

11

Life Cycle Nutrition: Infancy, Childhood, and Adolescence

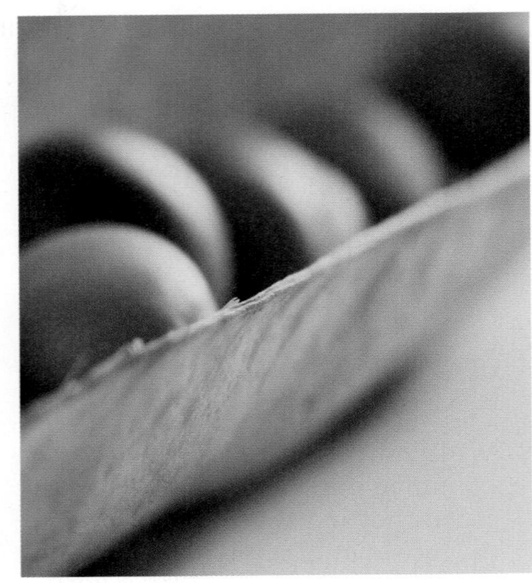

LEARNING OBJECTIVES

After completing this chapter, the student should be able to:

- Describe normal growth patterns and corresponding nutritional needs for a full-term infant, a toddler, a school-age child, and an adolescent.
- Explain why breast milk is uniquely suited to the human infant's capabilities.
- Discuss the rationale for the sequence in which semisolid foods are introduced into an infant's diet.
- List causes and treatments of five common nutritional problems of infancy.
- Summarize common nutritional problems of the preschool child.
- Relate ways in which a child can be encouraged to establish good nutritional habits.
- Identify areas of concern regarding the typical adolescent's diet.
- Devise a comprehensive plan to prevent obesity in a target population of children or adolescents.

Good nutrition is essential for infants and children. Because of public health efforts, U.S. infant mortality rates have decreased significantly. Of every 1000 infants born alive in:

- 1915, approximately 100 died before the age of 1 year (Centers for Disease Control and Prevention [CDC], 1999a)
- 1940, 47 died
- 2005, 6.87 died (CDC, 2008)

The goal of *Healthy People 2010* is to reduce the infant mortality rate to 4.5 per 1000 live births or less for all racial/ethnic groups (CDC, 2002). Infants of very low birth weight (<1500 grams or 3.3 lb) account for approximately two-thirds of the black–white disparity in infant mortality (CDC, 2002). Ninety percent of these very low birth weight infants survive long term compared with 50% in the 1970s (Hofman et al., 2004). Nourishing these tiny survivors is a formidable task.

This chapter focuses on periods of rapid **growth** during infancy, childhood, and adolescence. In addition to nutritional needs for all periods of growth, the chapter considers the stages of physical and **psychosocial development** for these ages, noting ways in which food relates to psychosocial development. Toward the end of the chapter is a discussion of overweight and obesity, major public health issues for children and adolescents that, unless checked, do not bode well for the health of Americans.

Psychosocial Development

American psychoanalyst **Erik Erikson** divided life into eight stages, each of which involves a psychosocial developmental task to be mastered and an opposite negative trait that emerges if the task is not mastered. Even if a developmental task is successfully mastered, a new situation may arise, challenging the person to reaffirm his or her mastery. Erikson's developmental tasks through adolescence appear in Table 11-1.

Nutrition in Infancy

Infancy, the first year of life, is a critical period for growth and development.

Growth

Growth is the progressive maturation and increase in size of a living thing. The only time humans grow faster than in infancy is the 9 months before they are born. An infant's birth weight should:

- Double by 4 to 6 months of age
- Triple by 1 year

From a birth length of about 20 inches, an infant grows to about 30 inches by age 1.

An infant's *rate of growth* is more significant than absolute values. The growth charts on DavisPlus or at http://www.cdc.gov/growthcharts reflect growth patterns of all children in the United States.

Breastfed infants initially gain weight more rapidly than formula-fed infants. At 2 to 3 months of age, the breastfed infant's rate of gain slows, which may evoke concern unnecessarily (Fry, 2003).

In 2006, the World Health Organization (WHO) released new standards for growth and development. The children measured for these standards were raised in an optimal environment (breastfed, nonsmoking home) for proper growth. The standards are applicable to all children regardless of ethnicity, socioeconomic status, or type of feeding (WHO, 2006). The reason for new charts was the concern that the previous charts, based largely on formula-fed infants, would be misinterpreted and lead to unnecessary supplementation (Sachs, Dykes, and Carter, 2006).

During the first few days after birth, an infant loses weight as he or she adjusts to his or her new environment and food supply. Among his or her adaptations is learning to feed compared to receiving a continuous supply of nutrients in utero. The amount of weight lost in these first few days should not exceed 10% of the birth weight. The newborn (or *neonate*, as an infant is called during the first 28 days after birth) usually returns to its birth weight within 14 days.

The period most critical to brain development extends from conception into the second year of life. Brain cells increase most rapidly before birth and during the first 5 or 6 months after birth. To attain maximum brain growth, the infant needs optimal nutrition.

TABLE 11-1 ■ Erikson's Theory of Psychosocial Development

STAGE OF LIFE	DEVELOPMENTAL TASK	OPPOSING NEGATIVE TRAIT
Infancy	Trust	Distrust
Toddler	Autonomy	Doubt
Preschooler	Initiative	Guilt
School-age child	Industry	Inferiority
Adolescent	Identity	Role confusion

Development

The gradual process of changing from a simple to a more complex organism is **development**. Becoming a mature individual involves psychosocial and physical changes, not only an increase in size.

Psychosocial Development of the Infant

The psychosocial developmental task of the infant is to learn to **trust** (Table 11-1). The parent who responds promptly and lovingly to the infant's cries is teaching the infant to trust. If the caregiver handles the infant inconsistently—gently one time and roughly the next—however, the infant learns to mistrust.

In situations where physical care is provided but a tender relationship does not develop, infants may actually suffer stunted physical growth. **Failure to thrive (FTT)** is a medical diagnosis for severely underweight infants. Although different parameters exist, weight gain at the 5th percentile is a common indicator (Olsen, 2006).

Some researchers suggest that the role of deprivation and neglect has been overstated and that undemanding behavior, low appetite, and poor feeding skills may contribute to the onset and persistence of failure to thrive (Wright and Birks, 2000). To feed successfully, the infant has to be calm but alert and has to learn to display cues to its needs to the caregiver (Chatoor, 2002). Careful assessment of parent-child interaction is required to diagnose feeding difficulties lest the wrong party be blamed for a poor outcome.

Physical Development

Development proceeds at a different pace in various tissues and organs. Proper feeding practices are based on the maturation rate of body organs. See Table 11-2.

Nutritional Needs of the Term Infant

For DRIs, see Appendix A. In general, infants' values are based on the contents of breast milk. In 2008, the American Academy of Pediatrics recommended that all infants receive a

TABLE 11-2 ■ Physical Characteristics of Infant Impacting Nutrition

SYSTEM	INFANT'S LIMITED CAPACITY	ADAPTATIONS AND MATURATIONS	ADJUSTMENT IN FEEDING	BY 1 YEAR OF AGE
Gastrointestinal	Salivary and pancreatic amylases inadequate to digest complex carbohydrates for several months	Has lingual lipase to digest fat, an enzyme lacking in adults.	Delay offering complex carbohydrates.	
	Intestine permits absorption of whole proteins.		Delay offering foods likely to be allergenic until 1 year old.	
	Stomach holds about 1 oz.		Frequent feedings	Stomach holds about 8 oz.
Nervous	Suckles with up-and-down motion of the tongue for 3 to 4 months.	**Rooting reflex** well developed. When the infant's cheek is stroked, the head turns toward that side to nurse.	Feed breast milk or infant formula. If semisolid food is offered at this time, the natural motion of the tongue tends to spit it out.	
		After 4 months, the infant can suck using orofacial muscles. The tongue moves back and forth instead of up and down.	Semisolid food is more likely to be swallowed than spit out.	
		At 6 months has hand-to-eye coordination to put food into mouth.	Offer appropriate finger foods.	
		At 7 months can chew appropriate foods.	Increase variety of food offered.	
Urinary	Young infant's kidneys have limited capacity to filter solutes.	By end of the second month of life, kidneys can excrete the waste of semisolid foods.	Delay semisolid foods at least till 2 months of age, preferably 4 to 6 months.	Kidneys at full functional capacity

daily intake of 400 IU of vitamin D beginning in the first few days of life (Wagner and Greer, 2008).

A normal pregnancy is 38 to 42 weeks. An infant born after a normal pregnancy is a **term infant**. Breast milk is the species-specific food for human infants. Its characteristics are the standard for infant formulas, which replicate many of the components of breast milk but that cannot supply all of its desirable qualities.

Energy and Macronutrients

Resting metabolic rates of infants are high as evidenced by:

- Normal pulse rate of 120 to 150 beats/min
- Normal respiratory rate of 30 to 50 breaths/min
- Large proportion of skin surface to body size requiring energy for temperature regulation

An activity such as crying may double the infant's energy expenditure.

Energy needs for the first 6 months of life are 108 kilocalories per kilogram of body weight per day. From 6 to 12 months of age, the energy need is 98 kilocalories per kilogram per day.

Table 11-3 lists the macronutrients of special importance for infants with comparisons of the relevant components of breast milk and cow's milk. Clinical Application 11-1 discusses a carbohydrate source that should not be given to infants. Box 11-1 identifies some research linking cognitive development to breastfeeding.

Micronutrients

The general recommendations for vitamin and mineral supplementation in infants are listed in Table 11-4. Despite the recommendation by the American Academy of Pediatrics to supplement breastfed infants with vitamin D, only 36.4% of pediatricians surveyed did so. Among parents of predominantly breastfed infants who indicated that their child's doctor recommended vitamin D, just 44.6% gave the supplement to their child (Taylor, Geyer, and Feldman, 2010).

VITAMINS

The routine administration of vitamin K to all infants is mandatory. Two infants who did not receive vitamin K after home deliveries developed intracerebral hemorrhage at 5 weeks of age. Despite surgery, both suffered permanent neurological damage (Hubbard and Tobias, 2006).

Illness and medications can also affect the production of vitamin K in the intestine. Gastrointestinal bleeding and intracranial bleeding occurred in infants treated with antibiotics for prolonged diarrhea (Bay et al., 2006).

MINERALS

Compared to cow's milk, breast milk contains:

- One-third the sodium, potassium, and chloride
- One-eighth the phosphorus of cow's milk, an amount that accommodates the limited function of the infant's kidneys

TABLE 11-3 ■ Macronutrient Needs of Term Infant

	NUTRIENT NEEDED	BREAST MILK	COW'S MILK	CONTRAINDICATIONS
Carbohydrate	Galactose is necessary for brain cell formation.	Breast milk contains amylase that is 40–60 times more active than that of cow's milk		Honey (Clinical Application 11-1)
Fat	Fat and cholesterol are necessary for rapidly growing brain and nervous system, bile, and hormones.	Provides 55% of kilocalories from fat as concentrated energy source. Contains lipase to begin digestion for the infant so about 95%–98% of the fat in human milk is absorbed.		Reduced-fat milks before age 2
	The developing nervous system needs **arachidonic** and **docosahexaenoic** (DHA) fatty acids, the main omega-6 and omega-3 fatty acids of the central nervous system.	These two fatty acids, essential for retinal and neural development are found in human milk.	Not present	
Protein		Human milk contains 70% whey (easily digested) and 30% **casein.** The major whey protein in breast milk is alpha-**lactalbumin,** with an amino acid pattern much like that of the body tissues.	18% whey, 82% casein	

Adapted from Breastfeeding (2004); Brown (2008); Lo (1997).

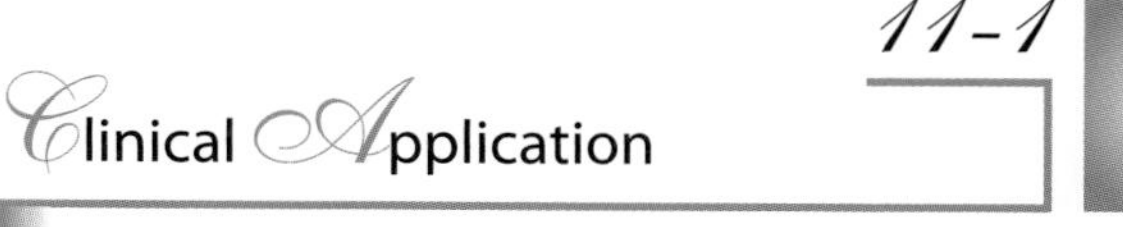

Honey Is a Danger to Infants

Infants should not be given honey until after their first birthday because honey frequently contains botulism **spores** acquired from plants or the soil. Up to 25% of honey products have been found to contain spores. Processing the honey does not destroy these spores.

Botulism spores may also be found in corn syrup and low-acid home-canned foods which should not be fed to infants (Hoecker, 2010).

Eighty to 110 cases of infant botulism occur annually in the United States (Arnon et al., 2006).

If the spores are ingested by an infant, they become active in the infant's intestinal tract and produce a neurotoxin that irreversibly binds to acetylcholine receptors on motor nerve terminals. Symptoms include:

- Constipation
- Weakness
- An altered cry
- Poor feeding
- A striking loss of head control (Heymann, 2004)

Unrecognized, the condition can quickly progress to respiratory failure. More than 70% of these infants will require mechanical ventilation (Cox and Hinkle, 2002). The nerve terminals regenerate as the child recovers. In adults and older children, natural defenses prevent the growth of the organism unless the person has abnormal gastrointestinal anatomy and microflora (Heymann, 2004).

Physicians are required to report all cases of infant botulism promptly to state and local health departments (CDC, 2003a).

Box 11-1 ■ *Research Linking Cognitive Abilities to Breastfeeding*

Early research associated breastfeeding with slightly enhanced performance on tests of cognitive development (AAP, 2005). Breast milk contains arachidonic (ARA) and docosahexaenoic (DHA) fatty acids, which accumulate during the brain growth spurt from the third trimester until age 2 (Fats and fatty acids, 2004).

Supporting the link of ARA and DHA to cognitive abilities are these studies:

- Adding ARA and DHA to infant formula supported visual acuity and IQ maturation at 4 years of age, similar to breastfeeding (Birch et al., 2007).
- In premature infants, additional ARA and DHA in their breast milk produced better scores on memory and problem-solving at 6 months of age than those of the placebo group (Henriksen et al., 2008).

Other researchers took a broader view, looking at maternal education.

- Increased verbal ability in 3-year-olds was associated with breastfeeding only in mothers with some post-secondary education (Gibson-Davis and Brooks-Gunn, 2006).
- Maternal intelligence predicted her choice to breastfeed more than any other factor and accounted for most of the child's increase in mental ability (Der, Batty, and Deary, 2006).

This issue is still under investigation. Adding ARA and DHA to infant formulas corresponds to other efforts to minic breast milk. Neither supplemented formula nor breastfeeding should be viewed as a magic elixir to boost intelligence.

These differences in mineral content affect the osmolality of the milk and the workload of the kidneys. See Clinical Application 11-2. *Unmodified* cow's milk is inappropriate for young infants.

Water

The infant's body is about 75% water. By 3 years of age, the body has developed so it has the adult

TABLE 11-4 ■ Vitamin–Mineral Supplementation for Infants

SUPPLEMENT	PRESCRIBED FOR	SITUATION	RATIONALE
Vitamin			
D	Breastfed infants Partially breastfed infants Formula-fed infants ingesting < 1 L of fortified formula	Beginning in the first few days of life	
K	All infants	Single intramuscular dose of vitamin K after the first breastfeeding and within 6 hours of birth	Until the infant's intestine becomes colonized with *Escherichia coli* from the environment, he or she is at risk for bleeding problems.
C	2-week-old formula-fed infants, if vitamin is not in formula	Synthetic preferable to juices Orange juice, especially, may be allergen	
B_{12} as cobalamin	Breastfed infant, if mother is strict vegetarian	See Chapter 10.	Growth failure and neurological impairment due to cobalamin deficiency occurred in breastfeeding infants of vegetarian mothers.
Mineral			
Calcium	Premature infants	See Clinical Application 11-5.	Breast milk contains about ⅙ to ¼ the calcium in cow's milk. 67% of breast milk calcium is absorbed vs. 25% of cow's milk calcium.
Phosphorus	Premature infants	See Clinical Application 11-5.	
Iron	Term infant, when birth weight has doubled Formula-fed premature, from onset Fortified human milk-fed premature, when full enteral feeding established	Iron-fortified formula is recommended.	Breast milk contains about 0.5 mg iron/L but 50% is absorbed. Just 10% is absorbed from cow's milk or fortified formulas.
Fluoride	All >6 months of age Children >3 years of age	If drinking water contains <0.3 ppm If drinking water contains <0.6 ppm	

SOURCES: American Academy of Pediatrics (2005; Appendix W, 2004); CDC (2003c); Chitambar and Antony (2006); Heird and Cooper (2006); Lo (1997); Schanler (1997); Wagner and Greer (2008).

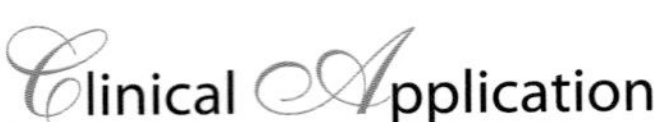

11-2

Renal Solute Loads

When selecting an infant formula, it is necessary to distinguish two measures of osmotic pressure. One is the osmotic pressure the formula presents to the gut. The other examines what remains to be excreted by the kidney after digestion, absorption, and metabolism have taken place.

These leftovers are excess electrolytes and byproducts of protein metabolism. The osmotic pressure of these leftovers presented to the kidney for disposal is called the renal solute load.

The accompanying table compares common infant feedings' intestinal osmolality and renal solute loads. Infant formulas change often in response to new scientific information, so the chart is an example only. The agency's dietitian or pharmacist should be consulted for the latest information. The standard of comparison is human breast milk.

Clearly, unmodified cow's milk would place the greatest burden on the infant's immature renal system. When fluid intakes are low or when extrarenal water losses are high, the infant may become dehydrated. His kidneys may be unable to retain enough water after excreting the renal solutes. The resulting negative water balance, if prolonged, can lead to serious dehydration. Strong epidemiological evidence shows that cow's milk or formulas with similarly high potential renal solute load increases infants' risk of serious dehydration (Ziegler, 2007).

MILK FORMULA	INTESTINAL OSMOLALITY (mOsm/kg)	RENAL SOLUTE LOAD (mOsm/L)
Human breast milk	300	101
Milk-based formula		
Similac with iron	300	125
Soy-based formula		
Isomil with iron	200	152
3.3% cow's milk	275	275

SOURCES: Klish and Montandon (1987); Ross Laboratories (2004); Thorp, Pierce, and Deedwanea (1987).

proportion of about 60% water (Gropper, Smith, and Groff, 2009). The daily turnover of water in the infant is approximately 15% of body weight.

Even in desert climates, an infant can be adequately hydrated on breast milk alone. An infant will regulate his or her intake of formula to obtain sufficient energy. This self-regulating mechanism is not perfect, however, because the infant may consume excess formula to quench its thirst.

The Breastfed Infant

Breast milk is designed for human infants and is the standard against which substitute milks are measured. Breastfeeding rates in the United States are at an all-time high (see Fig. 10-3), but compared with other countries, they are still low.

Even in this country:

- Breastfed infants are 21% less likely to die between 1 month and 1 year of age than those who never breastfed; however, the effects of breast milk and breastfeeding cannot be segregated completely from the family context (Chen and Rogan, 2004).
- Breastfeeding accounts for the race difference in infant mortality at least as well as low birth weight does (Forste, Weiss, and Lippincott, 2001).

Human breast milk banks make milk available for infants whose mothers do not produce enough milk. The goals of *Healthy People 2010* are to increase to:

- 75% the proportion of mothers who breastfeed in the early postpartum period
- 50% those who breastfeed until infants are 6 months old
- 25% those who breastfeed until infants are 1 year old (U.S. Department of Health and Human Services, 2005).

Later modifications to the goals include increasing to:

- 60% those who exclusively breastfeed until infants are 3 months old
- 25% those who exclusively breastfeed until infants are 6 months old (CDC, 2007)

The American Academy of Pediatrics (AAP, 2005) recommends exclusive breastfeeding (nothing but breast milk and vitamins, minerals, and medications) for the first 6 months of life.

Practices conducive to breastfeeding and lactation are covered in Chapter 10. Care of ill or frail infants must be individualized. An additional benefit to the infant is the analgesia provided by breastfeeding during painful procedures such as heelsticks, but such procedures on healthy term infants should be delayed until after the initial breastfeeding with skin-to-skin contact has been achieved (AAP, 2005).

Clinical Application 11-3 explains the procedures for storing human milk.

Composition of Breast Milk

Breast milk accommodates the infant's needs during the weeks an infant is nursing, even during the course of a single feeding. Breast milk varies from mother to mother and even in one mother with the time of day. It also varies with the lactation cycle. The variation in content also offers the infant a variety of taste experiences. See Table 11-5.

In general, a mother's active exercise program does not affect the volume or composition of breast milk

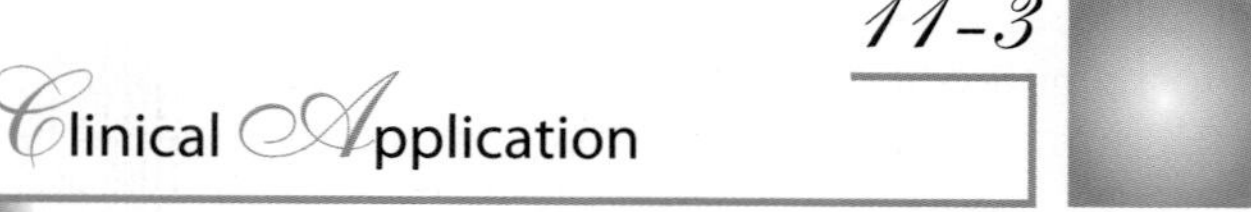

Storage of Human Milk

Careful collection and storage are necessary to preserve the sterility and quality of expressed human milk. The length of time that milk can be safely stored depends upon the type of container and the storage facility (Academy of Breastfeeding Medicine, undated).

Human milk banks in North America abide by national guidelines to screen and test donors and to pasteurize the milk (AAP, 2005). In 2005, 54% of milk donations were distributed to premature infants in neonatal intensive care units (Huiras, 2007).

TABLE 11-5 ■ Breast Milk Components

	SECRETED	APPEARANCE	COMPONENTS
Colostrum	2–4 days after delivery	Thin, yellow, cloudy fluid	High kilocalorie High protein Antibodies White blood cells Fat-soluble vitamins Minerals
Mature	72–96 hours after delivery As long as breastfeeding continues	Milky	High lactose High vitamin E Calcium:phosphorus ratio of 2:1 (prevents calcium deficient tetany) Antibodies (decreased at 3 months) Fore-milk (beginning of feeding): less fat Hind-milk (end of feeding): more fat to increase satiety At 3 months, fewer immunoglobulins

SOURCES: Brown (2008); *Merck Manual* (2005).

or infant weight gain (Brown, 2008). An experiment involving 24 women showed that moderate or even high-intensity exercise during lactation did not hinder infant acceptance of breast milk consumed 1 hour after exercise (Wright, Quinn, and Carey, 2002).

Unique Advantages of Breastfeeding

One well-documented advantage to breastfeeding that has not been duplicated by formulas is protection against infectious disease. Other advantages are limited improvement in the presentation of allergic disease and a possible negative association with obesity.

PROTECTION AGAINST DISEASE

In both developing and industrialized countries, breastfeeding reduces the incidence of gastrointestinal and respiratory diseases and otitis media (middle ear infection). Exclusive breastfeeding for 6 months instead of 4 months affords greater protection against gastrointestinal infection and respiratory tract infection including pneumonia and recurrent otitis media (Chantry, Howard, and Auinger, 2006).

Breast milk contains bioactive components that protect the infant from disease by:

- Direct action against microorganisms or
- Modulation of the immune system (Picciano and McDonald, 2006)

Among the infection-fighting agents in breast milk are immunoglobulin A (IgA) and leukocytes or white blood cells (WBCs). IgA, found also in tears and saliva, is thought to protect mucous membranes from viruses and bacteria (Van Leeuwen et al., 2006).

PREVENTION OF ALLERGIES

The young infant's gastrointestinal tract can permit the passage of whole proteins into the bloodstream. These proteins can stimulate an allergic response in susceptible infants.

Breastfeeding is protective against allergies for infants with at least one first-degree relative with allergic disease. Breastfeeding for at least 4 months (compared with feeding formula made with intact cow's milk protein) prevents or delays the occurrence of atopic dermatitis, cow milk allergy, and wheezing in early childhood (AAP, 2008).

If breast milk is unavailable or insufficient, infants at high risk of **atopy** may be fed special formulas. **Hydrolysis** splits whole proteins into smaller particles that are less likely to cause allergic reactions. Extensively hydrolyzed formulas are preferable to unhydrolyzed or partially hydrolyzed formulas in terms of the risk of some atopic manifestations (van Odijk et al., 2003). All hydrolyzed formulas do not protect equally against atopy (AAP, 2008).

Current evidence does not support a major role for maternal dietary restrictions during pregnancy or lactation as protective against allergies. In addition, little evidence backs the delayed introduction of complementary foods beyond 4 to 6 months of age as a strategy to prevent atopic disease (AAP, 2008).

NEGATIVE ASSOCIATION WITH OBESITY

The evidence that breastfed infants have a lower risk of later obesity than formula-fed infants is equivocal (Ryan, 2007). Reductions in risk of 13% to 20% have been reported (Koletzko, 2006; Owen et al., 2005; Singhal, 2007).

The mechanisms involved, although poorly understood, probably include the benefits of relative undernutrition and slower growth associated with breast rather than formula feeding. In both rich and poor countries, faster weight and length gains are associated with later obesity (Singhal, 2007).

In the United States, while rates of breastfeeding have risen slowly, childhood obesity rates have increased dramatically. Breastfeeding is just one of many factors involved in maintaining a healthy body weight (Ryan, 2007).

Genetic Abnormalities Affecting Breastfeeding

Among the conditions commonly included in newborn screening tests are two that have profound implications for the infant's nutritional intake. One affects carbohydrate metabolism and the other protein metabolism.

In **galactosemia**, the infant's lack of an enzyme to metabolize galactose is an absolute contraindication to breastfeeding. Galactosemia is inherited as an autosomal recessive trait. If untreated, the child will suffer growth failure, mental retardation, or death. Treatment involves a soy formula containing no lactose or galactose and lifelong avoidance of milk products.

The mother of an infant with **phenylketonuria** (see Clinical Application 5-2) often chooses to feed the child only the special formula. Breastfeeding the infant requires both limited amounts of breast milk and the special formula. To determine the amount of breast milk the infant may consume to keep his or her blood levels within the therapeutic limits requires constant monitoring and consultations, but it has been done successfully. Every state has at least one medical center for treating metabolic defects. The maternal and child health division of the state health department can assist with locating such a facility.

The Formula-Fed Infant

As good as it is, exclusive breastfeeding is not possible for all mothers and infants. Infant formula is the only food that is regulated by its own law, the Infant Formula Act of 1980, which sets minimum levels of 29 nutrients and maximal levels of 9 nutrients (Formula feeding, 2004). Formulas for full-term infants must contain 20 kilocalories per ounce. As much as possible, commercial formulas are designed to match the qualities of human breast milk.

Formulas contain more protein than breast milk. The cow's milk proteins do not contain the optimal amino acids for human infants. Enough protein is included in the formula to provide a sufficient distribution of amino acids.

The saturated fats of cow's milk are poorly digested by the infant. In formulas, vegetable oils replace the saturated fats.

Formula Preparations

Commercial formulas come in three forms: powder (to mix with water), liquid concentrate, and ready-to-feed. See Table 11-6.

Directions for preparing the formula will be given by the health-care provider. Commonly discussed issues include:

- Cleanliness/sterility of equipment
- Water to use for dilution:
  - Sterility
  - Fluoride content

TABLE 11-6 ■ Forms of Formulas

	ADVANTAGES	DISADVANTAGES
Liquid Concentrate	Relatively easy to prepare	Opened cans require refrigeration. Must be used within 48 hours.
Powder	Less waste Possible to prepare a small amount	Unsterile powder may be unsafe for premature infants.
Ready-to-feed	Most convenient No calculating or measuring	Most expensive. See Dollars and Sense 11-1.

Dollars & Sense 11-1

Cost of Different Preparations of One Brand of Infant Formula

	Package Size	Price	Cost per Prepared Ounce
Powder	12.9 oz	$13.76	$0.15
Liquid concentrate	13 fl oz	$4.34	$0.17
Ready-to-feed	32 fl oz	$6.48	$0.20

  - Possible lead contamination (see Clinical Application 8-8)
- Safe storage
- Use of correct strength formula. Formula too concentrated or too dilute can cause severe electrolyte imbalances. Some cases have been fatal.
- Safe heating of the formula before feeding the infant
- Discarding prepared bottles of formula unrefrigerated for 1 hour or partially consumed

Using a microwave oven for infant foods is not recommended. Heat may be unevenly distributed and continues to build even after the food has been removed from the oven.

Feeding Techniques

Approximately every 4 hours, the infant awakens for feedings. By the age of 2 to 3 months, the baby probably will have eliminated one feeding so the schedule is five times a day. By 6 months, most infants are feeding four times a day.

The baby is positioned in the crook of the arm, almost as if breastfeeding. The parent's or caregiver's touch is important to the infant's development. Correct techniques include the following:

- The nipple holes should be large enough for milk to drip out on its own without shaking the bottle.
- The nipple should always be filled with milk to prevent the infant from swallowing air while feeding.
- Daily formula intake for an infant should be 1.5 to 2 ounces per pound of body weight, but growth is a better measure of health than the amount of formula swallowed.
- A single feeding should not exceed 8 ounces.

Propping an infant with a bottle is never acceptable, because choking is a real hazard.

Special Formulas

Special formulas are available for infants who are allergic to cow's milk, those with galactosemia or lactose intolerance, and those with fat-absorption problems. See Clinical Application 11-4 for a brief description of such formulas, which are commonly soy-based. Rarely, soy proteins may also cause allergies (Klemola et al., 2005).

For a formula to be considered hypoallergenic, it should be well tolerated by at least 90% of individuals who are allergic to the parent protein from which that formula has been derived. Elemental formulas derived from synthetic amino acids are

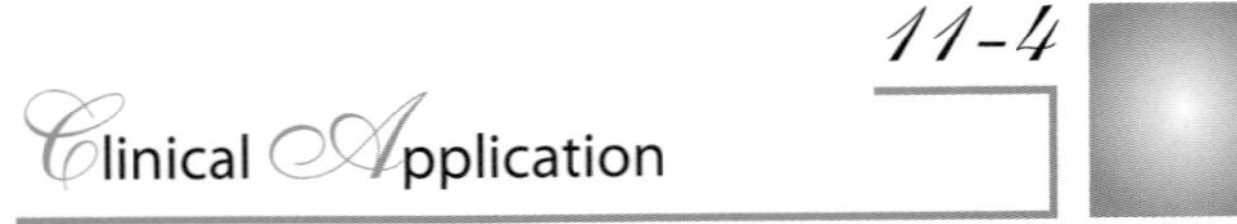

Soy Protein Formulas

The isolated soy protein formulas marketed today are all free of cow's milk protein and lactose and are iron-fortified.

The American Academy of Pediatrics recommends using soy protein-based formulas in term infants for:

- Galactosemia and hereditary lactase deficiency
- Those whose parents desire a vegetarian diet
- Secondary lactose intolerance following acute gastroenteritis

In contrast, the Academy *does not* recommend soy protein-based formula under the following circumstances:

- Preterm infants
- Cow's milk allergy
- Routine treatment of colic
- Healthy or high-risk infants to prevent atopic disease

SOURCE: Bhatia and Greer (2008).

well tolerated by practically all individuals, including those allergic to extensively hydrolyzed formulas (Bahna, 2008).

Palatability becomes an issue as the infant develops more discerning tastes. Hydrolysis produces bitter-tasting peptides. Soy formulas and rice formula were judged to have the best tastes, followed by the whey hydrolysates. The mixed hydrolysates and the casein hydrolysates had the worst tastes (Pedrosa et al., 2006).

The full-term infant's digestive, nervous, and urinary systems are immature—an even greater issue for premature infants. Clinical Application 11-5 summarizes some of the nutritional problems and appropriate interventions used for premature infants.

Hazards of Formula Feeding

On a few occasions, improperly manufactured formulas have been responsible for vitamin and mineral deficiencies in infants. This is an unacceptable, but fortunately rare, occurrence. A more common hazard, and one an individual nurse can monitor, is the improper preparation and use of formulas by the parent. Formulas can be:

- The wrong strength;
- Prepared with contaminated water, equipment, or hands
- Kept at feeding temperature too long. Body temperature is "just right" for bacteria to multiply, whether in the body or in a formula bottle.

Choice of Breast or Bottle

In the United States, infants can be well nourished whether breast- or bottle-fed. To raise a child successfully takes more than simply supplying the correct ratio of nutrients. The mother's informed decision should be supported and appropriate teaching provided.

An estimated 5% of women may be unable to produce a full milk supply because of anatomic or medical reasons. Moreover, because infants' sucking stimulates milk production, difficulty with the process may result in diminished milk supply.

Tragically, infants have died from malnutrition and hypernatremic dehydration due to breastfeeding failures (Neifert, 2001; Trotman et al., 2004). Inadequate breastfeeding or underfeeding caused hypernatremic dehydration in nine infants at one medical center in 4 years. At presentation, the affected infants ranged in age from 3 to 14 days and had lost from 12% to 29% of their birth weights (Wang et al., 2007).

Infants should:

- Be observed while suckling at 2 to 4 days of age by a knowledgeable health-care provider
- Have its weight monitored by the same health-care provider

All parents should be taught to expect the infant to have at least:

- Four good-sized bowel movements and
- Six saturated diapers per day

Most important, enthusiastic support for breastfeeding should never delay provision of formula when medically indicated.

Advancing the Diet

Teaching the infant to consume the foods he will receive throughout life is a gradual process. First semisolid foods are given to complement breast milk or formula. Eventually drinking from a cup will replace suckling.

Semisolid Foods

No proof exists of the folk wisdom that the early feeding of solid food to infants promotes their sleeping through the night. At 3 months, 75% of infants sleep all night, regardless of diet. If solid foods are introduced too early, the infant may develop allergies because of the permeability of the intestine.

The American Academy of Pediatrics supports exclusive breastfeeding (nothing but breast milk and vitamins, minerals, and medications) for 6 months

11-5

Clinical Application

Premature Infants

Premature infants are born before 37 weeks' gestation. By birth weight, premature infants are categorized as:

- Low-birth-weight (LBW)—less than 2500 g (5.5 lb) at birth
- Very low-birth-weight (VLBW)—less than 1500 g (3.3 lb)
- Extremely low-birth-weight (ELBW)—less than 1000 g (2.2 lb).

An infant can be both premature and LBW or VLBW. Not all premature infants weigh less than 2500 grams. Nor are all LBW infants premature, but birth weight is the most powerful single predictor of an infant's future health status. Infants weighing less than 2500 grams are 20 times more likely to die before their first birthday than normal-weight infants, and the mortality rates rise dramatically for VLBW and ELBW infants (CDC, 2002).

Maternal factors associated with prematurity include smoking, previous premature delivery, infection, and low BMI. A genetic variant has also been implicated. See Genomic Gem 11-1.

PROVIDING NOURISHMENT

- The infant's ability to coordinate sucking, swallowing, and breathing is not developed prior to the 32nd or 34th week of gestation. As a result, premature infants often require enteral or intravenous feeding. Enteral tube feeding will conserve energy even in an infant who is able to suck.
- Human milk from the infant's mother is the food of choice. Compared to term mothers' milk, preterm milk has more protein, sodium, and host defense factors but less calcium, phosphorus, and magnesium. Human milk fortifiers add protein, carbohydrate, vitamins, and minerals to the breast milk. See Figure 11-1. Moreover, the mother's enzymes and antibodies are still available to the baby.
- Special formulas for premature infants are designed to provide for the infant's growth needs despite the immature digestive system. If given 105 to 130 kcal/kg of body weight enterally, the infant will grow satisfactorily (Nutritional needs, 2004).
  - Ready-to-feed preparations should be used rather than powdered formulas that cannot be sufficiently sterilized.
  - Safe handling demands that prepared formula should not be at room temperature for more than 4 hours.
  - Formulas with 22, 24 and 28 kcal/mL are available. Their high osmolarity requires close attention to fluid and electrolyte balance (Brown, 2008).
- Because of low vitamin reserves, premature infants are given higher doses of supplemental vitamins than are term infants; plus the premature infants are given additional vitamins not contained in the standard infant multivitamin supplements (Nutritional needs, 2004).
- Because of poor bone calcification and muscle development, premature infants may need calcium, phosphorus, and sodium supplements. Rickets of prematurity can occur in the second postnatal month due not to the lack of vitamin D but to the lack of calcium and phosphorus. Human milk fortifiers and high-mineral containing formulas allow bone mineral accretion at or near in utero rates (Abrams, 2007).

FIGURE 11-1 Human milk fortifier, when *added to human milk*, increases the amount of protein, carbohydrates, and selected vitamins and minerals available to meet the needs of rapidly growing low-birth-weight infants. These are not nutritionally complete supplements.

TRACKING PROGRESS

Premature infants should not be evaluated against standards set for term infants.

- Premature infants should have their chronological age corrected by gestational age until age:
  - 18 months for head circumference
  - 24 months for weight
  - 40 months for length (Failure to thrive, 2004).
- Special growth grids for premature infants to 38-month gestational age are available.

NECROTIZING ENTEROCOLITIS

The most serious gastrointestinal disorder of neonates is necrotizing enterocolitis (NEC), an acquired injury to the bowel. This inflammatory bowel disease of neonates results in inflammation and bacterial invasion of the bowel wall (Thompson and Bizzarro, 2008). NEC causes significant morbidity and mortality in preterm infants, occurring in:

- 1% to 5% of all neonatal intensive care admissions and
- 5% to 10% of all VLBW (<1500 g) infants (Thompson and Bizzarro, 2008).

Established risk factors include:

- Preterm birth
- Hypoxic–ischemic events
- Formula feeding
- Abnormal bacterial colonization (Schnabl et al., 2008).

The precise etiology of this multifactorial disease process remains elusive. Consequently, treatments are symptomatic and surgical. The single most important predictor of outcome, besides gestational age, is whether the disease has progressed to a point requiring surgical intervention. Infants with NEC requiring operation have a high mortality (Henry and Moss, 2008).

Breastfeeding is the most effective preventative measure for NEC. Recent research has focused on duplicating the bioactive nutrients and trophic factors in human milk (Schnabl et al., 2008).

Genomic Gem 11-1
Possible Contributor to Premature Delivery

About one-half the cases of premature delivery have no identified cause. A variant has been found in the gene that codes for a protein that stabilizes collagen. One function of that protein would give strength to the amnionic membranes that encase the fetus. If the membranes are weak, they are more likely to rupture early and lead to preterm delivery (Hampton, 2006).

Black women are nearly twice as likely to give birth prematurely as white women. The variant described above is present in approximately 12.4% of black women and 4.1% of white women. This particular variant is responsible for approximately 12% of preterm births (Hampton, 2006).

One of the functions of vitamin C is to contribute to the synthesis of collagen. The genetic variant affecting collagen may help explain the effectiveness of vitamin C in maintaining the amnionic membranes. Pregnant women given 100 milligrams of vitamin C after the twentieth week of gestation had a 74% reduction in risk for premature rupturing of the membranes (Casanueva et al., 2005).

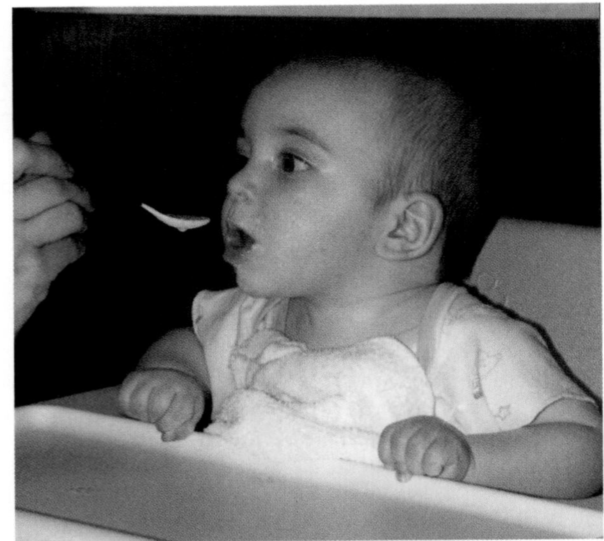

FIGURE 11-2 This 5-month-old baby is experiencing semisolid food for the first time. His readiness is clear. Notice how eager he is, how focused on the spoon.

TABLE 11-7 ■ Suggested Progression for Offering Foods to Infant at Low Risk of Allergies

AGE OF INFANT	FOOD	RATIONALE/PRECAUTIONS
4 Months	Infant cereal mixed with formula	Because of risk of allergies, rice offered first; wheat after age 12 months. Read labels: some mixed infant cereals contain wheat.
5–6 Months	Strained vegetables	Less sweet than fruits; thought less likely to be rejected if offered before fruit.
6–7 Months	Strained fruits	Will be well accepted; humans have strong preference for sweets.
6–8 Months	Finger foods (bananas, crackers)	Encourages self-feeding. Different textures may aid speech development.
7–8 Months	Strained meats	May be introduced earlier to add iron and zinc to the diet. Offer variety. (See Clinical Application 11-6.)
10 Months	Strained or mashed egg yolk	Start with ½ tsp. Due to possible allergy, delay egg white until 1 year old.
10 Months	Bite-sized cooked foods	Select appropriate foods. See Clinical Application 11-6.
12 Months	Foods from adult table	Select suitable foods, prepared according to baby's abilities.

while recognizing that infants are often developmentally ready for complementary foods between 4 and 6 months of age (Complementary feeding, 2004).

The infant should achieve voluntary control of swallowing at 3 to 4 months. Before being offered solid food, the infant should be able to control his or her head and trunk. With this ability, the baby can turn away when satisfied. By this time, the infant is drinking 8 ounces of formula or a similar estimated amount of breast milk, and yet becomes hungry in less than 4 hours.

In introducing solid food, it is best to follow the infant's lead. To avoid later feeding problems, solid foods should be started when the baby is interested. Babies ready for solid food are hungry and not fussy about tastes (Fig. 11-2). Children learn from adults; parents should avoid showing distaste for particular foods.

Waiting too long to introduce solid foods may delay the infant's acquiring the skill to manipulate the tongue and mouth appropriately. Early in the transition to semisolid foods, the amount consumed is likely to be small so the main source of nutrients continues to be milk.

FEEDING

New foods should be introduced one at a time and a week apart so that if a problem develops, the responsible food can be readily identified. A food should be tried for 3 to 5 days before the infant is permitted to reject it. Only a taste or two is sufficient for the first try.

A commonly used schedule for introducing new foods appears in Table 11-7. The baby's physician may modify it to meet individual needs. No evidence supports the superiority of a particular sequence of food introduction. In particular, infants might benefit from early introduction of infant meats containing iron and zinc to prevent iron deficiency (Complementary feeding, 2004). Food that the infant can chew and swallow safely should be offered (Clinical Application 11-6).

The parent should heat a small amount to serve the infant. Food that has been heated and not consumed should be discarded because of possible contamination with salivary enzymes and bacteria. Food that has been opened but not heated should be stored in the covered jar in the refrigerator and used within 3 days.

LEARNING ABOUT FLAVORS

Eating adult foods is a skill that babies must learn, but their culture affects the food choices they will be offered. The fetus will experience flavors from the mother's diet in swallowed amniotic fluid. Infants will later experience some of these flavors in breast milk that reflects the foods, spices, and beverages consumed by the mother (Mennella, Jagnow, and Beauchamp, 2001).

11-6

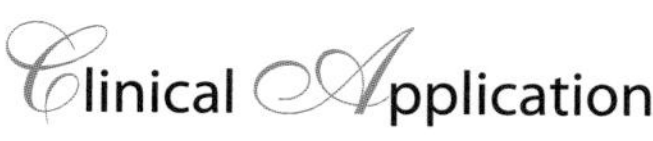

Avoiding Choking Accidents

Each year, several hundred infants, as well as older children, choke on food. On average, one death every 5 days is reported in children from infancy to 9 years of age.

- Hot dogs, or frankfurters, are involved most often. Hot dogs, apples, cookies, and biscuits cause choking most often in infants. Peanuts and grapes are the most dangerous for 2-year-old children, while 3-year-olds still face a risk from hot dogs.
- Other foods typically implicated in choking accidents appear in the table below by category. Because the child can safely eat many other foods, the prudent course is to avoid those foods when possible. If a choking incident occurs, any caregiver should be able to perform cardiopulmonary resuscitation (CPR) should it become necessary.
- Small children should always be supervised while they are eating, and they should be seated at a table to eat. Likewise, eating in a moving vehicle is discouraged. Special care is needed if local teething agents are used because of potential numbing of throat muscles (Feeding the child, 2004).

HARD FOODS	STRINGY FOODS	STICKY FOODS	PLUG-SHAPED FOODS
Apples	Beans	Bread	Grapes
Carrots	Celery	Chewing gum	Hot dogs
Cookies		Peanut butter	
Corn			
Hard candy			
Nuts			
Peanuts			
Popcorn			
Raisins			
Other raw vegetables			
Seedy items (e.g., watermelon)			

Weaning the Infant

Teaching the infant to use a cup is a gradual process. In most cases, the baby will show interest in the cup at 4 to 6 months. For these early attempts, and if the infant is not exclusively breastfed, water can be offered. If the mother decides to wean the child from breast or bottle before its first birthday, the replacement should be infant formula, not unmodified cow's milk.

The bottle-fed infant may not be ready to give up the bottle until 12 to 14 months of age. If bedtime bottles have not been used, weaning will proceed more rapidly. It is best to substitute the cup for the bottle for one feeding period at a time. After using the new schedule for 5 days or so, the new method is substituted for a second feeding.

Nutritional Problems in Infancy

Common problems of nutrition in infancy are summarized in Table 11-8. The table includes some home remedies, but if an infant does not improve rapidly from a nutrition-related problem, parents should seek medical attention.

Allergies

From 6% to 8% of children younger than 4 years old have food allergies that started in infancy (Brown, 2008). Most adverse reactions result from intolerances rather than food allergy (Story, 2008). The causes of food allergy are still unknown and no particular genes have been identified as associated with food allergy (Bjorksten, 2005).

IGE-MEDIATED ALLERGIES

Because true food allergies can have fatal consequences, identifying children with allergies is critical. An **allergen** is a substance that provokes an abnormal individual hypersensitivity or **allergy**. The steps in allergy production are illustrated in Figure 11-3. The food protein fragments causing an allergic reaction

TABLE 11-8 ■ Common Nutritional Problems in Infancy

PROBLEM	INTERVENTION	COMMENTS
Regurgitation of Milk	Handle baby gently. Burp well; sit up after feeding.	Very common for first 6 months; not serious unless vomiting is projectile or bile-tinged or baby has persistent respiratory symptoms or poor weight gain.
Constipation	½ oz prune juice with ½ oz water.	Rare in breastfed infants.
Burns to Mouth	Swirl formula after heating; test well.	Use water bath to heat. Formula warmed in a microwave oven continues to increase in temperature after removal.
Nursing-Bottle Syndrome	Do not use milk or juice as bedtime bottle. Do not put sweetener on pacifier.	See Chapter 3.

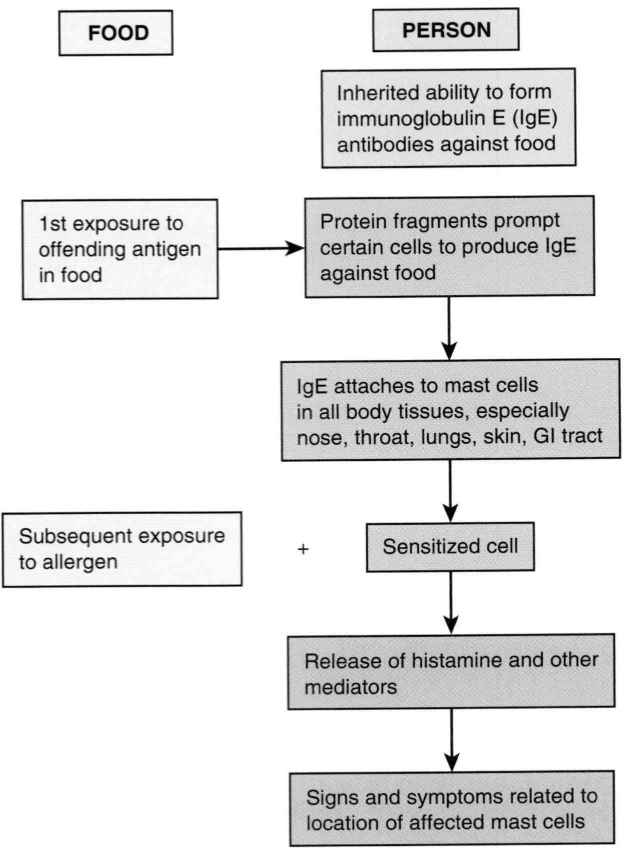

FIGURE 11-3 Development of an allergic reaction to food. (Adapted from Formanek [2001]; Taylor and Hefle [2006].)

are not broken down by cooking or digestive processes (Formanek, 2001).

The number of people with allergies is increasing rapidly both in developed and developing countries but not in underdeveloped areas. The fewer germs in the environment, the more time the immune system has to process and react to allergens. Growing up in a large family or in a day care center decreases the likelihood of developing an allergy (Formanek, 2001).

Common Food Allergens

As many as 90% of all IgE-mediated food allergies may be caused by eight foods or food groups. The eight major food allergens are:

1. Peanuts
2. Soybeans
3. Fish
4. Crustacean shellfish
5. Milk
6. Eggs
7. Tree nuts
8. Wheat (Taylor and Hefle, 2006)

In children, the most common allergenic foods are:

- Eggs
- Milk
- Peanuts
- Soybeans
- Wheat

Children typically outgrow allergies to:

- Eggs
- Milk
- Soy
- Wheat

but not to:

- Peanuts
- Tree nuts
- Fish
- Shrimp (Formanek, 2001)

Clinical Application 11-7 summarizes reports of fatal and near-fatal cases of **anaphylaxis following** ingestion of a food allergen. The seriousness of food allergies should never be underestimated.

Nonfood Transfers of Allergens

Allergens can be transferred by modes other than ingestion:

- Kissing: Twenty clients reported allergic reactions after kissing, one life-threatening and four even after the partner had brushed his teeth (Hallett, Haapanen, and Tueber, 2002).
- Inhalation:
  - Cooking vapors from legumes caused asthma (Garcia-Ortiz et al., 1995).
  - Weak associations were identified between asthma and unloading of soybeans from ships (Ballester et al., 1999).
  - Inhalation of seafood allergens through occupational exposure or through visiting an open-air fish market showed measurable fish allergen in the air (Taylor et al., 2000).
- Organ transplantation: A 60-year-old man with no history of nut allergy had an anaphylactic reaction to cashew nuts after receiving the liver of a 15-year-old atopic boy who died of anaphylaxis after peanut ingestion (Phan et al., 2003).

Allergens from dissimilar sources also can evoke an allergic response. Cautions pertaining to cross-sensitivity to latex among persons allergic to various foods appear in Clinical Application 11-8.

Diagnosis

Self- or parental-diagnosis is a common practice but prone to error. Misdiagnosis leads to elimination of the wrong food or too many foods. A 14-month-old boy developed rickets as a result of his parents' management plan for his eczema (Fox et al., 2004).

For infants, the timing of new foods is well advised. The signs and symptoms of food allergies may appear

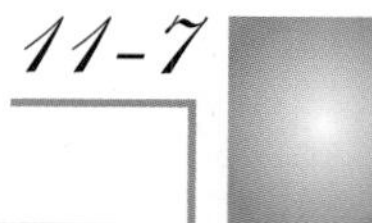

Clinical Application

Anaphylactic Reactions to Food

Allergy to food can be fatal. A comparison of six fatal and seven non-fatal cases of anaphylaxis is particularly enlightening. In all cases, the client was known to have asthma and to be allergic to some food.

- None of the clients were aware that the allergen was present in the foods consumed (candy, cookies, and pastry).
- Symptoms began soon after ingestion but in some cases abated before becoming severe.
- Three of the children who died and three who survived had injectable epinephrine prescribed. Only one (a survivor) used a dose.
- Mean time elapsed between ingestion of the allergenic food and a dose of epinephrine was:
  - 36 minutes in the survivors, all of whom had to have breathing tubes
  - 93 minutes in the deceased

Several recommendations came from this study:

- Epinephrine should be prescribed, kept available, and *used* for patients with IgE-mediated food allergies.
- Children and adolescents who have an allergic reaction to food should be observed for 3 to 4 hours after the reaction at a center capable of dealing with anaphylaxis.
- Parents of such children should be taught to ensure an appropriate, rapid response by schools and other institutions (Sampson, Mendelson, and Rosen, 1992).

Subsequent registries (between 1994 and 1999, 2001 and 2006) of 63 fatal cases of anaphylaxis caused by food allergies confirm those findings. Cases with sufficient retrospective data showed:

- 47 of 48 individuals were known to have asthma.
- 55 of 57 had allergies to foods.
- 7 of the 63 individuals are known to have received timely epinephrine, which did not save them but might have helped some of the others (Boch, Munoz-Furlong, and Sampson, 2001, 2007).

More education at all levels—physicians, clients, families, school personnel, restaurateurs, and the public—is required to combat these potentially preventable tragedies (Boch, Munoz-Furlong, and Sampson, 2007). Food allergies deserve more respect.

as long as 5 days after exposure to an allergen. Thus, allowing at least 5 days to elapse between new foods will increase chances of identifying allergens.

When allergy seems possible, a thorough history and a food diary may yield a list of suspected foods to test further. Skin tests and blood tests can confirm the diagnosis.

Treatment of Allergies

The key to treatment is avoidance of the allergen. Reading labels is likely to take over the lives of the family.

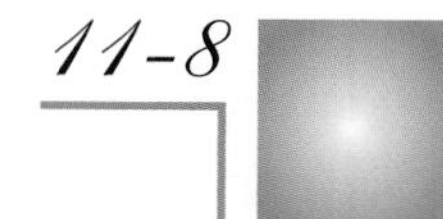

Clinical Application

Latex Allergies and Food Hypersensitivity

Individuals allergic to latex have demonstrated hypersensitivity to foods botanically unrelated to latex but that may share allergenic components. Authors of one study concluded that in most cases, sensitization to latex occurs via pollen or food (Ganglberger et al., 2001). Among the fruits and nuts identified as allergens are:

- Avocado
- Banana
- Chestnut
- Fig
- Kiwi
- Mango
- Melon
- Papaya
- Passion fruit
- Peach
- Peanut
- Pineapple
- Tomato (Brehler et al., 1997; SaraOclar et al., 1998).

Anaphylaxis occurred in many cases (Blanco et al., 1994; Cinquetti et al., 1995; Llatser, Zambrano, and Guillaumet, 1994). Researchers have identified components common to latex and some of the fruits (Delbourg et al., 1996; Latasa et al., 1995). Latex allergy should be ruled out in individuals allergic to any of those foods before performing clinical procedures using latex gloves.

Since the beginning of 2006, when the Food Allergen Labeling and Consumer Protection Act took effect, food labels are required to state clearly whether the food contains a major food allergen. The law identifies as a major food allergen as any of the eight listed as such above and any ingredient that contains protein derived from them. So if a product, for example, contains casein or whey, the label must include the word *milk*. The plain language declaration requirement also applies to flavorings, colorings, and incidental additives that are or contain a major food allergen (Bren, 2006).

The Food Allergy Network provides educational materials to assist in analyzing labels for ingredients with allergenic potential. Its Web site has notifications of products with ingredients not included on labels. For teachers and caregivers, the organization also has a model emergency plan in eight languages (About FAAN, undated).

Pharmacologic management of allergy signs and symptoms includes:

- Antihistamines that block histamine receptors in the tissues for mild to moderate symptoms

- Epinephrine (adrenalin) with bronchodilator and vasopressor actions for severe reactions; self-administered epinephrine can be life-saving.

Anaphylaxis guidelines suggest:

- Treatment with epinephrine
- Teaching about self-injectable epinephrine
- Referral to an allergist

Despite the above guidelines, chart reviews of 678 clients treated for food-related acute allergic reactions in 21 North American emergency departments found that:

- 16% received epinephrine (24% of those with severe reactions).
- 16% were given prescriptions for self-injectable epinephrine (Epi-pen).
- 12% were referred to an allergist (Clark et al., 2004).

As shown in Clinical Application 11-7, even if prescriptions have been filled, they are not always used appropriately.

Related Food Technology

In any single day, our immune systems are exposed to thousands of different proteins from the environment and the food we eat. The discrepancy between the vast numbers of proteins we encounter and the limited number that actually become allergens led to an allergy assessment strategy. This technique permits testing of biotechnology products for potential allergenicity before commercialization. As of 2007, no clinically documented food allergic reactions to biotechnology proteins in food crops were reported (Bannon and Martino-Catt, 2007).

The opposite actions are also possible, potentially improving the safety of plant-based foods. Genetic engineering has silenced the major allergen in peanuts and removed allergenic proteins from tomatoes (Singh and Bhalla, 2008).

COW'S MILK PROTEIN-SENSITIVE ENTEROPATHY

Up to 50% of pediatric cow's milk allergy is non–IgE-mediated (Maloney and Nowak-Wegrzyn, 2007). In this condition, the response of the immune system to a specific protein leads to inflammatory changes in the gastrointestinal tract (Garcia-Careaga and Kerner, 2005).

Symptoms resolve within 48 to 72 hours after eliminating cow's milk protein from the diet. Most infants tolerate cow's milk by their first birthday (Maloney and Nowak-Wegrzyn, 2007). The physician should be reminded of dietary limitations so that an appropriate time can be chosen to reintroduce the offending foods.

Colic

Infantile colic occurs in 10% to 25% of infants. Although the cause of colic is unknown, the condition is named for the presumed manifestation, spasms of the muscles of the colon. The abdomen is tense and the infant draws his or her legs up to its belly. He or she may cry for hours, starting late in the afternoon, just when caregivers are also tired and cranky. The classic definition of colic is the "Rule of Threes," crying for more than:

- 3 hours a day
- 3 days per week
- 3 weeks (Duro et al., 2002)

POSSIBLE CAUSES

Suggested causes fall into two main groups:

- Gastrointestinal (food protein hypersensitivity or allergy)
- Nongastrointestinal (parental or maternal–child interaction problems)

The various factors act together, leading to disturbances in infant gastrointestinal motility that manifests clinically as colic (Gupta, 2002).

Other physiological causes have been proposed:

- Abdominal distention resulting from swallowing air. Passage of flatus seems to relieve the pain.
  - If the infant is bottle-fed, the nipple holes may be too big or too small, increasing the amount of air swallowed.
  - The breastfed infant might be swallowing air because of incorrect nursing position.
- Carbohydrate metabolism may be immature, producing transient lactose intolerance.
  - Studies have shown a reduced crying time when lactase is added to formula or breast milk (Buckley, 2000).
  - A history of colic was associated with laboratory-tested carbohydrate malabsorption from apple juice (Duro et al., 2002).

TREATMENT OF COLIC

The following interventions have sometimes helped:

- Holding the baby upright
- Burping
- Providing warm water to drink
- Diluting the formula
- Offering cold formula
- Swaddling
- Carrying the infant
- Rocking
- Making soft repetitive sounds

For breastfed infants, a 7-day trial manipulating the mother's diet reduced the crying or fussing duration by 21%. Foods omitted by the mothers were cow's milk, eggs, peanuts, tree nuts, wheat, soy, and fish (Hill et al., 2005).

Even though their baby's condition is stressful for them, the parents should try not to be overly concerned. Most infants grow and gain weight despite colic.

The one proven treatment is time, as this behavior tends to dissipate by 6 months of age (Crotteau, Wright, and Eglash, 2006).

Diarrhea

Passage of more than three loose, watery stools a day distinguishes acute diarrhea. In developing countries, diarrhea is a common cause of mortality among children younger than 5 years old, with an estimated 2 million deaths annually. Among children in the United States, acute diarrhea accounts for:

- More than 1.5 million outpatient visits
- 200,000 hospitalizations
- Approximately 300 deaths per year (CDC, 2003b)

Seventy-five percent of an infant's body weight is water, 54% of it extracellular. For this reason, an infant is at high risk of rapid dehydration from diarrhea. The degree of dehydration can be estimated from the infant's weight loss:

- 3% to 9% weight loss = mild to moderate dehydration
- >9% = severe dehydration (CDC, 2003b)

CAUSES

Infants are subject to osmotic diarrhea. Overfeeding and food intolerances are common causes of diarrhea. Apple juice may produce diarrhea in infants because of carbohydrate malabsorption (see Colic).

The most common cause of infectious **enteritis** in human infants is **rotavirus.** Gastroenteritis caused by rotavirus results in about 20 to 60 deaths in the United States annually in children younger than 5 years old but 500,000 deaths in the same ages worldwide (CDC, 2006). Severe vomiting may accompany the diarrhea.

Children between 6 months and 2 years of age are most susceptible. By age 3, most children have antibodies against the virus. The fecal–oral route is its probable mode of transmission, but the virus survives for long periods on hard surfaces, in contaminated water, and on hands. Breastfeeding does not affect infection rates but may reduce the severity of the illness (Heymann, 2004).

Vaccines offer the best hope of reducing the burden of acute rotavirus gastroenteritis in both developed and developing countries (Dennehy, 2008).

PATHOPHYSIOLOGY

As a result of diarrhea, the wall of the intestine may become inflamed. The inflammation diminishes the amount of lactase produced, so the infant may exhibit a temporary lactose intolerance. Distension, cramps, and osmotic diarrhea ensue. In diarrhea caused by rotavirus, the virus damages the villous brush border, causing osmotic diarrhea, and also produces an enterotoxin that causes a secretory diarrhea (CDC, 2003b).

TREATMENT

Treatment should begin at home at the onset of the diarrhea. Caregivers should be instructed regarding signs and symptoms of dehydration and other parameters of treatment failure. The usual protocol is as follows:

- Oral rehydration solutions (ORS) should be used for rehydration, which should be accomplished in 3 to 4 hours.
- An age-appropriate, unrestricted diet should be given as soon as dehydration is corrected.
- For breastfed infants, nursing should be continued.
- For formula-fed infants, diluted formula is not recommended and special formula usually is not necessary.
- Additional ORS should be administered for ongoing losses through diarrhea.
- No unnecessary laboratory tests or medications should be administered (CDC, 2003b).

ORSs (see Chapter 8) are life-saving not only in developing countries but also in North America. Most infants who are vomiting can be rehydrated with oral fluids. They may have to be given 5 mL of ORS every 5 minutes, gradually increasing the amount (CDC, 2003b). Rehydration via a nasogastric tube may be used in an emergency room to rapidly correct dehydration (CDC, 2003b).

Ceralyte®, Oralyte®, and Pedialyte®, as well as store brands are available at nearly all drug stores and grocery stores. The CDC (1999b) advises parents to keep two bottles or packages of these products on hand to use when the child develops diarrhea, following the package instructions according to the child's age.

Sports drinks are not adequate substitutes for these solutions. Large amounts of fluids containing simple sugars, such as carbonated soft drinks, juice, and gelatin desserts, should be avoided because they might increase osmotic diarrhea. Liquids at room temperature are often better tolerated than warm or cold beverages.

A 1-year-old infant suffered from diarrhea for nine days due to:

- Original misdiagnosis
- Incorrect advice from an emergency room physician
- Misinformation found on an Internet site

Referral by his family physician to a pediatric enterologist and hospitalization under the ORS protocol for 2 days cured his diarrhea (Crocco, Villasis-Keever, and Jadad, 2002). Parents should be encouraged to challenge any advice, regardless of source, when it does not produce the desired results.

WHEN TO CALL THE PHYSICIAN

Parents should be instructed to call the primary health-care provider regarding an infant's diarrhea under the following conditions:

- Young or small infant
  - <6 months of age
  - <17.6 pounds in weight
- History of premature birth, chronic medical conditions, or concurrent illness
- Fever
  - >38°C (100.4°F) for infants ages <3 months
  - >39°C (102.2°F) for children ages 3 to 36 months
- Visible blood in stool
- High output, including frequent and substantial volumes of diarrhea
- Persistent vomiting
- Signs of dehydration
  - Sunken eyes
  - Decreased tears
  - Dry mucous membranes
  - Decreased urine output
- Change in mental status (e.g., irritability, apathy, or lethargy)
- Suboptimal response to oral rehydration therapy (ORT) already administered or inability of the caregiver to administer ORT (CDC, 2003b).

An emergency room randomized trial compared ORT with intravenous therapy. In moderately dehydrated children with gastroenteritis:

- ORT was as effective as intravenous (IV) therapy in achieving rehydration within 4 hours.
- ORT was initiated in an average of 19.9 minutes vs. 41.2 minutes for IV therapy.
- 31% of the ORT group required hospitalization vs. 49% of the IV therapy group (Spandorfer et al., 2005).

Risk factors for increased mortality from acute diarrhea in the United States are:

- Prematurity
- Young maternal age
- Black race
- Rural residence

The decision to hospitalize an infant should consider these factors along with degree of dehydration (CDC, 2003b).

Nutrition of the Toddler (Ages 1 to 3 Years)

The child's nutritional needs become more like those of adults after the first birthday. During the toddler years, growth is slower than during infancy, and although activity increases, the proportional need for kilocalories decreases compared with infancy. So the child's appetite slackens.

How and what the family eats will influence the child's habits and tastes for many years. Being forced to eat a distasteful food because "it's good for you" has imprinted permanent avoidance behaviors on some individuals. Conversely, some parents expand their repertory of menu choices to set good examples for their children.

Psychosocial Development

Autonomy or independence is the psychosocial developmental task of the toddler. Every 2-year-old knows the word *no.* One way parents can assist a toddler achieve autonomy is to encourage choices from acceptable food alternatives (Fig. 11-4). If parents insist that a child eat certain items or amounts, the child may learn to use food rejection as a means of gaining attention. Later, more serious eating problems may result from such interactions. The parent can, however, create structure in the child's day by insisting the child remain at the table during mealtime whether or not items are consumed.

Physical Growth and Development

During the toddler years, growth slows. The expected weight gain in the second year may be just 4 to 6 pounds. Height may increase by about 4 inches. By age 2, however, head circumference reaches two-thirds of its adult size. *See "Growth Charts" on DavisPlus or at http://www.cdc.gov/growthcharts.*

The toddler is aptly named. One of the skills acquired during this time is walking upright. As this

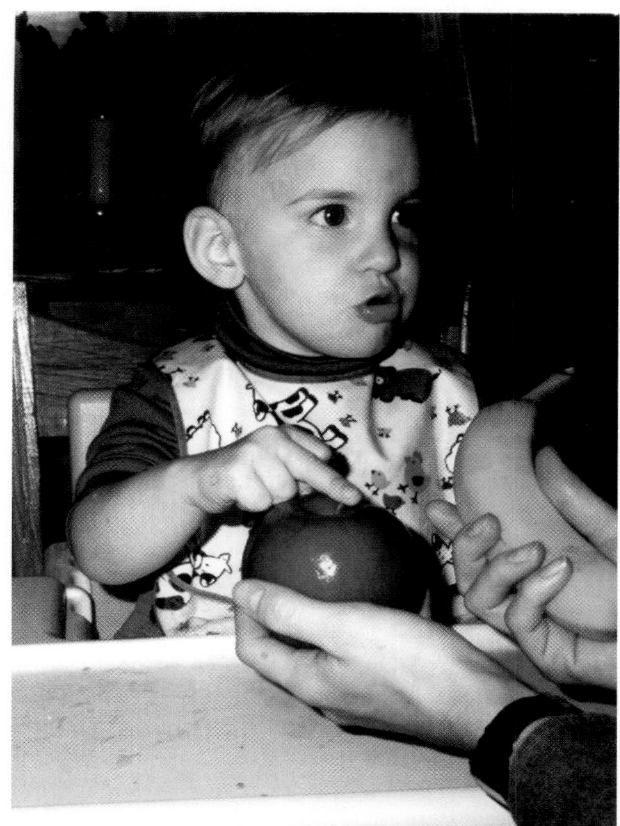

FIGURE 11-4 Autonomy is achieved in small steps. This 19-month-old girl is choosing her dessert.

skill is being perfected, the child's muscles of the back, buttocks, and thighs are enlarging. The bones are becoming more mineralized, and "baby fat" is disappearing.

Along with the gross motor skill of walking, the toddler's fine motor control improves. He or she is able to use eating utensils with more finesse. The spoon is likely to reach the mouth still filled with food. The toddler's mouth is more sensitive than an adult's mouth. Foods are eaten better at lukewarm temperatures rather than hot. Thus, dawdling at the table may have a physiological basis.

Nutrient Needs and Intake

For DRIs, see Appendix A. In 2008, the American Academy of Pediatrics recommended that all children receive a daily intake of 400 IU of vitamin D (Wagner and Greer, 2008).

The need for many nutrients increases proportionately with body size throughout the growth years. These needs, coupled with the toddler's poorer appetite, stretch parents' ingenuity and patience. See Table 11-9 for consumption patterns of 2- to 5-year-olds in 1999 to 2002.

According to the American Academy of Pediatrics, despite the toddler's poorer appetite, vitamin supplements are probably unnecessary for healthy children older than 1 year (Vitamins, 2004). See Dollars and Sense 11-2. Special circumstances may indicate a need for supplementation.

Food Likes

Toddlers like finger foods and can learn about texture by eating them. Toddlers prefer plain foods to most mixtures such as casseroles. Familiar combinations, such as macaroni and cheese, spaghetti, and pizza, however, may be relished. The parent should serve favorite foods occasionally but not exclusively so that new foods are given a fair trial (Cathey and Gaylord, 2004).

Mealtimes

Toddlers are learning social skills as well as good nutritional habits. Eating is a social experience for adults most of the time; toddlers appreciate company also. Visiting other homes might introduce food items and experiences not encountered at home.

TABLE 11-9 ■ 2- to 5-Year-Olds Consuming the Recommended MyPyramid Servings

FOOD GROUP	RECOMMENDED NUMBER OF SERVINGS	PERCENTAGE OF MALES	PERCENTAGE OF FEMALES
Grains	6	59	45
Vegetables	3	31	27
Fruit	2	48	42
Dairy	2	53	42
Meat: 2–3 years	3.3 oz	25	19
4–5 years	5 oz	25	19

Adapted from Cook and Friday (2005).

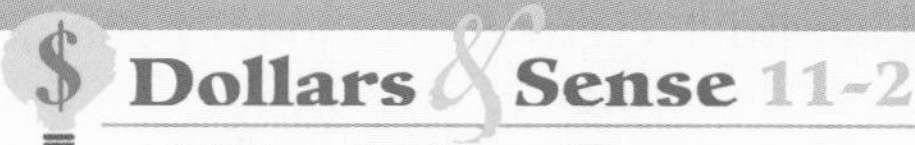

Children's Vitamins

Although the American Academy of Pediatrics does not recommend vitamin-mineral supplements for healthy children, many families provide them as insurance. If parents choose to give vitamin-mineral supplements to a child, they should be aware of the cost. For example:

Ages	Brand Name Product	Price/Daily Dose	Total cost
1–12 years	Children's chewable	$0.12	$501.88
12–18 years	Adult tablet	$0.07	$153.30
Total per child			$655.18

As with other financial decisions, families must decide on the best use of their funds. See Chapters 7 and 15 for quality issues.

Keeping to a regular schedule will help maintain the child's food intake. A 1-year-old's stomach holds just 1 cup, necessitating small servings. A serving is one-fourth to one-fifth the size of an adult's recommended serving. A good rule of thumb is to serve 1 tablespoonful for each year of age.

Eating regular meals and nutritious snacks helps to prevent fatigue and control the appetite. If high-sugar snacks are used to assuage hunger before a meal, however, the more nutritious foods at the meal may be taken poorly.

New Foods

After the pureed foods of infancy, parents will be pleased to offer more attractive plates of food to the toddler. Brightly colored foods are appealing. Nevertheless, chewing may not be well developed. Tough meat or very fibrous vegetables are not for the toddler.

Foods not recommended until after the first birthday can be gradually introduced if family history of allergies is not a concern. These foods include unmodified cow's milk, egg white, wheat, citrus fruits, seafood, chocolate, and nut butters. Parents should continue to introduce foods one at a time at weekly intervals and to watch for reactions.

Even very young children make their wishes known through body movements, pushing food away, closing their mouths, and turning away from the feeder. The astute parent will respond to these cues before the child resorts to crying to communicate distress.

Daily intake should include:

- One serving of a vitamin C-rich fruit or vegetable
- One serving of a green leafy or yellow vegetable
- Limited sugar
- Grams of fiber equal to child's age + 5 beginning at age 2

Parents should continue to avoid giving the toddler hazardous foods (Clinical Application 11-6). Sometimes chopping the food into very tiny pieces eliminates a choking hazard. Nevertheless, a toddler should not be left alone while eating.

Because the kidneys become mature at about age 1, the toddler can tolerate salt in moderation. Preference for salty foods is an acquired taste. Because of the association between salt and high blood pressure later in life, the prudent parent will discourage the consumption of heavily salted foods.

Nutritional Concerns

Toddlers are at risk for iron-deficiency anemia. Misguided food choices may lead to inadequate intakes of nutrients and interfere with growth and development.

Iron-Deficiency Anemia

Iron deficiency affects 2.4 million children in the United States. Childhood iron-deficiency **anemia** is associated with behavioral and cognitive delays. From 1999 to 2002, among 1- to 3-year-olds, the iron deficiency prevalence was:

- 12% in Hispanics
- 6% in whites
- 6% in blacks
- 20% in those who were overweight
- 7% for normal-weight toddlers (Brotanek et al., 2007)

In 2006, the rates were much higher for low-income children attending public health clinics:

- 14% among all attendees
- 17% in 6- to 17-month-olds
- 10% in 3- to 5-year-olds (Polhamus et al., 2007)

Overindulging in milk is thought to decrease the appetite for iron-rich foods, enriched cereals, meats, and some fruits and vegetables. Therefore, milk intake should be limited to 24 ounces per day for children ages 1 to 5 years. The term *milk anemia* refers to iron deficiency anemia caused by overconsumption of milk and underconsumption of iron-rich foods. Juice for toddlers should not exceed 6 ounces per day (Box 11-2).

Box 11-2 ■ *Recommendations for Juice Consumption*

For Infants

- No juice before 6 months of age
- No juice from bottles or covered cups that permit consumption throughout the day
- No juice at bedtime
- No unpasteurized juice

For Children and Adolescents

- Ages 1 to 6: Limit juice to 4 to 6 ounces per day
- Ages 7 to 18: Limit juice to 8 to 12 ounces per day
- Encourage consumption of whole fruits.
- No unpasteurized juice

Assessment and Interventions

- Determine amount of juice intake for children with overnutrition or undernutrition and those with chronic diarrhea or abdominal symptoms.
- Determine the amount and means of juice intake for children with dental caries.
- Teach parents the difference between juice and juice drinks.

SOURCE: Summarized from American Academy of Pediatrics (2001, Reaffirmed 2006).

Treatment of iron-deficiency anemia may include medication and ingestion of iron-fortified foods or foods naturally high in iron. Treatment should produce a normal hemoglobin level in 1 to 2 months, but replenishing iron stores may take 3 to 6 months (Deglin and Vallerand, 2009).

Vegetarian diets may pose a risk for iron deficiency in toddlers. The position of the American Dietetic Association (ADA) and Dietitians of Canada is that *well-planned* vegan diets are appropriate for all ages (italics added). Extremely restrictive diets such as fruitarian and raw foods diets, however, have been associated with impaired growth and are not recommended for infants and children (ADA, 2003).

Inadequate Intakes

To support brain growth and development, 1- to 2-year-old children should continue to drink whole milk. At age 2, fat intake should gradually be reduced to 30% of a child's intake (Feeding the child, 2004).

Cases of kwashiorkor and rickets have been reported in toddlers given a rice beverage and a soy beverage not formulated for children in place of milk (Carvalho et al., 2001).

Nutrition of the Preschool Child (Ages 3 to 6 Years)

This is a delightful time of enthusiastic learning, including food preferences. See suggestions for implementing the Food Pyramid for 2- to 6-year-old children in Table 11-10.

TABLE 11-10 ■ Food Pyramid for 2- to 6-Year-Olds

FOOD GROUP	NUMBER OF SERVINGS	SERVING SUGGESTIONS
Bread/Cereal	Six or more	Select whole-grain breads and iron-fortified cereals.
Fruit	Two or more	Include 4 oz of orange juice or other food high in vitamin C.
Vegetable	Three or more	Include one vegetable high in vitamin A. Crisp-cooked, warm rather than hot, vegetables preferred.
Meat	Two	Child-size servings of red meat are essential for RBC synthesis.
Milk	Two	Not to be overdone at expense of blood-forming nutrients. Low-fat milks are now permissible.

Psychosocial Development

Initiative is the psychosocial task to be mastered by the preschool child. Within their capabilities, children should be encouraged to set and achieve some goals of their own. Children can participate in planning and preparation of meals, and they should help in the kitchen, not just with cleanup. Preschool children can make gelatin desserts, fancy cookies, and showy relishes to foster a sense of accomplishment.

By making the meal a social time and eating slowly themselves, parents can encourage the same behavior in a child. Exemplifying good manners will be more productive than criticizing the child's manners.

Having company their own age is helpful. Children stay at the table longer and eat more in the company of their peers. Exchanging visits with a friend's child will begin to broaden the child's horizons.

Physical Growth and Development

From the third to the sixth year, a child continues to gain 4 to 5 pounds per year. A gain in height of about 2 inches per year is average so that by age 5, birth length will have doubled. Half the adult height is attained:

- In boys, by about age 2
- In girls, by about age 19 months (*Merck Manual*, 2009).

Adequacy of growth should be assessed every 6 to 12 months. Growth charts remain the standard against which a given assessment is judged. *See "Growth Charts" on DavisPlus or at http://www.cdc.gov/growthcharts.*

Nutrient Needs and Intake

For DRIs, see Appendix A. In 2008, the American Academy of Pediatrics recommended that all children receive a daily intake of 400 IU of vitamin D (Wagner and Greer, 2008).

Some children will consume more nutrients than reported in Table 11-9. More than 30% of children in the United States take dietary supplements regularly, most often multivitamins and multiminerals. Supplement use was associated with higher family income, a smoke-free environment, not participating in the Women, Infants, and Children program (WIC), lower child body mass index (BMI), and less daily television and computer use time (Picciano et al., 2007).

Preschool children are very active. A 3-year-old may need 1300 to 1500 kilocalories per day. Serving sizes for 4- to 6-year-old children are the same as those *recommended* for adults.

Developing Good Habits

The preschool child responds best to regular mealtimes. When the adult meal will be served late, the parents have to decide if it would be better to allow the child to socialize with adults at a late meal or to feed the child early.

Preschoolers cannot eat enough in only three meals to meet their needs. By age 3, a child is able to verbalize hunger. Some nutrient-dense, low-fat choices are:

- Cottage cheese
- Low-fat yogurt
- Fresh fruit
- Raw vegetables
- Low-fat milk
- Fruit juices
- Graham crackers
- Fig bars

Concentrated sweets such as candy and soda pop should be limited.

However, too much control is undesirable. Young children naturally obey inner cues of hunger and satiety. Parents who override those cues by insisting the child eat a given amount are teaching the child to overeat. It is better to acknowledge that the child cannot consume enough at mealtime and to provide healthy snacks.

Tableware should be appropriate for the preschool child. Unbreakable dishes that are designed for stability, with deep sides to permit scooping the food onto a spoon or fork, are practical choices. Small glasses and cups, also unbreakable, with a squat design and low center of gravity, will minimize accidents and mealtime tension.

It is not too early to emphasize the importance of cleanliness. Regularly washing hands before meals and brushing teeth after meals will cultivate good health habits.

New Foods

Parents should offer new foods one at a time in small amounts. Trying something new is most acceptable at the beginning of the meal when the child is hungriest. A taste or two is sufficient if new foods are offered at regular intervals. Often 8 to 10 tries are necessary before the child develops a taste for a new food.

Parents have the advantage of being able to select the food offered. Items the parents dislike will not grace the family table regularly, if at all. Children, too, should be permitted their preferences. If an argument over food develops into a power struggle, as sometimes happens, the child will not admit to liking the food, even when it turns out to be quite tasty. To stave off eating problems, parents choose what is available to eat but children choose whether to eat and the amount (Dietz and Robinson, 2005).

Nutritional Concerns

Preschool children should be monitored for problems. A nutrition screening tool, the PEACH Survey, for use with children up to 6 years old appears as Box 11-3.

In addition, dental caries and the nutritional quality in day care programs may be of concern.

Dental Health

The destruction of tooth enamel by dental caries (see Chapter 3) is a problem for all economic groups. The "baby" teeth, as well as the permanent teeth, deserve care and professional attention. For teeth to be correctly brushed, the parent may have to do it. Fluorosis (see Chapter 8) has occurred as a result of the overuse of supplements and the ingestion of fluoridated toothpaste. Children younger than 6 years are likely to swallow rather than to expectorate toothpaste. A pea-sized portion of toothpaste is sufficient. Regular dental checkups should be a part of the preschool child's routine.

Adequate dentition and good nutrition are mutually supportive. In a 9-year Iowa study, children of low socioeconomic status consumed more soda pop and powder-based beverages than children of high socioeconomic status. The group consuming more sweetened beverages also had significantly more decayed and filled surfaces on their teeth (Hamasha et al., 2006).

Childcare Programs

An estimated 12 million children 5 years old and younger are regularly in some form of child care delivered by persons other than their parents. The ADA (2005) has addressed meeting children's nutrition and nutrition education needs while in child care. Some pertinent recommendations are:

- If the child is in the program 4 to 7 hours per day, the child-care program should be responsible for meeting one-third of the child's daily nutritional needs.
- If the child is in the program 8 or more hours per day, it should be responsible for meeting one-half to two-thirds of the child's daily nutritional needs.
- The program should offer food to children 2 years of age and older every 2 to 3 hours during the active part of the day.
- Caregivers should not add extra salt or sugar to food.

Box 11-3 ■ *A Nutrition Screening Tool for Young Children*

The PEACH Survey is completed by a child's primary caregiver to help identify potential nutrition problems. The tool was validated on children from birth to age 5 years against a pediatric dietitian's assessment. *Yes* answers receive the points in the far right column. For instance, a child with a feeding tube would receive 4 points for that one *yes* answer. A score of 4 or more indicates a probable nutrition problem.

PEACH* Survey

Agency: ______________________ Date: ______________________

Child's Name: ______________________ Date of Birth: ______________________

Address: ______________________ Phone #: ______________________

Please circle YES or NO for each question as it applies to your child.

Does your child have a health problem (do not include colds or flu). If yes, what is it? YES NO 1

Is your child: Small for age: _____ Too thin? _____ Too heavy? _____

(If you check any of the above, please circle YES) YES NO 3

Does your child have feeding problems? If yes, what are they? YES NO 3

Is your child's appetite a problem? If yes, describe: YES NO 1

Is your child on a special diet? If yes, what type of diet? YES NO 2

Does your child take medicine for a health problem? (Do not include vitamins, iron, or fluoride.)

Name of medicine(s): YES NO 1

Does your child have food allergies? If yes, to what foods? YES NO 1

Does your child use a feeding tube or other special feeding method?

If yes, explain: YES NO 4

Circle YES if your child does not eat any of these foods: YES NO 1

Milk _____ Meats _____ Vegetables _____ Fruits _____ (Check all that apply)

Circle YES if your child has problems with: Sucking _____ YES NO 3

Swallowing _____ Chewing _____ Gagging _____ (Check all that apply)

Circle YES if your child has problems with: Loose stools _____ Hard stools _____

Throwing up _____ Spitting up _____ (Check all that apply) YES NO 3

Does your child eat clay, paint chips, dirt, or any other things that are not food? If yes, what? YES NO 2

Does your child refuse to eat, throw food, or do other things that upset you at mealtime? If yes, explain: YES NO 2

For infants **under 12 months** who are bottle-fed: Does your child drink less than 3 (8-ounce) bottles of milk per day? YES NO 1

For children **over 12 months:** (Check if applies and circle YES)

Is your child not using a cup? _____ Is your child not finger feeding? _____ YES NO 1

For children **over 18 months:**

Does your child still take most liquids from a bottle? YES NO 2

Circle YES if your child is not using a spoon. YES NO 2

*Parent Eating and Nutrition Assessment for Children with Special Health Needs

Total =

- Good institutional food management practices should be implemented, including good handwashing, adequate refrigeration, and proper storage of supplies.

Nutrition of the School-Age Child (Ages 6 to 12 Years)

A balanced diet suitable for healthy adults will also be good for a school-age child.

Diets should not be restricted because of the energy (kilocalorie), fat, or sugar content of any one food, nor should foods be labeled *good* or *bad*. In the first case, food may be regarded as medicine, and in the second, as "forbidden fruit." Neither viewpoint fosters positive attitudes.

Psychosocial Development

According to Erikson, the developmental task of the school-age child is **industry**. The school years are the years to build competence in many different skills. Making and keeping commitments is part of developing industry.

School-age children can participate in planning menus, shopping for food, preparing the meals, as well as cleaning up afterwards (Fig. 11-5). Limiting the child's role to washing the dishes or taking out the garbage will be more likely to foster a sense of inferiority than habits of industry.

Physical Growth and Development

The average yearly growth during the school years is 7 pounds and 2.5 inches (Brown, 2008). The growth is not evenly distributed throughout the year, reflected in an inconsistent appetite. A child's progress should be tracked on the CDC growth charts to determine if growth is within the normal range. *See "Growth Charts" on Davis Plus or at http://www.cdc.gov/growthcharts.*

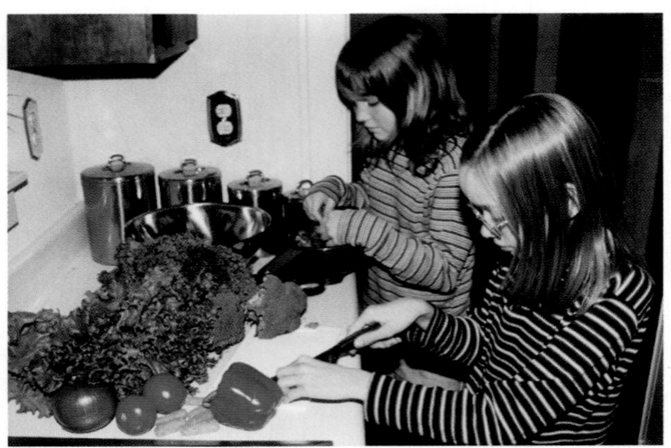

FIGURE 11-5 Preparing dinner for a friend can involve culinary practice.

Exercise can help the school-age child's growth and development by stimulating osteoblasts and expending energy to control weight. Activities that are likely to become lifetime interests should be especially encouraged. Unlike sports such as football that are played by few adults, tennis or similar skill sports may provide an outlet for a lifetime.

By school age, the effects of good or poor nutrition will begin to be apparent. The well-nourished child will display most of the qualities listed in Table 11-11.

Nutritional Needs and Concerns

For DRIs, see Appendix A. In 2008, the American Academy of Pediatrics recommended that all children receive a daily intake of 400 IU of vitamin D (Wagner and Greer, 2008).

See Table 11-12 for consumption patterns of 6- to 11-year-olds in 1999 to 2002.

Meal Patterns and Behaviors

A school-age child cannot consume all the needed nutrients in three child-sized meals. Healthy snacks are necessary to complement the main meals. Likewise, breakfast is essential and should contain one-fourth to one-third of the day's nutrients. A common choice for breakfast, ready-to-eat cereal, may be less nourishing if marketed for children than if marketed for adults. Sixty-six percent of children's cereals did not meet national nutrition standards, particularly regarding sugar content (Schwartz et al., 2008).

School-age children are generally so active that they may have trouble sitting still. Requiring them

TABLE 11-11 ■ Indications of Good Nutrition in the School-Age Child

General Appearance	Alert, energetic Normal height and weight
Skin and Mucous Membranes	Skin smooth, slightly moist; mucous membranes pink, no bleeding
Hair	Shiny, evenly distributed
Scalp	No sores
Eyes	Bright, clear, no fatigue circles
Teeth	Straight, clean, no discoloration or caries
Tongue	Pink, papillae present, no sores
Gastrointestinal System	Good appetite, regular elimination
Musculoskeletal System	Well-developed, firm muscles; erect posture, bones straight without deformities
Neurological System	Good attention span for age; not restless, irritable, or weepy

TABLE 11-12 ■ 6- to 11-Year-Olds Consuming Recommended MyPyramid Servings

FOOD GROUP	RECOMMENDED NUMBER OF SERVINGS	PERCENTAGE OF MALES	PERCENTAGE OF FEMALES
Grains	6	61	48
Vegetables	3	25	25
Fruit	2	26	26
Dairy: 6–8 years	2	53	40
9–11 years	3	39	30
Meat	5 oz	30	24

Adapted from Cook and Friday (2005).

to spend 15 to 20 minutes at the table for meals will increase the likelihood that they will eat a complete meal.

Concerning attention–deficit/hyperactivity disorder, little evidence supports dietary restriction as an effective treatment (Cormier and Elder, 2007; Cruz and Bahna, 2006). However, research is continuing into the influence of fatty acids and food additives on behavior (McCann et al., 2007; Sinn, 2008; Stevenson, 2006).

Eating dinner with the family was associated with improved diet quality for 9- to 14-year-old children. A survey of 16,202 children revealed that those eating family dinner more often consumed:

- More fruits and vegetables and
- Less fried food and soda than those who ate dinner with the family less often.

More than half of the 9-year-olds dined with the family every day, compared with about one-third of the 14-year-olds (Gillman et al., 2000).

Nutrition at School

Nutrition education continues in school, focusing on foods, not nutrients. Interactions with other children and school experiences expose a child to new foods and different cultures. A Food Guide Pyramid for older children is illustrated in Figure 11-6.

Curriculum innovations such as gardening projects can increase students' fondness for the produce grown. Researchers found that fourth graders who grew vegetables reported significantly greater preference for snow peas and zucchini than other comparable student groups. The gardening group maintained the difference 6 months after the intervention (Morris and Zidenberg-Cherr, 2002).

Because children need nourishment to learn and many come to school hungry, food assistance is available at school. Federally reimbursable school meals programs require participating schools to offer meals free or at reduced prices to eligible children. In 2007, 80% of children served by the School Breakfast Program received their meals free or at a reduced price. See Box 11-4 and Table 11-13 for requirements.

Nutrition in Adolescence

Adolescence is the period that extends from the onset of **puberty** until full growth is reached. For most individuals, adolescence occurs between the ages of 12 and 20. Adolescence is second only to infancy in the nutritional requirements necessary for growth and development.

Psychosocial Development

Achieving their own **identity** is the developmental task Erikson identified for adolescents, including accepting their capabilities. In this process, teenagers "try on" various identities. Adolescents pick up fads instantly and drop them just as suddenly. Food and eating fads are part of the same pattern.

Physical Growth and Development

The term *growth spurt* is accurate. Boys and girls differ in the timing and completion of the growth spurt. See Table 11-14. To track an adolescent's growth, BMI-for-age percentile charts (2- to 20-year-old boys and girls) are available on *DavisPlus or at http://www.cdc.gov/growthcharts.*

Approximately 40% of total bone mass is accumulated during adolescence (Baroncelli et al., 2005). During the peak of the adolescent growth spurt, the mineral and protein content of the body is increased as shown in Table 11-15. Iron and zinc can be obtained from body stores as well as food, but calcium must be acquired from dietary sources (Treuth and Griffin, 2006).

Nutritional Needs and Concerns

For DRIs, see Appendix A. In 2008, the American Academy of Pediatrics recommended that all adolescents receive a daily intake of 400 IU of vitamin D (Wagner and Greer, 2008).

See Table 11-16 for consumption patterns of adolescents in 1999 to 2002.

Calcium and Iron

Regarding nutrients, adolescent diets are lacking in calcium and for females, in iron. As a percentage of the RDA or AI, 12- to 18-year-old:

- Males consumed 91% of the AI for calcium
- Females consumed 65% of the AI for calcium

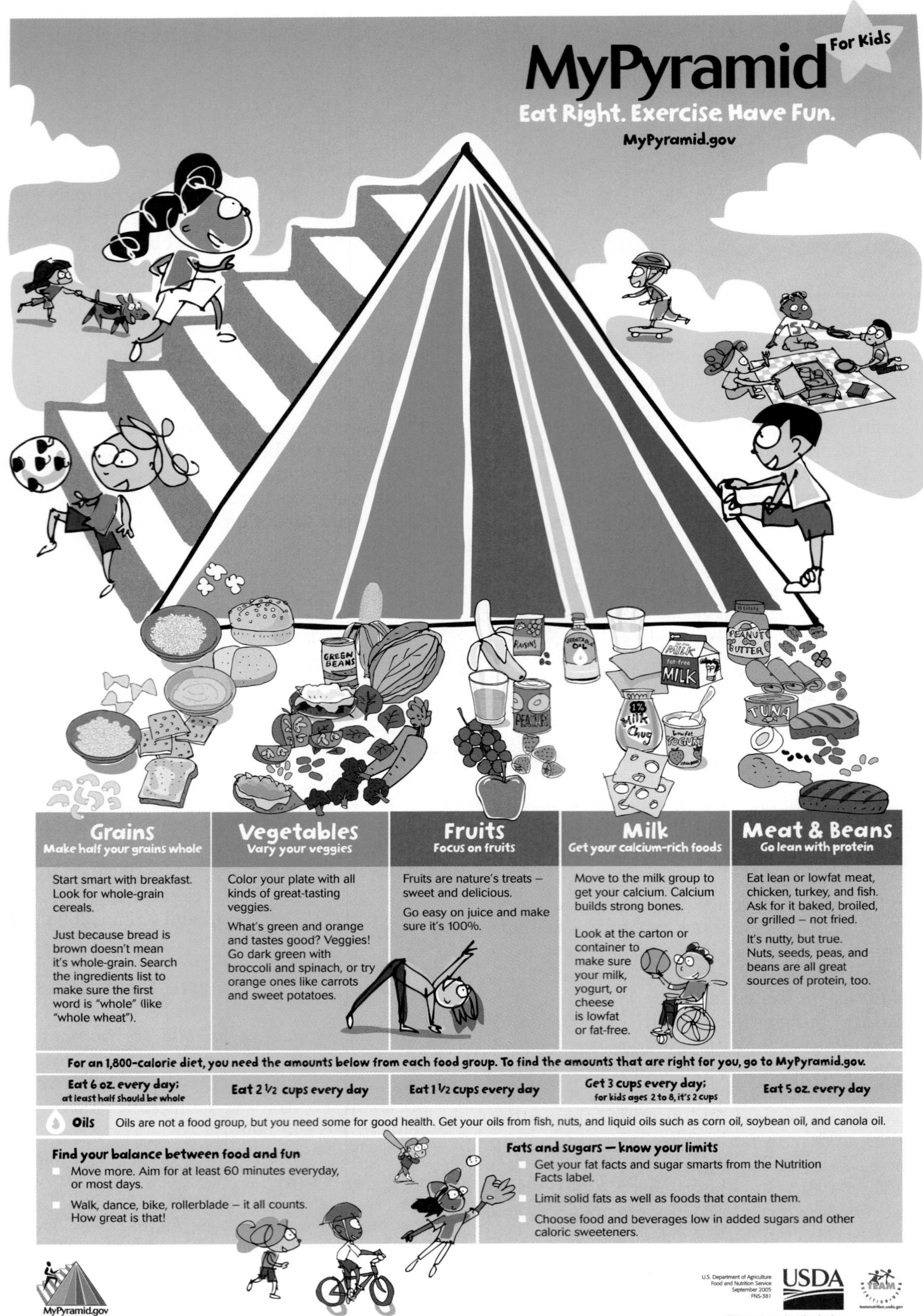

FIGURE 11-6 MyPyramid for Kids (2005) incorporates exercise. This version is designed for older children. A simpler version for younger children is also available from the U.S. Department of Agriculture.

Box 11-4 ■ *School Foods*

Federally funded school meals began in 1946 and specify nutritional content to be served. See Table 11-13.

Federal regulations prohibit access to foods of minimal nutritional value in food-service areas during meal times. However, potato chips, chocolate bars, and doughnuts are not so categorized and can be sold in the cafeteria or elsewhere at any time. At least 28 states and many school districts and schools have adopted more stringent regulations (CDC, 2005b).

Outside of meal times, many students have access to snack foods. A 2005 national study found vending machines were present in:

- 17% of elementary schools
- 82% of middle schools
- 97% of high schools.

To their credit, 15% of middle schools and 21% of high schools did not stock the vending machines with low-nutrient, energy-dense foods and beverages, commonly referred to as junk food (Finkelstein, Hill, and Whitaker, 2008).

The Institute of Medicine (2007) released standards for items available on school campuses but not part of the federally reimbursable school meals. The purpose of these stricter standards is to promote healthful eating habits. If followed, the standards would make a la carte cafeteria offerings, vending machine products, and fundraising items nearly conform to the Dietary Guidelines for Americans.

TABLE 11-13 ■ Federally Reimbursable School Meal Programs

	OPERATING SINCE	STUDENTS SERVED, 2007	NUTRITIONAL	REQUIREMENTS
School Breakfast	1975	10.1 million	¼ of RDAs/AIs for kilocalories, protein, calcium, iron, vitamins A and C	<30% of kcal from fat <10% kcal from saturated fat
National School Lunch	1946	30.5 million	⅓ of RDAs/AIs for kilocalories, protein, calcium, iron, vitamins A and C	<30% of kcal from fat <10% kcal from saturated fat

Adapted from U.S. Department of Agriculture (2008b, c).

TABLE 11-14 ■ Adolescent Growth Spurts

	Age in Years	
Status	**Boys**	**Girls**
Age in Years	12–17	9.5-14.5
Height Gain in Year of Peak Velocity	>10 cm (3.9 in.)	Possibly 9 cm (3.5 in.)
Age at Peak Growth Velocity	13–15	11–13.5
At Age 18	2.54 cm growth remains	Slightly less remaining growth than boys Growth 99% complete

Adapted from *Merck Manual* (2009).

TABLE 11-15 ■ Body Content Increases at Peak of Adolescent Growth Spurt

	AVERAGE DAILY INCREASE	
Addition to Body Content	**Boys**	**Girls**
Calcium*	400 mg	240 mg
Iron	1.1 mg	0.9 mg
Zinc	0.5 mg	0.3 mg
Protein	3.8 g	2.3 g

*Must be obtained entirely from dietary sources.
Adapted from Adolescent Nutrition (2004); Treuth and Griffin (2006).

TABLE 11-16 ■ Adolescents Consuming Recommended MyPyramid Servings

FOOD GROUP	RECOMMENDED NUMBER OF SERVINGS	PERCENTAGE OF MALES	PERCENTAGE OF FEMALES
Grains	6	64	48
Vegetables	3	38	34
Fruit	2	23	27
Dairy	3	32	17
Meat	5 oz	49	28

Adapted from Cook and Friday (2005).

- Females consumed 88% of the RDA for iron
- 18- to 19–year-old females consumed 74% of the RDA for iron (U.S. Department of Agriculture, 2008a)

Long term, deficiencies of those minerals may be manifested in osteoporosis or anemia. Short term, evidence suggests an influence of dietary factors on fracture occurrence. Although rates of fracture vary considerably with age, sex, and maturation, they peak in early puberty. At that time, rates of bone turnover are high, but bone mineral accrual lags behind gains in height and weight. Among the factors impacting pediatric fracture incidence are:

- Genetics
- Inadequate calcium intake
- Milk avoidance
- Excessive consumption of carbonated beverages
- Lack of weight-bearing physical activity
- Obesity
- High exposure to trauma (Goulding, 2007)

For all children and adolescents, breakfast, or lack thereof, impacts overall dietary intake significantly. See Box 11-5.

Overenthusiastic Weight Control

Because of the cultural value placed on thinness, adolescents, especially girls, may restrict their dietary intake to achieve a desired slim body. Some use unhealthy practices such as fasting, diet pills, laxatives, and vomiting to remain slim. **Anorexia nervosa** affects 0.5% to 1% of 14- to 18-year-old girls and is covered in Chapter 16. Subclinical problems may be manifested by excessive exercising, strict dieting, and occasional binging and purging (Treuth and Griffin, 2006). Participating in sports that value slimness is a risk factor for both girls and boys. See Box 11-6.

Some adolescents may adopt vegetarianism as a means to control weight and body shape rather than for ecological or spiritual reasons. Regardless of the reason they have become vegetarians, these adolescents should have their nutritional status and dietary intakes monitored.

Acne and Diet

Acne afflicts more than 17 million Americans with approximately 80% to 90% of adolescents affected (Marcason, 2010). The condition even persists into middle age in 12% of women and 3% of men (Cordain et al., 2002).

Acne is triggered by sex hormones stimulating the sebaceous glands. The skin becomes oilier and the ducts to the glands sometimes plug up, permitting the accumulation of harmful bacteria that produce inflammation. The sebaceous glands' production of sebum may be influenced by androgens and hormonal mediators that, in turn, may be stimulated by foods (Marcason, 2010).

Dietary components that have recently been revisited regarding acne are dairy products, high glycemic

Box 11-5 ■ *Breakfast versus No Breakfast Effects*

Among children and adolescents, breakfast or lack of breakfast appreciably impacts the day's nutritive intake. One significant predictor of adolescent breakfast eating was parental breakfast eating. In a national study, the proportions of children who had skipped breakfast the day they were surveyed were:

- 8% of 1- to 7-year-olds
- 12% of 8- to 10-year-olds
- 20% of 11- to 14-year-olds
- 30% of 15- to 18-year-olds.

Skipping breakfast is more prevalent in girls and children from lower socioeconomic backgrounds (Rampersaud et al., 2005).

On average, children who skipped breakfast did not make up the nutrient deficits during the remainder of the day. Breakfast skipping also has been associated with increased snacking and higher intakes of high-fat snacks (Rampersaud et al., 2005).

Conversely, children who ate breakfast tended to make better food choices throughout the day by consuming:

- More vegetables
- More milk
- Fewer soft drinks
- Fewer French fries

Overall, breakfast eaters have higher daily intakes of micronutrients and are more likely to meet the DRI standards than are children who skip breakfast (Rampersaud et al., 2005).

Box 11-6 ■ *The Female Athlete Triad*

Desire for athletic success, especially in sports or dance emphasizing body size, can lead to a trio of medical disorders. Alone or in combination, these disorders of the triad can negatively impact health and athletic performance (Beals and Meyer, 2007).

- Disordered eating—Over one-third of NCAA Division I female athletes reported attitudes and symptoms placing them at risk for anorexia nervosa. (See Chapter 16.)
- Menstrual dysfunction—22% of college females in aesthetic sports display **primary amenorrhea** compared to 7.4% of all college female athletes and fewer than 1% of non-athletes.
- Low bone mineral density—at all skeletal sites BMD is lower than average for amenorrheic athletes and anorexic women (Mandel, 2008). The incidence of stress fractures in female Division 1 collegiate athletes is double that of men (Feingold and Hame, 2006).

Female athletes should be screened for the triad before participating in sports and educated about the body's need for nutrients (Mandel, 2008). Monitoring weight, energy level, menstrual cycles, and bone mineral density may help to prevent the occurrence of stress fractures in female athletes (Feingold and Hame, 2006).

index foods, fat intake, and fatty acid composition (Marcason, 2010). On the one hand, some experts conclude that no clear proof exists as to whether culprit foods such as dairy products, chocolate, and fatty foods affect acne (Davidovici and Wolf, 2010). Others are convinced that dairy products and high glycemic index foods influence hormonal and inflammatory factors thus increasing acne prevalence and severity (Ferdowsian and Levin, 2010). The suggested link to dairy foods speculates that milk contains hormones and bioactive molecules (Marcason, 2010).

Another theory is that hyperinsulinemia initiates an endocrine sequence, affecting sebaceous glands (Thiboutot and Strauss, 2002). Recent trials have demonstrated decreased acne after 12 weeks on a low glycemic load diet. (See **glycemic index** in Glossary.) Foods with a high glycemic load, such as white bread or potatoes, cause a rapid rise in blood glucose. Foods with a low glycemic index, such as high-fiber cereals or beans, cause a more gradual change in blood glucose.

Young men with acne on the low glycemic load diet lost more weight and showed improved insulin sensitivity compared to the control group (Smith et al., 2007). Tests also showed changes in the fatty acid composition of skin surface triglycerides that may influence sebum production. Further research is needed to clarify the role of diet in sebum gland physiology (Smith et al., 2008).

Overweight in Children and Adolescents

Childhood overweight or obesity is increasing throughout the Western world as well as in China (Daniels et al., 2005). Box 11-7 describes the diagnosis and prevalence of overweight and obesity in children and adolescents in the United States.

Compared to normal weight children, those who are overweight or obese have:

- 10 times the risk for hypertension as young adults
- 3 to 8 times greater risk of dyslipidemias
- Twice the risk of diabetes (CDC, 2005a).

The estimated risk of obesity persisting into adulthood ranges from 20% for a 4-year-old to 80% for adolescents (AAP, 2003, Reaffirmed 2006). Overweight that begins before the age of 8 and persists into adulthood is associated with a mean BMI of 41 compared to a BMI of 35 for those with adult-onset obesity (Dietz and Robinson, 2005). Childhood overweight threatens to reverse the decreases in cardiovascular mortality of the last 50 years (Daniels et al., 2005).

Some of the factors contributing to overweight and obesity in children are:

- Unwise food choices (the "Fast Food Nation")
- Inactivity, with television and computer games replacing active play

Box 11-7 ■ *Overweight in Childhood and Adolescence*

Technically, obesity refers to fatness, often measured by skinfold thickness, not weight. However, BMI is used as a surrogate measure of obesity because its components, height and weight, are readily available data and the growth charts for comparison are easily obtained. *See "Growth Charts" on DavisPlus or at http://www.cdc.gov/growthcharts.*

A BMI between the 5th and the 85th percentile is considered normal for children and adolescents. Values over the 95th percentile have been variously defined in this population as overweight or obese. By late adolescence, the 95th percentile is about equal to an adult BMI of 30, signifying obesity.

The term *obese* may be used to convey the serious medical nature of the condition to parents (Daniels et al., 2005). However, other experts recommend the term overweight as less negative and therefore preferable (Dietz and Robinson, 2005).

Figure 11-7 illustrates the increasing prevalence of overweight since 1976 in both genders and in all age groups. Table 11-17 shows the prevalence in two recent **NHANES surveys** by gender, age and ethnic group. Clearly, the distribution varies by ethnicity but overall the percentage of children and adolescents with BMIs above the 95th percentile continued to increase.

TABLE 11-17 ■ Percentages of Children at or above the 95th Percentile, NHANES 2003–2006 (1999–2000)

	MALES			FEMALES		
Ethnic Group	**2–5 Years**	**6–11 Years**	**12–19 Years**	**2–5 Years**	**6–11 Years**	**12–19 Years**
Non-Hispanic White	11.1 (8.8)	15.5 (12.0)	17.3 (12.8)	10.2* (11.5)	14.4 (11.6)	14.5 (12.4)
Non-Hispanic Black	13.3 (5.9)	18.6 (17.1)	18.5* (20.7)	16.6 (11.2)	24.0 (22.2)	27.7 (26.6)
Mexican American	18.8 (13.0)	27.5 (27.3)	22.1* (27.5)	14.5 (9.2)	19.7 (19.6)	19.9 (19.4)

*Decreased in more recent survey.
SOURCE: Adapted from Ogden (2002); Ogden, Carroll, and Flegal (2008).

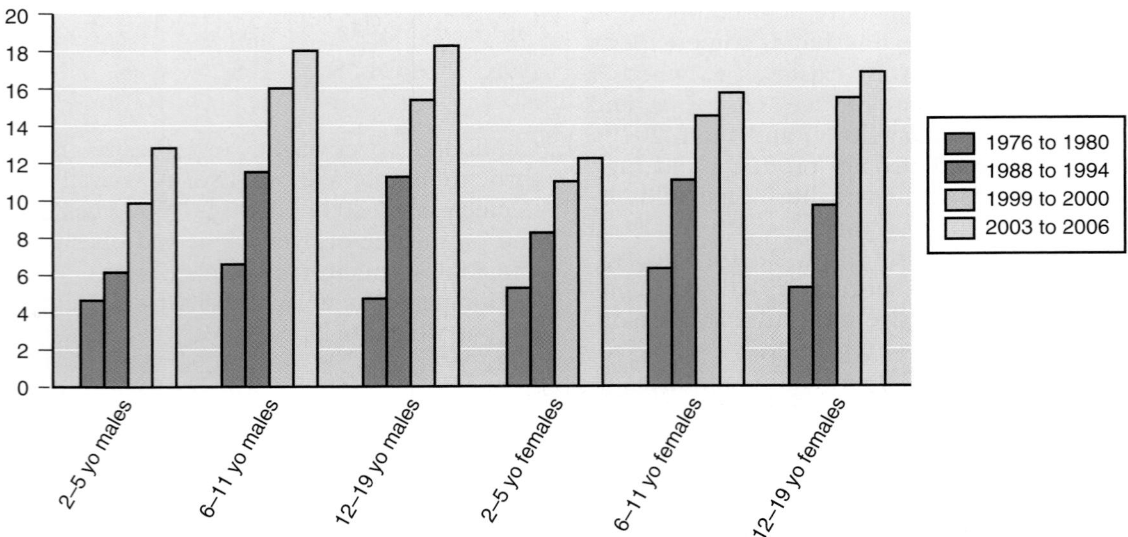

FIGURE 11-7 From 1976 through 2006, the percentages of males and females at or above the 95th percentile of BMI for age increased steadily in both sexes and in all age groups. (Constructed from data in Ogden [2002] and Ogden, Carroll, and Flegal [2008].)

- Decreased ability to self-regulate energy intake related to overcontrolling parents (AAP, 2003, Reaffirmed 2006)
- Inability of more than half of parents to see child as overweight (Parry et al., 2008)
- Failure of health professionals to communicate about overweight almost two-thirds of the time (CDC, 2005a)
- Genetics (see Genomic Gem 11-2)

Strategies to prevent overweight are listed in Table 11-18. These approaches cost less than treatment of established obesity and reach the greatest number of children.

Weight management is the subject of Chapter 16. Overweight children require careful supervision to maintain normal growth and development while reducing weight and adipose tissue. Treatment of obese children requires a multicomponent program encompassing diet, physical activity, nutrition counseling, and parent or caregiver participation (ADA, 2008).

The conditions permitting or encouraging overweight among youth have evolved over many years and have become embedded in the dominant culture that involves the food industry and marketing. No single change is going to reverse the trend. Multiple interventions and strategies are needed at all levels: individuals, families, schools, communities, and the nation.

Genomic Gem 11-2
It's in My Genes—Up to a Point

Up to 40% of variation in BMI is estimated to be genetic. Multiple genes are likely involved, including many affecting energy balance. Although obese parents produce the highest proportion of obese children, separating heredity from environment is problematic.

Evidence has emerged from family studies. The adult weight of adopted children is more strongly correlated with their biological parents than with the adoptive parents. Twins have similar BMIs, more so in identical than fraternal twins. This remains true whether the twins were raised together or apart (Hill, Catenacci, and Wyatt, 2006).

The 40% of BMI variance that is genetic may be treatable in the future. The 60% that is environmental can be modified with current information.

TABLE 11-18 ■ Strategies to Prevent Childhood Overweight

AGE GROUP	STRATEGY	BARRIERS	RATIONALE
Infant	Breastfeeding	Cultural norms about breastfeeding in general or in public or the workplace	Not proven to reduce obesity Many other health benefits May allow infant to control amount consumed better than with formula feeding
Toddler and Preschooler	Implement MyPyramid at home and in day care/preschool. Limit sweetened drinks. Begin 1% or fat-free dairy.	Parents/caregivers may be reluctant to change.	Need for full-fat dairy ceases at age 2
School-Age and Adolescent	Health curriculum Active, appealing physical education for all Offering healthy food and beverages in school	Ingrained curricular models Tendency to emphasize sports that for most youth are spectator events Advertising less healthy foods to youth	Gardening projects expand tastes for vegetables Include high-intensity activities such as endurance training and popular dance. Limit screen time. Limit carbonated beverages.
All Ages	Limit TV/computer game time to 2 hours/day. Eat breakfast daily. Encourage family meals. Serve recommended portion sizes. Calculate and plot BMIs yearly. Advocate for healthful food choices in restaurants. Discourage consumption of empty kilocalories. Expand access to supermarkets with reasonably priced produce. Provide safe environments for physical activity.		

Adapted from American Academy of Pediatrics (2003, Reaffirmed 2006); Daniels et al. (2005); Dietz and Robinson (2005); Davis et al. (2007); James et al. (2004); Mello, Studdert, and Brennan (2006); Morris and Zidenberg-Cherr (2002).

Keystones

- Breast milk is especially suited to the human infant, because the protein, fat, and carbohydrate in breast milk are tailored to the infant's digestive capabilities.
- After the age of 4 to 6 months, semisolid and then solid foods are added to the diet gradually, using carefully selected foods to avoid choking accidents.
- Nutritional problems in infancy include allergies, colic, and diarrhea, with the latter having the best documented treatment: oral rehydration therapy.
- Toddlers not only learn to accept new foods but also learn their culture's traditions surrounding food. Common nutritional problems for toddlers are iron deficiency and iron-deficiency anemia.
- Preschool and school-age children need healthy meals and snacks to sustain growth at a time when parents have less control over the child's eating while away from home.
- Most adolescents do not consume enough calcium to optimize their growth and development, and most girls lack iron in their diets. Self-prescribed reduction diets and poor choices of food are problems.
- Pediatric obesity is a major childhood health problem in the United States and the industrialized world, with the potential to spread in developing countries. Consequences are adult pathologies presenting decades early: hypertension, high blood cholesterol, and type 2 diabetes.

Ms. S is a school nurse in an inner-city high school. The principal asked for Ms. S's assistance in improving the students' nutritional and fitness states. A committee was formed that included students, teachers (classroom, home economics, and physical education), cafeteria and kitchen staff, parents, and a dietitian from a nearby hospital. The following plan reflects the program they devised after many meetings.

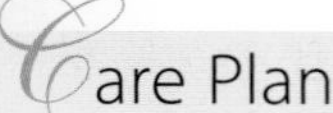

Care Plan

Subjective Data

Focus groups with students revealed their opinions of food and physical activity. ■ A school-wide survey solicited suggestions for classroom content, menu items, and physical activities.

Objective Data

Analysis of school lunch menus revealed an average fat content of 38% of kilocalories. ■ Vending machines in and around school offered only high-fat snacks or those with empty kilocalories. ■ Inspection of building usage identified 2 days after school when the gym was empty but other parts of the building were in use.

Analysis

Opportunity to improve students' nutrition and fitness

Plan

DESIRED OUTCOMES EVALUATION CRITERIA	ACTIONS/INTERVENTIONS	RATIONALE
Students will have increased opportunities to choose healthful foods in and around school.	Analyze sample lunch menus monthly to select areas to improve and to note progress.	Prioritizing changes is important to budget resources. Feedback to cafeteria staff will help maintain their interest and effort to improve.
	Include fresh fruit and vegetables on every lunch menu.	Fresh fruits and vegetables can offer vitamins, minerals, and fiber as well as decrease the dominance of high-fat items on the menu.
	Use student tasters to develop low-fat versions of popular dishes.	Palatability is critical in devising dishes the students will eat.
	Diversify contents of vending machines to include dairy products, fruit juices, cereal-and-dried-fruit snacks.	Items must be available to give students the opportunity to choose.
	Collaborate with biology teacher on fruit or vegetable growing as student projects.	Producing food items can stimulate interest in eating their own produce.
Students will demonstrate higher goals for their physical fitness.	Evaluate the place of physical education in the curriculum and campaign for needed changes.	To effectively prepare students for life requires offering skill development for an active life.
	Institute fitness testing in physical education classes.	Feedback to students allows them to track their progress.
	Ensure that 75% of time in physical education class is active.	Inactivity is a major contributor to overweight. Physical education class should not add to the problem.
	Institute activities students suggest, such as ethnic dances and games other than major sports in the United States.	Capitalizing on students' interests will recognize the value of their ideas. Later activities might broaden the scope to activities from other cultures.
	Arrange for supervised activities in the gym after school on the days the building would be open for other events. Vary the activities.	If community or volunteer leaders could be recruited, the cost would be minimized for the school and the students. A variety of activities would attract students other than the usual athletes who are active anyway.
Students will increase knowledge of healthful eating practices within time and budgetary constraints.	Design and promote a practical course in skills of modern life for both genders.	Practical courses will attract a different student than strictly academic courses do.
	Devise short instructional units on planning, purchasing, and preparing healthful food for classroom or after-school activity sessions.	Short units would give immediate feedback on the value of the information. Consuming the day's lesson is a bonus.
	Incorporate field trips to grocery stores as appropriate.	Expanding the students' perception of the choices open to them would offer the opportunity to increase variety in their diets.

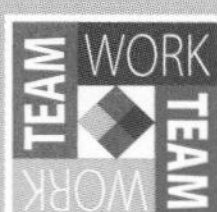

11-1

Community Committee Work

A committee was formed to improve the area surrounding the high school to permit opportunities for daily exercise for the students. Members included YMCA staff, neighborhood business owners, and city officials.

Subjective Parents described traffic congestion, lack of sidewalks and bike paths, and suspected undesirable activities occurring around the school.

Objective Police reports of auto-pedestrian accidents, assaults, thefts, and drug arrests indicated increased incidence compared to the district's other high schools.

Analysis School's environment a disincentive to walking or bicycling to and from school

Plan

Establish a Neighborhood Watch Program using business owners and nearby families.

Increase numbers of crossing guards and recruit volunteer monitors when students are coming and leaving school.

Improve traffic flow around the school.

Long term, construct bike paths and sidewalks to and from the surrounding neighborhoods

Critical Thinking Questions

1. What additional interventions might be used to improve nutritional intake and increase physical activity in these students?
2. Identify possible barriers to implementing the outlined program. Suggest strategies to overcome them.
3. It is possible that the committee's goals are not compatible with those of many of the students in this high school. How could the students be persuaded to value a more healthful lifestyle?

Chapter Review

1. A nurse in a clinic would identify which of the following infants as needing additional assessment of growth?
   a. Baby girl A, 4 months old, birth weight 7 lb 6 oz, present weight 14 lb 14 oz
   b. Baby boy B, 2 weeks old, birth weight 6 lb 10 oz, present weight 6 lb 11 oz
   c. Baby boy C, 6 months old, birth weight 8 lb 8 oz, present weight 14 lb 8 oz
   d. Baby girl D, 2 months old, birth weight 7 lb 2 oz, present weight 9 lb 10 oz
2. Which of the following are advantages of breast milk that formula does not provide?
   a. Less fat and cholesterol
   b. More antibodies and digestive enzymes
   c. More fluoride and iron
   d. More vitamin C and vitamin D
3. Which of the following foods would be appropriate for a 6-month-old infant?
   a. Cocoa-flavored wheat cereal, orange juice, and strained chicken
   b. Graham crackers, strained prunes, and stewed tomatoes
   c. Infant rice cereal, mashed banana, and strained squash
   d. Mashed potatoes, strained beets, and chopped hard-cooked egg
4. Families should be encouraged to provide fortified whole milk for children until the age of
   a. 18 months
   b. 2 years
   c. 36 months
   d. 4 years

Chapter Review—cont'd

5. Which of the following individuals is at greatest nutritional risk?
   a. 3-month-old infant being fed commercial formula
   b. 3-year-old child who drinks 3 cups of milk a day
   c. 8-year-old child who eats four chocolate chip cookies and drinks two glasses of milk after school
   d. 16-year-old girl who is pregnant and attempting weight loss

Clinical Analysis

1. Mrs. T is having her 2-month-old son checked in the well-baby clinic. She tells the nurse that the baby is not sleeping through the night yet. Mrs. T's mother advised her to start the infant on cereal to "fill him up" at bedtime. Despite the nurse's instructions, Mrs. T says she is going to try her mother's idea. Which of the following would be most important if Mrs. T chooses to start the cereal?
   a. Following the cereal with a bedtime bottle to wash it down
   b. Making cream of wheat very thin and feeding the baby with an eyedropper
   c. Putting infant cereal into a bottle and enlarging the nipple hole
   d. Using a spoon to feed the infant rice cereal mixed with formula
2. Ms. C has given a 24-hour dietary recall for her 18-month-old son. The nurse is alert to identify common causes of choking. To avoid choking accidents, which of the following groups of foods would be considered safest for a toddler?
   a. Apple quarters, green beans, and chicken noodle casserole
   b. Grapes, carrot strips, and macaroni and cheese
   c. Diced peaches, mashed potatoes, and spaghetti
   d. Watermelon chunks, cheese-stuffed celery, and sliced frankfurters
3. Ms. K has delivered a 3-lb 8-oz premature infant. She had planned to breastfeed. Upon which of the following statements should the nurse base her teaching?
   a. Human breast milk can be specially fortified for premature infants to increase its nutritive value.
   b. Because of their larger proportion of body weight as water, premature infants need supplemental water after every feeding.
   c. Formula feeding is advisable because room temperature feedings are better absorbed than those at body temperature.
   d. Breastfeeding a premature infant offers no advantage to the infant and is difficult for the mother because of the necessary supplements.

12

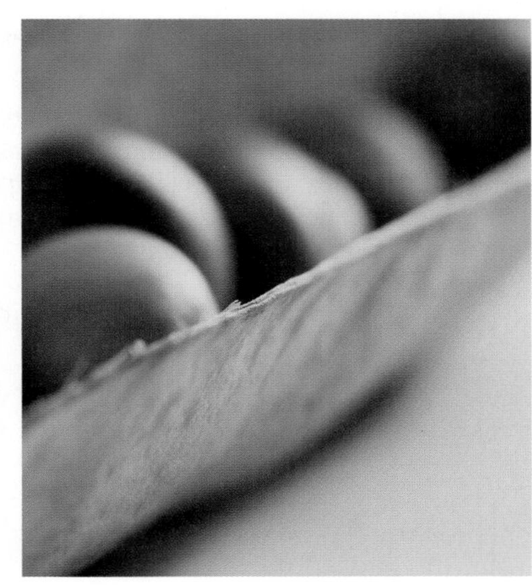

Life Cycle Nutrition: The Mature Adult

LEARNING OBJECTIVES

After completing this chapter, the student should be able to:

- Identify the foods and food groups most likely to be lacking or excessive in the diets of adults.
- Describe the changes in the older adult's body that affect nutritional status.
- Explain how a nutritional assessment of an older adult differs from that of a younger one.
- Illustrate ways in which food can be used to aid in the developmental tasks of adulthood.
- List several suggestions to improve food intake for older people in a variety of living situations.

The life cycle of human growth and development continues throughout the adult years. Both psychosocial and physical developments continue as a person matures. This chapter considers the impact on nutrition of the physiological and psychosocial changes that occur during young, middle, and older adult years. Because much of this book emphasizes the nutritional needs of young and middle-aged adults, the main focus of this chapter is the older adult. One major threat to health in adulthood is inactivity (Box 12-1), which can lead to overweight and obesity, the subject of Chapter 16.

Young Adulthood

Young adulthood spans ages 18 through 39. Not all 18-year-olds are adults, developmentally speaking; nor are all 40-year-olds middle-aged in thought or behavior.

Psychosocial Development

During the early years of young adulthood, the individual may be completing the adolescent task of identity. According to Erik Erikson, the developmental

Box 12-1 ■ *The Prevalence of Inactivity in Adults*

The *Healthy People 2010* initiative set a target of 20% of adults who report no leisure time physical activity. In 2004, only adults ages 18 to 29 achieved the goal. Overall, 31.9% of adults in the United States reported no leisure-time physical activity, a prevalence that steadily increases with age:

- Ages 18 to 29—19%
- Ages 30 to 44—22%
- Ages 45 to 64—25%
- Ages 65 to 74—28%
- Ages 75 and older—36%

A state-by-state report card showed the prevalence of inactivity ranged from 23.1% in Minnesota to 43.4% in Mississippi (CDC and The Merck Company Foundation, 2007c).

task of young adulthood is **intimacy** (Table 12-1). For example, people who delay commitment to a life partner until their 30s and 40s will probably be working at achieving intimacy; other 40-year-olds may be tackling the next task of generativity.

Nutrition in the Young Adult

Table 12-2 shows selected nutrients for which mean intake by age and gender is less than the DRIs.

Middle Adulthood

For this section, middle adult years are defined as those between ages 40 and 70 to match the DRI tables.

Psychosocial Development

Erikson's task of **generativity** involves serving as a mentor to the next generation. Teaching family members to prepare traditional foods, for example, may help a person achieve generativity.

Nutrition in Middle Adulthood

Table 12-2 shows selected nutrients for which mean intake by age and gender is less than the DRIs.

Older Adulthood

Changes in **life expectancy** and physiology affect the nutrition of older Americans.

Demographics of Aging

People are living longer. Older people constitute a larger proportion of the population. These trends are expected to continue, thus increasing the numbers of frail and dependent elderly.

Life Expectancy

In 1900, life expectancy at birth was 49 years. By 2003, however, life expectancy at birth was 77.6 years. By ethnic group, all values were record highs:

- 80.5 for white females
- 76.1 for black females
- 75.4 for white males
- 69.2 for black males (National Center for Health Statistics, 2005).

Compared to other countries, however, in 2004, the United States ranked 25th of 37 countries and territories for men's life expectancy and 23rd for women's life expectancy (Centers for Disease Control and Prevention [CDC], 2008b).

TABLE 12-1 ■ Erikson's Theory of Psychosocial Development in Maturity

STAGE OF LIFE	DEVELOPMENTAL TASK	OPPOSING NEGATIVE TRAIT	USE OF FOOD TO ACHIEVE TASK
Young Adult	Intimacy	Isolation	Arranging candlelight dinner
Middle Adult	Generativity	Stagnation	Teaching someone to prepare family favorite or ethnic dishes
Older Adult	Integrity	Despair	Using food fragrances or memories of food to reminisce

TABLE 12-2 ■ Mean Intakes of Adults Less than (X = <) DRIs

	YOUNG ADULT		MIDDLE-AGED		OLDER ADULT	
NUTRIENT	MALE	FEMALE	MALE	FEMALE	MALE	FEMALE
Fiber	X	X	X	X	X	X
Vitamin E	X	X	X	X	X	X
Vitamin K	X	X	X		X	X
Vitamin C				X		
Calcium		X	X	X	X	X
Iron		X		X		

Source: U.S. Department of Agriculture (2008).

Proportion of Population

Steady growth is seen in the proportion of the United States population older than the age of 65 years. It was:

- 4.1% in 1900
- 6.8% in 1940 (5 years after Social Security was enacted)
- 9.8% in 1970 (5 years after Medicare took effect)
- 12.6% in 2007 (range: 7% in Alaska to 17% in Florida) (U.S. Census Bureau, 2007).
- Estimated to be 20% by 2030 (71 million people) (CDC and The Merck Company Foundation, 2007a).

The increase in the aged population is evidence of successful public health efforts: improved sanitation, an increased concern for safety, and control of communicable diseases. Presently, the major causes of death in adults are heart disease, cancer, and stroke. All of them are linked to lifestyle, including diet.

Nursing Home Residency

Only about 5% of older adults live in nursing homes, but that proportion rises to 7.4% of persons age 75 and older and 16% of those 85 years old or older (El Nasser, 2007).

Psychosocial Development

Erikson's developmental task for older adults is **integrity**, in the sense of being whole or complete. Those who accomplish this task will look back on their lives as worthwhile.

A technique to help the older person achieve integrity is reminiscence. Asking an older person to recall special foods can stimulate reminiscence. Familiar food odors often will evoke memories.

Socially, older adults often must adapt to the loss of friends and relatives. The death of a spouse demands a tremendous adjustment. The accompanying depression and new responsibility for tasks the spouse performed may significantly affect an older person's food intake.

Physical Changes of Aging

Even without frank disease, the physical abilities of older adults diminish. "Middle-age spread" often gives way to dwindling bulk and waning strength.

The clinical guidelines on overweight and obesity in adults set a body mass index (BMI) of 25 as the upper limit of ideal weight for all adults regardless of age. Among men and women 65 years of age and older, however, a BMI in the overweight range is not associated with a significantly increased risk of mortality (Janssen and Mark, 2007). This finding does not negate the evidence linking overweight to arthritis, diabetes, coronary heart disease, and other conditions that may impact the older person's quality of life.

Integumentary System

Many changes take place in the skin as a person ages. As subcutaneous fat is lost, the skin becomes dry and wrinkled. Less elasticity is present to spring back after a pinch to the forearm, the usual site assessed for hydration status. The skin of the forehead or over the breastbone is a more reliable site in the elderly client than the forearm.

The older adult also loses some of the ability to synthesize vitamin D from sunshine, so that it may take twice as much sun exposure without sunscreens as necessary in a younger person to produce a given amount of vitamin D.

Sensory System

Four senses become markedly less acute as a person ages: vision, hearing, taste, and smell. Because the sense receptors do not deteriorate equally, some of the sense loss is attributed to changes in the central nervous system. Extensive variation exists among individuals.

EYES

Vision is often impaired. The older person sees reds, oranges, and yellows better than blues and violets. Clouding of the lens of the eye—cataract formation—decreases overall vision. Older eyes do not adjust well to glare such as is found in some supermarkets.

These vision changes may make grocery shopping burdensome. The fine-print labels on food items may be illegible to the elderly. Food preparation may become not only difficult but also hazardous if the person cannot see adequately. Colorful foods with visual appeal in meals for the elderly might stimulate the appetite and compensate for decreased taste sensation (Evans, Crogan, and Shultz, 2005).

EARS

The sound receptors in the inner ear deteriorate. First to be lost is the ability to perceive high tones. The older person with poor hearing usually hears men's voices better than women's. Hearing aids do not fully compensate for the hearing loss. In fact, they often magnify sideline noise to the point of distracting the wearer. The result may be social isolation when it becomes too laborious to interact with others. Socializing at meals may become embarrassing or frustrating, and older people may avoid such interaction.

NOSE AND TONGUE

For the sense of taste to function well, the sense of smell must also be intact. Food tastes bland when a person has a head cold. The sense of smell declines considerably after the seventh decade of life so that more than 75% of individuals older than the age of 85 years have major impairments (Boyce and Shone, 2006). Although the sense of smell is frequently more affected by aging than is the sense of taste, both faculties are important to help protect the person from noxious elements in the environment such as spoiled or burning food or gas leaks.

Chemical taste receptors are concentrated on the tongue's surface but also are located at the base of the tongue, on the soft palate, and in other areas of the nasopharynx. Saliva acts as a solvent to present the foods to the taste buds. If the mouth is dry, taste sensations are indistinct.

Taste receptors have been traditionally known to recognize sweet, sour, salty, and bitter sensations. Recently receptors have been identified for *umami*, a sensation described as savory or rich. It is caused by the amino acid glutamine in its free form and is associated with monosodium glutamate (MSG). Using MSG in foods such as soups permits a reduction in sodium content without altering palatability (Bellisle, 2008). Despite earlier reports, decades of research have failed to demonstrate a clear and consistent relationship between MSG ingestion and the development of the so-called "Chinese restaurant syndrome" comprising bronchospasm, urticaria, angio-edema, and rhinitis (Williams and Woessner, 2009). Neither have consistent data supported MSG as a trigger for asthma and migraine headache exacerbations or the existence of an MSG-sensitive subset of the population (Freeman, 2006).

Self-reported prevalence of diminished sense of taste was only 1.65% in a nationally representative sample. Whether or not this alone constitutes nutritional risk is questionable (Mattes, 2002). Both sex and age influence performance on taste tests, with older persons performing more poorly than younger ones and men typically scoring worse than women (Soter et al., 2008). Adequate individual assessment of intake should determine the causes of nutritional risk.

Reported sensory losses are uneven. Unlike sensitivity for sweet and sour that remains intact in older clients, the perceptivity for salt and bitter declines with age (Winkler et al., 1999). A possible physiological mechanism is suggested by discovering neurons that are sensitive to salts and acids also respond to bitter stimuli (Travers and Geran, 2009). If a person is oversalting his food as a result of a diminished taste sensation for salt, alternate seasonings that can be used to decrease sodium consumption are listed in Chapter 18. A technique to increase taste sensation in geriatric clients is including brushing the tongue as part of oral hygiene.

Gastrointestinal System

Particularly crucial to nutrition is gastrointestinal function. Hundreds of processes are required for the proper digestion, absorption, and metabolism of foods. Many functions of the gastrointestinal system decline significantly in older people.

DENTAL HEALTH

Older individuals are not immune to dental caries. In fact, when exposed by gum disease, the tooth root, lacking enamel, is particularly vulnerable to caries, causing increased occurrence in the elderly population. Contributing factors include:

- Inadequate oral hygiene
- Infrequent dental examinations and cleanings
- Salivary gland dysfunction
- Frequent snacking
- Removable partial dentures (*Merck Manual of Geriatrics*, 2005).

In contrast, adults who were free of root caries consumed 50% more cheese and 25% more milk than persons with caries (DePaola et al., 2006). Fluoride applied to the teeth or fluoridated water prevents caries among adults of all ages (Griffin et al., 2007).

The percentage of 65- to 74-year-old adults in the United States who were **edentulous** (having no permanent teeth) was:

- 55% in 1957
- 24% in 1999–2002 (12.4% in Connecticut to 42.9% in West Virginia) (CDC and The Merck Company Foundation, 2007b).

The major cause of tooth loss in the older adult is not dental caries but **periodontal disease,** which affects the gums (gingiva) and apparatus attaching the tooth to the jaw. Dentures, like hearing aids, only partially compensate, so that dentures are about 20% as efficient as natural teeth.

Furthermore, a denture cannot be effective if the underlying tissue is in poor condition. Persons with upper dentures that cover the palate containing taste receptors lose some taste sensation and are also subject to impaired swallowing.

Box 12-2 illustrates a self-administered dental screening form designed to alert older people to their need for dental care. It was validated with a clinical dental examination on 165 people 65 to 94 years old, correctly identifying 82% of those with dental disease. Notice that not all of the items are weighted equally.

The production of saliva decreases sharply in older adults, a condition called **xerostomia.** Chewing and swallowing become more difficult, and food intake may be affected. Also, with age, less mucus and smaller quantities of enzymes are secreted.

OTHER CONDITIONS

Atrophic gastritis, a chronic inflammation of the stomach lining with decreases in size of the glands and mucous membranes, occurs in 10% to 30% of the U.S. population older than the age of 50 (Bales and Ritchie, 2006). An extreme case is **achlorhydria,** the absence of hydrochloric acid in the stomach.

Either of these conditions may interfere with protein digestion and with vitamin and mineral absorption. Vitamin B_{12} may remain locked to the food protein, and less nonheme iron will be absorbed in the more alkaline environment. Heme iron does not require stomach acid, and thus is unaffected by atrophic gastritis (Bales and Ritchie, 2006).

Intestinal **motility** decreases because of lessened muscle tone. Medications may interfere with electrolyte balance, also diminishing muscle tone. Despite a decrease in size because of decreased hepatic blood flow, the aging liver appears to function relatively well (Anantharaju, Feller, and Chedid, 2002).

Box 12-2 ■ *The D-E-N-T-A-L Screening Survey Form*

Certain dental conditions interfere with proper nutritional intake and possibly dispose a person to involuntary weight loss. Please answer the following questions regarding your dental health by placing a check before the conditions that apply to you.

	Point Value
___ Dry mouth	(2)
___ Eating difficulty	(1)
___ No recent dental care (within 2 years)	(1)
___ Tooth or mouth pain	(2)
___ Alteration or change in food selection	(1)
___ Lesions, sores, or lumps in the mouth	(2)

If you have scored more than 2 points on this survey, you may have a dental problem that could be affecting your overall health and general well-being. We urge you to seek dental care as soon as possible for a check-up.

Source: Bush et al. (1996), with permission.

Urinary System

The size of the kidneys increases until 40 or 50 years of age but then decreases. Changes at the cellular level have been elucidated, including DNA mutations and the effects of oxidative stress (Martin and Sheaff, 2007).

The aging kidney loses some ability to concentrate urine and to conserve sodium. Mild hyponatrenia, the commonest electrolyte imbalance in the older population, is associated with gait and attention deficits, resulting in higher frequency of falls. In one study, asymptomatic hyponatremia attributed to diuretic or antidepressant drugs or to **idiopathic** syndrome of inappropriate secretion of antidiuretic hormone (**SIADH**) was associated with 9.2% of all bone fractures in ambulatory persons age 65 or older (Gankam Kengne et al., 2008).

This compromised kidney function makes urine samples less reliable for nutrient analyses in the elderly. Two laboratory tests frequently are used to assess renal function: **blood urea nitrogen (BUN)** and serum creatinine. An increase in the BUN level usually indicates a decrease in kidney function. It may also be elevated in dehydration or if excessive protein is presented to the liver for breakdown, as with a high-protein diet or with gastrointestinal bleeding. Because clients with even slightly elevated BUNs may not be able to excrete the waste products from protein metabolism, caregivers must be judicious about giving high-protein nutritional supplements to older people with elevated BUNs.

Creatinine, an end product of creatine metabolism, is excreted very efficiently by the healthy kidney. The amount of creatinine produced is proportional to the individual's skeletal muscle mass and remains fairly constant in the absence of extensive muscle damage. The serum creatinine test has the advantage over the BUN of being little affected by dehydration, malnutrition, or liver function.

Creatinine levels may not detect decreased kidney function, however, if a slow decline in renal function occurs simultaneously with a slow decrease in muscle mass, as occurs in the aging process. Consequently, both tests may be performed to obtain a more complete diagnostic picture.

Musculoskeletal System

The major loss of body mass in the older adult involves muscle mass. Between the ages of 25 and 75, the average person loses 15% of lean body mass, which for a man may represent 24 pounds of muscle that is replaced by 22 pounds of fat (Brown, 2008). Because muscle is a more metabolically active tissue than fat, energy needs decline with the diminished muscle mass. The losses are reversible, however. Even in the elderly, skeletal muscle protein anabolism can be stimulated by high biologic value protein foods (Symons et al., 2007).

Nutritional deprivation and catabolic states can affect the muscles of respiration in the chest and diaphragm. Because the older person relies more on the diaphragm than the chest muscles to breathe, a full stomach may impede breathing to a greater extent than in a younger person.

Perhaps more noticeable than the overall loss of muscle is the loss of height in older people. Although individuals vary widely, between the ages of 20 and 70, the average height loss is:

- 5.6 centimeters (2.2 inches) in men and
- 6.8 centimeters (2.7 inches) in women (Shils, 2006).

A major cause of this loss of height is osteoporosis. After age 30, bone loss occurs at a rate of about 0.3% to 0.5% per year. Beginning with menopause, bone loss accelerates in women to about 3% to 5% per year for 5 to 7 years (Raisz, 2008). In calculating the BMI, to avoid the influence of "shrinkage" in the height of aged clients, the use of the person's height at age 50 is recommended (Bales and Ritchie, 2006).

Older joint surfaces are roughened by arthritis. By age 50, half of all adults have some osteoarthritis. The resulting pain and stiffness impairs the use of the hands for opening jars, chopping raw foods, and cutting cooked foods at the table. Arthritis also can affect the mandibular joint of the jaw used for chewing.

Nervous System

For many people, deteriorating brain function is the most feared loss of old age, one that is shared by their loved ones, who may see the person gradually fade from the present with the onslaught of dementia. By the time a person reaches old age, the brain has endured a lifetime of stressors but some individuals weather the storms better than others. Some significant changes include:

- Brain shrinkage with increasing age with resulting changes at all levels from molecules to structure (Peters, 2006)
- Brain volume decreases about
  - 0.1% to 0.2% per year between the ages of 30 and 50 and
  - 0.3% to 0.5% per year after the age of 70, with the resulting space filled by the ventricular system (Esiri, 2007)
- Blood flow to the brain decreases because of narrowing of the arteries.
- Thirst sensation becomes less operative, increasing the risk of uncompensated dehydration. Mortality from heat stroke rises sharply in people older than 60 years.

Several factors influence brain function in the elderly. More years of education, physical exercise, and cognitive stimulation are positively related to better brain function. Nutritional factors of benefit to the aging brain include:

- Vitamins B_6, B_{12}, and folic acid
- High intake of polyunsaturated fatty acids (Esiri, 2007).

Dietary omega-3 fatty acids play a role in the prevention of some disorders including depression and dementia, particularly Alzheimer's disease. Deficiency of omega-3 fatty acids can prevent the renewal of membranes, thus accelerating cerebral aging (Bourre, 2005).

ALZHEIMER'S DISEASE

The prevalence of Alzheimer's disease increases from 1% at age 65 to approximately 40% to 50% by the age 95. Although the cause of the disease is not fully understood, genetics is known to affect its onset (Wang and Ding, 2008). See Genomic Gem 12-1.

Decreased brain levels of docosahexaenoic acid (DHA) are associated with aging (Uauy and Dangour, 2006). Consumption of omega-3 fatty acids (particularly DHA, for example, as obtained in one fish meal weekly) and antioxidants such as vitamin E appear to

Genomic Gem 12-1
Alzheimer's Disease

Although the cause of Alzheimer's disease has not been fully elucidated, gene mutations may complicate the relationship of nutrients to the risk of the disease. Likewise, genetics plays a role in its onset.

One variant of the apolipoprotein E gene, the *APO E2* allele, is overrepresented in centenarians and protects against Alzheimer's disease. This allele is suggested to influence successful aging (Esiri, 2007).

The mixed results in studies of vitamin E in relation to Alzheimer's disease may result from the varied genomes of the people recruited. Vitamin E from food has been associated with a reduced risk of Alzheimer's disease but only in people without a polymorphism in the apolipoprotein E gene, the *APO E4* allele (Ghosh, Skinner, and Laing, 2007). The same *APO E4* allele is associated with lower cognitive performance at age 11 and age 80 and is a risk factor for late-onset Alzheimer's Disease (Esiri, 2007).

Screening tests for persons at high risk of the disease are currently available and may help the clients and their families prepare for the hardships of life with Alzheimer's disease (Wang and Ding, 2008).

lower the risk of Alzheimer's disease. Confirmatory evidence from clinical trials is necessary to prove causation (Morris, 2009). Special concerns of nourishing clients with dementia are covered in Clinical Application 12-1.

PARKINSON'S DISEASE

Another neurological disease, more common in older people than in younger ones, is Parkinson's disease. In the United States, at least 500,000 people are thought to suffer from Parkinson's disease, and about 50,000 new cases, with an average age at onset of 60 years, are reported annually (National Institute of Neurological Disorders and Stroke, 2004). Early research indicates dietary vitamin E may protect against Parkinson's disease, but confirmation by randomized clinical trials is needed (Etminan, Gill, and Samii, 2005). See the section on vitamins under Nutrition in the Older Adult later in this chapter. Box 12-3 details some nutritional ramifications of the disease.

Clinical Application 12-1

Nutrition and Dementia

Care of clients with dementia challenges family and health-care providers because eating is recognized to be fundamental to life. Clients with dementia progressively lose the ability for self-care, including feeding. A simple tool to assess the client's level of functioning is the Eating Behavior Scale (below). The six items assessed direct the caregivers to an appropriate strategy to assist the client without usurping a task the client still can perform.

Managing the client's environment is a major part of the care of the client with dementia.

- Provide quiet, adequately lit dining rooms.
- Offer clients the same seats to achieve familiarity.
- Serve one course at a time.
- Supply appropriate but limited utensils, large-handled if necessary.
- Select dishes with high sides to enable the client to scoop up the food onto a spoon.
- Serve finger foods that are within the client's capabilities.

Clients with dementia must be reminded of the steps involved in self-feeding:

- Putting the food on the spoon
- Directing it to the mouth
- Swallowing

Verbal cues or guiding the client's hand can get him or her started or keep the process going. Despite the surroundings, common courtesies can be effective in reminding clients of social expectations and in maintaining their dignity. For example:

- Introducing the client to the other people at the table
- Providing a cup rather than a carton for milk
- Offering foods separately rather than mixing them all together (Kayser-Jones and Schell, 1997; Tully et al., 1997)

The effect of music in the dining room is the most researched intervention for dementia (Watson and Green, 2006). Selections with a slow tempo—at or below the human heart rate—tend to dampen environmental noises that might startle clients. Fewer incidents of agitated behaviors occurred during the weeks that music was played compared with weeks without music (Denney, 1997). Since staff also heard the music, perhaps some of the effect was obtained by relaxing them.

A multidisciplinary project to improve nutrition in clients with late-stage dementia not only achieved that but also decreased the distress of clients and nursing staff caused by the clients' swallowing problems. Among the interventions used were:

- Thickened liquids
- Three levels of dysphagia diets
- Daylong snacks
- Unbalanced diets if those were all that the clients would take, under the pragmatic principle that any food is better than no food (Biernacki and Barratt, 2001)

Tube feeding (see Chapter 14) has not been shown to improve the specific outcomes of survival, pressure ulcers, nutrition, and aspiration pneumonia in dementia clients (Garrow et al., 2007).

National Institutes of Health Warren G. Magnuson Clinical Center Nursing Department†

EATING BEHAVIOR SCALE (EBS)

Patient # _____	Admit date _____	Observation date ____
Observer initials _____	Meal start _____	Finished ______
Patient room _____	Day room _____	Time, minutes ______
Circle only one answer: ___	Maximum score = 18_____	Total = ______

OBSERVED BEHAVIOR	I.*	V.**	P.***	D.****
Was the patient—				
1. Able to initiate eating?	3	2	1	0
2. Able to maintain attention to meal?	3	2	1	0
3. Able to locate all food?	3	2	1	0
4. Appropriately using utensils?	3	2	1	0
5. Able to bite, chew, and swallow without choking?	3	2	1	0
6. Able to terminate meal?	3	2	1	0

Comments

____
____
____
____

*I. = Independent.
**V. = Verbal prompts.
***P. = Physical assistance.
****D. = Dependent.
†For printing, also available on DavisPlus.

Endocrine System

The average older person is slowing down. Resting energy expenditure (REE) decreases, especially in the brain, skeletal muscle, and heart. The older adult's REE may be 10% to 12% less than that of a younger person's. Lost muscle mass is replaced, if at all, by adipose tissue that is less active metabolically than muscle.

The pancreas often secretes inadequate amounts of insulin or the body loses its ability to utilize insulin, leading to diabetes mellitus (see Chapter 17). Receptors in the kidney for antidiuretic hormone (ADH) may function poorly to produce a less effective response. Levels of aldosterone also decrease with age. Both of these changes make maintaining correct fluid volume more difficult for an older person than for a younger one.

Box 12-3 ■ *Parkinson's Disease*

Parkinson's disease is a progressive neurological disorder characterized by degeneration of neurons in the area of the brain that controls movement. This degeneration causes a shortage of dopamine, a neurotransmitter or brain-signaling chemical (National Institute of Neurological Disorders and Stroke, 2004). Among the signs of the disease are:

- Tremors
- Rigidity
- Loss of facial expression
- Gait disorders.

The above signs could impact the ability to obtain, prepare, and consume food. Swallowing changes occur from the earliest stages of Parkinson's disease, even in clients without dysphagia (Miller et al., 2006).

An extensive Swedish case study of 10 women with Parkinson's disease illustrates some of the difficulty encountered by these clients with a median age of 75 years and median disease duration of 10 years. Five of the women lived with spouses; five lived alone.

	Married, Living with Spouse	Living Alone	Adaptation
Shopped for self	One woman	Two women	Shopped in early morning and in small shops to avoid tiring crowds and distances.
Cooked own meals	Three women	Three women	Simplified cooking and used ready-cooked foods.
Difficulty feeding oneself	Four women	Five women	Took small portions, especially with guests. Ate from packages. Used spoon or fork to avoid spills. Employed both hands to drink.
Swallowing problems	Three women	Three women	Thickened liquids for better control.
Deteriorated sense of smell	Four women	Five women	Imagined taste of familiar foods.

Despite these problems, three of the married women were overweight and one was obese. Of the four single women reporting food intake, three were of normal weight and one was morbidly obese with a BMI of 40 (Andersson and Sidenvall, 2001).

It can be readily seen that providing for nutritional needs for individuals with Parkinson's disease can be a day-in-day-out, all-day process. Other impairments of movement may impact clients in similar ways.

Cardiovascular System

As the older adult continues to age, cardiac output and heart rate decrease. In response to exercise, the heart rate does not increase as effectively as in youth, nor does it return to normal as rapidly. Because of this diminishment, the elderly are at risk for diseases of the heart. Dietary modifications for heart disease are included in Chapter 18.

A part of the cardiovascular system, the immune system, is less effective in the older person than in the younger one. In apparently healthy elderly, micronutrient supplements may enhance the immune response.

At greatest risk of immunodeficiency are persons with protein–kilocalorie malnutrition that is associated with increased complication rates (mainly infections) and death. Repeated challenges to the immune system can deplete body reserves, leading to lower nutritional status and increased fragility (Lesourd, 2006). Table 12-3 shows some of the effects of aging on **humoral** and **cellular immunity.**

TABLE 12-3 ■ Some Effects of Aging on Immunity

TYPE OF IMMUNITY	LYMPHOCYTES INVOLVED	FUNCTION	EFFECT OF AGING
Humoral	B-cells	Produce antibodies against foreign antigens.	Slightly fewer antibodies produced but less specific and less effective
Cellular	T-cells	Protect against viruses, fungi, malignant cells, and foreign tissue grafts without using antibodies. Autoimmune reactions are a dysfunction of this mechanism.	Declines with age but only after age 90 in very healthy people (Lesourd, 2006).

Nutrition in the Older Adult

Table 12-2 shows selected nutrients for which mean intake by age and gender is less than the DRIs. Food pyramids can be used for assessing and counseling.

Food Pyramids

MyPyramid can serve the older adult well because age and activity level are two of the data fields required for computation. Tables 12-4 and 12-5 compare MyPyramid recommendations for a woman with the same characteristics during three different decades of life. A greater proportion of adults age 65 or older eat five or more fruits and vegetables daily than do younger adults. Still, compliance varies:

- 19.5% in Mississippi meet the five-a-day recommendation
- 29.8% of 65+ adults overall
- 40.2% in Vermont (CDC and The Merck Company Foundation, 2007d).

A special Modified Food Guide Pyramid for People Over 70 Years of Age appears as Figure 12-1. Eight servings of water provide a foundation of the pyramid, and symbols for fiber have been added to emphasize the food groups that are good sources of fiber. A pennant at the top of the pyramid signifies

TABLE 12-4 ■ MyPyramid Daily Recommendations for an Elderly Woman*

	65 YEARS OLD	75 YEARS OLD	85 YEARS OLD
Grains	6 oz	5 oz	5 oz
Vegetables	2.5 cups	2 cups	2 cups
Fruits	1.5 cups	1.5 cups	1.5 cups
Milk	3 cups	3 cups	3 cups
Meat/beans	5 oz	5 oz	5 oz
Oils	5 tsp	5 tsp	5 tsp
Kilocalories	1800	1600	1600

*Calculated for a woman 5 ft 4 in. tall, 145 lb, exercising >30 min/day.

TABLE 12-5 ■ MyPyramid Weekly Recommendations for an Elderly Woman*

	65 YEARS OLD	75 YEARS OLD	85 YEARS OLD
Dark green vegetables	3 cups	2 cups	2 cups
Orange vegetables	2 cups	1.5 cups	1.5 cups
Dry beans and peas	3 cups	2.5 cups	2.5 cups
Starchy vegetables	3 cups	2.5 cups	2.5 cups
Other vegetables	6.5 cups	5.5 cups	5.5 cups

*Calculated for a woman 5 ft 4 in. tall, 145 lb, exercising >30 min/day.

calcium, vitamin D, and vitamin B_{12} supplementation (Russell, Rasmussen, and Lichtenstein, 1999).

Energy Nutrients and Energy Balance

Older adults need about 5% fewer kilocalories per decade after the age of 40. Small changes have been recommended in intakes from carbohydrates, fats, and protein. As with younger people, the simplest criterion for the suitability of intake is the maintenance of a healthy body weight. Energy expenditure varies within the elderly population.

CARBOHYDRATES AND FIBER

Older people should derive 50% to 60% of their kilocalories from carbohydrates. The RDA for carbohydrate, based on its role as primary energy source for the brain, is 130 grams per day, the same as for younger adults.

The AI for fiber is 30 grams per day for men 50 years and older and 21 grams for women in the same age group. Both of the values are less than recommended for younger adults. Like among younger adults, the mean amount actually consumed by older adults is less than the DRI (U.S. Department of Agriculture, 2008).

FATS

Fats should contribute 20% to 35% of the day's kilocalories. Limiting fats should also increase comfort, because fat absorption is delayed in older people, leading to a feeling of fullness. Particularly among the elderly, rigid application of diet rules may be inappropriate. Restricting fat by eliminating whole milk and eggs, which are easily eaten and relatively inexpensive, could endanger nutrition in the short term for uncertain long-term benefits.

PROTEIN

Mean nutrient intake data indicate the RDA for protein is exceeded by older adults (U.S. Department of Agriculture, 2008). Moderately increasing daily protein intake beyond 0.8 gram per kilogram of body weight may enhance muscle protein anabolism and reduce the progressive loss of muscle mass that accompanies aging. Some experts maintain that nitrogen balance studies indicate a protein intake of 1.0 to 1.3 grams per kilogram of body weight per day is required to maintain nitrogen balance in the healthy elderly (Morais, Chevalier, and Gougeon, 2006).

Although little evidence links high protein intakes to increased risk for impaired kidney function in healthy individuals, a prudent course would be to assess renal function of older individuals before

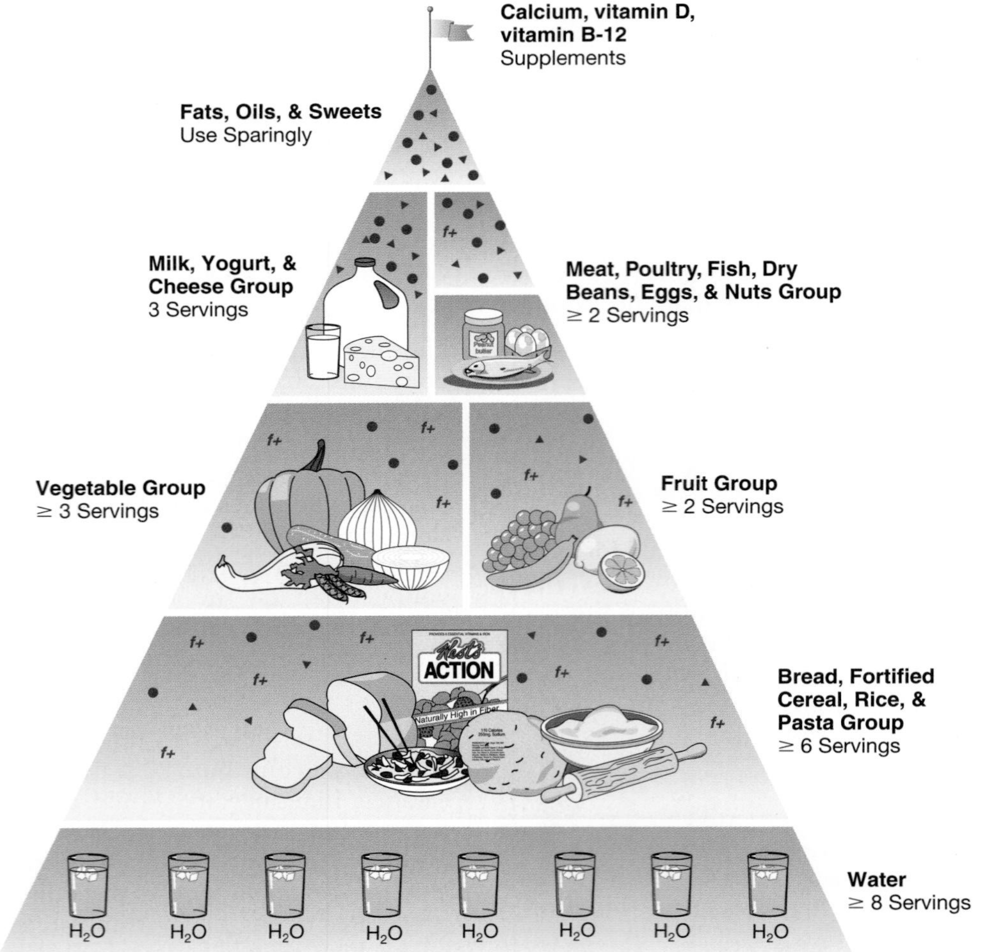

FIGURE 12-1 The Modified Food Guide Pyramid for People Over 70 Years of Age. (Reprinted from Russell, Rasmussen, and Lichtenstein, J Nutr 129:752, 1999, with permission of American Society for Nutritional Sciences.)

embracing a higher protein intake (Paddon-Jones et al., 2008).

Although serum albumin levels are used as a measure of body protein stores, for a given individual, serum albumin levels can indicate nutritional status, pathology, or both. The prevalence of malnutrition in hospitalized medical–surgical clients was reported to be 38% to 62%, depending on the criteria used, possibly testifying to the interconnectedness of disease and malnutrition (Heimburger, 2006). Protein–kilocalorie malnutrition has been reported in 30% to 50% of nursing home residents (Bales and Ritchie, 2006).

Protein status is an important component in the body's defense system. In seniors with protein–energy malnutrition (PEM), decreased functions in all aspects of immunity are strongly related to protein nutritional status. Refeeding can boost immune response in clients with inflammation but at a lower rate than in those without inflammatory responses (Lesourd, 2006).

EXERCISE

Older adults should have at least 30 minutes a day of moderate activity, which can be taken at one long or in two or three short sessions. For previously sedentary persons, an exercise routine should be introduced gradually after medical clearance is received. MyPyramid recommends men older than 40 years of age and women older than 50 years of age should check with their health-care providers before starting or increasing physical activity.

An objective of *Healthy People 2010* is for 30% of adults to perform strength training activities on two or more days per week. Strength training decreases muscle mass loss, functional decline, and fall-related injuries. In 2004, 22% of men and 18% of women achieved the goal, but only 14% of men and 11% of women older than the age of 65 did so (CDC, 2006).

Vitamins

The RDAs/AIs for vitamins D and B_6 are increased for older adults. The RDA for vitamin B_{12} specifies fortified foods or supplements as sources because of the possibility of malabsorption. Mean nutrient intakes from food for older adults are below the RDAs/AIs for vitamins E and K (see Table 12-2).

VITAMIN E

Besides functioning as a scavenger of free radicals, vitamin E has been linked to immune and cognitive functions. Oxidative stress has been shown to contribute to the etiology of dementia. Although antioxidant treatment has been demonstrated to be effective in cellular and animal research, only inconclusive results have been found with humans (Ancelin, Christen, and Ritchie, 2007).

One difficulty with pinpointing effects of vitamin E is its various forms with differing functions. Tocotrienols possess powerful neuroprotective, anticancer, and cholesterol lowering properties that are often not exhibited by tocopherols. At minute concentrations, alpha-tocotrienol, not alpha-tocopherol, prevents neurodegeneration. Thus, lumping all vitamin E effects into a judgment about "vitamin E" is not advised (Sen, Khanna, and Roy, 2006). In humans, combined intake of the 8 different forms of tocopherol reduces oxidative stress and inflammation to a greater degree than alpha-tocopherol alone (Morris, 2009).

VITAMIN K

Vitamin K can be depleted relatively more quickly than the other fat-soluble vitamins. Besides its role in blood clotting, vitamin K contributes to bone metabolism. Based on the current evidence from epidemiologic and intervention studies, insufficient evidence exists to recommend routine supplementation of vitamin K for optimal bone health (Francucci et al., 2007). However, vitamin K deficiency has been shown to contribute to the occurrence of hip fractures in elderly women. Therefore, supplementation is recommended in conjunction with drug therapy for established osteoporosis in clients with vitamin K deficiency (Iwamoto, Takeda, and Sato, 2006).

Outside of deficiency states, one might suspect the vitamin K antagonist, warfarin, would impinge on bone health. In elderly clients receiving warfarin, however, its use was not associated with increased risk of nonspine fractures (Mamdani et al., 2003; Woo et al., 2008).

Minerals

Calcium has been given an increased AI for older persons. Mean intake from food for men older than 70 years of age was 881 milligrams, for women 752 milligrams (U.S. Department of Agriculture, 2008). Those intakes are 73% and 63% of the respective AIs.

In the elderly, calcium was found to be equally bioavailable from skim milk, calcium-fortified orange juice, or calcium carbonate (Martini and Wood, 2002). Whether from food or supplements, calcium intake should be spread out throughout the day, with 600 milligrams or less being consumed at each meal.

Supplements, except calcium citrate, should be taken with meals to ensure an acid environment to optimize absorption (Kamel, 2006).

In contrast, sodium intake is more than double the AIs for older adults. See Table 12-6.

Water

No AI for water has been established for individuals older than the age of 30 years. Healthy older adults need enough fluid intake to produce about 1.5 liters of light yellow urine in 24 hours.

Loss of sphincter muscle tone in women and difficulty urinating in men may prompt older people to limit their fluid intake, a practice that is not recommended. Omitting fluids in the 2 hours before bedtime, however, may help decrease the frequency of nocturia and nighttime incontinence.

One of the early signs of dehydration in the elderly is confusion, which may be difficult to ascertain in clients with dementia or altered consciousness. Signs of dehydration in the elderly are listed in

TABLE 12-6 ■ Sodium Intake in Older Adults

	50–59 YEARS	60–69 YEARS	70+ YEARS
Adequate Intake	1.3 grams	1.3 grams	1.2 grams
Men's Actual Intake	4.0 grams	3.7 grams	3.1 grams
Women's Actual Intake	3.0 grams	2.6 grams	2.4 grams

Data from U.S. Department of Agriculture (2008).

Table 12-7. The increase in pulse rate on standing is an appropriate assessment technique for fluid volume status in the elderly except when heart disease and its treatments would block the physiological response.

Clients who are immobilized may need as many as 12 to 14 glasses of fluid per day. Immobility increases the calcium loss from bones. The calcium then circulates in the blood until the kidney excretes the excess. A large fluid intake dilutes the urine so that the calcium does not form stones. A determined effort to increase fluid intake in nursing home residents is recounted in Clinical Application 12-2.

TABLE 12-7 ■ Signs of Dehydration in the Elderly

BODY SYSTEM	SIGN
Skin and Mucous Membranes	Skin warm and dry Decreased turgor; pinch test may be more accurate over the sternum or on the forehead than on the hand. Furrowed tongue Elevated temperature
Cardiovascular	Elevated pulse
Urinary	Increased specific gravity Increased urinary sodium
Musculoskeletal	Weakness
Neurological	Confusion

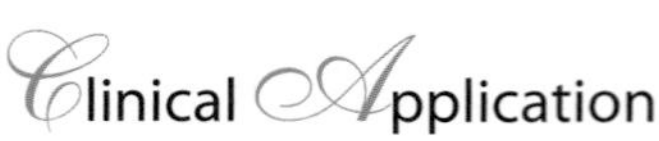

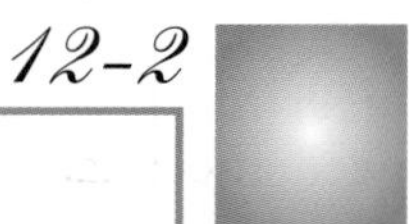

Designated Hydration Duties

A project using colorful beverage carts and designated hydration assistants attempted to increase nursing home residents' fluid intake by 8 ounces each midmorning and midafternoon. Providing choices of cold or hot beverages in colorful cups and assistance in drinking when needed had these results:

- Increased the residents' total body water as measured by bioelectrical impedance
- Decreased laxative use
- Increased the number of bowel movements
- Decreased the number of falls during the 5-week program

These results were obtained even though only 53% of residents consumed the desired 16 ounces of fluid every day. Measurements of total body water revealed these percentages of residents with below normal readings:

- 47% at the beginning of the project
- 6% at the end of the program, all of whom were in the late stages of dementia and had much difficulty swallowing (Robinson and Rosher, 2002)

Common Problems Related to Nutrition

Although arthritis, osteoporosis, and protein–kilocalorie malnutrition are not unique to the elderly, they do represent special concerns for geriatric clients. Constipation is a frequent complaint also and is covered in Chapter 20. A special food-based recipe to control the symptom of constipation that is effective in nursing home residents is given in Chapter 24.

Arthritis

This group of diseases is characterized by inflammation of various joints often accompanied by pain, swelling, stiffness, and deformity. **Arthritis** affects an estimated 21.6% of the adult U.S. population (46.4 million persons), and 8.3% (17.4 million people) reported arthritis limited their activities. Prevalence was high among:

- Women
- Older age groups
- Non-Hispanic whites
- Obese or overweight individuals
- Physically inactive persons (CDC, 2006).

OSTEOARTHRITIS

Formerly known as degenerative joint disease, **osteoarthritis** is characterized by progressive deterioration of cartilage in joints and vertebrae. Arthritis of the spine, hips, or knees is more likely to cause disability than that affecting other areas. Risk factors for osteoarthritis include:

- Aging
- Obesity
- Overuse or abuse of joints
- Trauma

Because the force exerted on the knees when walking may be up to six times the body weight, overweight people have a significantly increased risk of osteoarthritis of the knees. Thus, weight control has an important role in the prevention and treatment of osteoarthritis.

RHEUMATOID ARTHRITIS

In contrast to osteoarthritis, which is a local disease, rheumatoid arthritis is a systemic disease affecting about 2.1 million people in the United States. Because it is a systemic disease, some have tried to modify the disease effects through diet or supplements.

Omega-3 fatty acids, in addition to blocking the formation of inflammatory compounds from omega-6 fatty acids, produce compounds that are less inflammatory and less bioactive than the ones metabolized from omega-6 fatty acids. Consequently, fish oil supplements are now considered part of standard therapy for rheumatoid arthritis, conceivably permitting lower doses of drugs that have significant risks of toxicity (Morgan and Baggott, 2006).

In a small number of clients, food allergies may play a role in rheumatoid arthritis, but it is not a major factor for most. Likewise, a vegan diet may be helpful for a minority of clients with rheumatoid arthritis (Morgan and Baggott, 2006). A possible mechanism of action relates to eliminating sources of the omega-6 fatty acid arachidonic acid.

Osteoporosis and Fractures

Osteoporosis is covered in detail in Chapter 8. This section examines only the risks of and results of hip fracture (actually a fracture of the femur). Although half as common as reported vertebral fractures, hip fractures are much more likely to be diagnosed and treated. Clinically diagnosed vertebral fractures are estimated to represent just one-third of the total vertebral fractures.

INDIVIDUALS AFFECTED

One in three women and one in six men who reach the age of 90 will fracture a hip during their lifetime (*Merck Manual of Geriatrics*, 2009). Other facts about hip fractures include:

- About 76% of all hip fractures occur in women.
- More than 90% of hip fractures are caused by falling, most often by falling sideways onto the hip.
- About one out of five persons with hip fracture dies within a year of their injury.
- Up to one in four adults who lived independently before his or her hip fracture has to stay in a nursing home for at least a year after the injury (CDC, 2008a).

RISK FACTORS

Box 12-4 lists major risk factors for hip fractures. All these factors have been covered earlier or are self-explanatory, except height and **parity.**

Engineering analysis of the hip indicates greater resistance to fracture in shorter femoral necks, which occur in shorter people (Slemenda, 1997), although lower-extremity length is proposed as a better predictor (Opotowsky, Su, and Bilezikian, 2003).

Women who had never borne a child had a 44% increased risk of hip fractures, independent of hip bone mineral density, than women who had borne children, with each additional birth reducing hip fracture risk by 9% (Hillier et al., 2003). A proposed mechanism relates to changes produced in the pelvis by pregnancy. It can be readily seen that many clients have more than one of these risk factors.

Box 12-4 ■ *Risk Factors for Hip Fractures*

Among the risk factors for hip fractures are:

- Increasing age; 90% occur after 70 years of age (Wilkins and Birge, 2005).
- Female gender
- White race
- History of falls; risk is more strongly related to falls than to bone mass per se (Wilkins and Birge, 2005).
- Insufficient exercise
- Low BMI
- Being tall
- Never having borne children

NUTRITIONAL INTERVENTIONS

Once a fracture of the hip occurs, can dietary means improve outcomes?

- Compared with clients not receiving supplements, clients with hip fractures receiving a 10-day intravenous and oral supplement protocol had nearly optimal energy and fluid intakes as well as fewer complications and lower mortality rates than the control group (Eneroth, Olsson, and Thorngren, 2006).
- In Wales, employing dietetic assistants to provide nutritional support to hip fracture clients resulted in significantly better, but still inadequate, mean daily energy intake (1105 kilocalories vs. 756 kilocalories in 24 hours), significantly smaller reductions in mid-arm circumference as inpatients, and fewer deaths in the hospital and for 4 months afterward (Duncan et al., 2006).

PREVENTION

The most effective way to prevent fall-related injuries, including hip fractures, is to combine exercise with other fall prevention strategies. External hip protectors reduce hip fracture risk among elderly women with fall history and a BMI of 19 or less (Koike et al., 2009). Calcium and vitamin D given together reduce hip fractures and total fractures, and probably vertebral fractures, irrespective of age, sex, or previous fractures (DIPART Group, 2010).

Even after sustaining a hip fracture, only a minority of elderly clients receive treatment for osteoporosis to attempt to modify the risk of future fractures. Programs to improve osteoporosis testing and treatment after a fracture by reminders to physicians (Majumdar et al., 2007) or by outreach to clinicians and patients (Feldstein et al., 2007) increased such management. Still the goal was achieved for, at most, only 44% of the clients.

Compared with information-based strategies, direct interventions through a coordinated multidepartment post-fracture program at one hospital (Bogoch et al., 2006) and through outpatient fracture clinics (Kuo et al., 2007) improved osteoporosis management for 73% to 96% of identified clients.

Weight Loss and Protein–Kilocalorie Malnutrition

The older person's metabolic rate declines, primarily as a result of less lean body mass or muscle, so that loss of 5% or more of body weight requires aggressive intervention (Morley, 2006). The **anorexia of aging** is described in Box 12-5.

Studies of hospitalized older adults have reported between 50% and 80% are malnourished or at risk for malnourishment (DiMaria-Ghalili and Guenter, 2008). Malnutrition contributes to many complications of illness, such as infections, anemia, and pressure ulcers (Clinical Application 12-3).

Box 12-5 ■ *The Anorexia of Aging*

Humans and other animals of advanced age have reduced food intake. Physiological factors contributing to anorexia of aging include:

- Changes in taste and smell
- Delayed gastric emptying
- Altered digestion-related hormone secretion and hormonal responsiveness

Healthy elders have been shown to be less hungry at meal initiation and to become more rapidly satiated during a standard meal compared to younger adults.

Nonphysiological causes include:

- Social (poverty, isolation)
- Psychological (depression, dementia)
- Medical (edentulism, dysphagia)
- Pharmacological factors (Hays and Roberts, 2006).

Older persons eat more in social situations than when eating alone, even when the person delivering Meals on Wheels just sits with the recipient while dining.

Depression accounts for about 30% of the weight loss seen in the elderly (Morley, 2006), and recently widowed persons were shown to be at increased risk of weight loss compared with married individuals (Shahar et al., 2001). Older adults, who take more than 30% of all prescription drugs, are at increased risk of drug–nutrient interactions, the subject of Chapter 15.

In a chronic-care hospital and a home for the aged, analysis of a 28-day cycle of menus revealed that, even if the 2000-kilocalorie diets were entirely consumed, the diets would not supply enough vitamins and minerals to provide recommended intakes. In practice, long-term care residents more consistently consume between 1000 and 1500 kilocalories per day; therefore, Wendland et al. (2003) recommend vitamin and mineral supplements for all older long-term-care facility residents.

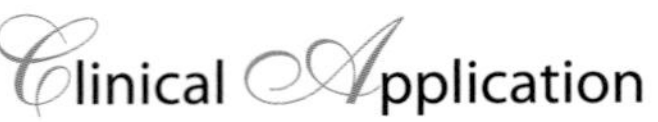

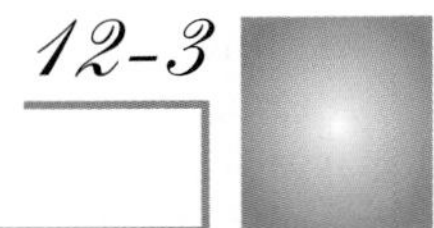

12-3

Nutrition and Pressure Ulcers

The basic cause of **pressure ulcers** is impaired circulation from the weight of the body on a bony prominence or by shearing forces from pulling on the skin that damages the underlying tissue. Risk factors include:

- Immobility
- Inactivity
- Incontinence
- Impaired consciousness
- Malnutrition

Progression of the ulcer from intact skin to an open, sometimes very deep sore increases the challenge to control infection, to replenish nutrient losses from the wound, and to promote healing. Copious wound drainage can result in a deficit of 100 grams of protein per day (Russell, 2001).

A systematic review concluded that enteral nutritional support, particularly high protein oral nutritional supplements, can reduce the risk of developing pressure ulcers by 25%. Although studies suggest oral nutritional supplements and enteral tube feeding may improve healing of pressure ulcers, further research is needed (Stratton et al., 2005).

In a small pilot study, a two-ounce serving of a 2-kilocalorie per milliliter supplement was given four times a day with medications. After 6 months, the pressure ulcers of the four residents who had them at the beginning of the study were healed. In addition, 89% of the residents gained weight (Doll-Shankaruk, Yau, and Oelke, 2008).

Nutritional support is only a part of the overall strategy to combat pressure ulcers. The other risk factors must be controlled and diligent nursing care provided to effectively prevent or treat this serious condition.

Food Insecurity

The main reason individuals do not consume enough protein or kilocalories is lack of money (Box 12-6). To rectify the situation for older adults, the federal government, with an amendment to the Older Americans Act, established meal programs for senior citizens. Low-cost meals are offered at central gathering places or are delivered to the homebound. Senior citizens participate in some 2200 such local meal programs (Fig. 12-2), which in 2002 served about 250 million meals to 2.6 million older adults (Brown, 2008).

Dietary Interventions

Enhancing well-consumed menu items with additional kilocalories and protein while maintaining the usual volume of food employs a "food-first" philosophy to counter weight loss. Clients may accept foods more readily than liquid supplements of which less than 50% are actually consumed (Castellanos, Marra, and Johnson, 2009). Milk-based supplements that are

Box 12-6 ■ *Food Insecurity*

Assessment of 189 community-dwelling older adults participating in congregate meals showed that 80.4% were food secure compared with the national rate for older adult households of 92.4% (Duerr, 2006b). Increasing frailty apparently increases food insecurity because only 74.8% of community-dwelling individuals participating in a home-delivered meals program were food secure (Duerr, 2006a).

Environmental Factor

Some elderly persons must choose between food and comfort. In low-income households, especially those consisting entirely of elderly persons, the incidence of food insecurity is correlated with heating and cooling costs:

- In high-cooling states, the risk of food insecurity was 27% higher in the summer than in the winter.
- In high-heating states, the risk of food insecurity was 43% lower in the summer than in the winter (Nord and Kantor, 2006).

Psychosocial Factor

Older adults are less likely than any other age group to use the federal Food Stamp Program. Just one in five impoverished American citizens older than the age of 65 years had received food stamps in 2003 (Fuller-Thomson and Redmond, 2008).

Assuming a client even has a household may be a mistake. Johnson and McCool (2003) identified many nutritional problems among older homeless women eating most of their food at shelters. The women's intake was inadequate for most nutrients because of limited consumption of fruits, vegetables, dairy products, and whole grains. Their intake of saturated fats and simple carbohydrates was high.

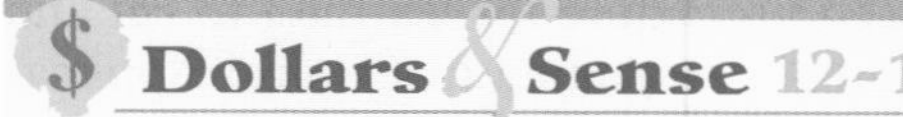

Dollars & Sense 12-1

Nutritional Supplements

Substituting Carnation Instant Breakfast® for Ensure® would save 55 cents per serving or $33 for 30 days assuming two servings per day. See calculations below.

To equal the kilocaloric content of Ensure requires a 10-ounce serving of modified Instant Breakfast instead of eight ounces of Ensure. The protein content of the Ensure and Instant Breakfast made with whole milk and ice cream are equivalent. The fat, saturated fat, cholesterol, and sodium contents are higher in the homemade recipe. Whether that intake would be a major concern for the client is a clinical judgment. Other nutrients have not been compared.

To implement the Instant Breakfast recipe also requires a refrigerator and freezer and a blender or shaker to mix the one package of instant breakfast, one cup of whole milk, and one-quarter cup of ice cream.

	Ensure	Carnation Instant Breakfast	Whole Milk	Ice Cream
Price	$7.99	$4.20	$3.09	$4.17
Package	6–8 oz bottles	10 packages of powder	1 gal	1.5 qt
Serving size	1 bottle	1 package	1 cup	¼ cup
Cost/Serving	$1.33	$0.42	$0.19	$0.17
Kilocalories	350	130	150	67
Protein	13 g	5 g	8 g	1 g
Total fat	11 g	0 g	8 g	3.5 g
Saturated fat	1.5 g	0 g	5.1 g	2.3 g
Cholesterol	10 mg	<5 mg	33 mg	15 mg
Sodium	220 mg	100 mg	120 mg	27 mg
Cost per prepared serving	$1.33	$0.78		

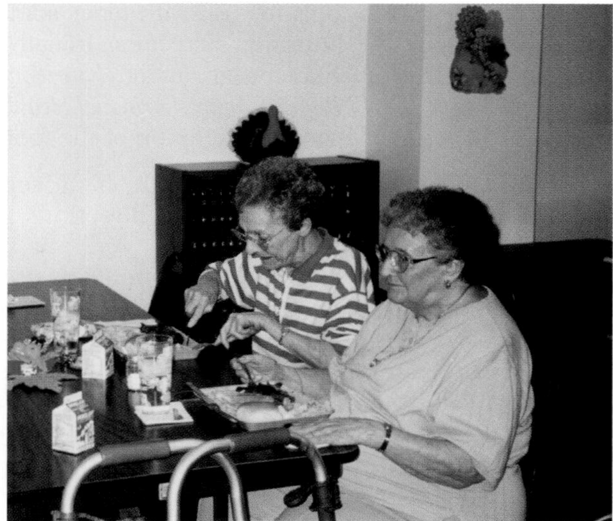

FIGURE 12-2 These women partake of an evening meal served at their place of residence under the auspices of the Older Americans Act and managed by a county agency.

both nutrient-dense and easy to consume might succeed for a person who is losing weight or one who cannot chew. Use of a nutrient-dense (120 kilocalories and 5 grams of protein in 60 milliliters) supplement four times a day for 4 weeks as part of medication administration resulted in significant weight gain in residents of a long-term care facility. Contributing to the positive outcome was a 7% increase in intake at meals, including 16% at the evening meal (Welch, Porter, and Endres, 2003).

A more economical choice than prepared supplements may be an instant breakfast preparation. A homemade supplement recipe using ice cream is given in Dollars and Sense 12-1. To prevent dampening of appetite at mealtime, liquid caloric supplements should be given at least 1 hour before a meal (Morley, 2006).

An unbalanced intake is better than no intake. Protein-kilocalorie malnutrition was reversed in one study by serving as much of a favorite food, ice cream, as the client wanted (Winograd and Brown, 1990).

To accommodate dentures, the person may reduce his or her intake of meats, fresh fruits, and vegetables. Assistance in selecting appropriate substitute items is in order. Just two dietary counseling sessions significantly increased fruit and vegetable consumption in edentulous denture-wearers (Bradbury et al., 2006).

A recommended procedure for learning to eat and drink with dentures is explained in Clinical Application 12-4.

Nutritional Care for the Elderly

Box 12-7 lists topics to consider in a nutritional assessment.

Assessment

When assessing the elderly, special care is necessary to ensure marginal deficiencies are detected before major problems occur. Body weight and its stability are critical data in nutrition screening, yet an investigation in three large medical centers revealed that just 65.7% of clients older than 18 years reporting being weighed at admission and only 67% of those not weighed had been asked about their weight.

Clinical Application 12-4

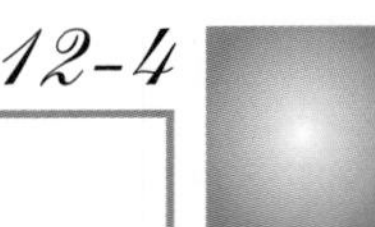

Learning to Eat with Dentures

Clients should learn to use dentures one step at a time:

1. Practice swallowing liquids with the dentures in place.
2. Practice chewing soft foods.
3. Learn and practice to bite regular foods.

Splitting the process into manageable units decreases frustration.

Box 12-7 ■ *Topics to Be Assessed in the Elderly***

Oral Cavity Function

- Difficulty tasting; changes in taste perception
- Bleeding gums; dry mouth
- Difficulty chewing; toothaches; poorly fitting dentures
- Foods client is unable to eat

Meal Management

- Who shops? Where? Ease of making food decisions?
- Transportation problems?
- Budgeting a concern? Knowledge to make informed choices?
- Who cooks? Knowledge and skill level?
- Refrigeration, storage, and cooking facilities?
- Ability to manage containers: jars, cans, bottles

Psychosocial Factors

- Where are most meals eaten?
- Mealtime companions
- Recent change in living conditions?
- Satisfaction with situation?

*In addition to the normal assessment, that is, appetite or weight changes and bowel habits.

More than one-fourth (25.9%) of documented weights in the nursing records differed by 5 pounds (2.27 kg) or more compared with measurements by research personnel (Jensen et al., 2003).

MINI NUTRITIONAL ASSESSMENT

The Mini Nutritional Assessment (MNA) tool for use with older adults features two parts. The first 6 items (Box 12-8) provide a screening score and the last 12 items an assessment score that determines if further action is needed. The screening portion has the advantage of incorporating alternative measures for height if the person cannot stand and compensatory calculations for clients with missing limbs. The entire tool is available in 15 languages. Both a guide to its use and an online scoring program are available (Nestle Nutrition Institute, undated).

An advantage of the MNA is its ability to detect malnutrition before changes in weight or serum protein levels appear (DiMaria-Ghalili and Guenter, 2008). A low MNA score was found to be predictive of adverse clinical events during hospitalization and of high mortality (Donini et al., 2003).

The MNA focuses on malnutrition and underweight. In the face of the obesity epidemic, however, scoring maximum points for a BMI greater than 23 without distinguishing abnormalities at the high end of the BMI scale has been questioned (Amella, 2008).

NUTRITION SCREENING INITIATIVE TOOLS

Nutritional assessment tools for use with older adults were developed by the Nutrition Screening Initiative. The first two instruments appear under *Nutritional Assessment Tools as "DETERMINE Your Nutritional Health" on DavisPlus*. The following is a description of the tools.

- Determine Your Nutritional Health is a self-administered checklist with scoring directions to evaluate risk.
- Level I Screening Tool is to be administered by professionals in health or social service programs and includes directions for appropriate referrals.
- Level II Screening Tool is for use in physicians' offices and health-care institutions and includes a clinical examination, skinfold measurements, and laboratory tests (Quinn, 1997).

Implementation

Some interventions are appropriate regardless of a client's living situation. Others are more focused on institutionalized elderly.

INDEPENDENTLY LIVING ELDERLY

Suggestions to increase the nourishment of elderly clients living in their own homes appear in Box 12-9.

Box 12-8 ■ *Geriatric Mini Nutrition Assessment*

Assessment	Score
Has food intake declined over past 3 months due to loss of appetite, digestive problems, or chewing or swallowing difficulties? 0 = severe loss of appetite 1 = moderate 2 = no loss	
Weight loss during last 3 months 0 = >3 kg (6.6 lb) 1 = unknown 2 = 1–3 kg (2.2–6.6 lb) 3 = no weight loss	
Mobility 0 = bed or chair bound 1 = able to get out of bed/chair but does not go out 2 = goes out	
Psychological stress or acute disease in past 3 months 0 = yes 2 = no	
Neuropsychological problems 0 = severe dementia or depression 1 = mild dementia 2 = no psychological problems	
BMI (Weight in kg/Height in m^2) 0 = <19 1 = 19–20.9 2 = 21–22.9 3 = 23 or more	
Score (Max 14): 12 or more = normal; 11 or less = possible malnutrition, continue assessing	

Alternative knee to heel height calculation: With knee at 90-degree angle, measure from bottom of heel to top of knee.
Men = (2.02 × knee ht, cm) – (0.04 × age, yr) + 64.19 = ht, cm
Women = (1.83 × knee ht, cm) – (0.24 × age, yr) + 84.88 = ht, cm

Amputees' BMI calculation: Increase scale weight by percentage below.
Single below knee, 6.0%   Single at knee, 9.0%
Single above knee, 15%   Single arm, 6.5%   Single below elbow, 3.6%

Source: Rubenstein et al. (2001). Reprinted with permission.

Box 12-9 ■ *Increasing Food Intake in Independently Living Elderly*

Prepare for Mealtime

- Suggest oral hygiene before meals to freshen and moisten mouth.
- Suggest smokers refrain for 1 hour before a meal to increase appetite.

Promote Social Interaction

- Encourage potluck meals with friends for those who live alone.
- Combine meals at the senior center with activities of interest.

Serve Food Attractively

- Suggest varying textures, colors, flavors.
- Suggest raw, crisp-cooked, or marinated vegetables to increase vegetable intake.
- Suggest using attractive dishes and flatware, centerpieces, tablecloths, or placemats.

Provide Nutrient-Dense Foods

- Help the client to select satisfactory meal-replacer supplements, whether commercial canned products or instant-breakfast powders.
- If additional kilocalories are needed, recommend whole milk for beverages and cooking instead of reduced-fat varieties.

Outside Help

- Obtain a home health aide to shop, do basic fix-ahead preparations.
- Provide Meals-on-Wheels for homebound.
- Refer to the social worker for food stamps, surplus commodity programs for those eligible.
- Recommend instructional materials on food purchasing, storage, cooking from county extension services.

Increasing physical activity according to the client's ability offers benefits beyond weight control. Physical activity helps to:

- Prevent heart disease and hypertension
- Improve bone mineral density
- Enhance balance and strength for activities of daily living
- Promote restful sleep

Many individuals, however, report never having been advised to exercise by their health-care providers. An intervention to enable the client to see improvement (or the need for improvement) is the keeping of an activity log.

The nurse's role in nourishing hospitalized older clients undergoing diagnostic tests is discussed in Clinical Application 12-5. Obtaining adequate food for such a client may tax the nurse's ingenuity because of timing and the need to entice a fatigued and perhaps fearful client to eat.

INSTITUTIONALIZED ELDERLY

Suggestions to increase the nourishment of institutionalized elderly appear in Box 12-10.

12-5

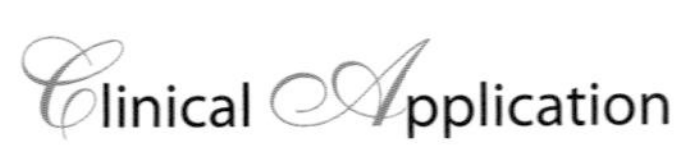
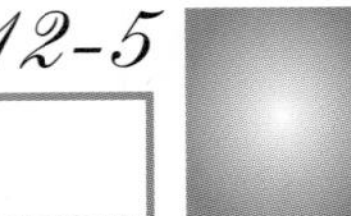

Clinical Application

Hospitalization of the Elderly

Except in obstetrical and pediatric practices, elderly clients dominate as consumers of health care. Eighty percent of the elderly, compared with 40% of individuals younger than the age of 65 years, have one or more chronic diseases. In many cases, elderly clients not only are admitted to the hospital undernourished but also their nutritive status worsens during hospitalization.

Serving no food to a client because of diagnostic tests is starvation. The conscientious nurse obtains meals or feedings for a client who is *nil per os*, or NPO (i.e., nothing by mouth) for breakfast and lunch. There is nothing magical about the times of 8 AM, 12 PM, and 6 PM for meals. The committed nurse will arrange for adequate nourishment for clients when their tests are completed and they are permitted to eat. Dietary personnel have no idea when an individual client is finished with tests for the day until notified by the nurse.

Box 12-10 ■ *Increasing Food Intake in Institutionalized Elderly*

Prepare for Mealtime

- Provide oral hygiene before meals to freshen and moisten mouth.
- Suggest smokers refrain for 1 hour before a meal to increase appetite.
- Manage the environment by removing unsightly supplies or noxious waste.
- Allow 60 minutes to elapse after a significant amount of supplement before serving the next meal.

Promote Social Interaction

- Encourage alert nursing home residents to choose compatible mealtime companions.
- Control the noise in the dining room to avoid overstimulating those with hearing aids.

Serve Food Attractively

- Vary textures, colors, flavors.
- To increase vegetable intake, offer raw, crisp-cooked, or marinated vegetables as appetizers.
- Provide enough nonglaring light so food can be seen clearly.
- Schedule special events such as musical entertainment to enhance interest in eating.

Provide Nutrient-Dense Foods

- Add powdered milk or ice cream to appropriate beverages and foods.
- Increase the eggs, milk, or cheese in recipes.
- When appropriate, offer 1 ounce of a nutritionally complete supplement every hour and use as "chaser" when administering medications.
- If additional kilocalories are needed, provide whole milk for beverages and use for cooking instead of reduced-fat varieties.

Providing nourishment for frail and ill elderly is a monumental task. In 2008:

- 41% of residents of long-term care facilities could eat independently (Centers for Medicare & Medicaid Services, 2008).
- 10% needed extensive help with eating.
- 14% were totally dependent upon caregivers (Stockdell and Amella, 2008).

To ease the mealtime burden of dependent clients, Medicare and Medicaid now permit long-term care facilities to use paid feeding assistants under certain conditions (Centers for Medicare, 2003).

When asked, nursing home residents recalled that food tasted really good when eating with family and friends, especially in childhood. When staff learn about residents' previously enjoyed foods and occasionally provide those favorites as special treats, residents maintain individuality within their peer group and among staff. Other suggestions to make mealtimes more homelike include:

- Buffet service
- Item selection that permits portion control
- Choice of accompaniments (Evans, Crogan, and Shultz, 2005)

When family members of nursing home residents were asked for preferred nutritional interventions, liquid oral supplements ranked nearly last on the list of choices. In order of most to least desirable, the family members preferred to:

1. Improve the quality of the food
2. Improve the quality and quantity of feeding assistance
3. Provide multiple small meals and snacks throughout the day
4. Place the resident in a preferred dining location
5. Provide an oral liquid nutritional supplement between meals
6. Provide a medication to stimulate appetite (Simmons et al., 2003)

Bolstering fluid intake in institutionalized elders takes planning. Frequent small drinks may be more acceptable to the client than trying to swallow large amounts with meals. Suggested strategies include:

- Giving clients a minimum of 180 milliliters of fluid with each medication pass
- Giving a resident 60 milliliters of fluid every time a provider enters the room
- Including variety of liquid refreshments at all activities
- Scheduling tea parties (Mentes and Iowa-Veterans Affairs Research Consortium, 2000)

Keystones

- The mean intakes of fiber and vitamin E are below the DRIs for all adults. Only young men have average intakes of calcium meeting the DRI. Mean intakes of iron are less than the DRI for young and middle-aged women.
- Aging affects almost all body systems, impacting food procurement, preparation, consumption, digestion, and metabolism.
- Supplements and fortified foods as sources of calcium and vitamins D and B_{12} are recommended for middle-aged and older adults in recognition of impaired absorption, metabolism, and synthesis as people age.
- Involuntary weight loss in the elderly should stimulate a broad search for causes: physical, environmental, financial, and social.
- Overweight increases the risk for certain diseases such as osteoarthritis and diabetes mellitus but a BMI in the overweight range is not associated with a significantly increased risk of mortality in individuals older than the age of 65 years.
- The most nutritionally vulnerable adults are nursing home residents who are unable to eat unassisted.

CASE STUDY 12-1

Mr. E is a 70-year-old widower who relies on public transportation. His home is two blocks from the bus route and eight blocks from the nearest supermarket. Mr. E has moderately painful knees from arthritis. He has been taking the bus to the supermarket every other day so that he could manage one package on the way home. He has confided to the nurse in his doctor's office that he is ready to "just give up. It's too much trouble to eat anymore." Mr. E's weight today is 160 lb, 5 lb less than last month.

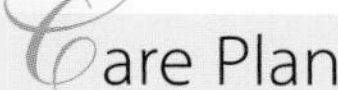

Care Plan

Subjective Data

Dependent on public transportation ■ Painful knees ■ Verbalized discouragement with procuring food

Objective Data

Weight loss of 5 lb in past month

Analysis

Lack of information concerning resources available to maintain senior citizens in their homes

Plan

DESIRED OUTCOMES EVALUATION CRITERIA	ACTIONS/INTERVENTIONS	RATIONALE
Mr. E will acknowledge need for assistance with meals by end of visit today.	Discuss Mr. E's weight change with him. Determine what kind of assistance he would accept.	Clients are likely to change behaviors only if the new behavior is acceptable to them.
Given several options of community support, Mr. E will select one and begin to implement the change within 3 days.	Describe Senior Citizen Nutrition Program, Meals on Wheels, home health aide shopping service, and door-to-door Care-a-Van service.	Clients may know about these programs but prefer to remain independent. Allowing the client some time to choose makes the choice more his own.
	Explore social support available from family and less-restricted friends.	
	Nurse to follow up with telephone call in 3 days.	Following up with a telephone call shows the nurse is committed to working through this problem with Mr. E.

During the follow-up telephone call, Mr. E said he would like information on the Senior Nutrition Program and the Care-a-Van Service.

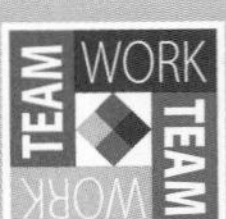

12-1

Senior Center Nutrition Coordinator's Notes

The following Senior Center Nutrition Coordinator's Notes are representative of the documentation found in a client's medical record.

The Nutrition Coordinator at the Senior Center interviewed Mr. E and introduced him to several "regulars" at his first noon meal at the Senior Center. On his card she noted:

- Regular diet, no allergies
- Enjoyed woodworking and card games in past
- Major difficulty—obtaining groceries
- Will try Care-a-Van instead of bus

Follow up with alternate grocery suggestions if plan is unsatisfactory. Encourage socialization.

Critical Thinking Questions

1. What additional data could be sought in a more comprehensive assessment?
2. What other areas could be investigated to help balance to Mr. E's need for assistance with his desire for independence?
3. As you read this case, how would you define the underlying problem?

Chapter Review

1. The RDA/AI for which of the following nutrients is increased for older adults compared to younger ones?
   a. Sodium
   b. Calcium
   c. Vitamin C
   d. Vitamin K
2. The decrease in gastric acid that accompanies aging causes concern for the absorption of which of the following nutrients?
   a. Carbohydrate and water
   b. Fat and cholesterol
   c. Vitamins A and E
   d. Vitamin B_{12} and iron
3. A nurse making a home visit routinely screens for dehydration in elderly clients. Which of the following would the nurse assess?
   a. Body temperature and urine-specific gravity
   b. Tongue condition, pulse rate, and muscle strength
   c. Skin turgor and heart and lung sounds
   d. Client's intake and output records
4. Which of the following conditions is likely to contribute to vitamin D deficiency in older adults?
   a. Atrophied skin, dislike for milk, and indoor life
   b. Lack of exercise, failing hearing and vision
   c. Slowed peristalsis, diminished secretion of intrinsic factor
   d. Achlorhydria and inability to chew meats
5. Ms. P is a 58-year-old retired cook who tells the clinic nurse she regrets not having had children and grandchildren. Which of the following activities might assist Ms. P to attain generativity?
   a. Editing a cookbook for her church group
   b. Taking a class in ethnic cooking in preparation for her next trip
   c. Serving on the Meals-on-Wheels advisory board
   d. Volunteering to teach a special recipe at a local school

Clinical Analysis

Ms. O is a 76-year-old retired schoolteacher who has been admitted to a long-term care facility after surgical repair of a fractured hip.

1. While performing the Geriatric Mini Nutrition Assessment for Ms. O, to calculate the most accurate BMI, the nurse would use the client's height
   a. Listed on her driver's license
   b. At age 50
   c. As determined in the supine position with a tape measure
   d. Using the alternative knee to toe calculation
2. Ms. O reports a weight loss of 4 lb in the 3 months before her injury. Her present weight is 125 lb. Which of the following nursing actions is appropriate at this point?
   a. Asking the physician to order an appetite stimulant
   b. Ordering balanced nutritional supplements three times a day
   c. Deferring action until the team conference next week
   d. Instructing the nursing assistants to feed Ms. O
3. Because Ms. O will have limited mobility, providing adequate fluid intake is necessary to prevent complications in the ___ system.
   a. Cardiovascular
   b. Endocrine
   c. Urinary
   d. Integumentary

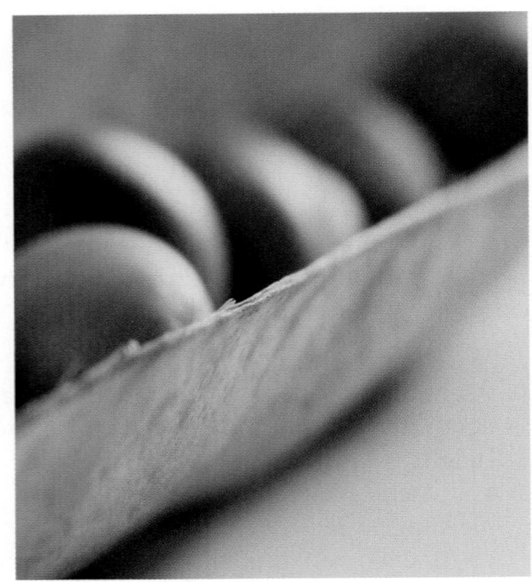

13

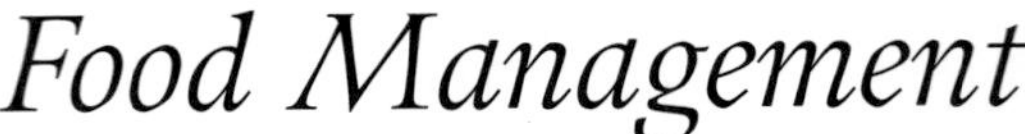

Food Management

LEARNING OBJECTIVES

After completing this chapter, the student should be able to:

- Describe the conditions under which microbiologic food illnesses can occur.
- Identify foods that are likely to harbor disease-producing microorganisms.
- Teach clients how to prevent foodborne illnesses.
- Discuss the information on food labels.

Effective meal management requires knowledge about food safety, including microbiological hazards, environmental pollutants, and natural food intoxicants. Reading food labels can help prevent nutritional hazards. How food is handled between the time it leaves the farm and the time it reaches the dinner table affects our health and well-being. How food crops are grown and animals are raised influences health as well. As health care moves from institutions to home care, health-care workers need to understand the vital importance of safe and nutritious food. See Box 13-1.

On average, each American eats more than 10,000 pounds of food each year. Considering the number of people involved in the growth, distribution, preparation, and service of food, our food safety record is excellent. The food supply in the United States is as safe, wholesome, and nutritious as any in the world.

Some food handling and consumption behaviors practiced 10 years ago are not considered safe today.

Box 13-1 ■ *YOPI*

Those most at risk:

Young, **o**ld, **p**regnant, and **i**mmunocompromised clients (YOPI)—25% of the United States population—are at the greatest risk for foodborne illness.

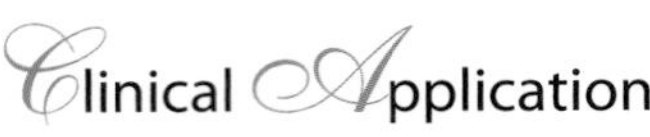

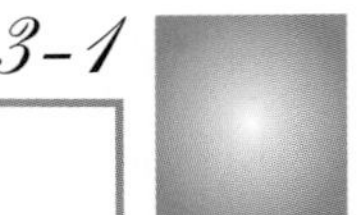

Clinical Application 13-1

Food Safety and Immunosuppressed Clients

All clients receiving an immunosuppressive agent need counseling on food safety and sanitation. These clients have an inability to fight infections, so a relatively small number of bacteria could cause illness. **Immunosuppressive agents** are medications that interfere with the body's ability to fight infections. These drugs are used in tissue and organ transplantation procedures, such as a kidney transplant. These are also used as part of the treatment of certain diseases like cancer.

New strains of pathogens, or disease-producing organisms, are continually evolving; in some cases, these organisms have proven resistant to antibiotics. The development of these resistant foodborne pathogens has been attributed to increased use of antibiotics in hospitals, outpatient facilities, and veterinary applications.

The most common foodborne illnesses occur when microbiological microorganisms that are naturally present in the environment contaminate food and are allowed to grow because of improper food handling. This chapter discusses many of the Food and Drug Administration's (FDA's) food safety concerns.

Microbiological Hazards

Many organisms in our environment cause disease, including bacteria and parasites, viruses, and fungi. These microorganisms may be carried from one host to another by animals; humans; inanimate objects including food; and environmental factors, such as air, water, and soil. Many microorganisms cause disease. Under certain conditions, food becomes a vehicle for disease transmission.

Most foodborne diseases infect the tissues of the digestive tract and cause gastric distress; symptoms range from mild to severe. See Box 13-2.

Bacterial Foodborne Disease

Bacteria are everywhere and account for 90% of all foodborne disease. Doorknobs, countertops, hands, eyelashes, mouths, some water supplies, and food are a few of the many places where bacteria can be found. Animal and human fluids and waste harbor bacteria and cause many foodborne illnesses.

The Centers for Disease Control and Prevention (CDC) reported the following to have contributed to the majority of foodborne illnesses in the United States during 2005 (www.cdc.gov/foodbornebreaks):

- Ground beef contamination with *Escherichia coli (0157 H), Salmonella, Cyclospora cayetanensis* or hepatitis A
- Bare-handed food contact by handler/worker/preparer
- Raw product/ingredient contaminates from animal or environment
- Allowing food to remain at room temperature or outdoor temperature for several hours
- Insufficient time and/or temperature during the initial cooking/heat processing

Box 13-2 ■ *Mild and Severe Symptoms of Foodborne Disease*

Mild symptoms include gastric and intestinal distress with:

- Abdominal pain
- Nausea
- Vomiting
- Diarrhea
- Cramps

Severe symptoms include:

- Dehydration
- Bloody stools
- Neurological disorders
- Death

Conditions for Growth

Bacterial growth refers to an increase in the number of organisms. Under ideal conditions, cell numbers can double every half hour: one cell becomes two, two become four, and four become eight (in an hour and a half). A single bacterium can multiply to 33 million after 12 hours. Although bacteria cannot be eradicated from our environment, bacterial growth can be controlled. For this reason, understanding the following conditions necessary for bacterial growth and microbiological food illness to occur is important:

- Source of bacteria—The bacteria must come in contact with the food.
- Food—The food must permit the bacteria to grow (increase in number) or produce a poisonous toxin. Bacteria grow in foods only within a certain pH range. This is reason vinegar and lemon juice are frequently used to preserve food, such as cucumbers (pickles) and cabbage (sauerkraut). These ingredients lower the pH so bacteria cannot grow.
- Temperature—The temperature must be favorable for bacterial growth. The temperature range in which most bacteria multiply rapidly is 40°F to 140°F—the range that includes room and body temperature (Fig. 13-1).

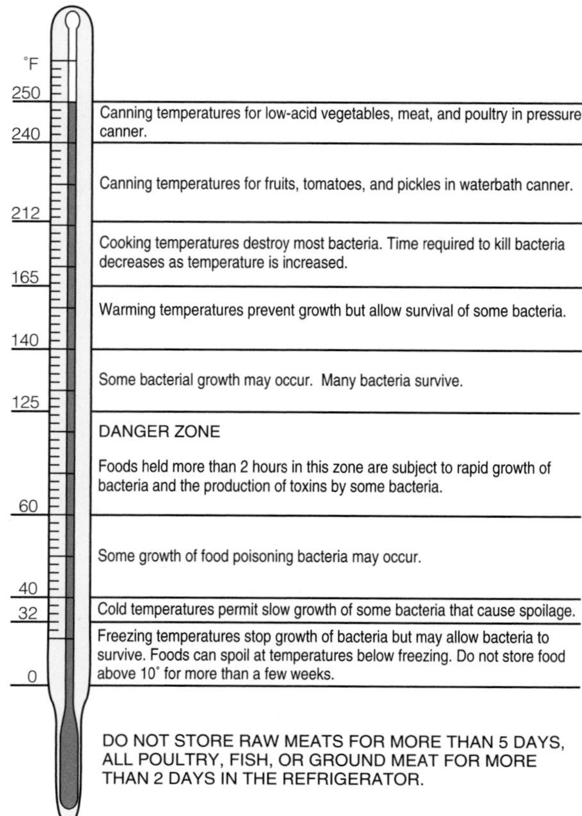

FIGURE 13-1 A temperature guide to food safety.

- Time—Enough time must elapse for bacteria to grow, produce a toxin, or both.
- Moisture—Bacteria need water to dissolve and digest food. Foods that contain water support bacterial growth better than do dehydrated foods. This is the reason dehydration is a food preservation method.
- Ingestion—An unsuspecting person must eat the food or drink the beverage that contains the toxin or bacteria.

Bacteria are frequently odorless, tasteless, and colorless; therefore laboratory analysis is the only way to tell whether a food will cause illness. Table 13-1 lists pathogens, common food vehicles, and symptoms.

Food Infections

A **food infection** is caused by eating a food containing a large number of disease-producing bacteria. Symptoms of such infections usually start 12 to 36 hours after consuming an offending food.

SALMONELLA

Salmonella infection, called **salmonellosis**, is the most common foodborne disease. It is transmitted by the consumption of contaminated foods or contact with an infected person. Some foods support the growth of *Salmonella* better than others. One study found that 20% of samples of ground meat obtained in supermarkets were contaminated with *Salmonella*. Other common food vehicles include raw eggs, unpasteurized milk, and poultry. See Dollars and Sense 13-1.

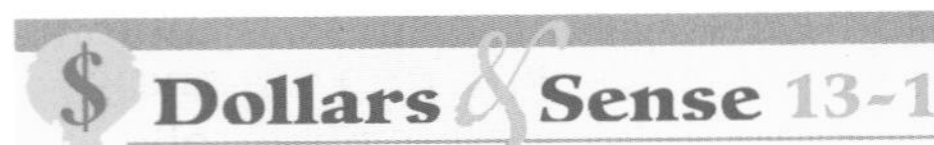

Preventing Illness

Prevention of foodborne illness is one of the most effective and simple ways to stretch your healthcare budget. *Salmonella* alone accounts for 1,397,187 cases with an Economic Research Service (ESR) cost of $2,544,394,344.00 (www.ers.usda.gov/data). That's an average cost of $18.20 per occurrence. ESR costs include forgone earnings, spending on medications, and long-term medical treatment. When in doubt, throw it out.

TABLE 13-1 ■ Pathogens, Common Food Vehicles, and Symptoms

PATHOGEN	COMMON FOOD VEHICLES (HAZARDOUS FOOD ITEMS)	SYMPTOMS
Salmonella	Raw eggs, raw milk, poultry, red meat, ground beef	May lead to sudden onset of headache, abdominal pain, diarrhea, nausea, and vomiting. Dehydration may be severe, and fever is usually present. May develop into septicemia. See Clinical Application 13-1.
Listeria	Soft cheeses, deli meats, pâté, burritos, ice cream	May lead to meningoencephalitis and/or septicemia in newborns and adults and abortion in pregnant women.
Escherichia Coli 0157:H7	Ground beef, other beef, raw milk, unpasteurized apple juice	May lead to acute hemorrhagic colitis (cramps, bloody diarrhea, nausea, vomiting, and fever). May result in hemolytic uremic failure or kidney failure.
Campylobacter Jejuni	Poultry, beef, raw eggs, water	May lead to an acute gastroenteritis of variable severity characterized by diarrhea, abdominal pain, malaise, fever, nausea, and vomiting. Guillain-Barré syndrome or meningitis has been seen in severe cases.
Norwalk Virus	Raw shellfish and salad ingredients in the United States; rehydrated cereals, grains, legumes, and nuts worldwide	May lead to nausea, vomiting, diarrhea, abdominal pain, headache, malaise, and low-grade fever. Usually a self-limited mild to moderate disease
Staphylococcus Aureus	Poultry, processed meats, cheeses, ice cream, mixed dishes such as potato salad, spaghetti	May lead to Ritter syndrome (an inflammatory skin disease seen in newborns, characterized by pustules that fill with a straw-colored fluid and become encrusted). Wide variety of syndromes with manifestations such as skin lesions, lung or brain abscess, and endocarditis.
Clostridium Botulinum	Improperly processed canned food; large masses of food with air-free center	May lead to acute bilateral cranial nerve impairment and descending weakness or paralysis. Double vision, dysphasia, and dry mouth may be present. Vomiting, diarrhea, or constipation may be present initially.
Typhoid Fever	Food, water, and people infected/contaminated with human feces	May lead to fever up to 104°F for about 7 days, followed by flat, rose-colored fleeting rash, abdominal pain, anorexia, and extreme exhaustion. Septicemia and internal bleeding are possible after about 14 days (Venes, 2005).
Clostridium Perfringens	Meats, gravies, and stews in large masses of food	May lead to abdominal cramping, diarrhea, vomiting, and fever are common. Incubation time between 8 to 16 hours

Typhoid fever is caused by one type of ***Salmonella*** bacteria. This illness is spread by food and water contaminated by feces and urine of carriers.

CAMPYLOBACTER

Another type of bacteria causing food infections is *Campylobacter jejuni,* which is carried in the intestinal tracts of cows, hogs, sheep, and poultry. Contaminated water or raw manure can spread the organism. For example, an animal can defecate in a vegetable garden and contaminate the produce.

Foods found to be contaminated with *Campylobacter jejuni* include raw milk, fresh mushrooms, and raw hamburger. ***Campylobacter*** can be controlled by keeping food below 40°F or above 140°F and by maintaining good food-handling practices.

LISTERIA

Another pathogen is ***Listeria.*** This organism is problematic because the bacteria can grow slowly at refrigerator temperatures (32°F to 34°F) and on moist surfaces. Cooking facilities must be kept clean and dry to prevent the growth of this organism. Chlorine (bleach), one tablespoon per gallon of water, is also effective in inhibiting *Listeria.*

According to the CDC, pregnant women are 20 times more likely than other healthy adults to get listeriosis (www.cdc.gov). Hormonal changes during pregnancy affect the mother's immune system, allowing for the increased susceptibility. Listeriosis can be transmitted to the fetus through the placenta, leading to premature delivery, miscarriage, stillbirth, or other serious health problems for the newborn. The USDA Food Safety and Inspection Service (FSIS) and the U.S. FDA provide guidelines for pregnant women. See Box 13-3.

Box 13-3 ■ *Food-Safety Guidelines for Pregnant Women*

Pregnant women should follow these safe-eating suggestions:

- Do not eat hot dogs, luncheon meats, or deli meats unless they are reheated until steaming hot.
- Do not eat soft cheeses such as feta, Brie, Camembert, blue-veined cheeses, and Mexican-style cheeses such as queso blanco fresco. Hard cheeses, such as mozzarella, pasteurized processed cheese slices, and spreads, cream cheese, and cottage cheese may be safely consumed.
- Do not eat refrigerated pâté or meat spreads. Canned or shelf-stable pâté and meat spreads may be eaten.
- Do not eat refrigerated smoked seafood unless it is an ingredient in a cooked dish such as a casserole. Canned fish such as salmon and tuna or shelf-stable smoked seafood may be safely eaten.
- Do not drink raw (unpasteurized) milk or eat foods that contain unpasteurized milk.

Food Intoxication

Food intoxication is caused by the consumption of a food in which bacteria have produced a poisonous toxin.

STAPHYLOCOCCUS AUREUS

One of the most common bacteria producing a poisonous toxin is ***Staphylococcus aureus,*** commonly referred to as staph. Staph have been reported to be in the nasal passages of 30% to 50% of healthy people and on the hands of 20% of healthy people. Infected cuts, boils, and burns harbor this organism.

Heat destroys the bacteria but not the toxins the bacteria already have produced. Because heat does not destroy the toxin, control of temperature alone will not provide protection. Prevention of staph poisoning must include good personal hygiene and keeping foods below 40°F or above 140°F.

CLOSTRIDIUM BOTULINUM

Another bacterium producing a toxin is ***Clostridium botulinum,*** and the resulting disease is **botulism.** The organism is found worldwide in soils and the intestinal tracts of domestic animals. Vegetables grown in contaminated soil harbor this organism. Botulin, the toxin produced by *C. botulinum,* is so poisonous that a single ounce is enough to kill the world's population. The spores of *C. botulinum* grow under anaerobic (without oxygen) conditions. Canned foods are processed to be anaerobic; thus, they provide an ideal medium for this bacterium's growth. Home-canned, nonacid fruits and vegetables, faultily processed commercially canned tuna, and improperly packaged smoked fish all have transmitted botulism.

Outbreaks of botulism can be avoided by the proper processing and preparation of susceptible foods. For each food, home canners should consult a reliable home-canning food guide regarding proper time, pressure, and temperature required to kill spores. As an additional precaution, all home-canned foods should be boiled for at least 10 minutes before serving to destroy botulinal toxins.

NORWALK VIRUS

This is another pathogen that can withstand freezing temperatures and chlorine solutions. This organism, however, is susceptible to high temperatures (above 140°F). The best insurance against this pathogen is to eat foods hot. Other control measures include good personal hygiene and the purchase of food and water from reliable sources.

Complicating Factors

The following complicate the risk of foodborne illness:

- The worldwide overuse of antibiotics. Antibiotics kill not only pathogens but also normal flora, which help keep the disease-producing organisms in balance.
- In the United States, the average age of the population continues to increase as life expectancy increases. Older people are more susceptible to pathogenic bacteria than younger people; fewer organisms are needed to produce symptoms in older people.
- Food production has become more centralized, an effect that has both good and bad ramifications. Food inspectors can more closely monitor the sanitation at food-processing plants, but a foodborne illness outbreak affects more people in wider geographical areas.
- As the population becomes highly educated about food safety, illnesses that in the past might have been dismissed as "stomach flu" are increasingly being identified as foodborne illnesses.
- Many foods are imported from countries whose regulatory procedures are not as stringent as those in the United States.
- Consumers are eating more meals away from home and using more convenience foods. Both behaviors increase the number of individuals involved in food handling and the time food is held in the danger zones. For example, a frozen convenience food is held in the temperature danger zone (between 40°F and 140°F) twice, once during assembly in the food-processing factory and a second time when the consumer is reheating it.
- Consumers are eating more raw food and more lightly grilled and sautéed foods, which are sometimes not cooked to proper temperatures.

Box 13-4 discusses how the simple behavior of frequent hand washing minimizes the risk of foodborne disease. Figure 13-2 pictures the correct amount of soap lather needed to cleanse hands.

Box 13-4 ■ *Hand Washing*

The best defense against foodborne disease is hand-washing and keeping the hands away from the mouth. Figure 13-2 demonstrates proper hand washing. Hands should always be washed:

- Before food preparation
- After food preparation
- After using the restroom
- Between touching another person's body including the hands and touching the mouth or eating
- After smoking
- Before smoking
- Between touching one person and then another person
- After covering the mouth when coughing or sneezing
- When visibly dirty
- After touching any surface area around any person who is visibly ill
- After changing an infant's diapers or touching any body secretion of another person

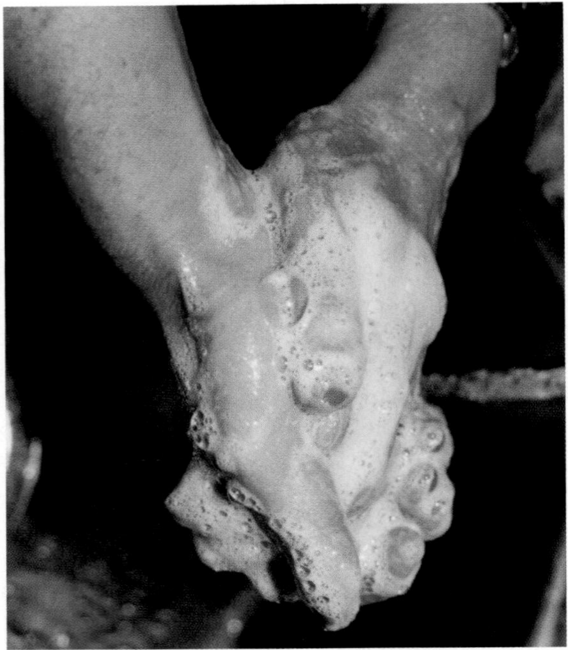

FIGURE 13-2 Amount of soap lather necessary to thoroughly cleanse the hands.

Infectious Agents

Mad cow disease, also known as **bovine spongiform encephalopathy (BSE),** is related to a disease in humans called Creutzfeldt–Jakob disease (variant CJD). Humans acquire this disease by eating beef that contains an infective agent (called a prion). A **prion** is a small protein that is resistant to most traditional methods that destroy a protein. BSE has been found in infected brain, spinal cord tissue, retina, dorsal root ganglia (nervous tissue near the backbone), distal ileum, and bone marrow in cattle experimentally infected by the oral route. Cattle acquire the infection when fed ground-up carcasses of animals, both sheep and other cattle, which contain the infected prion. Both the United States and Canada banned this feed practice for cattle in 1997, but the practice was not banned for poultry and hogs.

Variant CJD has been seen primarily in young adults and is characterized initially by psychiatric and sensory problems, followed by ataxia (defective muscular coordination), dementia, and myoclonus (caused by fungus). This disease is considered a fatal brain disorder (American Dietetic Association, 2003).

Parasitic Infections

A **parasite** is an organism that lives within, upon, or at the expense of a living host without providing any benefit to the host. Several parasites can live in animals that humans use for food. When a person eats an infected animal, he or she also consumes the parasite and the result is illness. Two common parasites are *Trichinella spiralis* and tapeworms.

TRICHINELLA SPIRALIS

Although the prevalence of this infection is low in the United States, it is significantly higher in people living in parts of Europe, Asia, and Southeast Asia.

Trichinella spiralis is a worm that becomes embedded in the muscle tissue of pigs. Pigs acquire the worm when fed meat from an animal harboring the worm in its muscle. The worm produces larvae that are protected from animal (including human) digestion. The larvae mature in the animal's stomach in 5 to 7 days. Adult worms then invade the lining of the small intestine, where they reproduce. The larvae enter the bloodstream of the animal and are carried to all parts of the body. They then penetrate the muscles, form cysts, and remain alive and infective for months. The cycle is completed when another animal eats the muscle containing the live *Trichinella spiralis* larvae.

When a human eats the larvae, usually in undercooked pork, he or she develops **trichinosis.** The symptoms of trichinosis usually appear 9 days after the ingestion of infected meat, but the time can vary from 2 to 28 days. This period of time is called the **incubation period**—the length of time it takes to show disease symptoms after exposure to the offending organism. The first symptoms, which mimic food poisoning, are nausea, vomiting, and diarrhea. When the larvae migrate into muscles, including the heart, systemic symptoms develop that include fever, swelling of the eyelids, sweating, weakness, and muscular pain. Death due to heart failure may occur.

TAPEWORMS

Humans acquire tapeworms through the ingestion of raw seafood or undercooked beef and pork. Hogs and steers become intermediate hosts when they graze on sewage-polluted pastures. Tapeworm infestation can occur when human wastes contaminate freshwater streams and lakes, animal pasture, or feed.

Symptoms of a tapeworm infection may be trivial or absent. In some people, the worms attach to the jejunum and hosts develop vitamin B_{12} deficiency, anemia, and massive infections with diarrhea. Obstruction of the bile duct or intestine can be another complication.

Viral Infections

A **virus** is a microscopic parasite that is entirely dependent on the nutrients inside host cells for its metabolic and reproductive needs. Viruses may invade the cells of people, animals, plants, and bacteria to survive and thereby cause disease. Food frequently serves as a vehicle for some viruses, including those that cause influenza and infectious hepatitis.

Food can become contaminated in its growing environment or during processing, storage, distribution, or preparation. Partly for this reason, the federal government requires all food-service workers to wear plastic gloves when handling food.

Some viruses are found in the intestinal tract of infected humans. If an infected person neglects to wash his or her hands after defecation and then handles food, the virus can contaminate the food and be passed on to unsuspecting consumers. The disease varies from a mild illness lasting 1 to 2 weeks to a severely disabling disease lasting several months.

HEPATITIS A VIRUS

The hepatitis A virus causes infectious hepatitis, a liver disease. This virus can be found in water that has been contaminated with raw sewage and in shellfish harvested from fecally contaminated water. During food processing, hepatitis A can be transmitted when polluted water is used or by fecal contamination from insects or rodents. Infected workers can transmit the virus through food they handle. The onset of viral hepatitis A is abrupt, with fever, malaise, anorexia, nausea, and abdominal discomfort. A few days later, the client may develop jaundice.

Substances Made Poisonous by Other Organisms

The consumption of toxic fish and plants can cause illness. Some molds can also produce disease (others are beneficial).

TOXIC SEAFOOD

The tissue of fish and shellfish can be naturally toxic to humans, even when the fish is fresh. The fish may not show any outward signs of illness, and there is usually no way to tell whether the fish is toxic. Because most fish toxins are stable to heat, cooking does not destroy them. **Paralytic shellfish poisoning** outbreaks have been reported involving the consumption of poisonous clams, oysters, mussels, and scallops.

Ciguatera poisoning is a serious human intoxication caused by ingestion of any of more than 400 species of marine fish (Shils, 2005). This intoxication results from eating certain fish that have consumed marine bacteria and algae associated with coastal reefs and nearby waterways. Fish eating the algae become toxic, and the effect is magnified through the food chain so that large predatory fish become the most toxic; this occurs worldwide in tropical areas. Coastal waters are routinely monitored for the presence of the organism that produces ciguatera. If excessive numbers of the organism are found, a "red tide" alert is made. The best prevention is to avoid eating fish caught during a red tide.

Scromboid fish poisoning is caused by the presence of undesirable bacteria. This poisoning occurs in fish such as tuna, mackerel, bonito, and skipjack. The bacteria produce a toxin on the flesh of fish after the fish have been caught. Scromboid fish poisoning can be prevented by the adequate refrigeration of freshly caught fish and the purchase of fish from reputable sources.

MOLDS

Molds are the most widely encountered microorganism, and are spread by air currents, insects, and rodents. Some molds are beneficial, such as those used to make some cheese and soy sauce. Like bacteria, molds are often involved in food spoilage. A number of molds grow well in cold storage but are easily destroyed by heating to 140°F or higher.

Molds grow on bread, cheese, fruits, vegetables, preserves, grains, and a wide variety of other products. ***Aspergillus*** molds produce a series of **mycotoxins** called **aflatoxins** that may be present in peanuts or peanut products, corn, and cottonseed meal (Shils, 2005). Many experts believe aflatoxins to be the most potent liver toxin known.

The best advice is to discard moldy bread because mold may have penetrated the entire item. Mold on natural cheese can be safely removed and the remainder of the cheese eaten, because the mold is not likely to have penetrated deeply.

Environmental Pollutants

Although environmental pollution is widespread, situations that pose a severe and immediate health danger are uncommon. The U.S. Environmental Protection Agency (EPA) regulates the use of **pesticides** and sets tolerance levels to provide a high margin of safety in food.

Chemical Poisoning

Chemical poisoning occurs when people eat toxic substances that may be intentionally or accidentally added to foods during growing, harvesting, processing, transporting, storing, or preparing foods. Two general types of chemical poisoning can occur. They are heavy metal and chemical-product contamination pesticides.

Heavy Metals

Several metals can be toxic. Metals in the soil come from rocks and minerals weathered by water erosion, metals as added ingredients or impurities in fertilizers, pesticides, manure and sludge, and airborne dust. Airborne dust comes from industrial and mining waste, fossil fuel combustion products, radioactive fallout, pollen, sea spray, and meteoric and volcanic material. This dust eventually settles to the ground and becomes part of the soil. Plants may grow normally but contain levels of selenium, cadmium, molybdenum, or lead that are toxic to humans.

The toxic action of metals is thought to be important in enzyme poisoning. For example, mercury, lead, copper, beryllium, cadmium, and silver have been found to inhibit the enzyme **alkaline phosphatase.** One function of alkaline phosphatase is in the mineralization of bone. Some diseases associated with the consumption of toxic minerals include rickets and bone tumors. Lead ingestion with a subsequent elevation of blood lead levels has been linked to toxic effects, including adverse neurologic, neurobehavioral, and developmental conditions.

Mercury is extremely toxic and is distributed worldwide. Episodes of serious poisoning include those in Minamata (1953 to 1960) and the Niigata area (1965) in Japan (Shils, 2005), in which large chemical plants poured industrial waste containing mercury into nearby bays. Area residents who ate fish from the bays complained of numbness of the extremities, slurred speech, unsteady gait, deafness, and visual disturbances. Mental confusion and muscular incoordination were apparent in all the clients. Because mercury can damage the fetal nervous system, the Food and Drug Administration has issued a consumer alert for pregnant women and women of childbearing age not to eat large fish types in which mercury may accumulate: shark, swordfish, king mackerel, and tilefish (Am Diet Assoc, 2003).

Chemical Products

Chemical foodborne illness is also associated with products such as detergents, sanitizers, pesticides, and other chemicals that may enter the food supply. After such toxins have been ingested, symptoms of chemical poisoning appear in a few minutes to a few hours, but usually in less than 1 hour. Nausea, vomiting, abdominal pain, diarrhea, and a metallic taste are common complaints with chemical foodborne illnesses. Death is possible. See Box 13-5.

Pesticides are chemicals used to kill insects or rodents, and when accidentally mixed with food, pesticides have caused poisonings in people. In addition, using pesticide-containing aerosols around foods and packaging materials and in food preparation areas can be dangerous. According to the Environmental Protection Agency (EPA), studies have linked pesticides to problems such as cancer, nerve damage, and birth defects.

Pesticide residues are of great concern to consumers. **Residues** are trace amounts of any substance remaining in a product at the time of sale. Three governmental agencies regulate products that enter the U.S. food supply:

- The Environmental Protection Agency (EPA)
- The Food and Drug Administration (FDA)
- The United States Department of Agriculture (USDA) Food Safety and Inspection Service (FSIS)

The EPA regulates the use of potentially harmful pesticides in food production. Included among the duties of the EPA is the establishment of tolerance levels for pesticides.

The FDA regulates animal drugs, including food additives, herbicides, and environmental contaminants. The FSIS sets tolerance levels for these chemical residues in edible foods. In setting a **tolerance level**, the FSIS determines the highest dose at which a residue causes no ill effects in laboratory animals. The tolerance level is then divided by a factor ranging from 100 to 1000 to account for possible differences between animals and humans.

The numbers used assume that humans are 10 times more sensitive than the most sensitive animal species tested. In addition, a further assumption is made that children and the elderly are 10 times more sensitive than others. This is the 100-fold safety factor (multiplying 10 times 10). Thus, a large margin of safety is built into residue limits for compounds involved in the production of human food.

The FSIS enforces the residue limits in meat and poultry. The FDA is responsible for foods other than meat and poultry. When an illegal residue is found, the FDA can conduct an investigation and the FSIS can detain future shipments from the violating producer.

Box 13-5 ■ *Chemical Poisoning*

Chemical poisoning can be prevented by:

- Using each product for its intended use and in the amounts recommended
- Reading product labels before use
- Keeping chemicals in their original containers
- Never storing or transporting chemicals in containers used to store food

They may be mistaken (especially by children) for food or beverages.

Natural Food Intoxicants

Many foods (unprocessed or uncooked) contain natural components that can harm health. All foods are made up of chemicals, some of which can alter the way the body uses nutrients. For example, phytates in grains decrease the bioavailability of zinc, calcium, iron, and manganese (Shils, 2005). **Bioavailability** is the rate and extent to which an active drug or nutrient or metabolite enters the general circulation, permitting access to the site of action (Venes, 2005). Another example are proteinase inhibitors in peas, peanuts, potatoes, and many varieties of beans, which block the activity of enzymes such as trypsin and chymotrypsin (Shils, 2005).

Healthy people in this country who eat well-balanced diets should not worry about natural food intoxicants. However, if an individual eats large amounts of a single food at one time, he or she may experience the effects of natural intoxicants. The best protection, therefore, against the effects of natural intoxicants is to eat a wide variety of foods.

Food Additives

Additives may be introduced into food deliberately or accidentally. An **additive** is a substance added to food to increase its flavor, shelf life, or characteristics, such as texture, color, and aroma, and other qualities. In the United States, the FDA regulates food additives under the authority of the Food, Drug, and Cosmetic Act of 1938 and amendments in 1958 and 1960. These amendments include the Delaney Clause, which bans the approval of an additive if it is shown to cause cancer in humans or animals. Before using a new food additive, a manufacturer must petition the FDA for approval. The manufacturer must prove the additive is not harmful to humans at expected consumption.

Two categories of food additives are not subject to the testing and approval procedure: *prior-sanctioned* and *GRAS* substances. The FDA before the 1958 Food Additives Amendment approved substances appointed as prior sanctioned. GRAS (generally recognized as safe) additives are those that have been used extensively in the past with no known harmful effects and are thought to be safe. Substances on the GRAS list have been under review since 1969. Substances on the GRAS list include sugar, salt, and vinegar.

Intentional Use

Additives are intentionally added directly to food during processing for four reasons:

1. To maintain or enhance a food's nutritional value. Vitamins, minerals, and fiber are examples.
2. To maintain a food's quality. Many additives are used to prevent the growth of microorganisms and extend a product's shelf-life. Some additives, called antioxidants, are used to prevent fats in food from deteriorating. Selected antioxidants may be effective in delaying proliferation of some cancers, mainly those related to fat metabolism, such as breast and prostate cancer.
3. To assist in processing, transporting, or holding a food. One additive that helps facilitate the processing of food is an **emulsifier,** to evenly distribute the molecules of two liquids that normally do not mix. Mayonnaise is an example of an emulsified product. Baking soda and baking powder are other commonly used additives. These substances cause such products as cakes to rise and improve their texture and volume.
4. To improve the way a food tastes, looks, or smells. Artificial colors, flavors, and sweeteners all fall into this category.

Types of common food additives are listed in Table 13-2.

Accidental Use

Some additives enter the food supply accidentally. For example, chemicals may enter food through contact with surfaces that have been cleaned with chemical solutions.

The Food Label

The FDA requires food labeling under the Federal Food Drug and Cosmetic Act and its amendments. Most prepared foods, such as breads, cereals, canned fruits and vegetables, snacks, desserts, and drinks, require a food label. Nutrition labeling for raw produce (fruits and vegetables) is voluntary. Recently, the USDA added a requirement that farm raised seafood must be labeled with the country of origin (www.USDA.gov). Figure 13-3 provides information on using the Nutrition Facts panel. The following list describes a food label's contents.

TABLE 13-2 ■ Common Food Additives

Acidity Control Agents	Influence flavor, texture, and shelf life	Sodium bicarbonate Citric acid Hydrogen chloride Sodium hydroxide Acetic acid Phosphoric acid Calcium oxide
Antioxidants	Prevent discoloration Protect fats from rancidity	Vitamin C Vitamin E BHT and BHA
Flavors	Food enhancers	Hydrolyzed vegetable protein Black pepper Mustard Monosodium glutamate
Leavening Agents	To make dough rise	Sodium acid phosphate Sodium aluminum phosphate Monocalcium phosphate Yeast
Preservatives	To extend shelf-life	Sulfur oxide Benzoic acid Propionic acid EDTA
Stabilizers and Thickeners	To enhance texture	Sodium caseinate Gum arabic Modified starch Pectin

1. *Standardized Format:* Every label has the same layout and design; the nutrition information is entitled "Nutrition Facts." Some very small packages may use a simplified format.
2. *Serving Sizes:* All serving sizes listed on similar products are stated in consistently used household and metric measures to allow comparison shopping.
3. *Daily Values:* The bottom half of the Nutrition Facts panel shows either the minimum or maximum levels of nutrients people should consume each day for a healthful diet. For example, the value listed for carbohydrates refers to the minimum level, whereas the value for fat refers to the maximum level.
4. *% Daily Values:* The figures for percentage of daily values are based on a 2000-kilocalorie diet; this schema makes it easier for consumers to judge the nutritional quality of a food.
5. *Health Claims:* A **health claim** describes the relationship between a food or food component and a disease or health-related condition. Food manufacturers are allowed to write health claims on food labels that show only a preliminary promise of disease prevention. The FDA tried at one time

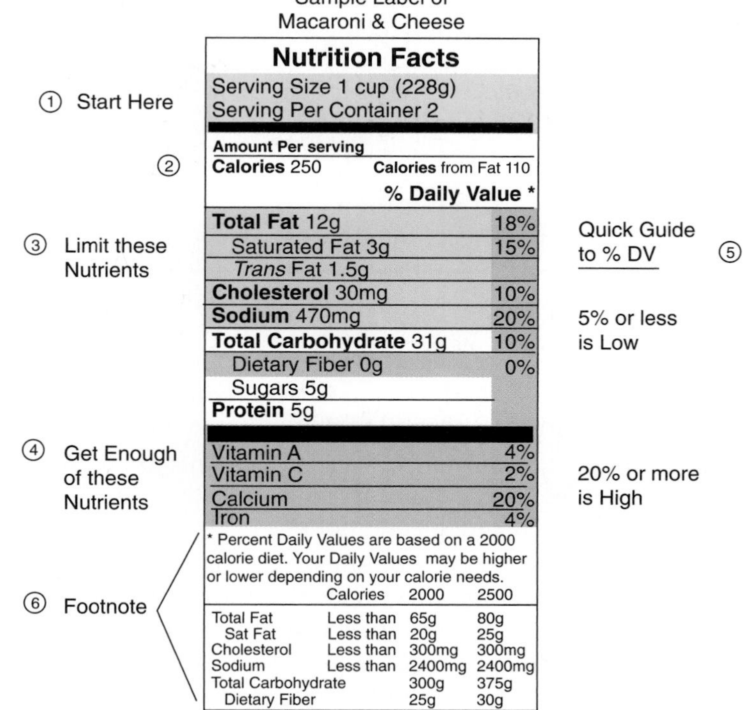

1. Start Here: The first place to start reading the Nutrition Facts Panel is the serving size and the number of servings in the package. Note how much you actually eat.

2. Calories: Displays the number of calories in the given serving size. The label also tells you how many calories are derived from fat.

3. Limit these nutrients: Eating too many of these nutrients may increase your risk of certain chronic diseases, such as heart disease, some cancers, and hypertension. Americans generally eat these nutrients in adequate amounts or too much.

4. Get enough of these nutrients: Americans often don't get enough of these nutrients.

5. Quick guide to % D.V.: % D.V. is based on 2000- and 2500-calorie diet.

6. Footnote: The D.V. are based on expert advice about some key nutrients that should be eaten daily.

FIGURE 13-3 Using the Nutrition Facts Panel on food labels. (*Source*: www.dietaryguidelines.gov)

to enforce more stringent regulations for health claims but the court ruled that this was a violation of free speech. The FDA has only limited control on a health claim printed on a food product.

6. *A Structure/Function Claim:* A **structure/function claim** describes the role of a nutrient or dietary ingredient intended to affect the structure or function in humans or characterizes the documented mechanism by which a nutrient or dietary ingredient acts to maintain such structure or function, e.g., "helps promote a healthy heart" or "helps support the immune system." Structure/function claims can be made without any scientific evidence to support the claim. The FDA has no regulatory control over a structure/function claim.
7. *Descriptors:* Terms like *low, high,* and *free* used on food labels must meet legal definitions: For example:

Free means less than 0.5 gram of fat per serving and tiny or insignificant amounts of cholesterol, sodium, and sugar.

Low indicates 3 grams of fat (or less) per serving; also low in saturated fat, cholesterol, and/or kilocalories.

Lean signifies less than 10 grams of fat, 4 grams of saturated fat, and 95 milligrams of cholesterol per serving. (*Lean* is higher in fat than *Low*.)

Extra Lean means 5 grams of fat, 2 grams of saturated fat, and 95 milligrams of cholesterol per serving. (*Extra Lean* is lower in fat than *Lean* but not as low in fat as *Low*.)

Light (Lite) denotes one-third fewer kilocalories or one-half the fat of the original or no more than one-half the sodium of the higher-sodium version.

Cholesterol Free means the item has less than 2 milligrams of cholesterol and 2 grams (or less) of saturated fat per serving.

High in a nutrient means the food must contain 20% or more of the Daily Value for that nutrient.

Good Source Of denotes that one serving of a food is considered to be a good source of a vitamin, mineral, or fiber, containing 10% to 19% of the Daily Value for that particular vitamin, mineral, or fiber.

8. Ingredients are listed in descending order by weight. The ingredients list is required on almost all foods, even some standardized ones like ice cream, mayonnaise, and bread.

Keystones

- The U.S. food supply is as safe, wholesome, and nutritious as any in the world, but there are no guarantees that all food purchased and eaten in the country is safe.
- Thousands of substances besides nutrients are present in foods. Most of these substances are harmless in the amounts typically eaten if the food item is selected, stored, and prepared under recommended conditions.
- Many foods contain toxic substances naturally. Only in recent years have we been able to detect and measure these toxic substances. The human body appears able to safely handle small amounts of some toxic substances without injury.
- The FDA ranks pathogenic (disease-causing) microorganisms as the most dangerous food-related public health threat. An individual is more likely to suffer from a foodborne illness due to microbiologic contamination than from any other source.
- Good food-handling methods can control most microbiologic hazards.
- Selecting a wide variety of foods, storing the foods appropriately, and preparing foods correctly all help prevent illness.
- Health-care workers should teach their clients about the use of food labels and the risks of microbiologic and residual chemical hazards of foods.

CASE STUDY 13-1

Ms. N is a 95-year-old woman who is 5 ft tall and weighs 122 lb (dressed without shoes). She has just been admitted to the nursing home. During the routine nursing admission process, Ms. N requested eggnog every night at 8:00 P.M. She stated she dislikes packaged mixes and would prefer her eggnog made with whole milk, ice cream, and a raw egg. Ms. N's physician has ordered eggnog at HS (Latin for hour of sleep, or just before bedtime) every day. Ms. N stated she has drunk a homemade eggnog every night for the past 50 years. The client's daughter has stated she makes her mother eggnog from raw eggs.

Care Plan

Subjective Data

Client stated she drinks eggnog made with a raw egg each day. ■ Client's daughter stated she makes her mother such a beverage.

Objective Data

Height: 5 ft, 0 in. ■ Weight: adm 122 lb ■ Age: 95

Analysis

Increased risk of infection related to consumption of raw eggs and client's advanced age.

CASE STUDY *(Continued)*

Plan

DESIRED OUTCOMES EVALUATION CRITERIA	ACTIONS/INTERVENTIONS	RATIONALE
The client will state that raw eggs can make one ill.	Provide verbal and written information to the client and the client's daughter on the relationship between food illness and *Salmonella* infections.	Elderly clients are particularly at risk for salmonellosis.
	Have the client and the client's daughter state that raw eggs are hazardous.	Verbal recognition of a hazard is the first step in behavioral change.
The client will accept and eat another item for her evening snack.	Request the dietitian provide client with a list of other alternatives for her evening snack and evaluate if client needs the snack.	Do not offer client an item that is not available from the Food and Nutrition Department. The client may need the nutrients in the evening snack.
	Chart acceptance or rejection of the snack.	Refusal to eat substitute snack defeats the purpose of sending the snack.

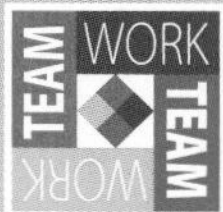

13-1

Dietitian's Note

The following Dietitian's Notes are representative of the documentation found in a client's medical record.

Subjective: Spoke with patient and her daughter. The risk of Salmonella foodborne disease with the consumption of raw eggs in an older adult was explained to client and her daughter. A 24-hour dietary recall cross-checked with a food frequency was completed. Client has been eating three times per day, accepts all major food groups, and denies food allergies. Usual intake consists of: 6 medium-fat meats, 5 starches (3 whole grain), 3 vegetables (including a source of vitamin A), 3 fruits (including a source of vitamin C), and 6 fats. Claims good dentition, denies nausea and vomiting (N/V), constipation, diarrhea

Objective: Albumin 3.7 mg/dL; body mass index 23; Height 5 ft, 0 in.; weight 122 lb

Analysis: Usual intake about 1400 to 1450 kcal with 67 grams of protein. No laboratory, diet history, and anthropometric evidence of nutritional risk.

Estimated kilocalorie needs based on maximum ideal body weight (IBW) of 110 lb or 50 kg and 25–35 kcal/kg max equals 1250–1750 kcal

Estimated protein need based on 50 kg and 0.8–1.2 g/kg equals 40–60 grams of protein per day.

Estimated kilocalories in homemade eggnog equals 275 kcal.

After explaining risk with the consumption of raw eggs, patient agreed to have one cup of hot cocoa and a banana for her evening snack as she would need the kilocalorie from these items to meet her estimated kilocalorie needs. Patient's protein intake more than exceeds estimated requirements.

Plan:

1. Follow-up in 3 days.
2. Order evening snack as described above.

Critical Thinking Questions

1. What other areas of the home might you inspect to minimize the risk of a foodborne illness?
2. What clients need to take extra precautions to prevent a foodborne illness?
3. Do you think it is within the scope of practice for a nurse when making a home visit to discuss unsafe food practices?

Chapter Review

1. Cold foods should be stored:
   a. At less than 50°F
   b. At less than 0°F
   c. At less than 40°F
   d. For no more than 6 hours outside the recommended temperature range.
2. The term *Low* on a food label means the product contains:
   a. Less than 3 grams of fat (or less) per serving; also low in saturated fat, cholesterol, or kilocalories
   b. ___ the fat of the original
   c. Less than 10 grams of fat, 4 grams of saturated fat, and 95 milligrams of cholesterol per serving
   d. More fat than a product labeled *Extra Lean.*
3. Foods commonly contaminated with *Campylobacter* are:
   a. Hard-cooked scrambled eggs
   b. Raw vegetables
   c. Canned foods
   d. Raw poultry
4. The best method to control the spread of foodborne illness is by:
   a. Wearing gloves when handling food
   b. Proper hand washing
   c. Taking food supplements
   d. Avoiding certain foods
5. Farm-raised seafood must be labeled with
   a. Country of origin
   b. Grams of mercury
   c. Kilocalories in one serving
   d. Grams of protein

Clinical Analysis

1. Mr. P has brought his 35-year-old male companion who has a history of AIDS to the ambulatory care clinic for treatment for a sudden onset of headache, abdominal pain, diarrhea, nausea, and vomiting. The nurse should:
   a. Document all food consumed during the past 7 days.
   b. Inquire about food practices in the home.
   c. Inspect Mr. P's passport for foreign travel in the past month.
   d. Document the client's immunization status.
2. You are on a committee to help plan the annual hospital picnic. One employee volunteers to make Texas-style chili at home and serve it at the picnic. You have a responsibility to:
   a. Inquire how the chili will be made, transported, and held at recommended temperatures
   b. Taste the chili on arrival at the picnic for safety
   c. Check the temperature of the chili on arrival at the picnic
   d. Review the recipe for the potential use of unsafe ingredients
3. Mr. J is an 85-year-old man recently discharged from the hospital for a partial bowel obstruction that he had surgically repaired. His wife is getting ready to serve him eggnog made with raw eggs. What would be the most effective way to determine if the client consumed any contaminated food?
   a. Ignore the situation because that is not the purpose of the visit.
   b. Inquire about any gastrointestinal pain Mr. J may have had.
   c. Instruct the wife about the safe preparation of eggs.
   d. Assess the amount of sugar used in the beverage.

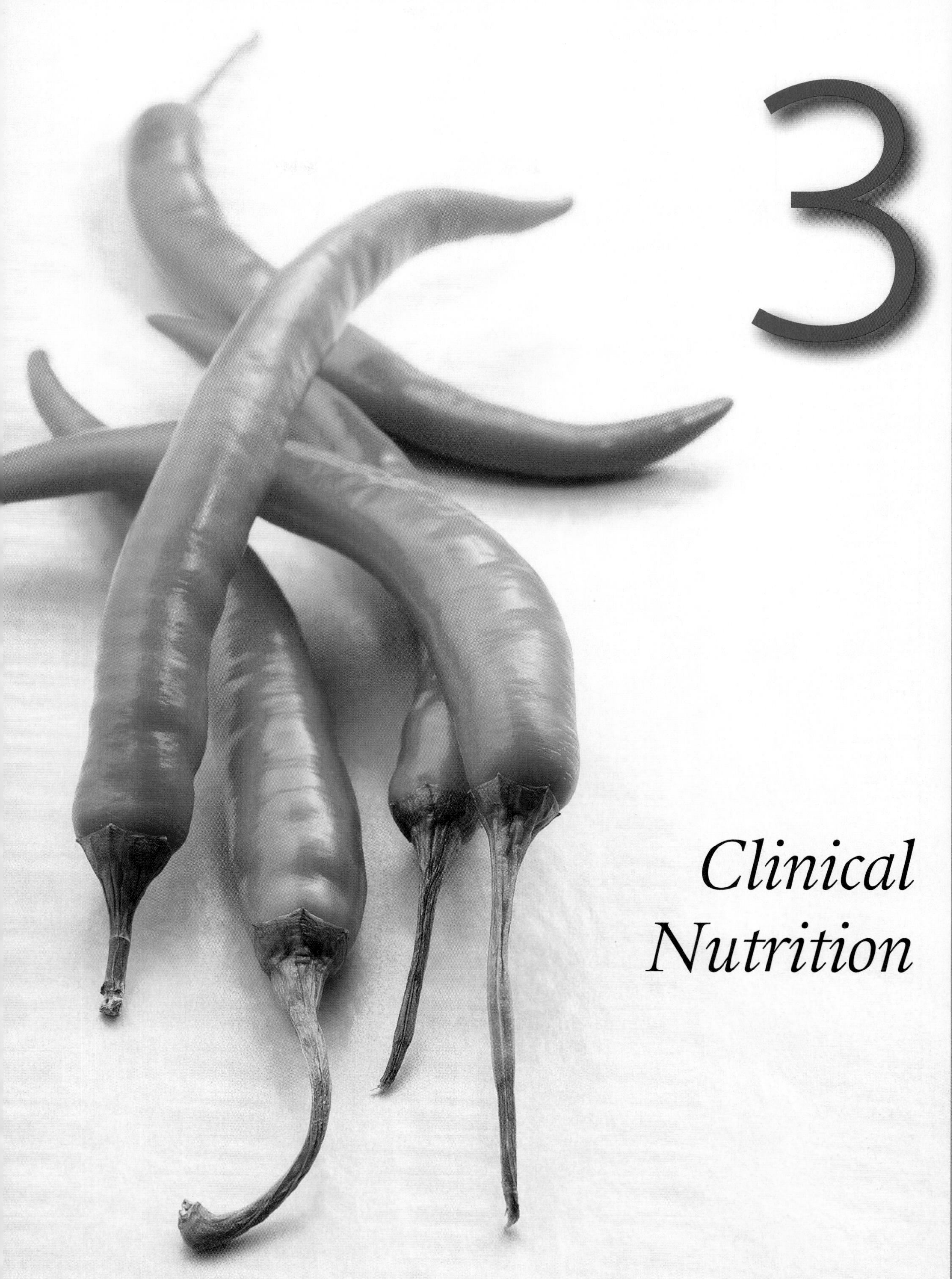

3

Clinical Nutrition

14

Nutrient Delivery

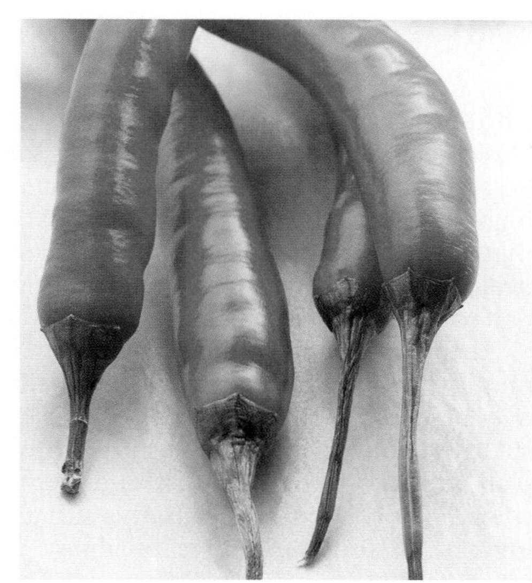

LEARNING OBJECTIVES

After completing this chapter, the student should be able to:

- Identify three routes used to deliver nutrients to clients and potential complications with two of these routes.
- Discuss the kinds of commercial formulas available for oral and tube feedings.
- Discuss why it is important to carefully control the concentration, rate of delivery, and volume of formula delivered to a client.
- List at least five reasons for the high incidence of malnutrition in institutionalized clients and the interventions nurses can perform to combat malnutrition.
- Describe suggested procedures for administering medications through feeding tubes.

This chapter introduces the methods commonly used to deliver nutrients to clients: oral and tube feedings, total parenteral nutrition (TPN), and peripheral parenteral nutrition (PPN). Food services in health-care facilities have two major functions: the preparation and delivery of nutrients to clients and the nutritional care of clients. The nutritional care of clients includes four areas:

1. Assessing the client's need for nutrients
2. Delivering nutrients to the client
3. Monitoring the client's nutrient intake
4. Counseling the client about nutritional needs

High-quality nutritional care saves the client and society health-care dollars and preventable hardship.

Food Service in Institutions

All members of the health-care team need to become familiar with some aspects of the food service in their place of employment. Specific personnel duties are typically related to meal-service schedules. The scheduling of diagnostic procedures, blood work, surgery, and administration of medications is dependent on when the client last consumed food.

Meal Service Patterns

Many institutions serve three meals to clients each day as well as several between-meal feedings. Feedings between meals are available for clients in need of extra nutrients, those who desire extra food, or those unable to consume sufficient kilocalories at the regular mealtimes. Some institutions offer a room service system and patients may order food whenever they desire. In this situation, specific procedures are necessary to ensure that medication administration is coordinated with meal delivery.

Nutritional Care Services

Institutions vary in the types of nutritional services they offer clients. A large teaching hospital or medical center frequently has nutrition professionals on staff who specialize in treating particular types of clients. A critical-care dietitian, for example, has special training to assess, plan, implement, and counsel clients in high-risk stages of trauma, disease, and conditions that affect nutritional support. In such settings, other health-care workers can rely on the critical-care dietitian to provide technical support.

At the other end of the spectrum, in a small community hospital or a long-term care facility, a dietitian may be present only part time or as a consultant. In such circumstances, other health-care workers must plan to make the best use of the dietitian's services when he or she is available. In this situation, the nursing staff assumes more responsibility for the nutritional care of clients.

Home- and community-based programs also provide nutritional care services. For example, hospice, home-care programs, and some governmental agencies deliver nutritional care services. Frequently, a dietitian is available through any of these programs for consultation. Third-party payers increasingly cover medical nutritional care.

Assessment, Monitoring, and Counseling

Nutritional care is a responsibility of many members of the health-care team. The nurse is usually the first member of the team to interview and assess the client, often before the physician visits the client. The physician and/or physician's assistant complete a physical examination of the client, order necessary treatments and diagnostic procedures, and provide either a diagnosis or tentative diagnosis. The diagnosis may change after the diagnostic tests are completed. The nurse, physician, or the physician assistant usually makes referrals to other team members. Institutions frequently require specific team members to assess each client. Figure 14-1 presents an overview of a nutrient-delivery decision-making tree.

Assessment

Clients found to be at a nutritional risk have a complete nutritional assessment, which usually includes the following items:

- Height, weight, body mass index (BMI), and weight history
- Laboratory test values
- Food intake information
- Potential food–drug interactions
- Mastication and swallowing ability
- Client's ability to feed him- or herself
- Bowel and bladder function
- Evaluation for the presence of **pressure ulcers**
- Food allergies and intolerances
- Any other factors affecting nutritional status, such as food preferences and cultural and religious beliefs about food
- Determination of body composition
- Presence of severe burns, trauma, infection, or other physiological stressors that increase nutrient needs and are likely to prolong hospital stay
- Learning barriers such as hearing, mobility, language, need for interpreter, vision, speech, reading/writing skills, inability to follow instructions, cultural and religious barriers, learning disability, learning readiness (requests, accepts, or avoids information), and preferred learning style

The American Society for Parenteral and Enteral Nutrition (A.S.P.E.N.) has defined nutrition assessment as a comprehensive approach to defining nutritional status that uses medical, nutrition, and medication histories; physical examination; anthropometric measurements; and laboratory data. In addition, A.S.P.E.N, defines any disorder of nutrition status including those resulting from deficiency of intake, impaired nutrient metabolism, or overnutrition as Malnutrition (A.S.P.E.N, 2008). In this context, nutrition assessment is much more than an initial client screening, as completed by nursing personnel. In this context, a nutritional assessment requires all members of the health-care team to deliver quality care.

Computer technology has greatly facilitated the client assessment process. Information may group clients such as all those with low blood albumins; on specific mediations; with low weight for height; and on NPO (nothing by mouth) or on inadequate diets for longer than 3 days, and so forth. The consolidation of this information allows for a greater number of clients to be identified and targeted for in-depth nutritional assessment and care.

Client care has also become standardized as a result of computer technology and the development of standards of practice. For example, a health-care organization may require clients with a blood albumin level of less than 3 mg/dL be evaluated by a registered dietitian within 24 hours of admission. A licensed speech pathologist may be required to evaluate all clients with dysphasia before the client is given any food or fluids. Or a registered nurse may be required to phone a physician immediately on receipt of data showing a potassium level greater than 5.0 mEq/L and document the phone call. The occupational therapist may be required to evaluate clients who are unable to feed themselves, and so forth.

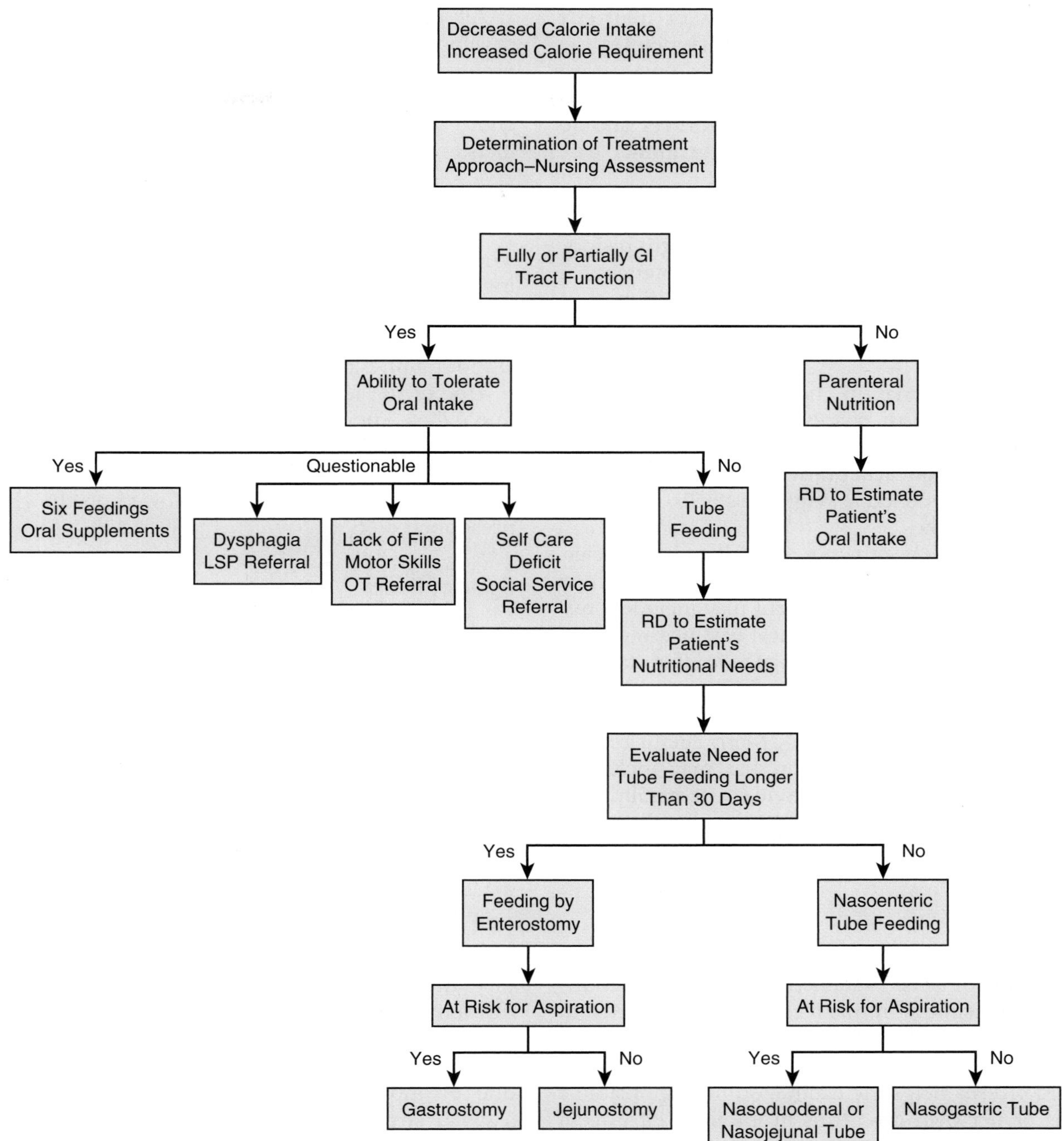

FIGURE 14-1 Nutrient delivery decision-making tree. OR = occupational therapist; RD = registered dietitian; LSP = licensed speech pathologist. (Adapted from Abbott Nutrition: Abbott Nutrition Pocket Guide 2008, Columbus, OH.)

Regulatory agencies of long-term care facilities require that clients have a nutritional assessment performed by a registered dietitian shortly after admission. An initial assessment or screening identifies clients at nutritional risk. An in-depth assessment as defined by A.S.P.E.N. requires a care plan by several team members who coordinate services.

Monitoring

All clients should be reassessed or monitored at appropriate intervals. Most organizations include the required frequency of client monitoring in their standards of practice. Some clients in hospital intensive care units require continuous monitoring. Other clients require daily, weekly, monthly, or quarterly reassessment as determined by preset guidelines.

The **client care conference** (interdisciplinary conference) is a productive means of monitoring clients. Before the conference, health-care workers should gather information on the client's nutritional care including:

- The client's initial nutritional assessment
- The client's present body weight and weight history
- A record of the client's recent food acceptances
- Any changes in the client's medical condition
- The client's diet order
- Family support (or lack of)

With this information, health-care workers can easily determine most changes in the client's nutritional status. Weight loss is readily identified. A review of the client's **food acceptance record,** if available, can verify whether such a weight loss is likely a result of poor food intake.

Clients whom health-care providers have determined to be at nutritional risk because of poor food intake should be treated; treatment may include a nutritional supplement, between-meal feedings, a change in the diet prescription, or a change in feeding status. If, for example, a client can no longer feed him- or herself, the client's feeding status would need to be changed from self-feed to assisted feeding. Many clients require aggressive nutritional treatment that may include a tube feeding, inserted either surgically or nasally, and/or parenteral feedings. Monitoring the client's weight, laboratory values, and food intake is an important part of delivering high-quality nutritional care.

Counseling

All clients should be evaluated for nutritional counseling. The assumption that a client is not expected to be discharged and therefore is not entitled to education is unjustifiable. Educating the client about nutritional concerns helps the client assume responsibility for his or her own care, thus promoting self-esteem and a sense of worth.

Diet Manuals

Current accreditation standards (both long-term and acute-care) require all health-care institutions to have a diet manual available to all team members. The diet manual defines and describes all diets used in the facility and includes information about the particular food service operation. What is included in a "soft diet" may vary slightly from one institution to another. For example, one soft diet may allow lettuce, whereas another may not.

All health-care professionals in a facility jointly develop and approve the diet manual. Regional food preferences and the unique training of the facility's medical staff and other professionals influence the choice of food items allowed or avoided on special diets.

Diet Orders

The physician or designee is responsible for prescribing a diet for the client. Just as a medication cannot be administered to a client without a medication prescription, food or fluids cannot be served to a client without a physician's written diet order.

One of the functions of the diet manual is to define a diet. The diet manual is the first place to look when clients request food items not being served to them. The diet manual may state, perhaps, that the food item is restricted or not allowed on the client's prescribed diet.

Special Diets

The purpose of a special or modified diet is to restore or maintain a client's nutritional status by manipulating one or more of the following dietary aspects:

- Nutrients such as protein, calcium, iron, sodium, potassium, and vitamin K may be increased, decreased, or eliminated.
- Kilocalories may be either restricted or increased.
- Texture or consistency of foods may be an issue. For example, only clear liquids may be served.
- Use of seasonings such as pepper may be restricted or eliminated.

All modified diets are variations of the general diet; the client nonetheless needs all the essential nutrients. For this reason, each modified diet must be carefully planned to provide each of the essential nutrients or a documented reason for not providing one or more essential nutrients. For example in a given situation for a specific client, a physician may think resuming oral nutrition is not medically indicated.

Common Diet Orders

Some common diet orders are for *clear liquid, full liquid, soft,* and *general* or *regular*. A clear-liquid diet is any transparent liquid that can be poured at room temperature. Gelatin, some juices, broth, tea, and coffee are clear liquids. A clear-liquid diet is nutritionally inadequate. Clear-liquid nutritional supplements, however, are available.

A full-liquid diet is any liquid that can be poured at room temperature. Milk, custard, thinned hot cereals,

TABLE 14-1 ■ Composition of Liquid Diets

DIET	PROTEIN (GRAMS)	FAT (GRAMS)	CARBOHYDRATE (GRAMS)	SODIUM (MEQ)	POTASSIUM (MEQ)	KILOCALORIES
Clear Liquid	5	Trace	70–95	65	20	375
Clear Liquid with Three 6-oz Servings of Citrotein®/Enlive®	30	1	140–165	80	30	750
Full Liquid	50	55	205	110	65	1500

Box 14-1 ■ *Clear-Liquid Diet*

Description

The clear-liquid diet provides energy and fluid in a form that requires minimal digestive action.

Indications

The clear-liquid diet is prescribed when it is necessary to limit undigested food in the gastrointestinal tract, before bowel surgery, diagnostic imaging procedures, and colonoscopic examination. A clear-liquid diet is also used during acute stages of illness to assist with fluid and electrolyte replacement and as a first step in oral alimentation after intravenous feeding, surgery, and gastrointestinal disturbances.

Adequacy

This diet is inadequate in all nutrients and should be used only in the short term.

Food Allowed	Foods To Avoid
Coffee and tea	All other food and beverages
Carbonated beverages such as 7-Up and ginger ale	
Fruit-flavored gelatin and popsicles	
Apple, grape, or cranberry juice	
Clear fat-free broth and bouillon	
Sugar	

Recommended to Enhance Nutrition

Nutritional supplements such as Enlive® (Ross) or Citrotein (Novartis)

High-protein broth and gelatin desserts are also available.

Sample Breakfast, Lunch, and Dinner Menu

Clear apple, grape, or cranberry juice
Broth
Flavored gelatin
Coffee or tea
Sugar
Clear-liquid complete nutritional supplement if client is on this diet for longer than two meals

all fruit juices, ice cream, and all items allowed on the clear-liquid diet are allowed on most full-liquid diets. The major difference between a clear-liquid and a full-liquid diet is that the latter contains milk and milk products (Table 14-1 and Boxes 14-1 and 14-2).

Box 14-2 ■ *Full-Liquid Diet*

Description

The full-liquid diet provides foods and beverages that are liquid or may become liquid at body temperature.

Indications

This diet is used as a progression between clear liquids and a soft diet and after oral surgery. Acutely ill clients with a chewing or swallowing dysfunction and clients with oral, esophageal, or stomach disorder who are unable to tolerate solid foods because of strictures or other anatomical disorders find this diet useful.

Adequacy

This diet can be adequate in all nutrients according to the Recommended Dietary Allowances. Special care needs to be taken to meet folacin, iron, thiamin, niacin, vitamin A, fiber, and kilocalorie allowances.

Foods Allowed	Foods Not Allowed
Beverages	
Any beverage that pours at room temperature	All others
Breads, cereals, and grains:	All others
Cooked refined cereals (thinned or strained) such as cream of wheat	
Fruits	
All fruit juices	All others
Vegetables	
Any vegetable juice	All others
Meats	
None	
Milk	
Any	
Fats	
Butter, margarine, cream, and oils	All others
Other	
Custard, ice cream, flavored gelatin, sherbet, sugar, and popsicles	All others and any made with coconut, nuts, or whole fruit

Special Notes

The use of a complete nutritional liquid supplement is often necessary to meet nutrient allowances for clients who follow this diet for longer than 3 days.

Continued

Box 14-2 ■ *Full-Liquid Diet—cont'd*

An oral supplement that contains fiber minimizes the potential for problems with constipation and abdominal cramping. However, liquid supplements with fiber are not indicated for all patients on full-liquid diets.

Sample Menu

Breakfast	Lunch and Dinner	Snacks
½ cup fruit juice	½ cup fruit juice	A complete nutritional supplement as needed to meet protein and kilocalorie allowances
½ cup cream of wheat	½ cup vegetable juice	
1 cup pasteurized eggnog	1 cup strained cream soup	
Coffee, cream, and sugar	½ cup custard	
	8 oz Ensure® or Sustacal® or similar product	
	Coffee as desired	

Soft diets vary greatly from one facility to another. For example, a mechanical soft diet is ordered when the client has only a few or no teeth (edentulous). A soft diet is ordered following surgery when easily digested foods are required. A facility that specializes in treating clients with eye, ear, nose, and throat disorders may have many types of soft diets. A pureed diet usually consists of foods that have been run through a blender or food processor to meet the consistency needs of the patient. Table 14-2 lists recommended foods on a pureed, mechanical soft, and soft diet.

A general or regular diet means that the client is on an unrestricted diet. Frequently, an *as tolerated* or *progressive* diet may be prescribed, which means that a clear-liquid diet is to be served initially and the diet advanced (full-liquid to soft to general) as the client is able to tolerate. The nurse is usually responsible for determining the client's tolerance for food just before tray delivery. This last-minute determination of client tolerance is necessary for many clients because of fluctuating medical status.

TABLE 14-2 ■ Consistency Modifications—Recommended Foods

FOOD GROUP	PUREED DIET	MECHANICAL SOFT DIET	SOFT DIET
Soups	Broth, bouillon, strained or blenderized cream soup	Broth, bouillon, strained or blenderized cream soup	Broth, bouillon, cream soup
Beverages	All	All	All
Meat	Strained or pureed meat or poultry, cheese used in cooking	Ground, moist meats, or poultry, flaked fish, eggs, cottage cheese, cheese, creamy peanut butter, soft casseroles	Moist, tender meat, fish, or poultry, eggs, cottage cheese, mild flavored cheese, creamy peanut butter, soft casseroles
Fat	Butter, margarine, cream, oil, gravy	Butter, margarine, cream, oil, gravy, salad dressing	Butter, margarine, cream, oil, gravy, crisp bacon, avocado, salad dressing
Milk	Milk, milk beverages, yogurt without fruit, nuts, or seeds, cocoa	Milk, milk beverages, yogurt without seeds or nuts, cocoa	Milk, milk beverages, yogurt without seeds or nuts, cocoa
Starch	Cooked, refined cereal, mashed potatoes	Cooked or refined ready-to-eat cereal, potatoes, rice, pasta, white, refined wheat, light rye bread or rolls, graham crackers as tolerated	Cooked or ready-to-eat cereal, potatoes, rice, pasta, white, refined wheat, light rye or graham bread, rolls, or crackers
Vegetables	Strained or pureed, juice	Soft, cooked, without hulls or tough skin as in peas and corn, juice	Soft, cooked, vegetables, limit strongly flavored vegetables and whole-kernel corn, lettuce and tomatoes
Fruit	Strained or pureed, juice	Cooked or canned fruit without seeds or skins, banana, juice	Cooked or canned fruit, banana, citrus fruit without membrane, melon, juice
Desserts	Gelatin, sherbet, ice cream without nuts or fruit, custard, pudding, fruit ice, popsicle	Gelatin, sherbet, ice cream without nuts or fruit, custard, pudding, fruit ice, popsicle	Gelatin, sherbet, ice cream without nuts, custard, pudding, cake, cookies without nuts or coconut, fruit ice, popsicle
Sweets	Sugar, honey, jelly, candy, flavorings	Sugar, honey, jelly, candy, flavorings	Sugar, honey, jelly, candy, flavorings
Miscellaneous	Seasonings, condiments	Seasonings, condiments	Seasonings, condiments

Diets for Diagnostic Procedures

Many diagnostic **procedures** requiring dietary preparation are performed in hospitals.

Poor Client Preparation

Poor dietary preparation can force a client to have an expensive procedure repeated or postponed (Fig. 14-2). Figure 14-2A is an x-ray film from a poorly prepared client. Feces in the colon block the view of structures within the colon. Figure 14-2B shows the colon of a well-prepared client. In the absence of fecal material, the entire length of the colon can be visualized.

Some x-ray procedures are not only expensive but also uncomfortable. The client must have the procedure repeated if necessary bodily structures cannot be visualized. Although the specific dietary preparation for x-ray studies of the colon may vary from one facility to another, dietary preparation usually is somewhat similar. The client should be instructed not to eat or drink anything after midnight on the day of the imaging study. In addition, the client may need to follow a clear-liquid diet for 12 to 48 hours before the x-ray procedure.

Many clients undergo x-ray studies as outpatients. The nurse or medical assistant working in a physician's office is usually responsible for dietary instruction before these procedures.

Misdiagnosis

Poor dietary preparation can lead to a misdiagnosis. For example, a blood sample for a fasting blood glucose (FBS) test should be drawn on a **fasting** individual; that is, one who has not had any food (nor, sometimes, fluid) by mouth for at least 8 hours before the blood draw. If the client eats before the procedure, his or her blood glucose level may be elevated, and this elevation may cause a misdiagnosis of diabetes. A misdiagnosis may cause a client unnecessary anxiety and expense.

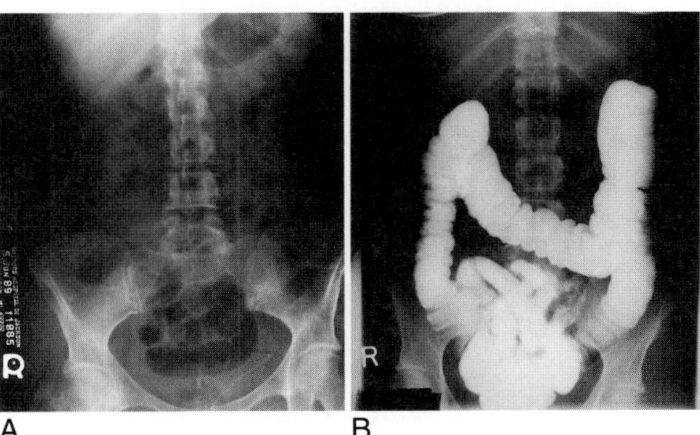

FIGURE 14-2 *A*, Image of a client who was poorly prepared for a barium enema. *B*, Image of a client who was adequately prepared for a barium enema. (Courtesy of Dr. Russell Tobe.)

Importance of Nutritional Care

Malnutrition associated with acute and chronic disease is common in hospital settings. **Acute** means that the illness has a rapid onset, severe symptoms, and a short course. **Chronic** means that the illness has a long duration.

The presence and importance of malnutrition has been increasingly recognized over the past 30 years. Malnutrition is one of the most common conditions affecting the care of hospitalized clients. Nutrition surveys in hospitals continue to suggest that upwards of 40% to 50% of patients, particularly those in intensive care units, have moderate to severe malnutrition (Pfau and Rombeau, 2000). Many patients come into hospitals malnourished, and their acute illnesses further worsen their malnutrition.

Malnutrition is associated with a 25% morbidity and a 5% mortality. **Morbidity** is defined as the rate of being diseased. **Mortality** is defined as the death rate. A malnourished client is thus more likely to be sicker and run a higher risk of death than a well-nourished client with the same diagnosis. Because malnutrition affects morbidity and mortality, it is also associated with a prolonged hospital stay.

Iatrogenic Malnutrition

The term **iatrogenic malnutrition** was first used in 1974 and is a less offensive phrase than induced malnutrition, that is, induced by a physician or an institution (Butterworth and Blackburn, 1975). Routine hospital practices such as extended periods of food or nutrient deprivation because of treatments, as well as diagnostic tests that interfere with the client's meal schedule or that cause a lack of appetite, are related to the high prevalence of malnutrition. Drug therapy may also affect a client's appetite. Some drugs cause drowsiness, lethargy, nausea, and anorexia. Problems related directly to an illness, such as pain, unconsciousness, paralysis, vomiting, and diarrhea, can also interfere with eating.

Today many institutions have written policies and procedures for members to follow to minimize the likelihood of iatrogenic malnutrition. The tasks team members should perform to combat institutional malnutrition are discussed in Clinical Application 14-1.

Methods of Nutrient Delivery

Nutrients can be delivered to the client orally in foods or supplements, by tube feeding, or parenterally through veins. An **enteral tube feeding** means the feeding of an appropriate formula or liquid via a tube to a client's gastrointestinal tract. A **parenteral feeding** designates any intravenous route.

Figure 14-3 shows two feeding pumps. The feeding pumps are set to deliver a given rate, volume, and amount of both enteral and parenteral feedings to a client. The importance of connecting the enteral feeding to the tube that leads to the client's gastrointestinal tract and connecting the intravenous solution to the tube that leads directly into the blood stream cannot be overemphasized. Although this is primarily a nursing responsibility, every trained team member should make a habit of checking tube connections every time a client with two different feeding routes is visited. The placement of a feeding tube into the wrong lead is called a misconnection.

Oral Delivery

Most institutionalized clients are fed orally. Whenever possible, the client should be encouraged to eat foods, because this is an optimal way for the client to not only obtain nutrients but also experience the normal psychological and physical pleasure associated with eating.

The Menu

An institution's menu can be selective or nonselective. A selective menu is similar to a restaurant menu; clients can choose the specific menu items that appeal to them. Clients eat best when they fill out their own menus or a significant other does so for them. Marking the menu is one way in which a client can participate daily in care planning.

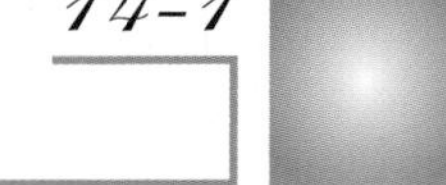

Clinical Application 14-1

Methods for Team Members to Combat Iatrogenic Malnutrition

Nursing actions can affect the nutritional health of institutionalized clients. The following behaviors minimize the likelihood of malnutrition:

- Recording height and weight
- Regular communication among nurses, physicians, dietitians, and other health-care workers
- Food tray viewing (monitoring) and documentation of client's food intake
- Good food sanitation for oral and enteral feedings
- Knowledge of the importance of good nutrition, nutritional supplements, and the composition of vitamin mixtures
- Monitoring the length of time clients are NPO, on liquid diets, and on intravenous feedings of only glucose
- Appreciation of the role of nutrition in the prevention and recovery from infection
- Recognition of the increased nutritional needs due to injury or illness
- Monitoring of stool frequency, urinary losses, losses by suction tubes, drainage, and so forth
- Recording of weight at regular intervals
- Monitoring of behavior patterns, vomiting, and any unusual comments clients make about food
- Monitoring of client fluid intake and output

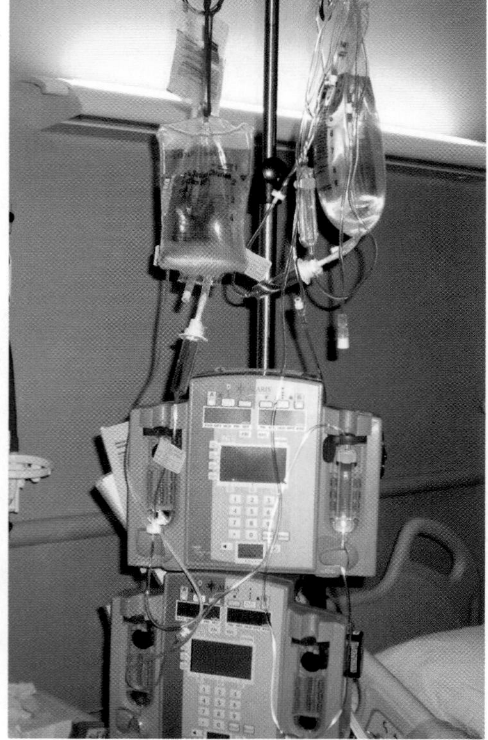

FIGURE 14-3 These two feeding pumps are set to deliver both a tube feeding and TPN simultaneously. The client also has lines running for medications. Note how confusing it is to misplace the lines.

Not all institutions have a selective menu. One kind of meal is prepared and served to all clients. Food and labor required for providing a selective menu is more expensive than for institutions providing a nonselective menu. However, many clients may fail to eat the food from a nonselective menu.

Eating Environment

Health-care workers need to create as pleasant an environment as possible immediately before and during mealtime. The room should be checked for objectionable odors, sounds, and sights. Obviously, a full bedside commode or an emesis basin nearby discourages eating. In addition, the client should be prepared to eat when the tray arrives. Cleaning the client's hands and face helps the client become more enthusiastic about eating. The client's bedside table should be cleared of all miscellaneous items, and unnecessary delays in serving the tray should be avoided. The client should be properly positioned to eat. This includes elevating the head of the bed (if his or her condition permits) and positioning the bedside table to the correct height.

Some clients may find the odor of food offensive. For these clients, it is best for the nurse not to uncover the food items directly in front of them, minimizing the risk of nausea.

Assisted Feeding versus Self-Feeding

Some clients must be fed. Food should be offered in bite-sized portions and in the order that the client prefers. Nurses or nursing assistants should check the temperature of all hot liquids against the inside of their wrists before offering them to the client. Clients should not be rushed. Talking with the client while feeding makes mealtime pleasant and signals to the client that he or she is not being rushed. Personnel are encouraged to sit while feeding the client, as this indicates a willingness to spend time with the client and encourages relaxation.

Some nursing personnel have found they can enhance a client's food intake by mimicking normal eating behavior:

- Sit behind the client.
- Place your right arm over the client's arm (if you and the client are right-handed).
- Place a fork or spoon with food in either the client's hand or your own hand (depending on the client's ability to do this maneuver).
- Guide the client's hand to his or her mouth.

In a long-term care facility, a client's ability to feed him- or herself should be reevaluated at regular intervals.

Assisting the Disabled Client

A client with a disability may require either total or partial assistance with eating. Partial assistance may include opening milk cartons and plastic bags containing condiments and eating utensils, buttering bread, and cutting meat. Visually impaired clients may be able to feed themselves when they know where the food is on the plate. The usual technique is to describe food placement in terms of hours on a clock face.

Some clients can feed themselves but may be very slow, clumsy, and messy. A large napkin under the chin may assist in cleanup. Offering hot beverages in small amounts may minimize the likelihood of an accident.

Sometimes the consistency or form of a food may influence whether clients can feed themselves. A thin liquid, for example, may cause some clients to choke. A thicker substance such as yogurt may be better tolerated. Some disabled people are able to manage finger foods such as french fries or hard-cooked eggs. Health-care personnel can learn the food tolerances and preferences of disabled clients by asking or observing. The physician should be notified if a client appears to be choking or coughing while being fed. A licensed speech pathologist (LSP) can be invaluable in determining the optimal solid food and liquid consistency to minimize the risk of aspiration.

Health-care workers should evaluate a client who cannot feed him- or herself and encourage clients to remain as independent as possible in all the activities of daily living, including eating. Some clients' inability to feed themselves may be related to neuromuscular disabilities. The occupational therapist has special training in the selection and fitting of eating devices to assist such clients.

Supplemental Feedings

Many clients are unable to consume sufficient kilocalories or nutrients because of anorexia or an increased need for nutrients. The first step is to offer these clients additional food at or between meals. Any between-meal feedings must adhere to the client's diet order. Closely monitoring a client's food intake including supplemental feedings is important. If the client will not accept supplemental feedings, another treatment approach may be needed.

Many clients accept liquid supplementation better than solids. Many debilitated clients seem to feel less full after drinking a beverage than after eating a comparable number of kilocalories and nutrients in foods. Liquid supplements can include:

- Milk
- Milk shakes

- Instant breakfast drinks
- Commercially prepared beverages

Many different commercially prepared liquid formulas are available. Four different types of supplements are used as oral feedings:

1. Modular supplements
2. Intact or "polymeric" formulas
3. Elemental or "predigested" formulas
4. Disease-specific formulas.

MODULAR SUPPLEMENTS

A **modular supplement** contains a limited number of nutrients. Polycose, for example, contains only carbohydrate. Microlipid is an example of a lipid supplement. Modular supplements for protein include Resource Beneprotein® and Pro-Mod Liquid Protein®.

Modular supplements are available in a liquid or powder form and can be added to foods, other types of oral supplements, or tube feedings. Sometimes modular supplements are readily accepted if mixed with food. For example, Resource Beneprotein® mixed with hot cereal and mashed potatoes does not change the taste of these foods and adds a significant amount of protein to a client's diet.

Some modular products available contain two nutrients. Resource Arginine® contains both the amino acid arginine and carbohydrate. Juven® is a modular supplement that contains two amino acids, a small amount of carbohydrate, and healthy body weight (HBW) that helps reverse muscle breakdown and increase protein synthesis. The manufacturers list these products as modular feedings because they do not contain all the essential nutrients.

INTACT OR POLYMERIC FORMULAS

An **intact** or **polymeric formula** is used when the gastrointestinal tract is functional and the client needs all of the essential nutrients in a specified volume. Dozens of such products are on the market. A complete supplement, such as Ensure®, Boost®, Jevity®, and Nutren Replete® should always be used when the formula is the sole source of nutrition.

Some complete nutritional supplements are also designed for tube feedings; the consistency and flavor of a feeding designed to be tube-fed will probably not be acceptable to the client when fed orally.

Commercial supplements should be used only after the client's requirements for nutrients have been assessed. Excess nutrients are rarely beneficial, and consuming too much of a feeding may be medically harmful. Many organs in the human body are in a stress situation in the poorly nourished client. Why subject the client's kidneys or liver to unnecessary work if the nutrients cannot be used efficiently? See Clinical Calculation 14-1.

ELEMENTAL OR PREDIGESTED FORMULAS

Another group of oral supplements includes **elemental** or **predigested formulas**. Examples of such formulas include Peptamen®, Vital®, and Vivonex®. The nutrients in these formulas are easier to digest or are already partially digested. For example, maltodextrins, corn syrup solids, oligosaccharides, and glucose polymers are rapidly hydrolyzed by maltase and oligosaccharidases, which are apt to be present in the small intestine in higher concentrations than lactase.

Protein is either partially or totally predigested. Partially predigested protein (small peptides) offer an advantage over totally predigested protein (single amino acids). Peptides and free amino acids do not inhibit each other's transport across the gastrointestinal tract, and absorption of nitrogen is actually improved by the inclusion of small peptides. Easier-to-digest fats include medium-chain triglycerides. Partially digested fats include monoglycerides and diglycerides.

Predigested formulas contain little lactose and residue and may be given orally or through a tube. These formulas are very expensive and are for use with clients with limited gastrointestinal function or metabolic disorders. Because the formulas are less palatable than **intact feedings**, client acceptance of oral feedings is sometimes a problem.

DISEASE-SPECIFIC FORMULAS

The last group of oral supplements includes special formulas designed for clients with specific metabolic problems such as kidney and liver disorders. These formulas are discussed in subsequent chapters.

Oral supplements are also used extensively to wean clients from tube and parenteral feedings. After a client ceases to consume foods orally, a transition period is always necessary to reacclimate the client to oral feedings. This process can sometimes take a couple days to months.

Enteral Tube Feeding

Tube feedings are the second way nutrients can be delivered to clients. With some medical conditions, oral feeding is impossible, insufficient, or impractical. Several common conditions in which a tube feeding is indicated are listed in Table 14-3.

Tube feedings, like oral supplements, can be made from table foods or purchased prepared. If the client's finances are tight and the client has no impairment of digestion and absorption, he or she can

14-1

Clinical Calculation

Calculating an Oral Supplement

1. Place the client on a kilocalorie count.
2. Estimate the client's kilocalorie requirement.
   - Calculate the client's ideal body weight (IBW). Females = 100 pounds for the first 5 feet and 5 pounds for each additional inch ± 10%; males = 106 pounds for the first 5 feet and 6 pounds for each additional inch ± 10%
   - Use maximum IBW for all further calculations except those (1) who are underweight then use their actual body weight (ABW) to prevent over feeding. (2) Use ABW for clients within their IBW range.
   - Divide the weight calculated in above to obtain the client's weight in kilograms.
   - Estimated energy needs for noncritical care clients are 25 to 35 kcal/kg; Energy needs for critical care clients are 20 to 30 kcal/kg.
   - Protein needs for noncritical care clients are 0.8 to 1.2 grams/kg; protein needs for critical care clients are 1.2 to 1.5 grams/kg
   - Fluid needs are 1 mL/kg or 30 mL/kg or as tolerated to maintain fluid status
3. Select an appropriate oral supplement for the client. Some hospitals allow clients to taste several supplements and choose the one most palatable to them.
4. Determine the difference between the client's recorded food intake and kilocalorie allowance.
5. Determine the kilocalorie concentration of the formula. This can be done by referring to either the appropriate table in the diet manual or the supplement's label. Usually formulas are between 1.0 and 2.0 kcal/mL.
6. Determine how many milliliters of formula are needed to meet the client's kilocalorie allowance.
7. Divide the total milliliters needed by the number of feedings to be offered.
8. Check to make sure the client's protein and fluid needs are within the desired range. If not, select a different supplement.

EXAMPLE

1. Assume that the client ate 550 kcal.
2. Assume that the client is a woman who weighs 132 lb and is 5 ft 2 in. tall. Client's IBW would be 100 lb + 10 lb for her additional 2 in. = 110; ± 10% = 100 to 120. She weighs more than her IBW, so use her maximum IBW of 120 to compute kilocalorie needs. 120 divided by 2.2 = 54.5 kg.
3. Client's estimated need for kilocalories is 25 to 35 kcal/kg × 54.5 kg = 1363 to 1908 kcal.
4. Assume that the client has tasted several supplements and prefers Boost Shake 1.0
5. The client's estimated range for kilocalories is 1363 to 1908.
   The client ate 300 kcal.
   The difference is a deficit of 1063 to 1608 kcal.
6. Boost Shake contains 280 kcal and 8 grams of protein in 240 mL.
7. The client stated she would prefer to drink this feeding five times per day, some on each tray, and during two between-meal feedings.
8. Assume from the client's recorded food intake that her diet contains about 10 grams of protein per day. A woman weighing 54.5 kg has an estimated protein allowance of 0.8 to 1.2 grams/kg.

   54.5 kg × 0.8 gram/kg = 43.6 g of protein to 54.5 × 1.2 grams/kg = 65.4 grams
   Subtract the 10 grams eaten from trays
   43.6 grams – 10 grams = 33.6 grams

   The supplement should provide at least 33.6 grams of protein and no more than 65.4 grams of protein (0.8 to 1.2 grams/kg of maximum IBW)
9. 5 cans of Boost Shake contains 1400 kcal and 40 grams of protein for a total of 1200 mL.
10. Eight grams of protein × 5 cans (240 mL each) = 40 grams of protein from oral supplement + 10 g of protein from food = 50 grams
11. Double check: Food intake of 300 kcal + 10 grams of protein + 1400 kcal from Boost Shake + 40 grams of protein from Boost Shake = 50 grams of protein total + 1700 kcal total + 1200 mL fluid total from supplement (client should be encouraged to drink at least 300 mL of water extra per day to meet her fluid needs). This information should be documented and verbally given to the nurse assigned to the client.

TABLE 14-3 ■ Conditions Indicating a Tube Feeding

CONDITION	EXAMPLES
Client has mechanical difficulties that make chewing and/or swallowing impossible or difficult.	Obstruction of the esophagus, weakness or nausea, mouth sores, throat inflammation
Client has an intestinal disease and cannot digest or absorb food adequately.	Malabsorption syndromes
Client refuses to eat or cannot eat.	Anorexia nervosa
Client is unable to consume a sufficient amount of food because of clinical condition.	Coma, serious infections, trauma victims, clients with large kilocalorie requirements

learn to prepare a tube feeding from table foods. Home-prepared tube feedings are less expensive than commercially prepared feedings but more prone to contamination. Many of the commercial products described in the previous section can be used for tube feeding.

The medical literature addresses tube feedings for clients with dementia (Climent, 2000; Vollman, 2000). Both articles advocate ending the use of stomach tubes to feed people with advanced Alzheimer's disease and other types of dementia. Patients with these conditions frequently pull the tubes out, leading nursing home and hospital staff to place the patients in restraints. An argument can be made that tube feedings deprive patients of the enjoyment that can be derived from eating and the social satisfaction that accompanies eating by hand. For this reason, most institutions have strict guidelines that all team members must follow before inserting a feeding tube into any patient. For these clients, surgically inserted feeding tubes placed directly into the stomach or small intestines are frequently used.

Gastrointestinal Function

The gastrointestinal tract should always be used to the extent possible. Oral supplements should be considered before tube feeding; tube feeding should always be considered before intravenous feeding. Tube feeding is safer, less expensive, and more physiological than intravenous feeding; in other words, it more nearly mimics normal feeding conditions. Nutrients should be supplied intact rather than predigested if the client has normal digestion. **Intact nutrients** are nutrients that are not predigested, so the body must keep producing the secretions and enzymes necessary for digestion, thereby forcing the gastrointestinal tract to function.

Tube Placement

Feeding tubes can enter the body through the nose or through a surgically made opening. A **nasogastric (NG) tube** runs from the nose to the stomach. A **nasoduodenal (ND) tube** runs from the nose to the duodenum. A **nasojejunal (NJ)** tube runs from the nose to the jejunum. These types of tubes are for short-term use because of client discomfort and tissue irritation.

When long-term tube feeding is needed or in clients with dementia or when a tube cannot be inserted through the nose (as in throat cancer), an **ostomy,** or surgically created opening, is created. An **esophagostomy** is a surgical opening into the esophagus through which a feeding tube is passed. A **gastrostomy** (called percutaneous endoscopic gastrostomy [PEG]) is a surgical opening in the stomach through which a feeding tube is passed; this is the most common tube insertion method.

PEG tube placement is used for clients who require a feeding tube long term. A PEG tube can be placed **percutaneously** with the aid of an **endoscope** or surgically if the patient is already undergoing abdominal surgery or has a condition that makes working with an endoscope difficult. Percutaneous endoscopic jejunostomy (PEJ) tube placement is generally reserved for clients who are not candidates for a PEG. For example, a client who has had a gastrectomy (stomach removal) procedure requires a PEJ tube placement. A PEJ tube is also indicated for clients prone to aspiration.

A critical responsibility of team members is assessment of feeding tube placement, especially with tubes inserted nasally. The most reliable method of determining tube placement is radiography. Tubes have been mispositioned in such dangerous locations as the lungs and even the brain (Metheny and Titler, 2001). Unfortunately, feeding tubes migrate (after x-ray exam) and may move out of the stomach or jejunum. Tube migration places the client at risk for aspiration because the tube may move into the trachea. The client is also at risk if he or she regurgitates the feeding. **Regurgitation** means to cause to flow backward. If the feeding backs up into the client's lungs, a lung infection can develop.

When a client has inhaled fluids regurgitated from the stomach, he or she may develop aspiration pneumonia. **Aspiration** is the state whereby a substance has been drawn up into the nose, throat, or lungs. Pulmonary aspiration is a common occurrence in hospitalized patients. Nonsurgically inserted enteral tube feeding increases the risk of aspiration and is associated with the development of nosocomial pneumonia, which significantly increases morbidity and mortality in critically ill patients.

In the past, many nurses were taught and institutions recommended tinting of enteral feedings with blue dye to promote early detection of aspiration. Every time the patient was suctioned, the specimen was inspected against a white background for the presence of dye. Blue dye was the favored color because blue is not found in secretions. It is now widely recognized that blue dye has toxic effects. These effects include lactic acidosis, altered mental status, hypotension, hyperthermia, and rapid death (Super, 2003). Another problem associated with the use of blue dye is bacterial contamination. The American Dietetic Association's evidence-based library states blue dyes should not be added to enteral nutrition for detection of aspiration. The risk of using the dye outweighs perceived benefits (www.adaevidencelibrary.com, 2008).

Contamination

Unfortunately, all tube feedings provide an excellent environment for growth of microorganisms. When a client's tube feeding becomes contaminated with bacteria, the client receiving the feeding may become ill and suffer from nausea, vomiting, or diarrhea. For this reason, many hospitals and nursing homes use only commercially prepared tube feedings, which are packaged under sterile conditions. However, commercially prepared formulas can become contaminated if they are not handled properly after opening.

To prevent contamination, first check the can for the correct product, flavor, expiration date, and any signs of contamination such as swelling. If the can is swollen, notify your supervisor. Do not administer a feeding from a damaged can. Other cans in the same shipment should be checked for contamination.

Good personal hygiene is important. The following recommendations help reduce contamination:

- Always wash your hands before opening the can.
- Wash the top of the can carefully before opening it.
- Shake the can well before opening it.
- Use a clean opener if one is needed.
- Transfer the formula into a clean container.
- Label any remaining formula carefully with the client's name, room number, the date the formula was opened, the amount in the container, the name of the product, and other pertinent information. Other information may include whether the formula is diluted or contains medications, vitamins, or other additives.
- Store the formula in the refrigerator in a covered container. When a new supply of formula is received, place it in the rear of the storage area so that the older formula is used first.
- Once opened, use or discard most formulas within 24 hours.

Administration

Tube feedings can be administered continuously, intermittently, or by **bolus**. Clogging of the tube occurs significantly more often with continuous rather than intermittent feedings.

CONTINUOUS FEEDING

Many professionals feel that **continuous feeding** is preferable to other methods. A continuous feeding is always recommended for formulas delivered directly into the small intestine. One recommended rate is 30 to 50 mL/h, increasing daily by 25 mL/h to the rate necessary to meet energy needs. This gradual increase in the formula's volume gives the client's gastrointestinal tract a chance to adjust to the formula and helps prevent many complications that occur in tube-fed clients. Safety precautions for continuous feedings include

1. Flushing the tube with water every 4 to 6 hours
2. Allowing no more than a 4-hour hang time for each bag of formula unless the formula is packaged in a sterilized delivery system

These procedures help prevent contamination and bacterial growth. An infusion pump is necessary for precise control of a continuous feeding.

INTERMITTENT FEEDING

An **intermittent feeding** means giving a 4- to 6-hour volume of feeding solution over 20 to 30 minutes. Clients tolerate intermittent feedings much better than bolus feedings because these feedings more closely approximate normal eating behavior. The tube needs to be flushed after each feeding to minimize bacterial growth and prevent contamination. Many mobile clients prefer intermittent feedings because they are not continuously attached to the feeding pump.

BOLUS FEEDING

Bolus feeding means giving a 4- to 6-hour volume of feeding solution within a few minutes. A client is thus fed only four to six times per day. Feedings given by this method are frequently poorly tolerated, and clients complain of abdominal discomfort, nausea, fullness, and cramping. Some clients, however, can tolerate bolus feedings after a period of adjustment in which the volume is slowly increased. Bolus feedings entering the intestines are usually poorly tolerated.

Clients on bolus feedings should not recline for at least 2 hours after the feeding. Tubes should be irrigated (flushed with water) after each feeding to prevent contamination. The patient with normal gastric function can usually tolerate 500 mL of formula at each feeding (Blouch and Mueller, 2004).

Potential Complications

Complications fall into three categories:

1. Mechanical,
2. Gastrointestinal
3. Metabolic.

Table 14-4 reviews these complications and lists system-specific prevention strategies.

Osmolality

The osmolality of a solution is based on the number of dissolved particles in the solution. The greater the

TABLE 14-4 ■ Feeding Complications and Prevention Strategies

COMPLICATION	PREVENTION STRATEGY
Mechanical	
Tube irritation	Consider using a smaller or softer tube. Lubricate the tube before insertion.
Tube obstruction	Flush tube after use. Do not mix medications with the formula. Use liquid medications if available. Crush other medications thoroughly. Use an infusion pump to maintain a constant flow. Feeding should not be started until tube placement is radiographically confirmed.
Aspiration and regurgitation	Elevate head of client's bed greater than or equal to 30 degrees at all times. Discontinue feedings at least 30 to 60 minutes before treatments where head must be lowered (e.g., chest percussion). If the client has an endotracheal tube in place, keep the cuff inflated during feedings. Test pH of aspirate with pH paper or meter: a. pH of tracheobronchial secretions is alkaline, >7.4 b. pH of gastric secretions is acidic, <5.0 c. As the tube moves from the acid stomach to the alkaline duodenum, pH will change from acid to alkaline.
Tube displacement	Place a black mark at the point where the tube, once properly placed, exits the nostril. Replace tube and obtain physician's order to confirm with x-ray imaging.
Gastrointestinal	
Cramping, distention, bloating, gas pains, nausea, vomiting, diarrhea*	Initiate and increase amount of formula gradually. Bring formula to room temperature before feeding. Change to a lactose-free formula. Decrease fat context of formula. Administer drug therapy as ordered, e.g., Lactinex, kaolin-pectin, Lomotil. Change to a formula with a lower osmolality. Change to a formula with a different fiber content. Practice good personal hygiene when handling any feeding product. Evaluate diarrhea-causing medications the client may be receiving (e.g., antibiotics, digitalis).
Metabolic	
Dehydration	Assess the client's fluid requirements before treatment. Monitor the client's hydration status.
Overhydration	Assess the client's fluid requirements before treatment. Monitor the client's hydration status.
Hyperglycemia	Initiate feedings at a low rate. Monitor blood glucose levels. Use hyperglycemic medication if necessary. Select a low-carbohydrate formula. Evaluate total kilocalories provided; overfeeding in a critically ill patient exacerbates hyperglycemia.
Hypernatremia	Assess the client's fluid and electrolyte status before treatment. Provide adequate fluids.
Hyponatremia	Assess the client's fluid and electrolyte status before treatment. Restrict fluids. Supplement feeding with rehydration solution and saline. Diuretic therapy may be beneficial.
Hypophosphatemia	Monitor serum levels. Replenish phosphorus levels before refeeding.
Hypercapnia	Select low-carbohydrate high-fat formula.
Hypokalemia	Monitor serum levels. Supplement feeding with potassium if necessary.
Hyperkalemia	Reduce potassium intake. Monitor potassium levels.

*The most commonly cited complication of tube feeding is diarrhea.

number of particles, the higher the osmolality. At a given concentration, the smaller the particle size, the greater the number of particles present.

Oral supplements and tube feedings with a high osmolality draw body fluid into the bowel, resulting in a fluid imbalance. The symptoms are diarrhea, nausea, and flushing. The osmolality of normal body fluids is approximately 300 mOsm/kg. Predigested nutrients have a higher osmolality than intact nutrients. An **isotonic** feeding has an osmolality of 300 mOsm, the same as body fluids. A high-osmolality feeding can provide a more concentrated source of nutrients than a feeding of lower osmolality.

Sensitivity to the osmolality of oral supplements and tube feedings varies from one individual to another. All clients need a period of adjustment to a high-osmolality formula. Most clients are able to eventually develop a tolerance to a high-osmolality formula; some clients, however, are more likely to develop symptoms of an intolerance. Such clients include those who:

- Are debilitated
- Have gastrointestinal disorders
- Are preoperative and postoperative
- Have a gastrointestinal tract that has not been challenged by food for a significant period
- Have newly inserted surgically placed tubes (PEG and PEJ)

Administration of Medications

To minimize or prevent complications, all health-care workers should be aware of potential drug–food interactions (see Chapter 15). Clinical Application 14-2 discusses suggested procedures for administering medications through feeding tubes. Medications can be physically incompatible with the tube feeding because of changes in the feeding's viscosity (thickness) or flow characteristics. Some medications may also cause the feeding to separate, granulate, or coagulate.

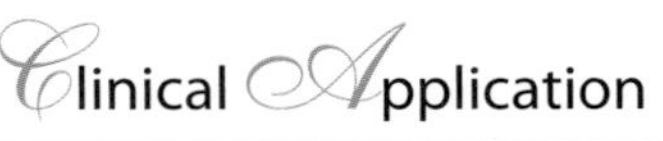

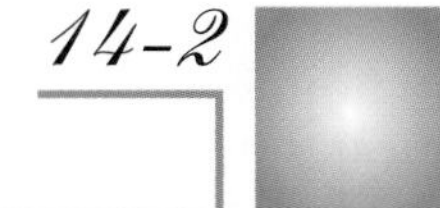

Procedures for Administering Medications Through Feeding Tubes

Procedures for the administration of medications through feeding tubes may vary slightly from one institution to another. The following procedures, however, are common:

- If possible, administer drugs in liquid form.
- If the drug is not available in liquid form, consult with the pharmacist; he or she may be able to procure a liquid form or similar drug provided by the American Society of Hospital Pharmacists in Pediatric Extemporaneous Formulation List of the manufacturer's suggestions.
- Exercise caution when calculating equivalent liquid doses. Many liquid dosage forms are intended for pediatric use, and the dose must be adjusted appropriately for adults.
- Administer crushed tablets only when no other alternatives are available.
- If administering crushed tablets, crush the tablet to a fine powder and mix with water. Do not crush any tablet on the list of oral drugs that should not be crushed. Do not crush drugs with a sustained-release action or an enteric coating. If in doubt, consult the pharmacist.
- Administer each drug separately. Do not mix all the medications for one dosing time. Flush with at least 5 mL (1 tsp) of water between each medication.
- Flush the tube with at least 30 mL of water before giving the medication and before restarting the tube feeding.
- To avoid causing gastric irritation and diarrhea, dilute drugs that are hypertonic or irritating to the cells that line the gastrointestinal tract, such as potassium chloride, in at least 30 mL of water before administration.
- If the medication is ordered to be added to the feeding, observe the feeding after the addition for any reaction or precipitation. Shake the solution thoroughly. Label the feedings with at least the name and amount of the drug added, the time, date, and your initials.
- Dilute drugs, such as indomethacin—which are usually administered with meals to avoid gastric irritation—with water before administration.
- Divide dosing schedules—if necessary—of sustained- or slow-release formulations of drugs used for once-daily dosing when administering in liquid form.

Monitoring

Nutritional status, fluid balance, and gastrointestinal tolerance should be monitored in tube-fed clients. Whether the client requires daily or weekly monitoring depends on client acuity, duration of feeding, and the practice in the facility.

Nutritional status monitoring begins with a comparison of the client's kilocalorie and protein allowances to the volume and composition of the nutritional product utilized. Initially the client's kilocalorie and protein allowances are not met because a tube feeding is usually started at a low volume to increase gastrointestinal tolerance. Changes in the client's medical status and treatment, physical activity, and tolerance to the tube feeding may continually alter the volume and kind of feeding the client requires. Thus, the kilocaloric and protein content of the tube feeding requires reassessment.

In stable clients, serum levels of sodium, blood urea nitrogen, hemoglobin, and albumin are indicators of fluid status. Urine osmolality can be used to monitor hydration status. Urine osmolality is normally 50 to 1400 mOsm, with a usual range 300 to 900 mOsm and an average of 850 mOsm. Decreased osmolality indicates overhydration, and increased osmolality indicates dehydration.

Fluid intake and output need to be recorded daily. Fluid intake should be at least 500 mL greater than output in clients who are neither overhydrated nor underhydrated. This 500-mL surplus is needed to cover insensible losses in feces and from the skin and lungs. Clinical signs of hydration status include skin turgor, presence of axillary sweat, condition of the mucous membranes, and the presence or absence of edema. Constipation is another possible sign of dehydration.

Gastrointestinal tolerance can be assessed by the absence or presence of diarrhea, bowel sounds, nausea, distension, and vomiting. The type of feeding delivered, the volume given, or the delivery rate can cause diarrhea. Diarrhea is frequently caused by medications. Antibiotics, laxatives, H_2 receptor blockers, and antacids with magnesium can cause stools to become watery. Medications that contain sorbitol can also have a laxative effect.

Gastric residuals are usually measured several times daily or about every 4 hours in clients at risk with tubes leading into the stomach. Because elevated residuals indicate delayed gastric emptying and a potentially increased risk for aspiration, feedings are advanced only when gastric residuals are less than 250 mL (www.adaevidencelibrary.com, 2008).

Measurement of gastric residuals in a stable alert client who has a well-established tolerance to the tube feeding is usually not necessary. Feedings continuously dripped into the intestines do not normally produce a gastric residue because there is no place for the fluid to collect. Gastric residue measurement is most relevant in critically ill patients and others at risk for gastroparesis (Blouch and Mueller, 2004).

Home Enteral Nutrition

With the increase in home-based health-care agencies, hospitals and nursing homes discharge many clients on enteral nutrition and follow the clients closely as out-patients.

Parenteral Nutrition

Parenteral nutrition in which nutrients are delivered to the client through the veins (intravenously) is the third means of feeding. **Peripheral parenteral nutrition (PPN)** means to feed the client via a vein away from the center of the body in a line terminating in a peripheral site (Fig. 14-4). In **total parenteral nutrition (TPN),** the client is fed via a central vein. Clients are also fed via a central line that has been inserted peripherally and threaded into the subclavian or jugular veins. This is called a **PIC line**.

The terminology is confusing. Therefore, note whether the line terminates peripherally or centrally. TPN, PIC lines, and PPN can be used to provide partial or total daily nutritional requirements. Clients

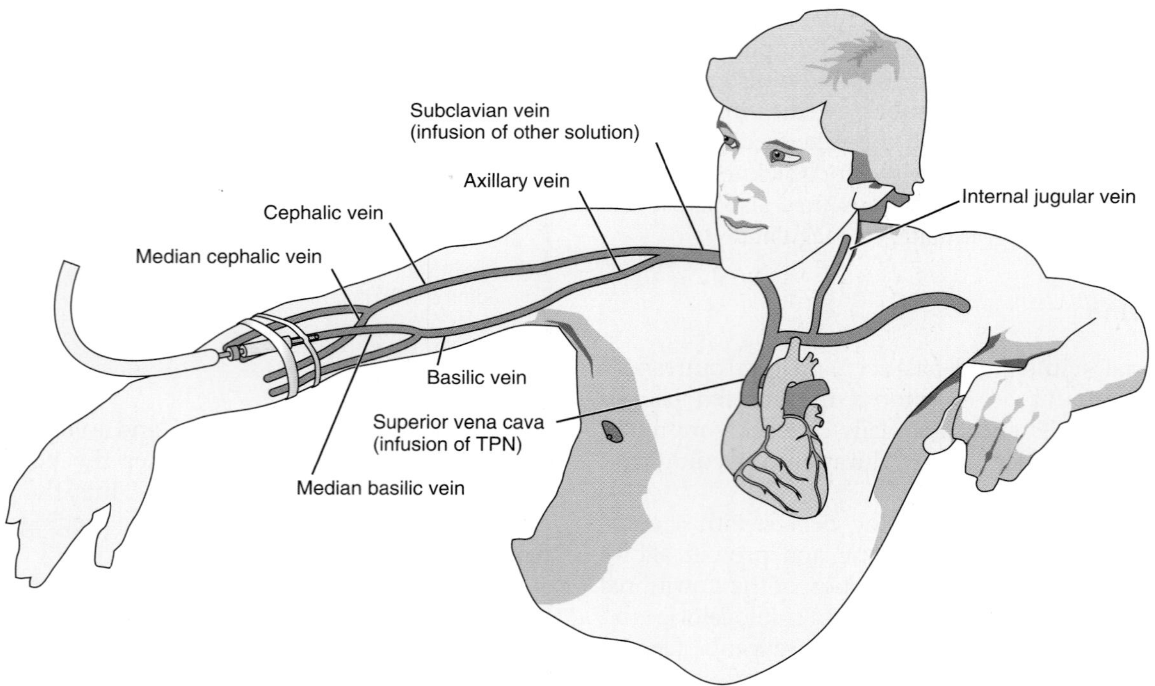

FIGURE 14-4 Correct placement of a peripherally placed central catheter (PICC).

who cannot or should not be fed through the gastrointestinal tract are candidates for TPN, PIC lines, and PPN. See Box 14-3 for appropriate indications for the use of PPN and TPN.

Peripheral Parenteral Nutrition

Intravenous (IV) feeding (peripheral parenteral nutrition [PPN]) is routine in some health-care institutions. IV solutions, usually containing water, dextrose, electrolytes, and occasionally other nutrients, are used to maintain fluid, electrolyte, and acid–base balance. Intravenous solutions do contain kilocalories. The calculation of the kilocalorie content of an intravenous solution is demonstrated in Clinical Calculation 14-2.

Amino acids and fat can be supplied peripherally. To prevent ketosis, intravenous lipid emulsions should contribute no more than 60% of the total kilocalories provided. Dextrose concentrations are limited to approximately 10%, because peripheral veins cannot withstand concentrations greater than 900 mOsmol/kg. Thus, PPN has often failed to provide adequate kilocalories and other nutrients for repair and replacement of losses. PPN has been used to supplement a partially successful enteral nutrition program.

A system for PPN (called all-in-one or three-in-one) has been developed that allows a higher osmotic load (1200 to 1350 mOsmol/L) to be delivered peripherally.

Box 14-3 ■ *Indications for PPN and TPN*

PPN

PPN is an effective method of nutritional support for clients who have mild to moderate nutritional deficiencies and who are unable to receive enteral nutrition or have an inaccessible or undesirable central venous route. Specifically, PPN is indicated for clients:

- Who are expected to be NPO for 5 days
- Who have inadequate GI function expected to last 5 to 7 days
- Who are making the transition to an oral diet or tube feeding
- In whom central venous access is contraindicated
- Who are malnourished and expected to be NPO for several days
- Who have energy and protein requirements that can be met with PPN (1800 kcal/day or less)

TPN/PIC

Potential candidates for TPN/PIC include clients who are anticipated to require nutritional support for longer than 10 days or who have an increased requirement for energy, such as clients:

- Who need preoperative preparation but are severely malnourished
- Who have postoperative surgical complications
- Who have inflammatory bowel disease
- Who have inadequate oral intake or malabsorption

14-2 Clinical Calculation

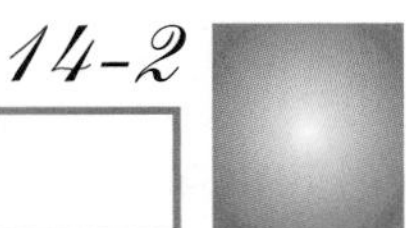

Calculating Kilocalories in IV Solutions

D_5W means 5% dextrose in water. The subscript following the D tells you the % of dextrose in the solution. Other common concentrations of sugar and water are $D_{10}W$ and $D_{50}W$.

A 5% concentration of dextrose means 100 mL of water contains 5 grams of dextrose. A 10% concentration of dextrose means 100 mL of water contains 10 grams of dextrose. A 50% concentration of dextrose means 100 mL of water contains 50 grams of dextrose. A simple proportion should be used to calculate the number of kilocalories in any given volume of a solution.

The formula is:

percent of concentration/100 mL =
× grams of dextrose/volume of solution client received

For example, a client has received 1000 mL of D_5W:

5% of dextrose/100 mL =
× grams of dextrose/1000 =
50 grams of dextrose

Proportions are solved by cross-multiplication and division: (5 grams × 1000 mL) divided by 100 mL = 50 grams of dextrose. One gram of carbohydrate given intravenously provides 3.4 kcal; thus, 50 grams multiplied by 3.4 kcal/grams = 170 kcal.

Lipids, amino acids, dextrose, electrolytes, trace elements, and vitamins are all incorporated into one container. Tolerance of this higher osmotic mixture in peripheral veins might be attributed to the buffering and dilution effects of intravenous fats in combination with the higher pH of the amino acid solutions and the addition of heparin to the mixture.

Total Parenteral Nutrition and PIC Lines

When nutrients are infused into a terminal central vein, parenteral nutrition is often referred to as total parenteral nutrition (TPN). The **superior vena cava,** one of the largest-diameter veins in the human body, is commonly used for TPN. Total parenteral nutrition can deliver greater nutrient loads because the blood flow in the superior vena cava rapidly dilutes these solutions 1000-fold. Concentrations for both dextrose and amino acids are determined by the client's needs. See Clinical Calculation 14-3 for an explanation and demonstration of the calculation of a sample TPN solution. A line inserted peripherally but threaded into a central vein is TPN.

INSERTION AND CARE OF A TPN LINE

A physician or trained registered nurse inserts the PIC line usually to the subclavian vein and into the superior

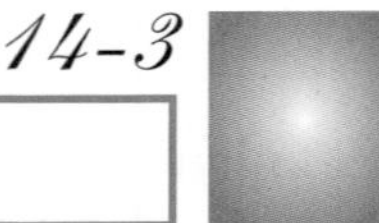

Clinical Calculation

Calculating TPN Solution/TPN Energy Nutrient Content (or PIC line)

TPN/PIC solutions are usually packed in 500-mL bags. Pharmacists prefer to use dextrose and amino acids in 500-mL bags and vary the concentration of the nutrients to achieve the appropriate nutritional parameters. For example, a 500-mL bag of dextrose mixed with a 500-mL bag of amino acids equals 1000 mL. Lipids are usually provided as 250 mL of 20% lipid (1/2 bag) or 500 mL (one bag) of 10% lipid.

The client's needs for kilocalories, protein, and fat can be accommodated by individualizing the concentration of each energy nutrient. For example, dextrose can be ordered from 5 to 70%, noted as D_5, D_{40}, D_{50}, etc. Commonly used concentrations of amino acids are 5%, 8.5%, and 10%.

NUTRITIONAL VALUES USED IN COMPUTATIONS OF TPN SOLUTIONS

Dextrose = 3.4 kcal/g
20% lipid = 2.0 kcal/mL
10% lipid = 1.1 kcal/mL
Protein = 4.0 kcal/gram
1 g of nitrogen = 6.25 grams of protein

Calculate the total kilocalories, nonprotein kilocalories, grams of nitrogen, calorie/nitrogen ratio, and % kilocalories from fat in 500 mL of D_{50}, 500 mL of 10% amino acids, and 250 mL of 10% lipid.

Dextrose	Percent concentration × volume = grams of dextrose	0.50 × 500 = 250 gram dextrose
	Grams of dextrose × 3.4 kcal/gram = kcal of solution	250 grams dextrose × 3.4 kcal/gram = 850 kcal
Amino acids	Percent concentration × volume = grams of protein	0.10 × 500 mL = 50 grams of protein
	Grams of protein × kcal/gram = protein kcal	50 grams of protein × 4 kcal/gram = 200 kcal
Lipids	kcal/mL × volume in mL = fat kcal	1.1 × 250 mL = 275 kcal
Total kilocalories	Add kilocalories from dextrose, protein, and lipid.	850 + 200 + 275 = 1325 kcal
Percent kilocalories from fat	Kilocalories from fat divided by total kcal = % fat kilocalories	275 divided by 1325 = 21% fat

vena cava. The line can be inserted at the client's bedside using strict aseptic technique. TPN solutions and PIC lines need to be sterile. The sterile mixtures consist of dextrose, amino acids, lipid emulsion, electrolytes, vitamins, trace elements, and other additives. The pharmacist usually prepares them in a sterile environment. Careful attention is required to provide vitamins and minerals to clients maintained on TPN/PIC lines to prevent problems such as Wernicke–Korsakoff syndrome (see Chapter 7).

TPN requires close monitoring and the therapy is very costly. The high cost is directly related to the number of highly trained health-care team members required to monitor the client, the laboratory work required for monitoring, and the cost of the solution. A nurse and a dietitian are typically responsible for assessing, monitoring, and educating clients destined for home parental nutrition. The clinical dietitian on the team usually has an advanced degree and special training. The dietitian is responsible for constant nutrition assessment, monitoring, interpretation of data, and calculating formula needs with the physician. The initials CNS (certified nutrition support) indicates the nurse, pharmacist, or dietitian has had advanced training in the delivery of nutrition orally, enterally, and parenterally.

MONITORING

Careful administration of the central lines solutions is important. Most institutions have a strict protocol that must be followed by all health-care professionals. A **protocol** is a description of the steps for performing a procedure. Protocols vary widely from one institution to another.

Most TPN protocols include:

- A slow start
- A strict schedule
- Close monitoring
- Instructions for increasing the volume
- Maintenance of a constant rate
- Instructions for a slow withdrawal

The solution may require adjustment, which can be made by increasing or decreasing any or all of the nutrients. All long-term TPN/PIC line patients should receive ongoing monitoring by a home-care clinician, including an assessment of micronutrient status, to ensure adequacy of the nutrition support regimen (Falk, 2002). Careful monitoring of the client's response to central line nutrition and taking corrective measures when needed are essential for safe administration of these solutions.

Many metabolic complications are possible with TPN. Rapid shifts of potassium, phosphorus, and magnesium from the intercellular compartment to the intracellular compartment result in a lowering of nutrient concentrations in the serum. As a result, initial laboratory tests rapidly fluctuate during the course of treatment. Immediate replacement of potassium, phosphorus, and magnesium is indicated if the corresponding laboratory values of these nutrients fall below normal.

Providing glucose in excess of kilocaloric needs can result in several problems, including carbon dioxide retention with respiratory difficulty. Too high a glucose content in solutions also leads to hyperglycemia. Therefore, glucose levels should be assessed regularly and insulin may be necessary. Liver function test results may become abnormal after an excess glucose load. Excess glucose may also lead to hyperlipidemia and fatty deposits in the liver. Elevated triglyceride levels may indicate too much glucose is being infused.

The avoidance of metabolic complications directly related to a glucose overload is one reason TPN clients need to be monitored closely. Such complications can be avoided by providing only an appropriate and not an excessive amount of kilocalories. In addition, an initial slow infusion at low concentrations prevents complications. Box 14-4 lists general recommendations for TPN monitoring.

TRANSITION AND COMBINATION FEEDINGS

Clients need a transition period from TPN to oral feedings. Some physicians prefer to wean clients from TPN by using tube feeding. This was the situation shown in Figure 14-2. The client has both an Enteral feeding line and TPN. Other physicians prefer to avoid the tube and wean clients orally. In the latter case, as the client's oral intake increases, the TPN solution is gradually withdrawn. Expect clients who have been on TPN for a significant time to experience some difficulty with oral feedings. They may need much encouragement to eat.

One of the problems with TPN is that the gastrointestinal tract does not have to work during TPN administration. Consequently, the gastrointestinal tract will have undergone some atrophy. Oral foods should be offered slowly during the weaning process. Some physicians avoid this problem by allowing some clients to consume a clear-liquid or light diet while on TPN, if their condition permits.

HOME PARENTERAL NUTRITION

Increasingly, clients are discharged on TPN. These clients need adequate follow-up by either the hospital or a community home-health agency. The pharmacist is responsible for the storage of TPN solutions in most institutions. Nurses involved in home parenteral nutrition need to be aware that vitamin degradation during the storage of total parenteral nutrition mixtures is significant and affects clinical outcome (Dupertuis, 2002). Factors affecting vitamin degradation include TPN bag material, temperature, and length of time between TPN compounding and end of infusion into the patient. The home-care nurse needs to work closely with the pharmacist and patient to minimize nutrient losses in TPN solutions.

Box 14-4 ■ *Monitoring TPN*

Initial Assessment

- Vital signs (respiration, pulse, temperature)
- Body weight and height
- Serum electrolytes, glucose, creatinine, blood urea nitrogen levels
- Serum magnesium, calcium, phosphorus levels
- Serum triglycerides and cholesterol levels
- Liver function tests
- Serum albumin and prealbumin
- Complete blood count
- Energy (estimated or measured), protein, fluid, and micronutrient needs

Routine Every 4 to 8 Hours

- Vital signs

Every 24 Hours

- Weight
- Fluid intake and output
- Serum electrolytes, glucose, creatinine, blood urea nitrogen levels; daily for 5 days or until stable; then twice a week

Weekly

- Serum ammonia, SGOT*, serum calcium, phosphorus, magnesium, total protein, and albumin
- Complete blood count
- Reassessment of actual oral, enteral, and TPN intake
  Other monitors may be indicated depending on the client's clinical condition.

*Serum glutamic oxaloacetic transaminase is a liver enzyme that reflects liver cellular damage when elevated (as opposed to liver obstructive disease).

Keystones

- The nutritional care of clients is a joint responsibility of all team members.
- How meals are distributed to clients and meal-service schedules are important for team members to know because they affect the administration of medications and the scheduling of clients for procedures.
- Nutritional care includes three areas: Assessing the client's need for nutrients, monitoring nutrient intake, and counseling clients about nutritional needs.

Continued

Keystones—cont'd

- Nutrition assessment is defined differently by various team members.
- Nutrients can be delivered to clients orally, via tube feeding, or parenterally.
- One principle is followed when selecting a feeding route: If the gastrointestinal tract works, use it to maximum capability.
- Oral feedings should be considered before tube feeding.
- Tube feeding should be considered before intravenous feeding.
- Intravenous feeding can be delivered peripherally or centrally.
- Clients on either tube feedings or intravenous feedings need to be closely monitored.

CASE STUDY 14-1

P was brought to the emergency room by ambulance; his mother accompanied him. The mother stated her son had been hit by a car while riding his bike. P is 11 years old, 4 ft 11 in. tall, and weighs 89 lb. The client's mother stated her son was well before the accident. In the emergency room, it was observed that both his eyes were surrounded by contusions and his throat and the left side of his face were swollen. Communication with the client was at first minimal because it was painful for him to speak. An intravenous solution of D_5W was started in the emergency room. He was also shown to have a fractured femur. Surgery was required to reset the bone. The physician determined that traction would be necessary. P was expected to require traction, and thus hospitalization, for 3 to 5 weeks.

Five days later, P is still having problems swallowing. He has not progressed beyond sips of clear liquids. The kilocalorie count shows an average daily intake of 395 kcal, with only 8 g of protein for the past 3 days. P appears to be in pain when he swallows and has choked twice on larger sips of the clear liquids. The client speaks only in single words or short sentences. It is still painful for him to talk. The swelling in his esophagus has decreased enough to allow the insertion of a small silicone feeding tube. The physician has ordered a nasogastric feeding tube with Nutren 1.0 Fiber. The order reads:

Day 1 Continuous drip 50 mL/h ½ strength
Day 2 Continuous drip 50 mL/h ¾ strength
Day 3 Continuous drip 50 mL/h full strength
Day 4 Continuous drip 84 mL/h full strength

Nutren 1.0 Fiber® contains 1.0 kcal/mL and 40 g of protein per 1000 mL. P may have ice chips and small amounts of clear liquids in addition to the tube feeding as desired. The physician states, "The client will remain on a tube feeding until he can consume his kilocalorie requirement orally. This client requires adequate nutrition to enable the femur to heal properly." P is not expected to be discharged on a home enteral tube feeding. His prognosis is good, and he is expected to make a full recovery.

The physician inserts the nasogastric tube because of the swelling in the esophagus and the danger of a perforation. The nurse assists at the client's bedside. The client holds the nurse's hand tightly as the tube is inserted. He has a worried look on his face, increased facial perspiration, and increased pulse/respirations during the procedure.

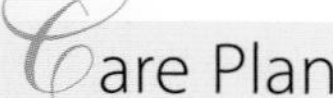

Care Plan

Subjective Data

Client held hand tightly during nasogastric tube insertion and appeared worried, apprehensive, and jittery.

Objective Data

Client is a trauma victim who showed increased perspiration and increased pulse/respirations during the tube insertion procedure.

Analysis

Child is showing signs and symptoms of anxiety related to feeding tube placement.

CASE STUDY *(Continued)*

Plan

DESIRED OUTCOMES EVALUATION CRITERIA	ACTIONS/INTERVENTIONS	RATIONALE
The client will state he needs the food in the tube feeding to heal his leg until he is eating better.	Explain enteral nutrition therapy procedures as performed.	A tube feeding is unfamiliar to most clients. Knowledge about the procedure may relax the client.
	As the client's condition permits, be available for listening and talking. Encourage the client to acknowledge and express feelings.	The client needs to vent his feelings about both the tube feeding and the situational crisis (the accident).

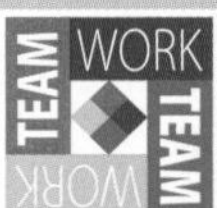

14-1

Dietitian's Notes

The following Dietitian's Notes are representative of the documentation found in a client's medical record.

Subjective: Client not able to provide much verbal information. Per client's mother, client was well nourished before accident. No food allergies, intolerances, or food dislikes. Client did not avoid any of the major food groups and ate at least four times a day.

Objective: 11-year-old child 4 ft 11 in. tall, weight 89 lb (40.4 kg). Client now being fed 84 mL of Enrich® per day every hour times 24 hours. No complaints of nausea, vomiting, last BM this B/N/

Analysis: Kilocalorie intake from tube feeding as ordered equals 2217 per day with 59.8 grams of protein. Client's estimated kilocalorie needs at 30 to 35 kcal/kg and 40.4 kg equals a maximum of 1414 kcal. Client's estimated protein needs are 1.0 to 1.5 g/kg actual body weight or 40.4 to 60.6. BMI = 17.9. Pt is just above the 50th%ile for BMI-for-age%ile. Laboratory values are all within normal limits.

Client is consuming some oral food each day—about 395 kcal and 8 grams of protein.

Plan: Recommend decreasing number of feedings from 24 hours to 14 hours per day. This would provide 1293 kcal, 1176 mL of fluid, and 46 grams of protein. Recommend flushing the tube feeding with 50 mL of water 4 times per day. Will closely follow prealbumin levels and reevaluate protein content of tube feeding (adding a protein supplement) if prealbumin below normal.

Critical Thinking Questions

1. What would you do if the client pulled out the tube after insertion?
2. How would you reassess the client's continued need for a tube feeding?
3. How should this client be monitored while on the tube feeding?

Chapter Review

1. Parental nutrition is usually indicated in the following situation:
   a. Rectal abscess
   b. Cancer esophagus
   c. Bowel obstruction
   d. Malnutrition

2. 1000 mL of a D_5W solution provides ___ grams of CHO and ___ kcal.
   a. 50 and 170
   b. 5 and 20
   c. 50 and 200
   d. 5 and 17

3. Careful administration of total parenteral nutrition includes all of the following except:
   a. A slow start
   b. Close monitoring
   c. Abrupt withdrawal
   d. A strict schedule

4. Among the following, diarrhea in a tube-fed client is most likely related to:
   a. A continuous-infusion feeding
   b. A contamination
   c. A fluid deficit
   d. Insufficient kilocalories

5. Which of the following is not a recommended procedure for administering medications through a tube feeding?
   a. Mix all of the medications together, crush thoroughly, mix with water, and add to the formula.
   b. If at all possible, use medications in the liquid form.
   c. Flush the tube with at least 30 mL of water before giving the medication and before resuming the tube-feeding formula.
   d. If a medication is ordered to be added to the formula, observe the feeding after the addition for any reaction or precipitation.

Clinical Analysis

1. Mr. J, 58 years old, visits his physician with a complaint of abdominal pain. He is scheduled for a diagnostic work-up, which will include a **barium enema** (x-ray study of his colon). Before this procedure, the nurse should instruct the client to:
   a. Eat a large breakfast on the day of the examination, such as orange juice, cereal, toast, scrambled eggs, and milk.
   b. Drink ample fluids on the morning of the examination, including at least 12 ounces of juice, 1 cup of gelatin, and broth.
   c. Take nothing orally after midnight on the day of the examination and consume only gelatin; clear broth; tea; coffee; and grape, apple, or cranberry juice on the day before the examination.
   d. Drink milk, juices, and coffee and eat only strained cream soups, ice cream, and gelatin on the day before the examination and take nothing orally after midnight.

2. Ms. L has a jejunostomy. She was discharged from the hospital last week after receiving instructions on home care from the nutrition support service. The local pharmacy is out of the Vivonex formula she has been instructed to use. As the nurse, you recommend that:
   a. She substitute Ensure®
   b. She substitute Polycose®
   c. She contact the Nutrition Support Service for instructions
   d. She substitute an intact or polymeric formula

3. Mr. W has been receiving a tube feeding of Ensure® via nasogastric tube for 3 weeks via a bolus infusion. He has just started to have loose stools (300 mL each × 6 today). You should first suspect the following to be responsible for the diarrhea:
   a. A new medication added to his treatment plan
   b. Bacterial contamination
   c. Intolerance to the bolus delivery method
   d. Lactose intolerance

15

Interactions: Food and Nutrients vs. Medications and Supplements

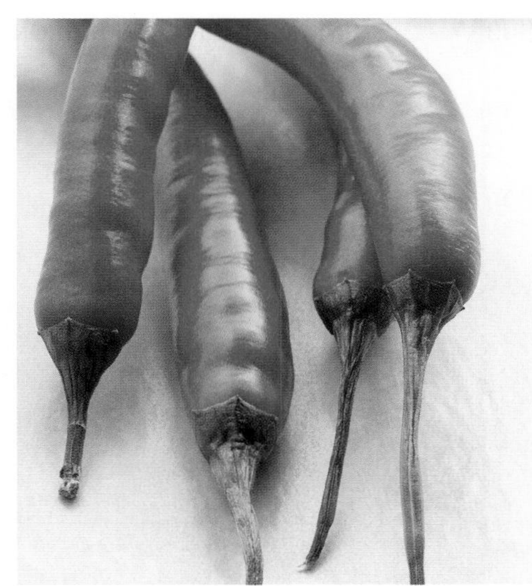

LEARNING OBJECTIVES

After completing this chapter, the student should be able to:

- Explain the importance of proper scheduling of medications in relation to food intake.
- Identify two groups of clients likely to experience food–drug interactions.
- Describe four ways in which foods, nutrients, drugs, and dietary supplements can interact and give an example of each.
- Discuss two potentially life-threatening food–drug interactions and design nursing interventions to avoid these events.
- Compare and contrast the regulatory processes for products sold in the United States as dietary supplements with those for products marketed as drugs.
- List examples of adverse effects from complementary medicines.
- Discuss the use of dietary supplements by athletes.

Drug–nutrient–supplement interactions encompass any alteration in the effect of one caused by the interplay with one of the others. Because medication or legal drug use is widespread in the United States, opportunities abound for such interactions. A population-based survey indicated that 81% of respondents used at least one medication the previous week, 50% took at least one prescription drug, and 10% took five or more prescription drugs. The most commonly used products were:

- Multivitamins (27% of adults)
- Herbal/natural supplements (22%)
- acetaminophen (19%)
- aspirin (18%)
- ibuprofen (17%) (Slone Epidemiology Center, 2006). See Figure 15-1.

About 25% of persons taking prescription drugs also take dietary supplements (Gardiner, Phillips, and Shaughnessy, 2008).

Some drugs interact with other drugs, foods, and nutrients in ways that can be beneficial or detrimental, enhancing or inhibiting the action of the other. In no sense is the information in this chapter exhaustive. Emphasis is placed on interactions that illustrate the range of known mechanisms and those that increase the risk of malnutrition or therapeutic failure. Pharmacists and dietitians use computer databases. In all cases, pharmaceutical resources should be consulted when administering medications.

A drug is a substance, other than a food, that is intended to affect a structure or function of the body. As used in this text, the term *drug* includes alcohol and both prescription and over-the-counter medications. As is the usual practice in medical literature, **generic names** are given for drugs.

Dietary supplements that may also interact with drugs and nutrients are included later in the chapter. Because of the lack of pre-marketing regulation and ongoing inspections of manufacturing processes, these substances invite special scrutiny when used by clients.

Since athletes may be tempted to try to gain a competitive edge by using supplements, information on

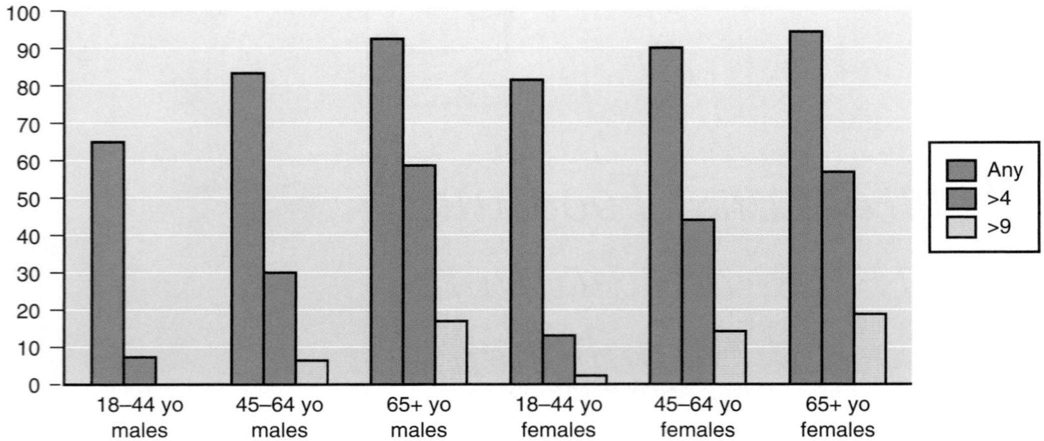

FIGURE 15-1 Percentages of adults who took at least 1, 5 or more, or 10 or more medications in the week surveyed. Medications included prescription, over-the-counter, vitamin/mineral, or herbal supplements. (Adapted from Slone Epidemiology Center, 2006.)

safety and effectiveness of some performance-enhancing supplements as well as food-based interventions for the athlete round out the chapter.

Mechanisms of Interactions

Both pharmacokinetics and pharmacodynamics can be involved in interactions with nutrients or supplements.

Pharmacokinetics is the study of the action of a drug, emphasizing absorption time, duration of effect, distribution in the body, and method of excretion. Among the considerations pertinent to pharmacokinetics are:

- **Half-life**—time for a drug's concentration, usually in plasma, to be reduced by one-half
- **Bioavailability**—proportion of the drug that reaches the systemic circulation. By definition, intravenous drugs and nutrients administered via total parenteral nutrition (TPN) are 100% bioavailable.
- **Presystemic clearance**—metabolism of orally ingested compounds before they reach the systemic circulation (formerly known as the **first-pass effect).**

Pharmacodynamics is the study of drugs and their actions on living organisms, and their physiologic or clinical effects. Pharmacodynamic effects of interactions that result in toxicities or treatment failures are major concerns of health-care providers.

For instance, *phenytoin*, a drug used to control epileptic seizures, is a folic acid antagonist that competes with the vitamin for binding sites. Its effects can be:

- Pharmacokinetic, resulting in lower serum levels of *phenytoin* or
- Pharmacodynamic if seizure activity increases.

The interaction works both ways, so that long-term *phenytoin* therapy also can cause folic acid deficiency (Chan, 2006). See Table 15-1.

Starting at the pharmacy and ending with excretion of the drug or its components, interactions are classified into one of four types. See Table 15-2.

Type I Interactions

Type I interactions usually occur outside the body:

- In the intravenous or TPN solution
- In the syringe where substances are admixed
- In tube feeding reservoirs
- In the respective tubings

For example, calcium phosphate precipitates in TPN has caused two deaths from microvascular pulmonary emboli (McKinnon, 1996; Mirtallo, 2004). In Europe, seven infants suffered adverse cardiopulmonary events and six of them died after intravenous administration of ceftriaxone and calcium-containing solutions, including one case involving TPN solution (U.S. FDA, 2009a). No one should rely on visual inspection to identify precipitates that may be

- Too small to be seen with the naked eye or
- Invisible in opaque solutions

Up-to-date references regarding compatibility should be consulted.

Clinical Application 15-1 offers some insight into the knowledge and skill necessary to administer TPN safely. Some of the considerations involved with appropriate administration of tube feedings in conjunction with oral medications appear in Chapter 14.

TABLE 15-1 ■ Nutrient–Drug Interactions

NUTRIENT	DRUG(S)	INTERACTION	INTERVENTION
Calcium	*ciprofloxacin* *norfloxacin* *ofloxacin* *tetracycline*	Combines with drugs, yielding insoluble compounds	Separate drug doses from calcium-containing foods
Folic Acid	*phenytoin* *aspirin*	Competition for binding sites Competition for binding sites	Monitor blood levels of vitamin and drug in long-term therapy. Monitor blood levels of vitamin in long-term therapy.
Iron	*ciprofloxacin* *norfloxacin* *ofloxacin* *tetracycline*	Combines with drugs yielding insoluble compounds	Separate drug doses from iron-containing foods.
Magnesium	*ciprofloxacin* *norfloxacin* *ofloxacin* *tetracycline*	Combines with drugs, yielding insoluble compounds	Separate drug doses from magnesium-containing foods.
Niacin	*isoniazid* *phenytoin*	Drug is structurally similar to niacin. Unknown mechanism	Observe for pellagra with long-term therapy. Observe for pellagra with long-term therapy.
Vitamin B_6	*levodopa*	Formation of a complex that makes vitamin unavailable (Type IIC interaction)	Monitor vitamin status with long-term therapy.
Vitamin B_{12}	*antacids* *nitrous oxide anesthesia*	Drugs neutralize gastric acid that normally facilitates separation of vitamin B_{12} from the foods containing it. Nitrous oxide oxidizes the cobalt atom in cobalamin to an inactive state.	Monitor vitamin status with long-term therapy. Rare event: occurred in client with long-term very restrictive vegetarian diet
Vitamin D	*carbamazepine* *corticosteroids* *phenobarbital* *phenytoin* *rifampin*	Interferes with vitamin D metabolism in Type III interaction Interfere with vitamin D metabolism in Type III interaction Interferes with vitamin D metabolism in Type III interaction Interferes with vitamin D metabolism in Type III interaction Interferes with vitamin D metabolism in Type III interaction	Monitor vitamin status with long-term therapy. Monitor vitamin status with long-term therapy. Monitor vitamin status with long-term therapy. Monitor vitamin status with long-term therapy. Monitor vitamin status with long-term therapy.
Zinc	*ciprofloxacin* *norfloxacin* *ofloxacin* *tetracycline*	Combines with drugs, yielding insoluble compounds	Separate drug doses from zinc-containing foods.

TABLE 15-2 ■ Classification of Interactions

	CHARACTERISTICS	POSSIBLE EFFECT	EXAMPLE	INTERVENTION
Type I	Usually occur when substances are in direct physical contact, i.e., in delivery device	Physical, biochemical reactions, i.e., oxidation, precipitation	Calcium phosphate precipitates in TPN solution.	Follow recommendations in the literature. Do not rely on visual inspection.
Type II	Limited to substances taken orally or administered enterally	Increased or decreased bioavailability	High-fiber meals decrease absorption of *digoxin*.	Administer *digoxin* 1 hour before or 2 hours after high-fiber meals.
A		Modified enzyme activity	Grapefruit juice inhibits intestinal isoenzyme CYP3A4, raising blood levels of many drugs.	Advise client not to consume grapefruit juice when taking these drugs orally. (See Table 15-3.)
B		Modified transport mechanism	Water-soluble formulations of vitamin E inhibit the transfer protein, P-glycoprotein, increasing blood levels of *cyclosporine* and *digoxin*.	Do not use water-soluble formulations of vitamin E with *cyclosporine*. Monitor blood levels regularly if used with *digoxin*.
C		Complexing or binding of substances	Calcium, iron, magnesium, and zinc bind with *tetracycline*, yielding insoluble compounds.	Separate drug doses from foods and tube feedings containing these minerals by 1 to 3 hours.
Type III	Occur after the substances have reached the systemic circulation	Changed cellular or tissue distribution	*Warfarin* interferes with synthesis of clotting factors.	Equalize amounts of vitamin K-rich foods eaten day-by-day.
Type IV	Affect disposition of substances by liver and kidney	Promoted or impaired clearance or elimination of substances	*Lithium* is excreted in tandem with sodium and water.	Monitor therapeutic effect and urine specific gravity.

Adapted from Chan (2006).

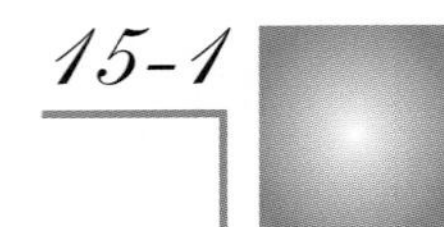

Preventing Drug Interactions with Total Parenteral Nutrition (TPN)

TPN is a complex formulation of dextrose, amino acids, fat emulsion, electrolytes, vitamins, and trace elements. Up to 38 additives may be included, each having individual characteristics that might contribute to interactions.

TPN is not recommended as a drug delivery vehicle because of limited or unreliable compatibility information. The preferred mode of medication administration is to separate the drugs from the TPN. Separation can be accomplished by using multiple-lumen catheters, alternating the TPN infusion with medication infusion, or, if possible, oral administration of medications.

Multivitamins should be admixed immediately before infusion. Thiamin and vitamin A are known to have a short stability in TPN. For example, night-blindness caused by vitamin A deficiency developed in a client whose TPN was admixed in the pharmacy and later delivered to the home.

Interactions may become apparent if changes are noted in the solution or if the catheter becomes plugged, but loss of effectiveness of the drug or the TPN can also occur without outward clues.

Source: Summarized from Mirtallo (2004).

Type II Interactions

Type II interactions occur with oral or enteral intake, producing increased or decreased bioavailability of either the drug or nutrient. Even 8 to 10 menthol cough drops daily interfered with warfarin's effectiveness (Coderre, Faria, and Dyer, 2010). Factors influencing Type II bioavailability include:

- Food intake
- Modification of enzyme activity or transport mechanisms
- Complexing or binding of drugs or nutrients so one or both are unavailable for absorption. See Type IIC interaction and Tables 15-1 and 15-3.

Drugs Taken on an Empty Stomach

Some drugs must be taken on an empty stomach. A strict protocol is used for *alendronate*, a bone resorption inhibitor given for osteoporosis. *Alendronate* must be taken first thing in the morning with plain water 30 minutes before any other medications, food, or beverages. Any intake other than water significantly decreases absorption. Moreover, the person must remain

TABLE 15-3 ■ Drug–Nutrient Interactions

DRUG	CLASSIFICATION	INTERACTION
alendronate	Bone resorption inhibitor	Any intake but water decreases absorption.
ampicillin	Anti-infective	Food, acidic juices, or carbonated beverages increase gastric degradation of drug.
atorvastatin	Lipid-lowering agent	Grapefruit juice increases bioavailability for several days in Type IIA interaction.
atovaquone	Antiprotozoal	Fatty meal increases the drug's solubility.
azithromycin*	Anti-infective	Food, acidic juices, or carbonated beverages increase gastric degradation of the drug.
captopril	Antihypertensive	Potassium-containing salt substitutes increase risk for hyperkalemia in type IV interaction.
ceftriaxone	Anti-infective	Calcium-containing IV products, including TPN, combine with the drug in a Type I interaction.
ciprofloxacin	Anti-infective	Taking on empty stomach maximizes absorption. Calcium, iron, magnesium, and zinc combine with the drug to form insoluble compounds in Type IIC interaction.
cloxacillin	Anti-infective	Food, acidic juices, or carbonated beverages increase gastric degradation of the drug.
cyclosporine	Immunosuppressant	Grapefruit juice increases bioavailability for several days in Type IIA interaction. Water-soluble formulations of vitamin E have increased blood levels of drug in Type IIB interaction.
diazepam	Anxiolytic, anticonvulsant	Grapefruit juice increases bioavailability for several days in type IIA interaction.
digoxin	Antiarrhythmic	High-fiber meal decreases absorption. Water-soluble formulations of vitamin E have increased blood levels of drug in Type IIB interaction.
enalapril	Antihypertensive	Potassium-containing salt substitutes increase risk for hyperkalemia in Type IV interaction.
erythromycin (some formulations)	Anti-infective	Decreased gastric acidity associated with milk, alcohol, or hot beverages causes early dissolution of enteric coatings.
felodipine	Antianginal, antihypertensive	Grapefruit juice increases bioavailability for several days in Type IIA interaction.
furazolidone	Anti-infective	Tyramine-containing foods may provoke hypertensive crisis in Type III interaction.
griseofulvin	Antifungal	Fatty meal taken with drug stimulates bile secretion and increases bioavailability of the drug.**
indinavir*	Antiretroviral	Food precipitates the drug.
isocarboxazid	Antidepressant	Tyramine-containing foods may provoke hypertensive crisis in Type III interaction.

TABLE 15-3 ■ Drug–Nutrient Interactions (Continued)

DRUG	CLASSIFICATION	INTERACTION
isoniazid*	Antitubercular	Food, acidic juices, or carbonated beverages increase gastric degradation of the drug. Vitamin B_6 complexes with the drug in Type IIC interaction: useful in drug overdoses and in minimizing drug side effects. Tyramine-containing foods may provoke hypertensive crisis in Type III interaction.
levodopa	Antiparkinson agent	High-protein diet may compete with the uptake of levodopa into the brain.
levothyroxine	Thyroid preparation	High-fiber diet requires higher doses to achieve the therapeutic goal. Large amounts of calcium, iron, magnesium, or zinc may bind levothyroxine and prevent complete absorption in a Type IIC interaction.
linezolid	Anti-infective	Tyramine-containing foods may provoke a hypertensive crisis in Type III interaction.
lisinopril	Antihypertensive	Potassium-containing salt substitutes increase the risk for hyperkalemia in Type IV interaction.
lithium	Mood stabilizer	Increased sodium and water intake increases renal excretion of the drug, decreasing its effect. The opposite is also true. (Type IV interaction)
lovastatin	Lipid-lowering agent	Grapefruit juice greatly increases bioavailability for several days in Type IIA interaction.
melphalan*	Antineoplastic	Competes with amino acids for absorption.
mercaptopurine*	Antineoplastic	Oxidized by food into inactive metabolites.
metformin	Antidiabetic	Decreased absorption with fiber intake†
midazolam	Anxiolytic, anticonvulsant	Grapefruit juice increases bioavailability for several days in Type IIA interaction.
nicardipine	Antianginal, antihypertensive	Grapefruit juice increases bioavailability over several days in Type IIA interaction.
nisoldipine	Antianginal, antihypertensive	Grapefruit juice increases bioavailability over several days in Type IIA interaction.
norfloxacin	Anti-infective	Taking on empty stomach maximizes absorption. Calcium, iron, magnesium, and zinc combine with drug to form insoluble compounds in Type IIC interaction.
ofloxacin	Anti-infective	Taking on empty stomach maximizes absorption. Calcium, iron, magnesium, and zinc combine with the drug to form insoluble compounds in Type IIC interaction.
penicillin V	Anti-infective	Food, acidic juices, or carbonated beverages increase gastric degradation of the drug.
phenelzine	Antidepressant	Tyramine-containing foods may provoke hypertensive crisis in Type III interaction.
phenytoin	Antiepileptic	Folic acid antagonist that competes with the vitamin for binding sites Tube feedings decrease serum levels of the drug.
procarbazine	Antineoplastic	Tyramine-containing foods may provoke hypertensive crisis in Type III interaction.
selegiline‡	Antiparkinson agent	Tyramine-containing foods may provoke hypertensive crisis in Type III interaction.
simvastatin	Lipid-lowering agent	Grapefruit juice greatly increases bioavailability for several days in Type IIA interaction.
tetracycline*	Anti-infective	Calcium, iron, magnesium, and zinc combine with drug to form insoluble compounds.
tranylcypromine	Antidepressant	Tyramine-containing foods may provoke hypertensive crisis in Type III interaction.
triazolam	Anxiolytic, anticonvulsant	Grapefruit juice increases bioavailability for several days in Type IIA interaction.
verapamil	vasodilator	Food delays but does not decrease absorption. Consistency in drug administration in relation to food is advised.
warfarin	Anticoagulant	Cranberry juice interferes with drug metabolism in Type IIA interaction. Large amounts of vitamin K-rich foods and beverages reduce anticoagulant effect in Type III interaction. Concomitant enteral feeding interferes with *warfarin* absorption, possibly through protein-binding in a Type IIC interaction.

*Risk of treatment failure if taken with food (Schmidt and Dalhoff, 2002).
**Risk of treatment failure especially in children if procedure not followed (Schmidt and Dalhoff, 2002).
†Akamine, Filho, and Peres (2007).
‡Transdermal preparation does not require severe dietary restrictions at certain doses (Chen and Swope, 2007; Robinson and Amsterdam, 2008).

upright for 30 minutes to facilitate passage through the pylorus and minimize risk of esophageal irritation.

In general, food stimulates gastrointestinal secretions that assist in dissolving solid forms of medication; however, certain drugs are best taken without food. Taking the following drugs with food risks treatment failure by various mechanisms. See Table 15-3.

- *ampicillin*
- *cloxacillin*
- *indinavir*, given for HIV
- *melphalan*
- *mercaptopurine,* given for leukemia
- *penicillin V*

Drugs Taken With Food

Meal intake usually stimulates gastric and intestinal secretions. Some nutrients and drugs are dependent on the normal acidity of the stomach for optimal utilization. See Figure 8-18. Disruption of the system can have undesirable consequences.

- Gastric acid and pepsin are required to split cobalamin from protein foods. Antacid medications have reportedly caused cobalamin malabsorption, resulting in megaloblastic anemia (Chan, 2006).
- Some drugs are **enteric coated** with an acid-resistant shell to protect the active ingredient from gastric acid and delay dissolution until the medication reaches the alkaline intestine (Fig. 15-2). Substances contributing to the early erosion of enteric coatings include:
    - Milk (see *erythromycin* in Table 15-3)
    - Alcohol
    - Hot beverages

Absorption can be delayed or decreased by food intake. Each interaction can impact administration schedules. See Box 15-1.

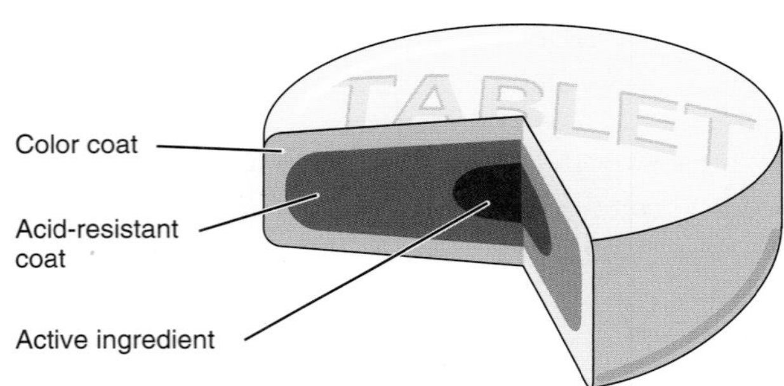

FIGURE 15-2 Enteric-coated tablet. Substances that penetrate the acid-resistant coating defeat the purpose of this type of tablet. (Reprinted from Clayton, BD, and Stock, YN: *Basic pharmacology for nurses,* ed 9. Mosby, St. Louis, 1989, p 56, with permission.)

Box 15-1 ■ *Delayed Versus Decreased Absorption*

Some drugs take longer to be absorbed if ingested with food but the total amount absorbed is unchanged. This delay is the case with *verapamil,* a vasodilator. Therefore, emphasis can be placed on consistency in drug administration in relation to food intake.

However, spacing of doses in relation to food and beverage intake becomes important when a smaller amount of the drug is absorbed in the presence of food than in an empty stomach. In such a situation, correct timing of medication and other intake is necessary. This decreased absorption is the case with *azithromycin.*

Also complicating the picture, not all drugs in a given class are equally affected by interactions with food. The total amount absorbed of the quinolones *ciprofloxacin, norfloxacin,* and *ofloxacin* is reduced if taken with food but absorption of other quinolones is not reduced by food (Chan, 2006).

Fiber intake with certain medications decreases drug absorption. See Table 15-3 for the following drugs.

- *Digoxin,* given for heart disease, is less well absorbed if taken with a high-fiber meal than with one containing a smaller amount of fiber (Deglin and Vallerand, 2009). See also Table 15-2.
- *Levothyroxine,* used to treat hypothyroidism, requires much higher doses if given with a fiber-enriched diet (Boullata, 2005).
- *Metformin,* an antidiabetic drug, reportedly shows decreased absorption with fiber than without it (Akamine, Filho, and Peres, 2007).

In contrast, meals containing fat favor absorption of certain drugs that require bile salts for optimal absorption. Fat also stimulates the release of cholecystokinin, which slows gastrointestinal motility, thus permitting the drug to remain in contact with the intestinal tissues for a longer time than otherwise. The extra intestinal exposure to the drug enhances its absorption.

See Table 15-3 for the following drugs affected by fat intake:

- *griseofulvin,* given for fungal infections of the skin such as athlete's foot
- *atovaquone,* given for *Pneumocystis carinii* pneumonia.

An example of a special intervention involving a high-fat diet to control epileptic seizures in children appears in Clinical Application 15-2.

Changes in Enzyme Activity (Type IIA Interactions)

Cytochrome P450 (CYP450) is a superfamily of more than 50 enzymes found mainly in the liver but also in the gastrointestinal tract, lungs, placenta, and kidneys (Lynch and Price, 2007). The three major families of isoenzymes are CPY1, CPY2, and CPY3 (Anderson, 2002) but the two enzymes most significant to drug metabolism are CYP3A4 and CYP2D6 (Lynch and Price, 2007). The isoenzyme CYP3A4, found in the small intestine, is known to play a major role in regulating the oral bioavailability of up to 70% of drugs. That function may have evolved to protect the body from toxins.

After uptake by the intestinal epithelial cells (enterocytes), many substances are metabolized by CYP3A4 or returned to the intestinal lumen by a transporter protein, **P-glycoprotein** (P-gp), thus limiting the amount of the substance available for absorption (Chan, 2006). Individuals show a wide variation in the amount of CYP3A4 in the liver and the intestine due to genetic, physiological, and environmental factors with resulting differences in the severity of interactions.

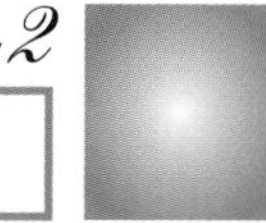

15-2

Clinical Application

The Ketogenic Diet for Seizure Control in Children

Some children with **epilepsy** that is poorly controlled with medication benefit from a high-fat, low-carbohydrate, ketogenic diet. Kilocalories and fluid are limited to less than the RDA. The diet is also inadequate in micronutrients so that supplementation and close monitoring of the child's growth are essential.

The mechanism of action is unknown and ketosis alone does not explain the anticonvulsant effect. Normally, the brain derives most of its energy from glucose. When deprived of its preferred fuel, the brain uses ketone bodies for energy, a process shown to be more effective in young animals than in old ones. In humans, the ketogenic diet is more successful in children younger than 8 years old than older children, but the diet is not universally helpful.

About one-third of children with intractable seizures become seizure-free on the ketogenic diet, one-third have seizures significantly less frequently, and one-third do not benefit (Papandreou et al., 2006). Some children in the study continued to receive medications for their epilepsy but in reduced amounts. Any reduction in medication improves the child's quality of life.

Unfortunately, the diet has several known complications: kidney stones, gall stones, anemia, and cardiac abnormalities. Nevertheless, the ketogenic diet provides an option for families with a child suffering from difficult-to-control seizures.

GRAPEFRUIT JUICE

An accidental discovery in 1989 that grapefruit juice, used to mask the taste of alcohol in a study, enhanced the absorption of *felodipine* has spurred research into the underlying mechanism. It appears that grapefruit juice's major effect is through the inhibition of intestinal CYP3A4 so that the oral bioavailability of affected drugs is increased dramatically, in some cases as much as fivefold, sufficient to cause drug toxicity and increased side effects or treatment failure.

Even when intake of grapefruit juice is stopped, the increased bioavailability of the affected drugs continues for 72 hours until the intestine can manufacture more of the enzyme. Individuals differ as much as eightfold in the amount of intestinal CYP3A4 expressed, and those with the greatest amount of the enzyme show the greatest effects on drug bioavailability (Sica, 2006).

Because most of the evidence has been gathered using grapefruit juice, disagreement exists as to whether the interaction with drugs is clinically significant with whole grapefruit, Seville oranges used in marmalade, or other products (Chan, 2006; Sica, 2006).

Applying this knowledge to clinical practice is complicated by the fact that even within a given class of drugs, not all agents are metabolized by CYP3A4, so some medications in the class are affected by grapefruit juice and others are not. These are some examples.

Of calcium channel blockers, given to manage hypertension and angina pectoris, grapefruit juice:

- Increases bioavailability of *felodipine, nisoldipine,* and *nicardipine* (see Table 15-3)
- Shows little interaction with *nifedipine* and *amlodipine,* presumably because they have a higher bioavailability compared with the first three (Dahan and Altman, 2004).

Similarly, grapefruit juice increases the bioavailability of the benzodiazepines:

- *diazepam, midazolam,* and *triazolam* (see Table 15-3)
- But not *alprazolam* (Dahan and Altman, 2004)

Likewise, differing effects with grapefruit juice are seen with statin drugs, given to lower cholesterol and prevent ischemic heart disease. See Table 15-3.

- *Simvastatin* and *lovastatin* had greatly increased blood levels when given with grapefruit juice;
- *Atorvastatin* showed a lesser effect than with the previous two drugs and
- *pravastatin* no effect (Dahan and Altman, 2004) because *pravastatin* is not exclusively metabolized by CYP3A4 (Schmidt and Dalhuff, 2002).

Cyclosporine, an immunosuppressive agent used to prevent rejection of transplanted organs, is metabolized by intestinal CYP3A4, and elevated blood levels have occurred when administered with grapefruit juice. Because *cyclosporine* has a narrow **therapeutic index** and serious side effects on the kidney and brain that high levels of the drug may evoke, avoiding grapefruit juice during oral therapy is well advised (Dahan and Altman, 2004). See Table 15-3.

CRANBERRY JUICE

A similar mechanism but a different isoenzyme is proposed to explain an interaction between the anticoagulant *warfarin* and cranberry juice. After a chest infection, a client subsisted almost solely on cranberry juice for 2 weeks while taking his prescribed medications, *digoxin, phenytoin,* and *warfarin.* He died of gastrointestinal and pericardial hemorrhage (Suvarna, Pimohamed, and Henderson, 2003). *Warfarin* is mainly metabolized by the cytochrome P450 isoenzyme CYP2C9, and cranberry juice contains flavonoids known to inhibit P450 enzymes.

Another case of a persistently elevated International Normalized Ratio (INR) used to monitor prothrombin time occurred in a client with a prosthetic mitral valve 2 weeks after the client began drinking cranberry juice. Subsequent symptoms included postoperative bleeding problems (Grant, 2004).

By October 2004, the regulatory agency in the United Kingdom had received 12 reports of possible interactions between *warfarin* and cranberry juice. Health professionals were advised to avoid cranberry products with *warfarin* unless the health benefits outweighed the risks (MHRA, 2008).

Subsequent case reports include evidence of:

- Pharmacokinetic effects in a man with an INR of 6.45 (therapeutic range of 2 to 3) without abnormal bleeding after drinking a half gallon of cranberry/apple juice in the week before the elevated INR (Paeng, Sprague, and Jackevicius, 2007)
- Pharmacodynamic effects in a client taking stable doses of *warfarin* who developed major bleeding and high INR values soon after starting daily cranberry juice with no other identifiable reasons for the high INR. Fortunately, discontinuation of the juice consumption resolved the problem (Rindone and Murphy, 2006). See Table 15-3.

Controlled studies on clients with atrial fibrillation and on healthy volunteers using 250 and 200 milliliters, respectively, of cranberry juice daily did not confirm a link between cranberry juice and *warfarin* (Li et al., 2006; Lilja, Backman, and Neuvonen, 2007) but some authors recommended cautioning clients and surveillance of INR values regardless (Li et al., 2006; Pham and Pham, 2007). The two controlled studies used a total of 17 subjects who likely did not encompass the range of genetic possibilities for metabolizing the juice and the drug. See Genomic Gem 15-1.

LICORICE

Clinical Application 15-3 describes interference with cortisol metabolism caused by licorice consumption.

Genomic Gem 15-1

Variants in CYP2C9

CYP2C9 enzyme, mainly expressed in the liver, is involved in the metabolism of about 10% of all drugs. A large variation among individuals exists in CYP2C9 activity, which accounts for differences in drug response and in adverse effects. Two common variants, found in between 7% and 10% of Caucasians and fewer Africans, decrease the activity of the enzyme. One of the variants has not been detected at all in Asians. This information can be implemented in drug development and in administering specific drugs to improve responses to the drugs and reduce costs (Ingelman-Sundberg et al., 2007). In addition, it is likely that genotyping of subjects used in drug–nutrient interaction studies would yield more conclusive findings than general population studies.

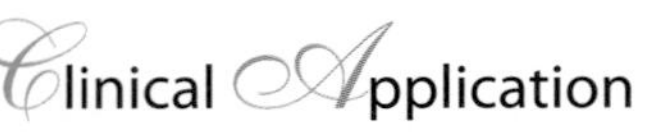

Clinical Application 15-3

Licorice Affects Cortisol Metabolism

Natural licorice, a flavoring agent, contains glycyrrhetinic acid, which when metabolized inhibits an enzyme that controls the conversion of cortisol to cortisone in the kidney. The result is the enhanced mineralocorticoid effect of cortisol, leading to hypokalemic hypertension (Mattarello et al., 2006). When eaten in excess, licorice can cause sodium and water retention, hypertension, hypokalemia, and alkalosis as shown in the following cases.

- Control of hypertension took 8 months in a 49-year-old woman who, unbeknownst to her physician, consumed large quantities of a licorice-flavored sweet (Dellow, Unwin, and Honour, 1999).
- Life-threatening hypokalemic paralysis occurred as a result of consuming licorice as a tea sweetener (a common custom among the Arab population) superimposed on long-term consumption of licorice candy (Elinav and Chajek-Shaul, 2003).
- Muscle weakness progressed to paralysis in an elderly Asian man with hypertension, hypokalemia, and metabolic alkalosis, attributed to a 3-year daily ingestion of tea flavored with natural licorice root (Lin et al., 2003).

These clients did not realize the risks of their habits. Besides these deliberate ingestions, however, a person may consume licorice unknowingly because it is used to flavor many foods, some chewing tobacco, chewing gum, alcoholic beverages, and some laxatives.

Changes in Transport Mechanism (Type IIB Interactions)

A nutrient can also inhibit P-glycoprotein as is the case with water-soluble formulations of vitamin E. Administration of this form of vitamin E to liver transplant recipients and healthy volunteers has been shown to increase *cyclosporine* bioavailability. By the same mechanism, vitamin E increases oral bioavailability of *digoxin* in young, healthy volunteers (Chan, 2006). See Table 15-3.

Hence, a client taking *cyclosporine* could be in major trouble if he concurrently consumes grapefruit juice and water-soluble vitamin E, both of which are readily available and for most people, innocuous. Such a situation demands vigorous and effective client education.

Complexing or Binding of Substances (Type IIC Interactions)

Well documented interactions involve antimicrobials, an oral anticoagulant, and an antiepileptic drug.

ANTIMICROBIALS

Tetracycline, an anti-infective agent, combines with calcium, iron, magnesium, and zinc to form insoluble compounds. The drug and the nutrient thus bound are both unavailable for absorption. For this reason, *tetracycline* should not be administered within 1 to 3 hours of:

- Taking iron supplements
- Eating iron-containing foods (red meat, egg yolks)
- Consuming milk, other dairy products or, calcium-fortified juices
- Taking antacids containing magnesium, aluminum, or calcium

Tetracycline should be taken without food or milk to avoid a high risk of treatment failure. Bioavailability of *tetracycline* is reduced

- Up to 57% when taken with food
- 65% with dairy products
- 81% with iron supplements

Even a small amount of milk in coffee or tea can reduce the drug's bioavailability by 49% (Schmidt and Dalhoff, 2002). See Tables 15-1 and 15-3.

Some *fluoroquinolones* react with metal cations in the same manner as does *tetracycline*. See *ciprofloxacin*, *norfloxacin*, and *ofloxacin* in Table 15-3 and the nutrients in Table 15-1. The bioavailability of *ciprofloxacin* was decreased by 28% when administered orally to normal subjects with Ensure® (Society of Hospital Pharmacists, 2005). Equal or greater impairment of absorption has been found with enteral feeding so that withholding tube feedings for 1 hour before and after the dose of medication is delivered is usually suggested.

Foods or supplements containing large amounts of calcium, iron, magnesium, or zinc also may bind *levothyroxine* and prevent complete absorption (Deglin and Vallerand, 2009).

Both the antituberculosis drug *isoniazid* and the anti-Parkinson agent *levodopa* form a complex with vitamin B_6. The kidney then excretes this complex in the urine rather than returning it to the bloodstream.

This interaction can be used therapeutically.

- Supplemental *pyridoxine* may be added to a *levodopa* regimen to prevent vitamin B_6 deficiency, also decreasing the effectiveness of *levodopa*.
- *Pyridoxine* supplementation can:
  - Limit the nervous system side effects of *isoniazid* (Boullata, 2005)
  - Intravenous *pyridoxine* is the treatment for *isoniazid* toxicity when it causes seizures unaffected by conventional antiepileptic drugs. In one case of attempted suicide, regional efforts were required to obtain sufficient supplies of IV pyridoxine (Morrow et al., 2006). See Tables 15-1 and 15-3.

ORAL ANTICOAGULANT

A significant difference in INR values has been demonstrated in intensive care clients receiving *warfarin* and enteral nutrition either continuously or paused for *warfarin* administration. Therefore, continuous enteral nutrition should be withheld for 1 hour before and after *warfarin* administration (Dickerson et al., 2008). See Table 15-3.

ANTIEPILEPTIC

Although the exact mechanism is unknown but bearing characteristics of a type IIC interaction, decreased serum levels of the antiepileptic drug *phenytoin* when administered with nasogastric feedings are well documented, as well as rebounding levels of the drug when the feedings are discontinued. Monitoring of serum *phenytoin* levels two or three times a week if administered with tube feedings is recommended (Chan, 2006). See Table 15-3.

Type III Interactions

Type III interactions occur after the nutrient or drug has reached the systemic circulation that delivers nutrients and drugs throughout the body to be metabolized by multiple organs. Two interactions with pharmacodynamic effects involve *warfarin* and *monoamine oxidase inhibitors* (MAOIs).

Vitamin K and Warfarin

The most commonly prescribed anticoagulant, *warfarin*, is given to prevent blood clot formation in clients with that history, other clotting disorders, and those with mechanical devices in the vascular system.

MECHANISM OF INTERACTION

Warfarin works by competing with vitamin K at its binding sites, thus inhibiting the synthesis of vitamin K–dependent clotting Factors II, VII, IX, and X, prolonging clotting time and "thinning" the blood.

Eating large amounts of foods high in vitamin K during anticoagulant therapy with *warfarin* decreases or may even negate the desired effect of the drug. Clients should not stop eating foods containing vitamin K, but they should avoid large variations in the amounts eaten. A problem might arise if they eat mounds of green leafy vegetables one day and then none for the following several days. See Table 15-4.

An experiment using diets that decreased vitamin K intake by 80% or increased it by 500% during a 4-day in-hospital stay demonstrated significant changes in the clients' INRs, thus supporting the

TABLE 15-4 ■ Diet for Oral Anticoagulant Therapy

AVOID	ONE SERVING PER DAY, 1 CUP RAW OR ½ CUP COOKED	CHECK WITH PRESCRIBER IF LARGE INCREASES OR DECREASES
Kale (except garnish)	Broccoli	Green vegetables
Parsley (except garnish)	Brussels sprouts	Garbanzo beans
Natto (Japanese) Swiss chard Purple laver Seaweed (Japanese)	Spinach Turnip or other greens	Lentils Canola oil Soybeans or soybean oil Products containing above oils Liver Green tea Cranberry juice/products

relevance of diet to therapeutic anticoagulation (Franco et al., 2004).

Even beverages such as green tea can be a significant source of vitamin K. A case of interaction with *warfarin* was reported in a 44-year-old client who had been stabilized on the drug but who later drank one-half to one gallon of green tea per day (Taylor and Wilt, 1999). Table 15-4 shows a diet for oral anticoagulant therapy. The items popular in Japanese cuisine are only examples. Culturally competent counseling of clients from different backgrounds requires specialized knowledge of food preferences. The key to effective oral anticoagulation is consistent intake of foods rich in vitamin K.

Overall, the influence of diet on the effectiveness of *warfarin* is less important than factors such as client age, physical health, and genotype of CYP2C9, the primary enzyme for the metabolism of *warfarin*. However, because the drug may be prescribed long term, all factors should be addressed to optimize and stabilize the therapeutic effect.

OTHER FACTORS AFFECTING WARFARIN

Abnormal intestinal function and pharmacokinetics of the drug also affect the effectiveness of *warfarin*.

Intestinal Conditions

Even a short-term change in physical health can affect *warfarin*'s pharmacodynamics, as has been reported in cases of diarrhea that may interfere with the absorption of dietary and **endogenous** vitamin K. Excessive anticoagulation has occurred in clients with:

- Protracted diarrhea (Roberge et al., 2000)
- Relapsing Crohn's disease symptoms but partly attributed to chronic malabsorption of vitamin K (Fugate and Ramsey, 2004).

Clients with inflammatory bowel disease have a greater incidence of vitamin K deficiency and malabsorption. Such clients may not absorb oral vitamin K, given to reverse elevated INRs, but may require parenteral products (Fugate and Ramsey, 2004).

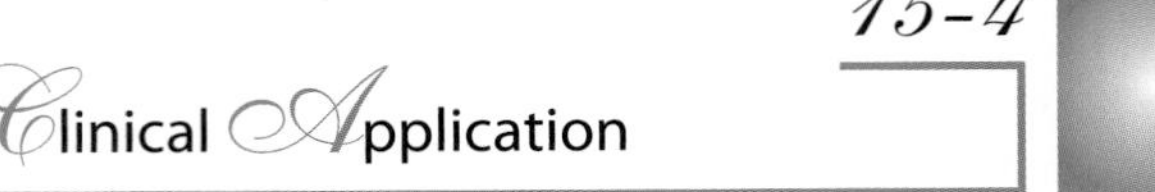

Vitamin K Deficiency in an Infant

Anti-infective drugs, besides fighting pathogens, destroy beneficial intestinal bacteria that synthesize vitamin K. Cerebral hemorrhage in a 4-month-old infant was attributed to isoniazid and rifampin therapy for congenital tuberculosis (Kobayashi et al., 2002).

Clients taking *warfarin* who experience diarrhea or decreased food intake should have their INRs monitored more frequently than usual and *warfarin* dosages adjusted accordingly. Note: Drugs other than *warfarin* may interfere with endogenous vitamin K. See Clinical Application 15-4.

Pharmacokinetics: Protein Binding

Warfarin is 99% bound to plasma proteins (Deglin and Vallerand, 2009). A client with low levels of serum albumin as a result of malnutrition or disease is at risk for drug toxicity with drugs that are usually highly bound to albumin. The drug that is bound to protein is inactive, whereas the unbound drug circulating in the blood is active and able to exert its intended therapeutic effect. Figure 15-3 sketches two consequences of the competition between drugs and foods or nutrients for protein binding sites.

Tyramine and Monoamine Oxidase Inhibitors

The usual abbreviation for this group of drugs is **MAOI (monoamine oxidase inhibitor)**. Several antidepressants are MAOIs, and some other drugs produce similar reactions with tyramine (see Table 15-5).

MECHANISM OF DRUG ACTION

MAOIs prevent the breakdown of **dopamine** and tyramine, chemicals necessary for proper functioning of the nervous system. The drugs' therapeutic effects

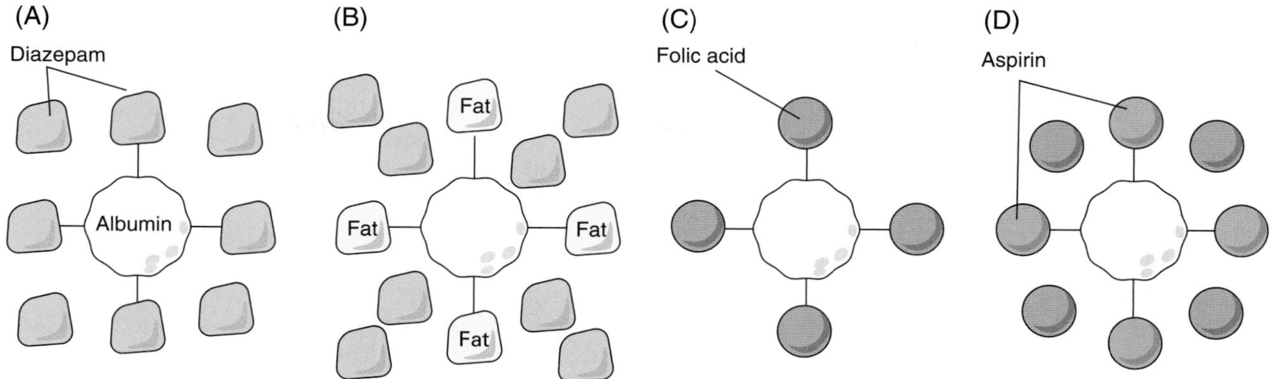

FIGURE 15-3 *A,* Four molecules of diazepam are bound to the albumin molecule, leaving the other four molecules of diazepam free to leave the bloodstream for the central nervous system. *B,* Fat displaces the diazepam from the albumin molecule so that all eight molecules of diazepam are immediately free to exert sedative effects on the central nervous system. *C,* Four molecules of folic acid are attached to the albumin molecule and able to circulate through the kidney intact. *D,* Aspirin displaces the folic acid from the albumin molecule, and the separate molecules of folic acid are likely to be excreted in the urine.

TABLE 15-5 ■ Tyramine-Restricted Diet

DESCRIPTION	INDICATION	ADEQUACY
Restricts food with naturally high levels of tyramine.	Used when clients receive drugs classified as monoamine oxidase inhibitors (MAOIs) and those with MAOI activity. **Antidepressants:** *isocarboxazid* *phenelzine* *tranylcypromine* **Anti-infectives:** *furazolidone* *isoniazid* *linezolid* **Antineoplastics:** *procarbazine* **Antiparkinson:** *selegiline*	Adequate in all nutrients according to the current Recommended Dietary Allowances if the individual makes appropriate food choices.
FOOD GROUP	**TO AVOID**	**TO USE MODERATELY**
Breads and cereals	None	None
Fruits and vegetables	Avocados Bananas Figs Broad (fava) beans Chinese pea pods Eggplant Fermented soy products Italian flat beans Mixed Chinese Vegetables Raspberries Sauerkraut	None
Dairy	Aged cheese (brick, blue, brie, cheddar, Camembert, Swiss, Romano, Roquefort, mozzarella, Parmesan, provolone) Sour cream Yogurt	Gouda cheese, processed American cheese
Meat and fish	Any canned meat Anchovies Beef or chicken liver Sausage (bologna, salami, pepperoni, summer) Fish (caviar, dried fish, salt herring)	
Beverages	Ale, beer, sherry, red and white wines	Coffee, colas, hot chocolate (1–3 cups per day)
Other	Chocolate, bouillon and other protein extracts, protein supplements, meat tenderizer, soy sauce, yeast concentrates	

are to increase the concentration of epinephrine, norepinephrine, serotonin, and dopamine in the central nervous system, thus counteracting depression.

In the peripheral nervous system, MAOIs also prevent the release of the norepinephrine that builds up in the nerves. The stores of norepinephrine become especially high in the nerves that regulate the size of blood vessels. The result is a decreased ability to constrict peripheral blood vessels. The vasodilation thus produced leads to hypotension.

To compound the situation, the drugs also inhibit the body's normal response to a low blood pressure, i.e., an increased heart rate. Thus, the individual displays the unusual combination of hypotension and bradycardia.

EFFECT OF FOODS ON MAOIs

Some foods contain **tyramine**, a metabolic intermediate product in the conversion of the amino acid tyrosine to epinephrine. Foods that contain degraded protein, such as aged cheese, are high in tyramine. When a client taking MAOIs consumes foods or beverages high in tyramine, the drugs prevent the normal breakdown of tyramine. The tyramine oversupply consequently leads to excessive epinephrine, producing hypertension. Sometimes the blood pressure is severely elevated, which can cause intracranial hemorrhage.

As with many substances, individuals' responses to tyramine vary. Four factors interact to determine the severity of reaction:

1. The amount of tyramine ingested
2. The type and dose of the MAOI
3. Client susceptibility
4. The time between the drug dose and a tyramine-containing meal

TYRAMINE-RICH FOODS

Many foods contain enough tyramine to create problems for clients receiving MAOIs. The amount of tyramine varies even in different samples of a particular food. Table 15-5 describes the tyramine-restricted diet. Because this interaction can be life-threatening, the best advice to give a client is to avoid all foods capable of causing problems, even though a small amount of the food, or a given batch of a product, might be safe. Less restrictive diets have been developed and may be used to increase compliance (Rapaport, 2007).

Newer formulations of MAOIs, such as *rasagiline* and transdermal (patch) *selegiline* are more selective in targeting the central nervous system and do not require severe dietary restrictions at certain doses (Chen, Swope, and Dashtipour, 2007; Robinson and Amsterdam, 2008). However, despite the well-documented selectivity of *rasagiline*, the manufacturer recommends virtually all of the dietary and drug restrictions of the nonselective MAOIs (Guay, 2006). The effects of nonselective MAOIs may persist for 2 weeks after they have been discontinued (Rapaport, 2007).

Protein Intake and Levodopa

Levodopa is given for Parkinson's disease. A high-protein diet may compete with the uptake of *levodopa* into the brain, and therefore may result in reduced *levodopa* effects (Khor and Hsu, 2007). Dietary recommendations may include limiting total protein to the RDA and taking higher protein foods with the evening meal rather than earlier in the day. See Table 15-3.

Vitamin D: Multiple Interactions

Corticosteroids increase the catabolism of the matrix of the bone, inhibit the osteoblasts from building new bone, and prevent the liver from processing vitamin D. When this lack of vitamin D results in insufficient calcium absorption by the intestine, parathyroid hormone causes withdrawal of calcium from the bones and osteoporosis results. Because of the seriousness of this adverse effect, monitoring of the client's vitamin D status should be ongoing during long-term corticosteroid therapy. See Table 15-1.

Phenytoin also interferes with the liver's processing of vitamin D. Clients receiving long-term therapy need an estimated 15 to 25 micrograms of vitamin D daily to prevent rickets or osteomalacia. Other medications that increase the metabolism of vitamin D, possibly resulting in low serum levels of the vitamin, include *carbamazepine, phenobarbital*, and *rifampin* (Linus Pauling Institute, 2008). See Table 15-1.

B Vitamins: Multiple Interactions

Water-soluble vitamins are particularly susceptible to drug interactions with long-term therapy. See Table 15-1 for interactions of drugs with niacin, folic acid, and vitamins B_6 and B_{12}. Documented cases of interactions include niacin and vitamin B_{12}.

NIACIN

Phenytoin has been related to pellagra in the following cases.

- A client with cerebral palsy receiving *phenytoin, valproic acid*, and *diazepam* for years was treated with multiple therapies from numerous physicians before the correct diagnosis was reached. Symptoms resolved in 2 months with niacin and multivitamin supplementation, and the cause was attributed to the anticonvulsants (Lyon and Fairley, 2002).

- Three weeks of *phenytoin* therapy was credited with causing a pellagrous dermatitis in a 3-year-old child that resolved within 3 weeks of niacin supplementation and within 2 weeks of replacing *phenytoin* with *carbamazepine* (Kaur et al., 2002).

The mechanism producing pellagra in those cases is unknown, possibly an alteration in absorption of vitamins or interference with synthesis of niacin from tryptophan.

Because *isoniazid* is structurally similar to niacin, the body recognizes it as niacin and reduces its production of the vitamin from tryptophan; thus, pellagra is also a complication of isoniazid therapy (Das, Parajuli, and Gupta, 2006).

VITAMIN B_{12}

An exceptional case of cobalamin deficiency is related to a client's dietary pattern predisposing to adverse effects from an inhaled anesthetic. The woman so affected had been a vegetarian for 10 years and for 5 years had restricted her intake to apples, nuts, and raw vegetables while avoiding legumes. (See Chapters 7 and 11 regarding vegetarianism and vitamin B_{12} deficiency.)

Nitrous oxide was one component of the anesthesia this client received to repair a traumatic hip fracture. Six weeks later, she was unable to walk and was diagnosed with degeneration of the spinal cord.

The deficiency in this case was caused by the known action of nitrous oxide to oxidize the cobalt atom in cobalamin to an inactive state, thus reducing the effectiveness of cobalamin-dependent enzymes. The client improved with cobalamin injections but still had some residual effects 1 year after anesthesia (Rosener and Dichgans, 1996).

Type IV Interactions

Interactions between drugs and nutrients can continue as the kidneys excrete waste products of metabolism.

Sodium, Fluids, and Lithium

Both sodium intake and increased fluid intake affect the mood stabilizer, *lithium,* given for manic episodes of manic–depressive illness. This drug is absorbed, distributed, and excreted with sodium and may result in the following scenarios.

- Decreased sodium intake with decreased fluid intake may lead to *lithium* retention manifested by slurred speech, decreased coordination, drowsiness, and muscle weakness or twitching.
- Increased sodium intake and increased fluid intake increase the excretion of *lithium,* thus worsening signs and symptoms of mania.

Use of loop diuretics or angiotensin-converting enzyme (ACE) inhibitors significantly increases the risk of hospitalization for lithium toxicity in the elderly (Juurlink et al., 2004). Because of the interaction with salt and water intake, clients who take *lithium* are taught to monitor the concentration or **specific gravity** of their urine. See Table 15-3.

Salt Substitutes and ACE Inhibitors

The ACE inhibitors lower blood pressure by preventing conversion of angiotensin I to angiotensin II, thereby decreasing aldosterone secretion and increasing excretion of sodium and water (see Fig. 8-17) and increasing retention of potassium. Clients receiving ACE inhibitors such as *captopril, enalapril,* and *lisinopril* should be monitored for hyperkalemia. See Table 15-3.

Hyperkalemia has been reported in two clients using salt substitutes containing potassium while receiving ACE inhibitors. In each case, serum potassium returned to normal after cessation of the salt substitute. One client had to be resuscitated after cardiac arrest before the contribution of a salt substitute to his hyperkalemia became apparent (Ray, Dorman, and Watson, 1999).

Folic Acid Displaced by Aspirin

Plasma proteins can bind with nutrients as well as drugs. When there are insufficient binding sites on the plasma proteins for all of the drug or nutrient, the excess accumulates in the bloodstream as free, small particles. The kidney is likely to excrete these small particles rather than to restore them to the bloodstream.

One common drug that interferes in this manner with a nutrient is *acetylsalicylic acid,* or *aspirin.* It displaces folic acid from its plasma protein. The kidney then excretes the folic acid in the urine (Fig. 15-3).

Dietary Supplements

Sales of dietary supplements amounted to $21 billion in 2007 (Saldanha, 2007). Herbals and natural supplements are used by 22% of adults in the United States. Among prescription drug users, 32% also take herbals or natural supplements (Slone Epidemiology Center, 2006).

A national survey found herbal/natural supplements to be used by:

- 16% of non-Hispanic whites
- 11% of Hispanics
- 6% of African Americans (Kelly et al., 2006)

Special Rules

The rules for labeling the nutrient content of foods and drugs in the United States are much more stringent than those applied to dietary supplements.

Before receiving permission to market a new drug, the pharmaceutical company must conduct rigorous tests on animals and on people in randomized, double-blind clinical trials. Randomization requires that participants be assigned by coin toss or equivalent unbiased method to receive the investigative drug or not. **Double-blind** trials are experiments in which neither the subject nor the investigator knows whether a subject is receiving the treatment or a **placebo**.

For foods, label information must be supported by research or scientific agreement, which is not the case with dietary supplements.

Because it is not required by law, research into the effectiveness and adverse effects of dietary supplements is limited. Most dietary supplements, because the evidence is inadequate to permit health or nutrient content claims, must use structure–function claims (Institute of Medicine, 2005). The standard for the structure–function claim for dietary supplements is simply that it be truthful and not misleading. See Box 15-2.

Areas of Concern

With botanical products, nature keeps some of the ingredients secret. Not all the constituents of these products have been identified, and they may exert more than one physiological effect in the human body. Therefore, when ingesting one of them, a person takes not only the active ingredient that is purported to have the desired medicinal effect but also other substances in the plant tissue as well.

Among those other substances may be defensive chemicals the plant has evolved to protect itself from predators. Despite a long history of use, little is known

Box 15-2 ■ *Regulation of Dietary Supplements*

Under the provisions of the Dietary Supplement Health Education Act of 1994, referred to as DSHEA, dietary supplements can be sold unless shown by the FDA to be unsafe, adulterated, or labeled in a misleading manner. The burden of proof in this case rests with the FDA, not with the manufacturer, and no prior notice from the manufacturer of intent to sell is required unless the product contains a new dietary ingredient. The Bioterrorism Act does require manufacturers to register with FDA before producing or selling supplements and in 2007, the FDA published comprehensive regulations for Current Good Manufacturing Practices for those who manufacture, package or hold dietary supplement products (U.S. FDA, 2009b).

Under DSHEA, a dietary supplement is defined as a product taken by mouth that

1. Contains a dietary ingredient: vitamin, mineral, herb; botanical, amino acid, enzyme, tissue; or a concentrate, metabolite, or constituent extract from the ingredients previously mentioned
2. Is in the form of a supplement (meaning tablet, capsule, softgel, gelcap, liquid, or powder)
3. Is not represented as a food or sole item of a meal or of the human diet (U.S. FDA, 2009b).

DSHEA does not limit the serving size or the amount of nutrients in any form of dietary supplement, but its regulations spell out the nature of the claims that can be made for a product on the label and its format. The following types of statements are allowed:

1. Health claims that have substantial scientific support or if limited support, the claim must contain qualifying statements
2. Nutrient content claims that describe the level of the nutrient or dietary ingredient in a product compared with an established daily value
3. Structure–function claims that describe the product's effect on structure or function of the body or on general well-being. These claims must also include the following information displayed prominently on the label:
   "This statement has not been evaluated by the Food and Drug Administration. This product is not intended to diagnose, treat, cure or prevent any disease."

Manufacturers of dietary supplements that make structure/function claims on labels or in labeling must submit a notification to the FDA that includes the text of the structure/function claim no later than 30 days after marketing the dietary supplement (U.S. FDA, 2003, Updated 2009).

For instance, a structure–function claim could state the product "helps to maintain bone health." If the label said the product is used to treat arthritis, it would be disallowed as a medical claim. Monitoring the system is incomprehensible. In the 10 years since the passage of DSHEA, the number of dietary supplement products on the market ballooned from an estimated 4000 to more than 29,000 (Atwater, Montgomery-Salguero, and Roll, 2005).

The FDA maintains a MedWatch program to receive information about possible adverse effects dietary supplements. Health care providers and consumers can report these events online by calling 1-800-FDA-1088. The identity of the patient is kept confidential.

DSHEA has supporters of the status quo (Bass and Marden, 2005) as well as those calling for regulation of dietary supplements in the same manner as pharmaceuticals (Cohen, 2005). Health-care providers should know the current system and be aware of changes in order to provide wise counsel to clients.

about the toxicity of botanical products. Most such knowledge comes from acute cases of toxicity sporadically reported, but recently some scientific studies have been conducted.

Manufacturers and distributors of dietary supplements must record, investigate and forward to the U. S. Food and Drug Administration (FDA) any reports they receive of serious adverse events associated with the use of their products that are reported to them directly. The FDA evaluates these reports and any other adverse event information reported directly to it by healthcare providers or consumers (U.S. FDA, 2009b).

Because the FDA's responsibility begins only after the products have been packaged and marketed, the maintenance of quality is the responsibility of the manufacturer. Cases of selenosis have been caused by a supplement containing more than 100 times the amount of selenium claimed on the label. One severely affected client had consumed 400 times the RDA for 7 weeks (Sutter et al., 2008). The affected products, distributed to 15 states, were voluntarily recalled (U.S. FDA, 2008a).

Besides the dearth of information and questionable manufacturing practices, issues of standardization, contamination, and interaction with other substances are major concerns.

Lack of Standardization

The potency of herbal products varies with the:

- Climate and soil conditions
- Life cycle of the plants from which they come

Great differences in the quantities of active ingredients have been found, depending on:

- The source
- The species and part of the plant used
- Storage conditions
- Time of harvest
- Method of processing
- Country of origin
- Inclusion of look-a-like plants

Without consistent products, research cannot be generalized as a basis for evidence-based practice.

Botanical products can come to market not containing the ingredients on the label. For example, analysis of:

- Echinacea preparations determined that labeled species content was correct in only 52% of the samples and 10% contained no echinacea at all (Gilroy et al., 2003).
- 54 samples of St. John's wort determined that just 2 of them (3.7%) contained active ingredients within 10% of the amounts stated on the label (Draves and Walker, 2003).

Discerning the species of a plant product by visual inspection is not always possible:

- Chinese star anise (*Illicium verum*) when used as a spice is on the Generally Recognized As Safe **(GRAS) List** but
- Japanese star anise (*Illicium anisatum*) causes neurological and gastrointestinal toxicities.

Seven infants, ages 2 to 12 weeks, were treated at Miami Children's Hospital for star anise poisoning. Symptoms included irritability, hyperexcitability, vomiting, abnormal eye movements, and seizures (Ize-Ludlow et al., 2004).

After approximately 40 individuals, including about 15 infants, became ill following ingestion of star anise teas, the FDA issued an advisory to not drink such beverages because the particular variety of star anise involved in these illnesses could not be identified (U.S. FDA, 2003).

Contamination with Dangerous Substances

Botanical products have been contaminated with toxic substances. The United States Pharmacopoeia (see Box 15-3) limits the presence of heavy metals in most oral pharmaceuticals to 30 parts per million (ppm), with lower limits for lead, arsenic, and mercury.

HEAVY METALS

In August through October 2005, one-fifth of both U.S.-manufactured and Indian-manufactured Ayurvedic medicines purchased via the Internet contained detectable lead, mercury, or arsenic. Among the metal-containing products, 95% were sold by U.S. Web sites and 75% claimed to use Good Manufacturing Practices. All metal-containing products exceeded one or more standards for acceptable daily intake of toxic metals (Saper et al., 2008).

From 1966 to 2007, 76 cases of lead encephalopathy potentially associated with traditional medicine were located:

- 5% in adults, at least one of whom had residual neurological impairment
- 95% in infants and young children of which 8 cases were fatal and at least 15 had residual neurological deficits (Karri, Saper, and Kales, 2008).

Those are only the cases in which the lead poisoning proceeded to encephalopathy. Young children and fetuses of pregnant women are at special risk for the toxic effects of lead, because these Ayurvedic products are used to treat infertility in women (Centers for Disease Control and Prevention [CDC], 2004).

Box 15-3 ■ *Standards for Health-Care Products*

The United States Pharmacopeial Convention (USP), a nongovernment, nonprofit organization, sets standards for drugs, dietary supplements, biologics, and other articles used in health care. Substances listed as USP meet standards of purity and strength as determined by chemical analysis or animal responses to specified doses. A zero tolerance policy for pesticides applies to food and botanicals.

A verification program for dietary supplements is available to assure consumers of the safety of the products they buy. Certain supplements with known safety concerns are excluded from the program:

- Ephedra
- Kava
- Comfrey
- Chaparral
- Aristolochia.

The USP mark on a product verifies the accuracy of the label, the strength and quantity of the contents, the lack of contaminants according to federal standards, and the use of good manufacturing practices (Srinivasan, 2006).

DRUGS

Dietary supplements have also been contaminated with prescription medications. Because of the special rules governing the industry, discovery of the contaminants frequently occurs long after the products are first marketed.

While studying natural anti-inflammatory substances in human placental blood, investigators detected an unknown substance. It was subsequently identified as the drug *colchicine* that is used to treat gout, traced to five women who consumed ginkgo biloba during pregnancy. Further searching located the drug in samples of ginkgo biloba distributed commercially in the area. This drug has the potential to be **teratogenic** (Petty et al., 2001).

In 2007 and 2008, two voluntary recalls of three dietary supplements involved contamination with the prescription drug *sildenafil*. The danger is a possible interaction with nitrates, found in some prescription drugs such as nitroglycerin, that would lower blood pressure to dangerous levels. The contamination was discovered by the FDA, not the manufacturer or distributor (U.S. FDA, 2007, 2008b).

Interactions With Other Drugs

Compared to the number of possible interactions between supplements and medications, only a small proportion have been examined or reported. Surveys have revealed significant proportions of clients consuming dietary supplements with prescription medications or without informing their primary providers.

- Of 458 outpatient veterans, 43% were taking at least one dietary supplement with prescription medications, of which 45% had a potential for a significant drug–dietary supplement interaction (Peng et al., 2004).
- Forty-five percent of children seen in the emergency department had been given an herbal product by their caregivers, of whom just 45% had discussed the herbal therapy with the child's primary health-care provider (Lanski et al., 2003).

So many botanical products have the potential to increase bleeding times that the American Society of Anesthesiologists suggests that all herbal medications be discontinued 2 to 3 weeks before elective surgery (Kaye, Kucera, and Sabar, 2004).

The most commonly cited substances in interactions from three categories are:

- Among supplements, St. John's wort
- Among drugs, *warfarin*
- Among foods, grapefruit juice

However, fewer than 15% of claimed interactions are well documented (Boullata, 2005). For examples of documented interactions see the section on Common Dietary Supplements.

Difficulty Obtaining Reliable Information

Supplement labels are often lacking needed information. For example:

- Experienced pharmacists could not discern ingredient information from some of the labels in one survey (Atwater, Montgomery-Salguero, and Roll, 2005).
- Analysis of labels on St. John's wort showed the vast majority did not adequately address clinically relevant safety issues. At best, 8% included information on pertinent drug interactions (Clauson, Santamarina, and Rutledge, 2008).

Moreover, available information regarding supplements may be misused. Often a consumer's source of information about a dietary supplement is the seller of the product.

- Analysis of 443 Web sites identified 55% that contained claims to treat, prevent, diagnose, or cure specific diseases despite the prohibition of such statements (Morris and Avorn, 2003).
- Editors of the *New England Journal of Medicine* linked a caution to a 1990 article on human growth hormone because an Internet seller referenced the article inappropriately in promotional materials. The caution reiterated the view in the 1990 editorial that use of human growth hormone in the elderly is not justified (Drazen, 2003).

Reliable information on the quality of dietary supplements is available via the Internet. The U.S. Food and Drug Administration maintains a Web site at http://www.fda.gov/Food/DietarySupplements/default.htm. Another source of information is Consumer Lab.com. Since its founding in 1999, Consumer Lab has published independent test results for more than 2,100 products, representing more than 350 different brands and nearly every type of popular supplement. Companies can have their products voluntarily tested for potential inclusion in its list of Approved Quality products (Consumer Lab, 2010).

Suggestions for clients regarding the use of dietary supplements can be found on DavisPlus.

Common Supplements

Knowledge and caution are necessary to weigh the risks and benefits of dietary supplements (see Fig. 15-4). See Table 15-6 for documented interactions between several of the most commonly used dietary supplements and drugs.

St. John's Wort

St. John's wort has been favorably compared to pharmaceutical antidepressants in some studies, but significant interactions with medications have been discovered. Drugs most prominently affected and contraindicated for concomitant use with St. John's wort are metabolized by both CYP3A4 and P-glycoprotein pathways (Mannel, 2004). Caution is indicated when St. John's wort and medications metabolized by CYP3A4 are used together (Boullata, 2005). See Table 15-6.

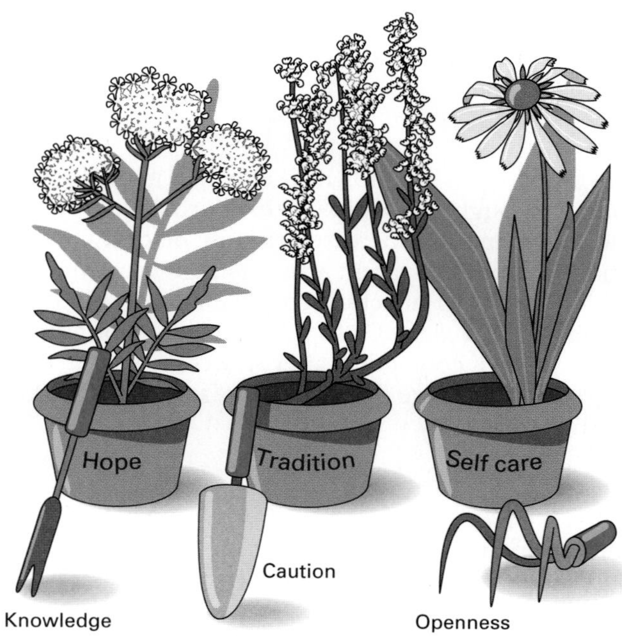

FIGURE 15-4 Because of cultural traditions, many people use botanical products as they seek a measure of self-care and hope. Those who use botanical products, however, need to cultivate knowledge and caution in their choices. They also should practice openness with their health-care providers.

TABLE 15-6 ■ Documented Dietary Supplement–Drug Interactions

DIETARY SUPPLEMENT	DRUG	DRUG CLASS	EFFECT
Garlic	*indinavir*	Antiretroviral	Decreased drug effect
	nelfinavir	Antiretroviral	Decreased drug effect
	saquinavir	Antiretroviral	Reduced plasma level of drug
	warfarin	Anticoagulant	Increased drug effect
Ginkgo Biloba	*aspirin*	Antiplatelet agent	Increased bleeding
	clopidogrel	Antiplatelet agent	Increased bleeding
	ibuprofen	Nonsteroidal anti-inflammatory agent (NSAID)	Increased bleeding
	nifedipine	Antihypertensive	Increased drug effects
	omeprazole	Antiulcer agent	Increased drug effects
	trazodone	Antidepressant	Increased drug effects
Ginseng	*phenelzine*	Antidepressant	Increased drug effect
	warfarin	Anticoagulant	Decreased drug effect
Glucosamine-Chondroitin	*warfarin*	Anticoagulant	Increased drug effect
St. John's Wort	*alprazolam*	Anxiolytic	Increased drug clearance and decreased drug effect
	cyclosporine	Immunosuppressant	Rejection of transplanted organs
	digoxin	Antiarrhythmic	Decreased drug level and effect
	indinavir	Antiretroviral	Decreased drug level and effect
	midazolam	Anxiolytic, sedative/hypnotic	Decreased drug level
	nifedipine	Antihypertensive	Decreased drug level
	Oral contraceptives	Hormonal contraceptive	Reduced bioavailability and contraceptive failure
	simvastatin	Lipid-lowering agent	Decreased drug effect
	warfarin	Anticoagulant	Increased drug clearance and decreased drug effect

Adapted from Boullata (2005); Knudsen and Sokol (2008).

Because St. John's wort is associated with increased metabolism of oral contraceptives, women should be cautioned that St. John's wort might interfere with contraceptive effectiveness (Murphy et al., 2005). However, just 50% of community pharmacists and 11% of health food store clerks identified the interaction when asked directly (Sarino et al., 2007).

Ginkgo Biloba

Ginkgo biloba is promoted to enhance mental functioning through improved cerebral circulation but its side effects include increased risk for bleeding. Interactions become apparent when ginkgo is combined with other drugs affecting coagulation. In one case, the addition of *ibuprofen* to a 2-year intake of ginkgo biloba extract concluded after 4 weeks with a fatal cerebral hemorrhage (Meisel, Johne, and Roots, 2003). See Table 15-6.

Ginseng

Three varieties of ginseng, Asian, American, and Siberian, have different properties and interactions. Persons taking American ginseng and *warfarin* should be monitored when changing herbal products or even using a new bottle of the same product (Gardiner, Phillips, and Shaughnessy, 2008). See Table 15-6.

Garlic

Garlic is promoted for cardiovascular health. For both high cholesterol and high blood pressure, the reported effects are small and probably not clinically relevant (Pittler and Ernst, 2007). However, garlic does increase bleeding risk with warfarin (Deglin and Vallerand, 2009).

Moreover, in another test, 21 days of garlic supplementation reduced plasma *saquinavir* concentrations in healthy volunteers. Other antiretroviral drugs have also been affected by garlic supplements (Boullata, 2005). See Table 15-6.

Glucosamine–Chondroitin

Glucosamine and chondroitin are substances found in the human body in and around cells of cartilage. Consumers sometimes take one or both supplements for osteoarthritis. Some experts believe that scientific studies have not conclusively proved the supplements' effectiveness (Dahmer and Schiller, 2008). However, a meta-analysis showed that after 2 to 3 years of daily consumption, glucosamine and chondroitin sulfate may delay radiological progression (joint space narrowing) in clients with osteoarthritis of the knee (Lee et al., 2010).

In addition, interactions associated with the supplements have been reported: Twenty reports of glucosamine or glucosamine-chondroitin use with *warfarin* were associated with increased INRs or increased bleeding or bruising. One report described an intraventricular bleed and subdural hematoma, which resulted in a persistent vegetative state (Knudsen and Sokol, 2008). See Table 15-6.

When Things Go Wrong

Untoward effects have occurred with dietary supplements even without drug interactions. Over 22 months, supplement use alone accounted for the most cases of fulminant liver failure referred to one transplant service, exceeding *acetaminophen* toxicity and viral hepatitis. Ten patients were recent or active users of potentially hepatotoxic supplements; seven of them had no other identified cause for hepatic failure (Estes et al., 2003). At another center, 19% of clients admitted to using herbal remedies combined with vitamins after liver transplantation (Neff et al., 2004).

Individuals have experienced spontaneous bleeding while taking ginkgo. Fifteen published case reports described a temporal association between using ginkgo and a bleeding event, but in 13 of the cases the clients had other risk factors for bleeding. In six cases, however, it was clear that when ginkgo was stopped the bleeding did not recur (Bent et al., 2005).

A Prudent Course

Clients at greatest risk from drug–dietary supplement interactions are:

- Children
- The elderly
- People with chronic diseases or impaired organ function
- People taking many medications
- Individuals with genetic variants in drug metabolism (Boullata, 2005)

The fact that many botanical products have been used for centuries does not negate their dangers. Clearly, "let the buyer beware" holds true. To protect clients, thorough assessment is vital. Often the use of dietary supplements does not come to light until late in the treatment cycle. Did health-care providers ask the clients about use of dietary supplements? If so, was it done in a manner that permitted them to reveal their practices without feeling ridiculed or condemned? Some items to consider when assessing diet supplement use are listed in Clinical Application 15-5.

Education is essential. Without disparaging a client's background, the health-care provider must counter the concept that "everything natural is safe." Substances strong enough to produce the effects attributed to

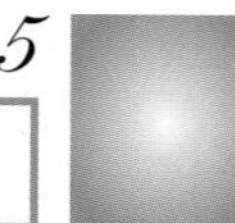

15-5 Clinical Application

Assessment for Dietary Supplement Use

Questions the nurse might ask to determine supplement use:

What kinds of herbal products, dietary supplements, or other natural remedies do you take?
Do you give any of them to children?
Do you find the recommended dose satisfactory?
Are you taking any prescription or over-the-counter medications for the same purpose? Or for opposite purposes?
Have you used this product before? For how long?
Where do you obtain these products?
Is anyone else in your household taking botanical products?
Are you allergic to any plant products?
Are you pregnant, planning to become pregnant, or breastfeeding?

dietary supplements are medicines, no matter what the law currently allows for distribution. Such substances should be treated with respect, including the use of childproof containers.

Enhancing Athletic Performance

Physical training and proper nutrition are vital for success in sports. Energy and macronutrient needs, especially carbohydrate and protein, must be met during times of high physical activity to maintain body weight, replenish glycogen stores, and provide adequate protein to build and repair tissue (Rodriguez, Di Marco, and Langley, 2009). Skeletal muscles and their metabolic energy pathways can be improved through training and proper nutrition.

Ergogenic Aids

An ergogenic aid is a means to increase work output or the potential of work output. For athletes the aid is any means of enhancing energy utilization, including energy production, control, and efficiency. Athletes in training, attempting to build a competitive edge, sometimes alter their dietary intake and consume various supplements.

Many athletic organizations prohibit the use of certain pharmacological, physiological, and nutritional aids. Before using any supplements, the athlete, with the advice of a health-care provider, parents, and coach, should evaluate the supplement carefully. The Consumer Lab screens for banned substances based on the Olympic Movement Anti-Doping Code or the codes of other sports associations (2008). Products that pass the screening are listed on its Web site.

Some ergogenic aids clearly fall into the classes of nutrients included in Chapters 3, 4, 5, 7, and 8 whereas others do not, although they may be substances with physiological functions. The ergogenic aids included in this chapter are categorized either as nutrients corresponding to those in the above listed chapters or as nonnutrients.

Nutrients

The Acceptable Macronutrient Distribution Ranges (AMDRs) are broad enough to cover the macronutrient needs of most active individuals, but alternate formulas based on body weight have been developed for athletes. See Clinical Calculation 15-1. These requirements can generally be met by dietary management without the need for supplements. In fact, the efficacy of most supplements available on the market is unproven (Hespel, Maughan, and Greenhaff, 2006).

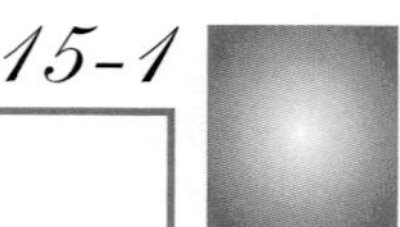

15-1 Clinical Calculation

Individualizing Macronutrient Recommendations for the Athlete

Depending on kilocalorie needs and the sport, endurance athletes may need these adjustments in diet.

	GRAMS/KILOGRAM BODY WEIGHT	SUGGESTED DISTRIBUTION RANGE
CHO	7–11	50%–70% of kcal
Protein	1.2–1.7	12%–20% of kcal
Fat	0.8–2	20%–30% of kcal

If an endurance athlete, 70 kg (154 lb), 5 ft 9 in., runs an average of 10 miles per day, lifts weights 3 or 4 times a week, and needs 3600 kcal/day, his suggested intake would be:

CHO

7–11 grams/kg = 490–770 grams/day = 54%–86% of kcal
7 grams × 70 kg = 490 grams; 11 grams × 70 kg = 770 grams
490 grams × 4 kcal/gram = 1960 kcal; 770 grams × 4 kcal/gram = 3080 kcal

$$\frac{1960}{3600} = 54\% \qquad \frac{3080}{3600} = 86\%$$

Protein

1.2–1.7 grams/kg = 84–119 grams/day = 9%–13% of kcal
1.2 grams × 70 kg = 84 grams; 1.7 grams × 70 kg = 119 grams
84 grams × 4 kcal/gram = 336 kcal; 119 grams × 4 kcal/gram = 476 kcal

$$\frac{336}{3600} = 9\% \qquad \frac{476}{3600} = 13\%$$

Fat

0.8–2 grams/kg = 56–140 grams/day = 14%–35% of kcal
0.8 grams × 70 kg = 56 grams; 2 grams × 70 kg = 140 grams
56 grams × 9 kcal/gram = 504 kcal; 140 grams × 9 kcal/grams = 1260 kcal

$$\frac{504}{3600} = 14\% \qquad \frac{1260}{3600} = 35\%$$

Adapted from Carlson (2008).

CARBOHYDRATE

Carbohydrate is the body's main dietary energy source for:

- Anaerobic (1 to 2 minutes) and
- Aerobic (more than 3 minutes) exercise.

Suggested daily intakes of carbohydrate per kilogram of body weight are:

- 5 to 7 grams for the average athlete in training (Williams, 2006)
- 7 to 11 grams for endurance athletes (Carlson, 2008)

Note that the latter amount might exceed the AMDR, which is designed for 97% to 98% of individuals of a given age, gender, or female reproductive status.

Distribution of intake is related to performance and recovery.

- Consumption of approximately 1 gram of carbohydrate per kilogram of body weight per hour during prolonged exercise such as a marathon appears sufficient to improve performance (Murray, 2007).
- Ingesting 1.2 to 1.5 grams of carbohydrate per kilogram of body weight per hour appears to maximize glycogen synthesis for 4 to 5 hours after exercise (Williams, 2006).

Recommended distribution of macronutrients for athletes (Clinical Calculation 15-1) clearly emphasizes carbohydrate intake. Elite Kenyan runners consume 75% of their kilocalories as carbohydrate (Carlson, 2008).

PROTEIN AND AMINO ACIDS

Exercise-induced muscle damage is commonly experienced after physical activity, and different studies showed that the amount of protein consumed seems to affect its magnitude (Borrione et al., 2009). The American College of Sports Medicine, the American Dietetic Association, and Dietitians of Canada concluded that protein requirements are higher in very active persons than in the general population. Suggested daily amounts are:

- 1.6 to 1.7 grams per kilogram of body weight in resistance athletes
- 1.2 to 1.4 grams in endurance athletes

These amounts are approximately 50% to 100% higher than the RDA, but well within the AMDR of 10% to 35% of daily energy intake (Williams, 2006).

A vegetarian diet per se is not associated with detrimental effects in athletes, but an optimal protein intake should be achieved through careful planning with an emphasis on protein-rich plant foods. **Rhabdomyolysis** has occurred in a young athlete following a poorly planned vegetarian diet (Borrione et al., 2009).

After resistance exercise, assuming positive nitrogen balance, the rate of resynthesis of muscle protein is elevated for 48 hours. The result is:

- Increased lean body mass
- Muscle hypertrophy

Ingestion of protein immediately after exercise seems optimal for anabolism (Ciocca, 2005); however, no studies have shown an advantage to ingesting protein supplements over natural, protein-containing foods (Duellman et al., 2008). In fact, endurance cycling performance was significantly impaired following a 7-day high-protein diet supplemented with whey compared with a 7-day high-carbohydrate diet containing equal kilocalories (Macdermid and Stannard, 2006).

Regarding specific amino acids for athletes, glutamine for improved immune function is not recommended by most experts. Neither are branched-chain amino acids effective in reducing fatigue as long as carbohydrate intake is adequate (Williams, 2006).

A comparison of sports protein supplements found on the Internet appears in Dollars and Sense 15-1. Not only does the price range from $1.44 to $5.19 per serving, not including shipping costs, but in addition the carbohydrate content varies from 4 to 48 grams per serving. Comparing the cost of 10 grams of protein to the real foods in Dollars and Sense 5-1, all the supplements would be more expensive than tuna, peanut butter, milk, American and cottage cheese, and eggs.

WATER

Normal hydration is the goal for athletes. Dehydration degrades aerobic exercise and mental performance in warm to hot environments. Fluids should be consumed during exercise to prevent excessive dehydration (loss of more than 2% of body weight).

Sweat losses vary depending upon:

- The activity
- Clothing
- Equipment
- Environmental conditions
- Individual differences in sweat rates

Serious athletes may sweat from 0.5 to 2 liters per hour. Some football players, often with large body weights, reportedly can lose 8 liters of sweat per day in hot weather.

Customized plans for fluid intake can be designed based on sweat rates estimated from weight lost during exercise. Replacing only the fluids lost is the goal. Skeletal muscle cramps are thought to be related to

Dollars & Sense 15-1

Comparison of Sports Protein Supplements

Product	Price	Package	Serving Size	Protein Grams/serving	Cho Grams/serving	Cost/serving	Cost/10 Grams of Protein*
A	$28.95	12 cans	11 oz	35	4	$2.42	$0.69
B	$34.50	24 cans	11 oz	30	48	$1.44	$0.48
C	$41.54	32 oz powder	4 oz powder	40	10	$5.19	$1.30

*Compare to Dollars and Sense 5-1.

dehydration, electrolyte deficits, and muscle fatigue (Sawka et al., 2007).

However, consuming excessive water can lead to electrolyte imbalances. During long events, an athlete's blood is shunted to the skeletal muscle with less blood flow to the kidneys. If fluids are over-consumed, the kidney may not be able to excrete the excess fluid producing dilutional hyponatremia (Sawka, 2007). For examples, see Chapter 8.

Nonnutrients

Among the ergogenic aids promoted for athletes, these aids perform as claimed: sodium bicarbonate, creatine, and caffeine. Glycerol has insufficient evidence to support claims (Williams, 2006). The United States Olympic Committee (USOC) has banned many drugs. The lists are accessible at its Web site: http://www.usoc.org.

BICARBONATE

Muscular activity generates lactic acid as a waste product with consequent lowering of blood pH. The ingestion of sodium bicarbonate before intense exercise could temper the metabolic acidosis that contributes to fatigue. Many studies have reported performance increases in laboratory-based cycling and running after sodium bicarbonate ingestion. Other studies have reported no benefit, and the incidence of negative side effects is high (Spriet, Perry, and Talanian, 2008). Most prevalent untoward effects, such as bloating and diarrhea, concern the gastrointestinal tract (Jenkinson and Harbert, 2008).

CREATINE

Creatine is a nonprotein substance synthesized in the body from the amino acids arginine, glycine, and methionine. When combined with phosphate, the resulting compound, phosphocreatine, serves as a storage form of energy that is released with anaerobic muscle contraction.

The majority of the experimental evidence suggests that creatine supplementation can improve short-term exercise performance, especially in sports that require repeated short-term sprints (Spriet, Perry, and Talanian, 2008). Creatine is effective for strength and power athletes but not for aerobic endurance athletes (Williams, 2006).

Few data are available on the long-term consequences of creatine supplementation (Persky and Rawson, 2007). One 27-year-old weight lifter had been taking creatine for 8 or 9 months. Four weeks after adding whey protein supplements, he developed acute liver injury that was reversed with intravenous fluids and discontinuation of the supplements (Whitt et al., 2008). Because of a lack of studies on growing adolescents, the use of creatine by adolescent athletes is not recommended (Patel, Torres, and Greydanus, 2005).

CAFFEINE

Available evidence supports moderate caffeine use (5 milligrams per kilogram of body weight) as an effective ergogenic aid for aerobic endurance events but the mechanism underlying improved performance is unknown (Williams, 2006). Caffeine is rapidly and completely absorbed by the gastrointestinal tract and is readily distributed throughout all tissues of the body (Magkos and Kavouras, 2005).

GLYCEROL

As an ergogenic aid, glycerol has been tested as a means of hyperhydration to prevent dehydration. Glycerol does have the capacity to enhance fluid retention and decrease urine output, which may give a performance advantage by offsetting dehydration (Nelson and Robergs, 2007).

However, for some sports, the increase in body weight from the retained fluid could be a disadvantage. Insufficient evidence exists to conclude glycerol is an effective ergogenic aid (Williams, 2006).

Advice for Athletes

The same advice given for the general dietary supplements applies to those marketed for athletes. Just because they are available over-the-counter does not assure safety. One 24-year-old man developed acute renal failure while taking creatine and multiple other supplements for bodybuilding. Fortunately, complete recovery followed discontinuation of the supplements (Thorsteinsdottir, Grande, and Garovic, 2006).

In addition, players must be cautious of inadequate product labeling and supplement impurities that may cause a positive drug test (Hespel, Maughan, and Greenhaff, 2006). Of 634 samples of nonhormonal supplements from 15 countries, 14.8% contained prohibited anabolic androgenic steroids not declared on the label (Geyer et al., 2004).

Athletes should seek advice from qualified nutritionists. Sports nutrition is a specialty practice for dietitians who often help professional and college athletes maximize their performances in their chosen activity through individualized nutrition prescriptions.

Some basic suggestions for fueling the body for high energy expenditure sports appear in Table 15-7. The timing and distribution of nutrients is intended to ensure adequate glycogen levels and to maximize protein synthesis and recovery.

Responsibilities of Health-Care Professionals

Preventing or modifying pharmacodynamic effects of drug–nutrient–supplement interactions is a team effort involving physicians, pharmacists, dietitians, and nurses. Health-care agencies often assign the client teaching to certain members of the team to ensure that no one will be missed. For instance, pharmacists may be responsible for teaching clients receiving *warfarin* therapy and dietitians for teaching those receiving tube feedings. Nurses often do the discharge teaching and follow-up with a telephone call to field questions after the client returns home.

Persons at highest risk for food and drug interactions are those who:

- Take many drugs, including alcohol
- Require long-term drug therapy
- Have poor or marginal nutrition

Polypharmacy, the concurrent use of a large number of drugs, is a risk factor for untoward reactions, particularly if the person is treated by many prescribers. The elderly are particularly vulnerable because they take more than 30% of prescription drugs that presumably are more potent than over-the-counter drugs. Of all age groups, the elderly are most likely to take many drugs. See Figure 15-1.

Regardless of the age of the client, each additional drug or nutritional supplement exponentially increases the potential for interactions (Chan, 2006). The elderly are likely to be on long-term regimens for chronic diseases, further increasing the risk of adverse effects, as exemplified in Figure 15-5. Other groups at risk of food and drug interactions are infants and adolescents because of high nutrient needs and immature detoxification systems. Clinical Application 15-6 reviews triggers that should prompt a further search for drug–nutrient interactions.

TABLE 15-7 ■ Exercise Fueling Basics for Athletes*

TIME	CHO	PROTEIN	FAT	WATER	EXAMPLE	RATIONALE
3–5 Hours Before Exercise; About ⅕ of Kilocalories for Day	60% of kcal	15%–20% of kcal	20%–25% of kcal			
45–60 Minutes Before Exercise	30–50 grams	10–15 grams	5 grams or less	2 cups	2 cups 1% fat chocolate milk 52 grams CHO 16 grams Protein 6 grams Fat	Tops off glycogen stores. Increases fluid absorption: 2.7 grams of water bound to 1 gram of glycogen
0–60 Minutes After Exercise and Every 2–3 Hours Thereafter	90–110 grams	15-30 grams	Modest	1 cup per pound of weight lost	2 cups granola, 1 cup skim milk with ¼ cup powdered milk (130 grams CHO, 30 grams protein)	Milk can help restore fluid balance also.

*Depending on athlete's size, the sport, environmental conditions, etc.
Adapted from Carlson (2008) and Sehnert (2008).

The consequences of improper scheduling of drugs and foods or nutrients can be:

- Treatment failure
- Toxicity
- Increased expense

In contrast, identifying the client's inherent ability to metabolize drugs offers exciting opportunities to individualize treatment and minimize interactions.

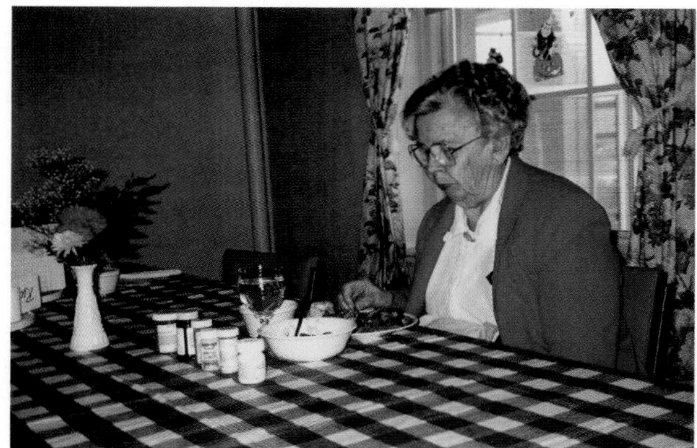

FIGURE 15-5 This woman has several risk factors for drug–nutrient interactions. She is elderly, is on a multiple-drug regimen, and takes some of her medications with a meal.

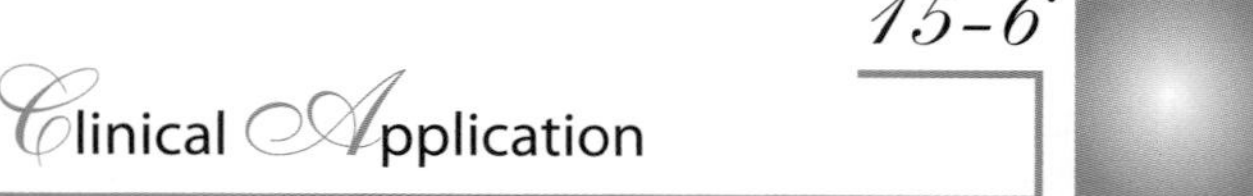

Screening Clients at Risk for Drug–Nutrient Interactions

Further nutritional assessment may be in order if a client:

- Reports a recent weight change.
- Abuses alcohol.
- Consumes a modified diet, prescribed or self-imposed, including one with significant changes in protein content.
- Receives tube feedings.
- Takes many medications or dietary supplements, some with meals, some known to interfere with nutrition.
- Shows worsening of signs and symptoms of disease.
- Displays laboratory values indicating nutrient depletion.

Keystones

- Persons at highest risk for food–drug interactions are those who take many drugs, including alcohol; require long-term medication therapy; have poor or marginal nutrition; or have immature or impaired metabolic systems.
- Interactions can take place in the delivery device or within the body by affecting bioavailability (antibiotics), cellular or tissue distribution (*warfarin*), or disposition by the liver or kidneys (*lithium*).
- The most commonly cited interactions, sometimes life-threatening, involve grapefruit juice, *warfarin,* or St. John's wort interacting with each other or with another drug.
- A tyramine-restricted diet may be necessary for drugs with MAOI properties to avoid hypertensive crises.
- Sodium and water intake are crucial components to control for effective *lithium* therapy.
- Persons taking dietary supplements should be aware of the risks associated with their production and should always inform their health-care providers of their use.
- Athletes should consume a healthy diet emphasizing appropriate proportions of carbohydrate and protein for their body and sport and avoid unproven dietary supplements.

CASE STUDY 15-1

Mrs. S, a 72-year-old client, is being seen by the home health nurse to reaffirm her suitability for independent living. She has a history of heart failure for which she has been successfully treated with *digoxin* 0.125 mg daily for the past 6 months. Mrs. S takes the tablet with her usual breakfast of orange juice, raisin toast, and tea.

Recently she has had difficulty with constipation. Obtaining information on bowel hygiene on her own, she decided to improve her nutritional intake by adding a high-fiber cereal to her breakfast.

After 1 week, her constipation has been relieved, but she now is becoming easily fatigued. When climbing a flight of stairs she finds it necessary to rest twice en route. The nurse asked Mrs. S to weigh herself. Mrs. S reported she had gained 5 lb in 2 weeks. Based on the above data and her observations, the home health nurse prepared a care plan. The portion of it pertinent to food and drug interactions appears below.

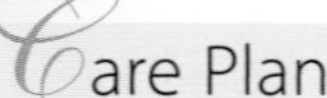

Care Plan

Subjective Data

Easily fatigued ■ Short of breath (SOB) <1 flight of stairs ■ History of constipation, relieved by addition of high-fiber cereal to diet ■ Medications: *digoxin*, 0.125 mg daily in morning with breakfast

Objective Data

Alert, oriented, cooperative. Vital signs normal except pulse 90 beats per minute. Weight gain: 5 lb over 2 weeks.

Analysis

Lack of information regarding self-care related to food–drug interaction as evidenced by beginning signs of heart failure

Plan

DESIRED OUTCOMES EVALUATION CRITERIA	ACTIONS/INTERVENTIONS	RATIONALE
Client will revise medication or meal schedule immediately to maximize effectiveness of *digoxin*.	Teach client to take *digoxin* 1 hour before or 2 hours after high-fiber meals.	High-fiber foods decrease the absorption of digitalis preparations.

Thinking Ms. S could benefit from more extensive education about the management of chronic heart disease, the nurse refers her to the Health Educator at the home health agency.

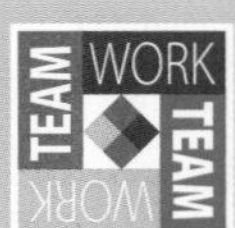

15-1 Health Educator's Notes

The following educator's notes are representative of the documentation found in a client's medical record.

Subjective: Believes her heart failure was a one-time event and was cured by hospitalization. Eager to do whatever she can to remain independent in her home.

Objective: Lives in two-story home, utilizing both floors.

Analysis: Could benefit from information on managing lifestyle to accommodate chronic heart disease.

Plan: Suggest she join the Living With Heart Disease group to learn about self-assessment techniques, when to call the doctor, and modifications to home and lifestyle to make the best use of her available energy.

Critical Thinking Questions

1. In what way might the scenario develop such that the nurse should contact the client's physician during the initial home visit?
2. From the little bit of information given about Ms. S's dietary intake, how might you approach improving her nutrition?
3. What additional assessment data on social resources could impact the resolution of this situation?

Chapter Review

1. Which of the following clients is at greatest risk for food–drug interaction?
   a. A 50-year-old man with no current disease who takes one baby aspirin daily to prevent heart disease
   b. A 75-year-old woman taking medication for several chronic diseases
   c. A 39-year-old man who usually consumes two cocktails before dinner
   d. A 25-year-old pregnant woman who is taking a prenatal vitamin supplement and calcium tablets
2. For which of the following items is there most agreement that athletes require increased amounts compared with more sedentary individuals?
   a. Creatine
   b. Glucosamine
   c. Glycerol
   d. Protein
3. Which of the following statements by a client prescribed simvastatin would indicate he understood the instructions?
   a. "One glass of grapefruit juice a day is as much as I can have."
   b. "I can have grapefruit juice for breakfast since I take the pill at bedtime."
   c. "I won't drink grapefruit juice while I am taking this drug."
   d. "I can start with 1 ounce of grapefruit juice and work up to 4 ounces over a month's time."
4. A client taking lithium is most likely to experience increased mania with:
   a. Decreased fluid intake and decreased sodium intake
   b. Decreased fluid intake and increased potassium intake
   c. Increased sodium intake and decreased potassium intake
   d. Increased sodium intake and increased fluid intake
5. Individuals taking the anticoagulant *warfarin* must be counseled to consume no more than one serving per day of:
   a. Broccoli or spinach
   b. Vegetable oils
   c. Kale and parsley
   d. Dried apricots and dates

Clinical Analysis

Mr. A is being admitted to a long-term care facility. He is a 45-year-old post-trauma client. The motor vehicle accident in which he became paralyzed below the waist also killed his wife and daughter. The accident occurred 6 months ago. In the meantime, he has been treated at a rehabilitation center. He is depressed and freely sharing his feelings of guilt and loss. The depression has interfered with his progress toward rehabilitation and also contributed to a 20-pound weight loss since the accident. After many trials of various antidepressants, he is now receiving phenelzine. The following questions relate to his care.

1. Close attention to Mr. A's diet is essential. Which of the following foods will he have to avoid completely?
   a. Baked beans, dates, and roast beef
   b. Sugar, molasses, and maple syrup
   c. Bologna, cheddar cheese, and wine
   d. Green beans, whole-wheat bread, and oranges

2. When teaching nursing assistants about the dietary restrictions needed by Mr. A, the nurse should be sure the nursing assistants understand that:
   a. The potential complication can be life-threatening.
   b. Mr. A is to be kept unaware of the seriousness of his condition.
   c. As time goes on, the forbidden foods can be added to the diet slowly, one at a time.
   d. If Mr. A does not cooperate in his dietary care, his paralysis is likely to worsen.

3. Maria G. is pregnant with her third child. She tells the clinic nurse that she takes some herbal products "to keep my strength up and get me through the day." Which of the following products would raise the greatest concern for the nurse?
   a. Natural vitamin C from rose hips
   b. Ginger
   c. St. John's wort
   d. Protein supplement for athletes

16

Weight Management

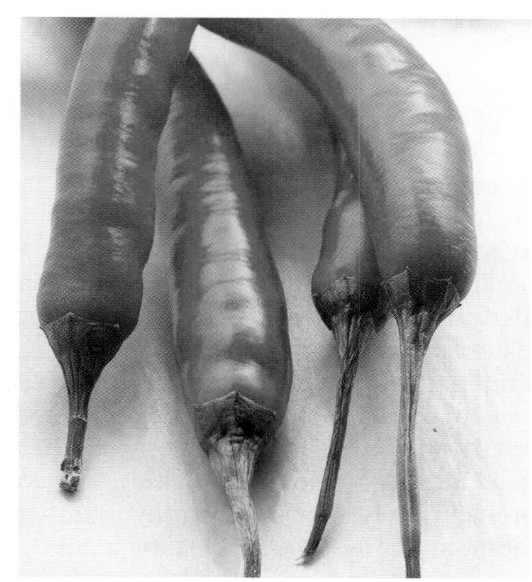

LEARNING OBJECTIVES

After completing this chapter, the student should be able to:

- List basic principles of energy imbalance.
- Discuss the effects of weight loss on the body.
- Identify the medical, psychological, and social problems associated with too much and too little body fat.
- Discuss the federal guidelines for the identification, evaluation, and treatment of overweight and obesity in adults.
- Describe the symptoms commonly exhibited by a client with anorexia nervosa and/or bulimia.
- Evaluate at least three fad diets used for weight reduction.

Weight management is a concern not only from a personal viewpoint but also from a societal perspective. Consequences of excessive body weight cause many individuals to suffer economically, socially, mentally, and physically. See Dollars and Sense 16-1.

Studies have repeatedly shown that at any one point in time more than 40% of the population describe themselves as trying to lose weight. Approximately 85% of those who lose weight will regain their original weight within 5 years. Although this sounds dismal, it also means that 15% of all people who lose weight are successful over the long term. Weight management, although difficult, is not impossible, and the financial and health benefits of weight control both to the individual and society are enormous.

> **Dollars & Sense 16-1**
>
> **Costs of Overweight and Obesity**
>
> According to a national study, costs attributed to both overweight and obesity (BMI 25 to 29.9) may have reached $92.6 billion in 2002 (CDC, 2009). Approximately one-half of these costs were paid for by Medicaid and Medicare. These costs do not include the indirect costs attributed to obesity such as absenteeism and decreased productivity.

Terminology and Classification

Historically the classification of people as underweight, normal weight, overweight, and obese has been a challenge for practitioners. Yet, how a person is classified is becoming more important. Third-party payers (insurance companies and state and federal governments) want an individual to meet specific criteria before they will grant financial approval for treatments. Percentage body fat is the true measure of how to classify clients but there are problems with this measurement. Therefore, body mass index (BMI) and waist circumference are the most commonly used methods for classifying clients.

Percentage Body Fat

An individual's percentage body fat is associated with her or his health risk. The most accurate definition for obesity is a body fat content greater than 30% to 33%.

The exact percentage is defined differently by various professional groups. The optimal fat content for females is 18% to 22%. The optimal fat content for males is 15% to 19%. However, percentage body fat is very expensive to measure accurately.

Techniques used to measure body fat involve underwater weighing, tissue x-ray exams, ultrasound, electrical conductivity, computed tomographic scans, and magnetic resonance imaging scans. Electrical impedance is used by some health-care workers but this method is gaining disfavor because of a lack of consistent results. Limitations include less accuracy in extremely obese persons; overhydration and underhydration; hormone abnormalities; and the need for a qualified technician. Thus, measurement of body fat is of limited usefulness for persons trying to lose weight. The other procedures previously mentioned are expensive and not available in clinical settings.

Body Mass Index

The National Institutes of Health (NIH) recommends and encourages all health-care professionals to use BMI to classify clients as underweight, normal weight, overweight, and obese in clinical settings. The classification of an individual as underweight, normal weight, overweight, and obese is defined according to BMI:

- Underweight <18.5
- Normal 18.5 to 24.9
- Overweight 25 to 29.9
- Obese >30

Individuals can calculate their own BMI using Clinical Calculation 16-1. Or they can use a Body Mass Index Chart (Table 16-1) to determine BMI without doing any calculations. The more complex calculation for BMI is weight in kilograms divided by height in meters squared.

Clinical Calculation 16-1

Steps in Calculating BMI

A BMI can be calculated in three easy steps.

1. Multiply weight in pounds by 703.
2. Multiple height in inches by height in inches.
3. Divide the product of step 1 by the product of step 2.

For example, for a 166-pound person who is 5 ft 6 in. or 66 in. tall:

1. 166 × 703 = 116,698
2. 66 × 66 = 4356
3. 116,698 divided by 4356 = 26.7

Although BMI correlates with the amount of body fat a person has, it does not measure body fat. Some athletes may have a BMI that identifies them as overweight but they do not have excessive amounts of body fat. The extra pounds are lean body mass acquired from rigorous training.

Similarly, a teen with a normal BMI may have all the health-related consequences of obesity if she has a high body fat content of greater than 33%. She may have a history of minimal physical activity and very poor food choices. The health-care professional should carefully evaluate the results of any BMI measurement along with other nutritional assessments (laboratory data, physical examination, and diet history).

Waist Circumference

Waist circumference is also used to classify fat distribution and central obesity. Women with a waist circumference greater than 35 inches and men with a waist circumference greater than 40 inches are at a higher health risk than those with a lower waist circumference (National Institutes of Health [NIH], 1998). NIH recommends waist circumference measurement for both the ease of measurement and low cost.

Prevalence and Incidence of Overweight and Obesity

The prevalence of obesity in the United States has had a startling increase since the mid-1970s. Figure 16-1 illustrates these trends more dramatically than words. **Prevalence** means the total number of cases of a specific disease divided by the number of individuals in the population at a certain time.

Many experts are concerned about the incidence and prevalence of obesity in the nation's children. **Incidence** is defined as the frequency of occurrence of any event or condition over time and in relation to the population in which it occurs. Asian children have the lowest incidence of obesity. Native American children have the highest incidence of obesity. Thus, one could conclude obesity is partially genetic in origin. Data from two NHANES surveys show (Centers for Disease Control and Prevention [CDC], 2008):

- For children 2 to 5 years, the prevalence of obesity increased from 5% to 13.9%
- For those ages 6 to 11 years, the prevalence increased from 6.5% to 18.8%
- For those ages 12 to 19 years, the prevalence increased from 5% to 17.4%.

TABLE 16-1 ■ Body Mass Index Chart

BMI	19	20	21	22	23	24	25	26	27	28	29	30	31	32	33	34	35	36
HEIGHT (INCHES)								**BODY WEIGHT (POUNDS)**										
58	91	96	100	105	110	115	119	124	129	134	138	143	148	153	158	162	167	172
59	94	99	104	109	114	119	124	128	133	138	143	148	153	158	163	168	173	178
60	97	102	107	112	118	123	128	133	138	143	148	153	158	163	168	174	179	184
61	100	106	111	116	122	127	132	137	143	148	153	158	164	169	174	180	185	190
62	104	109	115	120	126	131	136	142	147	153	158	164	169	175	180	186	191	196
63	107	113	118	124	130	135	141	146	152	158	163	169	175	180	186	191	197	203
64	110	116	122	128	134	140	145	151	157	163	169	174	180	186	192	197	204	209
65	114	120	126	132	138	144	150	156	162	168	174	180	186	192	198	204	210	216
66	118	124	130	136	142	148	155	161	167	173	179	186	192	198	204	210	216	223
67	121	127	134	140	146	153	159	166	172	178	185	191	198	204	211	217	223	230
68	125	131	138	144	151	158	164	171	177	184	190	197	203	210	216	223	230	236
69	128	135	142	149	155	162	169	176	182	189	196	203	209	216	223	230	236	243
70	132	139	146	153	160	167	174	181	188	195	202	209	216	222	229	236	243	250
71	136	143	150	157	165	172	179	186	193	200	208	215	222	229	236	243	250	257
72	140	147	154	162	169	177	184	191	199	206	213	221	228	235	242	250	258	265
73	144	151	159	166	174	182	189	197	204	212	219	227	235	242	250	257	265	272
74	148	155	163	171	179	186	194	202	210	218	225	233	241	249	256	264	272	280
75	152	160	168	176	184	192	200	208	216	224	232	240	248	256	264	272	279	287
76	156	164	172	180	189	197	205	213	221	230	238	246	254	263	271	279	287	295
BMI	37	38	39	40	41	42	43	44	45	46	47	48	49	50	51	52	53	54
HEIGHT (INCHES)								**BODY WEIGHT (POUNDS)**										
58	177	181	186	191	196	201	205	210	215	220	224	229	234	239	244	248	253	258
59	183	188	193	198	203	208	212	217	222	227	232	237	242	247	252	257	262	267
60	189	194	199	204	209	215	220	225	230	235	240	245	250	255	261	266	271	276
61	195	201	206	211	217	222	227	232	238	243	248	254	259	264	269	275	280	285
62	202	207	213	218	224	229	235	240	246	251	256	262	267	273	278	284	289	295
63	208	214	220	225	231	237	242	248	254	259	265	270	278	282	287	293	299	304
64	215	221	227	239	238	244	250	256	262	267	273	279	285	291	296	302	308	314
65	222	228	234	240	246	252	258	264	270	276	282	288	294	300	306	312	318	324
66	229	235	241	247	253	260	266	272	278	284	291	297	303	309	315	322	328	334
67	236	242	249	255	261	268	274	280	287	293	299	306	312	319	329	331	338	344
68	243	249	256	262	269	276	282	289	295	302	308	315	329	328	335	341	348	354
69	250	257	263	270	277	284	291	297	304	311	318	324	331	338	349	351	358	365
70	257	264	271	278	285	292	299	306	313	320	327	334	341	348	355	362	369	376
71	265	272	279	286	293	301	308	315	322	329	338	343	351	358	365	379	379	386
72	272	279	287	294	302	309	316	324	331	338	346	353	361	368	375	383	390	397
73	280	288	295	302	310	318	325	333	340	348	355	363	371	378	386	393	401	408
74	287	295	303	311	319	326	334	342	350	358	365	373	381	389	396	404	419	420
75	295	303	311	319	327	335	343	351	359	367	375	383	391	399	407	415	423	431
76	304	312	320	328	336	344	353	361	369	377	385	394	402	410	418	426	435	443
BMI	37	38	39	40	41	42	43	44	45	46	47	48	49	50	51	52	53	54

To use the table, find the appropriate height in the left-hand column. Move across to a given weight. The number at the top of the column is the BMI at that height and weight. Pounds have been rounded off.

Basic Science of Energy Imbalance

To understand the science of energy imbalance, think of the human body as a machine. Tens of thousands of researchers have spent years studying how the human body reacts to a kilocalorie imbalance. It is not adequate to say people weigh too much or to little because they overeat and do not exercise enough or vice versa. We need to ask: Why does someone's body seek or not seek food or exercise, when the human machine has adequate or inadequate energy available? What is not working? First, a brief outline of the science of energy imbalance follows.

Energy Imbalance

Energy imbalance results when the number of **kilocalories** eaten does not equal the number used for energy. An individual can determine whether food intake is meeting energy needs by monitoring his or her weight. If more kilocalories are eaten than are used by the body, weight gain will occur. If fewer kilocalories are eaten than are used by the body (and

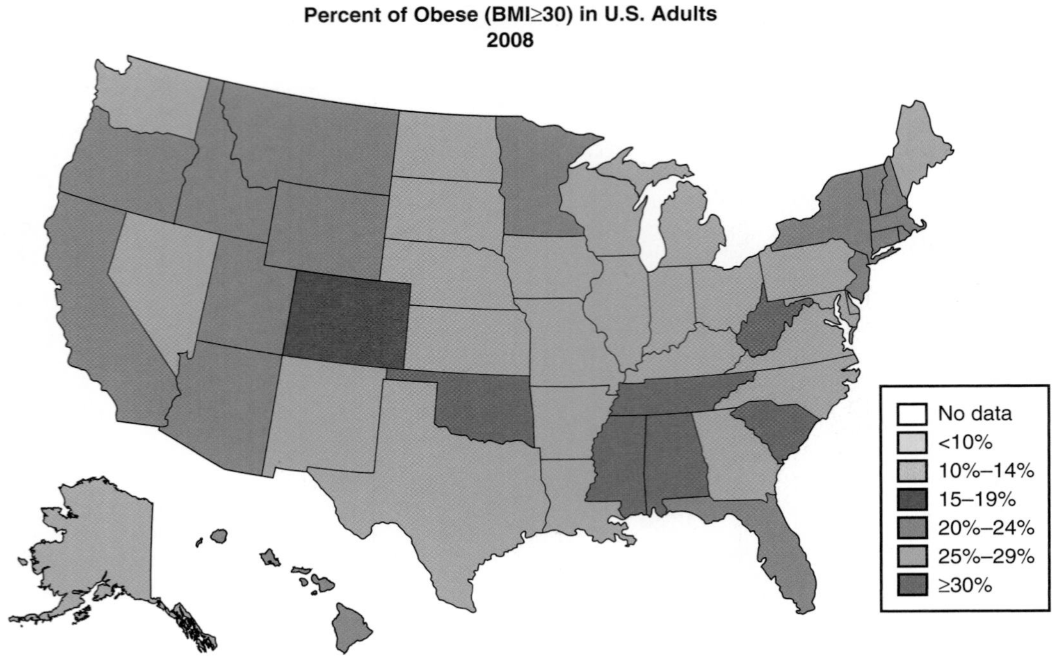

2008 State Obesity Rates

State	%	State	%	State	%	State	%
Alabama	31.4	Illinois	26.4	Montana	23.9	Rhode Island	21.5
Alaska	26.1	Indiana	26.3	Nebraska	26.6	South Carolina	30.1
Arizona	24.8	Iowa	26.0	Nevada	25.0	South Dakota	27.5
Arkansas	28.7	Kansas	27.4	New Hampshire	24.0	Tennessee	30.6
California	23.7	Kentucky	29.8	New Jersey	22.9	Texas	28.3
Colorado	18.5	Louisiana	28.3	New Mexico	25.2	Utah	22.5
Connecticut	21.0	Maine	25.2	New York	24.4	Vermont	22.7
Delaware	27.0	Maryland	26.0	North Carolina	29.0	Virginia	25.0
Washington DC	21.8	Massachusetts	20.9	North Dakota	27.1	Washington	25.4
Florida	24.4	Michigan	28.9	Ohio	28.7	West Virginia	31.2
Georgia	27.3	Minnesota	24.3	Oklahoma	30.3	Wisconsin	25.4
Hawaii	22.6	Mississippi	32.8	Oregon	24.2	Wyoming	24.6
Idaho	24.5	Missouri	28.5	Pennsylvania	27.7		

The data shown in these maps were collected through the CDC's Behavioral Risk Factor Surveillance System (BRFSS). Each year, state health departments use standard procedures to collect data through a series of monthly telephone interviews with U.S. adults. Prevalence estimates generated for the maps may vary slightly from those generated for the states by the BRFSS as slightly different analytic methods are used.

FIGURE 16-1 U.S. Obesity Trends 1986 to 2008 (www.cdc.gov/obesity/data/trends.html).

protein intake is adequate), weight loss will occur. (A low protein intake over an extended period will eventually lead to fluid retention and a subsequent weight gain from the fluid retained. In this situation, energy imbalance is difficult to ascertain by body weight alone.) Anyone can determine whether or not he or she is in energy balance by monitoring his or her weight over time. (This assumes normal hydration.)

There are two basic principles of energy imbalance. First, it takes a specific number of kilocalories to gain or lose a pound of body fat. Second, the body stores energy and uses stored energy in a highly specific manner.

The Five-Hundred Rule

To lose 1 pound of body fat per week, an individual must eat 500 kilocalories fewer per day than his or her body *expends* for 7 days. To gain 1 pound of body fat per week, the individual must eat 500 kilocalories more per day for 7 days than his or her body expends. The gain or loss of body fat need not occur during the course of a week; the kilocalorie surplus or deficit may occur over a month or year. The principle is the same. The total number of kilocalories required to gain or lose a pound of body fat is 3500. Too many kilocalories from any source of carbohydrates, fat, and/or protein promote weight gain. The five-hundred rule means that weight loss is independent of diet composition.

The key term here is *expend*. As you learned in the Energy Balance Chapter, the human body has some small subtle internal mechanisms that cause more or fewer kilocalories to be expended in some situations. The human body also has some small subtle internal mechanisms that cause the individual to eat more or less food in some situations.

Body Fat Stores

Excess kilocalories from any source (fat, carbohydrate, or protein) are stored as body fat in adipose fat tissue, which can accumulate in unlimited amounts. This accumulation can lead to overweight and, eventually, obesity. During a kilocalorie deficit, the body first seeks the energy necessary to sustain body functions in glycogen stores, which are limited. When a kilocalorie deficit occurs for longer than about 1 day, the body seeks the energy necessary to sustain its functions in both body fat stores (adipose tissue) and protein stores (organ and muscle mass). Weight loss always includes some loss of lean body mass (LBM). How much LBM is lost depends on how the weight loss is achieved.

Energy Imbalance and Body Composition

Weight loss affects body composition, and body composition affects health. The human body's two largest components (after water) are fat and lean mass that includes protein. Protein is stored primarily in muscle tissue, organs, and certain body chemicals. Preservation of lean body mass and of optimal health goes hand in hand. A loss of structural body content (e.g., heart and respiratory muscles, kidney, liver, body chemicals) is undesirable. Exercise can preserve and somewhat increase lean body mass. Weight gain increases body fat content. Weight loss decreases both body fat and lean body mass. An understanding of the difference between body fat content and lean body mass content is crucial to understanding the science of energy imbalance. The health benefits of weight loss are all related to a loss of body fat and not a loss of lean body mass. See Genomic Gem 16-1.

Genomic Gem 16-1

Obesity Genetic or Environmental?

Identical twins raised in different environments (adopted and nonadopted) have been studied extensively. Researchers concluded that adiposity heritability amounts to 77% for BMI and 76% of waist circumference (Wardle, 2008). This does not mean that a child with a high complement of susceptibility genes will inevitably become overweight, but his or her genetic endowment gives them a stronger predisposition. Our environment gives children unprecedented opportunities to overeat and be sedentary. Therefore, nutritious food should be provided to counterbalance the effect of genetics and help should be given to those who are more susceptible to obesity.

Loss of Fat versus Loss of Water and Protein

Most people, especially the overweight, can lose only about 2 pounds of body fat a week by eating less. Any weight loss beyond that is probably due to loss of water and/or lean muscle tissue. There is always some loss of body protein along with body fat during weight loss. This loss occurs because lean body mass is more metabolically active and therefore burns more kilocalories than fat tissue. The loss of body protein from reduced food intake is greater than the loss of body protein from a combination of reduced food intake and regular exercise. Thus, physical activity during weight loss protects lean body mass. Also, the greater the rate of weight loss, the more LBM is lost.

Severity of Obesity and LBM

Weight loss affects body composition of lean and obese people differently. The amount of lean body mass an individual loses during weight reduction depends on the degree of severity of the obesity. Obese animals tolerate starvation better than thin ones, and the same is true of humans. *Tolerate* means that they conserve body protein during weight loss. This means overweight and mildly obese individuals are at a higher risk of becoming protein-depleted during rapid weight loss. Rapid weight loss (0.5 to 1.0 pounds per day), if sustained for many weeks, is associated with an excessive loss of lean body mass and protein depletion of the heart. Malnutrition of the heart muscle can lead to sudden death. As an individual loses more and more fat during rapid weight loss, the ability to conserve lean body mass decreases. Thus, the length of time an individual diets as well as his or her beginning total body fat content has an impact on the amount of lean body mass lost.

Consequences of Obesity

Obesity can lead to many adverse consequences. For example, the distribution of body fat affects a person's susceptibility to medical problems, and the **psychological** ramifications of obesity are significant. Clients are commonly enmeshed in a tangle of societal, cultural, prejudicial and psychological issues. Many clients find great difficulty in breaking the cycle of behaviors that contribute to obesity. With an understanding of the issues, health-care providers can educate overweight and obese clients about the need for weight loss and encourage these clients to lose weight.

Social

The social consequences of obesity are connected to cultural expectations and the documented prejudice many obese people experience.

Cultural Expectations

Culture, in this context, refers to the convictions of a given people during a given period. Currently, many Americans perceive leanness as being attractive and desirable and fatness as being unattractive and undesirable. Yet what is and has been considered attractive has changed over time. Leanness has not always been the preferred body build. For example, during the 1800s, an overly fat body was considered the most attractive. Carrying excess weight meant that the person was well-to-do, that he or she could afford to overeat. Our society is slowly changing perceptions of what is attractive. For example, many perceive women with well-developed muscles as being more attractive than their lean, not-so-muscular counterparts. The increased numbers of female bodybuilders demonstrate this attitudinal shift.

In the United States, obese people have been under intense pressure to lose weight. Evidence of this pressure is the billions of dollars spent on weight-reduction programs and special foods each year. In an effort to be more attractive, many obese clients try to lose weight. Over time, however, most people regain the weight they have lost and commonly gain an additional few pounds. Thus, a self-defeating cycle begins. Clients generally need to be reminded that, although body weight is important, health and wellness are even more important.

Documented Prejudice

Several classic studies show that obese persons are the objects of prejudice and unfair discrimination. In a 7-year follow-up study of women 16 to 24 years old, obese women were less likely to have been married and had less schooling, lower incomes, and higher rates of household poverty than those with other chronic medical conditions (Canning and Mayer, 1966; Gortmaker et al., 1993).

Health-care workers should try to understand their own feelings about fatness, obesity, and obese persons. Sometimes, health-care workers unconsciously insult obese clients. For example, comments made in front of clients, such as "It will take three of us to move this client," are hurtful. Health-care providers should treat obese clients with respect, kindness, and patience.

Psychological

Obesity can be associated with a range of psychological problems, which may result from food restriction (Box 16-1). One important psychological consequence of obesity is body image disturbances.

Body Image Disturbances

Body image is the mental picture a person has of himself or herself. A disturbed body image can manifest itself in two ways. First, people with distorted body images are usually dissatisfied with their bodies. Chronic complaints, demands for extra attention, and frequent negative statements made by clients about the way they look may be signs of an underlying body image disturbance.

Box 16-1 ■ *Psychological Consequences of Food Restriction*

Food restriction, either voluntary or involuntary, has consequences. Xenophon in ancient Greece described a "ravenous hunger" in soldiers who had been deprived of food during a military campaign. During World War II, Keyes et al. studied the effects of semistarvation on subjects (Keyes et al., 1950). The effects of food restrictions in rats has also been studied. In many studies, the subjects responded to food deprivation with extraordinarily similar behaviors. First, restrained eaters did not necessarily have much, if any, long-term weight loss. Second, restraining one's eating made one highly susceptible to bouts of excessive eating even after restrictions were lifted. Third, study subjects exhibited **cognitive** and emotional changes when food was restricted, including heightened emotional responsiveness; cognitive disruptions, including distractibility; and a focus on food and eating (Polivy, 1996).

Health-care providers need to caution clients about the consequences of restrained eating. Overweight clients need to be helped to give up their crash diets and to be advised to eat balanced healthful diets that include whole grains, fruits, vegetables, and nonfat dairy products. Abandonment of the short-term "diet mentality" and adoption of long-term lifestyle changes will enhance physical and psychological well-being.

Second, persons with distorted body images frequently do not view their bodies realistically. For example, people may view themselves as having certain body parts larger than they actually are. A later section in this chapter discusses clients with anorexia nervosa, a mental health disorder, who frequently have body image disturbances. Very thin clients who have this condition frequently view themselves as overweight despite valid evidence to the contrary.

A classic study showed that body image disturbances are not found in emotionally healthy obese individuals (Stunkard and Mendelson, 1961). Body image disturbances are most common in young women of the middle and upper-middle classes who have been obese since childhood. Many of them have a generalized neurotic disturbance, and their parents and peers have criticized them for their obesity (Stunkard and Burt, 1967; Stunkard and Mendelson, 1961).

Medical

Obesity is considered a major health problem in the United States and is also considered a chronic medical condition. People who are overweight or obese are more likely to develop health problems such as:

- Hypertension
- Dyslipidemia (e.g., high total cholesterol or high levels of triglycerides)
- Type 2 diabetes
- Coronary heart disease
- Stroke
- Gallbladder disease
- Osteoarthritis
- Sleep apnea and respiratory problems
- Some cancers (endometrial, breast, and colon) (CDC, 2008)

The distribution of body fat affects risks. **Abdominal obesity**, in which excess weight is between the client's chest and pelvis, is more dangerous than gluteal-femoral obesity. Clients with abdominal obesity are said to be shaped like an apple and are especially vulnerable to chronic disease risks associated with excessive body weight.

In **gluteal-femoral obesity,** the excess weight is around the client's buttocks, hips, and thighs. Clients with gluteal-femoral obesity are said to be pear-shaped and are not as susceptible to chronic disease risks associated with excessive body fat.

Treating obesity is an important means of controlling some major chronic and degenerative diseases. For example, blood pressure levels can be reduced by a diet high in fruits and vegetables and low in fat. Up to 2½ cups of fruits and 4 cups of vegetables are recommended for a very active 18-year-old male. Up to 1½ cups of fruits and 2 cups of vegetables are recommended for a sedentary 65-year-old female.

Factors Influencing Food Intake

Lifestyle behaviors, appetite, satiety, and, questionably, macronutrient energy distribution influence food intake.

Lifestyle

These factors affect how much is eaten and influence kilocalorie consumption:

- Variety—The greater the variety of food served, the more kilocalories consumed.
- Taste—The better food tastes, the more is eaten.
- Weekend activity—Eating at regular times and planning non–food-related activities for weekends may assist in weight control.
- Skipping breakfast—People who regularly skip breakfast are more likely to be obese. Those eating four or more times daily are less likely to be obese. The fourth meal should be a small snack. Skipping meals is not a good weight-control strategy.
- Eating out—Eating meals away from home is associated with increased energy intake (CDC, 2008).
- Speed—The faster food is eaten, the more is consumed because it takes a little longer for satiety signals to reach the brain. The more foods need to be chewed, the fewer kilocalories are eaten because it takes time to chew the food.
- Soda intake—The consumption of sweetened soda is associated with a positive energy balance (CDC, 2008).
- Dietary fat—High dietary fat content of foods consumed is a risk factor for weight gain (Blundell and Stubbs, 2004).

Lifestyle behaviors that are responsible for *decreased* energy expenditure also increase body weight.

- Sedentary activities—The more hours spent watching television, the less time is spent being physically active. The same can be said for computer and video games.
- Changes in energy expenditure—Small daily decreases in energy expenditure, such as getting up to change the channels on the television and opening the garage door manually may be significant over the course of a year.

Physiology

Numerous hormones and neuropeptides that stimulate or inhibit food intake through central and peripheral mechanisms have been identified. Molecules that affect metabolic rates and energy expenditure are also an area of current research. Figure 16-2 illustrates multiple molecules and pathways involved in the internal regulation of food intake. In general, there is redundancy and counterbalance among these pathways so that, for instance, the inhibitory effect of one molecule is dampened by another. This intricate redundancy and counterbalance makes effective treatment of obesity complex. Perhaps as researchers learn more about the human energy balance system, more effective and safe treatments for imbalances may be available.

The brain, stomach, small intestine, and fat cells are all part of this complex energy balance system. The stomach, small intestines, and fat cells send messages to the brain to turn on or turn off eating. The triggers that influence food intake include satiety signals and hunger signals. When the brain, for instance, receives a satiety signal animals stop eating.

Neuropeptide Y is one example of a polypeptide in the brain that results in increased food intake. This chemical causes carbohydrate cravings, initiates eating, decreases energy expenditure, and increases fat storage. All of these actions favor positive energy balance and weight gain. Leptin, a protein made by fat cells, is a hormone that acts on the hypothalamus to decrease food intake. Interestingly, blood leptin levels increase in proportion to percentage of body fat (Colaizzo-Anas, 2007). Ghrelin is one example of a gastric-made polypeptide that stimulates growth hormone and regulates food intake. Release of ghrelin increases food intake.

This is a very short summary of the many ways the body has evolved to cope and survive during repeated cycles of feast and famine. Appetite can also be influenced by gastrointestinal distention to decrease food intake and contractions of an empty stomach to increase food intake. Satiety signals are sent from this area to the brain.

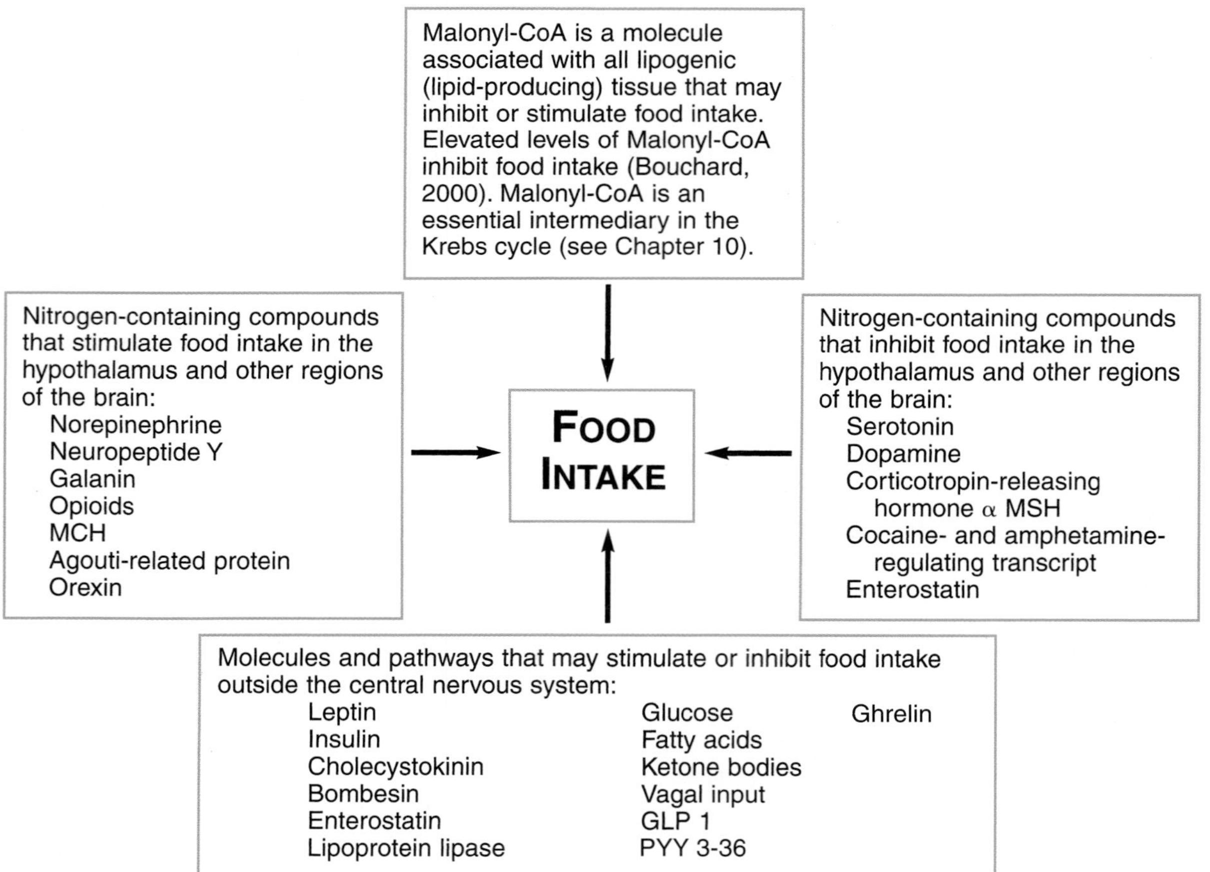

FIGURE 16-2 The hormones, molecules, and pathways that influence food intake through central or peripheral mechanisms. (Adapted from Bouchard, C: Inhibition of food intake by inhibitors of fatty acid synthase. N Engl J Med 343:25, 2000.)

Macronutrient Energy Composition

Researchers have conducted many studies on the role of macronutrient composition in energy balance. Following is a brief summary of this research. Protein seems to be more satiating than carbohydrate, which is more satiating than fat (Colaizzo-Anas, 2007). The brain appears to need some carbohydrate (delivered as glucose) for an individual to achieve satiety. In addition, fiber expands the stomach to assist in counteracting the release of polypeptides that increase food intake. In summary, eating a well-balanced meal that is planned to provide the energy nutrients within the accepted macronutrient distribution range (AMDR) is the best approach to weight management.

Glycemic Index

A low glycemic diet may also help with weight management, although studies are still producing conflicting findings. Some experts believe that eating carbohydrates that have a low glycemic index (GI) may result in a spontaneous reduction in food intake. GI is a measure of how much the blood glucose level increases after consumption of a particular food that contains a given amount of carbohydrate. A slice of white bread or glucose is the reference food. All other foods' GIs are set in comparison to white bread or glucose and are ranked according to their potential to raise blood glucose as compared with the reference white bread or glucose. Foods with a low GI are thought to promote satiety and decrease food intake. The glycemic index of mixed meals is not known. Following are some examples of the glycemic index of selected foods. Note: The reference food is white bread:

- White bread 100
- Glucose 138
- Fructose 26
- Honey 126
- Whole-wheat bread 100
- Rye (whole grain), pumpernickel 88
- Cornflakes 121
- Banana 84
- Baked potato 116
- Kidney beans, canned 74
- Ice cream 69
- Sucrose 83
- White rice, polished (boiled 10 to 25 minutes) 81
- Oatmeal 85
- All-bran 74
- Plum 34
- Sweet potato 70
- Lentils (green, canned) 74
- Skim milk 46
- Orange 59
- Orange juice 71
- Yogurt 52
- Soybeans (canned) 22

If the reference food is glucose, the numbers will be different, but not wrong. Many factors influence a food's GI. The rate of consumption and the time of day a food is eaten may increase or decrease a particular food's GI. Other components in a food besides carbohydrate influence a food's GI, including fat, fiber, and protein content and starch characteristics. How a food is prepared and processed influences GI. Physiological effects, including pregastric hydrolysis, gastric emptying rate, intestinal response, hydrolysis and absorption, pancreatic and gut hormone response, and colonic effects, influence a food's GI. Nondietary factors that influence a food's GI include medications taken, stress, physical activity, and overall health status.

Clinical use of GI as a guide to food selection may provide a health benefit and appears to be without adverse effects. Hints to incorporate the GI into the diet include these suggestions:

- Keep it simple—substitute whole grains and fresh fruits and beans for lower-GI foods.
- Focus on foods that contribute the most CHO, such as bread, breakfast foods, and potatoes.
- Do not worry about foods that contribute 5 or fewer grams of CHO in a serving. Some nutritionally dense foods, such as carrots, have a higher GI but contain a low amount of CHO in a serving.

Theories About Obesity

Theories about obesity are plentiful. Box 16-2 discusses one theory: the malfunctioning hypothalamus.

Efficient Metabolism

Some obese individuals actually require fewer kilocalories for normal body functions than do lean individuals. Some obese individuals, thus, use kilocalories very efficiently.

Brown Fat

Brown fat, a special type of fat cell, accounts for less than 1% of total body weight. Brown fat burns kilocalories and then releases the energy as heat. Energy released as heat is not stored as body fat. Some obese people may have defective brown fat or less brown fat than lean people.

Box 16-2 ■ *Can a Malfunctioning Hypothalamus Cause Weight Gain?*

The brain partially controls hunger and satiety. The hypothalamus, located in the brain, appears to be the center for weight control. A malfunctioning hypothalamus could cause an individual to receive incorrect hunger signals, thus stimulating continued eating and signaling weight gain. Appetite, satiety, and hunger may be incorrectly processed by a malfunctioning hypothalamus.

Various areas of the hypothalamus are sensitive to at least 13 neurochemicals, and these areas are involved in the regulation of hunger, eating, and satiety: The ventromedial nucleus and the lateral lobe in the hypothalamus are the two most significant areas.

- The ventromedial nucleus, which is activated by **serotonin** and antagonized by norepinephrine, mediates satiety.
- The lateral lobe, which is activated by norepinephrine and/or dopamine and antagonized by serotonin, mediates hunger and thirst.

Selective hypothalamic neurotransmitters are now being considered as medications to alter the brain sensation of hunger, appetite, and satiety. However, more research is necessary to understand better long-term and short-term effects of these medications.

Set Point Theory

The set point theory argues that each individual has a unique, relatively stable, adult body weight based on biologic factors. Hence, an obese person may have a higher set point than a lean counterpart.

Number of Fat Cells

Obese individuals have many more fat cells than do their lean counterparts. A kilocalorie deficit can reduce the fat in each cell but cannot break down the cell. Once manufactured, a fat cell exists until death. Empty fat cells release a chemical messenger that travels to the brain and sends a message to the reduced obese person to fill the depleted fat cells. As a result, the reduced obese person must learn to constantly ignore internal hunger signals. Ignoring such pains can be done for a short period, but long-term adaptation to hunger is difficult.

Enzymes in the Metabolic Chain

Lipoprotein lipase is an enzyme that is involved in the uptake of fatty acids for the manufacture of fat in individual fat cells. Research has shown that the activity of this enzyme increases during weight reduction. This action makes fat cells even more efficient in synthesizing fats.

Federal Guidelines

There are clear advantages to weight loss by overweight and obese clients. The primary reason should be to decrease the risk of disease. Treatment is also indicated for persons who have an obesity-related disorder. Options offered to clients should depend on their degree of overweight and obesity.

Advantages of Weight Loss

Federal clinical guidelines for identifying overweight and obesity in adults focuses on the medical benefits to be derived from weight loss. This panel recommends:

- Weight loss to lower blood pressure in overweight and obese persons with high blood pressure
- Weight loss to lower elevated levels of cholesterol, low-density lipoprotein cholesterol, and triglycerides, and to raise low levels of high-density lipoprotein cholesterol in overweight and obese persons with dyslipidemia (see Chapter 18)
- Some weight loss to lower elevated blood glucose levels in overweight and obese persons with type 2 diabetes.

Determining Overweight and Obesity

According to U.S. federal guidelines, practitioners should use the BMI and waist circumference to classify the degree of energy imbalance in clients. Body weight alone can be used to follow weight loss and to determine efficacy of treatment (NIH, 1998).

Treatment of Energy Imbalances

Federal guidelines address goals for weight loss, how to achieve weight loss, goals for weight maintenance, how to maintain weight loss, and special treatment groups.

Goals for Weight Loss

The initial goal of weight loss should be to reduce body weight by 10% from the baseline (current weight). With success, further weight loss can be attempted, if indicated. Safe weight loss occurs at about 1 to 2 pounds per week for a period of 6 months, with the subsequent strategy based on the amount of weight lost (NIH, 1998).

Achieving Weight Loss

The approach to weight loss should depend on professional evaluation and the client's BMI, waist circumference, and other factors (NIH, 1998). These are some of the weight-loss treatment options for clients:

- Dietary therapy (also called medical nutrition therapy)
- Physical activity
- Behavior therapy
- Pharmacotherapy
- Weight-loss surgery.
- Combined therapy (some or all of the above)

Diet Therapy

A weight-loss diet should be reduced in total kilocalories but adequate in all nutrients and should provide at least:

- 45% of kilocalories from carbohydrate
- 20% of kilocalories from fat
- 10% of the kilocalories from protein or 0.8 gram/kg whichever is higher.
- Remaining 25% of kilocalories open to negotiation with the client.
- 25 to 35 grams of fiber
- All essential vitamins, minerals, and fiber

The meal plan should be one the client can and will follow. When clients are given a standardized meal plan, weight loss is not usually successful. However, when behavior modification, nutritional counseling, and exercise recommendations support the meal plan, weight loss can be more successful.

Different clients need different types of dietary directions. A few clients want to be told what to eat and will follow through with appropriate behaviors. Some clients prefer receiving simplified instructions and do not want to learn a complicated diet. A MyPyramid Guide (US. Department of Agriculture [USDA], 2010) dietary plan may work well for the latter type of client (provided behavior modifications and the need for exercise are also discussed). Portion control must be emphasized.

A common tool used for teaching portion control and energy nutrient distribution is the American Diabetic and Dietetic Association's Exchange Lists. These lists provide detailed meal plans and clearly spell out portion sizes, making them an ideal guide for health-care employees when they serve and monitor weight-reduction diets.

Another advantage of the ADA Exchange Lists is that the system teaches clients the composition of foods, such as which foods contain sugar, which fat. The disadvantage to this meal planning system is that learning it takes a relatively long time, so some clients become discouraged. See the Exchange Lists in Appendix B. *Weight Watchers* uses a variation of this meal planning system with some success.

Sometimes clients are unable to make drastic changes in their food intake and become discouraged. In this situation, nutritional counselors should encourage clients to make major behavioral changes in their eating habits slowly. The goal in weight-reduction counseling is to help the client make permanent lifestyle changes.

Physical Activity

Population studies conducted in the United States, Great Britain, and France suggest that the rapidly increasing prevalence of obesity in recent decades may be largely due to increasing sedentary behaviors, perhaps to a greater extent than dietary excesses. Some nutrition counselors advocate a nondieting approach to weight control. Exercise and healthy eating is encouraged instead of adherence to a rigid diet plan.

Physical activity should be part of any comprehensive weight-loss and weight maintenance program because it:

- Modestly contributes to weight loss in overweight and obese adults.
- May decrease abdominal fat.
- Increases cardiopulmonary fitness.
- Increases lean body mass.

Initially, moderate levels of exercise for 30 to 45 minutes 3 to 5 days per week should be encouraged. All adults should set a long-term goal to accumulate *at least* 30 minutes or more of moderate-intensity physical activity on most, and preferably all, days of the week. Sixty minutes of daily exercise is needed by some people for long term weight management. See Genomic Gem 16-2.

To identify individuals at risk for heart disease, a physician should screen all clients before making exercise recommendations. Clients with known heart, lung, or metabolic disease should have a physician-supervised stress test before beginning an exercise program.

When following an exercise program, fluid intake should be adequate. Individuals should drink water before, during, and after exercise, and they should pay close attention to thirst to prevent dehydration.

Genomic Gem 16-2
Body Build and Propensity for Obesity

The propensity to be physically inactive may be at least partly determined by genetics. Individuals with certain body builds may be genetically predisposed to engage in less spontaneous physical activity and to have relatively low energy requirements. However, physical activity behaviors also influence whether we stay lean or become obese. For example, note these two studies:

1. One showed that within twin pairs, the twin who reported being more physically active was generally less obese than the more sedentary sibling (Samaras et al., 1999).
2. Another showed that physical activity in previously sedentary adults led to weight loss even when they were not dieting and had not been encouraged to lose weight (Stentz et al., 2004).

Four ounces of water every 15 minutes is usually sufficient, but when temperatures are very high, additional fluids may be necessary. During hot weather, the thirst mechanism may not be adequate to prevent dehydration in many elderly persons and in individuals involved in heavy exercise. Such persons need to drink water even if they are not thirsty.

One method to determine if fluid intake is adequate is to weigh oneself before and after exercise. One pound of water (sweat) weighs sixteen ounces or two cups. Therefore, for every pound of sweat lost during exercise, the person needs to drink 2 cups of water. Another indication that fluid intake is adequate is urine that is clear and has a minimal odor.

Behavior Modification

Behavior modification is a useful adjunct to weight loss and maintenance plans. A client's motivation to enter weight-loss therapy and his or her readiness to implement a plan require evaluation. Permanent weight loss can result only from a permanent change in eating and exercise behaviors. See Box 16-3 for common weight-reduction strategies.

Box 16-3 ■ *Behavior Modification Techniques to Share With Clients*

These behavior-change tips can help facilitate a weight-loss program.

Self-Monitoring

- Keep a food diary and record all food intake.
- Keep a weekly graph of weight change.
- Keep an exercise diary.

Stimulus Control

- At home, limit all food intake to one specific place.
- Plan food intake for each day.
- Rearrange your schedule to avoid inappropriate eating.
- Sit down at a table while eating.
- At a party, sit a distance from snack foods, eat before you go, and substitute lower kilocalorie drinks for alcohol.
- Decide beforehand what you will order at a restaurant.
- Save or reschedule everyday activities for times when you are hungry.
- Avoid boredom; keep a list of activities on the refrigerator.

Slower Eating

- Drink a glass of water before each meal. Drink sips of water between bites of food.
- Swallow food before putting more food on the utensil.
- Try to be the last one to finish eating.
- Pause for a minute during your meal and attempt to increase the number of pauses.

Reward Yourself

- Chart your progress.
- Make an agreement with yourself or a significant other for a meaningful reward.
- Do not reward yourself with food.

Cognitive Strategies

- View exercise as a means of controlling hunger.
- Practice relaxation techniques.
- Imagine yourself ordering a side salad, diet dressing, low-fat milk, and a small hamburger at a fast-food restaurant.
- Visualize yourself enjoying a fresh apple in preference to apple pie.

Pharmacotherapy

According to federal guidelines, approved FDA weight-loss medications may be used as part of a comprehensive weight-loss program, which includes diet and physical activity, for clients with a BMI equal to or greater than 30 and no concomitant obesity-related risk factors or diseases. For clients with a BMI equal to or greater than 27 and concomitant obesity-related risk factors or diseases, medications may also be indicated.

Medications should never be used without lifestyle modification. Medication therapy for obesity should be continually monitored for efficacy and safety and discontinued if the client does not lose weight. Table 16-2 lists weight-loss medications, actions, and adverse effects.

Surgery

Weight-loss surgery is an option for selected clients with clinically extreme or severe obesity (BMI ≥40 or ≥35 with comorbid conditions) when less-invasive methods of weight loss have failed and the client is at high risk for obesity-associated morbidity or mortality.

TABLE 16-2 ■ Weight-Loss Medications

DRUG	ACTION	ADVERSE EFFECTS
Sibutramine (Meridia)	Norepinephrine, dopamine, and serotonin reuptake inhibitor	Increase in heart rate and blood pressure, heart palpitations, and vasodilation Reports worldwide of deaths
Orlistat	Inhibits pancreatic lipase, decreases fat absorption	Decrease in absorption of fat-soluble vitamins Soft stools and anal leakage Possible link to breast cancer

Numerous surgical procedures are used to treat obesity. The removal of fat tissue through a vacuum hose is called **liposuction. Lipectomy** is surgical removal of adipose tissue. Both of these procedures are done more for cosmetic reasons than for weight control. A **jejunoileal bypass** involves the removal of a part of the small intestine. Clients lose weight after this procedure because they cannot absorb all the food they eat, although this places these clients at a nutritional risk. The jejunoileal bypass procedure is rarely performed currently; however, health-care providers are likely to encounter patients who have had this procedure.

Two of the most commonly performed surgeries for weight management are **gastric banding and gastric bypass (Roux-en-Y)**. Diagrams of these procedures are shown in Figure 16-3.

Gastric banding involves the placement of an adjustable band to create a small stomach pouch. When the stomach is smaller or reduced, only a limited amount of food can be consumed at one feeding. This induces weight loss from reduced kilocalorie intake. Before surgery, the surgeon specifies a diet and the client must make an enormous commitment to follow the diet exactly and choose foods very carefully The gastric band is adjusted by the surgeon for sometime after the initial procedure. Following is a description of a typical progressive diet plan—some surgeons use a variation:

Phase 1: 64 oz per day of sugar-free and noncarbonated clear liquids consumed in very small amounts immediately after the surgery; no straws

Phase 2: First week at home: 70 grams of protein daily in the form of full liquids; avoidance of empty kilocalories; no more than 8 oz per hour; vitamin and mineral liquid supplement; and two chewable sugar-free calcium carbonate tablets per day (usually requires drinking full liquids on the hour for 11 hours/day)

Phase 3: Pureed and crispy foods, defined as well-toasted bread, saltines, and melba toast; six small high-protein meals per day. Total amount of food at each meal not to exceed 6 oz; fluid goal is 64 oz per day; no fluid consumption with meals; no food particle larger than an M&M candy (usually requires eating or drinking on the hour for 11 hours/day)

Phase 4: Soft foods allowed usually 3 weeks after surgery; foods must be mushy in texture; 8 oz volume limit per meal; 70 grams of protein per day; no liquids with meals (usually requires eating or drinking on the hour for 11 hours/day)

Phase 5: Low-fat solids; 3 meals and 3 snacks per day; 70 grams of protein per day; no sugar or sugar-containing foods; no temperature extremes; no alcohol; 6 oz volume limit per meal; usually begins 4 weeks after surgery; no liquids with meals; no fried foods; 64 oz of fluid total per day

Each time the band is readjusted by the physician, the diet phase immediately following the adjustment is Phase 2.

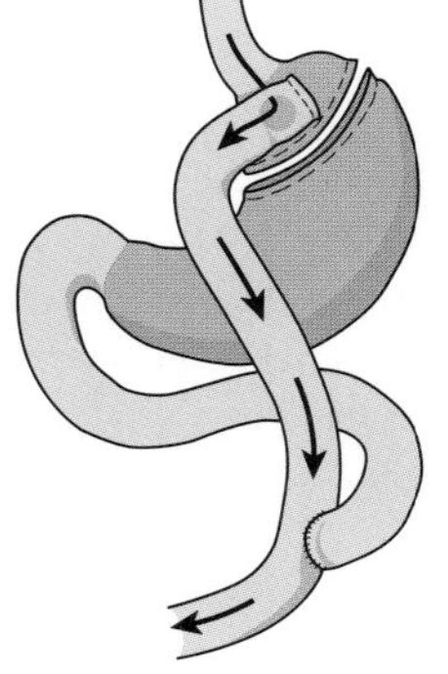

(a)

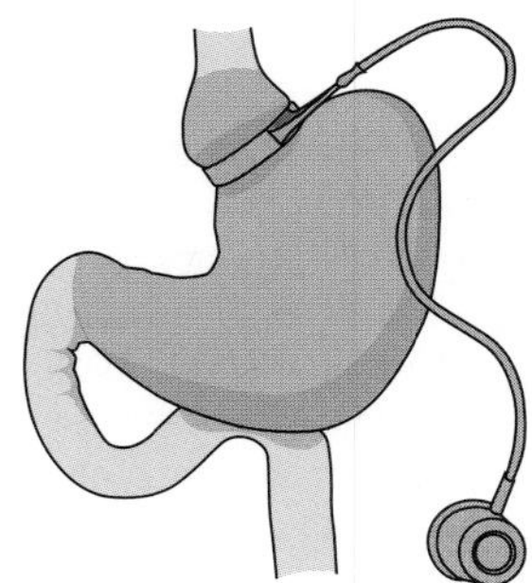

(b)

FIGURE 16-3 Surgery for weight loss. *A*, Roux-en-Y stomach bypass: large portion of stomach and duodenum are bypassed. *B*, Adjustable gastric banding: Stomach opening can be tightened or loosened over time to change the size of the passage.

Bariatric surgeons usually depend on team members to screen and monitor clients, who typically have several sessions with the team before the procedure is done. Most surgeons screen and monitor clients because the liability risk is great if clients are not screened and educated.

Clinical Application 16-1 discusses problems that clients often encounter after gastric surgery and suggests general guidelines for these clients to follow. Clients should be followed carefully postoperatively because of risks for deficiencies such as iron, folacin, and vitamin B_{12}. Clients are also at risk for maladaptive eating behavior. Clinical Application 16-2 discusses surgery guidelines for these clients post-surgery.

Expected results from gastric surgery procedures should always be explained to clients. No permanent effects can be promised, and having the surgery does not mean that afterward the client can overeat without weight gain. Ninety% of weight loss occurs in the first year, and clients typically begin to gain again in the second and third years. The client should view the procedure as a tool to be used in conjunction with behavioral training—the small pouch helps clients learn to reduce and slow down food intake. After the first year, because of pouch stretching or intestinal adaptation, much of the effect of the surgery can be negated and the lost weight may be regained. Gastric banding eliminates some but not all of the stretching challenge.

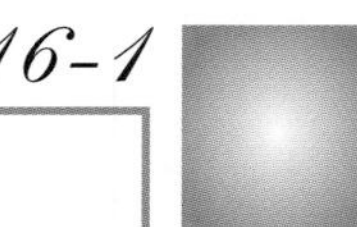
16-1

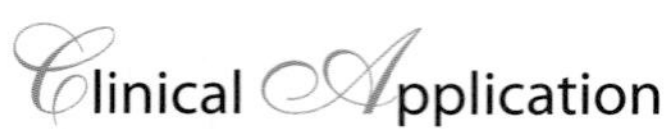
Clinical Application

Complications of Gastroplasty and Gastric Bypass

There are many potential acute complications of gastric surgery for weight reduction. These include:

- Nausea, vomiting, bloating, and/or heartburn: These signs and symptoms can be caused by overeating, not chewing food well, eating too quickly, drinking cold or carbonated beverages, using drinking straws, or eating gassy foods.
- Obstruction: An obstruction is the blockage of a structure. In this case, a blockage can occur close to the area stapled. A frequent cause of obstruction is poorly chewed food. The result is stomach pain, nausea, and vomiting.
- Dumping syndrome: Intake of concentrated sweets and large quantities of fluids causes quick dumping of food into the small intestine. Abdominal fullness, nausea, diarrhea 15 minutes after eating, warmth, weakness, fainting, racing pulse, and cold sweats are symptoms of this syndrome.
- Among the long-term risks is osteoporosis, due to decreased calcium absorption.

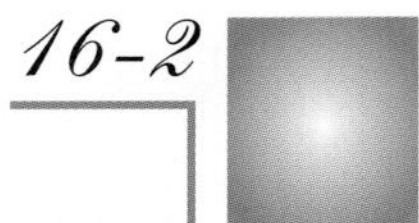
16-2

Clinical Application

Post Gastric Surgery Nutrition Guidelines

These strategies can help clients adjust after surgery:

- Eat three to six small meals per day.
- Eat slowly.
- Chew food thoroughly.
- Eat very small quantities.
- Stop eating when full.
- Drink most fluids between meals.
- Select a balanced diet.
- Take a multivitamin–multimineral supplement.
- Exercise regularly.

Weight-Loss Maintenance

Weight regains typically occurs after weight loss. A program of dietary therapy, physical activity, and behavior therapy enhances the likelihood of weight-loss maintenance. Drug therapy can also be used according to the guidelines published by the National Institutes of Health; however, drug safety and efficacy beyond 1 year of total treatment have not been established.

Research suggests, though, that frequent contacts between clients and practitioners increase the success of weight loss and maintenance therapies (NIH, 1998).

Obese clients who have successfully lost weight and kept the weight off report doing the following things (Foreyt, 2004). They:

- Include at least 30 minutes of moderate exercise each day.
- Have a strong social support network.
- Lost the weight gradually over a 6-month period.
- Have changed their attitudes toward their body weight.
- Have made realistic lifestyle changes.
- Eat smaller portion sizes.
- Avoid food high in fat.
- Eat a minimum of 35 servings of fruits and vegetables per week.
- Undereat 2 days per week.

They additionally report:

- Using nutritional portioned foods; Weight Watchers or Healthy Choice frozen dinners and diet beverages as meal replacements were widely used by successful dieters.
- Walking; it was the most frequently reported exercise.

- Taking part in structured programs; the more structured the weight-loss program was, the more successful the participants were.
- Keeping food records; 77% of clients who kept food records kept off previously lost weight versus 29% who did not keep food records.
- Referring clients to health-care professionals, including physicians and dietitians, when appropriate,
- Helping clients set realistic goals. See Box 16-5.
- In states that have regulations, assist in efforts to enforce these standards for safe weight loss.

The Role of Nutrition Educators

Appropriate roles for nutrition educators include:

- Providing accurate information
- Assisting children to prevent unhealthy weight gain. See Box 16-4.
- Warning against dangerous practices such as self-imposed starvation diets that eliminate one or more of the major food groups and encourage the intake of only one food group. See Table 16-3.
- Guiding clients to understand the risks and benefits of weight loss and weight-loss programs, products, medicines, procedures
- Teaching clients to evaluate the risks and benefits of surgery for themselves

Box 16-5 ■ *Realistic Goals*

Health-care and wellness professionals can assist clients in setting realistic goals for weight reduction and encourage loss of modest amounts of weight. Typically, clients have an unrealistic weight-loss goal. Despite considerable professional agreement that weight losses of 5 to 10% from baseline are successful for reducing comorbid conditions associated with obesity, obese patients often desire weight losses two to three times greater than this. For example, a weight-reduction diet may be planned to allow for a 1 pound per week weight loss. The client may expect to lose 5 lb per week. A female client may expect to be able eventually to wear a size 5 dress as a result of dieting. This expectation is not realistic for some clients with large bones.

Health-care workers provide a valuable service when they teach clients, especially those who are overweight, how to prevent weight gain.

Box 16-4 ■ *Weight Management in Children*

These are three ways in which individuals and communities can help children enjoy the physicial activities that can aid in weight management.

Develop appropriate activities—The enjoyment of physical activity should start young. Examples of appropriate activities for young children include ballet lessons, tricycle or bike riding, walking daily with a family member, swimming lessons, and sledding (see Fig. 16-2).

Develop play areas—Communities need to develop safe play areas for children. Local school districts should be encouraged to offer more opportunities for our young to be active in a noncompetitive environment.

Encourage noncompetitive activities—A totally sedentary child is uncomfortable in a competitive situation and will gain important health benefits from physical activity.

TABLE 16-3 ■ Weight-Loss Diets in the Popular Media

Fad diets come and go. Typically, fad diets limit a person to a few specific foods or food combinations, and do not provide kilocalories within the acceptable macronutrient range and the nutrient density so necessary for optimal health. For example, the brain needs sufficient carbohydrate for optimal function. One hundred and thirty grams of CHO is the average minimum amount of glucose used by the brain and the acceptable macronutrient range for CHO is 45 to 65% of kilocalories. The following describes three popular diets along with the diet author's rationale. These diets are not widely endorsed by the health-care community; however, health-care professionals should know what diets their clients may be following.

NAME OF DIET	RATIONALE OF DIET'S AUTHOR	DESCRIPTION
Atkins	Claims processed CHO and insulin rather than excess kilocalories are responsible for weight gain and obesity.	Restricts CHO and encourages protein with the use of vitamin and mineral supplements.
South Beach	The faster sugars and starches are absorbed, the more weight is gained. Low glycemic index meals suppress appetite and reduce food intake later in the same day in comparison to higher glycemic index meals (see below).	Three phases: ■ Severe CHO restriction for first 2 weeks ■ Reintroduction of "good CHO" (those with a low glycemic index, such as whole grains, fruits, vegetables) during phases 2 and 3 ■ Consistent meal times and plentiful water
Zone	Only through eating in the "Zone" can the body reach its physical peak. The author claims most people gain weight because they have an imbalance of energy nutrients. The kilocalorie intakes of the meal plans are between 1000 and 1700 kilocalories.	The zone is 40% CHO, 30% protein, and 30% fat All food is measured and only precise portion sizes are eaten. CHO serving sizes are small (⅛ cup of pasta).

Reduced Body Mass

Clients with a reduced body mass are as difficult, if not more difficult, to treat as overly fat clients. Body fat has important roles in insulation and protection of body organs. A client with a low body fat content usually has a loss of lean body mass as well, and loss of this functioning tissue concerns clinicians. Women cease to ovulate and menstruate when the percentage of body fat falls below a certain level. The client may experience cardiac abnormalities and become more prone to infections. These clients are at risk for osteoporosis in the long term.

Classification

A person with a BMI of greater than 18.5 should be evaluated before being classified as underweight. A man with a body fat content less than 15% and a woman with a body fat content less than 18% (if known) need to be evaluated and assessed before being classified as having a reduced body mass. The only reliable method to determine if the individual is at a nutritional risk is to do a complete nutritional assessment.

Consequences

Long-term follow-up of studies indicates that excessive leanness is associated with increased mortality and decreased life expectancy. However, the causes of mortality are different from those associated with excess weight. An excessively lean person is almost twice as likely to succumb to respiratory diseases such as tuberculosis. In addition, these clients have greater difficulty maintaining body temperature during cold weather. Infections and disturbances of the gastrointestinal tract are more likely in an underweight person, as is fragile bone structure and osteoporotic changes.

Causes

A person may be underweight because of genetic factors or because of a long-term or recent weight loss. A recent weight loss can often be related to a recent new medical diagnosis (such as trauma), a psychological diagnosis, or socioeconomic issues.

Rapid Loss Increases Risk

The greater the rate of weight loss, the more the client is at a nutritional risk. **Rate** means loss per unit of time. For example, a 20-pound weight loss in 2 weeks is an excessive weight loss. Such a client has lost a large amount of lean body mass. However, a 20-pound weight loss during a 20-week period could be attributed mostly to a loss of body fat with a minimal loss of lean body mass. If the client began with surplus body fat stores, a loss of 20 pounds may not place this client at a very high nutritional risk. If the client had a reduced body mass, even a slow weight loss may place him or her at a high nutritional risk. Laboratory data are useful to determine a client's nutritional risk level.

Not all changes in body weight are caused by insufficient kilocalorie intake. For example, a client may lose several pounds of body weight over the course of a single day as a result of diuretic therapy. The weight loss in this instance would be due to water loss and not to body fat or protein loss. See Box 16-6.

Eating Disorders

Eating disorders may be caused by psychological factors and may result in nutritional problems. Many experts are concerned about the prevalence of anorexia nervosa and bulimia. In the United States, as many as 10 million females and one million males are fighting a life-and-death battle with an eating disorder.

Anorexia Nervosa

Anorexia nervosa is a medical condition that results from self-imposed starvation. Symptoms include:

- Recent unplanned weight loss of 5% or more
- Decreased resting energy expenditure (ree)
- **Amenorrhea** (cessation of menstruation)
- Constipation
- Excessive hair loss
- Abnormal sleeping patterns
- Preoccupation with food
- Body image disturbance
- Misconception about physical status
- Intake of only 500 to 800 kilocalories per day
- Slow eating
- Increased physical activity
- Social isolation

Box 16-6 ■ *Is the Client Eating Enough?*

One method for determining whether a client is eating enough food is to monitor his or her food intake. Kilocalorie intake is monitored by recording actual food consumption and calculating the kilocalories eaten. Software programs, such as Food Processor or Diet Analysis, can assist with calculations.

- Intense fear of becoming obese
- Poor muscle tone

The disorder begins before age 20 in one-half of clients and before age 21 in three-fourths of clients. This disorder occurs 8 to 12 times more frequently in females than in males. The client may resort to a variety of devices to lose weight, including starvation, vomiting, and laxative use. The disorder may be life threatening.

Bulimia

Bulimia is more common than anorexia nervosa, especially during adolescence and young adulthood. The mean age for females at diagnosis was 23 years. An estimated 1.1% to 4.2% of females have bulimia nervosa in their lifetime. The condition is rare in males.

Bulimics binge and purge. **Binging** involves the consumption of as much as 5000 to 20,000 kilocalories per day. **Purging** is the intentional clearing of food out of the system by vomiting and/or using enemas, laxatives, and diuretics. Athletes such as ballerinas and gymnasts sometimes are bulimic. The female triad is a serious syndrome comprising three interrelated components:

- Disordered eating
- Amenorrhea
- Osteoporosis

Treating Eating Disorders

There are many approaches to treatment of eating disorders, including nutritional counseling, behavioral therapy, family therapy, and group therapy. It is important to help the client discover the reason he or she chooses to eat, not eat, binge, or purge. Some of these clients have symptoms including a fixation on food, weight, physique, or exercise. See Box 16-7.

Box 16-7 ■ *Treating Eating Disorders in the Hospital Setting*

Some clients are admitted to the hospital for treatment. Careful recording of kilocalories consumed is indicated. Sometimes nurses are asked to sit with these clients and watch them eat. These clients may attempt to hide food in their clothes, mouth, bedding, or anywhere else. It is sometimes necessary for the nurse to accompany these clients to the bathroom. Clients with eating disorders have been known to flush their food down the toilet. For these reasons, the physicians of such clients often order daily weighing.

Keystones

- Energy imbalance results from an inequality of energy intake and expenditure.
- The reason an individual eats more or fewer kilocalories than needed to maintain a stable body weight is only partially understood.
- Reasons a person may be in energy imbalance are both internal and external.
- Weight loss decreases *both* body fat and lean body mass.
- Care needs to be taken to minimize the loss of lean body mass during weight reduction.
- Exercise should be encouraged because it helps minimize the loss of lean body mass during weight reduction.
- Exercise, a well-balanced diet, and behavior modification are all essential components of a sound weight-reduction program.
- The prevention of energy imbalance is the key to decreased health-care costs nationally.
- Medications and surgical interventions may be indicated for individuals who meet the criteria set by the guidelines.
- Treating the client who has a reduced body mass is a concern for health-care workers.

CASE STUDY 16-1

The client arrives at the physician's office for a routine blood pressure check. Her blood pressure is 150/95. Her medications are 100 mg Lopressor daily and 150/12.5 Avalide daily. The client works nights as a cashier at a service station and days at a dry cleaner. Her BMI is 28. She recently had a stress test that was considered normal. The doctor would like the client to lose weight to help lower her blood pressure.

Care Plan

Subjective Data

Client stated, "I can barely afford my blood pressure medication, and the doctor has encouraged me to lose about 14 pounds. I know I need to eat less and exercise more. I need to spend less money on medications. I know I'm not too smart because I only completed the sixth grade in school." A food frequency record showed that this client usually eats four times each day. Her usual pattern includes 3 cups of low-fat milk, 8 starches (mostly refined), ½ cup of vegetables, 1 piece of fruit, 6 to 8 ounces of meat, 5 fats, 1 dessert, and an occasional beer. She eats fast food two nights each week and has pizza weekly for lunch. "I am desperate and will do anything to lose weight." The client has health insurance that will pay for one wellness program per year.

Objective Data

Blood pressure 150/95; height 5 ft 6 in.; BMI 28; waist circumference 36; stress test was normal.

Analysis

Energy imbalance; kilocalorie intake greater than kilocalorie expenditure. Overweight as evidenced by BMI of 28 and waist circumference of 36, probably contributing to hypertension.

Plan

DESIRED OUTCOMES EVALUATION CRITERIA	ACTIONS/INTERVENTIONS	RATIONALE
Increase physical activity.	Recommend Mrs. R monitor her exercise behaviors and try to walk at least 30 minutes three times per week and increase to 7 days per week as able.	Self-monitoring of lifestyle behaviors promotes behavioral change. The most sedentary individuals receive the most health benefit from even small amounts of exercise.
Consume foods in appropriate portions following the MyPyramid Guide.	Review food pyramid model with Mrs. R with emphasis on whole grains and fruits and vegetables and the avoidance of fats. Review portion sizes indicated on this teaching tool.	The MyPyramid Guide is a good tool to use for clients with a lower reading level and promotes a high-fiber, low-fat diet.
Client will state why a weight loss of 1 to 2 pounds per week may reduce her blood pressure.	Explain to the client that the rate of weight loss is important and why.	A 1- to 2-pound per week weight loss will minimize the loss of lean body mass. Self-starvation rarely results in long-term weight loss for overweight clients.
Refer client to the local hospital's Wellness center that incorporates diet, behavior modification, and exercise in the program.	Explain to the client why you are referring her to this particular program.	The best wellness programs include diet, exercise, and behavior modification.

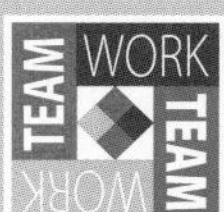

16-1

Follow-Up Note From Hospital's Wellness Program

Thank you for your referral to our program. Client has met with our registered dietitian, exercise physiologist, and psychologist in group sessions. She has attended most sessions and has done remarkably well. She has lost a total of 5 pounds at the rate of 1/2 to 1 pound per week for the last 8 weeks. We were also able to arrange a scholarship for her to attend the program for eight more weeks. She keeps very good food and exercise records. She has made several friends in the class and says she looks forward to this night out with her new friends. Thank you again for this referral.

Cordially,

Wellness Program Director

Critical Thinking Questions

1. What foods does this client need to eat less and what foods does she need to eat more?
2. What would you tell the client if after 1 week she gained a pound even though she had given up her daily dessert and had increased her vegetable intake to 5 servings each day?
3. What other dietary modifications would you recommend?

Chapter Review

1. To lose 2 pounds of body fat per week, an individual must eat ___ fewer kilocalories each day for 7 days without a change in energy expenditure.
   a. 1000
   b. 1500
   c. 2000
   d. 2500
2. A very rapid rate of weight loss (1 pound per day) in an adult who is slightly overweight:
   a. Usually encourages permanent changes in behavior
   b. May lead to sudden death in some clients
   c. Will preserve lean body mass
   d. Fosters long-term weight maintenance
3. An obese client should be enrolled in a weight-management program and meet the following criteria before medications are tried:
   a. BMI of 20 and a waist circumference of 30 inches
   b. In a male, waist circumference of at least 35 inches and a BMI of 27
   c. A BMI of 27 and no concomitant obesity-related risk factors
   d. In a female, a waist circumference of at least 35 inches and a BMI of 30 or greater
4. A client with anorexia nervosa:
   a. Has an increased resting energy expenditure
   b. Frequently complains of constipation
   c. Is not likely to have a body image disturbance
   d. Typically seeks the company of others
5. An elderly overweight smoker should first be encouraged to:
   a. Lose weight
   b. Quit smoking
   c. Lose weight and quit smoking using any means possible
   d. Be evaluated to determine if weight loss is indicated and bone health is adequate

Clinical Analysis

1. Mrs. R is a 40-year-old mother of three. She has arthritis in both knees. She weighs 180 pounds, has a medium frame, and is 5 ft, 3 in. tall. Her BMI is 32. Her physician has told her to lose weight to help reduce her knee pain. According to Mrs. R, she never thought she was overweight until she was 24 years old. At this time, her weight started increasing. When she weighed 140 pounds, she started to diet. One time she lost a total of 25 pounds, which she promptly regained plus an additional 5 pounds. The client described four additional **weight cycles.** Mrs. R claims she cannot exercise because "it is too painful on my knees." She has tried every conceivable type of diet, including a comprehensive medically supervised weight-control program. Mrs. R states that for the past year, no matter how little she eats, she cannot lose weight even on a 1200-kilocalorie diet. Mrs. R:
   a. Apparently knows a great deal about low-kilocalorie foods, because she has successfully lost weight before
   b. Knows very little about foods, because she always regained the weight she lost
   c. Lacks motivation, because she has an inability to follow through with the appropriate behavior
   d. Should be discouraged from further attempts to control her weight

2. Mrs. M had a slow weight gain for about 10 years. She asks for advice concerning how to best manage her weight. Mrs. M lives a sedentary lifestyle, eats three well-balanced meals each day, and enjoys going out to dinner with her husband one night each week. Her BMI is 27. Mrs. M would most likely benefit from:
   a. Decreasing her meal frequency
   b. Increasing her physical activity
   c. Taking a medication to lose weight
   d. Not going out to dinner with her husband each week

3. Mr. P wants to lose weight and has a BMI of 30 and a waist circumference of 41. Initially, the nurse should advise Mr. P to:
   a. Follow a 1200-kilocalorie diet.
   b. Ask his doctor for a medication to assist in weight reduction.
   c. Self-monitor and write down his food intake and physical activity.
   d. Refer the client to a surgeon for an evaluation.

17

Diet in Diabetes Mellitus and Hypoglycemia

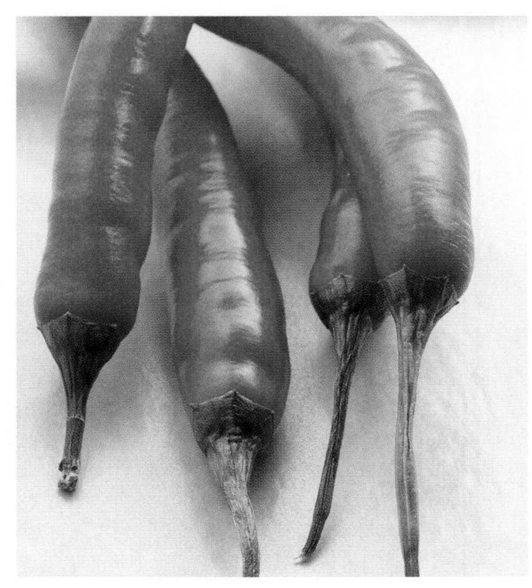

LEARNING OBJECTIVES

After completing this chapter, the student should be able to:

- Define and classify diabetes mellitus and describe the treatment for each type.
- Discuss the goals of nutritional care for persons with diabetes mellitus.
- List nutritional guidelines for people with diabetes for illness, exercise, delayed meals, alcohol, hypoglycemic episodes, vitamin and mineral supplementation, and eating out.
- Describe dietary treatment for reactive hypoglycemia as compared to diabetes mellitus.

This chapter introduces the importance of nutrition in diabetes and hypoglycemia. These two diseases are associated with insulin secretion and/or resistance to insulin accompanied by characteristic long-term complications. Diabetes mellitus is caused by the low secretion and/or utilization of insulin. Hypoglycemia is caused by excessive secretion of insulin. The Centers for Disease Control and Prevention (CDC) estimates the prevalence of diagnosed and undiagnosed diabetes in the United States for all ages in 2007 to be 23.6 million or 7.8% of the population—17.9 million people diagnosed, and 5.7 million undiagnosed (CDC, 2008). Nationally, diabetes is the seventh leading cause of death. Hypoglycemia is much rarer than diabetes mellitus. Nutrition is integral to the management of diabetes.

Definition and Classification

Diabetes mellitus is characterized by the passage of sweet urine, excessive urine production, thirst, excessive hunger, and, in some cases, weight loss. Diabetes mellitus can be defined as a group of disorders with measurable persistent hyperglycemia. **Hyperglycemia** means an elevated level of glucose in the blood. Definitions and classifications for the various subclasses of diabetes mellitus have been standardized.

Definition

Diabetes is diagnosed and defined by laboratory analysis. Fasting glucose levels of at least 126 milligrams per **deciliter** (mg/dL) are required for a diagnosis of diabetes in nonpregnant adults. Fasting is defined as no kilocalorie intake for at least 8 hours. A fasting blood glucose level 100 to 126 or greater is diagnosed as prediabetes or **impaired fasting glucose**. This must be confirmed as described. Casual or random blood glucose (RBG) greater than 200 mg/dL plus classic symptoms (increased urination, increased thirst, weight loss) is also an established method for diagnosing diabetes in adults and children. A random or casual blood glucose between 140 and 199 mg/dL is diagnostic of prediabetes. Random means the blood sample is tested without regard to time of day, prior diet, and physical activity. Refer to Clinical Application 17-1 for an explanation of other tests used for diabetes

17-1

Clinical Application

Laboratory Tests for Diabetes

Biochemical tests for diabetes include fasting blood sugar, glucose tolerance test, urine tests, and glycosylated hemoglobin.

FASTING BLOOD SUGAR

A measurement of a **fasting blood sugar (FBS)** is performed routinely on most diabetic clients. In preparation, the client should be instructed not to eat or drink for 8 hours before the test. Water is the exception, as it will not interfere with test results. The test ideally should be done after at least 3 days of unrestricted diet (≥150 grams of carbohydrate per day) and unlimited physical activity. The individual should remain seated and not smoke throughout the test. If the client usually takes insulin or a hypoglycemic agent, the medication should not be taken or given until the blood test is done. Normal FBS should be less than 100 mg/dL. A finding of 126 mg/dL is diagnostic of diabetes mellitus.

GLUCOSE TOLERANCE TEST

In the **glucose tolerance test,** 75 grams of anhydrous glucose dissolved in water is given orally or intravenously after a fasting blood sugar sample has been drawn. Blood samples are then drawn at specified intervals. The client's ability to process glucose can be evaluated by this means. A blood glucose value above or equal to 200 mg/dL at 2 hours and at least one other sample at less than 2 hours are required for the diagnosis in nonpregnant adults. A normal 2-hour blood sample would have an upper level of 140 mg/dL. Values between 140 and 199 mg/dL are indicative of impaired glucose tolerance or prediabetes. In the absence of unequivocal hyperglycemia, these criteria should be confirmed by repeat testing on a different day (American Diabetes Association, 2005).

Clients may need to discontinue certain drugs for 3 days before the test. Also, a high-carbohydrate diet of 300 grams of carbohydrate per day should be followed for the same period. The client should be given written instructions explaining the pretest dietary requirements. An inadequate diet before the glucose tolerance test may diminish carbohydrate tolerance and cause high glucose levels, creating a false-positive result. During the test, the client should be instructed not to have anything by mouth except water. Tobacco, coffee, and tea can alter the test results.

URINE TESTS

For most people, when blood glucose reaches 180 to 200 mg/100 mL, the kidneys begin to spill glucose into the urine. This point of spillage is called the **renal threshold.**

At one time, this test was assumed to reflect the glucose content of the blood, but the renal threshold varies from individual to individual. The renal threshold may also change in a given individual with decreasing kidney function. Although urine tests are used as screening tests, they are less reliable than the blood glucose tests available for home use.

URINE ACETONE

As a consequence of the body's inability to metabolize glucose, fat is partially broken down for energy. The intermediate products of fat breakdown are ketone bodies. These ketone bodies build up in the blood because the quantity of fat being catabolized exceeds the body's capacity to process these intermediate products effectively. As this occurs, ketone bodies begin to spill into the urine. One of the ketone bodies is acetone, which can be measured in urine. The presence of acetone in the urine is called **ketonuria,** a sign that the diabetes is out of control. Clients are typically taught to test for urinary ketones if their blood glucose level exceeds 240 mg/dL. When a client exhibits ketonuria, the physician and diabetes educator should be consulted for changes in the diet prescription or insulin dosage.

GLYCOSYLATED HEMOGLOBIN (A1C)

Glucose attaches to the hemoglobin molecule in a one-way reaction throughout the 120-day life of the red blood cell. In a high-glucose environment, a greater percentage of the hemoglobin is glycosylated. This blood test is performed on a random blood sample; the client does not have to fast. The result is not influenced by exercise or diabetic drugs. For good glycemic control, the AIC should be <7 (referenced to a nondiabetic range of 4.0% to 6.0% using a DCCT-based assay).

Because the **glycosylated hemoglobin** value reflects the average blood glucose level for the preceding 2 to 3 months, it is a good test of the effectiveness of long-term therapy. A client cannot follow the prescribed regimen for just a few days before a doctor's visit and claim otherwise. Glycosylated hemoglobin will be 4 to 8% of the total hemoglobin in adults without diabetes. In clients with diabetes, a value of 7% indicates good control of the disease, and greater than 8% is considered high.

An A1C is recommended at least two times a year for people in good control and more often if the 1cHbA is greater than 8% or when the treatment plan changes.

Classification

Diabetes has two major forms: **type 1 and type 2** (note the Arabic numerals). The American Diabetes Association recommends three additional categories to classify diabetes: secondary diabetes, prediabetes, and gestational diabetes.

Type 1

Type 1 diabetes has also been called **insulin-dependent diabetes mellitus (IDDM),** juvenile-onset diabetes, and type I diabetes. Clients with this disorder cannot survive without daily doses of insulin because the pancreas does not produce sufficient insulin for glucose uptake. This situation results in elevated blood glucose. After treatment starts, clients on medications that lower their blood glucose levels may have problems with too low a blood glucose level. These variations in blood glucose levels make clients prone to two conditions.

1. The first condition is **ketoacidosis.** The signs of ketoacidosis are hyperglycemia and excessive ketones. Ketoacidosis is discussed later in this chapter.

2. The second condition is **hypoglycemia,** or a low blood glucose level.

Type 1 diabetes can occur at any age, although its usual onset is during childhood. Five to 10% of people with diabetes have type 1. The onset of this disorder is usually abrupt, and the condition is difficult to control.

Type 2

Type 2 diabetes has also been called **non–insulin-dependent diabetes mellitus (NIDDM),** adult-onset diabetes, and type II diabetes. Persons with type 2 are not insulin dependent or prone to ketoacidosis. However, some of them do use insulin because of persistent hyperglycemia. Also, insulin is the preferred medication to treat persons with type 2 diabetes. Clients with type 2 diabetes can manufacture some insulin but do not make enough or cannot use insulin efficiently. Typically, the non–insulin-dependent diabetic client develops his or her condition after age 45. See Genomic Gem 17-1. Most of these clients are obese, and weight reduction usually improves their ability to process glucose. Ninety to 95% of people with diabetes in the United States have type 2. The prevalence is markedly increased among:

- Native Americans
- Native Hawaiians
- African Americans
- Hispanic Americans
- Pacific Islanders

The onset of this disorder is gradual. The condition is usually easier to control than type 1. Table 17-1 summarizes the differences between types 1 and 2.

Most diabetes results from a primary failure of insulin production or use, but diabetes can occur as a result of a variety of disorders, including:

- Pancreatitis
- Cystic fibrosis
- Surgical removal of the pancreas
- Cushing's disease
- Pharmacological doses of glucocorticoids (e.g., prednisone) or other hormones or drugs.

The term **secondary diabetes** is sometimes used when one of these disorders is responsible for hyperglycemia. The diabetes may be resolved if the cause is alleviated. If the cause is not correctable, secondary diabetes is treated similarly to other forms of diabetes.

PREDIABETES

Impaired glucose tolerance (IGT) and impaired fasting glucose (IFG) refer to a metabolic state intermediate between normal with glucose homeostasis and diabetes. The American Diabetes Association encourages the use of the term prediabetes. Individuals who have a fasting glucose level of greater than 100 mg/dL but less than 126 mg/dL on more than two occasions meet the criteria for IGT or IFG. IGT may represent a step in the development of types 1 and 2 diabetes. In fact, 25% of clients with IGT later develop diabetes mellitus.

GESTATIONAL DIABETES

Gestational diabetes (GDM) is glucose intolerance in pregnancy. Women who are diagnosed as diabetic before pregnancy are not classified as having gestational

Genomic Gem 17-1

Maturity-Onset Diabetes in the Young

Maturity-onset diabetes in the young (MODY) is a term used to describe a diabetes disorder that is found in clients younger than 25 years old. This condition is genetic. A parent with MODY has a 50% chance of passing on MODY to his or her children. Clients with MODY do not always need insulin treatment and often can be treated with oral agents and a weight-reduction diet

TABLE 17-1 ■ Insulin-Dependent and Non–Insulin-Dependent Diabetes Mellitus

	TYPE 1	TYPE 2
Cause	Beta cells damaged	Tissues resist insulin
Most Common Age at Onset	Younger than 20 years	Older than 45 years
Medication	1. Insulin injections OR 2. Insulin injections and oral agents 3. Insulin drip during critical illness	1. None OR 2. Oral agents OR 3. Some individuals may require insulin injections to attain optimal blood glucose levels. 4. Insulin drip during critical illness
Usual Body Build	Thin, underweight	Obese
Nutrition Therapy	Integration of insulin therapy, activity, and food intake Consistent timing of food intake	Achievement of near-normal glucose, lipid, and blood pressure goals Weight loss is desirable and possible with some clients.

diabetes. Clinical Application 17-2 discusses diabetes mellitus in pregnancy. A fasting plasma glucose level of greater than 126 mg/dL or a casual plasma glucose greater than 200 mg/dL meets the criteria for a diagnosis of diabetes (American Diabetes Association, 2008). The condition usually disappears after childbirth. However, women who have had gestational diabetes have a 40 to 60% chance of developing type 2 diabetes in the next 5 to 10 years (CDC, 2008).

Functions of Insulin

Every cell in the human body depends somewhat on glucose to meet energy needs. The brain and the rest of the nervous system depend almost exclusively on glucose for energy. Normally blood glucose levels decrease and increase within a given range pre- and post-feeding. Levels are lower before eating and higher after eating. Insulin is the only hormone that lowers blood glucose. A person normally secretes insulin in response to an elevated blood glucose level. Insulin decreases blood glucose by accelerating its movement from the blood into the cells. As glucose enters the cells, it may be metabolized to yield energy, may be stored as glycogen, or may be converted to fat (Table 17-2).

The ultimate fate of glucose once it is inside the cell depends on the body's need and the amount of glucose that enters the cell. The cells' energy needs will be met first. If cells have available glucose over and above immediate energy needs, the excess glucose is stored as glycogen. Insulin stimulates the storage of

Clinical Application 17-2

Diabetes in Pregnancy

Pregnancy raises blood insulin levels in all women. It is an adaptive mechanism. Early in pregnancy, the woman's body cells store energy. Later, the woman's tissues become insulin resistant so that the fetus can draw on energy stores when the woman is fasting.

When the pregnant woman has or develops hyperglycemia, the mother's blood glucose crosses the placenta but her insulin does not. Then the fetus produces more insulin, which increases his or her fat deposition. Women with diabetes have large babies for this reason.

Perinatal mortality of infants born to women with diabetes is higher than that of infants of women who do not have diabetes. Ketosis in early pregnancy can produce congenital malformations, central nervous system disorders, and low intelligence. With strict control of the diabetes, however, 97% of the fetuses survive, compared with 98 to 99% born to women without diabetes.

Insulin resistance is greater in the morning in pregnant women. For this reason, usually only 39 grams of CHO are planned for the breakfast meal. There is a heightened tendency for maternal ketosis during fasting, and the possible adverse effects of ketones on the fetus suggest that periods of fasting during pregnancy should be avoided. Small, frequent feedings throughout the day are recommended. A bedtime snack that contains between 15 and 45 grams of CHO is recommended to minimize an accelerated production of ketones, which has been known to occur during sleeping. Clients should be reminded not to skip meals. Following is a summary of these recommendations:

- Breakfast: 30 grams of CHO
- Lunch and dinner: 60 grams of CHO
- Snacks: between 15 and 45 grams of CHO (dependent on the client's energy allowance based on individual assessment)
- Recommend bedtime snack for all clients
- Include protein and fat at each meal (amount dependent on client's energy allowance based on individual assessment)

Nutritional regulation is central to management of diabetes in pregnant women. During pregnancy, the most commonly recommended kilocalorie distribution is 40% to 45% carbohydrate, 20% to 25% protein, and 30% to 40% fat. The treatment goal is to prevent hypoglycemia, defined as fasting plasma concentrations of 65 to 90 mg/dL and 2-hour postprandial plasma glucose levels of less than 140 mg/dL. Some medical experts believe that this goal is too rigid because hypoglycemia during early pregnancy may be **teratogenic** (causing abnormal development of the embryo). Hypoglycemic agents have been shown to cause significant risk to the fetus. In most instances, women are advised to discontinue use of hypoglycemic agents before conception. If medication is necessary to control hyperglycemia, insulin is safer for the fetus.

Early pregnancy loss and congenital malformations can be minimized by optimal medical care and client education before conception. Contraception, timing of conception, control of metabolic state, self-management techniques, assessment of diabetic complications, and other medical complications should be discussed with clients of child-bearing age. The desired outcome of glycemia control in preconception is to lower glycohemoglobin to achieve maximum fertility and optimal embryo and fetal development (American Diabetes Association, 1996a). Preconception counseling is best accomplished by a multidisciplinary approach including an endocrinologist; internist or family practice physician; obstetrician; and diabetes educators, including nurses, registered dietitians, social workers, and other specialists as necessary. Self-management skills essential for control during pregnancy include (Position Paper of the American Dietetic Association, 1996a):

- Using an appropriate meal plan
- Timing of meals and snacks
- Planning physical activity
- Choosing time and site of insulin injections
- Using carbohydrate and glucagon for hypoglycemia
- Reducing stress, coping with denial
- Testing capillary blood glucose
- Self-adjusting insulin doses

TABLE 17-2 ■ Metabolic Activities Promoted by Insulin

ACTIVITY	METABOLIC PATHWAY
Movement of glucose into cells	None
Energy production from glucose	Glycolysis
Manufacture of glycogen	Glycogenesis
Fat formation from carbohydrate and protein	Lipogenesis

Note: "Genesis" means building up.

TABLE 17-3 ■ Metabolic Activities Inhibited by a High Level of Insulin

ACTIVITY	METABOLIC PATHWAY
Movement of glucose from noncarbohydrate sources, e.g., glycerol and amino acids	Gluconeogenesis
Release of glucose from glycogen	Glycogenolysis
Breakdown of fat from adipose tissue	Lipolysis

glucose as glycogen. Once the glycogen stores are filled to capacity, any remaining glucose is converted to fat. The body can store about 0.4 pound of glycogen, which is equal to 800 kilocalories.

Insulin influences the metabolism of protein and fat, and stimulates entry of amino acids into cells and enhances protein formation. It also enhances fat storage in adipose tissue and indirectly inhibits the breakdown of fat for energy. If the body has ample glucose available for energy, protein and fat need not be broken down to meet energy needs. If the body does not have glucose available for energy, it will use dietary protein or break down internal body protein stores to meet its immediate need for energy.

Insulin levels fluctuate in the blood. Normally, blood insulin levels increase as the blood glucose level increases. A high level of insulin in the blood signals the cells not to break down stores for energy (Table 17-3). An anabolic, or building, state exists when metabolism is normal and glucose and insulin levels are high. Normally insulin levels decrease as the blood sugar level decreases. A low level of insulin in the blood indirectly signals the body to begin to break down body stores for glucose. Figure 17-1 illustrates glucose use by the cells.

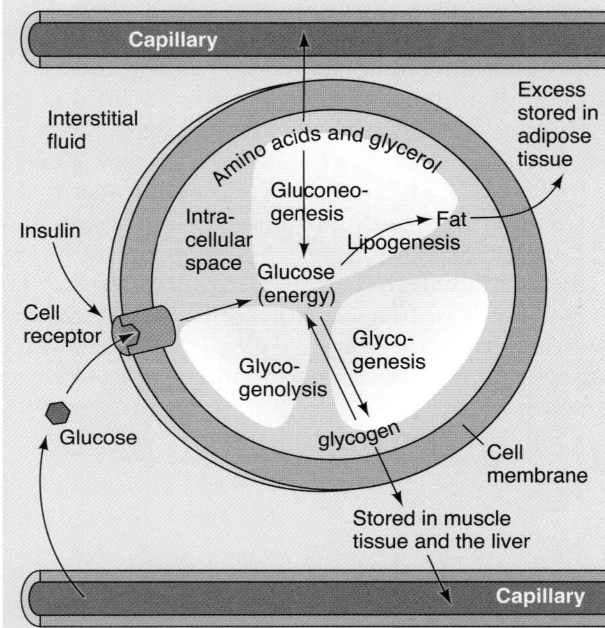

FIGURE 17-1 Insulin is necessary for glucose to gain entry into a cell. Once inside the cell, glucose can meet several fates: it can be burned as energy or stored as glycogen, or the glycerol portion of a fat molecule or some amino acids can be broken down into glucose. Some amino acids will be converted to glucose if the cell requires glucose.

Other Hormones

Glucagon and somatostatin assist in coordinating the storage and mobilization of the energy nutrients: carbohydrate, fat, and protein. Glucagon increases blood glucose levels and stimulates the breakdown of body protein and fat stores. Somatostatin acts locally within the islets of Langerhans to depress the secretion of insulin and glucagon. Evidence has shown that these hormones may not be at optimal levels in some clients with diabetes.

Cellular Sources of Glucose

Cells obtain glucose from both food that is eaten and internal glucose stores. Almost all carbohydrate eaten (except fiber), about 50% of protein eaten, and about 10% of fat eaten enter the blood as glucose. The internal body stores that can be converted to glucose are glycogen, some protein, and the glycerol portion of triglycerides. Body fat is stored as triglycerides in adipose tissue. To understand diabetes, it is necessary to know how the body coordinates all internal and external sources of glucose to maintain a normal blood glucose range.

Blood Glucose Curve

Given the vital need for every cell to have an uninterrupted supply of energy, the human body has evolved to allow an uninterrupted energy supply to reach cells without continuous eating. The blood glucose level increases after eating and decreases in the fasting state. Figure 17-2 illustrates the normal blood glucose curve.

Causes of Diabetes

The causes of diabetes include genetic factors, lifestyle, and viral infections. Some susceptibility to diabetes is genetic. However, not everyone with susceptible genes develops clinical diabetes. Before diabetes becomes apparent, this genetic susceptibility is often triggered by the individual's lifestyle or other environmental factors. A healthy lifestyle is particularly important for the *prevention* of diabetes in genetically susceptible clients. Excessive body fat, inactivity, and stress are risk factors for type 2 diabetes. A loss of body fat alone is sometimes sufficient to balance the insulin produced with a modified food intake. Sometimes emotional or physical stress is the stimulus that causes hyperglycemia. The body's stress response involves the release of epinephrine from the adrenal glands. One action of epinephrine is to raise the blood sugar level so the person has energy for the "fight or flight" response. See Genomic Gem 17-2.

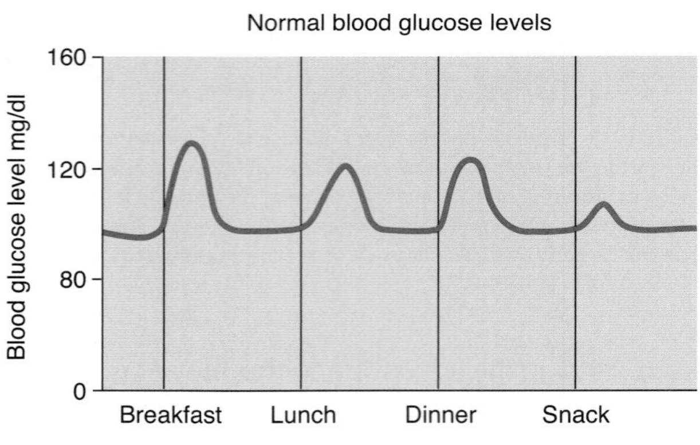

FIGURE 17-2 A person's blood glucose level normally goes up after food consumption and then down between feedings.

> **Genomic Gem 17-2**
> **Causal Connection**
>
> Links have been noted between viral epidemics and the onset of diabetes. This adds credence to the concept that a causal connection exists between viral epidemics and the onset of type 1 diabetes.

Signs and Symptoms

The classic triad of signs and symptoms includes:

1. **Polyuria** (increased urination)
2. **Polydipsia** (increased thirst)
3. **Polyphagia** (increased appetite and weight loss)

The triad is most commonly seen in type 1 diabetes. The following section describes these and other signs and symptoms commonly seen in persons with diabetes.

Classic Triad

In diabetes, glucose cannot optimally move from the intravascular space across a cell membrane into the intracellular space. This is why the diabetic person's blood glucose level remains elevated after eating. Under normal circumstances, the blood glucose level does not increase excessively because excess glucose undergoes glycolysis and is readily converted to adipose tissue or stored as glycogen inside the cell. As the glucose-rich blood circulates through the kidneys, these organs reabsorb as much glucose as they can. After this point is reached, glucose enters the urine. **Glycosuria** means an abnormally high amount of glucose in the urine. As the glucose exits the body in urine, water is pulled out also, as a result of the osmotic effect of glucose. This results in polyuria, or a large urine output. The large loss of water causes excessive thirst and polydipsia and prompts the person to drink fluids.

When glucose is not available for energy inside the cells, the body begins to break down protein and fat for energy. In untreated type 1 diabetes, the body's cells are starving. These starving cells send a message to the brain to turn on the person's appetite. The person responds by eating to satisfy the craving for food. The third symptom or sign of diabetes is **polyphagia**, an abnormal increase in appetite.

Other Signs and Symptoms

The abnormal carbohydrate metabolism of diabetes and its effects on the body's tissues cause other problems. Weight loss is more commonly seen in clients with type 1 diabetes than in clients with type 2. Clients with both types of diabetes may show these signs and symptoms:

- Blurred vision
- Fatigue
- Infection
- **Vaginitis** (inflammation of the vagina)
- Bladder infections

- Poor wound healing
- Impotence in men
- Kidney disorders

Complications

Both acute and chronic complications occur with diabetes mellitus. Acute complications require immediate care. Chronic complications include diseases of the eye, kidneys, heart, and nervous system. Chronic complications are responsible for the increased death rate among individuals with diabetes and the diminished quality of life that many of these clients experience.

Acute Clinical Situations

Three acute complications are seen in clients with diabetes:

1. **Diabetic ketoacidosis (DKA)**
2. Hyperglycemic hyperosmolar nonketotic syndrome
3. **Hypoglycemia**

Ketoacidosis

Individuals with type 1 diabetes who experience a profound insulin deficiency may progress to ketoacidosis. The three main precipitating factors in ketoacidosis are:

1. A decreased or missed dose of insulin
2. An illness or infection
3. Uncontrolled disease in a previously undiagnosed person

Ketoacidosis is a complex, life-threatening condition that demands emergency treatment. The predominant clinical manifestations and general principles of treatment are discussed next.

DEHYDRATION

Without insulin, glucose cannot be transferred across the cell membranes into the cells. A greatly increased number of glucose molecules (300 to 800 mg/dL) in the blood exert an osmotic effect, causing water to move from within the cells to the intravascular space and producing cellular dehydration. The body excretes the excess water, glucose, and electrolytes in urine.

ACIDOSIS

Unaware that the problem is not lack of glucose but lack of insulin, the body proceeds to increase blood glucose by mobilizing protein and fat from the tissues to be converted to glucose by the liver. Because the human body can use only the glycerol portion of the triglyceride molecule for glucose, the fatty acid portion is processed into ketones. Normally ketones are metabolized and excreted as carbon dioxide and water.

Under conditions of ketoacidosis, however, the body cannot metabolize this overload of ketones rapidly enough to maintain homeostasis, and thus the client has excessive ketones in the blood (ketonemia) and spills ketones into the urine (ketonuria). Acetone is one of the ketone bodies for which urine is tested. The ketone bodies are acid, and thus the term ketoacidosis.

Electrolyte Imbalances

Clients with severe ketoacidosis may excrete 6.5 liters of fluid and 400 to 500 milliequivalents of sodium, potassium, and chloride in 24 hours. A fluid loss of 15% of body weight is not unusual. Most critical in the treatment of electrolyte imbalances in diabetic ketoacidosis is the body's level of potassium. As the cells are being catabolized for fuel, the intracellular potassium is transferred to the intravascular space.

Serum potassium levels can be low, normal, or elevated in the person with ketoacidosis, depending on the body's current coping mechanism. Regardless of the serum concentrations of potassium and sodium, the pathological process of diabetic ketoacidosis depletes these electrolytes. Either hypokalemia or hyperkalemia can lead to cardiac arrhythmias and must be carefully managed in clients with ketoacidosis.

Treatment

Clients with severe diabetic ketoacidosis are critically ill. Treatment includes supplemental insulin, fluid and electrolyte replacement, and medical monitoring. Serum electrolyte levels change dramatically once treatment commences. Intensive care is necessary to provide the careful monitoring and frequent adjustments in therapy required as the fluids and electrolytes are being replaced. Intravenous regular insulin will permit the use of carbohydrate for energy and will halt the body's excessive use of fat, which has produced the ketone bodies. Insulin drives glucose back into the cells. Potassium, too, moves from the intravascular space to the intracellular space, necessitating frequent measurement of the serum levels of both glucose and potassium. When the client recovers, identification of the precipitating factor for the ketoacidosis and education focused on preventing additional occurrences are essential.

Hyperglycemic Hyperosmolar Nonketotic Syndrome

The four signs of **hyperglycemic hyperosmolar nonketotic syndrome (HHNS)** are:

1. Blood glucose level >600 mg/dL
2. Absence of or slight ketosis
3. Plasma hyperosmolality
4. Profound dehydration

This life-threatening emergency is usually seen in people with undiagnosed type 2 diabetes. HHNS is like DKA except that the insulin deficiency is not as severe, so increased **lipolysis** (the breakdown of body lipid stores) does not occur. Because these clients do not have symptoms of vomiting, nausea, and acidosis brought on by severe ketosis, as do clients with type 1 diabetes, they often do not seek prompt medical help. Their blood sugar levels are higher and their dehydration more severe than is seen in ketoacidosis.

In these clients, prolonged osmotic diuresis and dehydration secondary to hyperglycemia lead to decreased renal blood flow and allow blood glucose to reach very high levels. Medications that cause an increase in blood glucose levels, chronic disease, and infection may contribute to this condition. Treatment includes correction of the electrolyte imbalance, hyperglycemia, and dehydration.

Hypoglycemia

In both type 1 and type 2 diabetes, an individual can develop hypoglycemia. Hypoglycemia in type 2 diabetes is typically related to improper medication dosing. Hypoglycemia may be caused by:

- Too much insulin (accidental or deliberate),
- Too little food intake, a delayed meal,
- Excessive exercise,
- Alcohol (especially in the fasting state), and
- Medications such as oral hypoglycemic agents.

Symptoms may include:

- Confusion
- Headache
- Double vision
- Rapid heartbeat
- Sweating
- Hunger
- Seizure
- Coma

The treatment of hypoglycemia is discussed later in this chapter.

Chronic Complications

Clients with both type 1 and type 2 diabetes of sufficient duration are vulnerable to serious complications involving the eyes, kidneys, and nervous system.

Diabetic **retinopathy** is a disorder that involves the retina. Diabetes is a leading cause of blindness and of vision loss in the adult U.S. population. The blurred vision reported by these clients is related to retinopathy. These clients are also at a higher risk for cataracts.

Diabetic **neuropathy** is a chronic complication of diabetes mellitus. Clients may complain of a lack of sensation in their extremities. They may puncture, cut, or burn their feet and not feel any pain. A wound may become infected and heal poorly. Gangrene, or tissue death, may follow. The treatment for gangrene is amputation. **Neuropathy** can affect gastric or intestinal motility, erectile function, bladder function, cardiac function, and vascular tone.

Gastroparesis (paralysis of the stomach with delayed gastric emptying) may occur and alter the absorption of meals, which makes glycemic control problematic.

Cardiovascular disease is more common in clients with diabetes than in the non-diabetic population of the same age and gender. This is related in general to the fact that diabetes is a small vessel disease and the critical end arteries in the heart muscle are small vessels.

Diabetic **nephropathy,** or kidney disease, is another common complication in diabetic clients.

Tragically, some clients with diabetes do not take the threat of chronic complications seriously until much damage has occurred.

Treatment

The current medical goal is to *normalize* blood glucose throughout the day and to control blood pressure and blood lipids. A normal fasting blood glucose level is about 100 mg/dL before a meal and less than 140 mg/dL 2 hours after a meal. Realistic target levels for individuals with diabetes treated intensively are 70 to 140 mg/dL before meals, less than 180 mg/dL 2 hours after meals, and glycosylated hemoglobin within 1% of normal. A landmark study known as the Diabetes Control and Complications Trial (DCCT) in individuals with IDDM demonstrated that intensive control of blood glucose levels delays the onset and slows the progression of diabetic retinopathy, nephropathy, and neuropathy (Diabetes Control and Complications Trial Research Group, 1993). According to this study's results, people with type 1 diabetes who followed a tightly controlled regimen, compared with those who followed a standard regimen, showed reductions of approximately:

- 76% in progression of diabetic retinopathy
- 54% in albuminuria (albumin in the urine, which may be a sign of renal impairment)
- 36% in **microalbuminuria** (a more sensitive indicator of protein in the urine, which may be an early warning of renal impairment)

A tightly controlled regimen is not without problems, however. Among these is an increased incidence of insulin-induced hypoglycemic episodes. Clients undergoing intensive diabetes treatment do not face deterioration in the quality of their lives, even while the rigor of their diabetes care is increased (Diabetes Control and Complication Trial Research Group, 1996). This evidence has been further strengthened by a report from the United Kingdom Prospective Diabetes Study (UKPDS), which demonstrated that intensive therapy for type 2 diabetes significantly lowered the rate of diabetes-related events (UK Prospective Diabetes Study Group, 1998).

All health-care workers should assist the general population in the early detection of diabetes and prevention of complications. As Figure 17-3 emphasizes, the three cornerstones of the management of diabetes after diagnosis are:

1. Physical activity
2. Medication
3. Nutritional management

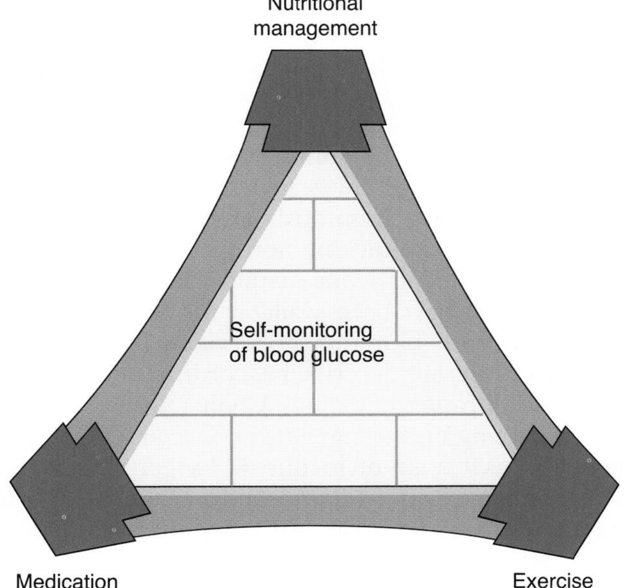

FIGURE 17-3 Nutritional management, medication, and exercise are the three components of treatment for diabetes. Each of these cornerstones has an influence on blood glucose levels. An individual can identify how each of these cornerstones impacts his or her blood glucose level by self-monitoring blood glucose.

Self-monitoring of blood glucose levels enables the client to assess how each of these factors interacts.

Self-Monitoring of Blood Glucose

Many individuals monitor their own blood glucose levels with a blood glucose meter. This procedure is called **self-monitoring of blood glucose (SMBG).** Individual response to medication, diet, and exercise can be determined with SMBG and can be performed using a single drop of blood. The client obtains the drop of blood from a finger with either a lancet or a spring-loaded device. The blood sample is placed in the meter, and the test results are available in less than 1 minute. The client can then adjust insulin dose and food and exercise behaviors accordingly. Many experts consider SMBG to be the most important development in diabetes management since the discovery of insulin. SMBG can also be done with a newer device that is easier to use because it does not require a skin prick and a drop of blood.

SMBG has allowed clients to try to normalize their blood glucose levels throughout the day. Health-care workers need to teach clients carefully how to interpret the results of SMBG. Continual reassessment of the client's technique and blood glucose records is necessary to guide treatment decisions. To evaluate the need for changes in diet or medications initially, monitoring should be done at least twice a day; four times a day for 3 days each week is preferable for clients who are stable. If near-normalization of blood glucose is the treatment goal, SMBG should be initially recommended four to eight times daily (before and 2 hours after each meal or snack). During acute illness, frequent self-monitoring is especially indicated. Once the blood glucose is stabilized, SMBG can be done less frequently.

Physical Activity

Exercise plays a key role in the management of diabetes. All individuals with diabetes who exercise should be encouraged to follow these guidelines:

1. Wear proper footwear, and use other protective equipment if necessary.
2. Avoid exercise in extremely hot or cold environments.
3. Inspect feet daily and after exercise for open areas, blisters, punctures, swelling, and redness; report any of these signs to the physician immediately.
4. Avoid exercise during periods of poor metabolic control (blood glucose levels that are <60 or >240 mg/dL levels).

5. Wear a diabetes ID badge or bracelet.
6. Carry a source of glucose in case of a decrease in blood glucose because exercise decreases blood glucose levels.

Exercise and Type 1 Diabetes

The American Diabetes Association strongly endorses an exercise program for people with type 1 diabetes because of the potential for improving cardiovascular fitness and psychological well-being. Exercise involves some risk for individuals with type 1 diabetes because it changes insulin requirements in sometimes unpredictable ways for more than 24 hours after the exercise. Retinopathy, neuropathy, and renal disease may worsen in some clients with type 1 diabetes who exercise. Blood pressure may also become elevated. For this type of client, self-monitoring of blood glucose should be incorporated into a modified exercise program tailored to individual needs and limitations. The client should demonstrate the ability to self-treat a hypoglycemic episode.

Exercise and Type 2 Diabetes

Physical activity is widely endorsed for persons with type 2 diabetes. Physical activity increases the number and binding capacity of insulin receptors, assists in lowering blood glucose levels, and reduces insulin requirements in persons who use insulin. Improved blood lipid levels occur in some clients who engage in regular exercise. This improvement helps delay or prevent the cardiovascular disease complications commonly seen in these clients. Exercise also assists in weight control and improves muscle strength and flexibility.

Exercise, SMBG, and Food Intake

Type 1 clients with diabetes who do exercise and all type 2 clients who engage in nonroutine exercise should monitor their blood glucose levels before, during, and after exercise. It is best to exercise 60 to 90 minutes after meals, when the blood glucose level is highest. If the blood glucose level is greater than 100 mg/dL before exercise, no additional food is usually needed if the planned exercise is of short duration and low intensity. Exercise of long duration and high intensity generally requires more kilocalories. Snacks that contain an additional 15 to 30 grams of carbohydrate-containing food should be ingested for every 30 to 60 minutes of exercise. Good choices for snack foods include:

- Fruit
- Starch
- Milk exchanges

To prevent wide swings in blood glucose levels, care should be taken not to overeat. Too much food will cause the blood glucose level to go up too high and subsequently to drop too low.

Medications for Diabetes

Two types of medications are used with diabetic clients:

1. Insulin
2. Oral hypoglycemic agents

Clients with type 1 diabetes require insulin. Clients with type 2 diabetes may not require any medication or may need to have an oral hypoglycemic agent or insulin prescribed. Frequently, clients with type 2 diabetes are able to discontinue the medication after a loss of body fat.

Insulin

Almost all the insulin used in the United States is human. Human insulin is manufactured by recombinant-DNA technology (biosynthetic). Human insulin **(Humulin)** produces few allergic reactions. Insulin cannot be taken orally because the gastrointestinal tract enzymes will digest it before absorption. Insulin must be administered by needle either **subcutaneously** (beneath the skin) or intravenously (IV). Only regular insulin is given IV. The substances used to delay absorption of intermediate- and long-acting insulins are not designed for IV administration. Regular insulin is usually administered IV only for the severely hyperglycemic or hospitalized client.

Insulin can also be administered with an insulin pump. These pumps are designed to provide a small inflow of insulin continuously and large inflows before eating, thus mimicking normal insulin secretion. Continuous subcutaneous insulin infusion (CSII) or insulin pumps have been available for nearly 25 years, but only recently have they been widely used.

Medications are described according to the onset, peak, and duration of action. A bolus dose of insulin is short acting and designed to cover needs for one meal. A basal dose of insulin is longer acting and usually injected once or twice a day. Table 17-4 lists the times of onset, peak, and duration of insulin. Variation in duration makes it possible to inject insulin in a pattern that is as close as possible to normal insulin activity. Ideally, the medication is planned around the diet, not vice versa. Most experts know that it is far easier to change a medication than a food behavior.

Oral Hypoglycemic Agents

Oral hypoglycemic agents lower blood glucose levels in type 2 diabetes. These drugs stimulate insulin release from the pancreatic beta cells, reduce glucose output from the liver, and increase the uptake of glucose in tissues. Many new oral agents are being prescribed in the United States, and many more are in development (Table 17-5). Recently, oral agents and insulin administered simultaneously have been used successfully to treat type 1 diabetes. Commonly prescribed oral hypoglycemic agents include glipizide, glyburide, glimepiride, metformin, acarbose, and tolazamide. Oral agents are used in combinations. Many of the oral agents work on different cell receptor sites. For example, metformin and acarbose can be added to sulfonylurea (e.g., glimepiride, glyburide) with an additional 0.5 to 2% reduction in HbA1C level (Zimmerman and Hagan, 1998).

TABLE 17-4 ■ Times of Onset, Peak, and Duration of Action for Insulins

	TIMES IN HOURS		
	Onset	Peak	Duration
Insulin Bolus (Short Acting)			
Humalog	5–15 minutes	1–2 hours	3½–5 hours
NovoLog	10–20 minutes	1–3 hours	3–5 hours
Regular	30–60 minutes	2–4 hours	6–8 hours
Basal (qd) Not Tx Intensively (2 x qd)			
Lantus*	1 hour	None	24 hours
NPH	1–1½ hours	4–10 hours	14–18 hours
70/30†	½ hour	2–3 hours and 4–10 hours	14–18 hours
Lente	1¼ hours	7–15 hours	24 hours
Ultralente	4–6 hours	10–16 hours	>36 hours

*Lantus is a long-acting insulin that is designed to be given at HS (Latin for hour of sleep and is commonly used to mean just before bedtime). Lantus has no pronounced peaks, with a relatively constant level over 24 hours. The FDA approved Lantus in early 2000.

†Mixture is 70% NPH and 30% regular.

Medical Nutritional Management of Diabetes

Diabetes is directly related to how the body uses food. Nutrition is thus an essential component of management for all persons with diabetes. Studies have shown that clients report improved health; better control of body weight; improved control of blood glucose, blood pressure, and lipid levels; and improved use of insulin when they adhere to dietary recommendations. The goals of nutritional care for persons with diabetes are the control and prevention of complications. This involves the promotion of normal nutrition and dietary modification to control blood glucose and lipid levels. Clients' nutritional goals need to be determined individually. There is **no** "diabetic diet" or "ADA diet," but several meal-planning approaches are widely endorsed by the American Diabetes Association and the American Dietetic Association. See Dollars & Sense 17-1.

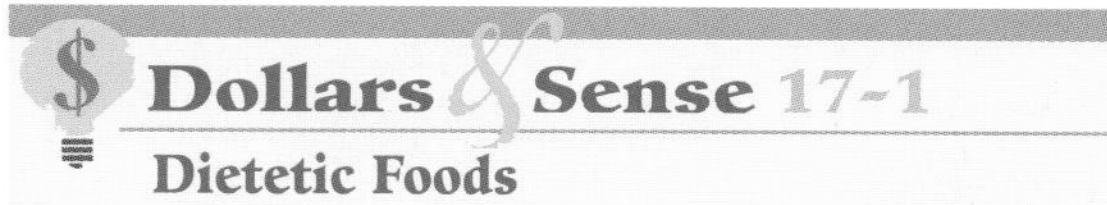

Dietetic Foods

Clients with diabetes do not need to buy special foods labeled "dietetic." Many clients find they actually save money because they eat less food on the prescribed meal plan.

TABLE 17-5 ■ Diabetes Oral Medications and Major Actions

CLASSIFICATION	MAJOR ACTIONS	GENERIC NAME (TRADE NAME)	COMMENTS
Sulfonylureas	Stimulate insulin release by the pancreas and may help decrease liver glucose production.	Glipizide (Glucotrol, Glucotrol XL) Glyburide (DiaBeta, Micronase, Glynase PresTabs) Glimepiride (Amaryl)	Glipizide must be taken on an empty stomach. Glyburide can be taken with food or on an empty stomach. Low toxicity. Use caution with elderly.
Biguanides	Decrease liver production of glucose. Increase glucose uptake into tissues.	Metformin (Glucophage)	Given in 2–3 doses per day with meals. Not metabolized.
Often used in Combination with Sulfonylureas Meglitinide	Stimulates immediate insulin release from pancreas as needed for meals.	Repaglinide (Prandin) Nateglinide (Starlix)	Given in 2–4 doses per day 15–30 minutes before meals.
Alpha-Glucosidase Inhibitors	Slow the rate of digestion of starches and complex sugars.	Acarbose (Precose)	Given in 3 doses per day with meals. 98% not absorbed. Rest excreted by kidneys.
Thiazolidinedione	Decreases insulin resistance.	Pioglitazone (Actos) Rosiglitazone (Avandia)	Clients need to be monitored for fluid retention and weight gain.

Nutritional Goals

The goal of medical nutritional therapy is to educate the client with diabetes so he or she can make changes in food and exercise habits that lead to improved metabolic control. Specifically, the client needs assistance with:

1. Attaining and maintaining near-normal blood glucose levels as feasible by the coordination of food intake, **endogenous** and **exogenous** insulin and/or hypoglycemic agents, and physical activity. This goal is a challenge in some clients who have fluctuating endogenous insulin production.
2. Attaining and maintaining optimal serum lipid levels and blood pressure
3. Providing adequate kilocalories to:
   - Attain and maintain a healthy body weight for adults and normal growth and development for children
   - Recover from illnesses
   - Meet the metabolic needs of pregnancy and lactation
4. Preventing and treating the acute and chronic complications of diabetes, such as renal disease, autonomic neuropathy, hypertension, and cardiovascular disease
5. Improving overall health through good nutrition. *MyPyramid, USDA Food Guide,* and *Dietary Guidelines for Americans* illustrate and summarize nutritional guidelines for all Americans, including people with diabetes.

Goal Priority

The medications prescribed, the type of diabetes the individual has, and the client's desire to change behavior determine goal priority. A high priority for the person taking insulin is to facilitate consistency in the timing of meals and snacks to prevent wide swings in blood glucose. This priority requires coordination among exercise, insulin, and food intake.

A high priority for the individual with type 2 diabetes is achieving glucose, blood pressure, and lipid goals. To achieve these goals, diet is a cornerstone of treatment. Weight reduction for these clients usually improves short-term glycemic levels and long-term metabolic control. The client's motivation to lose weight needs to be carefully assessed by the health-care educator.

Meal Frequency

Meal spacing is more crucial in type 1 than in type 2 diabetes. Consistent timing and meal size assist in stabilization of blood glucose levels in type 1 diabetes. In general, people with diabetes benefit from eating on a regular basis (every 4 to 5 hours) while awake.

Client Readiness to Change

Food behaviors are difficult to change. Although some clients with diabetes do successfully change or alter food behaviors to enhance their outcomes, many clients do not, will not, or cannot change harmful food behaviors. Modification of harmful behaviors involves progression through five stages: precontemplation, contemplation, preparation, action, and maintenance. Individuals typically recycle through these stages several times before terminating negative behaviors. Following is a brief description of stage:

1. *Precontemplation:* Individuals exhibit no intention to change behavior in the foreseeable future.
2. *Contemplation:* Individuals know they have a problem and they are seriously thinking about overcoming the harmful behavior but are not ready to take action.
3. *Preparation:* Individuals plan to take action in the near future, may have taken action unsuccessfully in the past, and may report small behavioral changes.
4. *Action:* Individuals modify their behavior, experiences, and environment to overcome the harmful behavior. This stage requires considerable commitment of time and energy.
5. *Maintenance:* Individuals continue to work to prevent relapse and to consolidate gains.

Health-care workers can assist clients in the precontemplation and contemplation stages by attempting to raise patients' consciousness about the benefits of behavioral change. Stimulus control and reinforcement also help patients become more aware of the need to alter behaviors (see Weight Management). The most difficult problems posed by clients for the health educator are at the precontemplation phase (Jacobson, 1993).

The health-care educator needs to consider carefully how much information the client desires and how ready he or she is to change behaviors. For example, an educational tool that takes 3 to 4 hours to review with a client is inappropriate for someone who is willing to devote just a few minutes to learning about his or her diet. In contrast, the client who wants to learn everything he or she can about self-care will not be satisfied with an elementary meal plan.

Survival Skills

The American Diabetes and Dietetic Associations recommend that the newly diagnosed client initially learn basic survival skills. DavisPlus contains a copy of Survival Skills or information the client needs to know immediately. After the client has demonstrated an understanding of this basic knowledge, a firm foundation has been set for the acquisition of additional, more individualized information. Individualized food and meal plans and insulin regimens provide flexibility to accommodate lifestyle, age, and overall health status.

Meal-Planning Approaches

Several meal planning tools are available for use with the newly diagnosed client including:

- *MyPyramid*
- *Dietary Guidelines for Americans*
- *The USDA Food Guide*

Any of these meal-planning approaches is considered survival-skill information. After the client understands the initial meal-planning approach, a more advanced approach should be considered. Many hospitals and private practitioners provide more comprehensive educational programs to achieve optimal blood glucose and lipid control. Two of the more widely used, more advanced meal-planning systems are discussed next. Figure 17-4 illustrates a dietitian providing nutrition counseling.

Energy Nutrient Distribution

Total energy requirements for an individual with diabetes do not differ from those for individuals without diabetes. Twenty-five to 35 kcal/kg, depending on the client's level of physical activity, nutritional status, desire for weight loss or gain, and body weight are usually a good starting point to estimate a need for kcal. The only way to more accurately determine a client's need for energy is by indirect calorimetry and this equipment is not widely available. The second best method to determine energy needs is for the client to eat a set amount of kcal for a few weeks and compare body weight before and after the given kcal level is consumed. If weight loss is desirable, the rate of loss should be 1 to 2 pounds per week.

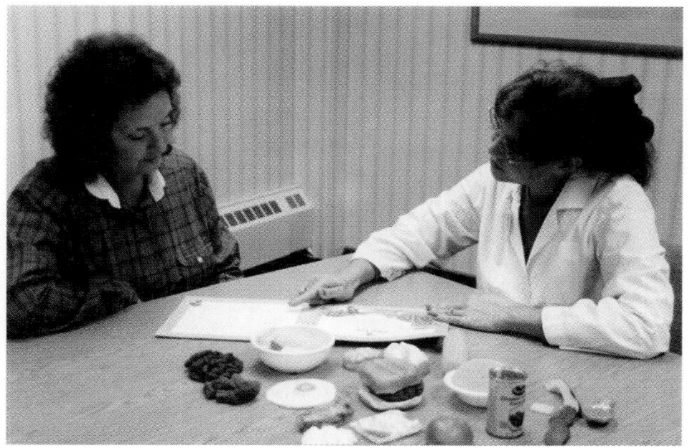

FIGURE 17-4 A diabetes educator providing nutritional counseling. The use of food models facilitates the learning process and teaches portion control.

The acceptable macronutrient distribution recommended for the general population is also recommended for clients with diabetes. The distribution of energy nutrients refers to the percentage of total kilocalories that should be derived from carbohydrate, fat, and protein as well as to the division of carbohydrate, fat, and protein among the day's meals/feedings. Clinical Calculation 17-1 shows how the percentage of energy nutrients is converted to grams of carbohydrate, fat, and protein and distributed throughout the day's meals/feedings.

Carbohydrate and Monounsaturated Fat

These two macronutrients are discussed together because they can to some extent be substituted for each other to supply energy. Carbohydrate and monounsaturated fat should ideally provide 60 to 70% of the total kilocalories. Dietary Guidelines for Americans recommends all people choose a variety of fiber-containing food, such as whole grains, fruits, and vegetables, because they provide vitamins, minerals, fiber, and other substances that optimize health. Considerations for a more definitive partitioning between carbohydrate and monounsaturated fat include:

- In weight-maintaining diets for type 2 clients with diabetes, replacing carbohydrate with monounsaturated fat reduces postprandial glycemia and triglyceridemia (Garg et al., 1994).
- Increased fat intake in ad libitum diets may promote weight gain and contribute to insulin resistance (Marshall, Bessesen, and Hamman, 1997).

The contribution of carbohydrate and monounsaturated fat to kilocalorie intake should be individualized based on nutrition assessment, laboratory results, and weight and treatment goals.

The American Diabetes Association published these general guidelines that pertain to carbohydrates (American Diabetes Association, 2008):

- A dietary pattern that includes CHO from fruits, vegetables, whole grains, legumes, and low-fat milk is encouraged for good health.
- Monitoring CHO, whether by carbohydrate-counting, exchanges, or experienced-based estimation, remains a good strategy in achieving glycemic control.
- The use of the glycemic index and load may provide a modest benefit over that observed when total CHO is considered alone.

Clinical Calculation 17-1

Distributing Energy Nutrients and Calculating a Diet

In the following example, an 1800-kcal diet is converted to 55% carbohydrate, 20% protein, and 25% fat.

1800 kcal × 0.55 = 990 kcal @ 4 kcal/gram = 248 grams of carbohydrate
1800 kcal × 0.20 = 360 kcal @ 4 kcal/gram = 90 grams of protein
1800 kcal × 0.25 = 450 kcal @ 9 kcal/gram = 50 grams of fat

In the following example, 248 grams of carbohydrate, 90 grams of protein, and 50 grams of fat are converted to a ⅕, ⅖, ⅕, and ⅕ distribution. Each fraction represents one meal; thus, ⅕ of the energy nutrients are to be provided each at breakfast, supper, and the evening snack; ⅖ of the energy nutrients are to be provided at the noon meal. Please note: ⅕ equals 20%, and ⅖ equals 40%.

248 grams of carbohydrate × 0.20 = 50 grams × 3 meals = 150
248 grams of carbohydrate × 0.20 = 99 grams × 1 meals = 99
90 grams of protein × 0.20 = 18 grams × 3 meals = 54
90 grams of carbohydrate × 0.40 = 36 grams × 1 meal = 36

Because only a small percentage of dietary fat enters the bloodstream as glucose, normally fat is not calculated into the distribution. Lunch (⅖ distribution) would contain about 99 grams of carbohydrate and 36 grams of protein. Each of the other meals (⅕ distribution) would contain about 50 grams of carbohydrate and 18 grams of protein.

The next step is to determine the number of exchanges to be provided from each of the six exchange groups. No exact method is used to determine this step. Usually the client is consulted to determine the amount of nonfat milk, fruits, vegetables, and so forth that he or she would be willing to consume. An effort should be made to calculate the diet with at least the recommended amount of food in the MyPyramid guide. Many health-care workers determine the amount of nonfat milk, fruits, and vegetables to be provided first. This calculation is followed by the grams of carbohydrate to be contributed by these groups. The remaining carbohydrate is then allocated to the starch group.

Protein is determined by first calculating the amount previously provided by nonfat milk, vegetables, and starches; the remaining protein is then allocated to meat exchanges. Fat is determined by first calculating the amount previously provided by the meat exchanges; the remaining fat is then allocated to fat exchanges. The calculations and meal plan for our sample 1800 kcal with 55% carbohydrate, 20% protein, and 25% fat with a ⅕, ⅖, ⅕, and ⅕ distribution appear in Table 17-6.

TABLE 17-6 ■ Sample 1800-Kilocalorie Diabetic Diet*

DIVISION OF ENERGY NUTRIENTS AND EXCHANGES

Exchange List	Number of Daily Exchanges	Protein (90 grams)	Fat (50 grams)	Carbohydrate (218 grams)	Breakfast	Lunch	Dinner	Bed-time
Skim milk	2	16	0	24	½	1		½
Starch	11	33	0	165	2	4	3	2
Fruit	3	0	0	45	1	1	0	1
Vegetable	3	6	0	15	0	2	1	0
Meat	5	35	25	0	1	2	1	1
Fat	5	0	25	0	1	1	2	1

MEAL PLAN AND SAMPLE MENUS

Meal Plan	Sample Menu 1	Sample Menu 2
Breakfast		
½ cup skim milk	½ cup skim milk	½ cup skim milk
2 starch	2 slices of toast	1 cup of oatmeal
1 fruit	½ cup orange juice	½ banana
1 meat	¼ cup low-cholesterol egg substitute	1 low-fat sausage link
1 fat	1 tsp margarine	2 pecans
Lunch		
1 skim milk	1 cup skim milk	1 cup skim milk
4 starch	1 cup brown rice	2 slices of bread†
		1 cup broth-type vegetable soup and 3 ginger snaps
1 fruit	1 apple	½ cup pineapple juice
2 vegetables	1 cup green beans	½ cup asparagus and 1 cup raw carrots
2 meat	2 oz stir-fried chicken	2 slices low-fat cheese†
1 fat	1 tsp oil	1 tsp margarine†

TABLE 17-6 ■ Sample 1800-Kilocalorie Diabetic Diet* (Continued)

MEAL PLAN AND SAMPLE MENUS		
Meal Plan	**Sample Menu 1**	**Sample Menu 2**
Dinner		
3 starch	1 large baked potato	¼ 10-in pizza, thin crust, and 2 bread sticks (4 × ½ in)
1 vegetable	½ cup broccoli[‡]	Sliced tomato
Free vegetable	Lettuce salad	Lettuce salad
1 meat	1 oz ground beef	(on pizza)
2 fat	2 tbsp sour cream[‡]	(on pizza)
	1 tbsp French dressing	1 tbsp French dressing
Free	Coffee	Diet soft drink
HS		
½ cup skim milk	½ cup skim milk	½ cup skim milk
2 starch	1½ oz pretzels	6 cups hot-air-popped popcorn
1 fruit	15 grapes	1 peach
1 meat	1 oz low-fat cheese stick	1 tbsp Parmesan cheese
1 fat	2 walnuts	1 tbsp lite margarine

*The calculations and meal plan based on 55% carbohydrate, 20% protein, and 25% fat with a ⅕, ⅖, ⅕, and ⅕ distribution.
†Cheese sandwich.
‡Potato toppings.

- Sucrose-containing foods can be substituted for other CHO in the meal plan, if added to the meal plan, covered with insulin or other glucose-lowering medications. Care should be taken to avoid excess energy intake.
- As for the general population, people with diabetes are encouraged to consume a variety of fiber-containing foods. However, evidence is lacking to recommend a higher fiber intake for people with diabetes than for the population as a whole.
- Sugar alcohols and nonnutritive sweeteners are safe when consumed within the daily levels established by the Food and Drug Administration (FDA).

Protein

The need for protein in the diabetic population is the same as for the general population if renal function is normal. Excessive dietary protein should be avoided. The concept that excessive dietary protein may have a health risk is discussed in Chapter 5. In addition, protein can increase insulin response without increasing plasma glucose concentrations. Therefore, protein should not be used to treat acute or prevent nighttime hypoglycemia (American Diabetes Association, 2008).

Fat

The primary goal regarding dietary fat in clients with diabetes is to decrease blood lipid levels. To achieve this goal, recommendations include:

- Limit saturated fat to <7% of total kilocalories.
- Intake of *trans*-fat should be minimized.
- Lower dietary cholesterol to <200 mg/day.
- Consume two or more servings of fish per week (with the exception of commercially fried fish filets) because these provide *n*-3 polyunsaturated fatty acids.

Some people with diabetes have better glucose control on high-monounsaturated-fat diets (40 to 45% of the kilocalories). If a diet is 40 to 45% fat, the carbohydrate content of the diet drops to 35 to 45%. Diabetes is a complicated disease, and clients with diabetes benefit from a highly individualized approach to diet manipulation. Some patients with hypertriglyceridemia and elevated low-density lipoprotein (LDL) cholesterol levels respond better to a 40 to 45% high-monounsaturated-fat diet (Nuttall and Chasuk, 1998). This is why the percentage of kilocalories from fat and the kind of fat consumed by persons with diabetes merit consideration. This concept requires rigid compliance. Individual evaluation by a registered dietitian is necessary to assess feasibility.

Not all clients with diabetes have these lipid abnormalities. In epidemiological studies, an increased plasma triglyceride and low HDL cholesterol have been associated with an increased risk for clinically apparent cardiovascular disease in people with diabetes. Overall, cardiovascular disease is at least two to three times more common in patients with type 2 diabetes (Nuttall and Chasuk, 1998).

Carbohydrate Counting

Carbohydrate counting is another frequently used menu-planning tool. Because CHO is the energy nutrient that has the greatest influence on blood glucose levels, some clients adhere to nutritional recommendations more closely with this approach and SMBG. Clients can readily see the effect that diet has on blood glucose levels throughout the day when combined with SMBG. The advantages of the carbohydrate-counting meal plan concept include:

- Single-nutrient focused
- More precise matching of food and insulin
- Flexible food choices
- A potential for improved blood glucose, and client-controlled treatment

Challenges for the client who uses this system may include:

- The need to weigh and measure food
- Maintenance of extensive food records
- Monitoring of the blood glucose before and after eating
- The need to calculate grams of carbohydrate consumed
- The need to maintain healthful eating and weight management

Knowledge of carbohydrate counting is often a prerequisite before consideration for insulin pump therapy. It is also a prerequisite for clients who want to learn how to calculate insulin:carbohydrate ratios. This type of teaching is usually done by a certified diabetes educator (CDE) and is considered advanced teaching.

The rationale for carbohydrate counting is a carbohydrate = a carbohydrate = a carbohydrate or one starch exchange = one fruit exchange = one milk exchange. One carbohydrate unit (or exchange) is about 15 grams of carbohydrate with an acceptable range of 8 to 22 grams per carbohydrate choice. Food labels, tables of food composition, and *Exchange Lists for Meal Planning* are some of the tools clients can use to determine the carbohydrate content of a particular food. Following is a typical meal plan for a client who has been taught to count carbohydrates:

Breakfast: 3 carbohydrates
Example: 1 whole bagel and 8 ounces (oz) skim milk
Lunch: 3 carbohydrates
Example: 8 oz regular cola, 1 fresh orange, and 1 slice whole-wheat bread
Dinner: 3 carbohydrates
Example: 1½ cups pasta
Snack: 1 carbohydrate (range, 8 to 22 grams)
Example: 8 oz skim milk

Protein and fat intake are not counted with this meal-planning system but should be given some consideration. Clients are usually counseled to eat about the same amount of protein each day and choose foods that are low in fat. For example, based on an individualized assessment, a client may be counseled to choose a food that provides approximately 3 grams or less of fat for each carbohydrate (15 grams). Thus, if a client is considering a canned entrée containing 30 grams of carbohydrate, he or she knows the food is not a good choice if it contains more than 6 grams of fat.

Exchange Lists

Exchange lists have been used for many years to teach clients portion sizes, food composition, and meal plan distribution. Many clients find this method of menu planning too complex to learn and difficult to implement. However, exchange lists are a good approach to meal planning if the client is highly motivated and the educator has sufficient time to spend with the client. Use of exchange lists are most widely taught in outpatient settings. Clinical Calculation 17-1 demonstrates how to distribute the energy nutrients and calculate a diet using the exchange system.

Special Considerations

Persons with diabetes frequently ask questions about nutritional problems related to vitamin and mineral supplementation, alcohol, acute illness, eating out, and delayed meals.

Vitamin and Mineral Supplementation

There is no clear evidence that people with diabetes benefit from vitamin or mineral supplementation solely because they have diabetes. Routine supplementation with antioxidants, such as vitamins E and C and carotene, is not advised because of lack of evidence of efficacy and concern related to long-term safety. Benefit from chromium supplementation in individuals with diabetes or obesity has not been clearly demonstrated and therefore cannot be recommended (American Diabetes Association, 2008).

Alcohol

Moderate use of alcohol does not adversely affect diabetes in well-controlled clients. Recommendations follow (American Diabetes Association, 2008):

- If people with diabetes choose to drink, daily intake should be limited to one drink per day or less for women and two drinks or less per day for men.

- To reduce nocturnal hypoglycemia in both insulin users and insulin secretagogues, people with diabetes who choose to drink should consume alcohol with food.
- In people with diabetes, moderate alcohol consumption (when ingested alone) has no acute effect on glucose and insulin concentrations but carbohydrate coingested with alcohol (as in a mixed drink) may raise blood glucose.

Nutrition During Acute Illness

Colds and flu-like symptoms can be fatal for some people with diabetes unless precautions are taken. Secretion of both glucagon and epinephrine increases during illness and contributes to an increase in blood glucose levels. This action may lead to a loss of glucose, fluid, and electrolytes. Dehydration, electrolyte depletion, and a loss of nutrients may follow. Acute illnesses can lead to DKA in type 1 and to HHNS in type 2 diabetes.

Dehydration is more rapid when electrolytes and fluids are not replaced. Vomiting, diarrhea, and fever all result in fluid loss. During acute illness, the individual should be instructed to monitor his or her blood glucose level every 2 to 4 hours until the symptoms subside. Urine ketone levels should be checked. The following guidelines are recommended by the American Diabetes Association (2008):

- Ingestion of 15 to 20 grams of glucose is the preferred treatment for hypoglycemia, although any form of CHO that contains glucose may be used.
- The response to treatment of hypoglycemia should be apparent in 10 to 20 minutes; however, plasma glucose should be tested again in 60 minutes, as additional treatment may be necessary.

Increased fluids reduce the risk of dehydration. Clients who are vomiting or nauseated and are unable to tolerate regular food should drink liquids that contain carbohydrate or electrolytes (Table 17-7). A general guideline is that approximately 15 grams of carbohydrate should be consumed every 1 to 2 hours. Some clients have an individually calculated sick-day menu based on the carbohydrate content of their regular diet.

Other meal-planning tips that may prove helpful during periods of acute illness include:

- Increasing water intake, even for clients who can eat regular foods
- Eating smaller, more frequent feedings
- Eating soft, easily digested foods

During acute illnesses, testing plasma glucose and urinary ketones, drinking adequate amounts of fluids, and ingesting carbohydrates are all important (American Diabetes Association, 2008).

TABLE 17-7 ■ Carbohydrate-Containing Foods for Sick Days

FOOD	AMOUNT	GRAMS OF CARBOHYDRATE
Regular cola	½ cup	13
Ginger ale	¾ cup	16
Milk	1 cup	12
Apple juice	½ cup	15
Grape juice	½ cup	15
Orange juice	½ cup	15
Pineapple juice	½ cup	15
Prune juice	⅓ cup	15
Regular gelatin	½ cup	20
Sherbet	½ cup	30
Tomato juice*	½ cup	5

*High in sodium.

Eating Out and Fast Foods

The best advice for persons with diabetes who enjoy eating out is that they know their meal-planning system and order small portions.

Hypoglycemia in Diabetes Mellitus

The immediate treatment goal for a glucose level of less than 60 mg/dL is to increase blood glucose to within a normal level as rapidly as possible. Take care not to overtreat hypoglycemia. If the client is monitoring his or her blood glucose level, at the first sign or symptom of hypoglycemia, he or she should measure the blood glucose level. If the blood glucose level is less than 60 mg/dL, 15 grams of carbohydrate should be consumed. Fifteen grams of carbohydrate are equal to:

- 2 to 3 glucose tablets
- 6 to 10 Lifesavers candies
- 4 to 6 ounces of fruit juice

Clients should be advised to carry a source of carbohydrate with them at all times. A snack should be consumed if a meal or snack is delayed (preplanned or not preplanned) by a half hour or more. At least one significant other should be instructed about hypoglycemia.

Teaching Self-Care

Persons with diabetes ultimately treat themselves. The better educated the individual is about diabetes, the greater the likelihood of his or her avoiding the acute and chronic complications of this disease. Many public health departments, hospitals, and clinics hold classes for clients with diabetes. Newly diagnosed clients with diabetes need to learn survival skills. Health-care workers often have to repeat instructions several times before the client understands the survival skills being taught.

Because of the genetic predisposition toward diabetes, many newly diagnosed clients have relatives who have suffered from the acute and chronic complications of diabetes. Hearing about such complications first hand often creates fear in newly diagnosed clients. They need time to accept their condition. Occasionally, it may take as long as a full year before clients can grasp the principles of self-care. This is especially difficult for children (see Clinical Application 17-3). During hospitalization, it is extremely difficult to effectively educate clients. Follow-up with a certified diabetes educator (CDE) and a registered dietitian (RD) is crucial.

Hypoglycemia, caused by increased endogenous insulin production (hyperinsulinism), is rarer than diabetes mellitus. Hyperinsulinism is most likely caused by islet cell tumors or, less often, by reactive hypoglycemia. Hypoglycemia that occurs 1 to 3 hours after a meal and resolves spontaneously with the ingestion of carbohydrate is often termed reactive hypoglycemia.

The dietary management of reactive hypoglycemia consists of avoiding simple carbohydrates and sometimes taking small, frequent feedings. The meal plans for diabetes offer a reasonable guide to meal planning. Table 17-8 is a 1-day meal plan for this type of diet.

TABLE 17-8 ■ Sample Meal Plan for Hypoglycemic Diet

EXCHANGE GROUP	SAMPLE MENU
Morning	
1 fruit	½ cup unsweetened orange juice
1 starch	¾ cup whole-grain cereal
1 meat	1 oz low-fat cheese
½ cup skim milk	½ cup skim milk
Free	Decaffeinated coffee
Mid-Morning	
1 meat	1 tbsp peanut butter
1 starch	4 whole-grain crackers
Noon	
Chef salad	
2–4 meat	2–4 oz lean meat
1 vegetable	Lettuce, tomatoes, and
1 fat	Dressing
1 fruit	1 small piece fresh fruit
1 cup skim milk	1 cup skim milk
1 starch	2 breadsticks (4 x ½ in.)
Mid-Afternoon	
1 meat	1 oz low-fat cheese
1 starch	4 whole-grain crackers
Evening	
2–4 meat	2–4 oz lean meat
1 starch	½ cup potato or pasta
1 vegetable	½ cup vegetable
1 fat	Lettuce salad with dressing
1 fruit	1 piece fresh fruit
Free	Decaffeinated coffee or tea
Bedtime	
1 starch and 1 meat	½ sandwich (1 slice whole-grain bread and 1 oz lean meat)
1 vegetable	Fresh vegetables
Free	Decaffeinated beverage

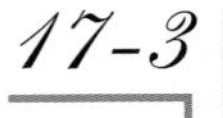

Clinical Application

Children with Diabetes

Kilocalorie allowances are based on a person's weight. As a rough estimate, a 1-year-old child needs 1000 kcal per day. For older children, 100 kcal per year of age are added to the daily intake. For a 9-year-old child, this would equal 1900 kcal. Typically, 55% of the total kilocalories should be consumed as carbohydrate. 1900 kcal multiplied by 55% equals 1045 kcal. To convert kilocalories from carbohydrate to grams of carbohydrate, divide by 4. 1045 kcal divided by 4 kcal/gram equals 260 grams of carbohydrate.

How these grams of carbohydrate are divided among the day depends on the child's prescribed medications and lifestyle. Let's assume the child eats three meals and two snacks (at mid-afternoon and bedtime) and takes one dose of basal insulin in the morning and three doses of regular insulin, one before each meal.

The diet could be planned to provide 20% of the carbohydrate at each feeding. Twenty% of 260 grams of carbohydrate equals 52 grams or 3½ carbohydrate choices. The child and the child's parents would be instructed to provide about 52 grams of carbohydrate at each feeding.

As long as the child eats balanced meals that provide all the essential nutrients, the source of the carbohydrate is not important. Scientific evidence has shown that the use of sucrose as part of the meal plan does not impair blood glucose control in individuals with type 1 and type 2 diabetes (American Dietetic Association, 2000). A typical menu for the child follows:

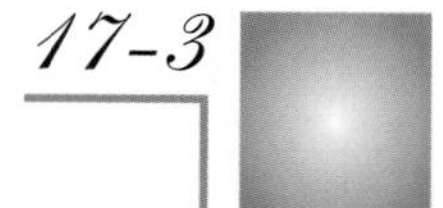

Clinical Application—cont'd

Acceptable Range, 46–60 per Meal or Snack

MEAL	GRAMS OF CARBOHYDRATE	MEAL	GRAMS OF CARBOHYDRATE
Breakfast		***Mid-Afternoon Snack***	
½ cup Honey Nut Cheerios	12 (package label)	¾ cup apple juice	23 (exchange value)
¾ cup skim milk	9 (exchange value)	13 animal crackers	25 (exchange value)
½ cup orange juice	15 (exchange value)	Total carbohydrates for snack	48
1 slice toast	15 (exchange value)	***Dinner***	
1 tsp peanut butter	0	15-in. cheese pizza	39 (table of food composition)
Total carbohydrates for meal	51	6 oz regular cola	20 (table of food composition)
Lunch		Total carbohydrates for meal	59
Ham and cheese sandwich with 2 slices of bread	30 (exchange value)	***Bedtime Snack***	
1 apple	15 (exchange value)	½ cup skim milk	6 (exchange value)
¾ cup skim milk	9 (exchange value)	Raw broccoli with dip	0 (free with this system)
Carrot sticks	0 (free with this system)	10 (1½ oz) whole-wheat crackers (no added fat)	30 (exchange value)
Total carbohydrates for meal	54	½ oz jelly beans	14 (table of food composition)
		Total carbohydrates for snack	50
		Total carbohydrates for the day	262

Keystones

- Diabetes mellitus is caused by an undersecretion or underutilization of insulin and/or receptor or postreceptor defects.
- Diabetes is actually a group of disorders with a common sign of hyperglycemia.
- The two major types of diabetes are type 1 and type 2. Impaired glucose tolerance or impaired fasting glucose, secondary diabetes, and gestational diabetes are other categories of this disease.
- Persons with diabetes suffer from acute and chronic complications.
- Treatment involves medication, nutrition management, and exercise.
- Nutrition is a fundamental part of treatment.
- Hypoglycemia, a rarer condition than diabetes, is caused by oversecretion of insulin and is also treated with dietary manipulation.

CASE STUDY 17-1

Mrs. S, a 45-year-old black woman, was admitted to the hospital with medical diagnoses of type 2 diabetes and cellulitis of the left leg. Her admitting height was 5 ft 5 in., and weight 200 lb (body mass index [BMI] = 33.5). Vital signs were temperature 98.6ºF, pulse 70 beats per minute, respirations 16 breaths per minute, and blood pressure 160/95 mm Hg.

Mrs. S reported a gradual increase in her weight since her third child was born 20 years ago. That baby weighed 12 lb. Two previous pregnancies produced infants weighing 10 and 11 lb. She has no known allergies. None of the children live at home. Mrs. S lives with her husband, who works as a construction laborer. She has been seasonally employed as a hotel maid at a nearby resort. Health insurance coverage is sporadic. They have a new insurance policy now.

Mrs. S is the oldest of six children. Her father died of a heart attack at age 60. Her mother died of a stroke at age 62 following 15 years of treatment for diabetes mellitus. The sister who is closest to Mrs. S in age developed diabetes mellitus 3 years ago and is being treated with oral medication. Their youngest sister was diagnosed as an insulin-dependent diabetic at age 18 after an episode of mumps.

Mrs. S reports a good appetite and a fluid intake of about 3 quarts per day. Her favorite beverage is iced tea with sugar and lemon. She does most of the grocery shopping and cooking.

Mrs. S hit her left ankle with the screen door about 2 months ago. The resulting sore has not healed but has gotten worse. Mrs. S knows that a sore that does not heal is a sign of cancer, which is why she sought medical attention. The ankle now has an open lesion 5 cm in diameter over the lateral ankle bone. The entire foot is swollen to twice the size of the right foot. The bandage over the sore had greenish-yellow drainage on it. A random blood glucose test in the doctor's office 3 hours after her last meal showed a glucose level of 400 mg/dL. Her urine glucose was negative for ketones. Before she left the office, the physician told Mrs. S she has type 2 diabetes mellitus. The physician prescribed the following care for Mrs. S:

- Bed rest with left leg elevated
- Bedside commode
- Diet assessment and teaching
- Multivitamin, 1 capsule daily
- Culture and sensitivity of drainage from left leg
- Cefuroxime, 250 mg, orally every 12 hours
- Warm, moist dressing to left leg ulcer four times per day
- Fasting blood sugar (FBS), electrolytes in AM
- Sliding scale insulin every 6 hours before meals as follows:
  - Blood glucose <400 mg/dL, 5 units
  - Blood glucose 350 to 399, 4 units
  - Blood glucose 300 to 349, 3 units
  - Blood glucose 250 to 299, 1 unit
  - Blood glucose 200 to 249, 1 unit
  - Blood glucose <199 no insulin

When asked, the physician stated, "I believe this patient's glucose will be ok at discharge and insulin will likely not be necessary."

The admitting nurse constructed the following Care Plan for Mrs. S.

Care Plan

Subjective Data

Family history of diabetes mellitus ■ Large appetite ■ Large fluid intake ■ Delay in seeking medical attention

Objective Data

Obesity: Ht 5 ft 5 in.; wt 200 lb ■ Newly diagnosed type 2 diabetes ■ Possible hypertension (only one reading given) ■ Open lesion 5 cm diameter over left lateral ankle; purulent discharge

Analysis

Lack of knowledge of disease process related to inappropriate self care as evidenced by elevated blood glucose levels and open lesion.

CASE STUDY *(Continued)*

Plan

DESIRED OUTCOMES EVALUATION CRITERIA	ACTIONS/INTERVENTIONS	RATIONALE
Client will verbalize self-care measures related to type 2 by hospital discharge.	Refer to dietitian for nutritional assessment and education.	One of the cornerstones of treatment of type 2 is weight loss. Clients with diabetes essentially need to learn to treat themselves as much as possible and know when to seek medical treatment.
	Review survival skills with client (see DavisPlus for client teaching tool).	The American Diabetes Association recommends all patients with diabetes learn survival skills.
Client will verbalize willingness to continue nursing/medical regimen after discharge.	Refer to social worker for sources of medical attention when uninsured.	Social workers are most familiar with community resources.
	Teach principles of wound care, including effect of high blood sugar on infection.	If Mrs. S understands that high blood sugar feeds the bacteria causing the infection, she may be more willing to work hard to control the diabetes.
	Reinforce dietitian's instruction. Have Mrs. S state the Dietary Guidelines and the reason why they are important.	Knowledge usually precedes behavior change.
	Have Mrs. S describe the meal plan she follows.	Short periods of instruction are most effective; frequent review of the material will help the client master it.
	Request physician's order for referral to outpatient diabetes clinic.	Insurance companies will more likely cover outpatient educational programs if ordered by a physician.

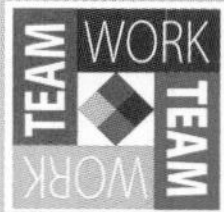

17-1

Dietitian's Notes

The following Dietitian's Notes are representative of the documentation found in a client's medical record.

Subjective: Spoke with patient, who was tearful throughout our session. Patient describes an uncontrollable thirst and hunger and inability to prepare food while her husband is at work. Claims her husband left her a thermos of coffee and snacks before he left for work. Snacks included bread, a jar of peanut butter, and a jar of jelly. Generally, she claims to have eaten both jars of peanut butter and jelly every day along with half the loaf of bread. She didn't eat the whole loaf because she knows too much bread is bad for anyone. For dinner, her husband usually brought home fast food from the burger store (hamburgers and French fries) or pizza. Denies daily consumption of milk, fruits, and vegetables.

Objective: Diagnosis: Type 2 diabetes (newly diagnosed) with open lesion over left ankle with drainage

Analysis: Inappropriate carbohydrate (CHO) intake related to diabetes and food and nutrition knowledge deficit as evidenced by blood glucose greater than 400 and diet history. Body mass index (BMI) 33.5. Ideal body weight based on maximum ideal body weight of 100 lb for the first 5 ft and 4 lb for each additional inch equals 120; plus or minus 10% equals 108 to 132 lb. 132 pounds divided by weight in kilograms (2.2) equals 60 kg, and this is the weight used to estimate kcal and protein needs.

Estimated kcal needs based on maximum ideal body weight and 25 to 35 kcal/kg equals 1500 to 2100. However, as weight loss is desirable for this client, would provide slightly less kcal to provide for a weight loss of about 1 lb per week. 1500 minus 500 kcal/day equals 1250 kcal/day. A 50% acceptable macronutrient distribution range was used to determine carbohydrate needs per meal: 10.5 exchanges/day or 3 per feeding and 2 for an evening snack.

Estimated kcal needs based on 1.0 kcal/kg equals 60 grams per day. Estimated protein needs on the high side to provide enough protein for wound repair.

Education: Reviewed carbohydrate counting with client. Will need much encouragement to follow through with healthful behavioral changes.

Plan:

1. Recommend to client 3 carbohydrate (CHO) exchanges per meal and 2 carbohydrate exchanges at bedtime.
2. Recommend referral to outpatient diabetes program for more intensive education.
3. Concur that social worker would be helpful to determine eligibility for home delivered lunch after discharge and transportation assistance to Outpatient Diabetes Program.

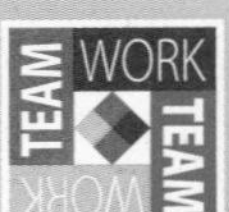

17-2

Social Worker's Notes

The following Social Worker's Notes are representative of the documentation found in a client's medical record.

Arrangements have been made for the client to receive a hot lunch daily and a cold boxed dinner 5 days per week after discharge. Will contact hospital meal delivery program and let them know when they should begin to send meals.

Arrangements have also been made to provide client with transportation to and from the Outpatient Diabetes Clinic after discharge.

Critical Thinking Questions

1. The client would like to learn how to monitor her own blood glucose levels (as the nurses do) before discharge. How would the nurse, in the role of client advocate, arrange for this to be done? Why is a physician's written order important?
2. The client's fasting blood glucose level has decreased steadily during her 3-day hospitalization. On the morning of discharge, the fasting blood sugar (FBS) was 150 mg/dL. The client stated, "It has come down enough. Now I don't need to worry about the diabetes any longer." How would you respond?
3. Why is a referral to a certified diabetes educator crucial for this client?

Chapter Review

1. If a client has a history of ketoacidosis, he or she most likely has which type of diabetes:
   a. Type 1
   b. Type 2
   c. Pituitary
   d. Gestational
2. The following statement is true:
   a. Acute illness lowers blood glucose levels.
   b. Fluid and electrolyte replacement is essential during episodes of acute illness in all persons with diabetes.
   c. Persons with diabetes who have an acute illness require a vitamin and mineral supplement.
   d. Persons with diabetes should never eat forms of simple sugar.
3. Dietary guidelines for people with diabetes include:
   a. One serving of alcohol daily
   b. Consume no more than 2000 milligrams of sodium each day
   c. Restrict fat intake to less than 10% of total kilocalories
   d. Consume at least 20 to 35 grams of fiber each day
4. For most clients, the cornerstone of treatment of type 2 diabetes is:
   a. Stress management
   b. Meal planning
   c. Strict adherence to five planned meals per day
   d. Hypoglycemic drugs
5. The diet for reactive hypoglycemia includes the following features:
   a. Small, frequent meals with restricted simple sugars
   b. Three meals with ample simple sugars and high complex carbohydrate
   c. Four to six small meals that are high in fat
   d. Three high-carbohydrate meals that are moderate in fat

Clinical Analysis

Ms. N, a 14-year-old, was diagnosed 1 year ago with type 1 diabetes mellitus. Her blood sugar levels have been stable on an intermediate-acting insulin and a 370-gram CHO diet. The teenager is now being seen in the doctor's office for routine follow-up. The nurse is reviewing Ms. N's knowledge of self-care.

1. To assess knowledge, the nurse asks how the client would handle a day when the client could not eat solid foods. Which of the following answers would show understanding of the usual procedure?
   a. Skip insulin that day.
   b. Call the doctor after missing one meal.
   c. Replace the carbohydrates in the meal plan with liquids containing equal amounts of carbohydrate.
   d. Take half her usual insulin dose and double the usual fluid intake.

2. The client plays volleyball for the high-school team and is moderately active during practices and games. Self-monitoring blood glucose (SMBG) records indicate a daily glucose level of between 120 and 140 mg/dL before the time she usually plays volleyball. Which of the following behaviors are appropriate for her before playing?
   a. No additional food is indicated.
   b. Increase intake by 15 grams of carbohydrate.
   c. Decrease intake by 15 grams of carbohydrate.
   d. Increase intake by one vegetable exchange and one fat exchange.

3. The client states, "I am getting tired of pricking my finger several times a day. Why can't I manage my diabetes with urine testing like my grandmother?" Which of the following responses by the nurse would be most appropriate?
   a. "The urine test is more accurate in older people."
   b. "The point at which sugar is spilled in the urine varies even for one individual. Therefore, the blood test is more accurate."
   c. "Urine tests are more costly."
   d. "The blood test is the newest thing. Your grandmother's doctor must be old-fashioned."

18

Diet in Cardiovascular Disease

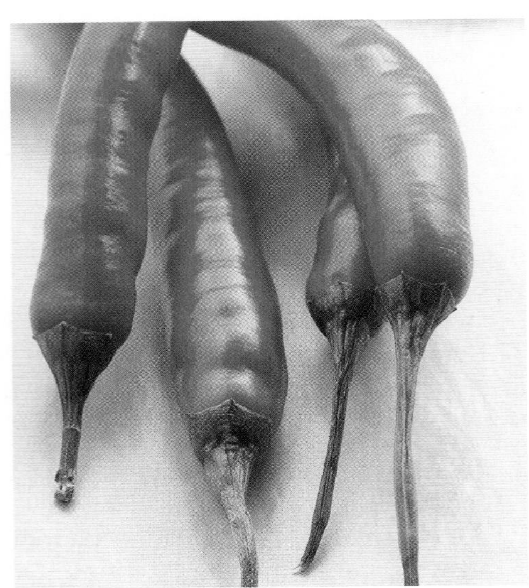

LEARNING OBJECTIVES

After completing this chapter, the student should be able to:

- Discuss the relationship between diet and the development of cardiovascular disease.
- Distinguish between type II and type IV hyperlipoproteinemias as to aggravating factors and the focus of dietary modifications.
- Identify strategies that are most likely to reduce the risk of cardiovascular disease.
- Compare and contrast dietary modifications for clients with myocardial infarction, heart failure, and stroke.
- Describe the 2-gram sodium diet.
- List several flavorings and seasonings that can be substituted for salt on a sodium-restricted diet.

The cardiovascular system includes not only the heart and blood vessels but the blood-forming organs as well. This chapter covers common diseases of the heart and blood vessels that can be influenced by dietary modification.

Occurrence of Cardiovascular Disease

Despite declines in recent years, heart disease and stroke remain the first and third leading causes of death in the United States, respectively. Of all U.S. deaths in 2005, heart disease accounted for 26.6% and stroke for 5.9% (National Center for Health Statistics, 2008). Death rates for heart disease are highest in Appalachia and the southern states (Centers for Disease Control and Prevention [CDC], July 1, 2008), while the southeastern United States has the highest stroke death rates, led by South Carolina, Alabama, and Arkansas (CDC, June 25, 2008).

Underlying Pathology

Two major pathological conditions contribute to cardiovascular disease:

1. Atherosclerosis, the most common form of **arteriosclerosis**
2. Hypertension, included here as contributing to pathology and later in the chapter as a risk factor for cardiovascular disease

Atherosclerosis

In **atherosclerosis** fatty deposits of cholesterol, fat, or other substances accumulate inside the artery, accompanied by inflammation. Initially, the deposited material, or plaque, is soft, but later it becomes fibrosed or hard. This disease process interferes with the pumping of blood through the artery in two ways:

- The deposits gradually make the lumen smaller and smaller.

- The fibrosis makes it progressively harder for the artery to constrict or dilate in response to the tissues' needs for oxygenated blood (Fig. 18-1).

When the lumen, or opening through the artery, is 70% blocked by atherosclerotic plaque, the person is likely to show symptoms of impaired circulation distal to the obstruction.

Hypertension

Blood pressure (B/P) is the force exerted against the walls of the arteries by the pumping action of the heart. Blood pressure is recorded in two numbers, for example, 120/80. The top number, **systolic pressure,** is the pressure when the heart beats. The bottom number, **diastolic pressure,** is the pressure between beats. Both pressures are reported in millimeters of mercury (mm Hg).

Diagnosis of Hypertension

Hypertension is defined as:

- Blood pressure of 140/90 or higher on at least three occasions on different dates, or
- Persons taking antihypertensive medication.

Several readings are taken on various days to eliminate the possibility of excitement or nervousness causing a transient elevation. Hypertension is classified as Stage 1 or 2 (Table 18-1). Blood pressure measurement should be part of a child's health assessment beginning at the age of 3 years. Almost 75% of the cases of arterial hypertension and 90% of the cases of prehypertension in children and adolescents are currently undiagnosed (Aglony, Acevedo, and Ambrosio, 2009).

A person with hypertension may not feel sick, so blood pressure screening is often offered as a community service (Fig. 18-2). Along with temperature, pulse, and respirations, blood pressure is a vital sign that is usually taken at every health-care visit.

Types of Hypertension

Depending on the cause, hypertension is labeled primary or secondary. About 90% of hypertensive clients have primary or **essential hypertension**. There is no single, clear-cut cause for this high blood pressure.

Secondary hypertension occurs in response to another event or disease in the body. One such event is pregnancy, during which hypertension may occur (see Chapter 10). Medications also can cause

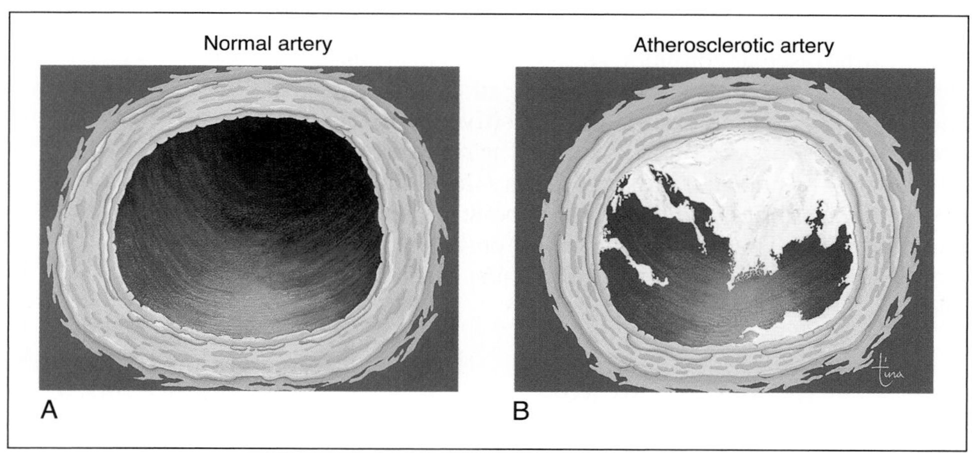

FIGURE 18-1 Cross-section of a normal coronary artery (A) and an atherosclerotic artery (B). Note both the narrowed diameter and the roughness within the lumen in the diseased artery. (Reprinted from Scanlon, VC, and Sanders, T: *Essentials of anatomy and physiology.* FA Davis, Philadelphia, 2007, p 280, with permission.)

TABLE 18-1 ■ Classification of Blood Pressure for Adults and Children

CLASSIFICATION	mm Hg SYSTOLIC	mm Hg DIASTOLIC	PERCENTILE DENOTING CLASSIFICATION IN CHILDREN AND ADOLESCENTS	ESTIMATED NUMBER OF U.S. ADULTS AFFECTED (MILLIONS)	
				Men	Women
Normal	<120	and<80	<90th		
Prehypertension	120–139	or 80–89	90th to 95th (Children) >120/80 (Adolescents)	41.9	27.8
Stage 1 Hypertension	140–159	or 90–99	95th to (99th + 5 mm Hg)	12.8	12.2
Stage 2 Hypertension	>159	or >99	>99th + 5 mm Hg	4.1	6.9

SOURCE: Adapted from National High Blood Pressure Education Working Group (2004); Qureshi et al. (2005); U.S. Department of Health and Human Services (2003).

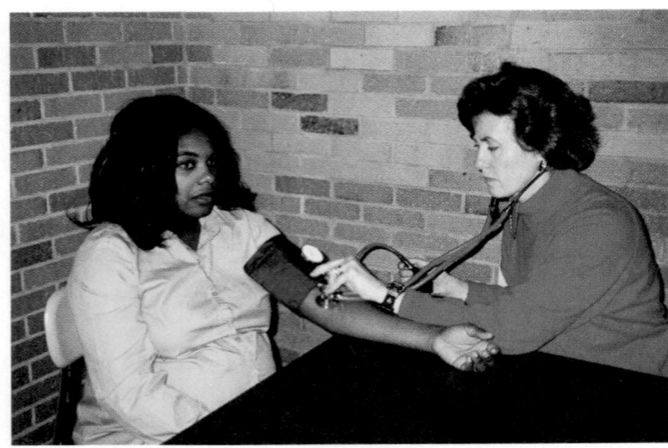

FIGURE 18-2 Hypertension is a silent killer. Blood pressure monitoring is a part of most health system visits.

secondary hypertension. Birth control pills that contain progesterone stimulate the production of renin (see Fig. 8–17), which may result in an elevation in blood pressure.

As mentioned in Chapter 15, the combined intake of monoamine oxidase inhibitors (MAOIs) and tyramine-rich foods or beverages can cause hypertension. Secondary hypertension also can result from diseases of the kidney, adrenal glands, or nervous system.

Positive Feedback Cycle

Many cardiovascular conditions have interlocking causative factors. The interaction between atherosclerosis and hypertension is an example of a **positive feedback cycle**. In this situation, the presence of the second condition worsens the first. Atherosclerosis narrows the lumen of the arteries, and the smaller opening increases blood pressure. Then the higher blood pressure forces more lipids into the arterial wall, worsening the atherosclerosis, and the cycle is repeated.

End Result of Pathology

Most affected people do not have either atherosclerosis or hypertension. More commonly, they have both conditions. Although many organs are likely to be damaged by atherosclerosis and hypertension, the major concern is the effect on the heart and brain, as described in the following sections on coronary heart disease and cerebrovascular disease.

Coronary Heart Disease

When the coronary arteries that supply the heart muscle with blood become blocked, the result is **coronary heart disease (CHD)** or coronary artery disease (CAD). If the blockage is temporary, due to increased activity and the body's increased demand for oxygen, the person may experience **angina pectoris,** or severe pain and a sense of constriction about the heart. Rest and the administration of vasodilating medications commonly produce relief, but changes in diet and lifestyle are necessary to stave off heart damage.

But if the vessel is blocked by atherosclerotic plaque, by a **thrombus** (blood clot), or by an **embolus** (a circulating mass of undissolved matter), the heart tissues beyond the point of obstruction receive no oxygen or nutrients. When this happens, the person exhibits signs and symptoms of a **coronary occlusion,** or a heart attack. When the blood supply cannot be restored quickly, myocardial cells in the affected area die. The medical diagnosis then becomes **myocardial infarction** (MI).

Heart Failure

When the heart cannot keep up with the demands on it, **heart failure** occurs. Causes may include:

- Atherosclerosis
- Hypertension
- Myocardial infarction
- Rheumatic fever
- A birth defect

The right side of the heart normally collects the blood returning from the body and pumps it to the lungs to excrete carbon dioxide and absorb oxygen. If the right ventricle is failing, usually due to lung disease, the blood backs up into the veins that empty into the right atrium, and the client has the signs of peripheral edema. If the client has excessive fluid volume and edema of the small bowel, the client suffers from anorexia and nausea.

The left side of the heart normally receives the oxygenated blood from the lungs and pumps it out to the body. If the left ventricle is failing, usually after a myocardial infarction, the blood that cannot be pumped effectively to the body backs up in the blood vessels of the lungs. Next, the fluid from the blood is forced into the lung tissue. The client will display shortness of breath and moist lung sounds and will expectorate frothy pink sputum.

In addition, if the heart cannot pump enough blood to maintain blood pressure, the body implements the renin response. Angiotensin II constricts the blood vessels, raising blood pressure. Aldosterone causes the kidneys to conserve sodium, and with it, water (see Fig. 8-17). More fluid fills the blood vessels. The higher blood pressure pushes this fluid out into the interstitial spaces, causing edema.

Obviously, one side of the heart cannot function long if the other side is failing. Therefore, the healthcare worker learns to look for early signs of heart failure in the extremities in right-sided failure or in the lungs in left-sided failure.

About 5.8 million people in the United States suffer from heart failure and about 670,000 new cases are diagnosed annually (CDC, 2010). Heart failure is associated with poor prognoses, reduced quality of life, and frequent hospitalizations (Varughese, 2007). It is the only cardiovascular disorder that is increasing in prevalence and incidence as the population continues to age. Early diagnosis is needed, when there may be no symptoms, since treatment can delay or reverse disease progression (Fonseca, 2006).

Clients often see heart failure as an acute disease that is resolved after they return home rather than the chronic disease it is. However, self-management at home is required and includes daily weighing so that a gain of 3 to 5 pounds triggers follow-up with the primary health-care provider for adjustment of therapy. Clients may need dietary prescriptions clarified or reinforced to limit water retention.

Hospitalized clients have lost fluid too rapidly when consuming a dietitian-managed intake even though they thought they were following the prescribed diet at home. Case management programs using pharmacists or nurses have decreased hospitalizations and improved quality of life in clients with heart failure but have not clearly improved survival. Other professionals or family and friends could be recruited to assist the client with self-management (Horowitz, Rein, and Leventhal, 2004).

Cerebrovascular Accident

When a blood vessel in the brain becomes blocked by atherosclerosis (ischemic stroke), the tissue supplied by that artery dies. This pathology causes about 87% of strokes or **cerebrovascular accidents (CVAs)** in the United States (American Heart Association and American Stroke Association, 2008). Strokes also can be caused by an embolus or by a ruptured blood vessel. Cerebrovascular accidents are usually secondary to atherosclerosis, hypertension, or a combination of both.

Each year, 780,000 strokes, 600,000 of them first attacks, occur in the United States. Blacks have almost twice the risk of first-ever stroke compared with whites (American Heart Association and American Stroke Association, 2008).

Stroke is called a "brain attack" and early treatment can minimize the long-term effects of ischemic stroke, but people often ignore initial signs and symptoms or fail to react appropriately. Analysis of 56,969 persons with strokes in 4 states, revealed that nearly 40% did not arrive at the hospital by ambulance, thereby limiting the possibility of definitive early treatment (George et al., 2009).

Individuals consuming more than five servings of fruits and vegetables daily had a 25% lower incidence of stroke than those consuming fewer than three servings (He et al., 2006). A diet with the following components will likely reduce the incidence of stroke (Ding and Mozaffarian, 2006):

- Low in sodium,
- High in potassium
- Rich in fruits, vegetables, whole grains, cereal fiber, and fatty fish

These are the same principles used to prevent cardiovascular conditions resulting from atherosclerosis. A heart-healthy diet may also be a head-healthy diet.

Risk Factors in Cardiovascular Disease

The occurrence of cardiovascular disease in a person cannot be predicted with certainty. Many attributes and behaviors interact to produce the illness. See Table 18-2.

Unchangeable Risk Factors

Risk factors that cannot be modified to prevent atherosclerosis and hypertension are:

- Age
- Gender
- Race
- Family history
- Personal medical history

Age, Gender, and Race

Hypertension usually develops at about age 50 to 60, and coronary atherosclerosis becomes problematic more frequently in individuals older than the age of 40.

Risk for coronary heart disease increases in men after age 45 and women after age 55. Until menopause, women have less atherosclerosis and coronary heart

TABLE 18-2 ■ Risk Factors for Cardiovascular Disease

UNCHANGEABLE	CHANGEABLE
Age	Hypertension
Gender	High blood cholesterol
Race	Obesity
Heredity	Diabetes mellitus
Family history	Physical inactivity
Prior medical history	Alcohol intake Cigarette smoking

disease than men, but women past menopause and younger diabetic women are stricken with coronary heart disease just as often as men are.

Native Americans and Alaska natives die from heart disease much younger than the rest of the population. Thirty-six percent of those natives die before 65 years of age compared with 17% for the U.S. population overall (American Heart Association, May 2008).

Family and Prior Medical Histories

A family history of premature coronary heart disease in a parent or sibling increases a person's risk of the disease. Premature coronary artery disease is a myocardial infarction or a coronary artery procedure before age 55 in men and 65 in women (Brunzell, 2007).

Of special concern are the inherited **hyperlipoproteinemias** (see Genomic Gem 18-1) resulting in increased lipoproteins and lipids in the bloodstream (Table 18-3). Type IV hyperlipoproteinemia is very common and is frequently associated with non–insulin-dependent diabetes mellitus (NIDDM). For functions and significance of the various lipoproteins, see Table 18-4.

Because all hyperlipoproteinemias are not the same, neither are the dietary treatments. Health-care providers should be informed about the differences and not assume that all clients with hyperlipoproteinemia receive the same diet prescription. For best results, the clinical dietitian individualizes the diet with the client.

Genomic Gem 18-1

Type II Hyperlipoproteinemia

Type II hyperlipoproteinemia results from a single gene defect in the cell receptor that binds circulating low-density lipoproteins. It is an autosomal dominant characteristic. Individuals with this defect have a rate of coronary heart disease 25 times that of the normal population. In addition, clients with the subgroup type IIA hyperlipoproteinemia generally develop heart disease 15 years earlier than the rest of the population. Some even suffer heart attacks in infancy and childhood.

Most common forms of cardiovascular disease are thought to result from many genes, acting alone or with other genes and environmental factors. The same haptoglobin phenotypes related to susceptibility to scurvy also show marked differences in susceptibility to atherosclerosis. This difference is attributable to variations in LDL oxidation (Delanghe et al., 2007). Because at least one-half the variation in serum cholesterol is genetic, determining the pathologic mechanisms could markedly improve diagnosis and treatment selection (Arnett et al., 2007).

Changeable Risk Factors

The major changeable risk factors for CAD are:

- Hypertension
- Elevated serum cholesterol
- Obesity
- Physical inactivity
- Diabetes mellitus
- Alcohol intake
- Cigarette smoking

Hypertension

Hypertension is a risk factor for CAD as well as the most important risk factor for stroke. Persons with normal blood pressure have about half the lifetime risk of stroke compared to those with high blood pressure (American Heart Association and American Stroke Association, 2008). See Table 18-1. For individuals who reach the age of 50 years, the lifetime risk of hypertension developing is 90% (Appel and Anderson, 2010).

HIGH SALT INTAKE

Blood pressure values increase with age everywhere but in extremely remote areas of the world and are

TABLE 18-3 ■ Inherited Hyperlipoproteinemias

				INCREASED PLASMA VALUES				
				Lipoprotein			Lipid	
Type	**Frequency**	**Inheritance Pattern**	**Aggravated by/Target of Control**	**Chylomicrons**	**VLDL**	**LDL**	**Cholesterol**	**Triglycerides**
I	Very rare	Autosomal recessive	Fat	X				X
IIA	Common	Autosomal dominant	Fat			X	X	
IIB	Common	Autosomal dominant	Fat		X	X	X	X
III	Uncommon	Multifactorial	CHO	Remnants			X	X
IV	Very common	Autosomal dominant	CHO		X			X
V	Rare	Autosomal recessive	Fat and CHO	X	X		X	X

SOURCE: Adapted from Dietary Management of Hyperlipoproteinemia (1980); Fauci et al. (1998).

TABLE 18-4 ■ Functions and Significance of Various Lipoproteins

LIPOPROTEIN	FUNCTION	CLINICAL SIGNIFICANCE
Chylomicrons	Transport exogenous triglycerides from intestines to blood stream	Formed in small intestine; present in blood only after a meal
VLDL	Main transporter of endogenous triglyceride	Synthesized by liver from free fatty acids, glycerol, and carbohydrate
LDL	Transports cholesterol to body cells	Evolves from VLDLs as body's cells remove triglyceride from them and attach cholesterol Carrier of about 60% of total serum cholesterol The higher the LDL level, the greater the risk of CHD Major target of cholesterol-reducing therapy
HDL	Transports cholesterol from body cells to liver to be excreted Inhibits atherosclerosis through anti-inflammatory, antioxidant and anti-thrombotic actions (Hausenloy and Yellon, 2008)	Synthesized by liver and intestines The higher the HDL level, the lower the risk of CHD Aerobic exercise increases HDL levels.

significantly related to salt intake. Approximately 30 to 50% of hypertensive persons and smaller percentages of normotensive people are salt-sensitive.

Although sodium has been identified as the major influence on blood pressure, it does not increase blood pressure when administered with anions other than chloride (Kotchen and Kotchen, 2006). Hypertensive clients most likely to benefit from salt restriction are those who:

- Are African American
- Are older than 65 years
- Have low plasma renin activity
- Have **polymorphisms** in angiotensin genes.
- Are taking antihypertensive medications

Because 75% of dietary salt is found in processed foods, a public health approach to reducing salt in those items is recommended because individual educational efforts have not been successful (Appel and Anderson, 2010).

LOW POTASSIUM AND CALCIUM INTAKES

Potassium influences blood pressure because it promotes urinary excretion of sodium. However, results of studies of potassium on blood pressure have been inconsistent. High potassium intake does produce a greater reduction in blood pressure in African Americans than in whites and in individuals with a high salt intake (Gropper, Smith, and Groff, 2009).

Calcium supplementation may result in small reductions in systolic but not diastolic blood pressure and is associated with reduced risk of hypertensive disorders of pregnancy (Gropper, Smith, and Groff, 2009). Individuals who benefit from oral calcium therapy are those who:

- Have low calcium intakes, especially less than 400 milligrams daily
- Have low serum calcium levels
- Are salt-sensitive (Gropper, Smith, and Groff, 2009)

Because results of calcium supplementation on blood pressure have been modest and inconsistent, calcium should not be recommended to prevent or treat hypertension (Kotchen and Kotchen, 2006).

Intake of certain foods has been correlated with disease occurrence, but individual nutrients have not shown an effect. Possibly the individual nutrient tested:

- Has a small effect alone but works in conjunction with other nutrients or
- The substance in the food causing the effect has not been identified.

See Table 18-5 for the decrease in cardiovascular disease risk attainable by controlling blood pressure.

Elevated Blood Cholesterol

Despite its categorization as a risk factor for cardiovascular disease, **cholesterol** serves vital functions in the body. Cholesterol is a component of:

- The nerve tissue of the brain and spinal cord
- The tissues of the liver, the adrenal glands, and the kidneys
- Bile

In addition, cholesterol serves as a precursor of adrenal hormones and the sex hormones.

Although some cholesterol contributes to a healthy body, blood cholesterol levels are measured to monitor risk, to promote health, and to prevent disease. See Boxes 18-1 and 18-2.

RELATIONSHIP TO DIET

About 1000 milligrams of cholesterol is processed in the body per day, but less than one-third of the body's store of cholesterol comes from the diet, exclusively from foods of animal origin. Nearly all of the body's tissues can synthesize cholesterol, with the liver and the intestine producing the greatest amount. Most

TABLE 18-5 ■ Lifestyle Changes Proven to Reduce Cardiovascular Disease Risk

BEHAVIOR	GOAL	APPROXIMATE LDL-C REDUCTION	APPROXIMATE SYSTOLIC B/P REDUCTION	APPROXIMATE ATHEROSCLEROTIC CARDIOVASCULAR DISEASE RISK REDUCTION
Optimize Diet	Consume <7% kcal as saturated fat (including <1% as *trans*-fat)	8–10%		>8–10%
	Consume <200 mg cholesterol daily	3–5%		>3%
	Consume 5–10 g soluble fiber daily	3–5%		>3%
	Limit sodium intake to 2300 mg daily		2–8 mm Hg	>5%
	Eat 5 servings fruit, vegetables daily		8–14 mm Hg	>10%
	Limit alcohol to 1 (women) or 2 (men) standard drinks per day		2–4 mm Hg	>3%
	Possibly consume plant sterol/stanol enriched foods, 2 g daily	6–10%		>6%
Other	10 lb weight loss	5–8%	5–10 mm Hg	>10%
	Moderate exercise 30 min daily		4–9 mm Hg	>10% (some due to B/P change)
	Smoking cessation			≥20%

Adapted from American Dietetic Association (2008a, c); Grundy (2006); Lichtenstein et al. (2006).

Box 18-1 ■ *Cholesterol Screening Goals*

A national health objective of *Healthy People 2010* is to increase to 80% the proportion of adults aged 20 years and older who have been screened for high blood cholesterol within the preceding five years. By 2003, only the District of Columbia and Massachusetts had achieved that objective (CDC, 2005b).

Between 1999 and 2002, approximately 63% of U.S. adults met the goal. Of those men were less likely than women and blacks and Mexican Americans less likely than whites to have had their cholesterol checked as recommended (Centers for Disease Control, 2005a).

Box 18-2 ■ *Screening Children's Cholesterol*

Universal screening of children's cholesterol is not recommended, but the need for screening is determined by family history of cardiovascular disease, lack thereof (i.e., adopted children), or presence of other risk factors. For these children, the first screening should take place after 2 years of age but no later than 10 years of age. Screening before 2 years of age is not recommended (Daniels and Greer, 2008).

Children who do have elevated serum cholesterol levels have to be managed carefully so that sufficient food is provided to support growth.

people can produce less cholesterol or increase its excretion in response to high levels of dietary cholesterol, but others respond weakly, a phenomenon that may be genetically based and seems to affect synthesis just by the liver and not by other tissues (Gropper, Smith, and Groff, 2009).

Consumption of substances other than dietary cholesterol can also influence serum cholesterol levels. *Trans* unsaturated fatty acids in vegetable oil products are a risk factor for cardiovascular disease because they raise low-density lipoprotein cholesterol (LDL-C) levels and lower high-density lipoprotein cholesterol (HDL-C) levels. See Table 18-5 for the decrease in cardiovascular disease risk attainable by controlling fat and cholesterol intake.

MEASUREMENT OF BLOOD CHOLESTEROL

Lipids such as triglycerides (the major form of dietary fat and of stored body fat) and cholesterol (a sterol with fat-like properties) cannot dissolve in water. To travel in the bloodstream they are bound to lipoproteins. See Table 18-4 for the functions and significance of the four main classes of lipoproteins: **chylomicrons, very low-density lipoproteins (VLDL), low-density lipoproteins (LDLs),** and **high-density lipoproteins (HDLs).**

Blood tests for serum cholesterol are reported as total cholesterol, LDL-C or HDL-C based on cholesterol's association with the two major transport lipoproteins. Serum cholesterol itself is neither good nor bad, but the lipoproteins are associated with greater or lesser risk of coronary heart disease.

Table 18-6 shows in a simplified form how the goals for LDL-C therapy are determined based on the risks of death from MI or CAD. A client may be prescribed pharmacological and nonpharmacological treatments. Therapeutic lifestyle changes (TLC) remain an essential modality in clinical management (Grundy et al., 2004). Table 18-7 details a cholesterol-lowering diet. Cholesterol-lowering medications are added to a healthy lifestyle, not substituted for it. LDL remains the target of therapy because a clinical trial testing the effects of an HDL-raising medication was stopped early because of adverse effects (Rader, 2007).

TABLE 18-6 ■ Serum LDL-C Goals Based on Risk of MI or CAD Mortality

Risk factors in Columns A and B are summed. Client's risk factors are located in Column C to determine a goal for his cholesterol level (Column D).

RISK FACTOR	POSITIVE (COLUMN A)	NEGATIVE (COLUMN B)
Cigarette Smoking	+1	
B/P >140/90 or Antihypertensive Drug	+1	
HDL-C <40 mg/dL	+1	
HDL-C >60 mg/dL		−1
Premature CHD in 1st-Degree Relative	+1	
Men ≥45 years; Women ≥55 years	+1	
Total	Add column A	Combine Column B with column A to determine risk factor count
	COLUMN C	**COLUMN D**
Classification of Risk	**If These Risk Factors Present**	**LDL-C (mg/dL) Goal**
High	CHD, other atherosclerotic disease and/or diabetes	<100
Moderate	Two or more risk factors	<130
Low	0–1 risk factors	<160

The table is a simplified example. Other factors may affect clinical judgment to set goals lower.
SOURCES: Expert Panel (2001); Goldberg (2008); Grundy et al. (2004).

TABLE 18-7 ■ Cholesterol-Lowering Diets

DESCRIPTION	INDICATION	ADEQUACY
These diets limit lipids and, for some clients, sugars.	These diets are prescribed when clients have elevated serum cholesterol. Consultation with a Registered Dietitian is encouraged to individualize a dietary plan.	The diets are adequate in all nutrients with the possible exception of iron because of the restriction on red meat. If the client is also on a sodium-restricted diet, imitation cheese, bacon, and eggs may exceed the prescription. Clients must be encouraged to consume enough energy to maintain a healthy body weight.
Food Group	**Recommended Foods**	
Milk	Skim milk, 1% milk, cultured buttermilk, evaporated skim or nonfat milk Nonfat or low-fat yogurt and frozen yogurt 1 or 2% fat cottage cheese Low-fat soft cheese: Farmer and pot cheese labeled no more than 2–6 g of fat/oz	
Breads, Cereals, and Starches	Breads (made without whole milk, eggs, or butter): whole wheat, rye, pumpernickel, pita, white, bagels, English muffins, sandwich buns, dinner rolls, rice cakes Low-fat crackers: Sticks, rye crisp, saltines, zwieback Hot cereals, most dry cold cereals Pasta: Noodles, macaroni, spaghetti Rice Dried peas and beans, split peas, black-eyed peas, chick peas, kidney beans, navy beans, lentils, soybeans, low-fat tofu	
Fruits and Vegetables	Fresh, frozen, canned, or dried prepared without butter, cream, or cheese sauce	
Meat, Poultry, Fish, Shellfish	Lean meat with fat trimmed: *Beef*—round, sirloin, chuck, loin *Lamb*—leg, arm, loin, rib *Pork*—tenderloin, leg, shoulder *Veal*—all except ground Poultry without skin Fish: Fresh or frozen cod, flounder, haddock, halibut, trout; fresh or canned-in-water tuna Shellfish: Clams, crab, lobster, scallops, shrimp	
Eggs	Egg whites, egg substitute	
Fats and Oils	Monounsaturated preferred (canola, olive, peanut oils) Low-fat dressings	
Desserts and Snacks	Low-fat frozen desserts: Sorbet, sherbet, Italian ice, frozen yogurt, popsicles Angel food cake Low-fat cookies: Fig bars, gingersnaps Low-fat candy: Hard candy, jelly beans Low-fat snacks: Pretzels, plain popcorn	
Beverages	Nonfat beverages: Carbonated drinks, juices, tea, coffee	

Obesity and Inactivity

The location of the body fat is significant: abdominal obesity is related to cardiovascular disease and diabetes mellitus more than is **gluteal-femoral obesity.** Abdominal obesity is associated with increased triglyceride levels and decreased HDL-C levels (Brunzell, 2007). The waist measurements at the umbilicus indicative of increased risk are:

- More than 40 inches in men
- More than 35 inches in women.

See Table 18-5 for the decrease in cardiovascular disease risk attainable by weight loss and increased physical activity. Note that weight loss contributes to improvement in both lipid level and blood pressure.

Lack of exercise contributes to many other risk factors for cardiovascular disease. For instance, activity is inversely related to blood pressure independent of being overweight in both sexes and across all ages. As well, increased physical activity has been accompanied by increased HDL-C levels with its attendant lessening of risk.

Diabetes Mellitus

Diabetic persons have a two to three times higher risk of atherosclerosis than other people. Diabetic women lose the preventive advantages usually associated with premenopausal women regarding cardiovascular risk.

Insulin is required to maintain adequate levels of **lipoprotein lipase,** an enzyme that breaks down chylomicrons. When lipoprotein lipase is inadequate, chylomicrons and VLDL particles accumulate in the blood. After the diabetes is controlled, serum lipid levels decrease.

Lipoprotein lipase activity is greater in physically active subjects and increases with exercise, a valuable concept in the management of type 2 diabetes. Another example of altered physiology is described in Box 18-3, relating undernutrition in utero to increased risk for diabetes mellitus and cardiovascular disease in adulthood

Metabolic Syndrome

A particular constellation of signs and symptoms labeled **metabolic syndrome** is used to designate a cluster of risk factors for cardiovascular disease. Clients with this condition display three or more of the following signs: glucose intolerance, hypertriglyceridemia, low HDL cholesterol, hypertension, and abdominal obesity (Expert Panel, 2001). Specific criteria are:

- Fasting blood glucose ≥100 mg/dL
- Triglycerides ≥150 mg/dL
- HDL-C <40 mg/dL in men; <50 mg/dL in women
- Blood pressure ≥130 mm Hg systolic; ≥85 mm Hg diastolic
- Waist circumference >40 inches in men; >35 inches in women

Metabolic syndrome is also called *insulin resistance syndrome* because that feature likely ties the signs together. Whether labeling this syndrome helps to prevent or treat cardiovascular disease better

Box 18-3 ■ *Fetal Nutrition and Cardiovascular Disease in Adulthood*

Environmental influences before and shortly after birth are generally accepted as important determinants of the risk of cardiovascular disease and diabetes mellitus in adulthood (Hofman, Jackson, and Knight, 2004). Programming of the fetus may result from adaptations invoked when the materno–placental nutrient supply fails to match the fetal nutrient demand (Godfrey and Barker, 2001). One example of such shunting is the diversion of fuels to the developing brain at the expense of the muscles and pancreas (Sperling, 2004).

Studies have connected low birth weight, thinness, and short body length at birth with high death rates from cardiovascular disease and high prevalence of type 2 diabetes mellitus (Barker, 1999). The associations are seen in small-for-gestational-age (SGA) babies, rather than premature infants, and are independent of social class or lifestyle. Babies who are thin at birth tend to be insulin resistant as adults and have a high prevalence of diabetes mellitus, hypertension, and hyperlipidemia as adults.

Research suggests that undernutrition during gestation alters the relationships between glucose and insulin and between growth hormone and insulin-like growth factors. In this way, the fetus adapts to its environment to permit survival, but its changed physiology makes the individual susceptible to cardiovascular disease in later life. See Genomic Gem 18-2.

Genomic Gem 18-2

Fetal Origins Hypothesis

Nutrient availability during fetal life can program the function of genes that lasts a lifetime by modifying which genes are expressed (can be turned on) and which remain inactive. The function of genes involved in cholesterol metabolism appear to be modified in males who weighed less than 7 lb at birth. In these men, HDL production decreases in response to high-fat, high-saturated-fat diets, the opposite response of that seen in men with higher birth weights (Brown, 2008).

An investigation of genes for type 2 diabetes and the metabolic syndrome attempted to relate fetal growth and genes to adult health outcomes. Small body size at birth and a particular polymorphism seemingly protected an individual against insulin resistance and type 2 diabetes in later life (Eriksson, 2008).

than evaluating individual risk factors is unclear (Gropper, Smith, and Groff, 2009). The focus of the American Heart Association is on controlling individual risk factors (Lichtenstein et al., 2006).

Alcohol Consumption

Moderate alcohol intake has been linked to lower occurrence of cardiovascular events. In small amounts, alcohol seems to cause vasodilation, whereas at high doses it acts as a vasoconstrictor. Current evidence does not justify encouraging non-drinkers to begin imbibing. See Table 18-5 for the decrease in cardiovascular disease risk attainable by controlling alcohol intake. See Dollars and Sense 18-1 for estimated savings from moderating alcohol intake.

Heavy doses of alcohol affect the brain long term as well as short term. Alcohol use is generally associated with an approximate dose-dependent risk for hemorrhagic stroke throughout the full range of intake (Mukamal, 2007).

Dollars & Sense 18-1

Drink Less, Save Money and Health

A couple drinks a bottle of wine (two glasses for her, four for him) every night with dinner and dines in a restaurant twice a week. Assuming modest tastes in wine, $8 per bottle at the grocery and $4.50 per glass in the restaurant, their current annual outlay is $2808 for restaurant wine and $2080 for home wine.

If they implemented the cardioprotective diet plan and reduced their alcohol intake by one-half, they would save $2444 in a year while lessening the risk of cardiovascular disease.

Cigarette Smoking

Among the major coronary risk factors, cigarette smoking has been shown to be harmful to the heart and blood vessels, whether from active or second-hand smoke. The exact toxic components among the thousands of pharmacologically active substances present in tobacco smoke and their mechanisms affecting cardiovascular dysfunction are largely unknown, but smoking does increase LDL-C (Ambrose and Barua, 2004).

CAD occurs about 10 years earlier in smokers than in nonsmokers (Brunzell, 2007). See Table 18-5 for the decrease in cardiovascular disease risk attainable by smoking cessation.

Dietary Measures in Prevention and Treatment

Major lifestyle changes proven to be effective in reducing cardiovascular risk appear in Table 18-5. Additional actions are listed in Table 18-8. Many of the recommendations in both tables were proven effective in controlling hypertension by the DASH (Dietary Approaches to Stop Hypertension) diet, which is still recommended for hypertension control (American Dietetic Association, 2008c). In uncomplicated Stage 1 hypertension, dietary changes serve as initial treatment before drug therapy (Appel et al., 2009).

TABLE 18-8 ■ Additional Dietary Changes That May Reduce Cardiovascular Risk

ACTION	RATIONALE	CONCERNS
Consume fatty fish (salmon, herring, trout, sardines, tuna) twice a week.	Omega-3 fatty acids are associated with a decreased risk of death from cardiac events.	Recommended for clients with and without CHD Beware of mercury hazards (see Chapter 10).
Consume 1 tbs canola or walnut oil, 0.5 tbs ground flaxseed.	Plant-based sources of omega-3 fatty acids	Conversion of ALA in the body produces modest amounts of DHA.
Take omega-3 supplements in consultation with physician.	If food sources unacceptable to client for lipid management	Especially for clients with documented CHD Do not appear to lower B/P
Substitute 25 to 50 grams of soy protein (isolated soy protein, textured soy, tofu) daily for animal protein.	Can reduce LDL-C by 4–24%	If not contraindicated by risks or harms FDA approved a health claim for soy foods Minimal evidence of direct cardiovascular benefit Indirect benefit if reduce saturated fat and cholesterol intake Isoflavones not proven to be beneficial
Consume 5 ounces of nuts (walnuts, almonds, peanuts, macadamia, pistachios, pecans) per week.	Contain beneficial fatty acids May reduce LDL-C 6–29%	Substitute for equal kcal from other sources to avoid weight gain.
Increase fruit and vegetable servings to 10 to 12 daily.	Good sources of antioxidants and potassium	Beta-carotene and vitamin C and E supplements have shown no cardioprotective benefit. Potassium intake $<$DRI is associated with increased B/P
Select whole oats and foods high in psyllium (e.g., Bran Buds).	Soluble fiber lowers serum LDL-C without affecting HDL-C and triglyceride concentrations.	FDA approved health claims for whole oats and foods containing psyllium seed husk. Consume adequate fluids.

Adapted from American Dietetic Association (2008a, c); American Heart Association (2008); Lichtenstein et al. (2006); Theuwissen and Mensink (2008).

Implementing Dietary Changes

The effect of dietary changes differs significantly among individuals, even though they may faithfully follow recommendations. Much more must be learned about gene–diet interactions before customized interventions are generally available.

The DASH Diet

An 11-week clinical feeding trial of individuals with systolic blood pressure of less than 160 mm Hg and diastolic pressures from 80 to 95 mm Hg showed that dietary modification is effective in reducing blood pressure. The three diets were:

- *Control Diet* was low in fruits, vegetables, and dairy products with fat content typical of the United States (given to all participants before randomization).
- *Fruits* and *Vegetables Diet* was similar to the *Control Diet* except that it provided more fruits and vegetables and fewer snacks and sweets.
- *Combination Diet* was rich in fruits, vegetables, and low-fat dairy foods and had reduced amounts of total fat, saturated fat, and cholesterol than either of the other two diets.

Weight reduction did not confound the results, because kilocalories were adjusted to maintain weight. Likewise, the three types of diets each contained about 3 grams of sodium, and individuals were permitted no more than three caffeinated beverages and no more than two standard alcoholic beverages per day. (See Box 18-4 for information on caffeine and heart disease.) Reported intakes of alcohol were similar across all the diets. After 8 weeks on the experimental diets, the reductions in blood pressure shown in Table 18-9 were obtained. Recently, an 8-year follow-up study showed significantly lower all-cause and stroke mortality in hypertensive adults who followed a DASH-like diet (Parikh, Lipsitz, and Natarajan, 2009).

An outstanding feature of this trial was its emphasis, not on limiting or restricting foods, but on increasing intake of certain foods. Commonly available foods, not specialty foods containing fat substitutes, were used throughout the trial.

Features of the DASH diet are shown in Table 18-10. The example is based on a 2000-kilocalorie diet. Individuals requiring more or less energy intake need to make proportionate adjustments.

Fruits and Vegetables, Not Supplements

Atherosclerosis is thought to be related to oxidative stress characterized by lipid and protein in the vascular wall (Bonomini, 2008). One of the earliest events

Box 18-4 ■ *Coffee and Heart Disease*

Coffee has over a thousand chemicals, many formed during the roasting process, that may have either beneficial or harmful effects on the cardiovascular system (Bonita et al., 2007). The evidence is mixed.

Higher Risk

Three or more cups of coffee per day was significantly associated with coronary heart disease (CHD) in case-control studies (Sofi et al., 2007). Randomized controlled trials have confirmed the cholesterol-raising effect of diterpenes present in boiled coffee, which may contribute to the risk of CHD associated with drinking unfiltered coffee. Discovery of a genetic polymorphism associated with a slower rate of caffeine metabolism provides evidence that caffeine affects the risk of CHD (Cornelis and El-Sohemy, 2007). See Genomic Gem 18-3.

Lower Risk

Antioxidants in coffee might contribute to the lower risk of CHD among moderate coffee drinkers (Cornelis and El-Sohemy, 2007). People ages 65 years or older consuming more caffeine had a lower risk of cardiovascular disease and heart disease mortality than those who consumed less caffeine. This was not true in persons with extreme hypertension or in younger individuals (Greenberg et al., 2007).

No Effect

A 20-year study of 128,000 men and women revealed no effect of coffee on CHD after adjusting for known risk factors (Lopez-Garcia et al., 2006). Neither was daily coffee consumption significantly associated with CHD in long-term prospective cohort studies involving 403,631 participants followed from 3 to 44 years (Sofi et al., 2007).

Clinical judgment on the issue of caffeine varies, so the protocol of the physician or the institution should be ascertained before providing caffeinated beverages to clients with cardiovascular diseases.

Genomic Gem 18-3
Variant Gene in Caffeine Metabolism

Evidence relating caffeine to myocardial infarction (MI) involves the cytochrome P450 gene CYP1A2 that accounts for about 95% of caffeine metabolism. See Chapter 15 for a discussion on isoenzymes.

In a Costa Rican population-based case-control study, individuals with a variant CYP1A2 gene who metabolized caffeine more slowly than normal had a 64% increased risk of nonfatal MI. Coffee intake of 4 or more cups per day (compared with less than 1 cup per day) was associated with an increased risk of MI. This relationship existed only among individuals with the slow caffeine metabolism allele, CYP1A2*1F, and only among those younger than 59 years of age. People younger than 59 years had twice the risk of nonfatal MI and those younger than 50 years had four times the risk of healthy controls (Cornelis et al., 2006).

TABLE 18-9 ■ Reduction in Blood Pressure Compared to Control Diet

	FRUIT AND VEGETABLE DIET		COMBINATION (DASH) DIET	
	Systolic	Diastolic	Systolic	Diastolic
Normotensive	2.8 mm Hg	1.1 mm Hg	5.5 mm Hg	3.0 mm Hg
Hypertensive	7.2 mm Hg	2.8 mm Hg	11.4 mm Hg	5.5 mm Hg

SOURCE: Adapted from Appel et al. (1997).

TABLE 18-10 ■ The DASH Diet

FOOD GROUP	DAILY SERVINGS	SERVING SIZES	EXAMPLES AND NOTES	SIGNIFICANCE OF FOOD GROUP TO DASH DIET
Grains and Grain Products	7–8	1 slice bread ½ cup dry cereal ½ cup cooked cereal, rice, or pasta	Whole-wheat bread, English muffin, pita bread, bagel, cereals, grits, oatmeal	Major sources of energy and fiber
Vegetables	4–5	1 cup raw leafy ½ cup cooked 6 oz juice	Tomatoes, potatoes, carrots, peas, squash, broccoli, turnip greens, collards, kale, spinach, artichokes, sweet potatoes, beans	Rich sources of potassium, magnesium, and fiber
Fruits	4–5	6 oz juice 1 medium fruit ¼ cup dried fruit ½ cup fresh, frozen, or canned fruit	Apricots, bananas, dates, oranges, grapefruit, mangoes, melons, peaches, pineapples, prunes, raisins, strawberries, tangerines	Important sources of potassium, magnesium, and fiber
Low-Fat or Nonfat Dairy Foods	2–3	8 oz milk 1 cup yogurt 1.5 oz cheese	Skim or 1% milk, skim or low-fat buttermilk, nonfat or low-fat yogurt, part-skim mozzarella cheese, nonfat cheese	Major sources of calcium and protein
Meats, Poultry, and Fish	2 or fewer	3 oz cooked meat, poultry, or fish	Select only lean; trim away visible fat, broil, roast, or boil instead of frying; remove skin from poultry	Rich sources of protein and magnesium
Nuts, Seeds, and Legumes	4–5 per week	1.5 oz or ⅓ cup nuts ½ oz or 2 tbsp seeds ½ cup cooked legumes	Almonds, filberts, mixed nuts, peanuts, walnuts, sunflower seeds, kidney beans, lentils	Rich sources of energy, magnesium, potassium, protein, and fiber
Fats and Oils	2.5	1 tsp	Canola, olive, peanut oils	Contain mainly monounsaturated fatty acids

Adapted from American Diabetes Association and American Dietetic Association (1995); National Institutes of Health (1997).

promoting atherosclerosis is the oxidation of low-density lipoprotein (LDL) that stimulates inflammatory and immunological mechanisms (Matsuura, 2008). Clinically:

- High levels of oxidized LDL have been associated with increased risk of future myocardial infarction, even after adjustment for LDL-C and other established cardiovascular risk factors (Holvoet, 2008).
- Metabolic syndrome is associated with a higher fraction of oxidized LDL and thus with higher levels of circulating oxidized LDL (Holvoet, 2008).

Hence, one might conclude that antioxidants would be effective in preventing atherosclerosis. Antioxidant-rich fruits, vegetables, and whole grains have been associated with reduced disease risk. However, beta-carotene and vitamin C and E supplements have not protected against cardiovascular events or mortality (American Dietetic Association, 2008a).

Reducing Saturated Fat Intake

About two-thirds of saturated fatty acids in the U.S. diet come from animal fats. Using nonfat or low-fat dairy products is an especially important strategy because milk fat contains more cholesterol-raising fatty acids than meat fat does (Grundy, 2006). Cooking methods also affect the fat in meat. For instance, warm water rinsing of cooked, crumbled ground beef containing 30% fat reduced its fat content by 33 to 52% (Love and Prusa, 1992). Other techniques to reduce fat in meat are shown in Figure 18-3.

Plant Sterols

Specialty foods containing plant sterols may be recommended *in prescribed amounts*. These foods are marketed as table spreads (butter substitutes), juices, yogurts, and salad dressings. **Plant sterols** (phytosterols) are

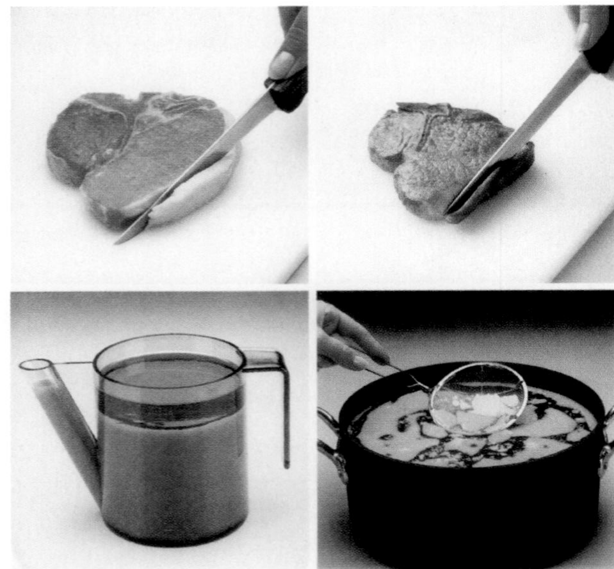

FIGURE 18-3 Selecting lean meat, trimming off visible fat, and skimming fat from meat juices reduce the amount of fat consumed. (From the National Live Stock and Meat Board, 444 North Michigan Avenue, Chicago, IL 60611, with permission.)

compounds that structurally resemble cholesterol but are not absorbed in the human body to any extent. In the gastrointestinal tract, plant sterols bind with bile and cholesterol, increasing their excretion in the feces (Gropper, Smith, and Groff, 2009). For maximum effectiveness, foods containing plant sterols should be consumed with other foods (American Dietetic Association, 2008a).

A rare autosomal recessive disorder is an absolute contraindication to the use of plant sterols. In this condition, *sitosterolemia*, both cholesterol and plant sterols are absorbed at a high rate and are not removed effectively by the liver, resulting in accelerated atherosclerosis and premature coronary artery and aortic valve disease. The possibility that plant sterols might be a risk factor for atherosclerosis in others is suggested by their presence in atheromatous plaque from individuals without absorption disorders (Patel and Thompson, 2006).

Despite their occurrence in foods, plant sterols are expected to act as drugs. Monitoring by the healthcare provider is in order.

Omega-3 Fatty Acids

Foods rich in marine omega-3 fatty acids, **eicosapentaenoic acid (EPA)** and **docosahexaenoic acid (DHA)**, result in:

- Decreased occurrences of arrhythmia and sudden death
- Lower plasma triglycerides
- Reduced blood clotting tendencies

One proposed mechanism for these beneficial effects was tested with people scheduled for carotid endarterectomy who received placebo, omega-6 fatty acids as sunflower oil, or omega-3 fatty acids as fish oil. Results indicated those receiving the fish oil had more stable plaque that incorporated omega-3 fatty acids, whereas the other two groups did not (Thies et al., 2003).

Fish containing omega-3 fatty acids include:

- Herring
- Mackerel
- Rainbow trout
- Salmon
- Sardines
- Swordfish
- Tuna

Commercially prepared fried fish are low in omega-3 fatty acids and high in *trans* fats. Fish oil has also been advocated as providing the benefits of omega-3 fatty acids without the risk of environmental toxins (Melanson et al., 2005).

In 2000, based upon supportive but not conclusive research that omega-3 fatty acids may reduce the risk of coronary heart disease, the FDA approved a qualified health claim for DHA- and EPA-containing supplements and in 2004 for foods that contain significant amounts of those omega-3 fatty acids. Foods specifically mentioned were salmon, lake trout, tuna, and herring. The FDA further recommends that consumers not exceed a total intake of 3 grams per day of EPA and DHA omega-3 fatty acids, with no more than 2 grams per day coming from a dietary supplement (U.S. Food and Drug Administration, 2004).

Clinical studies suggest that tissue levels of long-chain omega-3 fatty acids are depressed in vegetarians, particularly in vegans. Vegetarian diets, especially the vegan, are relatively low in α-linolenic acid (ALA) and provide little, if any, eicosapentaenoic acid (EPA) and docosahexaenoic acid (DHA).

Conversion of ALA by the body to the more active longer-chain metabolites is less than 5% to 10% efficient for EPA and 2% to 5% for DHA. Thus, total omega-3 requirements may be higher for vegetarians than for nonvegetarians. Moreover, the balance between omega-3 and omega-6 fatty acids impacts the conversion rate. Thus, it may be wise to consult a dietitian if the client:

- Is at risk for cardiovascular disease
- Has increased need for EPA and DHA (pregnant or lactating women)
- Is likely to poorly convert ALA to EPA and DHA (persons with diabetes or neurological disorders, premature infants, elderly)

Interventions might include careful selection of vegetable oils, use of marine plants or DHA-rich eggs, as well as supplements (Davis and Kris-Etherton, 2003).

More research is needed to show a cause-and-effect relationship between alpha-linolenic acid and heart disease (American Heart Association, 2008). Figure 18-4 shows fatty acids with their common food sources.

Psyllium

The FDA has permitted a health claim on the labels of foods containing psyllium seed husk (e.g., Kellogg's Bran Buds). The health claim states that the food, *as part of a diet low in saturated fat and cholesterol*, may reduce the risk of coronary heart disease.

To qualify, the food must provide at least 1.7 grams of soluble fiber in an amount customarily consumed. To obtain the result achieved in the controlled studies on which the FDA approval was based, a person would have to consume four servings per day (U.S. Food and Drug Administration, 1998).

Soy Protein

Clinical trials have shown that consumption of soy protein compared with other proteins such as those from milk or meat can lower total and LDL-C levels. The key is to replace some of the animal protein with soy protein.

In 1999 the FDA approved a health claim for soy-containing foods stating that including soy protein in a diet low in saturated fat and cholesterol may reduce the risk of CHD by lowering blood cholesterol levels. Because 25 grams of soy protein daily in the diet is needed to show a significant cholesterol-lowering effect, in order to qualify for this health claim, a food must contain at least 6.25 grams of soy protein per serving (U.S. Food and Drug Administration, 1999). Figure 18-5 shows the many choices available utilizing soy.

Because soy contains phytoestrogens, clients should discuss the feasability of adding soy products to their diets as a cardioprotective strategy with their health-care providers.

Not all research is easily or quickly interpreted. Clinical Application 18-1 describes the search for connections between diet and disease.

Sodium-Controlled Diets

Individuals with hypertension or heart failure may need to control their sodium intake. The preference for salty foods is learned and culturally transmitted, even though heavy salting is no longer necessary for preservation of food. After about three months on a sodium-restricted diet, most individuals lose their appetite for salt. Table 18-11 lists the legal definitions for sodium and salt descriptions on labels.

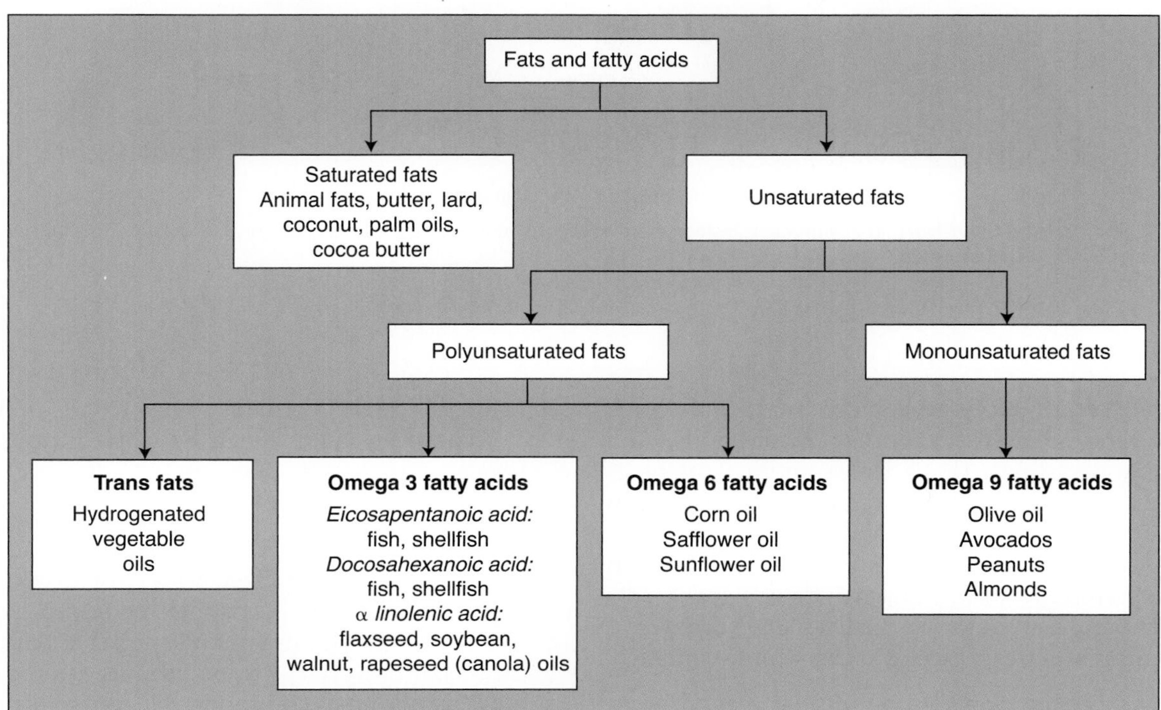

FIGURE 18-4 Fatty acids and their common food sources. Omega-3 fatty acids are particularly desirable in a heart healthy diet. (Adapted from Din, JN, Newby, DE, and Flapan, AD: Omega 3 fatty acids and cardiovascular disease—fishing for a natural treatment. BMJ 328:30, 2004.)

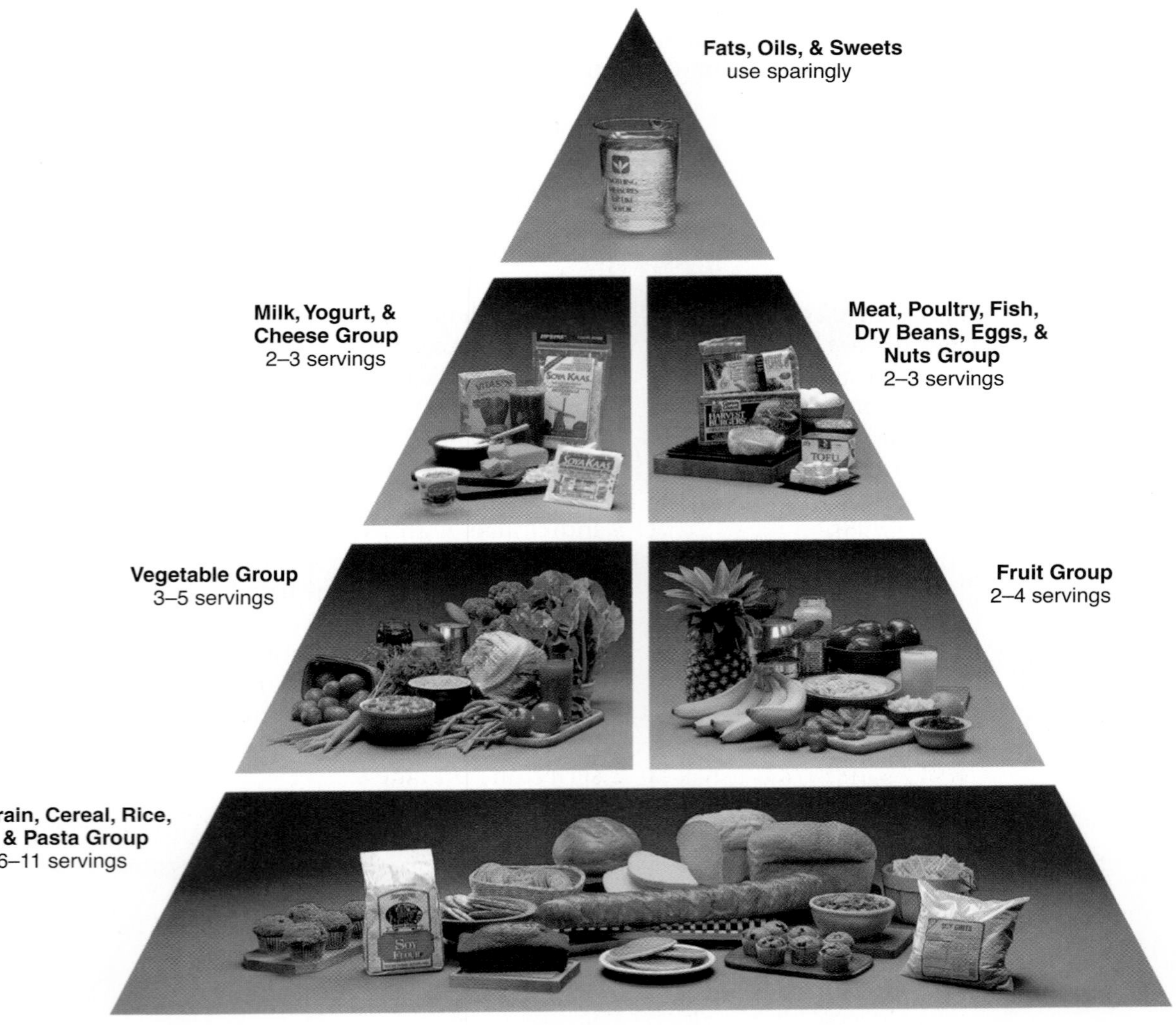

FIGURE 18-5 Daily Soyfood Guide Pyramid. Soy products include oil, milk, cheese, yogurt, beans, burgers, tofu, grits, and flour. (From Indiana Soybean Development Council, with permission.)

Unseen contributions to sodium intake may come from beverages, over-the-counter medications, and drinking water. Table 18-12 lists sodium content of beverages. Many toothpastes and mouthwashes contain significant amounts of sodium and should not be swallowed. Over-the-counter medications that may contain significant amounts of sodium include analgesics, antacids, antibiotics, antitussives, laxatives, and sedatives.

Softening water can increase its sodium content.

- Sodium in city water supplies has varied from 1.2 milligrams per liter in Seattle to 100 milligrams per liter in Phoenix.
- "Mineral waters" contain from 8 to 172 milligrams of sodium per liter. "Read the label" is appropriate advice.

Clients who require a diet containing less than 2 grams of sodium may elect to use bottled, distilled, deionized, or demineralized water for drinking and cooking in order to consume preferred sodium-containing foods. Some clients prefer a daily allotment of salt in a shaker to be used as desired. If this strategy is adopted, the foods high in sodium must be limited to a greater extent than for a standardized sodium-controlled diet.

18-1

Clinical Application

The Limits of Population Studies: An Historical Perspective

Research is sometimes misinterpreted or applied prematurely. Rarely does a single study merit widespread changes in diet in the pursuit of health.

FAT INTAKE

In the 1960s, Japan and Greece had the lowest rates of heart disease among seven countries. People in those two countries were very different in their fat consumption: 10% of kilocalories in Japan and 40% on the island of Crete. On the face of these findings, fat intake might be dismissed as relevant to heart disease. But the Greeks derived less than 10% of kilocalories from animal protein and 33% of their kilocalories from olive oil, which is 82% monounsaturated.

MULTIPLE CAUSATION

Since 1976, Spain has experienced a decrease in cardiovascular mortality, despite increased intakes of dairy products and meat, particularly pork and poultry. If attention focused only on those foods, the rationale for the decreased mortality would be missed.

Most of the decrease in cardiovascular mortality was due to a decline in stroke mortality. Improved hypertension control, including decreased intake of salt and salt-cured foods, is thought to have influenced this trend. Other contributing factors were increased consumption of fruit and fish, reduction in cigarette smoking, and expanded access to clinical care, including a major increase in the use of aspirin as a platelet inhibitor (Serra-Majem et al., 1995).

RED WINE

Consumption of red wine is credited with conferring some protection against coronary heart disease. The "French Paradox" refers to that country's second lowest coronary heart disease mortality rate among 21 countries, despite having the highest alcohol intake and the highest wine intake. Other studies have shown a maximum protective effect of alcohol against CHD at one to two drinks per day. Higher alcohol intake is progressively associated with higher risks of cardiovascular disease and other causes of mortality.

A 12-year study of French men indeed found a decrease in cardiovascular mortality of 30% associated with a daily intake of 48 grams of alcohol, mostly wine. In contrast, mortality by cancer and violent death was increased compared with that of abstainers (Renaud and Gueguen, 1998).

IRON

Men in eastern Finland have one of the highest recorded incidences of mortality from CHD. An association was reported between high levels of stored iron (as assessed by serum ferritin levels or ratio of serum transferrin receptor to serum ferritin) and increased risk for acute myocardial infarction (Salonen et al., 1992; Tuomainen et al., 1998). Iron overload thus was hypothesized to cause the higher occurrence of CHD in men compared with women. A study in Greece also correlated high dietary iron intake with increased risk of coronary artery disease in men and women 60 years of age or older (Tzonou et al., 1998).

A more detailed study found no association between total iron intake and risk of myocardial infarction after adjustment for age and gender, but the study did find high dietary intake of heme iron associated with occurrence of and mortality from myocardial infarction (Klipstein-Grosbusch et al., 1999). A reanalysis of Salonen's data associated increased iron intake with increased consumption of red meat (American Heart Association, 2000).

HOMOCYSTEINE

Thirty years ago, extensive atherosclerosis was found on autopsy of individuals with elevated plasma homocysteine levels due to errors of metabolism. This autosomal recessive genetic disease, homocystinuria, occurs in about 1 of 300,000 live births with a higher prevalence in Ireland and New South Wales (Refsum et al., 2004).

When untreated, homocystinuria results in thromboembolic events in 50% of the clients and a 20% mortality rate before the age of 30 (Nygard et al., 1997). Extending investigations to general populations found plasma homocysteine levels related to heart failure (Vasan et al., 2003), risk of stroke (Tanne et al., 2003), but also cancer mortality and all-cause mortality as well as cardiovascular mortality (Vollset et al., 2001).

Consequently, the early enthusiasm for reducing cardiovascular risk by reducing homocysteine levels has waned. Homocysteine appears to be a marker, rather than a cause, of cardiovascular disease. Therefore routine screening for and treatment of elevated homocysteine levels to prevent cardiovascular disease is not supported by the evidence (Wierzbicki, 2007). Clinically, there is little justification for using folic acid or B vitamins in patients with established cardiovascular disease, whether or not they have elevated homocysteine levels (O'Callaghan, 2007).

Thus, evidence accumulates slowly and must be interpreted cautiously. The many correlations found in large studies are often statistically significant but do not prove causation and may not be clinically useful. Advice to clients should be based, as much as possible, on randomized clinical trials, the "gold standard" of medical practice.

TABLE 18-11 ■ Labeling Regulations for Sodium Content Descriptions

TERM	LEGAL DEFINITION
Free	Less than 5 mg of sodium per serving
Salt Free	Must meet the criteria for free
Very Low* Sodium	Less than 35 mg of sodium per serving. For meals and main dishes: 35 mg or less per 100 g
Low* Sodium	Less than 140 mg of sodium per serving. Meals and main dishes: 140 mg or less per 100 g
Reduced or Less	This term means that a nutritionally altered product contains 25% less sodium than the regular, or reference, product. However, a reduced claim cannot be made on a product if its reference food already meets the requirement for a "low" claim.
Light in Sodium or Lightly Salted	May be used on food in which the sodium content has been reduced by at least 50% compared with an appropriate reference food.
Unsalted or No Added Salt	Must declare "This is not a sodium-free food" on information panel if the food is not sodium free.

*Synonyms for low include "little," "few," and "low source of."

TABLE 18-12 ■ Examples of Sodium Content of Beverages*

	REGULAR		DIET	
Beverage†	**Sodium (mg)**	**Kilocalories**	**Sodium (mg)**	**Kilocalories**
Club soda			75	0
Coffee	4	0		
Cola	15	151		
With aspartame			21	2
With saccharin			75	2
Gatorade	39	123		
Ginger Ale	25	125	130	4
Kool-Aid	0	150		
With aspartame			0	6
Lemonade	12	150		
Lemon-Lime Soda	41	149	70	4
Pepper-Type	38	151	70	0
Root Beer	49	152	170	4
Tea	2	0		

*Serving size is 12 fluid ounces.
†Sodium content may vary depending on the source of water.

Several salt substitutes are available. Many of them substitute potassium for sodium and may be unsuitable for clients with kidney disease or those taking potassium-sparing diuretics or angiotensin-converting enzyme (ACE) inhibitors. Clients should consult their health-care providers about using salt substitutes. These products are for table use only and are not appropriate for cooking because they turn bitter.

In clinical practice, diet orders such as "no-added-salt diet" or "low-sodium diet" require clarification. Usually, a facility's diet manual defines the terms. A "no-added-salt diet" may be calculated as 4 grams of sodium and a "low-sodium diet" as 2 grams in one facility but differently in another. Diet prescriptions should be written in milligrams of sodium to achieve the desired result. Table 18-13 describes diets with sodium controlled from 2 grams to 250 milligrams per day. Figure 18-6 shows some of the seasonings permitted on a sodium-controlled diet.

TABLE 18-13 ■ Sodium-Controlled Diets

DESCRIPTION	**INDICATION**		**ADEQUACY**	
These diets control sodium intake to prescribed levels.	Clients with hypertension, heart failure, fluid-retaining kidney or endocrine disease, or other edematous conditions.		The 500-mg and 250-mg diets may be deficient in some nutrients.	
Food Item or Group	**2 Grams of Sodium**	**1 Gram of Sodium**	**500 mg of Sodium**	**250 mg of Sodium**
Soups	Column A below	Column A below	Column A below	Column A below
Milk	2 cups Column B below	2 cups Column B below	1 cup Column B below	Column A below
Bread	3 slices Column B below	3 slices Column B below	Column A below	Column A below
Cereal	1 serving Column B below	Column A below	Column A below	Column A below
Fruits	Free	Free	Free	Free
Egg	1	1	1	1
Meat/Substitutes	6 oz	5 oz	4 oz	4 oz
Vegetables	Column A below	Column A below	Column A below	Column A below
Desserts	1 serving Column B below	Column A below	Column A below	Column A below
Fats and Oils	5 tsp Column B below	3 tsp Column B below	3 tsp Column B below	Column A below
Condiments	Column A below	Column A below	Column A below	Column A below
Food Group	**Column A Lower in Sodium than Column B**		**Column B Higher in Sodium than Column A**	
Soups	Unsalted broth and bouillon Low sodium canned soup Homemade soup made with allowed foods and milk allowance		Regular canned and frozen soups Dehydrated soup mixes Bouillon cubes and powder Consommé	
Milk	Commercially made low-sodium milk Low-sodium cheese		All milk from animals Yogurt Regular cheese Commercial milk products	
Breads and Cereals	Bread and crackers prepared without salt Rice, barley, and pasta without added salt Baked goods made without salt, baking soda, or baking powder Unsalted cooked cereal Puffed rice, puffed wheat, shredded wheat Cornmeal, cornstarch		Commercial mixes Frozen bread dough Instant rice and pasta mixes Regular crackers Instant and quick-cooking cereals Commercial stuffing and casserole mixes Self-rising flour and cornmeal Baked goods and quick breads made with salt, baking soda, baking powder, or egg white	

TABLE 18-13 ■ Sodium-Controlled Diets (Continued)

Food Group	Column A Lower in Sodium than Column B	Column B Higher in Sodium than Column A
Fruits	Fresh, frozen, dried, or canned fruit without added sodium All fruit juices	Crystallized or glazed fruit Maraschino cherries Dried fruit with sodium preservatives
Vegetables	Fresh, frozen without salt, low-sodium canned vegetables except those listed at right	Canned and frozen vegetables and juices Sauerkraut
Meat, Poultry, Fish, Shellfish	Fresh, frozen, or canned low-sodium meat and poultry Low-sodium luncheon meats Eggs Low-sodium peanut butter Fresh fish Canned low-sodium tuna and salmon	Real and imitation bacon Luncheon meat Chipped or corned beef Smoked or salted meat or fish Kosher meat Frozen and powdered egg substitutes Regular peanut butter Brains, kidney, clams, lobster, crab, oysters, scallops, shrimp, and other shellfish
Fats and Oils	Cooking oil Unsalted butter, margarine, salad dressings, and shortening	Salted butter and margarine Commercial salad dressings
Desserts and Miscellaneous	Alcohol Coffee, coffee substitutes Lemonade Tea Low-sodium candy Unflavored gelatin Jam, jelly, maple syrup, honey Unsalted nuts and popcorn	Salted popcorn, nuts, potato chips, snacks Instant cocoa or powdered drink mixes Canned fruit drinks Commercial pastry, candy, cakes, cookies, gelatin desserts
Condiments and Seasonings	Sweet: allspice, almond extract, anise seed, apricot nectar, baking chocolate, cardamom, cinnamon, coriander, ginger, lemon extract, lemon juice, mace, maple extract, mint, nutmeg, orange extract, orange juice, peppermint extract, pineapple, pineapple juice, unsalted pecans, vanilla extract, unsalted walnuts, walnut extract Tangy: Basil, bay leaves, caraway seeds, cayenne pepper, chili powder, chives, cloves, curry powder, dill weed, garlic, garlic powder (not salt), green pepper, horseradish without salt, marjoram, mustard powder (not prepared), mustard seed, onion powder (not salt) onions, oregano, paprika, parsley, pepper, poppy seed, rosemary, sage, savory, sesame seeds, tarragon, thyme, turmeric	Any salt Barbecue sauce Bouillon cubes or granules Catsup Chili sauce Tartar sauce Horseradish sauce Meat extracts, sauces, and tenderizers Kitchen Bouquet Gravy and sauce mixes Monosodium glutamate Prepared mustard Olives Pickles Saccharin, other sugar substitutes containing sodium Soy sauce Teriyaki sauce Worcestershire sauce

SAMPLE MENUS FOR 2-GRAM SODIUM DIET

Breakfast	Lunch and Dinner
½ cup orange juice	3 oz chicken breast, turkey, or fish baked in lemon juice
½ cup shredded wheat	Baked potato
2 slices toast	2 tsp spread
2 tsp spread	½ cup broccoli
1 tbsp strawberry jam	Tossed salad with homemade oil and vinegar dressing
1 cup 1% milk	1 dinner roll
Sugar	½ cup sherbet
Coffee	1 cup 1% milk (day's total = 2 cups)
	Tea

Modifications for Common Conditions

Persons with heart attacks, heart failure, or stroke may require modifications in diet. Referral to the dietitian may be in order.

Myocardial Infarction

After a heart attack, the client may be in shock. One adaptive response of the body is to slow gastrointestinal function. Thus the client may receive nothing by mouth while the shock persists. Fluid is given intravenously to maintain fluid balance and to keep an access site open for intravenous medications.

As the client recovers, the diet usually progresses from a 1000- to 1200-kilocalorie liquid diet to a soft diet of small, frequent meals. Large meals can increase the workload of the heart. The diet prescription begins to implement the principles of a cardioprotective diet. As soon as possible, client education should start.

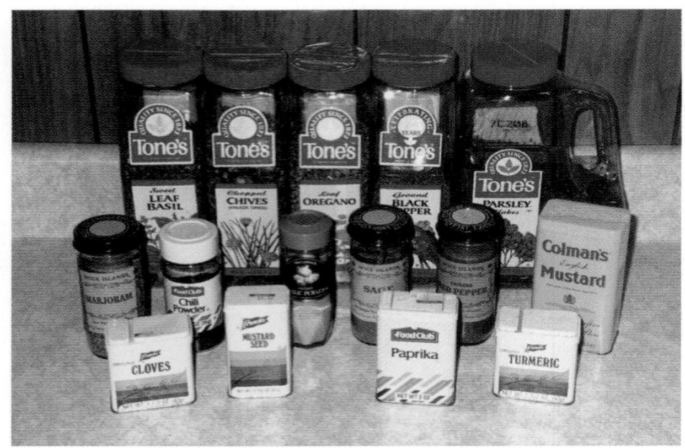

FIGURE 18-6 These are just a few of the many condiments and seasonings permissible on a sodium-restricted diet.

Heart Failure

For clients in heart failure, the diet order may read "as tolerated" but sodium and fluid restriction is common. Energy needs are increased due to the workload of the heart and respiratory system. Protein intakes of 1.12 to 1.37 grams per kilogram of body weight may be necessary to preserve body composition (American Dietetic Association, 2008b).

Food for the client with heart failure should be nutrient-dense, easily eaten, and easily digested. An hour's rest before meals conserves energy. Large meals, which would exert upward pressure on the chest, are undesirable. Liquid formulas, some special low-volume, nutrient-dense preparations, can be used to provide nutrients while moderating the feeling of fullness. It may be necessary to provide supplements of water-soluble vitamins and minerals that may be lost as excess fluid is excreted through treatment.

Stroke

Clients who have had a stroke may have trouble seeing their food as well as problems chewing, swallowing, and manipulating utensils. Generally, thicker, rather than thinner, liquids are easier to manage for a person with swallowing difficulty. Dry, chunky, or sticky foods are best avoided. Nurses feeding clients with hemiplegia should place the food on the unaffected side of the tongue. Turning the client's head toward the weak side while he is sitting upright may help with swallowing. In addition, stroke clients may be aphasic and unable to communicate their needs or desires. A speech therapist is skilled in assessing function and restorative therapy using adaptive devices for clients with dysphagia and aphasia.

Keystones

- Major changeable risk factors for cardiovascular disease are hypertension, hypercholesterolemia, obesity, physical inactivity, diabetes mellitus, alcohol consumption, and cigarette smoking.
- Dietary modifications in cardiovascular disease most often involve cholesterol-lowering or blood pressure-controlling measures.
- The major target of cholesterol-lowering measures is low density lipoprotein cholesterol (LDL-C).
- Lifestyle changes effective for hypertension control include reducing sodium intake and, if necessary, body weight.
- The most common inherited hyperlipoproteinemia is type IV, which requires restricted carbohydrate intake as well as controlled fat intake.
- Dietary treatment of chronic heart failure focuses on fluid balance and preventing malnutrition.

CASE STUDY 18-1

Mr. Z is a 59-year-old white man who was admitted to the acute-care hospital with a diagnosis of possible myocardial infarction. Subsequent testing proved Mr. Z did not have an infarction. His medical diagnoses are Stage 1 hypertension and myocardial ischemia. He is being readied for discharge to home.

Mr. Z is vice president for sales of a large manufacturing company. His business activities involve luncheon and dinner meetings at which alcohol consumption is common. He stated he has "at least one cocktail, usually two" with lunch and with dinner.

The clinical dietitian visited Mr. Z to evaluate his food behaviors as requested by the physician. After the dietitian left, Mr. Z said to the nurse, "That diet is impossible for my situation. She just doesn't understand the business world. I don't believe there's anything wrong with my heart, anyway. It was just indigestion."

Providing client care is a dynamic process. Based on the above information, the nurse added the following modifications to Mr. Z's care plan.

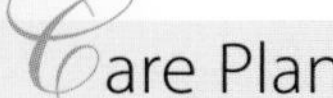

Care Plan

Subjective Data

Reported alcohol intake of two to four drinks per day ■ Perceived incompatibility of prescribed diet with current lifestyle ■ Stated disbelief in medical diagnosis

Objective Data

LDL-C 158; B/P 150/96; BMI 27

Analysis

Denial of illness and negative perception of treatment regimen as evidenced by statements to nurse.

Plan

DESIRED OUTCOMES EVALUATION CRITERIA	ACTIONS/INTERVENTIONS	RATIONALE
Client will acknowledge effect of lifestyle on health by hospital discharge.	Review pathophysiology of hyperlipoproteinemia and atherosclerosis with client.	Repeated information reinforces learning.
	Analyze with the client the possibility of partial compliance.	Perhaps the many changes required are overwhelming Mr. Z.
	Refer to clinical dietitian for repeat visit to prioritize actions and individualize diet plan.	One or two alterations might be acceptable as a starting point.
	Obtain the client's permission to discuss lifestyle changes with significant other.	Enlisting a support person might, over time, give Mr. Z reason to reconsider his options.
	Inform physician of extent of intended compliance with treatment regimen.	These statements will impact the success of treatment. It is appropriate to notify the physician and record it on the client's medical record.

The following day the physician showed Mr. Z his laboratory results and reviewed his diagnosis and risks. The clinical dietitian revisited Mr. Z and wrote the following:

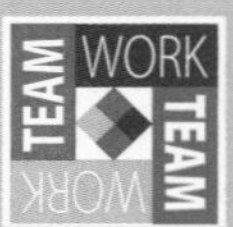

18-1

Dietitian's Notes

Subjective: Able to repeat the information given by physician. Does not smoke. Eats three servings of vegetables most days, some of them fried. No exercise program. Usually eats two weekday meals in a restaurant. Client consumes one to two servings of alcohol daily or twice daily. Client perceives that it is impossible to make dietary changes when he eats in restaurants.

Objective: B/P 150/96, LDL-C 158, HDL-C 36

Analysis: Harmful beliefs/attitudes about food or nutrition-related topics related to Stage 1 hypertension and myocardial ischemia as evidenced by client's reports.

Plan: Use local area restaurant menus to illustrate health meals—Done.

Obtain commitment to follow up with the outpatient dietitian. Appointment made.

Refer Mr. and Mrs. Z to Heart Healthy Support Group to help refocus Mr. Z's view of his health.

Critical Thinking Questions

1. How could additional assessment data regarding family history be helpful in interpreting this client's reaction? Would you expect his reaction to be different if the diagnosis of myocardial infarction had been confirmed?
2. What additional interventions have the potential to achieve the stated outcome after hospital discharge?
3. When more genomic information becomes available in the future, how might this scenario change?

Chapter Review

1. The DASH diet to reduce hypertension emphasizes:
   a. Increased amounts of fruits, vegetables, nuts, seeds, and legumes
   b. Specialty formulas as meal replacements
   c. Carbohydrate control and counting similar to that used in diabetes mellitus treatment
   d. Increased amounts of protein through low-fat dairy products and large servings of meats
2. The first action a hypertensive client should take to lower blood pressure is to:
   a. Restrict fluid to 1500 milliliters per day
   b. Eliminate saturated fat from the diet
   c. Lose weight if necessary
   d. Limit sodium intake to 1 gram per day
3. Lifestyle changes that are recommended to reduce cardiovascular disease risk limit saturated and *trans*-fat intake to ___ % of daily kilocalories and cholesterol to ___ milligrams per day.
   a. 45, 450
   b. 30, 300
   c. 15, 250
   d. 7, 200
4. Which of the following seasonings are permitted on a sodium-controlled diet?
   a. Catsup, horseradish mustard, and tartar sauce
   b. Chili powder, green pepper, and caraway seeds
   c. Celery seeds, seasoned meat tenderizer, and teriyaki sauce
   d. Dry mustard, garlic, and Worcestershire sauce
5. Which of the following lifestyle changes would have the greatest effect in reducing risk of atherosclerotic cardiovascular disease?
   a. Limiting cholesterol intake to the recommended amount
   b. Consuming plant sterols in recommended amounts
   c. Limiting alcohol intake to one (women) or two (men) standard drinks per day
   d. Eating five servings of fruits and vegetables daily

Clinical Analysis

Mr. T is a 55-year-old black man being seen in a health clinic for hypertension. His blood pressure was 152/98 3 months ago when he was first diagnosed. It has remained below that level but has not returned to normal. Today his blood pressure is 146/100.

Mr. T is 5 ft 9 in. tall and weighs 173 lb. He has a medium frame. When first diagnosed, he weighed 178 lb. A weight-loss diet with no added salt was prescribed, but progress has been slow.

Now the physician is prescribing a 2-gram sodium diet and starting Mr. T on a mild potassium-wasting diuretic. The clinic nurse is responsible for instructing the client.

1. Before he or she instructs Mr. T, which of the following actions by the nurse would best ensure his compliance with the diet?
   a. Doing a financial analysis to see if Mr. T can afford the special foods on his new diet
   b. Finding out which favorite foods Mr. T would have most difficulty giving up
   c. Listing the possible consequences of hypertension if it is not controlled
   d. Asking to see Mrs. T to instruct her on the preparation of foods for the new diet

2. Which of the following breakfasts would be best for Mr. T?
   a. Applesauce, raisin bran, 1% milk, and a bagel with cream cheese
   b. Canned pears, cornflakes, whole milk, and a cholesterol-free plain doughnut
   c. Cooked prunes, instant oatmeal, 2% milk, and raisin toast with margarine
   d. Orange juice, shredded wheat, skim milk, and whole-wheat toast with jelly

3. Mr. T has agreed to limit his alcohol intake to two drinks per week. He asks the nurse to recommend beverages compatible with his diet. Which of the following is the best choice?
   a. Tomato juice and bouillon
   b. Buttermilk and club soda
   c. Plain tea and fruit juice
   d. Gatorade and lemonade

19

Diet in Renal Disease

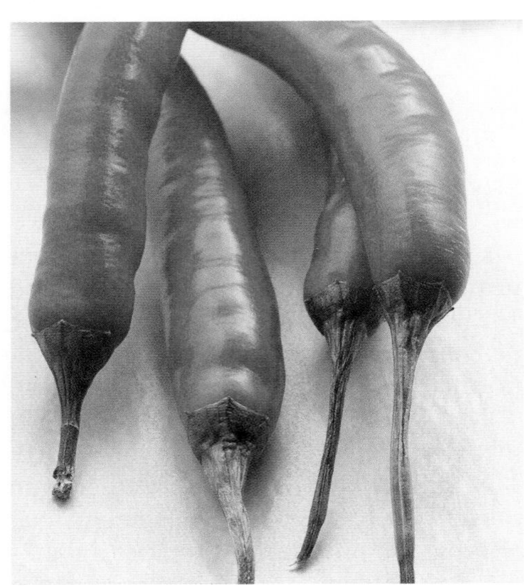

LEARNING OBJECTIVES

After completing this chapter, the student should be able to:

- Identify the major causes of acute and chronic kidney failure.
- List the goals of nutritional care for a client with kidney disease.
- List the nutrients commonly modified in the dietary treatment of chronic kidney disease (CKD).
- Discuss the relationship among kilocaloric intake, dietary protein utilization, and uremia.
- Discuss the nutritional care of clients with kidney disease in relation to their medical treatment.

Diet therapy for clients with kidney disease depends on an understanding of the normal function of the kidneys and basic concepts of pathophysiology of renal diseases. **Renal** means pertaining to the kidneys. The nutritional care of clients with renal disease is complex. These clients frequently must learn not just one diet in which one to seven nutrients are controlled but several different diets as their medical condition and the treatment approach change. The failure to adhere to necessary dietary changes can result in death. One aspect of working with clients with renal disease is that inattentiveness to dietary modifications can be measured objectively in weight changes or changes in blood chemistry.

Anatomy and Physiology of the Kidneys

No other organ in the human body can perform the multiple functions of the kidneys. These functions are possible because of the kidneys' internal structure.

Internal Structure

The functioning unit of the kidney is the **nephron.** Each kidney contains about a million nephrons. Figure 19-1 shows an individual nephron. Each nephron has two main parts. The first part, **Bowman's capsule,** is the cup-shaped top of the nephron. Inside Bowman's capsule is a network of blood capillaries called the **glomerulus** (plural, *glomeruli*). The second part of the nephron is the **renal tubule.** (A tubule is a small tube or canal.) The renal tubule is the rope-like portion of the nephron. This rope-like structure ends at the collecting tubule. Several nephrons usually share a single **collecting tubule.**

Functions

The kidneys assist in the internal regulation of the body by performing the following functions:

1. *Filtration:* The kidneys remove the end products of metabolism and substances that have accumulated in the blood in undesirable amounts during the

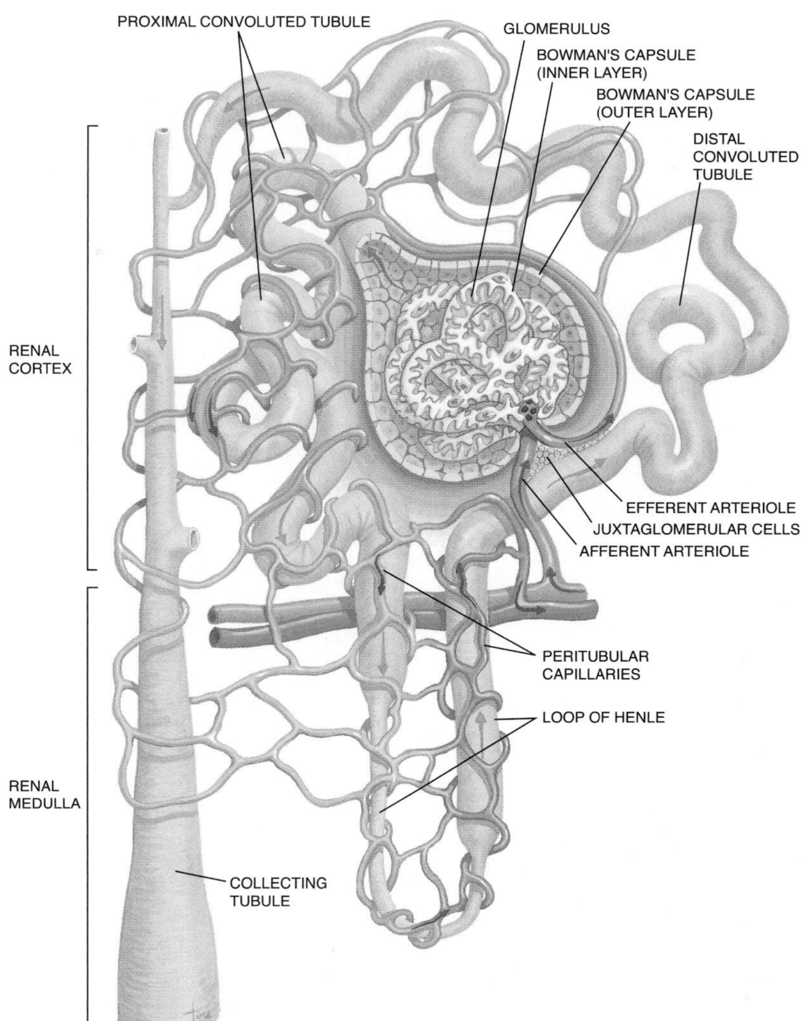

FIGURE 19-1 A nephron with its associated blood vessels. The arrows indicate the direction of blood flow. (Reprinted from Scanlon, VC, and Sanders, T: *Essentials of anatomy and physiology,* ed 5. FA Davis, Philadelphia, 2007, p 423, with permission.)

filtration process. Substances removed from the blood include:

- Urea
- Creatinine
- Uric acid
- Urates

Also filtered from blood are undesirable amounts of:

- Chloride
- Potassium
- Sodium
- Hydrogen ions

The **glomerular filtration rate (GFR)** is the amount of fluid filtered each minute by all the glomeruli of both kidneys and is one index of kidney function. This rate is normally about 125 milliliters per minute (Fig. 19-2).

2. *Reabsorption:* Previously filtered substances (e.g., water and sodium) needed by the body are reabsorbed into the blood in the tubules.
3. *Secretion of Ions to Maintain Acid–Base Balance:* Secretion is the process of moving ions from the blood into the urine. Secretion allows for the amount of a substance to be excreted into the urine in concentrations greater than the concentration filtered from the plasma in the glomeruli. The kidneys regulate the balance between bicarbonate and carbonic acid by the secretion and exchange of hydrogen ions for sodium ions.
4. *Excretion:* The kidneys eliminate unwanted substances from the body as urine.
5. *Renal Control of Cardiac Output and Systemic Blood Pressure:* The kidneys adapt to changing cardiac output by altering resistance to blood flow both at the beginning of the glomerulus and at the end.
6. *Calcium, Phosphorus, and Vitamin D:* The kidneys produce the active form of vitamin D, **calcitriol.** Activated vitamin D regulates the absorption of calcium and phosphorus from the intestinal tract

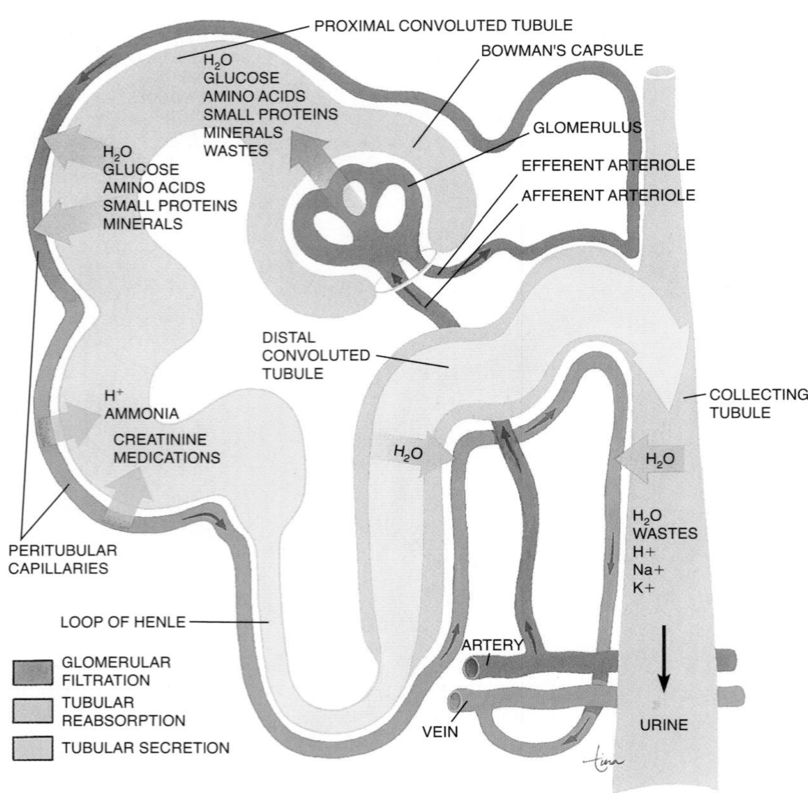

FIGURE 19-2 Schematic representation of glomerular filtration, tubular reabsorption, and tubular secretion. The renal tubule has been uncoiled, and the peritubular capillaries are shown adjacent to the tubule. (Reprinted from Scanlon, VC, and Sanders, T: *Essentials of anatomy and physiology,* ed 5. FA Davis, Philadelphia, 2007, p 426, with permission.)

and assists in the regulation of calcium and phosphorus levels in the blood.

7. *Erythropoietin:* The kidneys produce a hormone called **erythropoietin,** which stimulates maturation of red blood cells in bone marrow.

Kidney Disease

Because the kidneys perform so many different metabolic functions, kidney disease has serious consequences.

Causes

Renal disease can be caused by many factors, including:

- Trauma
- Infections
- Birth defects
- Medications
- Chronic disease (e.g., atherosclerosis, diabetes, hypertension)
- Toxic metal consumption
- See Genomic Gem 19-1.

> **Genomic Gem 19-1**
>
> **Genetic Mutations**
>
> Some kidney diseases are caused by errors in the genetic code. A genetic mutation can make it possible that a particular disease will happen. For example, high blood pressure is strongly associated with a selection of minor mutations plus lifestyle choices in diet and exercise and smoking, other environmental exposures, and kidney disease.

Diabetic nephropathy is the most common cause of renal failure. A physiological stress such as a myocardial infarction (MI) or an extensive burn can precipitate renal disease by decreasing the perfusion of the kidney or markedly increasing catabolism. Clinical Application 19-1 describes the renal response after MI and the effect of reduced renal blood flow. Catabolism causes an increase in nitrogenous products and potassium, which must be excreted and thus overworking the kidneys. Renal disease is a feared complication of many pathologies and treatments—including radiocontrast materials used in diagnostic procedures, some antibiotics, and some pain medications.

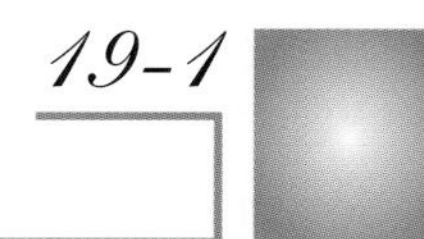

Clinical Application 19-1

Renal Response After a Myocardial Infarction

Immediately after a myocardial infarction (heart attack, or MI), blood flow through the systemic circulation is diminished. Systemic circulation refers to the blood flow from the left part of the heart through the aorta and all branches (arteries) to the capillaries of the tissues. Systemic circulation also includes the blood's return to the heart through the veins.

After a heart attack, blood flow to the myocardium, or heart muscle, is decreased and myocardial function is impaired. Less blood is thus delivered to the tissues. The kidneys sense the decreased cardiac output and try to compensate by reabsorption of additional water. This may lead to a fluid overload and edema. For that reason, most clients after a MI are on fluid restriction.

Three common conditions increase the risk of renal disease:

1. Obesity
2. Poorly controlled diabetes
3. Hypertension

Losing weight reduces the severity of diabetes and hypertension, the two leading causes of kidney failure, and helps prevent those conditions in people who have not developed them. Normalization of blood glucose and lipid levels along with blood pressure control also decrease the risk of renal disease. The Diabetes Control and Complications Trial (DCCT) and United Kingdom Prospective Diabetes Study (UKPDS) have definitively shown that intensive diabetes therapy can significantly reduce the risk of overt nephropathy in people with diabetes (American Diabetes Association, 2004).

Both systolic and diastolic hypertension markedly accelerate the progression of diabetic nephropathy, and aggressive antihypertension management is able to greatly decrease the rate of fall of GFR. For those reasons among others, all clients should be encouraged to follow their prescribed diets and faithfully take prescribed medications.

Glomerulonephritis

A general term for an inflammation of the kidneys is **nephritis.** This is the most common type of kidney disease. Inflammation of the glomeruli is called **glomerulonephritis,** which can be either acute or chronic. This condition often follows scarlet fever or a streptococcal infection of the respiratory tract. Young children and young adults are commonly victims. Symptoms include:

- Nausea
- Vomiting
- Fever
- Hypertension
- Blood in the urine **(hematuria)**
- Decreased output of urine **(oliguria)**
- Protein in the urine **(proteinuria)**
- Edema

Recovery is usually complete. However, in some clients the disease progresses and becomes chronic. This leads to a progressive loss of kidney function. Some clients develop **anuria,** which is a total lack of urine output. Without treatment, this condition is fatal.

Specific Tubular Abnormalities

A structural problem in the renal tubules may result in abnormal reabsorption or lack of reabsorption of certain substances by the tubules. The result of a tubular abnormality is ineffective cleansing of the blood.

Nephrotic Syndrome

The result of a variety of diseases that damage the glomeruli capillary walls is called **nephrotic syndrome.** Signs of nephrotic syndrome include:

- Proteinuria
- Severe edema
- Low serum protein levels
- Anemia
- Hyperlipidemia

Usually the higher the hyperlipidemia, the greater the proteinuria.

The disease is caused by the degenerative changes in the kidneys' capillary walls, which consequently permit the passage of albumin into the **glomerular filtrate.** Water and sodium are retained. Edema is sometimes so severe that it masks tissue wasting due to the breakdown of tissue protein stores. The degree of malnutrition is hidden until the excess fluid is removed.

Nephrosclerosis

A hardening of the renal arteries, known as **nephrosclerosis,** is caused by arteriosclerosis and results in a decreased blood supply to the kidneys. The condition is **hypertensive kidney disease** and can eventually destroy the kidney.

Progressive Nature of Kidney Failure

Kidney disease can be acute or chronic. The earliest clinical evidence of nephropathy is the appearance of low but abnormal levels (≥30 mg/day or 20 μg/min) of albumin in the urine, referred to as **microalbuminuria.**

In **acute renal failure,** the kidneys stop working entirely or almost entirely. Acute renal failure occurs suddenly and is usually temporary. It can last for a few days or weeks.

Chronic renal failure occurs when progressively more nephrons are destroyed until the kidneys simply cannot perform vital functions. Chronic renal failure occurs over time and is usually irreversible.

As individual nephrons are damaged, the remaining nephrons work harder to maintain metabolic homeostasis. As each functional nephron's workload is increased, the nephron becomes more susceptible to work overload and damage. The normal composition of the blood becomes altered when the remaining functional nephrons cannot assume any additional workload.

At such time, serum levels of **blood urea nitrogen (BUN), creatinine,** and uric acid become elevated. In some clients, even though the underlying condition (e.g., diabetes mellitus, hypertension) is treated, chronic renal disease may lead to **end-stage renal failure.** During end-stage renal failure, most or all of the kidneys' ability to produce urine and regulate blood chemistries is severely compromised.

Sodium Depletion

Often, the first sign of chronic renal failure is sodium depletion. This occurs when the kidneys lose their ability to reabsorb sodium in the tubule. Symptoms associated with sodium depletion include:

- A reduction of renal blood flow
- Dehydration
- Lethargy
- Decreased glomerular filtration rate (GFR)
- Uremia (see next section)
- Deterioration.

The client's blood pressure and body weight drop. Urine volume may be increased initially in chronic renal failure. A loss of body fat and protein content is responsible for the weight loss. The client's serum albumin level may fall as protein is lost in the urine.

Sodium Retention

As kidney function further deteriorates, some of these symptoms reverse. The kidneys lose the ability to excrete sodium. When this occurs, symptoms include:

- Sodium retention
- Overhydration
- Edema
- Hypertension
- Congestive heart failure (CHF)

The body can excrete little or no urine.

The GFR gradually declines in chronic renal failure. Chronic kidney disease has been formally classified into five stages based on the GFR. Table 19-1 lists the stages of chronic kidney disease (CKD) and describes each stage along with the corresponding GFR. Most clients with a GFR below 25 milliliters per minute will eventually require either dialysis or transplantation, regardless of the original cause of failure. Stages 1 through 4 represent kidney damage categories where medical and nutritional management can impact and potentially delay progression to Stage 5 (Beto and Bansal, 2004).

Progression to Uremia

If the client progresses to stage 5 CKD, **uremia** develops. Uremia is the name given to the toxic condition associated with renal failure. Uremia is produced by retention in the blood of nitrogenous substances normally excreted by the kidneys. The uremic client manifests many symptoms in virtually every body system as toxic waste products build up in the blood. The client may complain of:

- Fatigue
- Weakness
- Decreased mental ability
- Twitching and cramping muscles
- Anorexia
- Nausea
- Vomiting
- **Stomatitis,** an inflammation of the mouth
- Taste changes, especially for meats

TABLE 19-1 ■ Stages of Chronic Kidney Disease and Glomerular Filtration Rate (GFR)

STAGE		GFR
1	Some kidney damage with normal or elevated GFR	≥90
2	Kidney damage with mildly decreased GFR	60–89
3	Moderately decreased GFR	30–59
4	Severely decreased GFR	15–29
5	Kidney failure	<15 Dialysis, transplant, hospice, or palliative care Diet may provide comfort.

To complicate matters further, gastrointestinal ulcers and bleeding are common. All of these symptoms have a direct effect on the client's willingness to eat.

Halting the Progression

Health-care professionals have known for many decades that clients with chronic renal disease who have sustained a loss of GFR may continue to lose renal function until they develop terminal renal failure. Much research is ongoing to find a way to halt the progression of chronic renal failure. Among the nutrition-related causes of progressive renal failure are:

- A high-phosphorus diet
- A high-fat or high-cholesterol diet
- A high vitamin C intake, glycemic control
- A vitamin D overdose

Protein restriction and phosphate lowering may have benefits in selected patients (American Diabetes Association, 2004).

Individuals with diabetes who have early stages of chronic kidney disease should eat no more than 0.8 to 1 gram protein per kilogram of adjusted body weight. This may actually improve measures of renal function. For this reason, dietary intervention is now instituted when microalbumin appears in the urine. Aggressive antihypertensive treatment and the use of angiotensin-converting enzyme (ACE) inhibitors will slow the rate of progression of nephropathy. If the client progresses to stages 3 or 4 CKD, reduction of protein to 0.8 gram/kg will improve albuminuria, but not GFR (American Diabetes Association, 2004).

Treatment of Renal Disease

Renal functions cannot be assumed by another organ. There is no cure for chronic renal failure. However, many clients can be treated with dialysis (an artificial kidney) or a kidney transplant. Artificial kidneys have been widely used since the 1960s to treat clients with severe kidney failure.

Dialysis

Dialysis means the passage of solutes through a membrane. Two functions of the kidneys are:

1. The removal of waste products
2. The regulation of fluid and electrolyte balance

By removing waste products from the blood and assisting in the maintenance of fluid balance, dialysis reduces the symptoms of:

- Uremia
- Hypertension
- Edema
- The risk of CHF

Dialysis is usually started when GFR is less than 15 mL/minute when the client develops symptoms of severe fluid overload, high potassium levels, acidosis, or uremia. Dialysis cannot restore the lost hormonal functions of the kidney. In addition, dialysis cannot correct the anemia that occurs because of a lack of erythropoietin. Some dialysis clients still need treatment for hypertension.

Hemodialysis

During **hemodialysis,** blood is removed from the client's artery through a tube, is forced to flow over a semipermeable membrane where waste is removed, and then is rerouted back into the client's body through a vein. Before dialysis can be initiated, an access site that allows blood to be removed from the body and returned back to the body at the time of dialysis must be surgically created. Ideally, this access will be a **fistula** created several months before dialysis is anticipated.

Figure 19-3 illustrates a client undergoing a hemodialysis treatment. A solution called the **dialysate** is placed on one side of the semipermeable membrane, and the client's blood flows on the other side. The dialysate is similar in composition to normal blood plasma but may be manipulated to remove varying amounts of waste products. The client's blood has a higher concentration of urea and electrolytes than the dialysate has, so these substances diffuse from the blood into the dialysate. Sodium modeling may be used during dialysis. Modeling involves changing the concentration of sodium in the dialysate, which can improve the amount of fluid removed during the treatment. The composition of the dialysate varies according to the client's requirements.

Unit staff usually administers in-center hemodialysis treatments 3 to 4 hours three times per week. Home hemodialysis is becoming more widely used in the United States. The client and a care partner learn to do the procedure in their own home. In-home treatment regimens vary from 3 to 6 days per week for 2 to 4 hours per treatment. Nocturnal hemodialysis may be done at home or in a center. These treatments are long, slow daily or every other day for 6 to 8 hours while the client sleeps. Dialysis is not as effective as normal kidney function because blood cleansing occurs only when clients are attached to

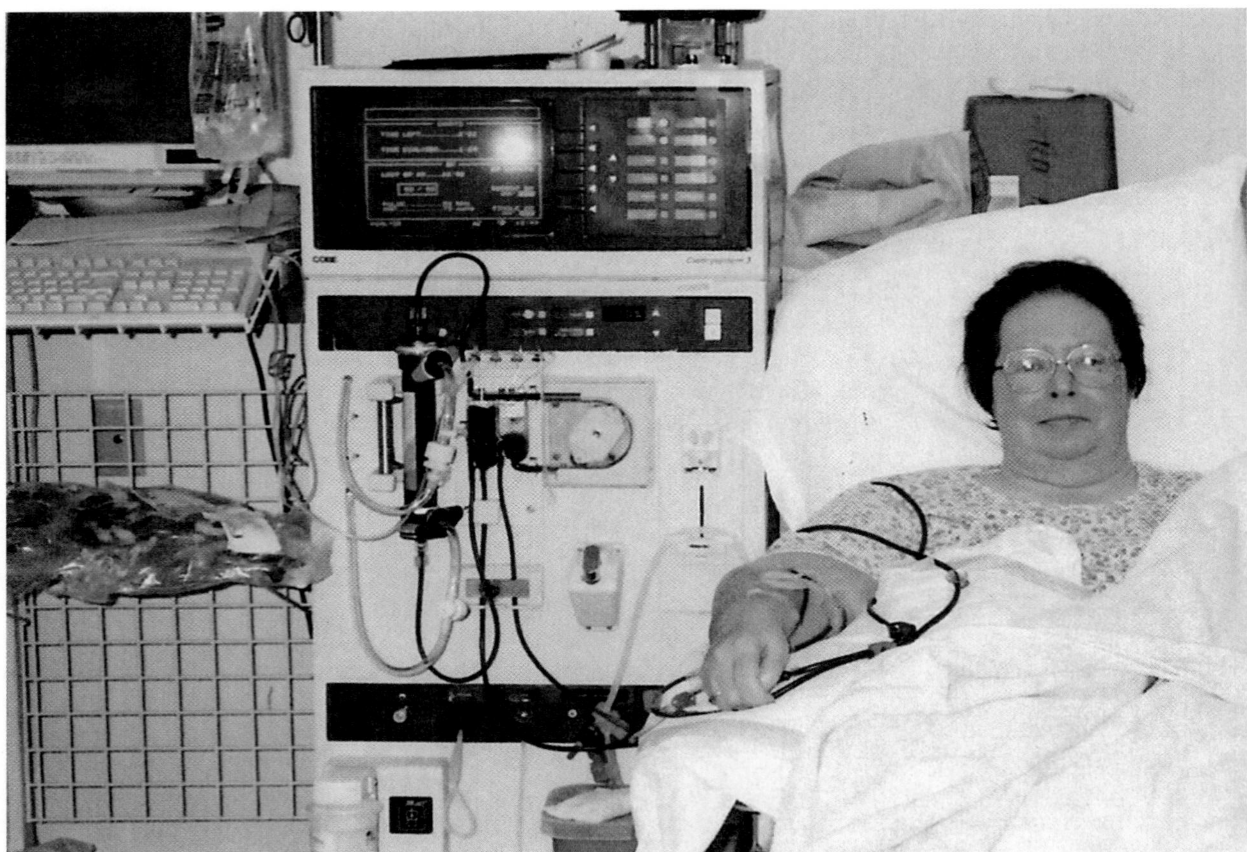

FIGURE 19-3 Client undergoing hemodialysis at dialysis center.

artificial kidneys. Normal kidneys clear the blood 24 hours a day, 7 days a week.

Peritoneal Dialysis

The **peritoneum** is the lining of the abdominal cavity. During **peritoneal dialysis,** the dialysate is placed directly into the client's abdomen by means of a soft permanent catheter implanted between the abdominal wall and the peritoneum. The dialysate enters the body through a permanent catheter placed in the abdominal cavity. The peritoneum thus functions as the semipermeable membrane, allowing waste products and excess fluid to pass from blood into the dialysate. Various glucose concentrations are used in the dialysate to manipulate the amount of fluid removed.

The most common types of peritoneal dialysis are **continuous ambulatory peritoneal dialysis** (CAPD) and **continuous cycling peritoneal dialysis** (CCPD). One study showed that patients receiving peritoneal dialysis rate care higher than those receiving hemodialysis (Rubin et al., 2004). The advantage of peritoneal dialysis is that the client's blood levels of sodium, potassium, creatinine, and nitrogen stay within a more stable range and allow for a more liberal diet than in hemodialysis. Large shifts in fluid balance are also avoided. However, part of the glucose in the dialysate is available to the client as calories. The higher the glucose concentration used, the more calories are absorbed. The decision about which treatment is best is based on the client's medical condition, lifestyle, and personal preference. For example, a client with poor personal hygiene would not be a good candidate for peritoneal dialysis because of a high risk for infection.

CONTINUOUS AMBULATORY PERITONEAL DIALYSIS

Clients choosing CAPD are dialyzing constantly. In this method the client instills 1.5 to 3 liters of dialysate into the abdominal cavity via a catheter. The fluid remains in the cavity for 4 to 6 hours while the client continues with activities of daily living. During this time, waste products and excess fluids diffuse through the peritoneal membrane into the dialysate. The dialysate is then drained and discarded, then replaced with fresh solution in a process called an **exchange.** Each exchange takes 30 to 40 minutes and clients will do 4 to 5 exchanges daily to achieve good dialysis.

CONTINUOUS CYCLING PERITONEAL DIALYSIS

CCPD is a process in which the "exchanges" described above are done during the night by means of a machine. The machine automatically fills and drains the dialysate. This process takes 10 to 12 hours, so is done during sleeping hours. Clients will often do one CAPD exchange during the day in addition to the CCPD.

Kidney Transplant

Although kidney transplant can restore full renal function, it is considered a treatment, not a cure. Immunosuppressants to prevent rejection of the transplanted kidney are necessary. Some commonly used immunosuppressants are azathioprine, corticosteroids, and cyclosporine. These medications have many side effects, including diarrhea, nausea, and vomiting, which influence nutrient intake and absorption.

Nutritional Care

The nutritional needs of clients with renal diseases are changing constantly. The reason for the change is that the disease state and treatment approach are not static. Clients with kidney disease require constant assessment, monitoring, and counseling. In addition, providing quality nutritional care to these clients, who frequently must be coaxed to eat, is challenging. Anorexia, nausea, and vomiting are frequent complaints, particularly in the hospital.

Client–nurse interactions are important because nurses can influence and enhance patient adherence to prescribed diets. One study showed that 81.4% of hemodialysis patients have difficulty following dietary modifications and 74.6% fluid restrictions (Kugler, Vlaminck, and Maes, 2005). Close communication among all members of the health-care team is vital to meeting the dynamic nutritional needs of these clients.

Malnutrition

Malnutrition in hemodialysis clients is associated with increased mortality and morbidity. Moderate to severe malnutrition is estimated to be about 34% in clients on hemodialysis. Among the reasons for the malnutrition are:

- Increased catabolism
- Metabolic derangement
- Decreased food intake
- Low economic status

These approaches may be used to treat the protein-energy malnutrition in such clients:

- Oral supplements
- Tube feedings
- Intravenous feedings
- Intradialytic parenteral nutrition

Intradialytic parenteral nutrition involves the administration of lipids, glucose, and amino acids into the peritoneal cavity.

Goals of Nutrition Therapy

Well-planned nutritional management is a fundamental part of any treatment plan for renal disease. Every client with renal disease requires an individualized diet based on the following goals:

- Attain and maintain optimal nutritional status.
- Prevent net protein catabolism.
- Minimize uremic toxicity.
- Maintain adequate hydration status.
- Maintain normal serum potassium levels.
- Control the progression of renal osteodystrophy (discussed later).
- Modify the diet to meet other nutrition-related concern, such as diabetes, heart disease, gastrointestinal tract ulcers, and constipation.
- Retard the progression of renal failure and postpone the initiation of dialysis.

No single diet is appropriate for all renal clients. Every client requires individual assessment and every client's diet will likely change over time.

Dietary Components

Several basic components need to be monitored and, if possible, controlled in renal diets:

- Kilocalories
- Protein
- Sodium
- Potassium
- Phosphorus and calcium
- Fluid
- Saturated fat and cholesterol
- Iron, vitamins, and minerals

The need to restrict or encourage the consumption of any of these nutrients changes according to the client's medical status and treatment approach. For example, at one time, client control of his or her potassium intake may not be necessary, but at another time, control may be vital.

Kilocalories

Clients with renal disease need additional kilocalories. Clients on high-kilocalorie diets are usually given all the simple carbohydrates and monounsaturated and polyunsaturated fats they will eat. *Trans*-fats are minimized. The end products of fat and carbohydrate catabolism are carbon dioxide and water. Neither of these dietary constituents imposes a burden on the client's compromised excretory ability.

Inadequate nonprotein kilocalories, however, will encourage tissue breakdown and aggravate uremia. Clients with renal insufficiency need 35 to 40 kcal/kg per day. The use of a specialized oral supplement such as Suplena®, a low-protein, high-calorie product by Abbott Laboratories, is one example of an appropriate oral supplement for clients who are unwilling or unable to eat enough food. An adequate intake of kilocalories is crucial to the success of the dietary treatment.

In addition, individuals with diabetes mellitus and renal diseases need good control of blood sugar levels. Diets for renal disease are typically high in simple sugars, and clients must learn how best to distribute the sugars through the day for optimal blood glucose control. In some cases, the primary nutritional goal is to decrease uremia, and blood glucose control may become less important.

Some renal clients require an alternate feeding route to attain and maintain optimal nutritional status. Accordingly, some physicians order tube feedings or a peripheral intravenous infusion of lipids to supplement oral feedings. Tube feeding products and total parenteral nutrition solutions for renal clients are commercially available.

Protein

In renal clients, a primary goal of nutritional therapy is controlling nitrogen intake. Control may mean increasing or decreasing dietary protein as the client's medical condition and treatment approach change. In addition, the kind of protein fed to the client may be important. At least 50% of the dietary protein should be of high biological value (National Kidney Foundation, 2002). Because animal products contain all the essential amino acids, examples of foods containing protein of high biologic value include:

- Eggs
- Meat
- Dairy products

A vegetarian diet has been proven beneficial for patients with renal failure. Human and animal models suggest that some plant proteins may increase survival rates and decrease proteinuria, glomerular filtration rate, renal blood flow, and histological renal damage compared with nonvegetarian diets.

Vegetarian diets by nature are high in potassium and phosphorus because of all the vegetables, whole grains, and fruits they contain. The client's goal is to eat the right combination of plant proteins while keeping potassium and phosphorus under control. A referral to a renal dietitian is indicated for these patients.

Protein restrictions are effective only if the client also consumes adequate kilocalories. Beginning renal insufficiency is usually called a predialysis and requires a restriction or modification of protein intake. Some physicians believe it is more difficult to clinically raise a depressed albumin than to clear the blood of the toxic products of protein metabolism through dialysis. Because of the danger of tissue catabolism, a diet that provides less than 40 grams of protein per day is rarely indicated.

The treatment approach influences protein requirements. Hemodialysis clients need increased protein because hemodialysis results in a loss of 1 to 2 grams of amino acids per hour of dialysis. A client on CAPD has an even higher protein need because he or she dialyzes continuously. During dialysis, protein passes out of the blood with the waste products and into the dialysate fluid. When the dialysate fluid is discarded, a significant amount of protein is lost. A high-protein diet is necessary to replenish the losses.

Sodium

The desirable sodium intake for renal clients depends on individual circumstances. Serum sodium is not a reliable indicator of sodium intake in CKD. Dietary levels of sodium are based on blood pressure and fluid balance and are also influenced by comorbidities such as congestive heart failure (National Kidney Foundation, 2002). Most clients require between 1 and 3 grams of sodium per day. The sodium intake of many clients with renal failure must be restricted to prevent sodium retention with consequent generalized edema. Clients need to know that high sodium intake influences thirst and therefore fluid intake. In a few situations, clients are advised to avoid water treated with a water softener.

The disease that precipitated renal failure plays a role in determining the need for sodium restriction. Because glomerulonephritis, for example, is more likely to produce hypertension and fluid retention, sodium restriction is often necessary. Low levels of sodium, absence of edema, and normal or low blood pressure commonly characterize other renal diseases, such as pyelonephritis. **Pyelonephritis** is an inflammation of the central portion of the kidney. In this situation, sodium intake may be higher than in the other groups of diseases but is individualized according to needs.

Potassium

Dietary potassium, like sodium, must be individually evaluated. **Hypokalemia** (low blood potassium level) must be avoided because it may introduce cardiac arrhythmias and eventually cardiac arrest. Boxes 19-1 and 19-2, respectively, list foods high and low in potassium. Salt substitutes are very high in potassium and should be avoided by renal clients. In addition, a water softener may be a source of dietary potassium. The need to restrict potassium generally increases in clients with decreased urinary output.

ACE inhibitors have been shown to reduce the level of albuminuria and the rate of progression of renal disease to a greater degree than other hypertensive agents that lower blood pressure by an equal amount (American Diabetes Association, 2007). Use of ACE inhibitors may exacerbate hyperkalemia in clients with advanced renal insufficiency; therefore, when used, serum potassium levels should be monitored.

If a client's potassium level is elevated, dietary potassium intake should be minimized. The recommended intake is 2.0 to 3.0 grams per day for most patients. In cases of anuria or when serum potassium exceeds 6.5 mEq/L, a dietary intake of 20 to 25 mEq/L (about 780 to 975 mg K) is suggested. This suggestion is for the acute, critical-care patient because of its poor palpability. When urinary output is 100 to 500 mL and serum potassium is 5.5 to 6.5, a 40- to 60-mEq (about 1563 to 2345 mg K) intake is suggested.

Fundamental to understanding medical nutritional therapy for clients with renal disease is that over-restricting a client's diet is never appropriate because of the danger of tissue catabolism and malnutrition. Before reducing diet, check the client's medications to

Box 19-1 ■ *High-Potassium Foods*

Clients should avoid these high-potassium foods in excess of ½ cups per day* or in the amount calculated by a dietitian.

Dairy Products

As calculated*

Meats

As calculated*

Starches

Bran cereals and bran products

Fruits

Orange, fresh
Mango, fresh
Nectarines
Papayas
Dried prunes
Avocado
Bananas

Vegetables

Bamboo shoots, fresh
Beet greens
Baked potato, with skin
Sweet potato fresh
Spinach, cooked
All others if eaten in excess of allowance*

Others

Chocolate, cocoa
Molasses
Salt substitute
Low-sodium broth
Low-sodium baking powder
Low-sodium baking soda
Nuts

*Dairy foods and meat products contain not only considerable potassium but also phosphorus and protein that need to be carefully planned in the diets of many clients.

Box 19-2 ■ *Low-Potassium Foods and Beverages**

Low-Potassium Foods

Bean sprouts, canned
Gum drops
Hard, clear candy
Nondairy topping
Honey*
Jams and jellies
Jelly beans
Lollipops
Marshmallows
Suckers
Sugar
Lifesavers
Chewing gum
Poly-Rich (nondairy creamer)
Cornstarch

Low-Potassium Beverages

Carbonated beverages
Lemonade
Limeade
Cranberry juice
Popsicles (1 stick—60 mL of fluid)
Hawaiian punch†
Kool-Aid†

Low-Potassium Unsweetened Beverages

Diet carbonated beverages
Diet lemonade
Diet Kool-Aid†

*Diabetics should not freely eat foods with sugar.
†These beverages are low in potassium but are often high in phosphorus and need to be restricted in many renal clients with a phosphorus dietary restriction.

be sure he or she is not on potassium supplements. If the client is undergoing hemodialysis, also check the potassium level of the dialysate to see that all potassium that can be safely removed is being removed.

The potassium content of fruits and vegetables varies according to the form and the preparation method. For example, ½ cup of canned pears in heavy syrup has about 80 milligrams of potassium, and one fresh pear has about 210 milligrams. Potassium is water soluble. For this reason, some renal clients on low-potassium diets are taught to use large amounts of water to prepare vegetables and to discard the water after cooking to decrease the vegetable's potassium content. Unfortunately, the process also decreases water-soluble vitamins. For this reason, most renal clients need vitamin supplements. Clients should eat fruits or vegetables in the form given on the list.

Phosphorus, Vitamin D, and Calcium

In the body, phosphorus, vitamin D, and calcium are all normally balanced. In clients with kidney disease, vitamin D cannot be activated, a situation leading to a low serum calcium level. At the same time, the kidneys cannot excrete phosphorus, a situation leading to an elevated serum phosphorus level.

When serum calcium level drops, calcium is released from the bones because of the increased secretion of **parathyroid hormone (PTH).** PTH is secreted in an effort to correct the calcium imbalance. This chain of events may lead to renal **osteodystrophy** and **vascular calcification,** which are complications of chronic renal disease. **Renal osteodystrophy** leads to faulty bone formation. **Vascular calcification** contributes to the high incidence of cardiovascular disease seen in clients with CKD.

Control of blood levels of calcium and phosphorus involves several treatment approaches. First, clients with hypocalcemia and secondary hyperparathyroidism are given activated vitamin D orally or, if they are on hemodialysis, intravenously during their treatment. Activated vitamin D cannot be given when serum calcium or phosphorus levels are very high or vascular calcification may result.

High phosphorus levels must be controlled with the initiation of dietary phosphorus restriction. Phosphorus is found mainly in:

- Dairy products
- High-protein foods
- Whole grain products
- Inorganic phosphate additives. See Box 19-3.

The use of phosphate additives to meats, beverages, convenience foods, and many others has more than doubled in the past 10 years and will likely continue to increase. Clients must learn how to read the ingredient label to avoid as many phosphate additives as possible. Though the amount added to a given food is

Box 19-3 ■ *Foods High in Phosphorus*

Dairy Foods	Meats	Nuts and Seeds
Milk	Sardines	Almonds
Cheese	Herring	Cashews
Cocoa	Smelt	Coconut
Condensed milk	Liver	Pecans
Evaporated milk	Sweetbreads	Walnuts
Cottage cheese	Tripe/menudo	Peanuts
Yogurt	Egg yolk (more than 2 per day)	Peanut butter
Custard		Pumpkin seeds
Ice cream		Sunflower seeds
Pudding		
Cream soups		
Grains	**Dried Beans**	**Other**
Bran	Navy beans	Cola drinks
Bran flakes	Kidney beans	Chocolate
Bran muffins	Lima beans	Toffee
Brown rice	Pinto beans	Caramel
Raisin bran	Lentils	Fudge
Whole wheat	Black-eyed peas	Mushrooms
Biscuits	Soybeans	Molasses
Waffles		Raisins and dates
Pancakes		Other dried fruits
Cereals with nuts		Casseroles with cheese or cream soup
Cheese crackers		
Cheese curls		

small, these additives are 100% absorbed, while organic phosphates found naturally in foods have a much lower absorption rate. Almost all clients with chronic renal disease, especially in stages 4 and 5, need to watch their phosphorus intake.

Phosphate binders may be added to a client's regimen if dietary modification does not produce desired results. Phosphate binders are medications that bind phosphorus in the GI tract, allowing the resulting complex to be eliminated in the stools. These medications *must* be taken while a client eats his or her meals. A **calcimimetic** may also be added to the treatment regimen. This medication acts directly on the parathyroid gland to reduce the release of PTH.

Fluid

Some predialysis (renal insufficiency) and most dialysis clients generally must restrict fluid intake because their kidneys can no longer excrete excess fluid. Table 19-2 lists guidelines for distributing fluids between meals and medications. Clients on hemodialysis are restricted to 500 to 1000 milliliters plus 24-hour urinary output. This fluid restriction allows for fluid gain of 2 to 2½ kilograms between dialysis treatments. Predialysis clients do not generally have fluid restrictions unless their clinical condition indicates a need. For clients on CAPD, fluid restriction is "as tolerated" according to their daily weight fluctuations and blood pressure.

Saturated Fat and Cholesterol

Clients with renal disease frequently have hyperlipidemia. High serum lipid levels increase the progression of renal disease, which contributes to an increased risk of cardiovascular disease. Total cholesterol levels may be increased up to tenfold. This increase is thought to be a problem especially in clients with nephrotic syndrome, diabetes, or an **LCAT deficiency.** LCAT is an enzyme that transports cholesterol from tissues to the liver for removal from the body. Most clients with an LCAT deficiency develop progressive glomerular injury.

Significant hypertriglyceridemia is commonly present in clients with a history of renal disease. The nutritional care of clients with elevated triglycerides includes a modified fat diet, modification of carbohydrate intake and encouragement to increase exercise—as tolerated and with their physician's knowledge. Clients are counseled to avoid saturated fat, trans fat and to increase their intake of monounsaturated fat.

Thirty to thirty-five percent of the total kilocalories are provided as fat because excessive carbohydrate could worsen the hypertriglyceridemia (Moore, 2009). Simple sugars and alcohol are usually limited for the same reason. Including omega-3 fatty acids to lower the levels of high triglycerides may be helpful. The literature suggests a beneficial effect of omega-3 fatty acids, particularly from fish, and suggests that further studies are warranted (National Kidney Foundation, 2002).

Iron

Anemias in clients with renal disease may be due to:

- A lack of the kidney's production of erythropoietin
- A decreased oral iron intake, which commonly occurs as a result of dietary restriction
- Blood loss

Epoetin alfa, a pharmaceutical form of erythropoietin, may be used to increase red blood cell production and thereby correct the anemia. The treatment for iron-deficiency anemia is oral or parenteral iron and an increase in dietary sources of iron.

TABLE 19-2 ■ Guidelines for Fluid-Restricted Clients

IF THE FLUID RESTRICTION IS	USE THIS AMOUNT OF FLUIDS WITH MEALS	USE THIS AMOUNT OF FLUIDS WITH MEDICATIONS
1000 mL (4 cups)*	600 mL (2½ cups)	400 mL (1½ cups)
1200 mL (5 cups)	700 mL (3 cups)	500 mL (2 cups)
1500 mL (6 cups)	1000 mL (4 cups)	500 mL (2 cups)
2000 mL (8 cups)	1000 mL (4 cups)	1000 mL (4 cups)

All foods contain some fluids, but it is especially important to count the following as part of the fluid allowance:

Milliliters of Fluid per ½ Cup					
Water	120	All juices	120	Watermelon	100
Coffee	120	Soda-pop	120	Sherbet	65
Tea	120	Ice	60	Ice cream	40
Sanka	120	Gelatin	100	Ice milk	40
Milk	120	Soup	120	Popsicle	80

*All cup measures are approximations.

A diagnosis of iron-deficiency anemia can be made by a laboratory measure of ferritin. **Ferritin** is the storage form of iron found primarily in the liver. A small amount of ferritin circulates in the blood and reflects the amount of iron in body stores. A laboratory value of less than 12 micrograms per liter suggests iron deficiency. KDOQI recommends that CKD clients have a serum ferretin of 100 to 800 thus ensuring adequate iron for erythropoietin-stimulated production of red blood cells. Higher levels of ferritin may indicate that inflammation or infection is present (National Kidney Foundation, 2002).

Nutritional therapy with iron supplements consists of 210 milligrams of ferrous iron salts per day divided among three to four doses. Absorption is enhanced when iron supplements are taken on an empty stomach or with vitamin C, though megadoses of vitamin C should be avoided because oxalosis may be induced, leading to kidney stones. In dialysis units, iron is commonly administered by IV. Patients should not take oral iron if receiving IV iron.

Vitamin and Mineral Supplementation

Unless supplements are given, chronically uremic patients are prone to deficiencies of water-soluble vitamins. Losses are most notable with pyridoxine, ascorbic acid, and folic acid. Supplementation of these nutrients is recommended for clients on dialysis. Fat-soluble vitamins are not lost in the dialysate, and supplementation is not indicated except with vitamin D for another reason (see previous discussion). Because the body's ability to excrete excess fat-soluble vitamins is compromised, toxicity is a potential problem.

Teaching the Renal Diet

In 1993 The American Dietetic Association and the National Kidney Foundation introduced the National Renal Diet, a uniform renal diet that could be used across the country. The second edition, introduced in 2002, included more simple lists with more emphasis on clients' involvement in determining and managing their own diets. The edition starts with survival information and allows the dietitian to introduce new topics as client interest and blood chemistries indicate the need for further diet modification and teaching.

The importance of individualizing medical nutrition therapy for the client with chronic kidney disease cannot be overemphasized. Regular contact with a renal dietitian increases the client's ability to change established behaviors and also allows for the most liberal diet possible. Table 19-3 shows the guidelines

TABLE 19-3 ■ Selected Nutritional Parameters for Varying Levels of Kidney Failure

NUTRITIONAL PARAMETER	NORMAL KIDNEY FUNCTION	STAGES 1–4 CHRONIC KIDNEY DISEASE	STAGE 5 HEMODIALYSIS	STAGE 5 PERITONEAL DIALYSIS	TRANSPLANT
Calories (kcal/kg per day)	30–37	<60 years: 35 ≥60 years: 30–35	<60 years: 35 ≥60 years: 30–35	<60 years: 35 including calories from dialysis	Initial: 30–35 Maintenance: 25–30
Protein (grams/kg per day)	0.8	0.6–0.75 50% HBV	1.2 50% HBV	1.2–1.3 50% HBV	Initial: 1.3–1.5
Fat (percent total kcal)	30%–35% Patients considered at highest risk for cardiovascular disease: emphasis on <10% saturated fat, PUFA, MUFA, 250–300 mg cholesterol/day				
Sodium (mg/day)	Unrestricted	2000	2000	2000	Unrestricted; monitor medication effect
Potassium (mg/day)	Unrestricted	Correlated to laboratory values	2000–3000 (8–17 mg/kg per day)	3000–4000 (8–17 mg/kg per day)	Unrestricted; monitor medication effect
Calcium (mg/day)	Unrestricted	1200	≤2000 from diet and medications	≤2000 from diet and medications	1200
Phosphorus (mg/day)	Unrestricted	Correlated to laboratory values	800–1000, adjusted for protein	800–1000, adjusted for protein	Unrestricted unless indicated
Fluid (mL/day)	Unrestricted	Unrestricted with normal urine output	1000 + urine output	Monitored; 1500–2000	Unrestricted unless indicated

Meant as guidelines only for initial assessment; individualization to patient's own metabolic status and coexisting metabolic conditions is essential for optimal care.
HBV = high biological value; PUFA = polyunsaturated fatty acids; MUFA = monounsaturated fatty acids.
SOURCE: Reprinted from Beto, JA, and Bansal, VK: Medical nutrition therapy in chronic kidney failure: Integrating clinical practice guidelines. J Am Diet Assoc 104:407, 2004. Copyright 2004, with permission from the American Dietetic Association.

for medical nutrition therapy of renal patients by treatment approach.

Nutrient Guidelines for Adults With Renal Disease

The nutritional care of renal clients is complex. Table 19-4 summarizes the nutrient control and the rationale for nutrient control by the stage of renal disease.

Renal Disease in Children

Growth failure is commonly seen in children with chronic renal failure treated with dialysis, but it is not an inevitable complication. Inadequate kilocaloric consumption and metabolic acidosis are reasons for the poor growth. These children usually need to have their sodium, potassium, and protein intake rigidly controlled, and this control may contribute to poor food intake. Anorexia and emotional disturbances are also contributing factors. Continually reinforcing the rationale for medical nutrition therapy and providing meal and snack ideas and emotional support can help to improve adherence.

Suggestions for improving children's intake include:

- Involving the children in selecting and preparing foods (insofar as possible)
- Serving meals in an appealing, attractive manner (e.g., serving contrasting colors and textures of foods, using decorative tableware and dishes)
- Serving small, frequent meals
- Ensuring that the child has someone with him or her at mealtime
- Planning special mealtime events such as picnics (even if they are held in the hospital playroom)

Kidney Stones

Kidney stones may be found in the bladder, kidney, ureter, or urethra. During urine formation, the urine moves from the collecting tubules into the renal pelvis. From the **renal pelvis,** the urine moves down the **ureter** and into the urinary bladder. Finally, urine passes from the bladder down the urethra and exits the body.

A stone, also called a **urinary calculus,** is a deposit of mineral salts held together by a thick, syrupy substance. A urinary calculus can block the movement of urine from the body. Symptoms of a blockage include:

- Sudden severe pain with chills
- Fever
- **Hematuria** (blood in the urine)
- An increased desire to urinate

A kidney stone can also pass out of the body with the urine.

Causes

The cause of most kidney stones is unknown. Some possible causes include:

- An abnormal function of the parathyroid gland
- Disordered uric acid metabolism (as in gout)
- An excessive intake of animal protein
- Immobility

At higher risk for kidney stones are men, people with a sedentary lifestyle, Asians, and whites. Typically, kidney stones occur in clients who are between ages 30 and 50. A determination of the stone's composition may lead to a restriction of dietary substrates (the substance acted on). Frequent dietary substrates of kidney stones are oxalic acid and purines. Decreased fluid intake and strongly concentrated urine or low urine volume are risk factors.

TABLE 19-4 ■ Stages of Chronic Kidney Disease, Nutrient Modification, and Rationale

STAGE	NUTRIENT MODIFICATION	RATIONALE
1	CHO control if indicated	Control blood glucose levels.
2	Sodium	Control blood pressure.
	Evaluate lipid levels and need to modify diet	CVD risk reduction
	Potassium	Begin to monitor to minimize cardiac complications.
		Continue modifications of stages 1 and 2.
3	Phosphorus	Begin to monitor and treat as indicated to maximize bone health.
4	RDA for protein	Promote adequate and not excessive protein intake.
	Potassium	Monitor monthly to avoid cardiac complications.
		All the above may slow the progression of kidney disease.
5	Highly individualized	As indicated by treatment approach, usual food intake, and laboratory values.

Treatment

All clients with kidney stones should drink sufficient water to keep the urine volume above 2 liters per day. About 3000 milliliters or 13 cups of water per day are necessary to produce this amount of urine. The primary reason for increasing fluid intake is to prevent formation of concentrated urine, in which crystals are more likely to combine and precipitate.

Oxalates

Calcium oxalate is the most common constituent of kidney stones. Some individuals are genetically susceptible to stone formation. A diet excluding foods high in oxalates (see Table 19-5) is frequently prescribed for clients with kidney stones if laboratory analysis shows removed or passed stone is high in oxalates. All stone formers may benefit from reduction of dietary oxalates, but especially hyperoxaluric stone formers (Massey, 2003).

Calcium

Historically, if laboratory analysis of a surgically removed or passed stone was found to be high in calcium, a low-calcium diet was prescribed (600 milligrams per day). Today, health-care professionals know that kidney stones are not usually caused by dietary calcium. In most individuals, kidney stones are of less concern with an increased calcium intake than with a decreased intake. A high-calcium diet binds the oxalate of dietary origin in the gastrointestinal tract and prevents its absorption, thereby reducing urinary oxalate formation.

Uric Acid Stones

Stones composed of uric acid are sometimes a complication of **gout,** a hereditary metabolic disease that is a form of arthritis. One symptom of gout is inflammation of the joints. The metabolism of uric acid is related to dietary **purines,** a product of protein digestion. Thus, a purine-restricted diet is commonly prescribed for gout. Table 19-6 shows purines in foods. Many physicians do not prescribe a low-purine diet for gout because the condition can be more effectively controlled by medications.

Clinical Application 19-2 summarizes the recommendations for medical nutrition therapy for kidney stones.

TABLE 19-5 ■ Foods High in Oxalic Acid

	mg/100 grams
Beverages	
Coffee, instant dry	143.0
Tea, brewed	12.5
Fruits	
Blackberries, raw	12.4
Gooseberries, raw	19.3
Plums, raw	11.9
Grains	
Bread, whole-wheat	20.9
Vegetables	
Beets, raw	72.2
Beets, boiled	109.0
Carrots, boiled	14.5
Green beans, raw	43.7
Green beans, boiled	29.7
Rhubarb, raw	537.0
Rhubarb, stewed	447.0
Spinach, boiled	571.0
Miscellaneous	
Cocoa, dry	623.0
Ovaltine, powder	45.9

SOURCE: Values taken from Pennington, JA, and Douglass, JA: *Bowes and Church food values of portions commonly used*, ed 18. Lippincott Williams & Wilkins, Philadelphia, 2004.

TABLE 19-6 ■ Purines in Food

GROUP A: HIGH CONCENTRATION (150–1000 mg/100 grams)	
Liver	Sardines (in oil)
Kidney	Meat extracts
Sweetbreads	Consommé
Brain	Gravies
Heart	Fish roes
Anchovies	Herring
GROUP B: MODERATE AMOUNTS (50–150 mg/100 grams)	
Meat, game, and fish other than those mentioned in Group A	
Fowl	Asparagus
Lentils	Cauliflower
Whole-grain cereals	Mushrooms
Beans	Spinach
Peas	
GROUP C: VERY SMALL AMOUNTS NEED NOT BE RESTRICTED IN DIET OF PERSONS WITH GOUT	
Vegetables other than those mentioned above	
Fruits of all kinds	Coffee
Milk	Tea
Cheese	Chocolate
Eggs	Carbonated beverages
Refined cereals, spaghetti, macaroni	Tapioca
Butter, fats, nuts, peanut butter*	Yeast
Sugars and sweets	
Vegetable soups	

*Fats interfere with the urinary excretion of urates and thus should be limited when attempting to promote excretion of uric acid.

SOURCE: From Venes, D (ed): *Taber's cyclopedic medical dictionary*, ed 21. FA Davis, Philadelphia, 2010, p 1943. Used with permission.

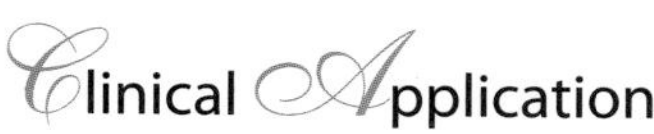
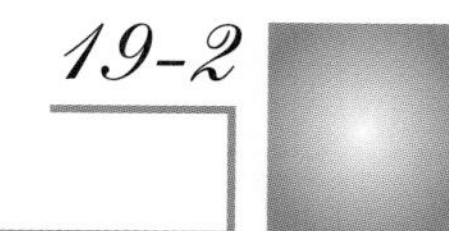

Clinical Application 19-2

Recommendations for Medical Nutrition Therapy (MNT) for Kidney Stones

GOALS	AVOID OR LIMIT
Ample hydration: 3–4 liters per day	Grapefruit juice
Urine volume goal: 2.0–2.5 liters per day	Limit soft drinks containing phosphoric acid
250 mL of fluid at each meal, between meals, at bedtime, and when arising to void at night. At least one-half fluid taken as water.	
Moderate amounts of tea (about 2 cups per day) diluted, and with milk	
Good voiding habits	Urinary tract infections
Adequate calcium intake (check RDA for age and sex appropriate recommendations)	Vitamin D supplementation
	Calcium supplementation unless recommended by physician

From Mehta, M. Nutrition and nephrolithiasis. Renal Nutr Forum 23, 2004. Used with permission from the Renal Dietitians Dietetic Practice Group of the American Dietetic Association.

Surgery

Surgery is sometimes necessary to remove large kidney stones. Surgical removal of the stones prevents infection, reduces pain, and prevents a loss of kidney function.

Urinary Tract Infections

One form of **urinary tract infection (UTIs)** is **cystitis,** an inflammation of the bladder. This condition is prevalent in young women. Recurrent UTI means that the individual has three or more bouts of infection per year. A general nutrition measure includes acidifying the urine by taking large doses of vitamin C. Regular intake of a cranberry juice beverage also reduces the frequency of urinary tract infections. Cranberry juice contains a substance with biologic activity that inhibits the growth of *Escherichia coli* in the urinary tract. Clients with UTIs should be encouraged to drink ample fluids.

Keystones

- The basic functional unit of the kidney is the nephron.
- Millions of nephrons work together to form urine and remove unnecessary substances from the blood.
- Glomerular filtration rate (GFR) is a measure of kidney function.
- The kidneys also are the site where vitamin D_3 (calcitriol) and erythropoietin are activated.
- Kidney failure can be acute or chronic. Chronic renal disease is progressive. Treatment for kidney failure is dialysis or a kidney transplant.
- Nutritional management of clients with renal disease is a fundamental part of treatment.
- Clients with kidney disease require constant assessment, monitoring, and counseling.
- The dietary components that may need modification are kilocalories, protein, sodium, potassium, phosphorus, fluid, cholesterol, and saturated fat.
- Vitamin and mineral supplements are often prescribed.
- Frequently, the diet these clients follow must be modified as their medical condition and treatment changes.
- Some nutritional intervention is necessary for clients with kidney stones and UTIs.
- The fluid intake of these clients should be high.

CASE STUDY 19-1

Mr. U is a 55-year-old man who works full-time and has a sedentary lifestyle. He is 5 ft 10 in. tall, has a medium frame, and weighs 68 kg. His ideal and usual weight is 76 kg. During the past 6 to 9 months, he has been anorectic and has had intermittent nausea and episodes of vomiting. He receives 4 hours of hemodialysis 3 times per week. His predialysis blood chemistry values were:

- Blood urea nitrogen, 63 mg/dL
- Sodium, 135 mmol/L (135 mEq/L)
- Potassium, 4.0 mmol/L (4.0 mEq/L)
- Phosphorus, 2.0 mg/dL
- Calcium, 9.0 mg/dL
- Albumin, 3.3 g/dL
- Urine output ranges between 800 and 1000 mL per day.

On arrival in the hemodialysis unit today, the client complained of hopelessness and a fear of dying. He complained he cannot meet the nutritional goals set by the dietitian because he just keeps getting "sick and sicker and is afraid of dying."

The client's medical record lists religious preference as Catholic.

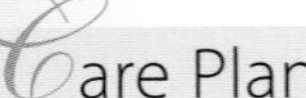

Care Plan

Subjective Data

Client complains of anorexia, nausea, and vomiting, a lack of hope, and a fear of dying.

Objective Data

Client tearful today. Documented history of anorexia, emesis, and nausea. His body weight is stable.

Analysis

Anorexia, nausea, and vomiting likely related to fear as evidenced by statement "I have given up hope and am afraid of dying.

Plan

DESIRED OUTCOMES EVALUATION CRITERIA	ACTIONS/INTERVENTIONS	RATIONALE
The client will maintain a sense of purpose despite fear.	Assist the client/family to identify areas of hope in life.	Clients and family members who can list foods and fluids that are better tolerated will provide hope.
Involve the client actively in his own care.	Explain to the client that despite his uncomfortable symptoms, his body weight is stable.	It is more effective to begin every counseling session with a review of the client's positive behaviors.
Seeks information to reduce fear.	As client has an ongoing relationship with the Dietitian, he or she may be able to expand clients repertoire of food and fluid related coping mechanisms.	Dietitians in hemodialysis centers visit clients at least monthly and frequently more often.
Help client expand spiritual self.	Ask the client if he would like you to arrange a visit from a Catholic priest or his designee.	Helping a client connect to his spiritual self helps maintain a sense of purpose despite fear.

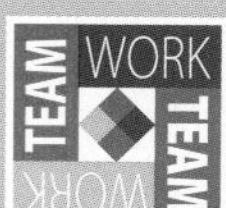

19-1

Dietitian's Note

The following Dietitian's Notes are representative of the documentation found in a client's medical record.

Subjective: Visited client per nursing request today. Client asked for specific information to decrease vomiting and nausea and increase food intake. He describes his food intake as sporadic. Lately food intake has been less than he would like. He states that he has not missed any days of work due to illness. Client states his wife has been especially helpful with meal preparation and grocery shopping but nothing sounds good to him. Usually eats/drinks ½ cup dairy, 4 starches, 2 vegetables, 5 meats, 3 fruits, and 6 fats. However, he is discouraged when he cannot rigidly follow this pattern everyday.

Objective: Weight stable at 76 kg; Compazine (for nausea) 2 times per day as needed; Albumin 3.3 g/L; BUN 63 mg/dL; Phosphorus 2.0 mg

Analysis: Client is eating about 66 grams of protein on the days when he is not experiencing nausea and vomiting. Phosphorus of 2.0 may be related to too many phosphate binders and not eating enough. Recommend that client try eating an extra egg or two each day on the days he is not nauseated. Also, recommended he sip four cans of Nepro (Abbott) on days he cannot eat and just to try a few sips every hour on the hour. Four cans of Nepro (Abbott) would provide 960 mL and 1700 kcal, and 76.2 grams of protein. Client was reminded that this would use 960 mL of his fluid allowance. Client appeared relieved to have a plan he could follow on days when he was not "up to eating."

Plan:

- Recommended client take one less phosphate binder per day until his next treatment
- Will speak again with client during his next hemodialysis treatment and provide positive reinforcement
- Client needs more kcal.

Daily Renal Diet Plan Goals

NUTRIENT	LEVEL	RATIONALE
Energy (kcal)	2300–2700	30–35 kcal/kg HBW*
Protein (grams)	91	1.2 grams/kg HBW
Sodium (mg)	2000	Control fluid weight gain
Potassium (mg)	3000	≤40 mg/kg HBW
Phosphorus (mg)	1080 mg	10–12 mg/kg of protein
Fluid (mL)	1500–1750	750 mL plus urine output

*Healthy body weight (may be called standard body weight or ideal body weight).

Critical Thinking Questions

1. Explain the relationship of each dietary modification to the signs and symptoms Mr. U is experiencing.
2. Mr. U eats only about half his needed kilocalories. What should you do?
3. Mr. U develops a stomach ulcer. What should you recommend?
4. Mr. U decides he would like to try CAPD. How would his diet probably change?

Chapter Review

1. Which of the following is a nutritional goal for a child with renal failure?
   a. Maintain current hydration status.
   b. Promote normal growth and development.
   c. Maximize uremia.
   d. Stimulate client well-being.
2. Kidney disease cannot be caused by:
   a. Consumption of toxic metals
   b. Consumption of 1 to 3 liters a day of water
   c. Infection
   d. Trauma
3. Kilocalories usually need to be increased in protein-restricted diets because an adequate kilocalorie intake:
   a. Assists in the control of serum potassium
   b. Is necessary to prevent renal anemia
   c. Controls and prevents osteodystrophy
   d. Spares protein
4. The ____ intake from food is not monitored in renal clients.
   a. Vitamin D
   b. Fluid
   c. Protein
   d. Sodium
5. The most important nutritional consideration in treating clients with kidney stones is to:
   a. Limit calcium intake.
   b. Restrict all end products of protein metabolism.
   c. Restrict all food sources of calcium, oxalic acid, and purines.
   d. Increase fluid intake.

Clinical Analysis

1. Bill, age 10, has acute glomerulonephritis. His mother explains that Bill had a streptococcal infection 1 week before the illness. When planning Bill's care, the nurse recognizes that he needs help in understanding his diet. Bill's restrictions will include:
   a. A low-fat diet
   b. A calcium restriction
   c. Measuring urine output (if any) daily and planning his fluid intake
   d. A high-protein diet
2. Mr. Jones, a 49-year-old mechanic, has been admitted to the hospital with diagnosis of renal failure. Mr. Jones has been following a 40-gram protein, 2-gram sodium, 2-gram potassium, 1000-milliliter fluid restriction for the past 5 years. Mr. Jones is scheduled for surgery tomorrow to have a permanent fistula implanted for hemodialysis. Mr. Jones's nutritional needs will change after he is maintained on hemodialysis to:
   a. More oranges, bananas, and baked potatoes
   b. More lean meat, eggs, fish, low-fat dairy products, and peanut butter
   c. Less starches, breads, and cereals
   d. Less margarine, oil, and salad dressings
3. Mr. Jones is found to have an elevated serum phosphorus level after 6 months on hemodialysis. He should:
   a. Restrict his intake of dairy products and peanut butter
   b. Restrict his intake of red meats
   c. Increase his intake of sugar, honey, jam, jelly, and other simple sugars
   d. Discontinue his phosphate binders

20

Diet in Gastrointestinal Disease

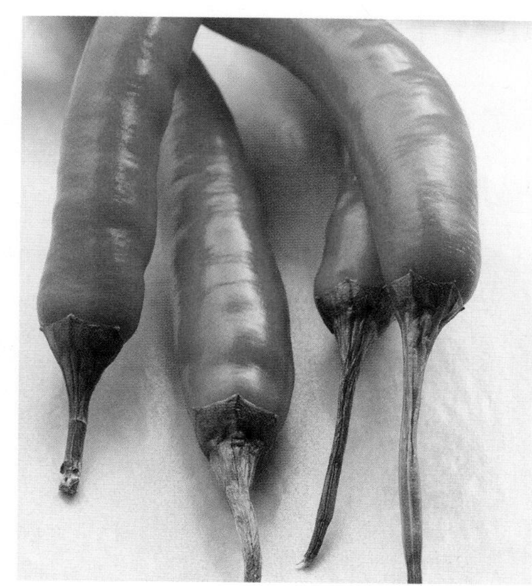

LEARNING OBJECTIVES

After completing this chapter, the student should be able to:

- Distinguish between the dietary preparation for gastrointestinal surgery and the dietary preparation for surgery on other body systems.
- Identify nutritional deficiencies that may accompany diseases or treatment of the gastrointestinal tract.
- Relate the pathophysiology of cirrhosis of the liver to the associated signs and symptoms.
- List several nutritional consequences of alcoholism.
- Discuss dietary modifications for common gastrointestinal diseases treated medically and surgically.

The gastrointestinal tract functions both as a barrier to substances from the environment and as an entry point for nutrients and other substances. Many disorders that affect the gastrointestinal tract and its accessory organs (liver, gallbladder, and pancreas) influence the nutritional status of clients. Most surgical procedures impact gastrointestinal tract function and require special dietary measures, both preoperatively and postoperatively. This chapter covers dietary modifications for surgical clients and for clients with common gastrointestinal disorders and diseases.

Dietary Considerations With Surgical Clients

Because of its role in tissue building and healing, protein is crucial in surgical clients. Protein depletion increases the risk of:

- Infection because the body cannot manufacture enough white blood cells
- Shock because low serum albumin prevents the return of interstitial fluid to the blood vessels
- Wound dehiscence because local edema persists and interferes with healing

Nutritional support is effective for malnourished surgical clients or those whose oral intake will be compromised after surgery. Although combination indices are available, preoperative albumin level is the single best indicator of postoperative complications and mortality after general surgery. A low albumin level may also be caused by liver disease, inflammation, or increased blood volume rather than malnutrition. A good screening technique for malnutrition is a thorough history and physical examination that identifies unintentional weight loss (Kudsk and Sacks, 2006). Clinical Application 20-1 relates one possible cause of malnutrition in surgical clients.

Persons with gastrointestinal disease are at special risk when facing surgery because such diseases interfere with nutrition. In cases involving gastrointestinal surgery, the gastrointestinal tract is incised and sutured, so postoperative feeding is postponed to allow for healing. If the gastrointestinal tract is permanently modified, specialty nutritional care is needed to optimize use of the remaining organs.

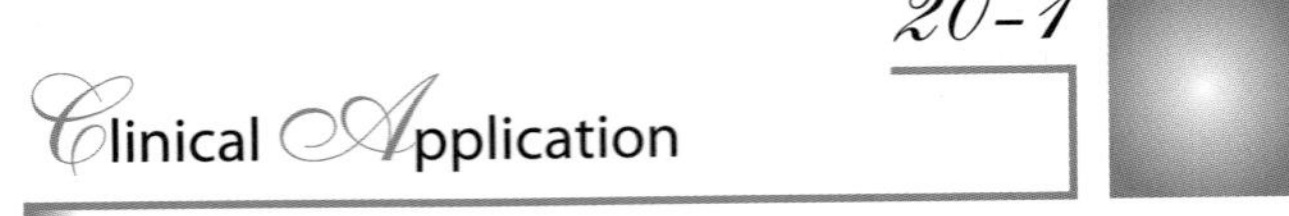

Surgical Clients With Rampant Dental Caries

Within a period of weeks, three clients on a gynecological surgical unit suffered postoperative wound disruptions. Each disruption was a **dehiscence,** a separation of the wound edges. Dehiscence occurs most frequently between the fifth and twelfth postoperative days. Risk factors for dehiscence include:

- Obesity
- Malnutrition
- Dehydration
- Abdominal distention
- Infection
- Increased abdominal pressure from improper deep breathing and coughing.

All three clients had at least one of the risk factors. One client ran a postoperative fever, which could have been caused by infection or dehydration. The other two clients had such severely carious teeth it would have been difficult for them to chew in the months before surgery. They probably were malnourished. Marked dental caries suggest a need for a thorough nutritional assessment. Carious teeth can cause and be caused by poor eating habits.

Surgical clients with liver disease also need special attention. The liver has many functions, some of which are listed in Table 20-1. Because of the liver's role in metabolizing and detoxifying drugs, clients with liver disease must be carefully managed when surgery is necessary. Moreover, some anesthetics, analgesics, and anti-infectives are toxic to the liver.

Preoperative Nutrition

Before elective surgery is undertaken, nutritional deficiencies should be identified and corrected. Many obese clients are instructed to lose weight to reduce the risks of surgery. If the client is anemic, an iron preparation may be prescribed. Other nutrients can be provided as needed. At least 2 to 3 weeks are required for objective evidence of the effectiveness of nutritional therapy.

Preoperative fasting protocols have been liberalized based on research showing slight risk of pulmonary aspiration with modern anesthetics. Guidelines for anesthesia administration to healthy individuals scheduled for elective procedures permit greater

TABLE 20-1 ■ Examples of Liver Functions

RELATED TO	PRODUCES/PROCESSES	STORES	BREAKS DOWN
Carbohydrate	Glucose from galactose and fructose Glucose from glycogen Glucose from glycerol and protein	Glycogen	
Fat	Fat from glucose Cholesterol Fatty acids and glycerol from cholesterol, phospholipids, and lipoproteins Lipoproteins Water-soluble bilirubin (from fat-soluble) Bile	Fat	
Protein	Albumin Some globulins Prothrombin Fibrinogen Transferrin Enzymes to convert ammonia to urea		
Vitamins	Retinol-binding protein Other transport proteins Activates thiamin Activates vitamin B_6 Processes vitamin D	A, D, E, K Thiamin Riboflavin B_6 Folic acid B_{12} Biotin	
Minerals		Iron	Worn-out red blood cells
Other			Acetaminophen Alcohol Aldosterone Bacteria Barbiturates Estrogen Glucocorticoids Morphine Progesterone Some anesthetics

oral intake than in the past (see Table 20-2). The guidelines do not supplant the need for individual assessment. Nor do they apply to individuals with gastrointestinal motility or metabolic disorders, individuals with potential airway problems, or women in labor. A review of studies permitting oral intake up to 2 hours before surgery found just one incident of regurgitation or aspiration in 2543 children (Brady et al., 2009) and no evidence suggesting a shortened fluid fast results in an increased risk of aspiration, regurgitation, or related morbidity in adults compared with fasting from midnight (Brady, Kinn, and Stuart, 2003).

TABLE 20-2 ■ Fasting Recommendations to Minimize Aspiration Risk

ORAL INTAKE	MINIMUM FASTING TIME	COMMENT
Clear liquids	2 hours	No alcohol
Breast milk	4 hours	
Infant formula and nonhuman milk	6 hours	
Light meal	6 hours	Example: toast and clear liquids
Regular meal including fat or meat	8 hours	Fat and meat delay gastric emptying

Adapted from American Society of Anesthesiologists (1999).

Surgery of the gastrointestinal tract demands additional bowel preparation. Anti-infectives such as neomycin that remain mainly in the bowel may be given to kill intestinal bacteria. A low-residue diet for 2 to 3 days will minimize the feces left in the bowel. **Residue** is the total solid material in the large intestine after digestion. A low-residue diet usually consists of foods that are easily digested and absorbed. Table 20-3 details a low-residue diet.

Postoperative Nutrition

Intravenous fluids are continued after surgery. The usual minimum replacement is 2 liters of 5% glucose in water in 24 hours. This amount contains 100 grams of glucose and delivers 340 kilocalories. Although this will not meet a person's resting energy expenditure,

TABLE 20-3 ■ Low-Residue Diet

DESCRIPTION	INDICATIONS	ADEQUACY
The low-residue diet limits milk and milk products and excludes any food made with seeds, nuts, and raw or dried fruits and vegetables. The purpose of the diet is to decrease colonic contents.	The diet can be used for severe diarrhea, partial bowel obstruction, and acute phases of inflammatory bowel diseases. Preoperatively the diet is used to minimize fecal volume and residue. Postoperatively the diet is used in the progression to a general diet. Long-term use of the diet is not recommended because it may aggravate symptoms during nonacute phases of disease.	Strict reduction in milk and milk products, vegetables, and fruits may necessitate supplementation of calcium, vitamin C, folate, and other nutrients.
Food Group	**Choose**	**Decrease**
Milk	2 cups/day Mild cheese	Strong cheese
Breads and Cereals	White bread Refined cereals: cream of wheat, cream of rice, puffed rice, Rice Krispies, corn flakes Crackers without whole grains or seeds Rice, noodles, macaroni, spaghetti	Whole-grain breads Bread made with seeds, nuts, or bran Cracked-wheat bread Whole-grain rice or pasta
Fruits	Juice without pulp Ripe banana Cooked or canned apples, apricots, Royal Anne cherries, peaches, pears Strained fruit	Prunes and prune juice Fruits not on "choose" list Dried fruit
Vegetables	Juice without pulp Lettuce Cooked or canned asparagus, green and wax beans, beets, carrots, eggplant, pumpkin, spinach, acorn squash, seedless tomatoes, tomato sauce or puree, white or sweet potatoes without skin Strained vegetables	Vegetables not on "choose" list Dried peas and beans Potato skins or chips Fried potatoes
Meat, Poultry, Fish, Shellfish, Eggs	Lean tender meat without grease: ground or well-cooked (roasted, baked, or broiled) beef, lamb, ham, veal, pork, poultry, organ meats, fish Eggs except fried	Tough, fried, or spiced meats Fried eggs

continued

TABLE 20-3 ■ Low-Residue Diet (Continued)

DESCRIPTION	INDICATIONS	ADEQUACY
Fats and Oils	Smooth peanut butter Butter, oils Cream (deduct from milk allowance) Margarine	All other nuts Coconut Olives
Desserts and Miscellaneous	Plain dessert made with allowed foods: fruit, ices, sherbet, ice cream, gelatin Candy: gum drops, hard candy, jelly beans, plain chocolate, marshmallows, butterscotch Honey, sugar, molasses Salt, pepper, ground seasonings Plain gravy Milk sauces (deduct from milk allowance) Mayonnaise Coffee, decaffeinated coffee Jelly Tea Soda	Popcorn Seeds of any kind Whole spices Chili sauce Rich gravy Vinegar Alcohol Jam, marmalade

SAMPLE MENU

Breakfast	Lunch/Dinner
Strained grapefruit juice	Baked halibut with clear lemon juice
Cream of wheat	Twice-baked potato (no onions)
Poached egg	Candied sweet potato (no nuts or whole spices)
White bagel with butter and honey	Canned pear and banana on lettuce
½ cup milk	French bread and spread
Coffee	Rice pudding (no raisins; deduct milk from allowance)

it will prevent ketosis. Previously well-nourished adults generally have nutrient reserves for 3 to 4 days of semistarvation. To prevent excessive muscle protein from being used for energy, adequate nourishment should be delivered to the client within 3 days. In general, 25 kilocalories/kilogram of body weight per day is an acceptable and achievable intake.

To avoid abdominal distention, oral feedings traditionally have been delayed until peristalsis returns but scientific evidence supporting this practice is lacking (Charoenkwan, Phillipson, and Vutyavanich, 2007). A sure sign of peristalsis is the passage via the rectum of **flatus** (gas). Ambulation as permitted helps clients pass the flatus and avoid uncomfortable distention.

Paralytic ileus is a complication of abdominal surgery and other traumatic events or diseases. Peristalsis ceases and secretions and gas accumulate in the bowel, leading to distention and vomiting. Removal of secretions by suction is the usual treatment.

A review of studies testing the traditional practice of delaying oral intake until peristalsis returns found no significant differences in postoperative complications in major abdominal gynecological surgery clients. The women fed within 24 hours of surgery experienced more nausea but also were discharged from the hospital earlier than those treated traditionally (Charoenkwan, Phillipson, and Vutyavanich, 2007).

Clients are usually progressed from clear liquids to full liquids, a soft diet, and then a regular diet as soon as possible (see Chapter 14). The progression time varies with the client and surgical procedure. It may be hours or days. If "diet as tolerated" is ordered, the client should be asked what foods sound appealing. Sometimes, a full dinner tray when the client does not feel well "turns off" the small appetite he or she has.

After gastrointestinal surgery, oral food and fluids are deferred longer than with other surgeries to allow healing. Giving the exact amount of food or fluid prescribed is important. More is not better if the client's stomach or intestine has been sutured. It is not advisable to give red liquids, such as gelatin or cranberry juice, after surgery on the mouth and throat so that vomitus is not mistaken for blood or vice versa.

Surgical removal of a part of the gastrointestinal tract, such as the stomach, duodenum, jejunum, or ileum, may result in malabsorption of specific nutrients. Similarly, realignment of parts of the tract can interfere with the digestive processes. (See Fig. 20-1.)

Note that bile salts are absorbed in the ileum. Although the loss of bile salts in the feces may seem harmless, the body ordinarily recycles these salts

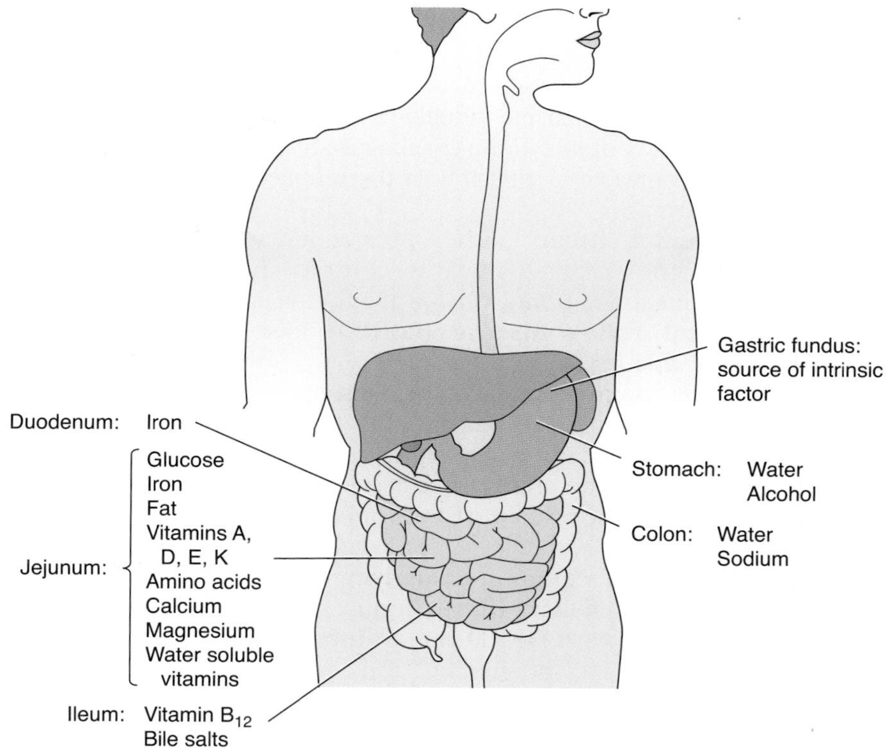

FIGURE 20-1 The chief sites of absorption for various nutrients. Disease or resection of an area will increase the risk of deficiency of specific nutrients. (Adapted from Scanlon, VC, and Sanders, T: *Student workbook for essentials of anatomy and physiology*, ed 4. FA Davis, Philadelphia, 2003, p 283, with permission.)

over and over in the management of fats. Prolonged impaired absorption of bile salts can result in failure to absorb fat and fat-soluble vitamins.

Disorders of the Mouth and Throat

Varied conditions such as dental caries, oral surgery, surgery of the head and neck, fractured jaw, cancer chemotherapy or radiation therapy can cause difficulty with chewing and swallowing. Special feeding techniques and scrupulous oral hygiene may be required. Often the client requires a feeding tube, as covered in Chapter 14. Suggestions to manage dysphagia are described in Chapter 9 and interventions for anorexia appear in Chapter 21. Box 24-2 summarizes the dietary management of many symptoms.

Disorders of the Esophagus

Its sole purpose is to conduct food to the stomach, but the esophagus sometimes malfunctions. Achalasia, gastroesophageal reflux, and hiatal hernia are types of esophageal disorders.

Achalasia

Failure of the gastrointestinal muscle fibers to relax where one part joins another is called **achalasia.** When it occurs in the **cardiac sphincter,** which separates the stomach from the esophagus, the condition is termed *cardiospasm.* Current evidence suggests that a viral infection or some other environmental factor causes inflammation of the esophagus provoking an autoimmune response in susceptible individuals who may be genetically predisposed to react (Park and Vaezi, 2005).

Very hot or cold foods may trigger esophageal spasm, and anxiety seems to aggravate the condition. Symptoms are described as "something sticking in my throat" and a feeling of fullness behind the sternum (breastbone). Vomiting may occur with achalasia, and aspiration of vomitus can cause pneumonia.

In mild cases, avoiding spicy foods and minimizing dietary bulk may be effective. Diets for these clients require much individual attention. Rarely does one achalasia client have intolerances for the same foods as another client. Plenty of liquids with small, frequent meals may help. Treatment of severe cases involves stretching the cardiac sphincter or surgically incising it to enlarge the passage.

Gastroesophageal Reflux Disease

Some regurgitation of stomach contents into the esophagus occurs in normal individuals. Usually the presence of stomach contents in the esophagus stimulates esophageal contractions that return the refluxed material to the stomach.

If excessive reflux occurs, either in frequency or volume, or if the esophagus fails to contract in response to stomach contents, the individual has **gastroesophageal reflux disease (GERD)** (also called *acid-reflux disorder*).

Regurgitation is common in infancy and disappears with age, often to reappear in old age due to poor muscle tone of the cardiac sphincter. In infants, usually no treatment is undertaken unless there is evidence of aspiration of food into the respiratory tract or of failure to thrive.

In adults, the most common underlying cause of gastroesophageal reflux is hiatal hernia. Other conditions associated with GERD due to increased abdominal pressure are pregnancy and obesity. Body mass index is associated with symptoms of gastroesophageal reflux disease in both normal-weight and overweight women. Even moderate weight gain among persons of normal weight may cause or worsen symptoms of reflux (Jacobson et al., 2006).

The stomach is normally protected from hydrochloric acid by a thick layer of mucus. Because the esophagus is not so protected, repeated bouts of gastroesophageal reflux can lead to esophagitis and ulcer formation that, when healed, may cause a stricture at the site of the scar tissue.

The prominent symptom of gastroesophageal reflux is heartburn with pain occurring behind the sternum. Sometimes the pain radiates to the neck and the back of the throat. Lying down or bending over may increase reflux and aggravate the pain. If the passage becomes narrowed, dysphagia may become bothersome.

Treatment involves several conservative measures:

- Small, frequent meals
- Normal amounts of dietary protein, the nutrient that is associated with tightening the cardiac sphincter

In addition, avoidance of these foods and behaviors that relax the sphincter can be helpful:

- Fat and chocolate
- Peppermint and spearmint
- Caffeine, alcohol, and smoking

A client might eliminate decaffeinated coffee and pepper because they stimulate gastric secretions. Likewise, acidic juices, such as citrus and tomato juice, also may be irritating.

Timing of intake is an important self-care strategy. Clients who ate dinner less than 3 hours before bedtime had more than 7 times the occurrence of GERD as those whose elapsed time was 4 hours or more (Fujiwara et al., 2005). Table 20-4 details a diet for gastroesophageal reflux.

TABLE 20-4 ■ Diet for Gastroesophageal Reflux and Hiatal Hernia

DESCRIPTION	INDICATIONS	ADEQUACY
The diet is designed to minimize reflux through timing of intake, texture control, limiting fat, and exclusion of sphincter relaxants and gas-forming foods. Adjunctive treatment involves positioning.	Esophageal reflux, hiatal hernia, esophageal ulcers, esophagitis, esophageal strictures, heartburn	The diet may not meet the RDAs for vitamin C and iron in the premenopausal woman.
LIFESTYLE CHANGES	**CHOOSE**	**DECREASE**
Meal Pattern	Six small meals Chew thoroughly. ½ cup liquid with meals Other liquids >1½ hours after meals >½ hour before meals	Eating within 3 hours of bedtime
Adjunctive Therapy	Sit upright 2 hours after meals. Relax at mealtime. Elevate head of bed 6 inches. Consider weight loss if needed.	Lying down in the hour after eating
Food Group		
Milk	Skim milk, buttermilk, evaporated skim milk Skim milk cheese Cottage cheese Low-fat yogurt	Other milk Hot chocolate

TABLE 20-4 ■ Diet for Gastroesophageal Reflux and Hiatal Hernia (Continued)

Food Group		
Breads and Cereals	White and whole-grain breads Plain rolls, biscuits, and muffins Plain crackers Any cereals except those on "decrease" list Rice Pasta	Pancakes, waffles, French toast Doughnuts, sweet rolls, nut breads Granola-type cereals with nuts and/or coconut
Fruits	Mild juices Any fruits except those on "decrease" list	Avocado Raw apples and melons Orange, grapefruit, and tomato juices
Vegetables	Any vegetables except those on "decrease" list	Creamed or fried vegetables Hashed brown potatoes Broccoli, Brussels sprouts, cabbage, cauliflower, cucumber, dried peas or beans, onions, green pepper, rutabagas, sauerkraut, turnips
Meat, Poultry, Fish, Shellfish Eggs	6 oz/day: lean beef, pork, ham, lamb, liver, veal, fish, skinless poultry Eggs	Sausage, bacon, frankfurters, luncheon meats, canned meats and fish, duck, goose
Fats and Oils	3 tsp/day: oil, butter, margarine, mild salad dressing 2 tbsp of the following may substitute for 1 tsp of fat: light cream, sour cream, nondairy cream Vegetable pan sprays as desired Low-fat salad dressings	Fried foods Gravies and sauces Cream Salad dressing Shortening, lard, or oils in excess of allowance Nuts, peanut butter
Desserts and Miscellaneous	Plain cakes and cookies Gelatin, popsicles Sherbet and pudding made with skim milk Caffeine-free carbonated beverages Decaffeinated tea Fat-free broth, bouillon, consommé Soup made from allowed foods Cream soup made with skim milk Sugar, honey, syrup, molasses Jam, jelly, preserves Plain candy Salt Condiments and spices in small amounts Vanilla Vinegar	Ice cream, ice milk Pie, pastry Butter cake and icings Chocolate, coconut, cream, cream cheese, whipped cream, nuts, peppermint, spearmint Caffeinated beverages Decaffeinated coffee Tea Alcohol Potato chips Candy containing chocolate, nuts, coconut, or peppermint Popcorn Snack chips Pickles, relish Catsup, chili sauce Mustard Steak sauce

SAMPLE MENU

35 Minutes Before Each Meal or Snack	
2 glasses of water	
Breakfast	**Lunch/Dinner**
½ banana	3 oz skinless chicken breast baked in lemon juice
½ cup oatmeal	½ baked potato with 1 tbsp sour cream
½ cup skim milk	½ cup whole-kernel corn
1 slice toast with jam	3 small celery sticks
	Hard roll with 1 tsp spread ½ cup decaffeinated tea
Midmorning Snack	**Midafternoon/Evening Snack**
½ cup pineapple juice	1 cup low-fat yogurt
3 graham crackers	

Hiatal Hernia

The *esophageal hiatus* is the opening in the diaphragm through which the esophagus is attached to the stomach. A ***hiatal hernia*** is a protrusion of the stomach through the esophageal hiatus into the chest cavity (Fig. 20-2). The symptoms of hiatal hernia are similar to those of gastroesophageal reflux, and its medical treatment is the same. Persistent symptoms despite conservative treatment might lead the client to elect surgical repair of the hernia.

Disorders of the Stomach

Disorders of the stomach often require diet modification and, in some cases, surgery. The following sections concern two common disorders, gastritis and peptic ulcers, and one disorder mainly associated with diabetes mellitus, delayed gastric emptying. Also included is an exaggerated physiological response that can cause problems for older adults, postprandial hypotension.

Gastritis

Inflammation of the stomach is ***gastritis***. Common causes of gastritis are the chronic use of aspirin and alcohol abuse. Symptoms of gastritis are:

- Anorexia
- Nausea
- A feeling of fullness
- Epigastric pain

Signs of gastritis are vomiting and eructating (belching).

Figure 20-3 illustrates the abdominal quadrants and regions used to record signs and symptoms revealed during the assessment process.

More often than not, discovering which foods are responsible for the pain and discomfort of gastritis is a trial-and-error process. Tolerances vary from

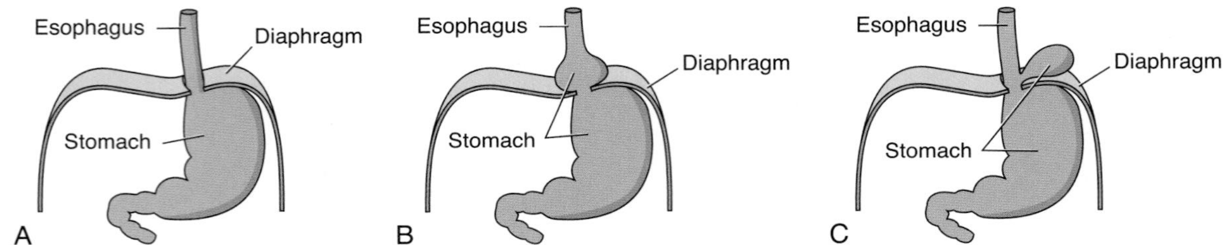

FIGURE 20-2 In hiatal hernia, the upper part of the stomach squeezes into the chest cavity through the esophageal opening in the diaphragm. *A*, Normal anatomy. *B*, Sliding hiatal hernia. *C*, Paraesophageal or rolling hiatal hernia. (Reprinted from Williams, LS, and Hopper, PD: *Understanding medical-surgical nursing*, ed 3. FA Davis, Philadelphia, 2007, p 672, with permission.)

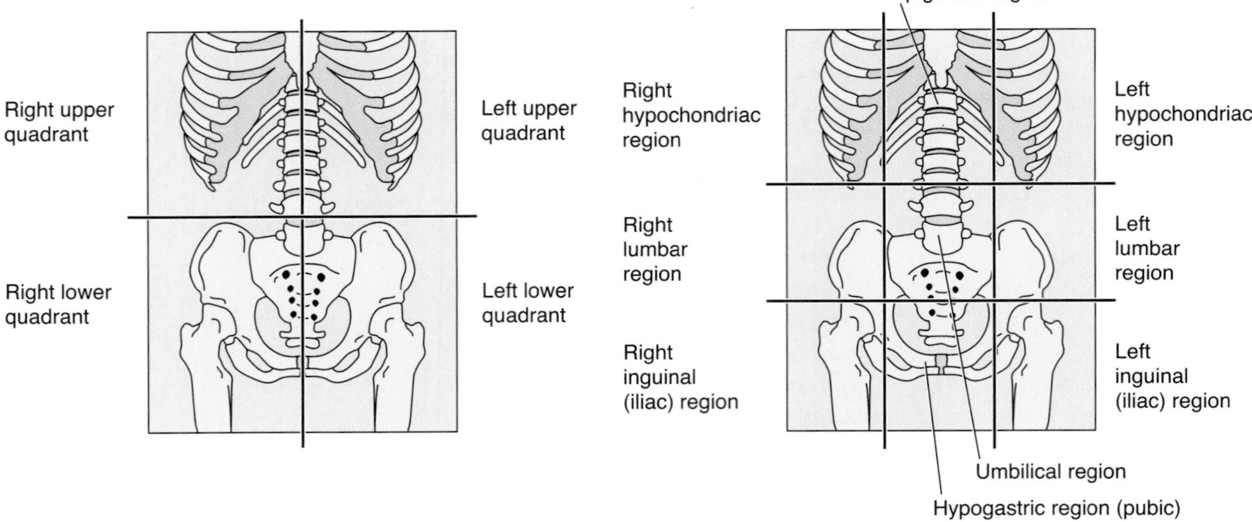

FIGURE 20-3 Abdominal quadrants and regions of the abdomen are used to describe locations of signs and symptoms. (Reprinted from Venes, D [ed]: *Taber's cyclopedic medical dictionary*, ed 21. FA Davis, Philadelphia, 2010, p 4, with permission.)

person to person. Suggested dietary treatments for gastritis are given in Box 20-1. Prolonged or recurrent gastritis deserves medical attention to diagnose and treat the underlying problem.

Delayed Gastric Emptying

This condition can be associated with certain prescription drugs as well as the use of alcohol, tobacco, and marijuana. Delayed gastric emptying can occur in anorexia nervosa and in malnutrition, but up to 50% of clients with diabetes may be affected, with no clear association between length of disease and symptoms such as **postprandial** (after eating) abdominal pain, nausea, vomiting, and bloating.

When delayed gastric emptying occurs with diabetes, it is termed *diabetic gastroparesis.* It can accompany both insulin-dependent and non–insulin-dependent diabetes (Intagliata and Koch, 2007). Treatment of delayed gastric emptying focuses on the cause of the disorder: removing offending drugs, intervening appropriately in malnutrition, and controlling hyperglycemia in clients with diabetes.

Dietary interventions include:

- Eating small, frequent meals
- Replacing solids with liquids such as soups (which leave the stomach sooner than solids)
- Reducing the fat ingested (which remains in the stomach longer than carbohydrate or protein)
- Decreasing fiber intake (Parkman, Hasler, and Fisher, 2004)

In severe cases, medications may be prescribed and stimulatory techniques may be implemented.

Peptic Ulcers

Gastric (stomach) and duodenal ulcers are called *peptic ulcers,* and they form when the mucosa is insufficiently resistant to stomach acids. If just the superficial cells are involved, the lesion is called an **erosion.** If the muscular layer of the stomach or duodenum is involved, the person has an **ulcer.**

Pathophysiology

The most relevant organic etiologies for peptic ulcers are infection with *Helicobacter pylori* and use of nonsteroidal anti-inflammatory drugs (NSAIDs). The latter account for more than 50% of peptic ulcers (Cohen, 2007). Between 5% and 20% of clients with peptic ulcer, however, do not have an identifiable organic etiology. In these patients, particularly, and in ulcer patients in general, psychosocial factors may play a significant role (Jones, 2006).

Helicobacter pylori is a key pathogen in gastroduodenal inflammation and peptic ulcers. About half of the world's population is infected with *Helicobacter pylori,* a gastric bacterium typically acquired in early childhood, and, unless treated, persists throughout life (Kivi and Tindberg, 2006). The organism is found in 20% to 30% of adults in developed countries; however, only a minority of these people develop duodenal ulcers (Heymann, 2004). See Genomic Gem 20-1.

Signs and Symptoms

A burning, cramping epigastric pain when the stomach is empty characterizes duodenal ulcer. This pain

Box 20-1 ■ *Dietary Treatment for Gastritis*

Do

- Eat at regular intervals.
- Eat in a relaxed manner.
- Chew food, especially fibrous food, slowly and thoroughly.

Avoid

- Foods that cause pain
- Foods that cause gas, especially vegetables in the cabbage family (broccoli, cauliflower, and Brussels sprouts)
- Gastric irritants such as caffeine and alcohol
- Nonsteroidal anti-inflammatory drugs (NSAIDs) such as aspirin
- Strong spices, including nutmeg, pepper, garlic, and chili powder

Genomic Gem 20-1

Gastroduodenal Disease

The irregular incidence of gastroduodenal disease despite infection of large numbers of people with *Helicobacter pylori* points to a genetic causality. Since the mid-20th century, gastroduodenal disease has been known to be related to blood type:

- Blood type O with duodenal ulcers
- Blood type A with gastric ulcers and gastric cancer (Gillen and McColl, 2005).

Likelihood of significant gastric disease depends on genetic polymorphisms influencing the virulence of the organism. Similarly, the specific disease pattern depends on genetic polymorphisms in the person governing his immune response (Gillen and McColl, 2005).

One hypothesis under investigation is the association of:

- Proinflammatory polymorphisms that predispose to gastritis of the stomach body, low acid secretion, and cardia cancer/gastric ulcer risk
- Less-inflammatory polymorphisms that may predispose to antral gastritis, acid hypersecretion, and duodenal ulcer risk (Gillen and McColl, 2005)

occurs 2 to 4 hours after eating or at night and is relieved by antacids or food.

With gastric ulcer, the burning, gnawing epigastric pain occurs 1 to 2 hours after meals and may be worsened by ingesting food (Williams and Hopper, 2007).

One-fourth of ulcer clients experience bleeding, which occurs more often with duodenal than with gastric ulcers. If the blood is vomited immediately after bleeding begins, it is bright red. If it stays in contact with digestive juices for a while, the vomitus is brown-black and granular, resembling coffee grounds. The medical term for this is *coffee-ground emesis*. Other symptoms of peptic ulcer are nausea, anorexia, and sometimes weight loss.

Complications

Hemorrhage is a complication of peptic ulcers. Scar tissue from a healed ulcer can restrict the gastric outlet, causing pyloric obstruction. If the ulcer continues to erode through the entire stomach or intestinal wall, the result is a **perforated ulcer.** Leakage of gastrointestinal contents into the sterile abdominal cavity causes **peritonitis**, an inflammation of the peritoneum (the lining of the abdominal cavity).

Treatment

Medical treatment for *H. pylori* infection includes combinations of antibiotics and other drugs. Only if such treatment proves ineffective is surgery considered. A dietary approach has also been investigated. In asymptomatic clients with *H. pylori* infections, bifidobacterium- and lactobacillus-containing yogurt twice daily for 6 weeks effectively suppressed the infection (Wang et al., 2004). Other regimens supplementing medication treatment with yogurt have reported improved outcomes (Kim et al., 2008; Sheu et al., 2006). See Box 20-2.

Box 20-2 ■ *Probiotics and Prebiotics*

Fermented foods have been considered health-promoting for centuries. More than 2000 years ago, Plinius the Old recommended fermented milk to treat acute gastritis (Vandenplas et al., 2007).

Probiotics are live microbial foods or supplements that improve the microbial balance of the intestine. Only small percentages of the ingested organisms reach the ileum alive. They do not colonize the colon because they are undetectable within a few days of ceasing intake (Vandenplas et al., 2007). Despite the health benefits attributed to probiotics, only specific strains have been tested. Results cannot be generalized to other strains.

Suggested modes of action are by:

- Producing bactericidal substances
- Competing with pathogens and toxins for adherence to the intestinal epithelium
- Regulating immune responses
- Enhancing intestinal barrier function (Vanderpool, Yan, and Polk, 2008).

Probiotic supplementation may benefit both children and adults with irritable bowel syndrome and adults with ulcerative colitis. It also can reduce the risk of travelers' diarrhea in adults, but does not affect its duration (Lomax and Calder, 2009). Under certain conditions, particular probiotics are beneficial for managing antibiotic-associated diarrhea, necrotizing enterocolitis (see Clinical Application 11-5), and infectious diarrhea (Wolvers et al., 2010).

Special caution is urged when introducing new and potentially infectious agents to immunologically immature infants (Kliegman and Willoughby, 2005). Similarly, cautious use of probiotics is warranted around children at increased risk for infections or those with compromised gut integrity (Vandenplas et al., 2007).

Probiotics are found in fermented or aged milk and milk products, other fermented products, breast milk, and supplements. Food sources of probiotics not only enhance the probiotic's stability by buffering stomach acid but also contain other nutrients. The most reliable food source is yogurt labeled "live and active culture." To earn this seal, the product must contain at least 100 million bacteria per gram of yogurt at the time it is made and must not have been heat treated because heat kills the bacteria. Many yogurts contain both starter cultures and additional bacteria presumed to be probiotic. Most labels do not differentiate the amounts of the bacterial strains contained in the product, making it difficult to choose a proven product for a given condition (Douglas and Sanders, 2008). Administration of bacteria-derived probiotics should be separated from antibiotics by at least two hours (Willams, 2010).

Prebiotics are nondigestible food ingredients that encourage the growth of favorable microorganisms. Prebiotics are specialized ingredients that target specific bacteria, not food fiber in general. Some foods that could be prebiotic sources are artichokes, bananas, garlic, onions, and wheat (Douglas and Sanders, 2008).

MEDICAL

Before the advent of anti-ulcer medications, clients with peptic ulcers were usually advised to take antacids every 2 hours, alternating with milk and cream. Later research demonstrated that milk is a potent *inducer* of gastric acid secretion. An additional adverse effect of this treatment was milk alkali syndrome (see Chapter 8).

New medications have revolutionized the treatment and are almost always effective without a drastic change in diet. In addition to antibiotics to eradicate *H. pylori*, commonly prescribed medications are:

- *cimetidine, ranitidine*, and *famotidine*, which block histamine-stimulated gastric acid secretion
- *omeprazole*, which suppresses gastric acid production

Despite reports from individual clients connecting certain foods to epigastric pain, no evidence indicates that dietary intake causes peptic ulcers. Neither does diet, including alcohol and coffee in moderation, influence healing (Stenson, 2006). A generally healthy diet while avoiding items causing distress is advised for these clients.

Cigarette smoking is a risk factor for developing peptic ulcers and related complications. Also, smoking impairs ulcer healing and increases recurrence (Cohen, 2007). Consequently, peptic ulcer clients should be advised not to smoke.

SURGICAL

When surgery is necessary, the ulcer is removed and the remaining gastrointestinal tract is sutured together. Surgical procedures designed to eliminate the diseased area include gastroduodenostomy (stomach and duodenum anastomosed) and gastrojejunostomy (stomach and jejunum anastomosed). **Anastomosis** is the surgical connection between tubular structures. Figure 20-4 illustrates these two procedures.

After gastric surgery, parenteral and tube feeding are used singly or in combination. If tube feeding is used, the tube must be inserted beyond the area that was resected (removed). Nutritional care includes delivering nutrients to ensure maximal utilization of the remaining functions of the gastrointestinal tract. After a client is advanced to an oral diet, he or she may experience **dumping syndrome,** a complication of a surgical procedure that removes, disrupts, or bypasses the pyloric sphincter. Clinical Application 20-2 describes the dumping syndrome in more detail. Table 20-5 depicts a diet to prevent or treat dumping syndrome.

Long-term nutritional consequences of reconstructive surgery for peptic ulcer include iron-deficiency anemia and osteomalacia. The deficiency of iron is related to decreased gastric acidity and decreased absorptive capacity of the duodenum. Clients have increased risk for osteomalacia after peptic ulcer surgery with a fracture rate two to three times that of the general population. The mechanism for developing osteomalacia is not completely understood, although the duodenum is a major site for calcium absorption (Stenson, 2006).

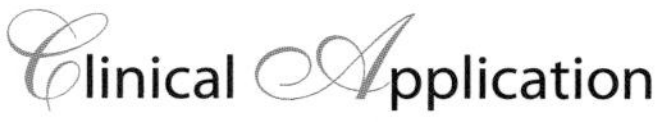

20-2

Clinical Application

Dumping Syndrome

The pyloric sphincter normally allows only small amounts of gastric contents into the duodenum at a time. After the pyloric sphincter is surgically removed, a concentrated liquid is suddenly "dumped" into the intestine. The concentrated contents then pull water from the bowel wall just as in osmotic diarrhea. Local effects are:

- Hyperperistalsis
- Diarrhea
- Abdominal pain
- Vomiting 30 to 60 minutes after a meal.

Systemic effects that relate to insufficient fluid volume include:

- Weakness
- Dizziness
- Sweating
- Hypotension
- Tachycardia
- Palpitations

The dumping syndrome is most often associated with a total gastrectomy or a partial gastrectomy involving resection of two-thirds of the stomach. The same signs and symptoms can occur in a client receiving a tube feeding if the nasogastric tube is accidentally carried down into the duodenum.

Dietary treatment of the dumping syndrome attempts to delay gastric emptying and to distribute the increased osmolality to the bowel over time. This can be achieved by:

- Limiting the intake of simple sugars that increase the osmolality of the gastric contents
- Consuming small frequent meals to reduce the intestinal load
- Limiting fluids with meals
- Avoiding very hot or cold foods that stimulate peristalsis

A nondietary intervention also helps. Lying down for 30 to 60 minutes after eating retains the meal in the stomach longer.

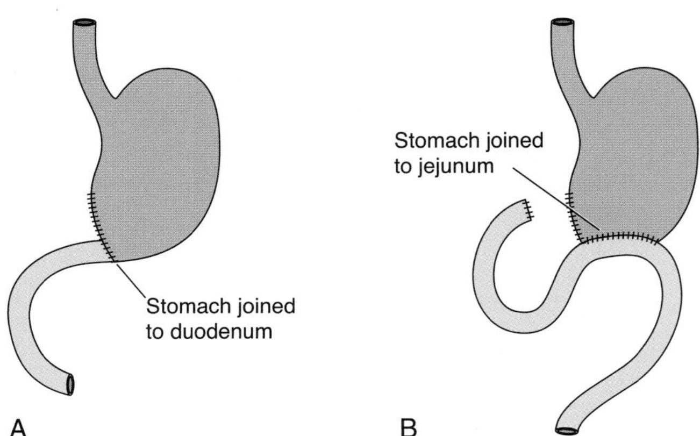

FIGURE 20-4 Common gastric resection procedures. *A*, Gastroduodenostomy or Billroth I procedure. *B*, Gastrojejunostomy or Billroth II procedure. (Reprinted from Williams, LS, and Hopper, PD: *Understanding medical-surgical nursing*, ed 3. FA Davis, Philadelphia, 2007, p 681, with permission.)

Postprandial Hypotension

Hypotension after a meal occurs in approximately 40% of nursing home residents (Gentilcore et al., 2006). Postprandial hypotension is a drop in systolic blood pressure of 20 mm Hg or more within 75 to 120 minutes after the beginning of a meal. Symptoms include:

- Dizziness
- Fatigue
- Weakness

TABLE 20-5 ■ Diet for Dumping Syndrome

DESCRIPTION	INDICATIONS	ADEQUACY
This diet consists of six small feedings, high in protein and low in simple sugars.	This diet and adjunct therapy, used after surgical removal of the pyloric sphincter or other treatments that speed gastric emptying, is designed to prevent rapid emptying of hypertonic gastric contents into the small intestine. Examples of such operative procedures include vagotomy, pyloroplasty, hemigastrectomy, total gastrectomy, esophagogastrectomy, Whipple's procedure, gastroenterostomy, and gastrojejunostomy. As the body adapts to its new condition, specific foods may be tolerated later in convalescence.	Deficiencies secondary to surgery or malabsorption may require supplementation. Among the nutrients likely to be needed are the vitamins B_{12}, D, and folic acid and the minerals calcium and iron.
LIFESTYLE CHANGES	**CHOOSE**	**DECREASE**
Meal pattern	Six small servings Eat slowly and chew thoroughly	Fluids with meals
Adjunctive therapy	Lie down for ½ hour after meals	
Food Group		
Milk	LactAid Aged cheese (>90 days)	Milk if lactose intolerant*
Breads and Cereals	White, whole-wheat, rye, Jewish, Italian, and Vienna breads* Rolls, crackers, biscuits, and muffins (milk-free)* Any cooked or dry cereal, milk-free* Rice, noodles, spaghetti, macaroni	Frosted breads Sweet rolls, doughnuts, coffeecake Bread made with milk (unless tolerated)* Sugar-sweetened cereal Cereal containing milk*
Fruits	Fresh, frozen, or unsweetened canned fruits, banana Juices, fresh, frozen, canned, unsweetened, between meals only	Sweetened canned or frozen juices and fruits, dried fruit Raw fruits unless tolerated Juices with meals
Vegetables	Any as tolerated Juices between meals only	Those causing discomfort Juices with meals
Meat Group	Any as tolerated	None
Fats and Oils	Milk-free margarine if lactose intolerant* Oils Vegetable shortening	Any containing milk unless tolerated*
Desserts and Miscellaneous	Artificially sweetened gelatin Angel food and sponge cakes Salt, pepper, spices as tolerated Mustard, catsup, pickles, relishes as tolerated Artificially sweetened beverages Decaffeinated tea and coffee, herbal tea Dietetic jam and jelly	Sugar-containing cakes, pies, cookies, ice cream,* sherbet* Seasonings that cause discomfort Caffeine-containing beverages Sugar, honey, syrup, molasses Jam, jelly Candy
SAMPLE MENU		
30 Minutes Before Breakfast	**30 Minutes Before Lunch**	
Decaffeinated beverage	1 cup LactAid®	
Artificial sweetener		
Breakfast	**Lunch/Dinner**	
½ banana	3 oz roast pork	
1 egg, poached	Barley with butter	
1 tsp milk-free margarine	½ cup squash	
Dietetic jelly	½ cup fruit cocktail, drained	
1½ Hours After Breakfast	**1½ Hours After Meal**	
Orange juice	Decaffeinated beverage	
	Artificial sweetener	
Midmorning Snack		
1 slice whole-wheat toast		
Dietetic jam		

*If lactose restriction is necessary.

- Light-headedness
- Disturbed speech
- Vision changes

The most severe hypotension occurs in individuals with neurological, cardiovascular, or renal diseases. Complications include higher incidence of coronary events, stroke, and total mortality (Malozemoff and Gentlemen, 2004). Normally the body compensates for the increased blood flow to the digestive tract following meals, but in the elderly the mechanisms maintaining adequate circulation to the rest of the body become less effective. Greater effects are seen when the stomach empties more rapidly.

To prevent postprandial hypotension, a person should:

- Limit carbohydrate intake.
- Take frequent small meals.
- Lie in a semirecumbent position for 90 minutes after eating.
- Avoid excessive exercise for 2 hours after meals.
- Schedule antihypertensive medications between rather than just before meals (Malozemoff and Gentlemen, 2004).

Special dietary additives or medications to delay gastric emptying are sometimes prescribed.

Disorders of the Intestines

To obtain satisfactory diagnostic radiographic or endoscopic studies of the bowel, it must be emptied. This is usually accomplished by a low residue/clear liquid diet followed by laxatives. Explaining the procedures and the necessity for them helps to gain the client's cooperation. For inpatients, the nurse should ensure that the client receives maximum nourishment when tests are completed for the day. Frequently, another series of tests is scheduled for the next day.

Problems With Elimination

Several problems with frequency and consistency of bowel movements are common. These include irritable bowel syndrome, diarrhea, and constipation.

Irritable Bowel Syndrome

As many as 20% of adult Americans have symptoms of irritable bowel syndrome (IBS), making it one of the most common disorders diagnosed by doctors. Women are diagnosed more often than men. About 50% of those affected show symptoms before the age of 35 (National Digestive, 2007).

The most common signs and symptoms of **irritable bowel syndrome** are:

- Cramping
- Abdominal pain
- Bloating
- Constipation
- Diarrhea

No specific cause for IBS has been identified. One theory is that people who suffer from IBS have a colon, or large intestine, that is particularly sensitive and reactive to certain foods and stress. The immune system, which fights infection, may also be involved (National Digestive, 2007).

Treatment for IBS is symptomatic. Offending foods should be identified and avoided. Exclusion diets are time-consuming and not completely effective in identifying triggers, but excluding foods based on elevated antibody levels improves symptoms. Antibodies to milk, eggs, wheat, beef, pork, and lamb have been elevated in IBS clients (Zar et al., 2005).

Additional strategies include:

- Stress management techniques
- Bowel hygiene principles
- Possibly a high-fiber diet to avoid constipation and increased pressure on the walls of the intestine

Clients should be reassured that IBS does not permanently harm the intestines, is unrelated to inflammatory bowel diseases, and does not lead to cancer (National Digestive, 2007).

Diarrhea

Passage of liquid or unformed feces, diarrhea, is an important cause of morbidity and mortality in the elderly and in children (see Chapter 11). Most instances of diarrhea in adults are self-limiting and resolve without treatment or the need for extensive medical workup. In many cases, the cause of diarrhea cannot be found. If an adult is in little jeopardy from an electrolyte imbalance, self-treatment for diarrhea following the conservative regimen listed in Table 20-6 is appropriate.

Medical consultation becomes important if diarrhea:

- Lasts for more than 3 days,
- Causes severe pain in the abdomen or rectum,
- Provokes a fever of 102 degrees or higher,
- Produces blood in the stool or black, tarry stools, or
- Is accompanied by signs of dehydration.

In addition to these concerns, if a client has medical conditions for which fasting, dehydration,

TABLE 20-6 ■ Self-Treatment for Diarrhea*

TIME	ORAL INTAKE	COMMENTS
First 12 hours	Water or oral hydration solutions at room temperature	Easily absorbed fluids to maintain hydration
Second 12 hours	Clear liquids, no caffeine or extremes of temperature	If up to 5% body weight lost; if more than 5% lost, seek medical attention
		Very hot, very cold, or caffeinated beverages stimulate peristalsis
Third 12 hours	Full liquids	Experiment with milk in case lactose intolerance has developed
Fourth 12 hours	Soft diet	Include applesauce or banana for **pectin;** rice, pasta, and bread without fat (digested by enzymes usually unaffected by gastroenteritis)
By 48th hour	Regular diet	Seek medical treatment if diarrhea has not resolved and regular diet is not tolerated. Other reasons for medical attention: dehydration, abdominal distension, fever, bloody stools.

*Appropriate for healthy adults.

or infectious disease is a hazard, a physician should be consulted.

TRAVELER'S DIARRHEA

Travelers' diarrhea affects more than 10 milion people per year (Singh and Redfield, 2009). An estimated 40% of travelers to developing nations will become ill with diarrhea (Koo and DuPont, 2006). Destination is the most significant risk factor for developing traveler's diarrhea. Regions with the highest risk are Africa, South Asia, Latin America, and the Middle East. Other risk factors are:

- Immunocompromised states
- Lowered gastric acidity
- Genetic susceptibility (Yates, 2005)

See Genomic Gem 20-2.

Traveler's diarrhea is transmitted by food and drinks contaminated with bacteria, viruses, or parasites. To minimize risk, people should avoid:

- Drinking tap water and ice made from it
- Foods washed in water and served raw
- Unpasteurized milk
- Sauces and salsas
- Uncooked seafood
- Raw or poorly cooked meats
- Foods from street vendors (especially risky)

Usually safe foods and beverages include:

- Carbonated bottled beverages (if the seal is intact)
- Food cooked and served piping hot
- Dry foods such as bread and cereal

Some experts advise all people who travel to high-risk areas to take curative antimicrobial agents with them for self-treatment of illness (DuPont, 2005). In all cases of infectious diarrhea, good handwashing for 30 seconds is likely to remove 95% of transient organisms and decrease the likelihood of transferring them to another (Musher and Musher, 2004).

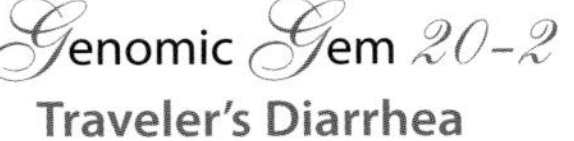

Traveler's Diarrhea

Traditional risk factors do not explain the individual differences in susceptibility to traveler's diarrhea among visitors to developing countries. Single-nucleotide polymorphisms of the genes encoding for lactoferrin and interleukin-8 (IL-8) have been linked to susceptibility to traveler's diarrhea.

In contrast, persons with mutations of the *FUT2* gene are immune to norovirus infection. The recognition of individual variations in susceptibility to traveler's diarrhea will aid in customizing prophylactic medication regimens and standby treatments (Cabada and White, 2008).

OTHER CAUSES

Diarrhea may be iatrogenic (produced by treatment) accompanying tube feeding or antibiotic therapy. Fiber supplementation of enteral feedings reduced stool frequency and yielded more solid stools than standard formulas in hospitalized geriatric clients (Vandewoude et al., 2005).

Probiotics have accelerated recovery from acute infectious diarrhea and have prevented antibiotic-associated diarrhea but optimal species, doses, and clinical conditions need further research (Sartor, 2005). See Box 20-2. An often overlooked cause of diarrhea, celiac disease, is covered in Clinical Application 20-3 and Genomic Gem 20-3.

Constipation

Each person develops a usual bowel pattern, so that a bowel movement every day or every second or third day may be perfectly normal for a given individual.

Constipation refers to a decrease in a person's normal frequency of defecation, especially if the stool is hard, dry, or difficult to expel. Changes in bowel habits should be investigated thoroughly to discover

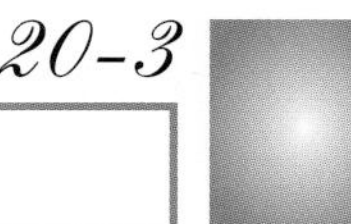

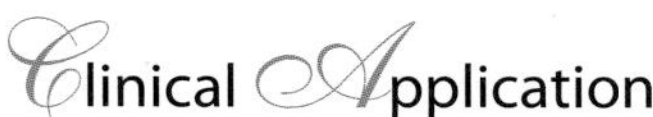

20-3 Clinical Application

Case Finding and Diagnosis: Celiac Disease (Gluten-sensitive enteropathy, Nontropical Sprue)

This illness is classically diagnosed in a child who presents with steatorrhea after gluten-containing cereals (wheat, rye, barley) are added to the diet. Oats may be problematic because they can pick up gluten from other grains during milling. Population studies have revealed 1% of both 7-year-olds and adults have celiac disease. Since the peak age of diagnosis is the fourth and fifth decades, these findings suggest the disease goes undetected for many years (Green and Jabri, 2006).

At presentation:

- Younger children are seen with diarrhea and failure to thrive.
- Older children are seen with short stature, anemia, neurological problems, and even constipation.
- Adults present with anemia or are discovered through endoscopies to evaluate symptoms not suggestive of celiac disease. A prior diagnosis of irritable bowel syndrome is common (Green and Jabri, 2006) and routine screening for celiac disease in clients with symptoms of IBS is recommended (Jadallah and Khader, 2009).

Gluten sensitivity also has a skin manifestation, *dermatitis herpetiformis*, affecting approximately 25% of clients with celiac disease (Collin and Reunala, 2003).

Several serological tests for antibodies are available for screening but no single test is diagnostic. The gold standard for definitive diagnosis is a biopsy of the small intestine. In all cases, the client should consume a gluten-containing diet until the diagnostic testing has been completed.

Genomic Gem 20-3

Celiac Disease

Celiac disease occurs in 10% of first-degree relatives (parent, sibling, child) of those with the disease but in 70% of the identical twins of clients with the disease. Although about 30% to 40% of Caucasians carry the essential genetic factors, fewer than 3% develop the disease (Green and Jabri, 2006).

Celiac disease is polygenic. Both human leukocyte antigen (HLA) and non-HLA genes have been linked to the disease. The HLA genes confer up to 40% of the risk with the remainder attributed to the non-HLA genes (Green and Jabri, 2006). Because only a few genetically susceptible individuals develop celiac disease, its etiology is considered to be multifactorial involving a combination of:

- Genetic predisposition
- Ingestion of gluten (see Chapter 9)
- An autoimmune response that produces chronic inflammation of the small intestine

or rule out disease. Medications that commonly cause constipation include opiates, iron, and anticholinergic agents (Lacy, 2007).

After disease conditions have been ruled out, a search for deficits in the following areas may suggest some of these changes:

- Gradually increase dietary fiber.
- Drink adequate water.
- Exercise regularly.
- Have a warm drink with breakfast.
- Evacuate at a regular time (usually after a meal to take advantage of the body's programming).

In some cases of fecal impaction, the client may experience diarrhea. Clinical Application 20-4 explains this paradox.

Inflammatory Bowel Diseases

The two most common inflammatory bowel diseases (IBDs) are **Crohn's disease,** also known as *ileitis* or *regional enteritis*, and **ulcerative colitis**. The two diseases share some similar characteristics but have some major differences. See Tables 20-7 and 20-8.

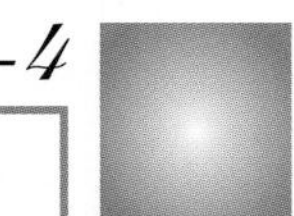

20-4 Clinical Application

Distinguishing Diarrhea From Fecal Impaction

If a client usually is constipated and then has diarrhea, the nurse should check the rectum for impacted stool. The stool will be dry and hard and the client will not be able to pass it unassisted. The diarrheal stool is passed around the impaction.

As in many cases, prevention is preferable to diagnosis and treatment. Institutionalized clients should be monitored for elimination problems. Frequency and consistency of bowel movements should be charted.

TABLE 20-7 ■ Similarities Between Crohn's Disease and Ulcerative Colitis

Etiology	Unknown
Theories	Autoimmune interaction of genetic susceptibility and environment
Likely stimulus of autoimmunity	Common, nonpathogenic microorganisms of intestinal tract
Familial links	About 20% of IBD clients have first-degree relative with IBD (see Genomic Gem 20-4)
Signs and symptoms	Diarrhea, abdominal pain Weight loss Decreased bone mineral density
Associated conditions	Arthritis, eye inflammation

Genomic Gem 20-4

Inflammatory Bowel Disease

Identical twins more often have IBD, especially Crohn's disease, than do fraternal twins. A susceptibility gene for Crohn's disease encodes an intracellular receptor that regulates immediate immune response to microbes. Mutations of this gene are neither necessary nor sufficient for the development of Crohn's disease, however.

Environmental factors contribute to the complex etiology of IBD. For instance, Asian immigrants to England experience increased ulcerative colitis after relocating. Some scientists suggest that smoking may be an environmental factor that determines whether a predisposed individual develops Crohn's disease or ulcerative colitis (Griffiths, 2006).

TABLE 20-8 ■ Differences Between Crohn's Disease and Ulcerative Colitis

	CROHN'S DISEASE	ULCERATIVE COLITIS
Location	Anywhere in gastrointestinal tract, most often terminal ileum	Large intestine
Distribution	Diseased areas alternate with healthy tissue	Usually starts in rectum and spreads upward in continuous pattern
Lesions	Involves all layers of intestinal wall	Confined to mucosal and submucosal layers
Associated Conditions*	Skin problems, kidney stones, gall stones	Osteoporosis, liver disease
Environmental Factors	Associated with smoking	Associated with nonsmoking
Complications	Fistula, obstruction, stricture	Toxic megacolon
Prognosis After Surgery	Disease recurs†	Cured

*It is not known why these problems occur outside the intestine. Scientists think these complications may be the result of inflammation triggered by the immune system. IBD treatment resolves some of these problems (National Digestive, 2006b).

†Postoperative maintenance is disappointing. Smoking cessation is the only effective measure (Cottone, Orlando, and Modesto, 2006).

General goals for nutritional care of IBD clients include:

- The prevention and correction of malnutrition
- The prevention of osteoporosis
- In children, the promotion of optimal growth and development (O'Sullivan and O'Morain, 2006)

Box 20-3 provides some facts about IBD in children. Table 20-9 lists general uses of nutritional modalities for IBD.

In general, clients with Crohn's disease are more affected by the foods they consume than are clients with ulcerative colitis. Clients who have either Crohn's disease or ulcerative colitis have reported that bananas, carrots, potatoes, rice, roast chicken, and water did not worsen their symptoms and made them feel good (Joachim, 2000).

Measures to decrease inflammation and balance the intestinal microbes are under investigation.

- Fish oil supplementation in clients with IBD incorporated omega-3 fatty acids into gut mucosa and modified inflammatory mediator profiles. Clinical outcomes vary but some trials reported improved gut histology and decreased disease activity (Calder, 2008).
- Probiotic bacteria have been effective in ulcerative colitis and refractory pouchitis (Leenen and Dieleman, 2007).

Box 20-3 ■ *Inflammatory Bowel Diseases in Children*

Twenty-five percent of IBD presents in childhood (Beattie et al., 2006). Investigation of growth retardation should consider IBD as a cause. In Crohn's disease, growth retardation may precede clinical evidence of bowel disease (Shamir, Phillip, and Levine, 2007).

Treatment with TPN or enteral formulas is effective in restoring growth. The method most commonly used is overnight nasogastric tube feeding that allows normal daytime activities. Fortunately, children become adept at swallowing the catheters (Griffiths, 2006).

TABLE 20-9 ■ Nutritional Care in Inflammatory Bowel Disease

	CROHN'S DISEASE	ULCERATIVE COLITIS
Prevention	Diet irrelevant	Diet irrelevant
Enteral Feeding*	Primary therapy in active disease and in children with impaired growth	Not proven as primary therapy
TPN	In acute disease to improve nutritional status In chronic disease, for clients with a very short gut	In acute disease to improve nutritional status

*May promote mucosal healing better than TPN (Griffiths, 2006).

Nutritional Therapy

Beyond general goals, the nutritional care of clients with IBD must be individualized according to the nutritional status of the individual, the location and extent of the disease, and the surgical and medical treatments. To maintain nutritional status, foods should not be eliminated from the diet without a fair trial. Restrictions should be limited to foods that produce gas or loose stools. Suspected foods should be tried in small amounts to determine tolerance levels.

CROHN'S DISEASE

No one diet has been proven effective for preventing or treating Crohn's disease. A food-symptom diary followed by a customized elimination diet for 2-4 weeks is one management technique (Brown and Roy, 2010) and a small 2-year study demonstrated a semi-vegeterian diet to be significantly better than an omnivorous diet in preventing relapse (Chjiba et al., 2010). A nutritional intervention based on circulating IgG antibodies against food antigens showed significantly decreased stool frequency but the mechanisms by which IgG antibodies might contribute to the disease are unclear (Bentz et al., 2010). When clients experience a flare in disease, foods such as bulky grains, hot spices, alcohol, and milk products may increase diarrhea and cramping (National Digestive, 2006a).

ULCERATIVE COLITIS

Dietary modification is usually based on client tolerance and avoidance of irritating foods. Despite clients' beliefs that food affected their disease course, no reported dietary behavior reduced the incidence of relapse of the illness (Jowett et al., 2004a).

Relapse from remission in ulcerative colitis has been linked to intakes of certain foods. Individuals in the highest third of consumption of the following items (versus the lowest third) had these increased risks of relapse:

- Meat consumption 3 times
- Red and processed meats 5 times
- Protein 3 times
- Alcohol 2.7 times

High sulfur or sulfate intakes were also associated with 2.8 and 2.6 times the risk of relapse (Jowett et al., 2004b). A suggested mechanism relates to colonic bacteria producing hydrogen sulfide from sulfur-containing amino acids (Magee et al., 2000; Tilg and Kaser, 2004). Clients with ulcerative colitis showed a fundamental difference in gut sulfide metabolism compared to those without that diagnosis (Ohge et al., 2005) and evidence implicates sulfate-reducing bacteria (SRB) as an environmental factor in ulcerative colitis (Rowan et al., 2009).

Surgical Treatment

Surgery may be recommended when IBD becomes medically unmanageable. The portion of the bowel that is inflamed can be surgically resected. This results in a shorter gut that may create additional nutritional hazards for the client (Clinical Application 20-5).

A **colectomy** is the surgical removal of part or all of the colon. Other surgical procedures include ileostomy and colostomy, which may be either permanent or temporary.

In an **ileostomy,** the end of the remaining portion of the small intestine (the **ileum**) is attached to a surgically established opening in the abdominal wall called a **stoma,** from which the intestinal contents are discharged.

In a **colostomy,** a part of the large intestine is resected and a stoma is created in the abdominal wall.

Clients who have surgery to divert intestinal contents through the abdominal wall often suffer psychological trauma in addition to the physical change.

20-5

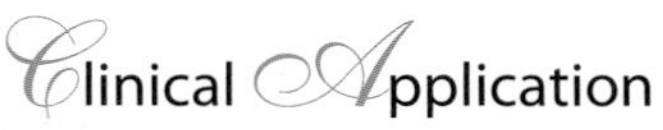

Short Bowel Syndrome

Because the small intestine is 16 to 20 feet long in the adult, up to 50% can be removed without dire consequences. Depending on the site of resection, the remaining bowel adjusts by becoming longer, thicker, and wider to increase its absorptive capacity. This process may take up to 6 months, however, and occurs only if the client receives food or tube feedings that stimulate gastrointestinal function. In cases in which the ileocecal valve or 80% of the small bowel is removed, the body cannot completely compensate for the loss.

Less than 200 cm (78.74 in.) of functioning small intestine constitutes short bowel syndrome (Matarese et al., 2005). Treatment of short bowel syndrome is intensive and requires ongoing consultation with an expert dietitian. Early nourishment is provided by TPN. When enteral feeding begins, elemental formulas may be chosen because they are completely absorbed in the proximal small intestine. When food is taken, it should be eaten as small low-fat meals, with medium-chain triglyceride products replacing regular fats. Liquids should be isotonic and taken between meals (Parrish, 2005).

ILEOSTOMY

An ileostomy produces liquid drainage containing active enzymes, which irritate the skin. In addition, nutrient losses are great. A loss of as much as 2 liters of fluid per day immediately after surgery is possible. Clinical Application 20-6 describes innovations for controlling ileostomy drainage.

Over time, the bowel adapts to some extent, and drainage decreases to 300 to 500 milliliters. This amount, however, is more than the 100 to 200 milliliters of water lost in the normal stool. Additional nutrient losses in ileostomy clients include sodium, potassium, and vitamin B_{12}.

COLOSTOMY

In contrast to an ileostomy, a colostomy after the convalescent period may be so continent that a dry dressing is all that is necessary to cover the stoma. The client may do daily irrigations or not, as the surgeon

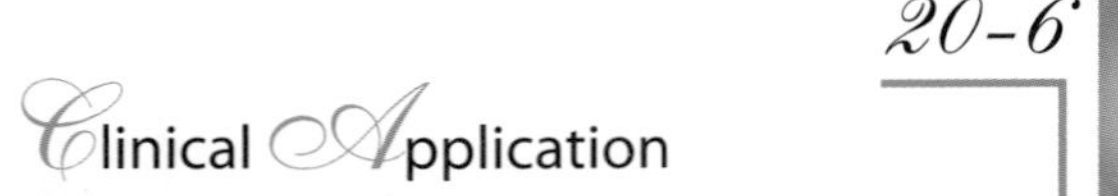

20-6 Clinical Application

Continent Ileostomies

Ordinarily if an ileostomy is performed, the client must wear an appliance to contain the drainage. Other procedures afford a measure of control of the drainage.

Continent ileostomies sometimes can be constructed from the remaining intestine, creating an intestinal reservoir or pouch just inside the abdominal wall. The pouch is emptied by inserting a catheter into the stoma several times a day.

Sometimes an ileoanal anastomosis is done so that the anal sphincter can be used to control elimination. Even after the bowel adapts to its shorter length, the client has 7 to 10 bowel movements per day.

It is important for all healthcare providers to know which procedure has been performed so that the surgeon's and client's expectations can be reinforced when teaching the client.

suggests. Sometimes, after the initial learning process, the client knows best.

DIETARY GUIDELINES FOR OSTOMY CLIENTS

A soft or general diet is usually served to ostomy clients after recovery from surgery with restrictions based on individual tolerance. Stringy, high-fiber foods are initially avoided until a definite tolerance has been demonstrated and then are best tried in small amounts one at a time. Stringy, high-fiber foods include:

- Celery, corn, cabbage, coleslaw, peas, sauerkraut, spinach
- Coconut, dried fruit, membranes on citrus fruits, pineapple
- Popcorn, nuts, seeds, and skins of fruits and vegetables.

In addition, some clients avoid **cruciferous** vegetables, fish, eggs, beer, and carbonated beverages because they produce excessive odor. Certain foods may be therapeutic because they thicken the stool: cheese, creamy peanut butter, marshmallows, pasta, pretzels, white bread, and white rice (Willcutts, Scarano, and Eddins, 2005).

Clients with ostomies should be encouraged to:

- Eat at regular intervals.
- Chew food well to avoid blockage at the stoma site.
- Drink adequate amounts of fluid.
- Avoid foods that produce excessive gas, loose stools, offensive odors, or undesirable bulk.
- Avoid excessive weight gain.

Diverticular Disease

A **diverticulum** (plural: diverticula) is an outpouching of intestinal membrane through a weakness in the intestine's muscular layer (Fig. 20-5).

One-third of the U.S. population will develop diverticula by age 60 and two-thirds by age 85 (Strate et al., 2008).

Diverticulosis

The presence of diverticula is called **diverticulosis**. A common location is the point at which a blood vessel enters the intestinal muscle. A proposed causative factor in diverticulosis is the increased force needed to propel insufficient intestinal contents through the lumen.

Frequently a person with diverticulosis has no signs or symptoms. After a diagnosis of diverticulosis, a high-fiber diet of 30 grams per day is advised. This should be accompanied by an adequate fluid intake.

Diverticulitis

When diverticula become inflamed, the condition is termed diverticulitis. At most, 10% to 25% of individuals with diverticular disease will develop diverticulitis. Risk factors, in addition to advancing age, are obesity and red meat intake. The known risk factors poorly identify those at increased risk, however, and

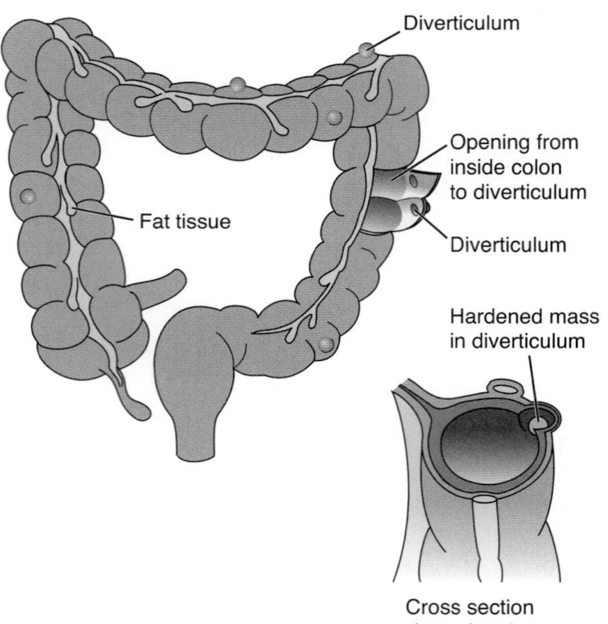

FIGURE 20-5 Diverticula of the transverse and descending colon. (Reprinted from Venes, D [ed]: *Taber's cyclopedic medical dictionary*, ed 21. FA Davis, Philadelphia, 2010, p 678, with permission.)

the predisposing pathophysiology is incompletely understood (Korzenik, 2006).

Signs and symptoms of diverticulitis, with the exception of fever, occur in the abdomen. The client complains of:

- Cramps
- Pain in the lower left quadrant
- Dyspepsia
- Nausea and vomiting
- Distention and flatus
- Alternating constipation and diarrhea

The inflammation can lead to abscesses, adhesions, or fistulas. A scarred intestinal wall can cause an obstruction. Hemorrhage is possible. Rupture of a diverticulum can initiate peritonitis that is a surgical emergency.

Initial therapy for uncomplicated diverticulitis is supportive, including monitoring, bowel rest, and antibiotics. While the inflammation is severe, elemental or predigested formulas or a low-fiber diet is given. After that, a high-fiber diet as for diverticulosis is prescribed. Clients should receive detailed instructions on the incorporation of fiber into the diet after they have followed a low-fiber diet: Fiber should be reintroduced gradually to avoid the abdominal cramping, bloating, and gas pains that can occur with drastic changes in fiber intake.

Dietary restrictions have customarily been placed on hard foods and small seeds because of the possibility of lodging in a diverticulum. Small seeds had been implicated in diverticular complications but blueberry and strawberry intake were not so related in a large study. Neither were foods traditionally excluded from the diet—nuts, corn, and popcorn—associated with risk of diverticulosis or with diverticular complications (Strate et al., 2008).

Diseases of the Liver

Some of the many functions of the liver are listed in Table 20-1. Major liver diseases, hepatitis and cirrhosis, often require careful nutritional management.

Hepatitis

Inflammation of the liver, or **hepatitis**, can result from viral infections, alcohol, drugs, or toxins. Acetaminophen poisoning accounts for approximately 50% of acute liver failure cases in the United States and Great Britain (Hinson, Roberts, and James, 2010). The overdose may be a deliberate suicide attempt or accidental, sometimes involving multiple drugs containing acetaminophen. Other hepatotoxic substances including alcohol contribute additively to the risk of acetaminophen toxicity (Deglin and Vallerand, 2009).

Three common viral infections are hepatitis A, hepatitis B, and hepatitis C. Table 20-10 compares the three types by mode of transmission, high-risk populations, and vaccine availability. Notable epidemics involved:

- Hepatitis A, transmitted by green onions, infected 601 persons of whom three died and one survived after a liver transplant (Wheeler et al., 2005). Hepatitis A is also discussed in Chapter 13.
- Hepatitis B caused two fatalities among 30 cases in three long-term care facilities in different states. Sadly, breaks in aseptic technique were responsible. At one of the facilities, 89% of the residents whose blood glucose was tested by the nursing staff developed acute hepatitis B compared with 0% in residents who performed their own fingersticks (Centers for Disease Control and Prevention [CDC], 2005).
- Hepatitis C caused six cases of acute disease and a search for other victims among 40,000 persons undergoing endoscopy at a free-standing clinic. The break in technique involved inappropriate reuse of syringes on individual persons and use of medication vials intended for single-person use on multiple persons (CDC, 2008a).

Signs and Symptoms

Regardless of type or cause, symptoms are:

- Anorexia
- Nausea
- Epigastric discomfort
- Fatigue
- Weakness

Signs of hepatitis are vomiting, diarrhea, and jaundice caused by the inability of the liver to convert fat-soluble bilirubin to a water-soluble (conjugated) form. The degree of jaundice gives a rough estimate of the severity of the disease. Physical examination shows an enlarged and tender liver and an enlarged spleen.

Treatment

No current medications can cure hepatitis, but combinations of interferon and antiviral drugs are being tested in efforts to modify its course. The cornerstones of treatment are:

- Bed rest
- Abstinence from alcohol
- Optimum nutrition to permit the liver to heal

Convalescence may take from 3 weeks to 3 months. Clients on bed rest, especially debilitated clients, are

TABLE 20-10 ■ Common Types of Viral Hepatitis

	HEPATITIS A	HEPATITIS B	HEPATITIS C
Usual Mode of Transmission	Fecal–oral: contaminated water, shellfish, raw produce Rarely, blood products, parenteral equipment	Body fluids Inanimate objects contaminated with body fluids including medical equipment, razors, toothbrushes, acupuncture and tattoo needles Virus is stable on environmental surfaces at least 7 days	Parenteral equipment Rarely, sexual contact or perinatal transmission
High-Risk Populations	Household and sexual contacts of acute cases Contacts with diapered children in day care Travelers to areas with endemic disease Men who have sex with men Injecting drug users	Household and sexual contacts of infected persons, including perinatal Injecting drug users Heterosexuals with multiple partners Men who have sex with men Long-term international travelers in close contact with local people Health-care and public-safety workers exposed to blood in their work Hemodialysis clients	Individuals who share injecting equipment Health-care workers using parenteral equipment (needle-stick accidents)
Vaccine	Yes; products vary by manufacturer; none recommended for infants	Yes; believed effective for 15 years; WHO recommends universal infant vaccination with first dose within 24 hours of birth	No; the 6 genotypes and approximately 100 subtypes of the virus impede development of effective vaccines.

Adapted from CDC (2008b); Heymann (2004); Wheeler et al. (2005).

more susceptible to pressure ulcers than the average client because of decreased synthesis of albumin and the globulins. If the client abstains from alcohol, the hepatitis is often reversible.

Nutritional Care

A high-kilocalorie, high-protein, moderate-fat diet is frequently prescribed for hepatitis clients:

- Up to 400 grams of carbohydrate provides energy intake.
- Up to 100 grams of protein promotes healing.
- Up to 35% of kilocalories in fat utilizes a dense energy source. Emulsified fats in dairy products and eggs may be better tolerated than other fats.
- Up to 3 to 3.5 liters of fluid intake per day.

Coaxing a person with hepatitis to accept such a substantial meal pattern is an enormous task because of the anorexia and nausea that accompany the disease. Because the nausea is often less in the morning than later in the day, hepatitis clients should be encouraged to eat a big breakfast. Polymeric oral feedings that are high in kilocalories and protein are widely used for between-meal feedings.

Cirrhosis of the Liver

In **cirrhosis,** the liver becomes scarred and ineffective at regeneration. Cirrhosis is most frequently caused by hepatitis C or alcoholism but can result from other insults. The major nutritional effects of alcoholism are summarized in Clinical Application 20-7, and its connection to mortality is described in Clinical Application 20-9.

Several barriers interfere with alcoholism case-finding:

- Alcoholism's multiple and varied manifestations
- The health-care provider's personal definition of alcoholism
- Denial by the client and family

The CAGE questionnaire shown in Clinical Application 20-10 is a brief, effective screening tool to identify possible alcohol abusers. In over 30,000 veterans, brief alcohol screening questionnaires predicted hospitalizations within 3.75 years for alcohol-related gastrointestinal conditions (Au et al., 2007).

Pathophysiology

Alcohol needs no digestion. It is absorbed rapidly, 20% from the stomach and 80% from the small intestine. Immediately after absorption, alcohol is carried throughout the body. In the liver, it is metabolized at the rate of ½ ounce of alcohol per hour. This refers to the alcohol content, not the whole beverage. This rate cannot be rushed, and giving coffee or other stimulants to an inebriated person induces not sobriety but merely alert intoxication.

If the liver is not able to repair the damage caused by alcohol, dying liver cells are replaced by scar tissue. Figure 20-6 traces the path from cell death to several cardinal signs of cirrhosis.

Because the liver has multiple functions, one pathological change reinforces another. Depressed plasma

Clinical Application 20-7

Nutritional Effects of Alcoholism

Alcoholism is a disease of alcohol consumption that produces tolerance, physical dependence, and characteristic organ pathology in the body. Countering some erroneous beliefs, alcoholism is found in individuals who:

- Consume as little as 3 to 5 ounces of whiskey per day
- Are obese, usually early in the disease
- Continue to function in several roles at work and in the family
- Are affluent.

In the United States, alcoholism is the single most important factor in nutrient deficiencies. Alcohol can damage the liver even in well nourished people (Lieber, 2006). Associating the numerous functions of the liver with the fact that alcohol is toxic to all body cells, the nutritional havoc accompanying alcoholism becomes obvious. Vitamin deficiencies in alcoholics, in order of frequency are:

- Folic acid
- Thiamin
- Vitamin B_6
- Niacin
- Vitamin C
- Vitamin A

Thiamin deficiency is almost synonymous with alcoholism. Alcohol impedes the intestinal absorption of thiamin and in severe liver disease the metabolism and storage of thiamin is decreased. See Chapter 7 for information on beriberi. Wernicke–Korsakoff syndrome (Clinical Application 20-8) is a neurological complication of thiamin deficiency.

These are examples of vitamin malnutrition associated with alcoholism:

- Scurvy in the United States is almost exclusively seen in alcoholics.
- Abnormal adaptation to darkness occurs in 50% of alcoholics with cirrhosis and 15% of those without it (Lieber, 2006).
- One-half of alcoholics show bone loss related to reduced intake and faulty metabolism of calcium and vitamins D and K.

Iron and zinc are the trace minerals most often deficient in alcoholics. Potassium, phosphorus, and magnesium are the most common major mineral deficiencies in alcoholics. Electrolyte status should be monitored during treatment. (See refeeding syndrome in Chapter 22.) Examples of mineral malnutrition associated with alcoholism include the following concerns:

- Anemia or bone marrow abnormalities have been found in 75% of clients hospitalized with alcoholism. Increased iron is absorbed through the damaged intestine but low folic acid levels prevent normal red blood cell production.
- Low iron levels may occur due to gastrointestinal bleeding.
- Up to 50% of alcoholic clients are deficient in zinc that has been associated with changes in smell, taste, and protein metabolism. Zinc is needed for the conversion of vitamin A to a functional form in the retina and has been used to treat nightblindness not responsive to vitamin A (Lieber, 2006).
- Magnesium blood levels are low in alcoholics. Neuromuscular excitability in acute alcohol withdrawal resembles signs of magnesium deficiency. Replacement may be required in individual cases but most clients can replenish magnesium stores with a normal diet (Lieber, 2006).

Awareness of the wide range of nutritional effects of alcoholism should stimulate case-finding. Interruption of the downward spiral in health caused by alcohol can literally be lifesaving.

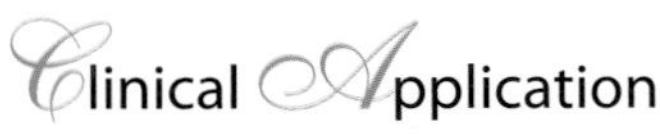
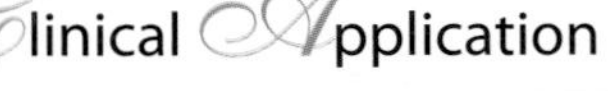

Clinical Application 20-8

Wernicke–Korsakoff Syndrome

Wernicke–Korsakoff syndrome, a disorder of the central nervous system, is caused by thiamin deficiency. It is diagnosed mainly in alcoholics but also occasionally in malnourished clients with no history of alcohol abuse, including women with hyperemesis gravidarum. (See Chapter 10.) In one study, half the clients with Wernicke–Korsakoff syndrome were not alcoholics and two of the nonalcoholics were diagnosed with Wernicke–Korsakoff syndrome only at autopsy (Ogershok et al., 2002).

Clients with Wernicke–Korsakoff syndrome display:

- Disorientation
- Memory dysfunction
- **Ataxia**
- Weakness of the muscles that control the eyes, producing
  - Double vision (*diplopia*)
  - Abnormal movements of the eyeball (*nystagmus*).

Residual impairments such as nystagmus or ataxia affect about 60% of the clients. Of 49 individuals with Wernicke's encephalopathy complicating hyperemesis gravidarum, just 29% achieved complete remission (Chiossi et al., 2006).

An understanding that thiamin is essential to energy production from glucose is critical for health-care providers. Administering a simple solution of glucose intravenously can precipitate symptoms of Wernicke–Korsakoff syndrome if the client is thiamin-deficient.

20-9

Clinical Application

Alcohol Contributes to Mortality

Excessive alcohol consumption is the third leading preventable cause of death in the United States and is associated with multiple adverse health consequences, including:

- Liver cirrhosis
- Various cancers
- Unintentional injuries
- Violence

In 2001, excessive alcohol use was responsible for approximately 75,000 preventable deaths, including:

- 13,674 from motor vehicle accidents, all of which were attributable to binge drinking (more than five drinks per occasion for men or four for women)
- 7655 homicides
- 6969 suicides
- 4766 due to falls (CDC, 2004).

Clients treated in general hospitals are unlikely to be diagnosed with an alcohol use disorder even when arriving at the hospital with a blood alcohol greater than 0.3 gram/dL, more than three times the legal limit (Bostwick and Seaman, 2004; Smothers, Yahr, and Ruhl, 2004).

Alcohol can be immediately lethal if a large quantity of ethanol (or a smaller quantity of alcohols not intended for beverages) is consumed in a short time.

Alcohol poisoning is especially heart-breaking when it kills a young person whose companions let the victim "sleep it off" through ignorance or fear of retribution. Teaching young people about the hazards of alcohol and counseling adult clients about the responsible use of alcohol are appropriate health-teaching functions in all settings.

20-10

Clinical Application

CAGE Questionnaire for Identifying the Alcohol Abuser

The CAGE questionnaire is a screening instrument to identify a need for a diagnostic workup. Its advantages are its simplicity and its proven accuracy in clinical studies. It also focuses on the behavioral effects of drinking rather than on the number of drinks consumed (O'Brien, 2008). The four questions are:

C—Have you ever had a need to CUT BACK on your drinking?
A—Have people ANNOYED YOU with criticism about your drinking?
G—Have you ever felt GUILTY about your drinking?
E—Have you ever needed to start the day with a drink? (an EYE-OPENER)

A score of 2 to 3 "yes" answers indicates a high index of suspicion and a score of 4 is virtually diagnostic for alcoholism (O'Brien, 2008).

protein production, as evidenced by decreasing albumin levels, indicates a poor client outcome.

The signs and symptoms of cirrhosis appear in Box 20-4. Esophageal varices occur in approximately one-half the clients with cirrhosis. One of the most serious complications of portal hypertension is variceal hemorrhage that occurs in about one-third of people with esophageal varices (Smith, 2010). Despite improvements in therapy, variceal hemorrhage is associated with a mortality of at least 20% at 6 weeks (Longacre and Garcia-Tsao, 2006). The end result of cirrhosis is liver failure, which can lead to hepatic coma.

Dietary Treatment

Avoidance of alcohol and excess fat and ingestion of four to six meals per day containing carbohydrates and protein are the most common recommendations (Tsiaousi et al., 2008). A precarious balance is required to provide protein yet avoid precipitating hepatic encehalopathy (Clinical Application 20-11). Sometimes only minimal amounts of protein can be ingested without altering the client's mental state (Lieber, 2006).

Table 20-11 displays various protein-controlled diets that assume the client tolerates fats. Extensive low-protein exchange lists have been developed to treat liver failure. The dietary management of these clients, particularly those with end-stage liver disease, is complex and constantly changing, requiring the continuing services of an expert dietitian.

Because of the high risk of vitamin deficiencies, cirrhosis clients are given pharmaceutical supplements. Up to five times the RDA of water-soluble vitamins may be necessary.

Monitoring the improvement or progression of ascites includes measuring abdominal girth and daily weighing. If the client has ascites without peripheral edema, a reasonable treatment goal for weight loss is 0.5 kilogram (1.1 pounds) per day. If both ascites and peripheral edema are displayed, the goal for weight loss is 1 kilogram per day.

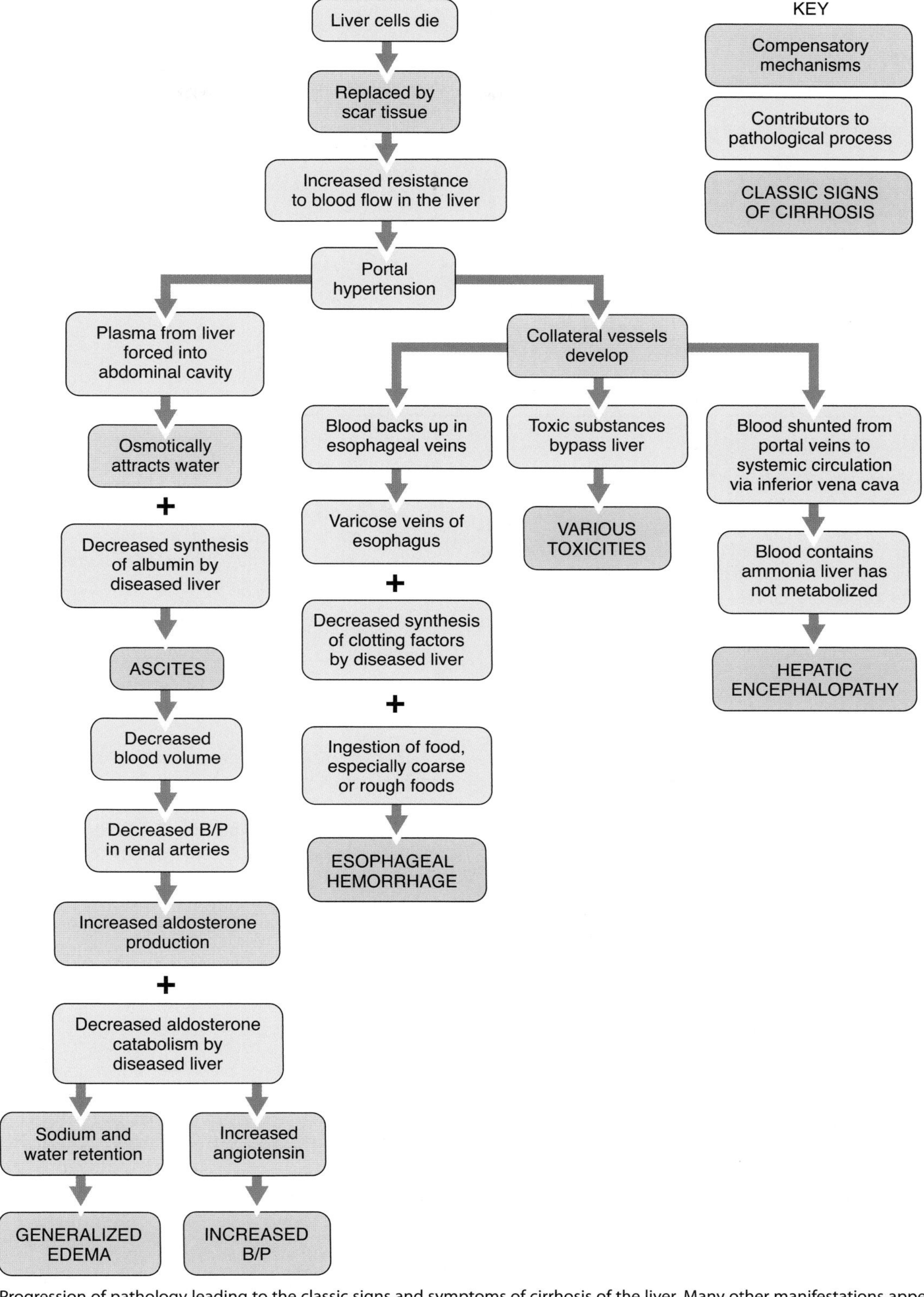

FIGURE 20-6 Progression of pathology leading to the classic signs and symptoms of cirrhosis of the liver. Many other manifestations appear given the multiple functions of the liver.

Box 20-4 ■ *Signs and Symptoms of Cirrhosis*

Symptoms

- Anorexia
- Epigastric pain
- Nausea that worsens as the day goes on

Signs

- Abdominal distention
- Vomiting
- Steatorrhea
- Jaundice
- Ascites
- Edema
- Gastrointestinal bleeding

Clinical Application 20-11

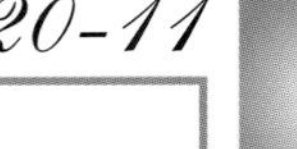

Hepatic Encephalopathy

Ammonia plays a key role in the pathogenesis of hepatic encephalopathy possibly involving oxidative/nitrosative stress and a low-grade cerebral edema (Haussinger and Gorg, 2010). Ammonia is produced by intestinal bacteria and by digestive enzymes breaking down protein. Even if the person consumes no protein foods, the bacteria work on the cast-off cells of the gastrointestinal tract and on the blood from gastrointestinal bleeding, which is common in alcoholic cirrhosis. Ordinarily, the liver degrades ammonia to urea, which is excreted in urine by the kidneys, but in liver failure, blood ammonia levels rise. Ammonia is toxic to all cells, including those of the liver and the brain.

Some signs of hepatic encephalopathy can be observed before the onset of coma, including:

- Personality changes
- Irritability
- Weakness
- Apathy
- Confusion
- Sleepiness

More specific signs are:

- *Asterixis*, involuntary jerking movements of the hand when the arm is outstretched,
- *Fetor hepaticus*, a fecal odor to the breath, and
- Finally, coma.

Primary treatment of hepatic encephalopathy is administration of lactulose. This drug, given orally or by enema, acidifies the large intestine. The change in pH causes ammonia to be converted to ammonium ions, which are not absorbed but eliminated in the feces. If lactulose is not sufficient, the antibiotic neomycin (that remains in the lumen of the intestine) may be added to decrease the bacteria present (Heidelbaugh and Sherbondy, 2006).

The goal of nutritional management of patients with hepatic encephalopathy should be to promote protein synthesis by supplying ample amounts of amino acids, while instituting other measures to reverse the ongoing catabolism.

Clients with cirrhosis hospitalized for encephalopathy received standard treatments for hepatic encephalopathy but were randomized to receive

- A low-protein diet with progressive increments or
- A normal protein diet for 14 days.

The outcome of hepatic encephalopathy was not significantly different between the two groups (Cordoba et al., 2004).

Early research suggested a benefit to altering the ratio of **aromatic** to **branched-chain amino acids** (BCAA). The influence of BCAA supplementation on hepatic encephalopathy could be more effective in chronic hepatic injury with hyperammonemia and low concentrations of BCAA in blood than in acute hepatic illness with inflammatory complications and enhanced protein turnover (Holecek, 2010). Although administering branched chain amino acids may benefit some clients, their routine use is not recommended (Lieber, 2006). In addition, long-term compliance is poor because of unpalatability (Cabre and Gassull, 2005).

If enteral feeding is necessary and branched-chain amino acids are selected as therapy, special preparations low in aromatic amino acids are available. Two of them are Hepatic-Aid II® and Travasorb-Hepatic®.

Aspartame (NutraSweet®) also contains phenylalanine, an aromatic amino acid. If the branched chain theory holds, it, too, should be avoided.

Gallbladder Disease

On the underside of the liver is a small pouch-like organ called the **gallbladder**. Its function is to concentrate and store bile until needed for digestion. The liver secretes 600 to 800 milliliters of bile per day that the gallbladder reduces to 60 to 160 milliliters.

The presence of gallstones is called **cholelithiasis**. About 10% to 20% of people in most Western countries have gallstones. About 50% to 70% are asymptomatic at the time of diagnosis, which may have been

TABLE 20-11 ■ Protein-Controlled Diets for Liver Disease

DESCRIPTION	INDICATIONS	ADEQUACY
Although not the main therapy, these diets are prescribed to help attain and maintain normal amino acid balance, reduce blood ammonia levels, and improve clinical status. In addition to protein, sodium and fluid may be restricted. Branched-chain amino acids that are chiefly metabolized in skeletal muscle may be given as a supplement.	These diets are used in severe liver disease such as acute hepatitis, advanced cirrhosis, or intractable hepatic encephalopathy.	The diets may not meet the RDA for B-complex vitamins (especially folic acid), calcium, and iron. Supplemental vitamins may be prescribed.
20-GRAM PROTEIN DIET (RARELY USED. MOST CLIENTS CAN TOLERATE AND NEED 40 TO 60 GRAMS.)		
Meal Plan	**Sample Menu**	
Breakfast		**40-GRAM PROTEIN DIET TO 20-GRAM PROTEIN DIET ADD:**
½ cup milk	½ cup whole milk	½ cup milk
1 Fruit	½ cup orange juice with 2 tbsp modular carbohydrate supplement*	2 meat exchanges
2 Starches	½ cup Cream of Wheat with 1 tbsp modular carbohydrate supplement and 1 slice of toast with 1 tbsp margarine and jelly	1 starch exchange
		60-GRAM PROTEIN DIET TO 20-GRAM PROTEIN DIET ADD:
Fat (as tolerated)	2 tbsp cream	2 cups milk
Beverage	As tolerated and per fluid restriction	3 meat exchanges
		1 starch exchange
		1 vegetable exchange
Lunch		
		80-GRAM PROTEIN DIET TO 20-GRAM PROTEIN DIET ADD:
2 Starches	1 cup rice with ¼ cup unsalted tomato sauce and 1 tbsp olive oil	
Vegetable	½ cup green beans with 1 tsp margarine	
Fruit	½ cup canned peaches with 1 tbsp modular carbohydrate supplement	2 cups milk
		5 meat exchanges
Beverage	As tolerated and per fluid restriction	4 starch exchanges
		1 vegetable exchange
Dinner		
2 Starches	1 baked potato with 2 tbsp sour cream and 1 slice of bread with 1 tsp margarine and jelly	
Vegetable	½ cup mushrooms (for potato topping)	
Fruit	½ cup strawberries with 1 tbsp modular carbohydrate supplement	
Beverage	As tolerated and per fluid restriction	

*Polycose®, Sumacal®, and Moducal® are all modular carbohydrate supplements.

made incidentally during an abdominal ultrasound exam. Asymptomatic gallstone disease has a benign natural course, as only about 10% to 25% progress to symptomatic disease (Sakorafas, Milingos, and Peros, 2007). Gallstones have reached epidemic proportions in North and South American Indian populations, accompanied by an increased risk for gallbladder cancer (Shaffer, 2005).

Most gallstones form when bile is too scant or too concentrated or contains excessive cholesterol. When the gallbladder becomes inflamed from irritation by stones (90% of the cases), parasitic infection, or prolonged fasting associated with total parenteral nutrition (TPN), the condition is labeled **cholecystitis**.

Causative Factors

The only established dietary risk is a high caloric intake (Shaffer, 2006). Women are three times more likely than men to have gallbladder disease. For both men and women, nuts seem to have a protective effect in that consumption of 5 or more ounces of nuts per week was associated with decreased risk of symptomatic gallstones in men and with decreased risk of cholecystectomy in women (Tsai et al., 2004a, 2004b).

Other risk factors for gallbladder disease include:

- Ileal disease or resection
- Long-term TPN

- Multiple pregnancies
- Oral contraceptive use

A long fast between the evening meal and the first meal of the next day is a modifiable risk factor. Two health-promoting practices include:

- Taking a light bedtime snack or
- Drinking two glasses of water on arising if breakfast will be delayed.

Either practice stimulates the gallbladder to empty, thus decreasing the likelihood of very concentrated bile.

Symptoms and Treatment

The cardinal symptom of gallbladder disease is pain after ingestion of fat caused by spasms of the gallbladder. The pain is located in the right upper quadrant and often radiates to the right shoulder.

Asymptomatic gallstones are usually just observed. Surgery is the preferred option to treat symptomatic gallbladder disease, but medical management may be recommended for individuals who are poor surgical risks.

Dietary Modifications

During an acute attack, a full-liquid diet with minimal fat is recommended. For chronic gallbladder disease, the client should limit fat and obese clients should lose weight. Some clients obtain relief with the restriction of dietary fat; others do not. A reasonable approach to fat restriction is to:

- Select skim milk dairy products,
- Limit fats or oils to 3 teaspoons per day, and
- Consume no more than 6 ounces of very lean meat per day.

Another approach is to eliminate foods that cause symptoms. Clients usually can identify foods that cause them pain. Fried foods are the worst offenders. Gas-forming foods also are often poorly tolerated. Table 20-12 identifies some foods that are low in fat and some that are high in fat.

Dietary factors that may prevent the development of gallstones include polyunsaturated fat, monounsaturated fat, fiber, and caffeine. A vegeterian diet is also associated with decreased risk (Gaby, 2009).

TABLE 20-12 ■ Comparison of Fat Content of Selected Foods

LOW-FAT FOODS	FAT (GRAMS)	HIGH-FAT FOODS	FAT (GRAMS)
Starch/Breads			
Angel food cake, 1⁄12	<1	Pecan pie, ⅛ of pie	24
Italian bread, 1 slice	<1	Bread stuffing, ½ cup	13
English muffin, 1	1	Danish pastry	12
Raisin toast, 1 slice	1	Croissant, 1	12
Pancake, 4-inch, 1	2	Glazed raised doughnut, 1	13
Meats, Fish, and Poultry			
Beef round, 3 oz lean roasted	9	Beef prime rib, 3 oz lean only	24
Chicken breast, 3 oz roasted, without skin	9	Chicken, deep-fried thigh, 1	14
Boiled ham, 3 oz	9	Spare ribs, 3 oz	24
Tuna, ½ cup water-packed	6	Tuna, ½ cup oil-packed, drained	24
Fruits and Vegetables			
Banana, 8¾ inch long, 1	1	Avocado, 1	30
Raisins, 1 cup	1	Coconut, dried, 1 cup	50
Potato, baked, 1	<1	French fried potato, 2 × 3½ inches, 15 pieces	12
Onion, raw, sliced, 1 cup	<1	French fried onion rings, 4	10
Milk Products			
Cottage cheese, 1%, ½ cup	1	Cottage cheese, 4%, ½ cup	5
Mozzarella, part skim, 1 oz	5	Cheddar, 1 oz	9
Skim milk, with added milk solids, 1 cup	1	Whole milk, 1 cup	8
Frozen yogurt, low-fat, 1 cup	4	Ice cream, regular, hard, vanilla, 1 cup	14
Fast Foods*			
Arby's			
Junior Roast Beef sandwich	10	Beef'n Cheddar sandwich	20
McDonald's			
Hamburger	9	Quarter pounder with cheese	26
Subway			
6-inch Roast beef	5	6-inch tuna	31
Wendy's			
Chicken Grill sandwich	7	Spicy Chicken Fillet sandwich	16

*Check with the restaurant. Recipes may be revised.

Medical and Surgical Interventions

Several procedures have been devised to treat gallstones without the traditional large incision. One technique involves agents to dissolve the stones, some taken orally and some injected directly into the gallbladder. Another method is to break up the stones using shock waves through a procedure called *lithotripsy*.

Clients and physicians still may opt for removal of the stones through an incision, a *cholecystotomy*, or for removal of the gallbladder, *cholecystectomy*, through a laparoscope or the traditional abdominal incision.

After traditional cholecystectomy, the client may initially receive nothing by mouth or clear liquids. Then the diet is progressed as tolerated. Following laparoscopic cholecystectomy, clients may receive a general diet immediately.

Later in convalescence, balanced meals should be well tolerated because bile enters the duodenum continuously. Clients who become nauseated and suffered pain after eating certain foods preoperatively, however, may continue to avoid them postoperatively because of the association.

> **Genomic Gem 20-5**
> **Pancreatitis**
>
> Hereditary pancreatitis is an autosomal dominant disorder caused by mutations in a trypsinogen gene. These individuals suffer recurrent attacks of acute pancreatitis beginning in childhood or adolescence. Frequently, the disease becomes chronic.
>
> Up to 37% of clients with idiopathic chronic pancreatitis have mutations on the cystic fibrosis gene. Other mutations have also been identified (Lieber, 2006).

Diseases of the Pancreas

In addition to the endocrine secretions, insulin, glucagon, and somatostatin, the **pancreas** secretes amylase, lipase, trypsin, and chymotrypsin. Because of those many secretions, diseases of the pancreas create major nutritional consequences. Two important disorders of the pancreas are pancreatitis and cystic fibrosis.

Pancreatitis

Normally, the pancreatic enzymes necessary for digestion are inactive in the pancreas and become activated only on entering the duodenum; otherwise, the active enzymes would digest the pancreas itself.

In **pancreatitis,** the retained pancreatic enzymes become activated and do digest the pancreatic tissue. In severe cases, the enzymes escape into the general circulation causing inflammation in distant organs.

The most common cause of acute pancreatitis is a gallstone impacting the distal common bile-pancreatic duct (Wang et al., 2009) whereas alcohol remains the main factor associated with chronic pancreatitis (Pezzilli, 2009). Pancreatitis can also be hereditary. See Genomic Gem 20-5.

Acute Pancreatitis

The characteristic symptom of acute pancreatitis is excruciating pain in the left upper quadrant. Nausea and vomiting accompany an attack. Laboratory tests reveal elevated levels of serum amylase and lipase.

Eighty percent of clients with acute pancreatitis have mild cases and relatively benign courses. Several systems for rating severity of disease are based on compilations of multiple laboratory findings (Despins, Kivlahan, and Cox, 2005). Nutritionally, mild pancreatitis may be treated with:

- Nothing by mouth to avoid stimulating the pancreas
- Intravenous fluids
- Clear liquids after pain has been controlled for 24 hours
- Nasojejuenal feedings only if necessary
- Soft to general diet over 3 or 4 days if satisfactory progress.

In a small percentage of patients, the disease develops into severe pancreatitis. These clients display an intense systemic inflammatory response and often develop multiple organ failure. Because mortality and morbidity rates are directly related to negative nitrogen balance, improving nutrition is a high priority that requires constant monitoring and adjusting.

The goal of nutritional support is to meet the elevated metabolic demands as much as possible without stimulating pancreatic secretion and self-digestion. The more distally the feeding enters the gut, the less it stimulates pancreatic secretions. Clients with acute severe pancreatitis should receive enteral nutrition early because it modulates the stress response, promotes more rapid resolution of the disease process, and provides better outcomes to the extent that enteral nutrition is the new "gold standard" in these cases (McClave et al., 2006).

Studies have shown that enteral nutrition is less expensive than TPN when treating acute pancreatitis. (See Dollars and Sense 20-1.) Further, enteral feeding was associated with decreased:

- Septic complications
- Surgical interventions
- Total hospitalization time (Ioannidis, Lavrentieva, and Botsios, 2008).

$ Dollars & Sense 20-1

Enteral Feeding Versus TPN

In a randomized comparative study, clients with acute pancreatitis were initially treated with a 48-hour fast with intravenous fluids and analgesics. After 48 hours, clients who were improving were started on oral feeding. The remaining clients, most of whom had biliary pancreatitis, were randomized to receive nasojejunal or parenteral feeding. Here are the findings.

	Enteral	TPN
Duration of feeding	6.7 days	10.8 days
Estimated nutritional requirements met	54%	88%
Metabolic and septic complications	Lower	Higher
Savings per patient	$2362	

SOURCE: Abou-Assi and Craig (2002).

In addition, enteral nutrition is more effective than TPN in:

- Controlling blood glucose (Petrov and Zagainov, 2007)
- Suppressing the inflammatory response
- Reversing multiple organ failure

Topical nutrients from feedings maintain mucosal health and gut function while stabilizing the intestinal flora (Hegazi and O'Keefe, 2007).

TPN still may be used to advantage as a back-up source of nutrition and for clients who cannot tolerate enteral feedings, for instance in paralytic ileus. Other antiinflammatory agents are under investigation:

- Amino acids arginine and glutamine
- *n*-3 fatty acids
- Prebiotics and probiotics (Hegazi and O'Keefe, 2007).

Chronic Pancreatitis

The most common cause of chronic pancreatitis is alcohol abuse with an average elapsed time between heavy alcohol consumption and chronic pancreatitis of 18 years. For whatever reason, clients rarely have both alcohol-induced liver disease and pancreatitis (Raimondo and Scolapio, 2006). Overall causes of chronic pancreatitis are distributed as follows:

- 70% are related to alcohol ingestion.
- 20% are idiopathic.
- 10% are hereditary or occur with cystic fibrosis, hypertriglyceridemia, or other conditions (Pandol and Cohen, 2007).

Most often, these clients present with dull abdominal pain that is intermittent and aggravated by food. Because fat malabsorption does not occur until pancreatic enzyme secretions are reduced by 90%, steatorrhea is a late-appearing sign (Raimondo and Scolapio, 2006).

General dietary management principles include:

- Total abstinence from alcohol
- Intake of energy nutrients:
  - 1 to 1.5 grams of protein per kilogram of body weight daily
  - 30% of kilocalories from fat (or less to minimize steatorrhea)
  - 40% to 60% of kilocalories from carbohydrate
- Serum glucose maintained at <200 mg/dL with insulin if necessary to reduce risk of infection
- Supplements
  - Pancreatic enzymes with meals to improve protein absorption and decrease steatorrhea
  - Antioxidant supplementation (selenium; methionine; vitamins A, C, and E) to reduce inflammation and pain
- Serum levels of fat-soluble vitamins and vitamin B_{12} monitored every 6 months (Raimondo and Scolapio, 2006).

Cystic Fibrosis

Originally considered a disease of childhood because of limited life expectancy, **cystic fibrosis** is increasingly seen in adults. Median survival is 36.9 years and 43% of cystic fibrosis clients are age 18 years and older (Boyle, 2007). Affecting multiple organ systems, cystic fibrosis is characterized by:

- Pulmonary dysfunction and infection
- Pancreatic impairment
- Elevated sweat chloride
- Male infertility

As indicated in Genomic Gem 20-6, multiple possibilities for developing the disease lead to variations in disease severity. In 5% of individuals, diagnosis is made after the age of 16 years (Boyle, 2007).

Case Finding

As of July 2008, 44 states (compared to 9 states in 2004) and the District of Columbia had programs to screen all newborns for cystic fibrosis (Medical News Today, 2008). Early diagnosis from screening produces long-term improvements in height for age and reductions in chronic malnutrition. Screening tests are not perfect, however, and the variable expression of the disease merits investigation if the clinical signs and symptoms warrant, even if the screening test was negative.

Genomic Gem 20-6
Cystic Fibrosis

More than 1500 mutations have been identified in the cystic fibrosis transmembrane conductance regulator gene (*CFTR*), not all of which result in cystic fibrosis. The CFTR protein is a chloride channel in the epithelial tissue of most of the lumens of the body where it significantly affects secretions and sodium and water balance.

Cystic fibrosis is an autosomal recessive disease that affects the following proportions of live births:

- 1 in 3200 white births
- 1 in 9200 Hispanic births
- 1 in 10,000 Asian births
- 1 in 15,000 black births (Boyle, 2007).

Another gene has been identified as modifying lung disease severity in cystic fibrosis (Drumm et al., 2005).

A genetic test has been developed but its widespread use has uncovered surprising relationships:

- Everyone with classical cystic fibrosis does not have mutations of *CFTR*.
- People with the same *CFTR* mutations have different disease courses.
- The frequency of cystic fibrosis mutations varies with ethnicity.
- Not all persons with two mutations in their *CFTR* gene have classical cystic fibrosis (Feetham, Thomson, and Hinshaw, 2005).

Pathophysiology

The chief cause of morbidity and mortality in cystic fibrosis is obstruction of exocrine glands with thick mucus. In the lungs, the stagnant secretions become a hospitable environment for bacteria; as a result, lung infection is the most common cause of death.

Obstruction by viscid material in the lumen of the glands interferes with the digestive secretions of the pancreas. The result is fat and protein malabsorption, leading to stunted growth (deficit in height for age).

The sign of cystic fibrosis related to the gastrointestinal tract is the passage of bulky, fatty, foul-smelling feces caused by the impaired fat digestion. By age 18 to 24 years, 20% to 30% of individuals with cystic fibrosis display hyperglycemia or diabetes mellitus (Boyle, 2007).

The sweat of a cystic fibrosis client has more sodium chloride than normal. A sweat chloride level greater than 60 milliequivalents per liter is diagnostic of cystic fibrosis, but other criteria in combination also can be used in doubtful cases. During fever or hot weather, the high sodium chloride content of the sweat causes increased losses and increased risk of electrolyte imbalance.

Treatment

Supportive care is the foundation of cystic fibrosis treatment. Pulmonary congestion and infections are treated as required. Because morbidity and mortality are directly related to nutritional status, achieving adequate nutrition is a vital goal. Malnutrition may hasten deterioration of lung function and improved nutritional status does increase muscle strength (Cooper and Heird, 2006). Cystic fibrosis clients have specific physiological changes related to nutrition:

- About 90% of cystic fibrosis clients have pancreatic exocrine insufficiency and require enzyme supplements (Boyle, 2007).
- Resting energy expenditure is 25% to 80% greater than normal due to the work of breathing.
- Riboflavin needs are increased because of the client's high-energy expenditure. Riboflavin deficiency manifested as stomatitis in three children, 2 to 10 years old, with cystic fibrosis. In addition, the children had deficiencies of thiamin, pyridoxine, and iron (McCabe, 2001).
- Fat-soluble vitamins are poorly absorbed.
  - Up to 50% of clients have vitamin A deficiency; 18% have visual defects.
  - Frequent courses of antibiotics interfere with synthesis of vitamin K.
  - Osteoporosis is widespread due to vitamin D malabsorption, lack of sunlight, and liver impairment.
- Iron and zinc deficiencies are common (Suckling, Johnson, and Chin, 2006).

Nutritional care is ongoing for cystic fibrosis clients. Some considerations to be incorporated in planning include providing:

- Sufficient energy and protein intake to support growth
- Gastrostomy feedings delivered continuously overnight or by bolus in daytime
- Appetite stimulants (Boyle, 2007)
- Supplemental pancreatic enzyme therapy to control symptoms and permit adequate food intake
- Adequate salt intake
- Vitamin/mineral supplements: fat-soluble vitamins in water-soluble forms
- Carbohydrate as simple sugars in lieu of starches that require amylase
- Possible inclusion of high-fat formulas that produce less carbon dioxide than carbohydrate to decrease the work of the lungs (Cooper and Heird, 2006)

Those are just the nutritional considerations. Clients with cystic fibrosis also may have extensive pulmonary medications to take and treatments to perform.

Keystones

- Dumping syndrome and postprandial hypotension require similar dietary interventions. Meals should be dry, frequent, and low in simple sugars. Lying down after eating helps retain stomach contents for a longer time.
- For gastroesophageal reflux (GERD) and hiatal hernia, meals should be frequent with limited liquid and fat. Remaining upright after eating encourages movement of stomach contents into the duodenum.
- Celiac disease and cystic fibrosis are seen in adults as well as children. A gluten-free diet is key to controlling intestinal damage in celiac disease. Adequate intake and pancreatic enzyme supplements are used to prevent malnutrition in cystic fibrosis.
- Inflammatory bowel diseases (Crohn's disease, ulcerative colitis) are treated individually, eliminating foods that cause problems. If a surgical stoma is constructed, the client may avoid stringy, high-fiber foods and those producing excessive odor.
- Keys to treating hepatitis and cirrhosis are abstinence from alcohol and optimum nutrition. Clients often have the best appetite at breakfast.
- Cholecystitis is treated medically with a low fat diet. To prevent cholelithiasis, eating breakfast or drinking two glasses of water on arising empties the gallbladder of concentrated bile that results from a long overnight fast.
- Acute pancreatitis is treated by fasting followed by enteral feeding into the jejunum. Clients with chronic pancreatitis should partake of a balanced diet with the exception of increased protein. Pancreatitis clients should abstain from alcohol.

CASE STUDY 20-1

An outpatient, Ms. C, a 40-year-old white woman, has just been evaluated for right upper quadrant pain. The pain occurs after meals and radiates to the right shoulder. Ms. C has noticed her stools have become pale gray in the past 2 months. Ms. C is 5 ft 4 in. tall, has a medium frame, and weighs 151 lb.

Ultrasound examination of the gallbladder showed the presence of numerous stones. None is obstructing the duct system yet.

Ms. C is a single parent of four children, ages 4 to 17, and is employed as a secretary. If surgery does become necessary, she would like to delay it until the youngest child is in school. For that reason, she is electing medical management.

Usual food intake: No breakfast; coffee and doughnut mid-morning; "this week's special" lunch meat sandwich and chips at noon; casseroles for dinner.

Stated she does not know much about nutrition, that she shops as her mother did, and that she cooks food her children will eat. Rarely buys fruits or vegetables because of the cost.

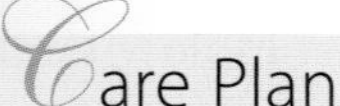

Care Plan

Subjective Data

Pain in right upper quadrant immediately after eating ■ Pale stools for 2 months by history ■ Usual intake: high-fat, low-fiber ■ Admitted lack of knowledge about nutrition

Objective Data

Gallstones per ultrasound ■ 115% of healthy body weight

Analysis

Lack of information related to prescribed low-fat diet for cholecystitis as evidenced by self-report

CASE STUDY *(Continued)*

Plan

DESIRED OUTCOMES EVALUATION CRITERIA	ACTIONS/INTERVENTIONS	RATIONALE
Client will verbalize foods to avoid to maintain low-fat diet by end of teaching session.	Explain low-fat diet, adapting to client's lifestyle. Provide written instructions for client to take home.	Having written instructions available as a teaching tool structures the session and may stimulate questions the client would not think of otherwise. Taking the material home will reinforce the instruction.
Client will state means to modify meals to accommodate prescribed diet by end of teaching session.	Explore Ms. C's preferences for adding fiber to her diet.	Soluble fiber will combine with cholesterol, which comprises most gallstones, and carry it out of the body. Building on the client's choices increases the chances of compliance.
	Obtain client's reaction to diet and offer alternatives to her present meal pattern.	Considering the client's wishes affirms her status as an individual. Personalizing the diet for her circumstances will increase the chances of success.
	Suggest Ms. C either eat breakfast or drink two glasses of water first thing in the morning.	Either of these actions will stimulate the gallbladder to empty the concentrated bile that has accumulated overnight.
Client will accept referral to social worker to maximize nutrition for self and family.	Make appointment with social worker for Ms. C before she leaves today.	Completing arrangements before the client leaves avoids the possibility of procrastination.

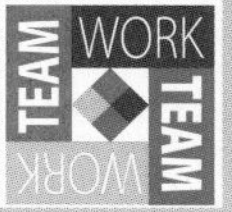

20-1

Social Worker's Notes

The following Social Worker's Notes are representative of the documentation found in a client's medical record.

Referred by Nurse instructing client on low fat diet for cholecystitis

Subjective: Head of household of 5; divorced 6 months; ex-husband unemployed and behind on child support

Objective: Earning slightly more than minimum wage per paycheck stub

Analysis: Eligible for Head Start and Food Stamp programs

Plan: Identify barriers to participation; assist with applications; encourage attendance at nutrition education sessions provided by Head Start

Critical Thinking Questions

1. How important is dietary modification for the children? How might the interventions be modified for them?
2. If Ms. C were not in such a dire financial situation and ineligible for assistance, what other approaches to improving the family's nutritional intake could be tried?
3. Critique the use of "lack of information" as a long-term evaluative criterion.

Chapter Review

1. Which of the following foods is allowed for a preoperative client on a low-residue diet?
   a. 8 ounces of milk with each of the three main meals
   b. Minestrone soup containing peas and lentils
   c. Broiled ground beef patty on a white bun
   d. A fresh fruit salad
2. The American Society of Anesthesiologists' guidelines suggest which of the following intakes is permissible for healthy individuals undergoing elective procedures?
   a. Water and apple juice until 1 hour before the procedure
   b. Plain tea and unbuttered toast with clear jelly 6 hours before scheduled surgery
   c. Infant formula or breast milk 4 hours before an elective procedure begins
   d. Light meal containing meat at 5 AM before a procedure scheduled for noon
3. Clients who have had resection of the ileum should be monitored for:
   a. Iron-deficiency anemia
   b. Fat-soluble vitamin deficiency
   c. Calcium and phosphorus deficiency
   d. Vitamin B_{12} deficiency
4. A client with cirrhosis of the liver should be asked if he or she experienced ___ before ordering a diet.
   a. Headache
   b. Vomiting of blood
   c. A recent course of antibiotic therapy
   d. Hives
5. Which of the following meal components is likely to lessen symptoms of the dumping syndrome?
   a. Mashed fresh strawberries
   b. Orange sherbet
   c. Salt-free tomato juice
   d. Whole-wheat toast with dietetic jelly

Clinical Analysis

Mr. W is a 55-year-old white man admitted to the acute care unit for jaundice and ascites secondary to cirrhosis of the liver. He has gained 15 pounds in the past 3 weeks, and his serum sodium is 125 mEq/L. He is a diagnosed alcoholic who has been through a detoxification program several times in the past 5 years. The dietitian has instructed Mr. W on a 1000-milligram sodium diet with a fluid restriction of 1000 milliliters per day.

1. When the nurse does the beginning of shift assessment, Mr. W says he tried "cutting down on salt" when he started gaining weight, but it didn't work. Which of the following statements best reflects a good understanding of Mr. W's pathology and treatment?
   a. Just cutting out added salt is not enough, because many foods are naturally high in sodium.
   b. Fluids are always restricted with a low-sodium diet.
   c. The ascites is caused by the inability of the liver to produce water-soluble bilirubin.
   d. Besides retaining sodium, Mr. W has ascites due to decreased blood pressure in the liver.
2. Mr. W vomits immediately after his next meal. The physician then orders a hydrating solution of 5-percent dextrose in water intravenously. If thiamin is not included in that order, the nurse should inquire about it because:
   a. Thiamin is necessary to predigest the dextrose for immediate absorption.
   b. Intravenous glucose without thiamin in the cirrhosis client can precipitate the Wernicke–Korsakoff syndrome.
   c. Thiamin prevents folic acid stores from being diluted by the hydrating solution.
   d. Deficiency of thiamin causes delirium tremens.
3. Mr. W's condition worsens. He is placed on a 40-gram protein diet. Mrs. W has been told the purpose of the protein restriction. The next day, Mrs. W asks the nurse, "If protein breakdown is causing the problem, why is he getting any at all?" Which of the following responses by the nurse would be most accurate?
   a. Some protein is necessary to spare glucose for basic energy needs.
   b. If the body receives no protein, it will destroy its own tissue to obtain it.
   c. The proteins in this diet are predigested and more easily absorbed than most.
   d. Protein is needed to feed the bacterial flora in the intestine.

21

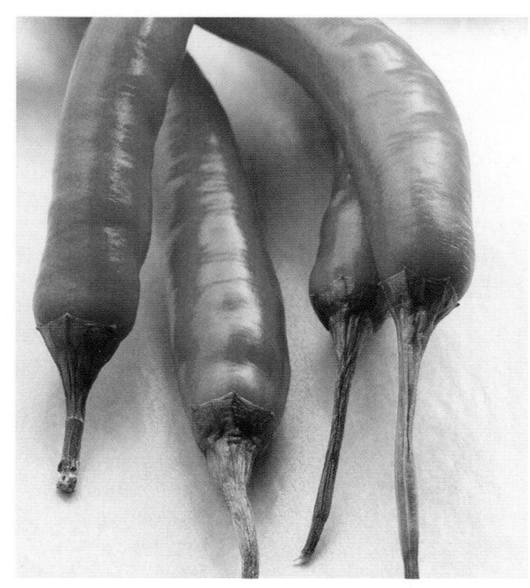

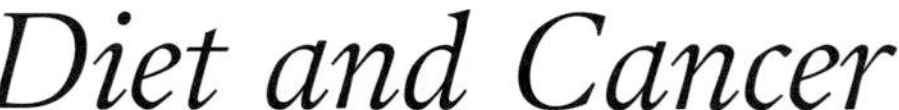

Diet and Cancer

LEARNING OBJECTIVES

After completing this chapter, the student should be able to:

- List several correlations between dietary intake and cancers of specific sites.
- Interpret dietary guidelines for the prevention of cancer.
- Identify reasons that population correlations may not apply to subgroups or to individuals.
- Discuss measures to increase oral intake for clients with cancer.
- Describe cachexia and the challenges of managing the condition.

Cancer has been known and described for thousands of years. Amazingly, one substance now linked to prevention was used as a treatment in ancient Rome, where crushed cabbage leaves were applied to cancerous ulcers (Albert-Puleo, 1983). Now cabbage is one of the cruciferous vegetables in the diet associated with reduced risk of cancer.

Definitions and Statistics

Cancer means "crab," for the creeping way in which it spreads. Cancer is a general term for more than 100 types of malignant neoplastic disease.

Terminology

A **neoplasm** is a new and abnormal formation of tissue (tumor) that grows at the expense of the healthy organism.

- **Benign** tumors are localized but potentially dangerous if located in vital organs.
- **Malignant** (cancerous) tumors infiltrate surrounding tissue and spread to distant parts of the body.
- **Sarcomas** arise from connective tissue, such as muscle or bone, and are more common in young people.
- **Carcinomas** occur in epithelial tissue, including cancers of the lung, breast, prostate, and colon, and are more common in older people.

Characteristics common to all types of cancer are uncontrolled growth and the ability to spread to distant sites (**metastasize**). Clinical Application 21-1 summarizes the transformation of normal cells into cancer cells.

Incidence and Mortality

In the United States, more than 30% of the 569,490 projected 2010 cancer deaths are attributed to smoking and an estimated 33% are due to physical inactivity and poor nutrition (American Cancer Society, 2010). Cancer is the second most common cause of death in the United States after heart disease.

The incidence of the three most common cancers for men (prostate, lung/bronchus, colorectal) and women (breast, lung/bronchus, colorectal) of different ethnicities is illustrated in Figure 21-1. Those cancers account for an estimated 50% of the new cases and of the deaths of men and women. Cancer mortality is highest in African Americans and lowest in Asian

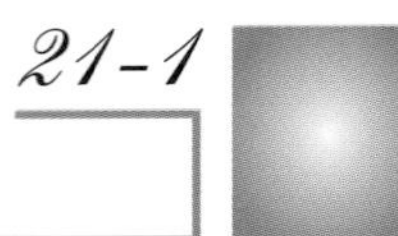

Transformation of Normal Cells Into Cancer Cells

Cancer is basically uncontrolled replication of cells. Normal cells divide in the processes of growth and maintenance but stop dividing at appropriate points.

Apoptosis, a process of programmed cell death, is necessary to the maintenance of healthy tissue. Apoptosis eliminates single cells that are aged, dysfunctional, damaged by external stimuli, and thus potential cancer cells (Martin, 2007). When this housekeeping process fails, cancer may result.

Transformation of normal cells into cancer cells is a two-step process:

1. The first step is **initiation.** In this step, physical forces, chemicals, biologic agents, or errors in replication alter a cell's DNA.
2. The second step is **promotion** which activates the altered genes, allowing uncontrolled cell growth.

The time between initiation and promotion in some cases is 10 to 30 years but may be shorter if a mutated gene is inherited from a parent. See Genomic Gem 21-1.

Substances that enhance the expression of the altered gene are called promoters. They must be present at high levels for a prolonged period. Promoters are tissue specific, such as saccharin for cancer of the urinary bladder (in rats) and bile acids for colon cancer. In contrast to initiation, which results in permanent change, the process of promotion is reversible. Reducing exposure to high levels of promoters allows the body to repair the damaged cells.

Genomic Gem 21-1
Growth and Suppression of Malignant Cells

Protooncogenes support the growth and division of normal cells. When a protooncogene's DNA is altered and the gene is activated, it is called an oncogene. Only one of the two alleles of a gene needs to be converted to an oncogene to cause malignant transformation. Thus, the oncogene is dominant over its corresponding protooncogene.

Other genes called **tumor suppressor genes** act to inhibit the growth of malignant cells. A tumor suppressor gene can function even if one of its alleles is mutated. The cause of the mutation may be spontaneous or inherited. If the mutation is inherited, the person is vulnerable to the loss of protection should the paired allele also mutate.

Many inherited cancers involve tumor suppressor gene mutations. Familial breast cancer and Wilms' tumor of the kidney are examples (Rathkopf and Schwartz, 2006).

American/Pacific Islanders. For each of the ethnic groups, mortality from these three cancers is higher among men compared with women (American Cancer Society, 2008).

Clients who are alive and without recurrence of cancer 5 years after diagnosis are considered cured. This is termed the *5-year survival rate*. Depending on the site in which the cancer occurs, survival rates vary greatly. Differences in survival, stage at diagnosis, and risk of death have been identified in racial/ethnic minorities, the medically underserved, and older adults for cancers of the lung, colon and rectum, prostate, and female breast (Sloane, 2009). The factors that drive these disparities as well as the causes of cancer are complex and often incompletely understood.

Certain cancers appear in great numbers in particular countries. Clinical Application 21-2 summarizes some of these findings. Residents of a given country experience similar environmental factors, including diet. They also may have **genes** that are similar compared with those found in people elsewhere. This chapter:

- Describes some examples of the associations that have been found between diet and cancer
- Explains some of the variability of effects of diet due to differences in the human phenotypes
- Shows the difficulty of generalizing dietary behaviors to adopt or to avoid with the goal of preventing cancer

Diet and Cancer Development

Cancer is considered to be a chronic disease of the genome that may be influenced at many stages by nutritional and metabolic factors. These factors may affect prevention, progression, and treatment of the disease (Go et al., 2005).

Diet is estimated to contribute to 35% of all human cancers and up to 80% of breast, colon, and prostate cancers (Go et al., 2005). Containing thousands of bioactive molecules, diet has the capacity to alter gene and protein expression (Martin, 2007). Developing personalized nutrition for cancer prevention and therapy will require:

- Understanding genotypes and phenotypes
- Identifying bioactive food components that can favorably intervene in cellular processes (Milner, 2008)

Unlike cancer chemotherapy drugs that affect the whole body, many bioactive food components selectively target cancer cells (Stan et al., 2008).

Until the era of personalized nutrition arrives, the American Cancer Society has issued general recommendations to decrease cancer risk (Box 21-1). The guidelines are consistent with those of the American Heart Association, American Diabetes Association, and the U.S. Department of Health and Human

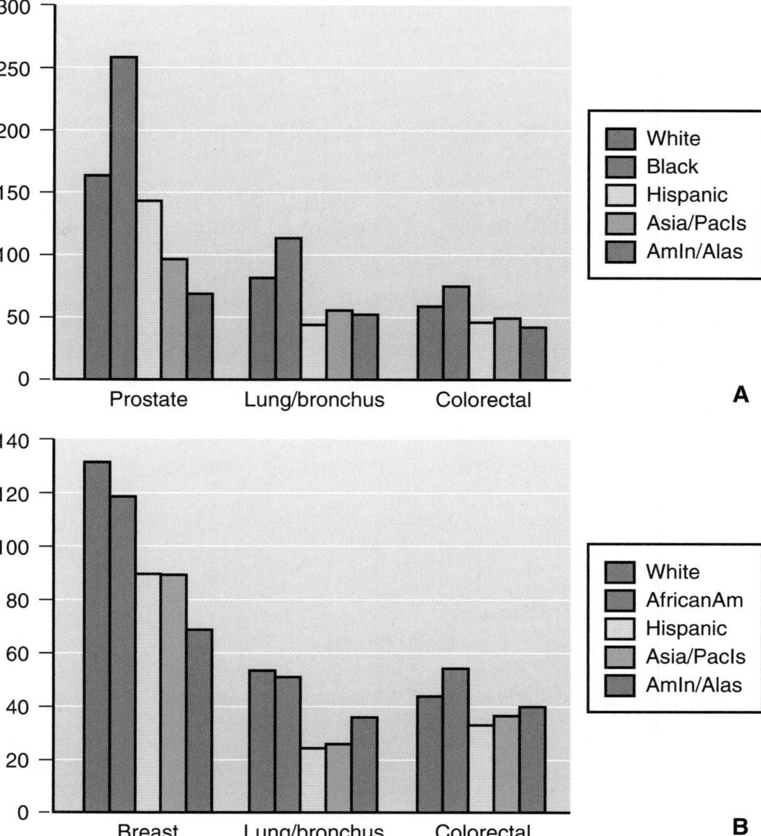

FIGURE 21-1 The three most common cancers for men (*A*) and women (*B*) in the United States, 2000–2004. These are age-adjusted rates per 100,000 persons. The race/ethnicity groupings are white, African-American, Hispanic, Asian/Pacific Islander, and American Indian/Alaskan native. (Data derived from American Cancer Society, 2008.)

Clinical Application 21-2

History of Diet–Cancer Links in Various Populations

Particular cancers occur with greater frequency in some countries than in others. When this difference was first noted, the search began for dissimilarities in environment that could explain the differences. Because hereditary factors can confound the results when comparing dissimilar populations, the study of generations of immigrants is especially enlightening.

- In Japan, the incidence of stomach cancer is higher and the incidence of prostate and colon cancer is lower than those in the United States. In second-generation Japanese immigrants to the United States, however, the distribution of cancers becomes similar to that of other Americans.
- Similar findings are reported in Polish men for prostate cancer.
- Migrants from Asia to the West who maintain their traditional diet do not have an increased risk of prostate cancer, attributed in part to phytoestrogens in vegetarian Asian diets (Vij and Kumar, 2004).
- Presumed adoption of a Western diet affects cancer development. Age-adjusted breast cancer incidence rates per 100,000 Japanese women were
  - 14 in Japan
  - 44 in Hawaii
  - 57 in Los Angeles (Tomlinson, 1994)
- Breast cancer rates remain low in first-generation Asian Americans but increase in their descendants to approach the rates of the U.S. population.
- Colon cancer rates start to increase in first-generation Asian immigrants to the United States, suggesting a shorter latency period than for breast cancer (Li and Pawlish, undated).

Stomach and esophageal cancers are common where nitrates and nitrites are prevalent in food and water and where cured and pickled foods are popular. These areas include China, Japan, and Iceland but the association has also been related to consumption of certain items in other countries.

- High consumption of processed meat, but not of other meats (i.e., red meat, fish and poultry), was associated with about a 50% increased risk of stomach cancer in 61,433 Swedish women followed for 18 years (Larsson, Bergkvist, and Wolk, 2006).
- Changing the staple diet of Black South Africans from sorghum to maize (corn) caused an epidemic of squamous carcinoma of the esophagus attributed to fungi growing freely on maize that contribute to the production of nitrosamines (Isaacson, 2005).

Services. The New American Plate (Fig. 21-2) exemplifies the guidelines.

Dietary Habits Linked to Cancer

Table 21-1 shows four dietary conditions that are convincingly related to cancers arising in specific organs. Many other items have been studied that may be related to particular cancers but the evidence is not as strong as for the ones listed. Numerous factors can impede certainty in nutrition research:

- Inconsistent results from small studies or varying designs
- Isolated nutrients or foods studied, thus oversimplifying the nutritive process
- Interventions too small, durations too short to produce an effect
- Individuals assumed to be equal in specific characteristics who are not (Genomic Gem 21-2)

Box 21-1 ■ *Recommendations to Decrease Cancer Risk*

For Community Action

- Increase access to healthful foods in schools, worksites, and communities.
- Provide safe, enjoyable, and accessible environments for physical activity in schools, for transportation, and for recreation.

For Individual Choices

- Maintain a healthy weight throughout life.
- Adopt a physically active lifestyle.
- Consume a healthy diet, emphasizing plant food sources.
- If alcohol is chosen, limit consumption.

Adapted from American Cancer Society (2010).

Obesity

In the United States, overweight and obesity contribute to 14 to 20% of all cancer-related mortality. Risk factors for breast cancer include weight gain after age 18 and, for postmenopausal breast cancer, overweight or obesity (American Cancer Society, 2010).

Obesity is associated with adverse outcomes in both pre- and post-menopausal women with breast cancer. Evidence suggests that weight management should be a strategy to prevent both the occurrence and recurrence of breast cancer as well as its mortality (Carmichael, 2006).

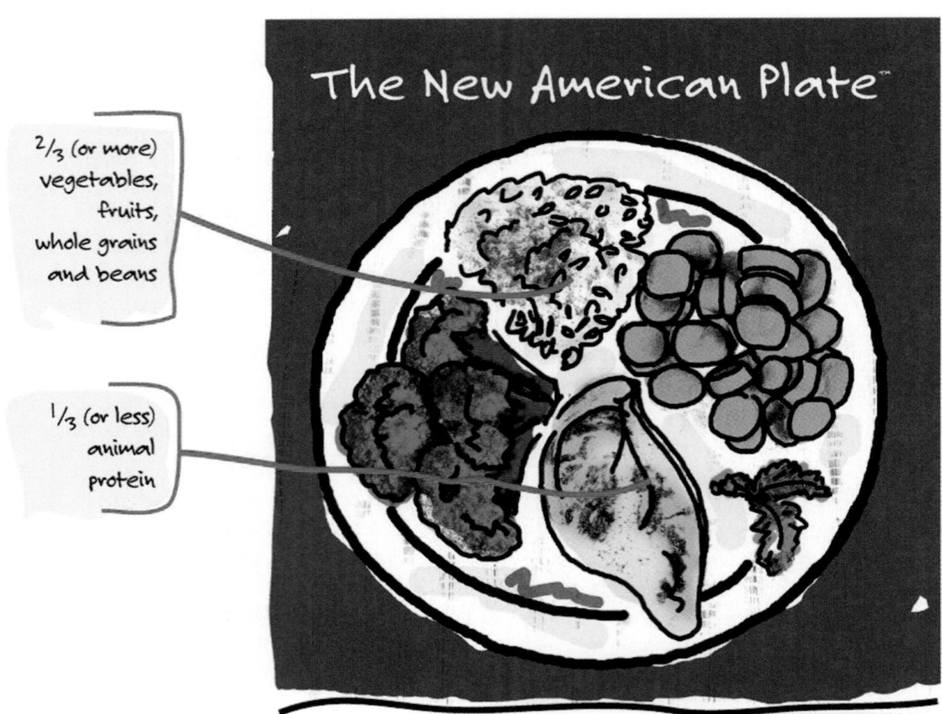

FIGURE 21-2 Vegetables, fruits, whole grains, and beans cover two-thirds (or more) of the New American Plate with the remaining one-third (or less) of the plate reserved for fish, poultry, meat, and low-fat dairy foods. (The New American Plate® is a registered trademark of the American Institute for Cancer Research, 2000. Reprinted with permission.)

TABLE 21-1 ■ Dietary Habits Convincingly Linked to Particular Cancers

CANCER SITE	OVERWEIGHT-OBESITY	RED OR PROCESSED MEAT	ALCOHOL	SALT-PRESERVED FOODS
Breast	X-postmenopausal		X	
Colon	X	X		
Endometrium	X			
Esophagus	X		X	
Kidney	X			
Larynx			X	
Liver			X	
Mouth			X	
Pharynx			X	X
Prostate		X		
Stomach				X

Data from Kushi et al. (2006); Willett and Giovannucci (2006).

Genomic Gem 21-2
Individual Differences in Metabolism

Many studies have related diet to risk of cancer, but frequently the follow-up intervention studies did not show the expected protection against cancer, possibly because the biological diversity of the participants was not controlled. Individuals vary in their metabolizing enzymes to activate potential **carcinogens** and in opposition, to counter oxidative stress and to repair damaged DNA.

Researchers have demonstrated genetic differences in enzymes that catalyze the formation of **carcinogens**. People who were classified as *slow acetylators* of the NAT2 enzyme had a decreased risk of colorectal cancer because of reduced activation of carcinogens (Dong et al., 2008).

The carcinogen does not have to be consumed. Even exposure to cooking oil fumes containing relatively high amounts of heterocyclic amines has been related to a greater than twofold increase in lung cancer in never-smoking females with NAT2 *fast acetylator* genotype (Chiou et al., 2005).

Genetics also impacts the mobilization of the body's defenses. Variation in enzymes involved in the metabolism of antioxidants may modify their effectiveness, perhaps increasing the amounts required for some individuals. Thus, the protective effect of cruciferous vegetables against colorectal cancer has been demonstrated in individuals lacking a particular gene (Reszka, Wasowicz, and Gromadzinska, 2006).

Contrary to earlier reports, little evidence supports the view that fat intake per se, except saturated fat, increases cancer risk. All fats are kilocaloric-dense, however, and may contribute to overweight and obesity (Kushi et al., 2006).

Red or Processed Meat

One of several suggested mechanisms for increased risk of colorectal cancer among people who eat the most red or processed meats is the formation of heterocyclic amines (HCAs). These carcinogens are produced by high-temperature cooking of muscle meats. Frying, broiling, and grilling are the least desirable methods to cook meat, poultry, game, and fish. One kind of HCA has been on the Department of Health and Human Services' list of cancer-causing agents since 2002 and three more HCAs that arise from grilling meat were added to the list in 2005 (American Institute for Cancer Research, 2005).

The amount of HCAs can be reduced by:

- Low-temperature, high-moisture cooking, such as stewing and pot-roasting
- Pan frying at lower temperatures and turning ground beef patties every minute (Salmon, 2000)
- Marinating grilled meats, to reduce HCAs by 92% to 99% (American Institute for Cancer Research, 2002)

Alcohol

Risk for the cancers associated with alcohol (Table 21-1) increases significantly with the consumption of more than two drinks per day. The risks are equal whether the drink is 12 ounces of beer, 5 ounces of wine, or 1.5 ounces of liquor. Moderate alcohol intake has been consistently associated with a 30% to 50% increase in breast cancer risk (Terry et al., 2007). Women at high risk of breast cancer might reasonably consider abstaining from alcohol (Kushi et al., 2006). The mechanism by which alcohol is related to breast cancer is unknown but possibilities include:

- Alcohol-induced increases in circulating estrogens or other hormones
- Reduction of folate levels, or
- Direct effect of alcohol or its metabolites on breast tissue.

Alcohol intake plus tobacco use increases the risk of cancers of the mouth, larynx, and esophagus far more than either practice alone (American Cancer Society, 2010).

Salt-Preserved Foods

Studies in other countries link diets containing large amounts of foods preserved by salting and pickling to increased risk of stomach, nasopharyngeal, and throat cancer (Kushi et al., 2006). Evidence suggests that the risk for gastric cancer may be decreased with a high intake of fruits and vegetables, particularly fruit. However, which constituents in fruits and vegetables play a significant role in gastric cancer prevention is not clear. Vitamin C is a plausible candidate, supported by a relatively large body of epidemiological evidence (Tsugane and Sasazuki, 2007).

No evidence suggests that moderate levels of salt used in cooking or flavoring foods affect cancer risk (Kushi et al., 2006).

A Diet to Prevent Cancer

First, implement the USDA Dietary Guidelines (see Chapter 1), minimizing consumption of red and processed meat, limiting alcohol, and avoiding excessive salt. Second, maintain a healthy weight,

Third, include a variety of vegetables and fruits in the 5-a-day plan. A logo developed for a California program to increase intake of fruits, vegetables, and fiber is shown in Figure 21-3. That campaign used broadcast and print media and point-of-sale reminders, posters, and recipes to educate consumers (Foerster et al., 1995). Inadequate consumption of fruits and vegetables is an important behavioral risk factor for multiple types of cancer. Nevertheless, adherence to the National Cancer Institute guidelines to eat between five and nine servings of fruits and vegetables daily is remarkably low (Cerully, Klein, and McCaul, 2006).

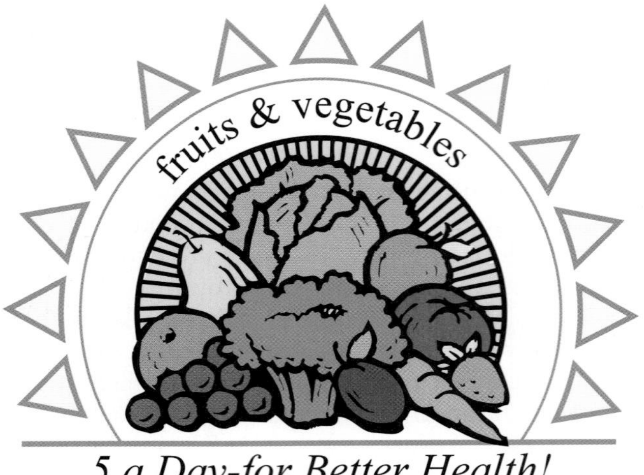

FIGURE 21-3 National 5-a-Day program logo. The program logo and slogan are registered service marks. To use them, food industry and state health authority partners sign a license agreement to follow guidelines that maintain the scientific integrity of all messages and other communications to the public. (Reprinted from Foerster, SB, et al: California's "5 a Day—for Better Health" campaign: An innovative population-based effort to effect large-scale dietary change. Am J Prev Med 11:124, 1995, with permission.)

Greater consumption of vegetables and fruits is associated with a decreased risk of lung, esophageal, stomach, and colorectal cancer (Kushi et al., 2006). Isolating the effects of vegetables and fruits from lifestyle is also problematic. People who eat a large amount of vegetables and fruits also tend to eat less meat and to be physically active.

Studies on cells and in animals supported the roles of many components of vegetables and fruits in cancer prevention (Birt, 2006). Human studies, however, have not shown the clear reduction in risk one might expect. Among the difficulties associated with such research is selecting appropriate components to test from the many nutrients and phytochemicals contained in vegetables and fruits. Research is continuing with particularly promising vegetables, fruits, and plant products such as the following.

Cruciferous Vegetables

In experimental animals, cruciferous vegetables (broccoli, cabbage, cauliflower, Brussels sprouts) have been shown to inhibit chemically induced colon cancer. However, the results of recent epidemiological cohort studies have been inconsistent. Possible explanations for the failure of epidemiological studies to detect an effect include:

- Assessment of intake is subject to large measurement errors.
- Interaction between diet and genotype is not considered.
- Care of vegetables after harvest, including cooking, affect bioactive components (Lynn et al., 2006).

Soy Products

The benefit of soy to reduce cancer risk has limited support. Soy contains phytochemicals with weak estrogenic activity. Short-term intervention studies suggest soy possibly stimulates breast tissue, evoking concerns of possible adverse effects in breast cancer clients. Not enough clear evidence exists on which to base guidelines for clinical use, although raising patient awareness of the uncertain effect of phytoestrogens is recommended (Velentzis et al., 2008).

Tomato Products

Dietary intake of tomatoes and tomato products containing **lycopene** has been shown in cell culture, animal, epidemiological, and case-control studies to be inversely associated with the risk of prostate cancer. Lycopene acts as an antioxidant to prevent free-radical damage to cells (Ansari and Ansari, 2005):

- Higher tomato sauce intake was inversely associated and positive family history directly associated with prostate cancer (Giovannucci et al., 2007).
- Increased intake of lycopene and tomato product intake was associated with a decreased risk of prostate cancer only in men with a family history of the disease (Kirsh et al., 2006).

Lycopene is more available for absorption in cooked products than in fresh tomatoes. Cooking breaks open the tomato cells and evaporates water to increase the concentration of lycopene.

In response to petitions for qualified health claims, however, the FDA found no credible evidence to support an association between lycopene intake and a reduced risk of prostate cancer. Further, the FDA found very limited evidence to support an association between tomato consumption and reduced risks of prostate cancer (Kavanaugh, Trumbo, and Ellwood, 2007).

Balance, Moderation, and Variety—Again

Population studies that found links between vegetable and fruit intakes and decreased cancer cases investigated whole foods. Whether the specific components can be proven to prevent cancer remains to be seen. For most people, including generous amounts of plant products in the diet is a healthful strategy. The notable exception involves soy and breast cancer survivors.

Consumption of vegetables and fruits is especially important if they replace other more kilocaloric dense foods. If the produce is fried or served with rich sauces, or the fruit is converted to high-kilocaloric beverages, the goal of reaching and maintaining a healthy weight will be thwarted.

As noted in Clinical Application 21-3, the best intended use of supplements can result in surprising adverse effects. Taking a single nutrient in large amounts clearly is harmful for some groups.

In 2003, the U.S. Preventive Services Task Force concluded that:

- Evidence is insufficient to recommend for or against the use of supplements of vitamins A, C, or E; multivitamins with folic acid; or antioxidant combinations for the prevention of cancer or cardiovascular disease.
- Recommendation is warranted against the use of beta-carotene supplements, either alone or in combination, for the prevention of cancer or cardiovascular disease.

Clinical Application 21-3

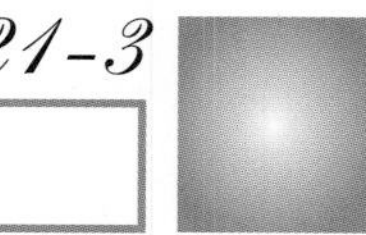

More Is Not Better: Beta-Carotene and Lung Cancer

Carotene, the precursor of vitamin A, is present in many green and deep-yellow vegetables. Vitamin A helps to maintain epithelial tissue, protects against oxidation, may influence host **immune** defenses, and assists in the control of cellular differentiation, a process that is faulty in the rapidly growing cancer cell.

Observational studies found people with lower rates of lung cancer:

- Consumed more fruits and vegetables
- Had higher serum beta-carotene concentrations

Connecting knowledge about the functions of vitamin A and observational findings, researchers designed clinical trials using supplements. In Finland, when testing beta-carotene and vitamin E as cancer-preventive agents for lung cancer, the intervention produced surprising findings:

- A 16% *increase* in lung cancer, and
- An 8% *increase* in total mortality in the beta-carotene group (Alpha-Tocopherol, 1994).

In another trial, beta-carotene and retinol were given to men and women who had been heavy smokers and to men with extensive occupational asbestos exposure. The results were similar:

- A 28% higher than expected incidence of lung cancer, and
- A 17% higher mortality (Omenn et al., 1994, 1996).

This research showed that beta-carotene can have pro-oxidant effects under certain conditions, such as high oxygen pressures and oxidative stress found in the lungs of smokers (Kamat and Lamm, 2002).

The fact that beta-carotene *supplements* were associated with increased morbidity and mortality from lung cancer, however, should not deter someone from consuming vegetables rich in this nutrient.

Box 21-2 outlines some of the factors to consider when confronted with research findings concerning nutrition. There are no guarantees, even with an optimal diet and favorable lifestyle, that an individual will not develop cancer.

Nutrition for Cancer Clients

Overall, in Westernized countries, nearly half of current cancer diagnoses end in cure and the other half end in death (Baracos, 2006). More than 10 million people in the United States are cancer survivors, a title that remains with them for life. Sixty-five percent of Americans diagnosed with cancer live more than 5 years (Doyle et al., 2006).

Box 21-2 ■ *Research Findings: Probabilities, Not Certainties*

There is a natural progression in research from descriptive to experimental studies that reflects increasing certainty that the findings display reality. Unfortunately, the significance and practical applications of research results are often overstated and publicized in the general press before being reviewed and replicated by other scientists. A single study may be interesting but should not be the basis for radical behavior changes. Peer scientists should examine all research for its strengths and weaknesses. Possible shortcomings affecting all research include:

- Inaccurate measurements. Recall data from questionnaires, although showing statistical differences in large studies, may not accurately reflect dietary intake or other behaviors. Even blood levels may be insensitive to small differences and may not correlate with cellular levels in certain organs.
- Imperfect statistical controls. Although extraneous variables are often held constant by statistical manipulation, the process is not perfect and all extraneous variables may not have been considered.
- Incorrect assumptions. An underlying physiological basis for a given effect increases the credibility of research. New methods to test physiological effects often challenge earlier assumptions and conclusions. For instance, the mechanism supporting the value of cranberry juice in decreasing bladder infections was determined to be inhibition of *Escherichia coli.* The earlier anecdotal evidence regarding cranberry juice was dismissed by scientists who assumed that the mechanism of action would have to be acidification of urine, and cranberry juice did not make that much difference in pH.

The following table lists some types of studies (descriptive, correlational, and experimental), their distinguishing qualities, and examples of individual studies focusing on nutrition and cancer.

Type of Study	Characteristics	Application to Nutrition	Limitations	Example
Descriptive (Observational)	Reports naturally occurring events.	Examines a population in relation to presence of risk factors, average intake of nutrients, cancer rates and mortality, utilization of health care, etc.	Cannot establish causation. Diet is just one of many influences on health outcomes. Even less certainty results if the population is diverse (Heaney, 2000).	No association between vitamin A or retinol intake and the risk of hip or total fractures was observed in 75,747 postmenopausal women (Caire-Juvera et al., 2009).
Correlational	Compares phenomena in groups with particular outcomes.	Determines the existence of systematic relationships between consumption of specific foods or supplements and cancer occurrence.	Correlation does not establish causation. An untested variable may be causing the relationship.	
Cross-Sectional	Compares behavior of different groups using the same measures at one point in time.		The point in time may not be typical.	Total preformed retinol intake exceeded the DRI tolerable upper intake level in 78% of children with cystic fibrosis (CF) and pancreatic insufficiency in 13 U.S. CF centers (Graham-Maar et al., 2006).
Case Control	Compares reported behavior by case clients with reported behavior by a control group of similar people without the illness.		Controls may differ from cases in significant ways that were not considered and in ability to recall behavior accurately.	Latinas with type 2 diabetes reported consuming artificially sweetened desserts and beverages more frequently than did the control group (Fitzgerald et al., 2008).
Prospective (Cohort)	Measures phenomena of interest in a large population. Much later compares those with a particular outcome to those without it in relation to the earlier determined practice.	Determines usual diet and other pertinent traits of large group of people at Point A. Waits until illness of interest develops in an adequate number of the people. Compares the groups with disease and without it in relation to the early diet.	Requires very large groups to obtain sufficient cases. May take years for illness of interest to develop, and diet may have changed in the interim.	After a mean follow-up of 8.9 years, a significant reduction in the risk of gastric adenocarcinoma was associated with high adherence to a relative Mediterrean diet among 449 cases from the 485,044 subjects studied (Buckland et al., 2010).
Experimental	Compares results of an intervention administered to one group but not to another.	Administers vitamin or specific food to one group, placebo or none to another. Measures changes in illness, symptoms, blood levels.	Component selected for intervention may not be the one that gave the effect when whole foods were investigated.	

Box 21-2 ■ *Research Findings: Probabilities, Not Certainties (Continued)*

Type of Study	Characteristics	Application to Nutrition	Limitations	Example
Cell and Tissue Cultures			Laboratory results may not be duplicated in animals or humans.	In vitro exposure of human peripheral blood mononuclear cells to watercress extract, increased gene expression for 2 detoxification enzymes, offering an explanation of the mechanism by which cruciferous vegetables can reduce cancer risk (Hofmann et al., 2009).
Animals			Very large doses may be used that are unrealistic to extrapolate to humans.	Compared to other formulas, glyceollin-enriched soy protein produced antiestrogenic effects when fed to female postmenopausal macaques given estradiol (Wood et al., 2006).
Humans			Difficult to shield participants from knowing their intervention or control status. May take a long time to see an effect. Ethical considerations limit the withholding of treatment from the control group.	Fifty-one men and women were fed a diet containing the adequate intake of choline (control) for 10 days, then a choline-deficient diet for up to 42 days. All subjects when fed the choline-deficient diet had twice as much lymphocyte DNA damage as when they were fed the control diet (da Costa et al., 2006).

In summary, careful reading of research reports is required to make wise judgments about the applicability to health practices. Occasionally, an intervention trial is terminated early to permit an obviously effective treatment to be extended to the control group, as in the folic acid–neural tube defect study (MRC Vitamin Study Research Group, 1991), or to prevent harm, as in the beta-carotene/vitamin A–lung cancer trial (Redlich et al., 1998).

Even in these rare situations, the complete reasons for the effect shown by the overwhelming evidence are not always clear. A broad perspective is necessary to guide a person's behavior toward healthy choices for a lifetime.

Regardless of the stage of the disease and because of the lack of contradictory data for cancer survivors, the Dietary Guidelines for Americans (see Chapter 1) are usually recommended. At the very least, adherence to the Guidelines may reduce the risk of second cancers.

Exceptions to the Dietary Guidelines' nutritional and physical activity recommendations due to the client's current condition are made on an individual basis.

Lifestyle Factors Affecting Recurrence and Survival

Determining exactly when a cancer's aberrant cell division began is difficult because of:

- Cancer's long development time
- The complex interaction between cancer cells and the body's defenses

Equating the beginning of the cancer with the date of diagnosis is incorrect. Consequently, it may be too much to expect that lifestyle changes would make a major difference in the client's outcome. Nevertheless, obesity, physical activity, and diet do influence recurrence and survival.

Obesity

Increased body weight has been associated with increased death rates for all cancers combined. Individuals who are obese at the time of diagnosis clearly have a greater risk for recurrence of breast cancer. For women diagnosed with early-stage breast cancer, weight management is considered a standard of care. Overweight women should be encouraged to lose weight after active therapy. Even during therapy, a modest weight loss program of 1 to 2 pounds per week could be prescribed and closely monitored with the approval of the physician (Doyle, 2006).

Cancer at other sites is also influenced by obesity:

- Pre-diagnosis obesity is also associated with poorer outcomes in clients with colorectal cancer. An increasing percentage of body fat resulted in an increase in disease specific deaths (Haydon et al., 2006).
- Obesity may promote the development of a more aggressive form of prostate cancer, resulting in higher recurrence rates and higher mortality rates, although the mechanism is unclear (Amling, 2005).
- Obesity profoundly increases the incidence of endometrial cancer (predominantly through the effects of unopposed estrogen) and may modestly increase the incidence of premenopausal ovarian cancer (Modesitt and van Nagell, 2005).
- Obesity has been consistently linked to an increased risk of cancers of the gallbladder, kidney, and pancreas (Hsing, Sakoda, and Chua, 2007).

Physical Activity

The impact of physical activity after a diagnosis of cancer impacts recurrence and survival of clients with breast cancer or colorectal cancer.

- Higher levels of physical activity after treatment were associated with a 26% to 40% reduction in breast cancer recurrence, breast cancer mortality, and all-cause mortality (Doyle et al., 2006).
- Prediagnosis physical activity was not predictive of mortality in women with colorectal cancer. However, women who increased their activity over prediagnosis levels decreased their risk of death by about 50% compared with those with no change in activity (Meyerhardt et al., 2006).

Food and Nutrients

Investigations of the effects of food and nutrients on recurrence and survival have reported mixed results.

- Diet after diagnosis of prostate cancer may influence clinical outcomes because consuming more tomato sauce or fish lowered the risk of disease progression (Chan et al., 2006).
- Vitamin D seemed to extend the 5-year recurrence-free survival period in clients with non–small cell lung cancer. Those who:
  - Had surgery during the summer, with the highest vitamin D intake, achieved a 56% survival.
  - Had surgery during winter, with the lowest vitamin D intake, a 23% survival (Zhou et al., 2005).
- Clients with colon cancer who consumed the highest level Western diet (high intakes of meat, fat, refined grains, and desserts) had a recurrence rate 2.9 times as high as those consuming the lowest level Western diet (Meyerhardt et al., 2007).

In contrast, adopting a healthy diet after diagnosis may have helped survivors of early stage breast cancer in other ways but not with recurrence or survival. Adoption of a diet very high in vegetables, fruits, and fiber and low in fat did not reduce additional breast cancer events or mortality during a 7.3-year follow-up (Pierce et al., 2007).

Providing Nutritional Care

Unintended weight loss is a classic warning sign of cancer. Involuntary loss of more than 10% of body weight signifies significant malnutrition (Shattner and Shike, 2006). More than 50% of clients sustain substantial weight loss and have poor nutritional status at the time of diagnosis (Doyle et al., 2006). Nutritional care for these clients focuses on:

- Reversing nutrient deficiencies
- Preserving lean body mass
- Promoting healing
- Minimizing nutrition-related side effects of therapy

The three major therapies for cancer—surgery, chemotherapy, and radiotherapy—may all interfere with normal nutrition. A thorough nutritional assessment should be conducted while treatment is being planned. The client's current nutritional status is considered as well as anticipated effects of treatment. Particularly when the cancer involves or impinges on the gastrointestinal system, early nutritional support may be advised.

Optimal nutrition may enhance medical treatment, although conclusive evidence is lacking.

- A review of studies of pelvic radiotherapy found no evidence to support the effectiveness of nutritional interventions in controlling bowel symptoms. Further research was recommended into:
  - Low-fat diets
  - Probiotic supplements
  - Elemental diets (McGough et al., 2004)
- Prophylactic endoscopic gastrostomy tube placement in clients receiving chemoradiotherapy for unresectable head and neck cancer resulted in:
  - Only 2.8% mean loss of weight during treatment
  - One-third of the clients with no evidence of disease at the last visit
  - Eventual removal of tube in 82% of clients with no evidence of disease (Wiggenraad et al., 2007)

Caution may be necessary with particular nutrients:

- High levels of folate may interfere with the desired anticancer action of methotrexate.

- No clear scientific conclusion has been reached regarding antioxidants during therapy.
  - Some experts believe antioxidants could be used by the tumor cells to repair damage by treatments.
  - Some experts believe the benefit to bolstering normal cells would outweigh the theoretical assistance to the cancer cells.

Nevertheless, a prudent course would be to confine antioxidant intakes to the RDAs when receiving therapy (Doyle et al., 2006).

Modalities of nutritional support for cancer patients are shown in Table 21-2. Enteral and parenteral nutrition are covered in detail in Chapter 14. Suggestions to mitigate costs of enteral nutrition appear as Dollars and Sense 21-1. Care of the client with terminal illness is the subject of Chapter 24.

Common Nutritional Problems

Some nutritional problems in cancer clients are due to the disease, and others are due to treatment modalities. Common problems affecting the consumption of meals and nourishment of cancer clients are early satiety and anorexia, taste alterations, local effects in the mouth, nausea, vomiting, diarrhea, and altered immune response. Cachexia is a wasting condition seen in cancer and other diseases.

Early Satiety and Anorexia

Although they may look starved, cancer clients may take a few bites of food and declare that they are full. They may say that they have no appetite at all. The main source of this symptom is the cancer itself, by mechanisms that are beginning to be understood. Control of the disease improves the appetite.

Sometimes, though, the physical pressure from the tumor or third-space fluid accumulation may give a feeling of fullness. Relieving that problem may improve food intake.

Some additional factors may interfere with appetite. The psychological stress of dealing with cancer may produce anxiety or depression. The person may be grappling with a body image change or may be going

TABLE 21-2 ■ Nutritional Therapies for Cancer Clients

	INDICATIONS	CLINICAL RESULTS	PRECAUTIONS
Oral	Impaired GI tract Special metabolic needs	Improved long term oral intake	Dietitian's conversion of prescribed diet to acceptable meal plan critical to success.
Enteral	Obstruction/defect in GI tract Limited absorptive capacity Chemoradiotherapy for head and neck cancer	Decreased infectious complications No effect on survival Prevents dehydration and interference with treatment due to inflammation of the mouth	Monitor swallowing ability to discontinue artificial feeding when appropriate.
TPN	Intensive anticancer therapy Intolerance of oral/enteral feedings >7 days Malnourished clients before chemotherapy or surgery Bone marrow transplant clients Severe GI injury in clients with cured/controlled cancer	Improved nutrient laboratory values Decreased infectious complications in severely malnourished clients	Routine use in chemotherapy clients gives no advantage in response to therapy, complications, or mortality
Pharmacotherapy			
Appetite Stimulants	Megestrol Cyproheptadine	Weight gain	
Antiemetic Drugs		Adequate control in 70%–90% of clients	Clients often do not mention nausea unless specifically asked.
Antidepressant Drugs	Major depression occurs in about 25% of cancer clients	Relieved anorexia Possible weight gain	

Adapted from Schattner and Shike (2006).

Dollars & Sense 21-1

For individuals receiving enteral nutrition at home, a bit of shopping among store brands at drug store chains may produce significant savings. Look for products containing the same kilocalories per milliliter as prescribed.

Food stamps can be used for payment.

Although it is possible to make a homemade solution from pureed foods, it is not recommended. Cancer patients may be immunocompromised. The commercially prepared solutions are less subject to contamination than a homemade feeding.

through the grieving process for the loss of a body function or the potential loss of life itself.

INTERVENTIONS

- Encourage eating whether hungry or not.
- Exercise appropriately before meals.
- Serve small, frequent, attractive meals.
- For inpatients, serve favorite foods from home or a family-shared meal.
- For children, serve food in shapes or decorated with the child's name.
- Vary supplement flavors to prevent taste fatigue.
- Offer 1 ounce of a complete supplement every hour.
- Add nutrients to regular foods.
  - 1⅓ cups (or whatever amount satisfies) of instant dry skim milk powder in 1 quart of liquid milk increases the nutrient density, with little or no change in palatability.
  - 1 tablespoon of dry skim milk powder in mashed potatoes or puddings.

Taste Alterations

Cancer clients may have changes in taste perceptions, particularly a decreased threshold for bitterness. Accordingly, they will often say that beef and pork taste bitter or metallic. Some clients report a decreased sensation of sweet, salty, and sour tastes, and they desire increased seasonings. These taste changes are caused by the cancer and the various modes of therapy.

INTERVENTIONS

- Provide oral hygiene before meals to freshen the mouth.
- Offer lemon-flavored beverages to improve taste sensations.
- Cook in a microwave oven or in glass utensils to minimize the metallic taste.
- Offer plastic table service if metal utensils are a problem.
- Serve eggs, fish, poultry, and dairy products that may be better received than beef or pork.
- Serve meat cold or at room temperature to lessen the bitter taste.
- Add sweet sauces and marinades to the meat to improve its palatability.

Local Effects in the Mouth

Clients being treated with radiation for head and neck cancers often experience inflammation or ulcers in the mouth, decreased and thick saliva, and swallowing difficulty. Any of these may interfere with nutritional intake.

INTERVENTIONS

- For all: Provide oral hygiene, before and after meals.
- For mouth ulcerations, try the following strategies:
  - Serve soft, mild foods.
  - Top foods with sauces, gravies, and dressings, which may make foods easier to eat.
  - Serve cream soups and milk, which provide much nutrition for the volume ingested.
  - Serve cold foods, which have a somewhat numbing effect and may be better tolerated than hot food.
  - Include liquids with meals to help wash down the food.
  - Introduce drinking straws, which may detour liquids around mouth ulcerations.
  - Avoid these irritants (a highly recommended strategy): hot items, salty or spicy foods, acidic juices, and alcohol (even in mouthwash).
  - If necessary, seek an anesthetic mouthwash, which can be prescribed. If the mouth is anesthetized, clients should be instructed to chew slowly and carefully to avoid biting their lips, tongue, or cheeks.
- For dry mouth try the following strategies:
  - Include adequate hydration to help keep the mouth moist.
  - Present food with lubricants, such as gravy, butter, margarine, milk, beer, or bouillon to aid intake.
  - Consider synthetic salivas, but they have caused allergic reactions (Kandala and Playfor, 2003). In addition, many clients prefer sips of water to the synthetic products.
  - Offer sugarless hard candy, chewing gum, or popsicles to stimulate saliva production.
- For swallowing difficulty, try the following strategies. (See the section on dysphagia in Chapter 9.)
  - Advise the client to make swallowing a conscious act (inhaling, swallowing, and exhaling) to lessen the risk of choking.
  - Suggest experimenting with head position, which may ease the dysphagia. Tilting the head backward or forward may help.
  - Serve foods that are nonsticky and of even consistency to minimize swallowing difficulty. Lumpy gravy and mixed vegetables, for example, are hard to manage.
  - Suggest dunking bread products in beverages to help lubricate the passage.
  - Refer to a speech therapist as necessary

Nausea, Vomiting, and Diarrhea

This triad of symptoms often accompanies radiation treatment or chemotherapy, as well as certain types of tumors. Since the gastrointestinal tract cells normally are replaced every few days, these rapidly dividing cells are more vulnerable to the cancer treatments than other body cells. Not all clients suffer these side effects to the same extent, and the effects generally cease when the treatment is completed.

Radiation enteritis involves injury to the intestine. Clients at greater risk of radiation enteritis are those:

- Who are thin
- Who have had previous abdominal surgery
- Who have hypertension, diabetes mellitus, or pelvic inflammatory disease; or
- Who receive chemotherapy along with the radiation

Estimated prevalence of chronic radiation enteritis after therapy is 5% to 15%. Some clients are disabled by diarrhea but reluctant to seek help. Thorough assessment of clients after therapy is also essential (Abayomi et al., 2005).

INTERVENTIONS

- For nausea and vomiting, try the following strategies:
  - Offer the client dry crackers before arising.
  - Serve liquids 30 to 60 minutes after solid food.
  - Limit fats in the diet to promote gastric emptying. Teach the client to eat slowly and chew thoroughly.
  - Suggest the client rest after eating.
  - Recommend the client save favorite foods for times of feeling well to avoid food aversion.
  - Instruct the client to take antiemetics and analgesics as prescribed. Pain causes nausea also.
  - Advise the client or caregiver to minimize strong cooking odors by
    - Selecting milder foods
    - Ventilating the kitchen
    - Preparing food in a microwave oven or by boil-in-bag methods
    - Scheduling meals at times of the day when nausea is least
- For diarrhea, try the following strategies.
  - Add pectin-containing (apple, banana) foods to the client's intake
  - Implement a low-residue diet
  - Test for and treat lactose intolerance
  - Consult with a dietitian about special feedings.

Altered Immune Response

Sometimes, antineoplastic agents also suppress the client's immune system. Clients receiving them are at risk for overwhelming infections from organisms that would not affect other persons. Clients receiving radiation therapy or radiation as part of bone marrow transplantation also are at high risk for infections and need to be protected from all organisms, even those that are harmless to most healthy people.

Clinical Application 21-4 relates the role of the aging immune system to cancer.

INTERVENTIONS

Depending on the client's condition the following strategies may be used.

- Institute protective isolation to minimize exposure to microorganisms.
- Restrict the following foods because of inadequate means to disinfect them:
  - Fresh fruits and vegetables
  - Raw and undercooked entrees
  - Smoked and pickled fish
  - Unpasteurized foods
  - Yogurt—may be off limits because of the possibility of translocation of bacteria from the intestine to the bloodstream.

Other measures are similar to those taken to protect AIDS clients and are included in Chapter 23.

Cachexia

A state of malnutrition and wasting is called **cachexia.** Frequently seen in cancer clients, it is also associated with other advanced diseases. Cachexia is

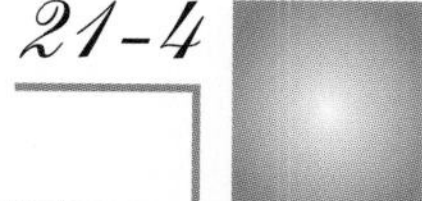

Role of the Immune System in Cancer

The immune system can recognize and eliminate tumor cells, but the tumors also can interfere with and evade immune responses by multiple mechanisms. The increased incidence of cancer in AIDS clients and in organ transplant clients on immunosuppressive drugs demonstrates the consequence of a weakened immune system.

Part of the body's immune defense is provided by certain white blood cells called **T-lymphocytes.** These cells have the task of recognizing foreign materials, including cancer cells, as "non-self" and acting to destroy the invaders. Some of the T-lymphocytes develop into killer cells, which bind to the foreign cell membrane and release lysosomal enzymes into the cancer cell to destroy it.

The T-lymphocytes mature in the **thymus** gland in the chest, hence the name, thymic lymphocytes. Contributing to the development of cancer in the elderly is the deterioration of the immune system, since the thymus gland begins to shrink at sexual maturity and by age 50 only 10% of the original gland remains.

characterized by muscle loss and alterations in fat and carbohydrate metabolism. Figure 21-4 shows a woman with cachexia.

Cachexia appears to be mediated by circulating catabolic factors, either secreted by the tumor alone or in concert with host-derived factors (Esper and Harb, 2005). The result is inefficient utilization of whatever nutrients are supplied to the client. The metabolic derangements are not reversed by TPN, thereby limiting its effectiveness in clients with active malignancies. In clients whose cancer has been cured or is well controlled, but in whom residual effects on the gastrointestinal tract preclude enteral feeding, long-term TPN is beneficial (Shattner and Shike, 2006). Research is ongoing to identify the catabolic mediators and design measures to counteract them.

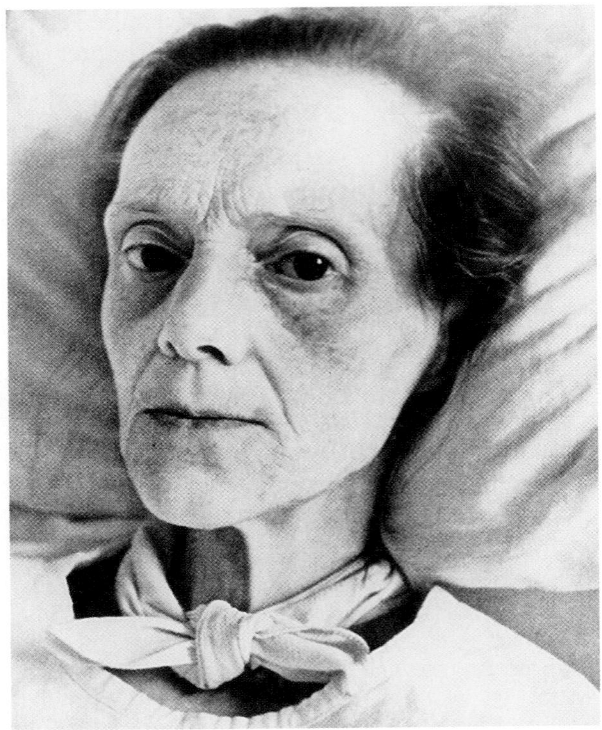

FIGURE 21-4 This woman is cachectic, showing signs of malnutrition and wasting. (Reproduced from *Nutrition Today*, 16(3), cover, © Williams & Wilkins, 1981, with permission.)

INTERVENTIONS

Depending on the cachectic client's condition and wishes and the provider's judgment, the following strategies to improve nutrition may be implemented.

- Appropriately treat symptoms interfering with nutritional intake. See Chapter 24.
- Possibly use selected antidepressants to rally the depressed client's mental state as well as improve appetite and produce weight gain.
- Try appetite stimulants to improve the quality of life in certain instances.
  - Megestrol, a progestational agent, has improved appetite and ameliorated weight loss in some cachectic clients.
  - Cyproheptadine, an antihistamine, has improved appetite with inconsistent effects on weight loss (Shattner and Shike, 2006).
- Consider using nutritional substrates, such as branched-chain amino acids or eicosapentaenoic acid to interfere with the mechanisms responsible for the metabolic alterations (Muscaritoli et al., 2008).

Dietary management of a long list of symptoms common in terminally ill clients is included in Chapter 24. The Charting Tip in Box 21-3 advocates forethought when documenting cancer clients' at-home treatments and diet plans.

One should not expect identical disease outcomes in different people. Just as human beings vary in characteristics, so do cancers differ from one another. Much of the difference in treatment outcomes for clients with cancer stems from variations in tumor biology. Those differences dictate spread of the tumor and its sensitivity to treatments (Burstein and Schwartz, 2008).

Box 21-3 ■ *Charting Tip*

When admitting a client who provides much of his or her own care at home, try to learn all about treatments and dietary preferences and document them. If the client becomes less self-sufficient after surgery or after beginning cancer therapy, the staff will not have to ask multiple questions before providing care. Recording this information ensures that others besides the nurse who obtained it will be able to meet the client's needs.

Keystones

- Cancer is the result of normal cells reproducing uncontrollably both at the site of origin and in metastatic sites of the body.
- Cancer develops in two steps: Initiation that alters a cell's genes and promotion that then activates the altered genes to begin their unruly growth.
- The best dietary advice to prevent cancer: Avoid obesity, stay physically active, and limit intakes of alcohol and red and processed meats.
- Nourishing clients with cancer (1) achieves or maintains optimal nutrition to improve outcomes of therapy and (2) adapts to changes in the gastrointestinal tract due to the disease or its treatment.
- Common problems associated with nutritional intake in clients with cancer are early satiety and anorexia, taste alterations, local effects in the mouth, nausea, vomiting, diarrhea, and altered immune responses.
- Cachexia is a wasting condition caused by profound changes in metabolism, not merely inadequate intake. Controlling the cancer is the best method of reversing cachexia.

CASE STUDY 21-1

Ms. Z is a 67-year-old white widow who had a lumpectomy for breast cancer yesterday. If no complications arise, she is scheduled for discharge tomorrow. The nurse providing her morning care asked how she felt.

"Terrible."

"Do you need something for pain?"

"No, I had something a little while ago. I'm just overwhelmed. This happened so fast. I don't know how I'm going to manage all I have to do. The doctor said I was a good candidate for lumpectomy but I don't know how I will get to radiation therapy. He also said I should lose weight. What good will that do—I've already got cancer!"

"Had cancer. It's gone, remember?"

The nurse continued to explore Ms. Z's risk factors conversationally. She eats the typical Western diet, red meat about every other day, a glass of wine, maybe two, daily with dinner. It was a habit she and her husband had until his death from prostate cancer 9 months ago. Ms. Z is 5 ft 6 in. tall and weighs 165 lb. She has no children, no relatives in the area, and no church affiliation.

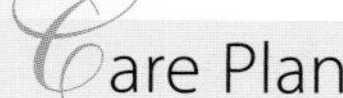

Care Plan

Subjective Data

Uncertain of ability to obtain radiation treatment ■ Lacks information about risk factors for breast cancer ■ Feeling overwhelmed; widowed <1 year

Objective Data

Wrist measurement 5.5 in. ■ Admission weight 165 pounds, height 5 ft 6 in. ■ 125% healthy body weight (130 lb)

Analysis

Lack of resources related to procuring cancer treatment; lack of information related to breast cancer prevention

(Continued on the following page)

CASE STUDY *(Continued)*

Plan

DESIRED OUTCOMES EVALUATION CRITERIA	ACTIONS/INTERVENTIONS	RATIONALE
Client will formulate plan to attend radiation therapy by discharge.	Refer to social worker to be seen today.	Ensuring that client has a bridge to continuing therapy will increase likelihood of completing the regimen.
Client will acknowledge three risk factors for breast cancer pertinent to her situation.	Teach that obesity, red/processed meats, and alcohol are recognized risk factors for breast cancer.	Acknowledging personal risk factors for breast cancer is the first step to changing behavior.
	Point out that -Diet is only one of many possible factors leading to cancer. -Diet is not clearly linked to breast cancer recurrence. -Her unaffected breast has been subjected to the same risk factors as the operated breast.	Recognizing the many factors that play a role in developing cancer should alleviate regrets and guilt about the cause of her cancer.
	Present or review information on a healthy diet according to the American Cancer Society.	Focusing on what can be done now and in the future to change her risk factors offers a measure of control to the client and encourages a positive outlook.

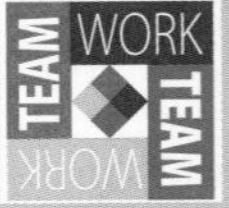

21-1

Social Worker's Notes

The following Social Worker's Notes are representative of the documentation found in a client's medical record.

The social worker, after interviewing Ms. Z, wrote the following:

Subjective: Lacks transportation to radiation therapy. Widowed, without social support system in place. States the doctor recommended weight reduction.

Objective: Coherent. Ready to accept advice.

Analysis: Immediate need is transportation to and from radiation therapy.

Secondary need is social support system to cope with diagnosis and lifestyle changes.

Plan: Set up transportation with American Cancer Society. Recommend follow-up with support group at ACS.

Critical Thinking Questions

1. What additional assessment data might impact the design of Ms. Z's care plan?
2. Was the nurse's statement, "Had cancer. It's gone..." a wise reply? Why or why not?
3. Do you think there is a relationship between Ms. Z's cancer and that of Mr. Z's illness and death?

Chapter Review

1. Research has identified which of the following factors as possibly explaining the conflicting results reported concerning dietary intakes and cancer development?
   a. Erroneous classification of the tumor types
   b. Genetic differences in the metabolism of the people studied
   c. A time frame that extends over too many years
   d. Too large a sample of people recruited to the study
2. Cruciferous vegetables that are thought to protect against cancer are:
   a. Corn, lima beans, and peas
   b. Carrots, green beans, and tomatoes
   c. Brussels sprouts, bean sprouts, and water chestnuts
   d. Broccoli, cauliflower, and cabbage
3. Which of the following foods is likely to be well received by a cancer client with mouth ulcerations?
   a. Hot chicken noodle soup
   b. Orange juice with orange sherbet
   c. Vanilla milkshake
   d. Soda crackers with cream cheese
4. Which of the following is the best advice to increase oral intake for a chemotherapy client who suffers from nausea and vomiting?
   a. Drink plenty of fluids with the meal.
   b. Eat high-fat, high-protein meals.
   c. Take only foods that are well liked.
   d. Eat slowly and chew thoroughly.
5. If visitors brought all of the following to a client in protective isolation, which should the nurse question?
   a. Fruit basket
   b. Homemade vegetable soup
   c. Apple pie
   d. Malted milk and French fries

Clinical Analysis

Ms. R is a 70-year-old widow under treatment for breast cancer. She is being cared for by her daughter, Ms. S, with assistance from a home health-care service. Despite fairly good oral intake at the daughter's urging, Ms. R continues to lose weight and now carries 95 lb on her 5-ft, 4-in. frame. Her main complaint regarding food is its bitter taste.

1. Ms. S asks why her mother continues to lose weight when she is taking half the meals and more than half the supplements offered. Which of the following replies by the nurse would be most appropriate?
   a. "Your mother must be too active and using more calories than she is taking in."
   b. "Probably the medications are dehydrating her. We should increase her fluid intake."
   c. "Frequently the tumor short-circuits the body's metabolism so that nutrients cannot be used normally."
   d. "She doesn't take in enough protein to prevent loss of muscle. We should try supplements of amino acid powders."
2. Ms. S expressed interest in learning what she could do to lessen her own chances of developing a malignancy of the breast. Which of the following suggestions have the best evidence for preventing breast cancer?
   a. Limit intake of red, processed, or charbroiled meats.
   b. Maintain a normal weight and minimize or avoid alcohol intake.
   c. Gradually increase fiber intake to 25 grams per day, accompanied by adequate fluid intake.
   d. Eat a variety of colorful fruits and vegetables every day.
3. Which of the following interventions could alleviate the bitter tastes Ms. R is experiencing?
   a. Serving meats cold or microwaved in glass dishes
   b. Limiting the intake of dairy products
   c. Avoiding sauces and marinades that could increase the bitter taste
   d. All of the above

22

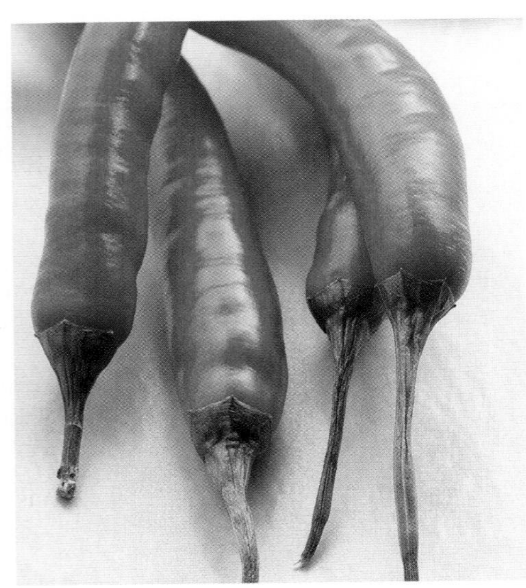

Nutrition in Critical Care

LEARNING OBJECTIVES

After completing this chapter, the student should be able to:

- List four hypermetabolic conditions that increase resting energy expenditure and hence kilocaloric requirements.
- Describe how metabolism differs in starvation and hypermetabolism.
- Discuss the effects of impaired respiratory function on nutritional status and appropriate nutritional therapy.
- List six recommendations for the safe refeeding of malnourished clients.

Patients admitted to critical care units have life-threatening injuries and illnesses. Acute conditions may include severe burns, trauma, and infections. The most likely chronic conditions related to admission to critical care units are respiratory and cardiac problems. This chapter focuses on clients admitted with respiratory problems. Chapter 18 focused on cardiac care. The body responds to life-threatening injuries and illnesses with a hypermetabolic response. The provision of nutritional care for these patients is a challenge. Either under- or overfeeding these patients may result in a loss of lean body mass and death, respectively.

Stress and Critical Care

Metabolically the body responds to starvation by decreasing energy expediture and to hypermetabolism by increasing energy expenditure. Some of the major complications seen in critical care include:

- Inflammation
- Sepsis (blood infection)
- Gastrointestinal (GI) effects
- Wounds
- Fluid imbalances
- Multisystem organ failure

The Stress of Starvation

The physical stress of starvation alters nutrient needs. Biologically, our bodies evolved to cope with periods of feast or famine. Our response to the stress of starvation evolved slowly over the course of millions of years. The human body's response to food deprivation allowed a person to survive despite inadequate food for longer periods than after other physical assaults.

Uncomplicated starvation means that the client is experiencing food deprivation without an underlying disease state. During uncomplicated starvation, clients expend about 70% of the kcalories they normally need to maintain body weight. Because of the biochemical adaptation to starvation, these clients require fewer kcalories than is normal for their height and weight.

The breakdown or catabolism of nutrient stores to meet energy needs characterizes our initial response to starvation. Every cell within the human body needs a constant supply of energy to function.

During starvation, a series of four chemical reactions occurs to meet each cell's energy needs:

1. ***Glycogenolysis*** is the breakdown of glycogen (the liver's carbohydrate stores). This breakdown releases glucose into the bloodstream. However, the body's limited glycogen stores last only a few hours.
2. ***Gluconeogenesis*** is the production of glucose from noncarbohydrate stores (only the glycerol portion of triglycerides and amino acids derived from proteins in muscle and organ mass). The primary source of glucose in early starvation is the increased rate of gluconeogenesis, which causes a reduction of lean body mass (LBM).
3. ***Lipolysis*** is the breakdown of adipose tissue for energy. This breakdown releases free fatty acids into the bloodstream. In prolonged starvation, adaptive mechanisms conserve body protein stores by enabling a greater proportion of energy needs to be met by increased fatty acids, with a decreased requirement for glucose.
4. ***Ketosis*** is the accumulation of ketone bodies: acetone, beta-hydroxybutyric acid, and acetoacetic acid. Ketosis results from the incomplete metabolism of fatty acids, generally from carbohydrate deficiency, and occurs commonly in starvation. The body utilizes some ketone bodies for energy during prolonged starvation to meet the central nervous system's need for glucose. This use of ketones reduces, but does not eliminate, the need for glucose.

Prolonged starvation, in sum, is characterized by decreased energy expenditure, diminished gluconeogenesis, and increased ketone production (Winkler and Malone, 2004). These chemical reactions are summarized in Figure 22-1.

Each body cell needs glucose, fatty acids, or the end products of fatty acids and amino acids for energy. Body cells need fuel constantly. Amino acids can be utilized for energy, but only after the liver converts them into glucose or fat. Specific organs have a preference for glucose as a fuel source. (The medical literature uses the word *preference* in this context; the word *affinity* may be substituted for preference.)

The brain, for example, prefers glucose for energy. Some cells can also utilize ketone bodies for energy. The brain will use ketone bodies but prefers glucose. For the most part, the human body can use only a very small part of the fat molecule, the glycerol portion, to manufacture glucose. Therefore, after the

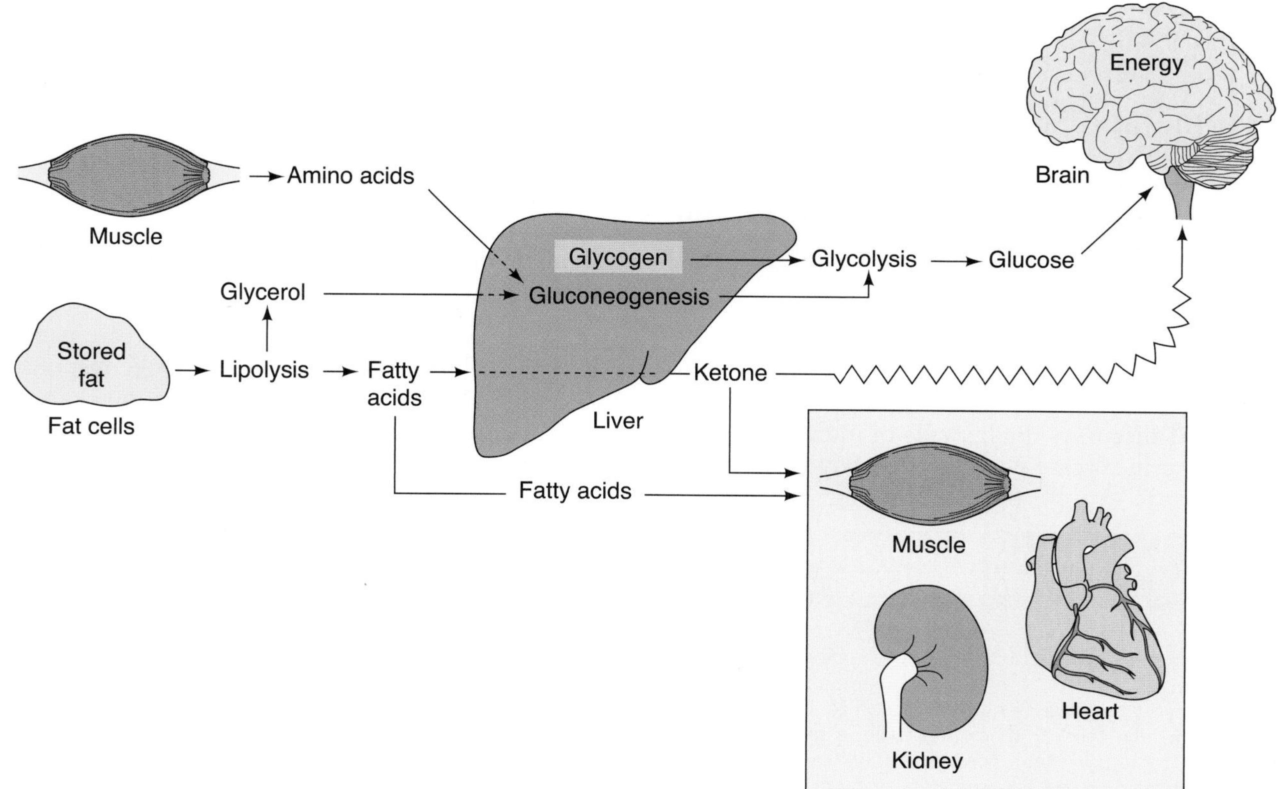

FIGURE 22-1 Origin of fuel and fuel consumption during starvation. The primary source of glucose in early starvation (after the depletion of glycogen stores) is the increased rate of gluconeogenesis. In prolonged starvation, adaptive mechanisms conserve protein by enabling a greater proportion of energy needs to be met by ketone bodies, with a decreased requirement for glucose.

liver's glycogen stores are depleted, body protein stores must be continually broken down to supply the brain with glucose during starvation.

The heart, kidney, and skeletal muscle tissues prefer fatty acids and ketone bodies for their fuel sources. As a result, even if a starving person is fed glucose (as in intravenous feeding), some fat is still needed to prevent the breakdown of adipose tissue. A balance of the end products of fat and carbohydrate metabolism is necessary for survival.

In prolonged starvation, most body organs switch to a less-preferred fuel source. Even the brain increasingly uses more ketone bodies for energy after adaptation to starvation than before. The breakdown of muscle tissue continues in prolonged starvation but at a much lower rate. The human body also becomes more efficient in reusing amino acids for protein synthesis. Thus, urea nitrogen excretion decreases during prolonged starvation.

The rate of tissue breakdown in prolonged starvation also decreases because the metabolic rate and total energy expenditure decrease to conserve energy and prolong life. The catabolic or starved individual spontaneously decreases physical activity, increases sleep, and has a lower body temperature. All of these adaptations during prolonged starvation serve one purpose—to prolong life. The human body gets "more miles per gallon" as a result of individual body organs switching to a less preferred fuel source.

Hypermetabolism

An abnormal increase in the rate at which fuel or kcalories are burned is called **hypermetabolism**. Characteristics of this condition are:

- An increased metabolic rate
- Negative nitrogen balance
- Hyperglycemia
- Increased oxygen consumption

Box 22-1 discusses the benefits of intensive insulin therapy in critical care clients. The body increasingly uses protein obtained from internal body stores (lean body mass) to meet energy needs and depletes lean body mass. A loss of 40% of lean body mass is fatal (Demling and DeSanti, 2001).

Box 22-1 ■ *Intensive Insulin Therapy in Critically Ill Patients*

Hyperglycemia and insulin resistance are common in critically ill patients because of hormonal response to a severe stress. Even if a patient has not had diabetes before the stressor, hyperglycemia frequently becomes problematic. Intensive insulin therapy to maintain blood glucose at or below 110 mg per deciliter reduces morbidity and mortality among critically ill patients in the surgical intensive care unit (Van den Berge, 2005). This level of glucose control is possible only with close monitoring and an insulin drip.

Hormonal Response

The stress response in hypermetabolism is also mediated by hormones. The catecholamines, glucagon, and cortisol oppose insulin and are typically referred to as counter-regulatory hormones. Collectively these hormones influence glucose and fat metabolism by causing the breakdown of glycogen and amino acids to produce glucose and triglycerides from body fat stores. The body produces glucose so it has the fuel to respond to stress. Two other hormones, aldosterone and antidiuretic hormone, also respond to stress, and result in the retention of both water and sodium.

Metabolic Response

The metabolic response of the immune system to infection or injury is called the **inflammatory response.** The signs and symptoms of inflamation include:

- Swelling
- Redness
- Heat
- Pain

C-reactive protein (CRP) is released by the liver during acute phase of the inflammatory response and alters:

- Metabolism
- Heart rate
- Blood pressure
- Body temperature
- Immune cell function

CRP is frequently measured in critical care patients. One practical application of this metabolic response is that an individual's kcalorie and protein intake may be sufficient but their pre-albumin level remains depressed. The negative nitrogen balance seen cannot be prevented because metabolic processes during stress promote protein breakdown. The inflammatory response needs to run its course before anabolsim begins again.

Early Feeding

When to start nutritional rehabilitation of the critical patient is under debate. Some physicians keep clients NPO for the first 24 to 72 hours, and others initiate tube feedings within 4 hours following a burn injury. Here, an important consideration is that **peristalsis,** the wavelike motion that propels food through the GI tract, ceases in some burn clients. Until peristalsis returns, the client's stomach should not be the site of choice for a tube feeding.

In addition, the client may have an ileus caused by muscle paralysis or an obstruction. Physicians who do feed clients early insert the feeding tube into the client's intestines past the ileus and deliver a very slow, continuous-drip feeding. The slow, continuous drip minimizes the likelihood of the feeding collecting in the intestines.

Some institutions have a policy of measuring gastric residual volume (GRV) in clients with gastric tube feedings. To measure stomach contents that have not been absorbed, the nurse will periodically suction the stomach's gastric contents. If the GRV is greater than 250 mL in two separate measures, consideration should be given to moving the feeding tube down gastrointestinal tracts into small intestines.

If the critically ill client is adequately fluid resuscitated, then enteral nutrition should be started within 24 to 48 hours after surgery or admission to the critical care unit. Enteral nutrition is associated with a reduction in infectious complications and may reduce length-of-stay (www.adaevidencelibrary.com) as opposed to parenteral nutrition.

Although early enteral feeding offers many advantages, in many cases it is not medically feasible. A functioning GI tract is a prerequisite to enteral feeding. These conditions preclude the use of enteral feedings:

- Low mesenteric blood flow (commonly referred to as the peritoneal fold that encircles the small intestine)
- Severe tachycardia
- Hypotension
- A volume deficit
- Multisystem organ failure

For these clients, intravenous nutrition is obligatory. Clinical Calculation 22-1 demonstrates the calculation of a sample total parenteral solution.

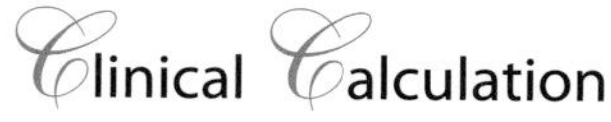

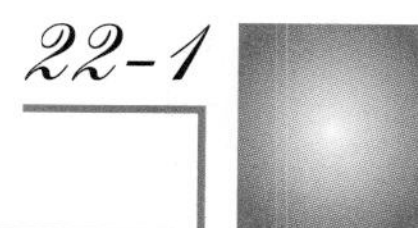

Calculating a Sample TPN Solution

These are the steps for calculating the total kcalories and grams of protein in the following TPN solution: 500 cc D_{50}, 500 cc amino acids 10%, 250 cc lipid 10%.

DEXTROSE

D_{50} = 0.50 × 500 mL = 250 grams of dextrose
250 grams × 3.4 kcal/gram = 850 kcal

AMINO ACIDS

500 mL × 0.10 = 50 grams of protein
50 grams of protein × 4 kcal/gram = 200 kcal

LIPIDS

250 mL × 1.1 kcal/mL = 275 kcal

TOTAL KCALORIES

850 from dextrose + 200 from protein + 275 from lipid = 1325 kcal

Examples of Hypermetabolism

Cancer, major surgery, burns, infections, and trauma are the physical stressors that have the greatest impact on metabolism. The needs of clients with cancer are described in Chapter 21. This section of this chapter focuses on the nutritional needs of clients experiencing surgery, burns, infections and fevers, and trauma. Nutritional support during extreme stress is needed to decrease the length of the stress, prevent complications, and minimize suffering.

SURGERY

Uncomplicated minor surgery increases the surgical client's kilocaloric requirement by only 5%. Surgery needed to repair soft tissue trauma requires a 14% to 37% increase in kcalories. A surgical client with complications may require a large increase in kcalories.

BURNS

Major burns are the most extreme state of stress a client can sustain and produce a hypermetabolic state that raises kilocaloric needs higher than those of most other stresses. Kilocaloric requirements may be as high as 8000 calories per day. Even a client who was well nourished before becoming burned may rapidly develop protein–calorie malnutrition. The degree to which the metabolic rate increases is directly related to the body surface area burned. The percentage of body surface area burned is determined by totaling the percentages in Figure 22-2A. Figure 22-2B illustrates first-, second-, and third-degree burns. Burn clients may remain in a hypermetabolic state for many weeks.

An increase in waste products in some clients with burns requires an increase in fluids. Extra fluids help the kidneys eliminate waste products. Capillary permeability is increased in burn clients; thus, plasma proteins, fluids, and electrolytes escape into the burn area and interstitial space. This shift reduces the volume of plasma, so fluid volume needs to be replaced.

Burn clients are particularly susceptible to **sepsis,** the state in which disease-producing organisms are present in the blood. Major sepsis further increases a client's metabolic rate. Clients with Foley catheters and intravenous lines are at risk for sepsis. Sepsis, of course, is not limited to burn clients; surgical and trauma clients may also suffer from sepsis.

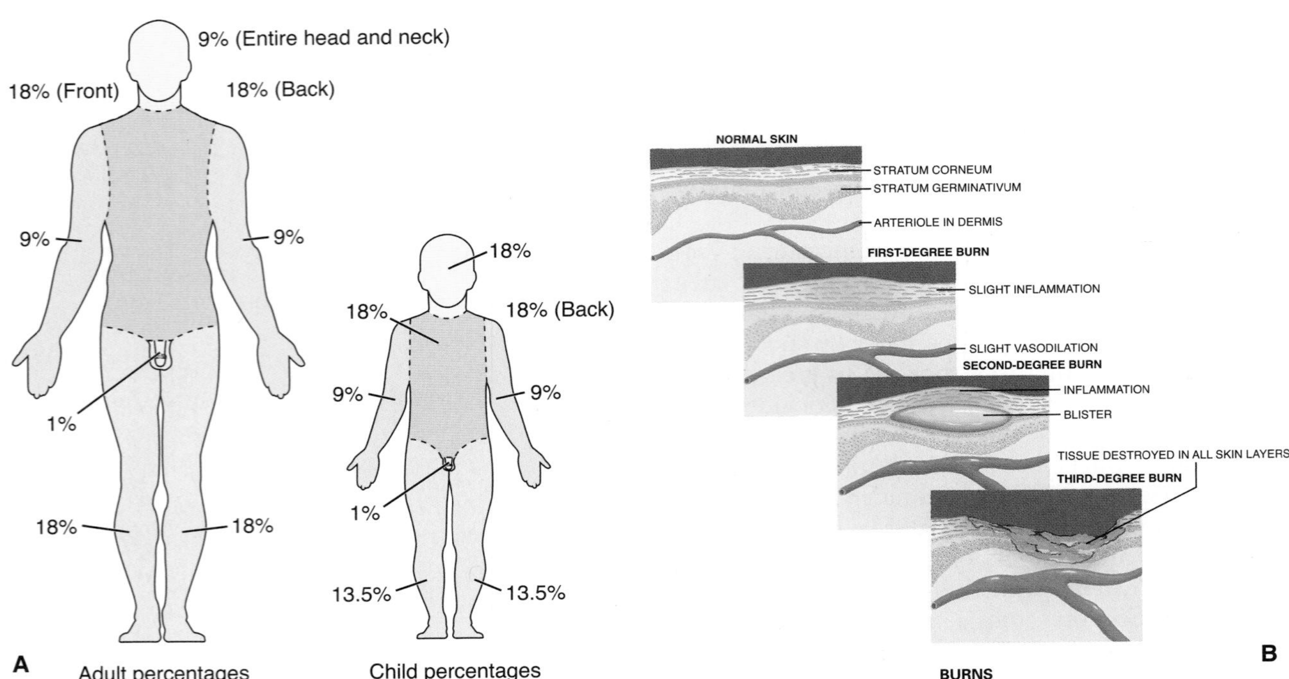

FIGURE 22-2 *A*, The percentage of body surface area burned is determined by comparing the body surface area of the client's burns to the percentages given in the chart. For example, if a client has extensive burns over both legs, the total body surface area burned would be 36% (18% for the first leg plus 18% for the second leg). (Reprinted from Venes, D [ed]: *Taber's cylopedic medical dictionary*, ed 21. FA Davis, Philadelphia, 2010, by Beth Anne Willert, MS, Illustrator, with permission.) *B*, Burns are classified as first-degree, second-degree, and third-degree. (Reprinted from Thomas, CL [ed]: *Taber's cylopedic medical dictionary*, ed 18. FA Davis, Philadelphia, 1997, p 278, by Beth Anne Willert, MS, Illustrator, with permission.)

For all burn clients, a nutritional assessment is essential to minimize complications and allow nutritional therapy to be evaluated effectively. The food intake of these clients should be monitored and documented. The kcalories and grams of protein consumed or taken intravenously should be monitored per the facility's policy.

A high-protein, high-kcalorie diet is ordered for most burn clients as soon as oral intake is medically feasible. Often the diet is initially offered in six small meals. Complete nutritional oral supplements are commonly used to increase the client's kilocaloric and protein intake. The protein content of the diet can be increased by providing a between-meal feeding high in protein, a serving of two eggs at breakfast, and a 4-ounce serving of meat at both lunch and supper. If the client drinks a full 8 ounces of milk with each meal, this further increases the protein content of the diet.

TRAUMA

Trauma is a physical injury or wound caused by an external violence. Stab and gun-shot wounds, multiple fractures, and injuries acquired in motor vehicle accidents are examples of trauma. Victims of traumas may become hypermetabolic, depending on the severity of the injury, and vitamin and mineral supplements may be necessary.

Vitamin C plays a role in wound healing, and its administration restores healing. Vitamin C functions as a cofactor in the hydroxylation of proline into collagen and enhances cellular and humoral response to stress. Doses as high as 100 to 200 mg a day of vitamin C for stage I or II pressure ulcers and 1000 to 2000 mg for stage III and stage IV, or for highly stressed, malnourished, cigarette smokers, and seriously injured patients have been recommended (Steckmiller, Cowan, and Johns, 2007).

Vitamin A, calcium, and zinc are also important in wound healing. Vitamin A enhances fibroplasia and collagen accumulation in wounds. Calcium is needed for calcium-dependent collagenases, iron for the formation of collagen, and zinc as a cofactor for enzymes responsible for cellular proliferation.

INFECTIONS AND FEVER

Malnutrition decreases resistance to infection, and infection aggravates malnutrition by depleting body nutrient stores. Fever characteristically accompanies infection but can also result from a variety of causes. The body needs extra kcalories and fluids during fever because it takes more energy to support the higher metabolic rate. Infection may result in:

- Decreased food intake and absorption of nutrients
- Altered metabolism
- Increased excretion of nutrients

Extra protein is also needed to produce antibodies and white blood cells to fight the infection. Perspiration entails a loss of fluids from the body, and many clients with fever have increased perspiration. Fluid may also be lost in vomiting and diarrhea and needs to be replaced.

Protein and Kcalorie Needs

The patient with hypermetabolism has an increased need for protein. Kcalorie intake should maintain energy balance without overfeeding. Many critical care patients have GI problems and poor food intake.

Protein

Injury or illness requires active protein formation. These states all require a constant supply of protein:

- Surgical wound healing
- Tissue repair
- Replacement of red blood cells and plasma protein lost in hemorrhage
- The immune response to infection

A hypermetabolic client may lose as much as 3 kg of lean body mass (LBM) per day (Mason and Epstein, 2003). The extent of hypermetabolism and catabolism depends on the degree of injury and patient response to the injury.

PROTEIN NEEDS

The protocol for calculating a patient's protein requirement varies from institution to institution. For noncritical care patients 0.8 to 1.2 grams of protein per kg of ideal body weight (IBW) or actual body weight (ABW) formula is often used. For critical care patients 1.2 to 1.5 grams of protein/kg of protein are recommended (Schwartz and DiMaria, 2007). Many researchers believe this recommendation needs to be reevaluated and increased.

URINE ASSESSMENT OF PROTEIN STATUS

Total urinary excretion of nitrogen increases with the client's stress level. Urinary creatinine measurements may be used to estimate muscle protein reserves. One problem common to the use of all urinary measurements is the completion of an accurate 24-hour urine collection. Nurses are typically responsible for collecting a 24-hour urine specimen from the client. If even one voiding is discarded, the measurement will be inaccurate.

Kcalories

Clients who are hypermetabolic have an increased need for kcalories. Patients lose weight because an increased need for energy coupled with a possibly inadequate energy intake and/or protein intake promotes weight loss.

KILOCALORIE NEEDS

Energy expenditure is the number of kilocalories that an individual uses to meet the body's demand for fuel. The gold standard for measuring energy expenditure is indirect calorimetry (see Chapter 6). However, many facilities lack the equipment and trained personnel to complete this procedure. Each organization usually has a protocol to follow to calculate the number of kilocalories to be initially delivered via nutritional support. The patient is then monitored closely to determine metabolic response to the initial kilocalorie estimate.

Kcalories are typically calculated by either kcal/kg or one of several different predictive formulas. Two of these formulas are discussed below. The first method is outlined in Clinical Calculation 22-2. Clinical Calculation 22-3 presents guidelines to follow for parenteral feedings.

Propofol is a commonly used medication to sedate mechanically ventilated patients. This medication is administered parenterally in a 10% fat emulsion. It is important to consider the number of calories derived from fat in this medication and include them when assessing the total overall kcalories the patient received.

Clinical Calculation 22-2

Calculating Kcalories

Kcalories are typically estimated using the following:

If overweight, use maximum IBW:
If underweight use actual body weight (ABW):
If within the IBW range use ABW:
Ideal body weight is calculated based on the following:

F = 100 pounds for 5 feet and 5 pounds for each inch over 5 feet + or – 10%
M = 106 pounds for 5 feet and 6 pounds for each inch over 5 feet + or – 10%

Energy needs are calculated as follows:

Critical care: 20–30 kcal/kg* (25–35 for ventilated patients)

*Noncritical care: 25–35 kcal/kg.

22-3

Clinical Calculation

Parenteral Guidelines for Macronutrients

Parenteral guidelines for macronutrient distribution include:

DEXTROSE

1. Initiate at 3 grams/kg or 300 mL of D_{70} (210 grams).
2. Maximum of 5 grams/kg in stressed patients
3. Maximum of 7–8 grams/kg in nonstressed patients
4. Assess tolerance with repeated blood glucose monitoring

LIPIDS

1. Initiate with 30% of total kcalories as fat.
2. Maximum of 0.5–1.0 gram/kg in stressed patients
3. Maximum of 2.5 grams/kg in nonstressed patients
4. Maximum of 40%–50% of total kcal in any patient
5. Assess tolerance with triglyceride levels and if greater than 300 mg/dL, hold lipid

PROTEIN

1. Give full protein requirement the first day in patients without hepatic or renal impairment.

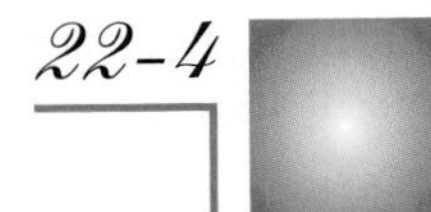

22-4

Clinical Calculation

Calculating Kilocaloric Needs Using the Harris-Benedict Predictive Equation

MALE CLIENT

Energy Need = REE × Activity Factor × Stress Factor

Step 1: Use the following **Harris–Benedict equation** to calculate the male client's resting energy expenditure:

REE = 66 + (13.7 × weight in kg) + (5 × height in cm) – (6.8 × age)

Step 2: Multiply an activity factor by the client's REE (Table 22-2).

REE × Activity Factor

Step 3: Multiply the answer obtained in step 2 by the appropriate stress factor (Table 22-1).

REE × Activity Factor × Stress Factor

FEMALE CLIENT

Energy Need = REE × Activity Factor × Stress Factor

Step 1: Use the following Harris–Benedict equation to calculate the female client's resting energy expenditure:

REE = 655 + (9.6 × weight in kg) + (1.7 × height in cm) – (4.7 × age)

Step 2: Multiply an activity factor by the client's REE (Table 22-2).

REE × Activity Factor

Step 3: Multiply the answer obtained in step 2 by the appropriate stress factor (Table 22-1).

REE × Activity Factor × Stress Factor

EXAMPLE CALCULATION

Assume you need to estimate the kcalorie need of a 154-lb (70-kg) man who is 5 ft 5 in. (165 cm) tall and 25 years old. Assume he is confined to bed and has a fractured long bone.

Sample calculation for step 1:
70-kg man who is 165 cm tall and 25 years old

REE = 66 + (13.7 × 70) + (5 × 165) – (6.8 × 25)
REE = 66 + 959 + 825 – 170
REE = 1680

Sample calculation for step 2:

REE × Activity Factor
1680 × 1.2
2016

Sample calculation for step 3:

Answer from step 2 × Stress Factor
2016 × 1.35
2721.6 = client's estimated energy need

EQUATIONS

Two different equations to predict kcalorie need are discussed.

Harris–Benedict Equation

Although the Harris–Benedict equation is still widely used to estimate resting energy expenditure (REE) for critically ill clients, the American Dietetic Associations' (ADA) Evidence-Based Library discourages its use. The rationale for this policy is that this equation has been found to be less accurate than other equations. However, because this formula has been used for some time, it is still loaded on many software programs. Because of the continued use in many institutions, a brief explanation of the equation is presented in Clinical Calculation 22-4. The Harris–Benedict equation is accurate in 60% of subjects within 100% of RMR when multiplied by a factor of 1.2 when actual body weight is used and 1.3 when adjusted body weight is used (www.adaevidencelibrary.com).

Stress Factors

When using the Harris–Benedict equation, the use of stress factors is common. Research has shown that different types of stress increase kilocaloric needs differently. A stress factor is a number assigned to a given pathological state to predict how much a client's kilocaloric need has increased as a result of the type of stress the client is experiencing.

Table 22-1 lists various types of physical stress and the stress factor used for each disease state. Stress factors are used most often with the Harris–Benedict equation. The Ireton-Jones, 1992 equation considers stress factors in the equation.

As the table shows, a client with burns over 50% of the body has a stress factor of 2.0. This means kilocaloric need is twice (200%) his or her resting

TABLE 22-1 ■ Stress Factors Used to Determine Kilocalories with Harris–Benedict Equation

STRESSOR	FACTOR
Uncomplicated minor surgery	1.05
Starvation	0.70
For each degree F above 98.6	1.07
Cancer	1.1–1.45
Soft tissue trauma	1.14–1.37
Skeletal trauma (fracture)	1.35
Burns (10%–30% of body surface area)	1.5
Burns (30%–50% of body surface area)	1.75
Burns (≥50% of body surface area)	2.0
Peritonitis	1.2–1.5
Major sepsis	1.4–1.8

TABLE 22-2 ■ Activity Factors Commonly Used to Calculate a Client's Activity Kcalories

For a client confined to bed	0.2, or 20%
For a client out of bed	0.3, or 30%

energy expenditure. In contrast, the stress factor after minor surgery is 1.05. This means a client who has had minor surgery needs only 5% more kcalories than his or her REE. Depending on the physical activity of the client, a factor for this is sometimes used. Stress factors are convenient to use in estimating kilocaloric needs when using predictive equations for clients with multiple stressors.

Ireton-Jones, 1992

Another equation considered slightly more accurate by the American Dietetic Association is the Ireton-Jones, 1992 version. Clinical Calculation 22-5 provides the formula used to estimate energy expenditure with this equation. This equation includes stressors for the ventilator dependant, burned, and trauma client.

Predictive equations are used to initially determine a client's kcaloric goal rate. Without indirect calorimetry, the best method to determine if too much or too little energy is being given to a patient is to closely monitor body weight, laboratory values (especially pre-albumin), nutritional intake, and sometimes blood gases at predetermined intervals.

Vitamin and Mineral Needs

Recommendations for vitamins and mineral supplementation for clients with greater than or equal to 20% of total body surface area burned include the following supplements (Gottschlich, 2007):

- One multivitamin daily
- 500 mg of vitamin C twice daily
- 10,000 IU of vitamin A daily
- 40 to 50 mg of zinc daily

The B vitamins help release the chemical energy stored in foods. Whenever a client requires increased kcalories, the need for the B-vitamin complex automatically increases. When anabolism or the building of body tissue is indicated, vitamin C requirements are increased.

Hypermetabolic clients usually need to build up depleted tissue stores. Catabolism with a loss of lean body mass increases the loss of potassium, magnesium, phosphorus, and zinc (Winkler and Malone, 2004). These may be provided in the diet or, more commonly, intravenously. Critically ill patients may have increased micronutrient needs, but research is lacking to make specific recommendations.

Clinical Calculation 22-5

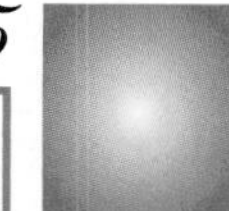

Ireton–Jones (IJ), 1992 Equation

An explanation of the equation components is followed by example equations.

(A) = Age in years
(W) = Weight in kilograms
(S) = Sex; male = 1; female = 0

DIAGNOSIS OF TRAUMA
(T) = present = 1; absent = 0

DIAGNOSIS OF BURN
(B) = present = 1; absent = 0

BODY MASS INDEX (BMI) >27
(0) = present = 1; absent = 0

Equations predict within 10% of resting energy expenditure (RMR) in 72% of obese subjects and 52% in nonobese subjects.

CLIENT WHO IS BREATHING SPONTANEOUSLY

$$IJ_{(s)} = 629 - 11(A) + 25(W) - 609(0)$$

CLIENT WHO IS VENTILATOR DEPENDENT

$$IJ_{(V)} = 1925 - 10(A) + 5(W) + 281(S) + 292(T) + 851(B)$$

Gastrointestinal Complication

Ulcers and some intestinal diseases are aggravated by stress. A client may report that he or she has specific food intolerances when under stress but that the same food is easily tolerated at other times. This change is partially due to impairment of GI function during episodes of stress and the use of some medications. Decreased motility can cause the development of anorexia, abdominal distention, gas pains, and constipation.

These symptoms may contribute to food intolerances or reduced food intake. Fear, anger, and worry also stimulate the hypothalamus to activate the autonomic nervous system, which depresses secretions, inhibits peristalsis, and slows propulsion of food by increasing sphincter tone (Bray, 2000). Thus, the effects of stress, including food intolerances, can vary not only from person to person but also in the same person at different times depending on the extent of autonomic nervous system activation.

Food Intake

The volume of food a client consumes and the desire to prepare food are influenced by stress. The time at which food is eaten also may be important. The best approach is to offer small frequent meals or oral nutritional supplements between meals.

Nutrition and Respiration

The scientific literature addresses the relationship between good nutrition and respiration:

Respiration refers to the exchange of gases (oxygen and carbon dioxide) between a living organism and its environment. The air or oxygen inhaled and the carbon dioxide exhaled is the act of ventilation.

Ventilation means breathing.

Pulmonary means concerning or involving the lungs.

Chronic obstructive pulmonary disease (COPD) refers to a group of lung diseases with a common characteristic of chronic airflow obstruction. COPD has become the fourth leading cause of death in the United States.

Respiratory failure is an acute or chronic disease caused by an imbalance between the amount of gases entering the lungs and the demand of body cells for gases, resulting in tissue hypoxia.

Acute respiratory failure is an imbalance caused by a disease that affects ventilation in a client who has a healthy lung and normal alveoli.

Chronic respiratory failure results from a disease in the bronchial structures or functioning (alveoli) structures of the lung. The primary reason for admission to a critical care unit is respiratory insufficiency or failure (Society of Critical Care, 2006). Malnutrition is commonly seen in clients with respiratory diseases.

Effects of Impaired Nutritional Status on Respiratory Function

Poor nutrition is related to inadequate pulmonary function in five important ways:

1. First, clients with respiratory diseases or inadequate respiratory function frequently have an inadequate food intake, which is related to anorexia, shortness of breath (SOB), or GI distress. Shortness of breath during food preparation and consumption of meals may limit kilocaloric intake. Inadequate oxygen delivery to the cells causes fatigue. Impaired GI tract motility is common in clients with respiratory diseases (see the following section).
2. Second, kilocaloric requirements are often increased in clients with pulmonary disease. Impending pulmonary failure can result in as much as 25% of resting energy expenditure related to the work of breathing compared to 2% to 3% normally (Schwartz and DiMaria, 2007). As a result of the combined effects of decreased food intake and increased energy requirements, weight loss is commonly seen in these clients.
3. The third important relationship between nutrition and pulmonary function is the effect of catabolism. When kilocaloric intake is decreased, the body begins to break down muscle stores, including those of the respiratory muscles. A loss in the lean mass of any muscle affects the muscle's function. The lung's structure itself is thus affected as a result of catabolism. Malnutrition may also result in decreased lung-tissue cell replacement or growth.

   GI distress is common in clients with pulmonary disease and is related to malnutrition. A loss of GI structure including muscle mass may lead to hemorrhage and paralytic ileus. **Paralytic ileus** is the temporary cessation of peristalsis and contributes to decreased food intake and the feeling of anorexia. In addition, paralytic ileus may lead to a translocation of bacteria. Decreased peristalsis in the GI tract fosters the movement (translocation) of bacteria from the GI tract into the bloodstream. This translocation, in turn, leads to sepsis, or blood-borne infection, a sometimes fatal complication.
4. The fourth relationship between nutrition and pulmonary function is that malnutrition increases the risk of respiratory tract infections. Lung infection is frequently the cause of death in pulmonary clients. In severe malnutrition, the body decreases the production of antibodies, which are necessary to fight infection. Also, as a result of starvation, the lungs decrease production of pulmonary phospholipid (a fat-like substance). Phospholipids assist in keeping the lung tissue lubricated

and help to protect the lungs from any inhaled disease-producing organisms.

5. The fifth relationship between nutrition and pulmonary function is that improved nutritional status has been shown to be associated with a better ability to wean clients from ventilators. A ventilator is a machine that provides gases under pressure to clients who are unable to breathe on their own because of an insufficient number of ventilations or inspired volume amounts for cellular respiration.

   Clients on ventilators do not have to use their respiratory muscles to breathe. Active muscle movement stimulates muscle growth through protein stimulus. This is the same principle that applied to physical exercise increasing muscle size. To some extent, all the respiratory muscles **atrophy,** or waste away, due to inactivity while a client is artificially breathing.

Clients on ventilators are usually weaned slowly from these machines as their conditions improve. Some experts have attributed clients' ability to be successfully weaned from ventilators to an increase in protein synthesis. Good nutrition stimulates respiratory muscle growth. By correcting for infections, inflammations, and injuries, avoiding iatrogenic complications, and devoting careful attention to nutritional status, patients with chronic critical illnesses can potentially overcome their pulmonary conditions and debilitated states, to fully recover (Mechanick and Brett, 2005).

In mechanically ventilated patients, there are good data to indicate that once a patient is extubated, swallowing dysfunction and a real risk of aspiration is present in most patients and may last up to several days. Patients who have been intubated for more than 48 hours are especially prone to aspiration (Ajemian et al., 2001).

Nutritional Therapy

Respiratory disease can affect food intake and nutrient utilization. Many clients with respiratory diseases also have problems with water balance.

Energy Nutrient Utilization

Care must be taken not to overfeed clients with reduced respiratory function. Excess intake can raise the demand for oxygen and the production of carbon dioxide beyond the client's capacity. The total number of kcalories fed to the pulmonary client should be closely monitored. A nutritional assessment helps estimate the client's kilocaloric need and assists in therapy. Patients with demonstrated carbon dioxide retention (critical $P_{CO_2} < 20$ or > 60) are especially at risk if excessive kcalories are delivered (Schwartz and DiMaria, 2007).

Several companies market complete nutritional supplements targeted to clients who need a greater percentage of kcalories provided from fat. However, recent data suggests no conclusive benefit for the routine use of high-fat formulas in mechanically ventilated patients (Schwartz and DiMaria, 2007). Most experts now believe that it is the total number of kcalories provided, not the energy nutrient distribution, that most influences patient outcomes.

Research has shown that in individuals with COPD, the presence of lower body mass index (BMI; <20 kg/m^2) may be as high as 30%, and the risk of COPD-related death doubles with weight loss (www.adaevidencelibrary.com). This means these patients require close monitoring with appropriate follow-up. Too many kcalories may increase carbon dioxide production and too few kcalories may result in a weight loss and contribute to a decreased body mass with a subsequent poor outcome. Kcalories are typically given on the low side of the 25 to 35 kcal/kg initially and increased slowly.

Vitamins and Minerals

Clients who have had a poor nutrient intake are at risk for nutrient deficits. Even if intake is adequate, nutritional depletion may occur in severe COPD patients, resulting in a need for supplementation of vitamins and minerals. Specific nutrients depleted in pulmonary disease include:

- Iron
- Vitamin A
- Vitamin C
- Vitamin E
- Selenium (Peters and Thomas-Peters, 2005)

Usually electrolyte levels are closely monitored in ICU patients because of fluid imbalances and the occurrence of **respiratory acidosis** and **respiratory alkalosis**. Some patients' intravenous solutions require daily manipulation to correct imbalances of electrolytes.

An adequate intake of vitamins A and C is essential for helping to prevent pulmonary infections and decrease the extent of lung tissue damage. The diet should include foods high in vitamin A, such as:

- Fortified milk
- Dark green or yellow fruits and vegetables
- Some breakfast cereals (check the label)
- Cheese
- Eggs

The diet should include foods high in vitamin C, such as:

- Citrus fruits and juices
- Strawberries
- Fortified breakfast cereals (check the label) should also be included.

Sources of vitamins A and C should be carefully chosen to ensure that they do not contribute to gas production.

Low bone density is problematic in many patients with COPD. Among the reasons for this are glucocorticosteroid therapy, reduced physical activity, a history of tobacco use, an inadequate calcium and vitamin D intake, and the pulmonary disease process itself.

Fat

Acute respiratory distress syndrome (ARDS) is often caused by conditions such as pneumonia and is characterized by a rapid onset of dyspnea and severe deficits in gas exchange. O_2 saturation reflects the percentage of hemoglobin saturated with oxygen and is an indicator of inadequate oxygen delivery to tissues. Normal oxygen (O_2) saturation in adults is usually 95% to 100% in adults and 95% in the elderly. Critical O_2 saturation is $\leq$75%. A fluid-restricted nutrient formulation should be used in patients, with ARDS whose hemodynamic status necessitates fluid restriction (Schwartz and DiMaria, 2007).

Water, Phosphorus, and Magnesium

Water balance and serum phosphorus levels need to be closely monitored. Clients with COPD and acute respiratory failure often need fluid restriction. Fluid restriction assists in the control of **pulmonary edema** or a movement of fluid into interstitial lung tissue.

Low serum phosphorus levels or hypophosphatemia are often seen in clients who are respirator-dependent. Phosphorus leaves the intracellular space and moves into the extracellular space during starvation. Serum phosphorus levels are in the normal or near-normal range at this point.

With refeeding, phosphate moves back into the intracellular space. At this point, the serum phosphorus level may drop below normal. If this occurs, it is crucial that the client receive phosphate replacement. Because acute hypophosphatemia has been reported to cause respiratory failure, serum phosphorus levels should be monitored in all clients receiving aggressive nutritional support. A magnesium deficiency appears to cause a loss of muscle strength (American Dietetic Association, 2000) and should, therefore, be monitored closely.

Feeding Techniques

Many of these clients lack the energy to eat. Complaints of fatigue are common. The GI distress experienced by these clients contributes to the anorexia. Foods from the cabbage family such as broccoli, cabbage, and Brussels sprouts may produce gas and contribute to gastrointestinal distress. Small, frequent feedings of foods with a high nutrient density should be encouraged. Serving food items that require little or no chewing may help with difficulties in chewing and swallowing and breathlessness.

Refeeding Syndrome

Refeeding is the reintroduction of kcalories and nutrients by oral or other routes. **Refeeding syndrome** is a detrimental state that results when a previously severely malnourished person is reintroduced to food and nutrients improperly. Complications with refeeding can occur regardless of the route by which nutrients are delivered:

- Oral,
- Enteral, or
- Parenteral.

The term *refeeding syndrome* has been used to describe a series of metabolic and physiological reactions that occur in some malnourished clients when nutritional rehabilitation is begun. Improper refeeding of a chronically malnourished client can result in congestive heart failure (CHF) and respiratory failure. Clients at risk include those with:

- Alcoholism
- Chronic weight loss
- Hyperglycemia, or insulin-dependent diabetes mellitus

Included also are clients on:

- Chronic antacid or
- Diuretic therapy

Elderly persons living alone who choose not to eat or are unable to eat because of progressive infirmity are likely candidates. Any incompetent mentally or physically challenged adult or abused child who has not been eating, either by choice or because of neglect, is also likely to experience refeeding syndrome.

Starvation leads to both a loss of the lean body mass in the heart and respiratory muscles and decreased insulin secretion. When carbohydrate intake is low, the pancreas adapts by decreasing insulin secretion. With the reintroduction of carbohydrates into the diet, insulin secretion will increase. The increased insulin secretion is associated with increased sodium and water retention.

Other hormones are also activated with carbohydrate feeding. As a result of hormone action, increases in metabolic rate, oxygen consumption, and carbon dioxide production occur. The net effect of these metabolic changes is an increased workload for the cardiopulmonary system. Refeeding may increase the work of the cardiopulmonary system beyond its diminished capacity (due to the loss of lean body mass) and cause CHF and respiratory failure.

Starvation also leads to an increase in extracellular fluid and an increased loss of intracellular phosphorus, potassium, and magnesium. The degree of intracellular loss of these minerals reflects the degree of loss of lean body mass. Before refeeding, serum phosphorus and magnesium levels may remain in the lower range of normal, whereas the intracellular and total body stores of these minerals are depleted.

After refeeding, these minerals are redistributed from the extracellular to the intracellular compartments. Repeated laboratory measurements taken after refeeding is started may show low serum levels of phosphorus, magnesium, and potassium. Failure to correct for these mineral deficiencies may be fatal for the client.

Principles of Safe Refeeding

Health-care workers need to be aware of the dangers of refeeding a severely malnourished or starved client. Starved or severely malnourished clients may be seen in outpatient settings as well as in hospital intensive care units and long-term care facilities. The recommendations in Clinical Application 22-1 may help health-care workers avoid the refeeding syndrome.

Refeeding the malnourished client requires a team effort. A careful diet history taken by the dietitian can assist in the identification of clients likely to become victims of refeeding syndrome. Indications of a significantly altered status include changes in:

- Taste,
- Appetite,
- Intake,
- Weight, or
- Consumption of a special diet.

Correction of electrolyte abnormalities by the physician before implementing nutritional support can prevent death. Careful observation and monitoring by the nutritional support service can identify early signs of this syndrome. Open and prompt communication among all health-care team members may be crucial to the client's survival.

Clinical Application 22-1

Recommendations for Refeeding the Malnourished Client

These six points are broad guidelines for working with malnourished clients.

1. Health-care professionals need first to recognize clients at risk. Refeeding syndrome occurs in:
   - Clients with frank starvation, including war victims undergoing repletion
   - Chronically ill clients who are malnourished
   - Clients on prolonged intravenous dextrose solutions without other modes of nutritional support
   - Hypermetabolic clients who have not received nutritional support for 1 to 2 weeks
   - Clients who report prolonged fasting
   - Obese clients who report a recent loss of a considerable amount of weight
   - Chronic alcoholics
   - Clients with anorexia nervosa
2. Health-care workers practicing in outpatient settings not directly under the supervision of a physician need to develop a referral plan in the event they suspect a client is a likely candidate for refeeding syndrome. These clients require the expertise of a physician.
3. A physician needs to test for and correct all electrolyte abnormalities before initiating nutritional support, whether by the oral, enteral, or parenteral route. Many physicians depend on other health-care workers to assist in the monitoring of:
   - Serum phosphorus
   - Magnesium
   - Potassium values

For nurses practicing within hospitals, this means notifying the physician on receipt of laboratory test results showing low serum levels of these minerals. It is especially important to notify the physician before implementing changes in:

- Tube feedings,
- Oral diets, or
- The rate of intravenous nutrition.

4. The physician needs to restore circulatory volume and to monitor pulse rate and intake and output before initiating nutritional support.

Continued

Clinical Application—cont'd 22-1

Again, many physicians depend on nurses and other health-care workers to assist in monitoring these signs.

5. The kilocaloric delivery to a previously starved client should be slow. Tube-fed and parenterally fed clients who have been previously malnourished need to be closely monitored for the following items:
   - Rate
   - Total volume
   - Concentration of kcalories delivered

   These items should be increased one at a time:
   - Concentration
   - Volume
   - Rate of kilocaloric intake
6. Stepwise advancement to a higher kcalorie intake should not occur unless the client is metabolically and physiologically stable.
7. Electrolytes should be monitored before nutritional support is started and at designed intervals thereafter.

Keystones

- Hypermetabolism differs from starvation in that resting energy expenditure (REE) increases during hypermetabolism and decreases during a prolonged state of starvation.
- Major surgery, severe infections, fever, major burns, and severe trauma are all examples of hypermetabolic states.
- Respiratory status profoundly affects nutrient need and utilization as well as food intake.
- Nutritional support can decrease catabolism of the respiratory muscles, improve immune function, minimize carbon dioxide production, and improve the likelihood of successfully weaning clients who are on mechanical respirators.
- Refeeding a previously starved client involves some risks. Refeeding may increase the work of the cardiorespiratory system beyond its diminished capacity and cause congestive heart failure and respiratory failure.

CASE STUDY 22-1

Mr. X is a 48-year-old man who was admitted to the intensive care unit (ICU) with a diagnosis of bilateral pneumonia that was resistant to a 10-day prior course of antibiotic therapy. On admission, the patient presented in acute distress: clammy to touch; weak; and unable to sit on examination table without assistance and support. Recumbent vital signs revealed the following: blood pressure 110/65; pulse 120 and weak; respiratory rate 28 breaths per minute and shallow; and sublingual temperature of 102.5°F. Medical history obtained from patient was unremarkable and, in particular, no history of prior respiratory distress, smoking, or exposure to inhalation of toxic substances such as asbestoses.

His O_2 saturation was 50 on admission and his Pco_2 53. Imaging studies showed diffuse bilateral pulmonary infiltrates and small to moderate bilateral plural effusions. His albumin level was 2.5. Based on these findings and the blood gases, mechanical ventilation was instituted.

Mr. X is 5 ft 11 in. tall and weighs 140 lb (63.6 kg). His BMI is 19.5. He reported a 9-lb weight loss over the past 3 weeks. He admits to living a sedentary lifestyle and a poor food intake. He states that his wife died about 6 months ago and since then he has quit eating much. Mr. X admits his personal hygiene has also been poor. The neighbor brought him to the hospital and stated Mr. X appeared to have lost "a lot of weight."

An orally placed feeding tube with the tip placed in the duodenum was inserted and placement was confirmed by diagnostic imaging. His kilocaloric need was estimated to be 1590 to 2226 based on 25 to 35 kcal/kg and his actual body weight. His protein needs were estimated to be 1.2 to 1.5 grams/kg or 75.8 to 95.4 grams/day, also based on his actual body weight.

CASE STUDY *(Continued)*

The dietitian recommended a formula with a 1.5 kcal/mL concentration. A 24-hour continuous feeding of 1435 total milliliters at 59 mL per hour was recommended as a goal. An initial rate of 20 mL per hour with a gradual increase of 10 mL every 8 hours as tolerated was set until the goal rate was reached. In addition, 750 mL water would be needed to meet fluid needs and should be used to flush the tube, as tolerated by the patient.

On the third day of his hospital stay, the patient's phosphorus, potassium, and magnesium, which had been in the normal range on admission, dropped below normal. These electrolytes were replaced intravenously by physician's order. The patient remained and tolerated the tube feeding without problems for the next 6 days.

The physician started to wean the patient from the mechanical ventilator 24-hours ago as his pneumonia related-symptoms responded well to the intravenous antibiotic treatment. The client states he does not know why he got so ill.

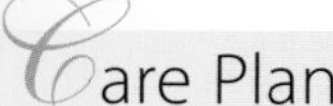

Care Plan

Subjective Data

Denies knowledge of the relationship among lifestyle behaviors and infection ■ Reported significant weight loss and very poor food intake and sedentary behaviors

Objective Data

BMI = 19.5 on admission ■ Mechanical ventilation for the past 8 days second to pneumonia ■ Tube feeding well tolerated since admission ■ On admission visually presented with dirty hands, soiled clothing, and body odor

Analysis

Client's condition related to poor personal hygiene as a result of grieving and knowledge deficit

Plan

DESIRED OUTCOMES EVALUATION CRITERIA	ACTIONS/INTERVENTIONS	RATIONALE
Expresses feelings about loss	Actively listen to the patient, particularly when he mentions his wife.	Patient needs much assistance learning to ask for help.
Seeks social support	Offer social services referral.	The social worker will be able to determine patient's eligibility for treatment and match Mr. X's financial resources to specific doctors or programs.
States that good nutrition and moderate exercise, and proper hygiene are important for disease resistance	Explain the relationship among lifestyle behaviors and resistance to infectious disease.	Knowledge is the first step to behavioral change.
	Offer patient a referral to the dietitian to discuss healthful eating and easily prepared meals.	The dietitian has reliable educational materials suitable for most populations.

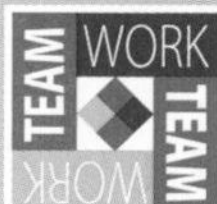

22-1

Social Worker's Notes

The following Social Worker's Notes are representative of the documentation found in a client's medical record.

Met with client per physician and nursing request. Although we did discuss his wife's death, client did not express grief or sadness. Also, phoned client's next closest relative, a sister living out-of-state. She indicated concern with her brother's inability to move forward with his life. She claims that before her sister-in-law's death, her brother was a well-groomed, cheerful person. At first, she denied any family history of mental illness. After some discussion, she admitted that her mother had committed suicide when she and her brother were very young. Long-term counseling and possibly medication are indicated. Mr. X has mental health coverage. Recommend referral to psychiatrist and possibly discharge to outpatient mental health program per the psychiatrist's evaluation.

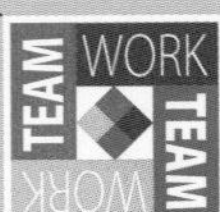

22-2

Dietitian's Follow-up Notes

The following Dietitian's Notes are representative of the documentation found in a client's medical record.

Spoke with client initially one day after his present hospital admission to assess his nutritional needs and write recommendations. At that time, client was tearful about his poor health habits. He did not mention much about his deceased spouse except to say she died 6 months ago. Concur with social worker's note. Client does not presently appear able to meet his own nutritional needs on discharge. Will defer education until after psychiatrist's evaluation. In the meantime, client is consuming sips of clear liquids only as he is still in the process of being weaned from the ventilator. The client agreed to try a complete liquid supplement, a few sips every hour. The client needs much encouragement.

Critical Thinking Questions

1. After 2 days of monitoring the patient's kcalorie and protein intake and despite encouragement to eat from the nurses and the dietitian, the patient refuses to eat much food. His kcalorie intake is less than 500, with only 12 grams of protein. What would you recommend?
2. The patient's physician has ordered a fluid restriction of 800 mL every day plus output. The patient is angry and wants more fluids. How would you handle this situation?
3. You question the client's mental competence. What should you do?

Chapter Review

1. The following is true about clients who have a life-threatening injury or illness:
   a. Their resting energy expenditure is about 70% of the kcalories normally needed to maintain body weight.
   b. They have a decreased need for fluids.
   c. Biologically, their organs do not adapt to their increased need for kcalories by switching to a less preferred fuel source.
   d. They need 0.8 to 1.2 grams of protein per kilogram of actual body weight.
2. Which of these conditions does not increase a client's resting energy expenditure?
   a. Infection
   b. Chronic obstructive pulmonary disease
   c. Starvation
   d. Burn
3. A burn client's need for kcalories is related to:
   a. The amount of protein eaten
   b. The total body surface area burned
   c. The volume of food tolerated
   d. Existing nutrient stores
4. Malnutrition is commonly seen in clients with pulmonary disease for all but one of the following reasons. Identify the exception.
   a. Many of these clients have a decreased food intake.
   b. Many of these clients expend more kcalories to breathe.
   c. Many of these clients have impaired gastrointestinal tract function.
   d. Many of these clients have an extraordinary ability to fight infection.
5. Experts advocate the following when refeeding a malnourished client:
   a. Immediately pushing kcalories and protein to replenish lost stores
   b. Progressing the rate, volume, and concentration of a tube feeding as rapidly as possible
   c. Full participation of all members of the health-care team to manage commonly seen metabolic abnormalities
   d. Correction of the hyperphosphatemia seen during the refeeding of a malnourished client

Clinical Analysis

1. Mr. X is suffering from second- and third-degree burns over 40% of his body. His physician has decided to use topical agents and leave the wound open to air. In the first 30 to 40 days postburn, the health-care team is planning nutritional support. The best supplemental feedings for the client would be:
   a. A high-fat feeding such as a milkshake made with ½ cup skim milk and 1 cup of ice cream
   b. A high-carbohydrate feeding such as soda with added honey
   c. A polymeric (complete nutritional) supplement that is acceptable to the client
   d. High-kcalorie desserts such as apple pie, cake, and ice cream

2. Mrs. J is an alcoholic who has previously reported that she has not eaten "food" for at least the last 3 months. She stated that her sole source of kcalories has been alcohol. After her treatment for alcohol withdrawal on another unit, she was transferred to the unit where you work. The physician has ordered a high-kcalorie, high-protein diet. So far, she has eaten 100% of the three high-kcalorie, high-protein trays she has received while on your unit. While reviewing the client's laboratory values, you notice her serum phosphorus, magnesium, and potassium levels have just recently decreased. Mrs. J's depressed phosphorus values may be related to:
   a. A movement of phosphorus into the extracellular space
   b. A total compartmental depletion of phosphorus
   c. A lack of phosphorus in Mrs. J's present dietary intake
   d. A movement of phosphorus into the intracellular space

3. Mr. C is a heavy smoker. He was recently admitted to your unit with carbon dioxide retention and a diagnosis of chronic obstructive pulmonary disease. He complains of gas pains. The client will not derive benefit from:
   a. Caffeinated beverages
   b. Broccoli, onions, peas, melons, and cabbage
   c. Six small meals
   d. Custard, hot cooked cereals, bananas, ground meats, and mashed potatoes

23

Diet in HIV and AIDS

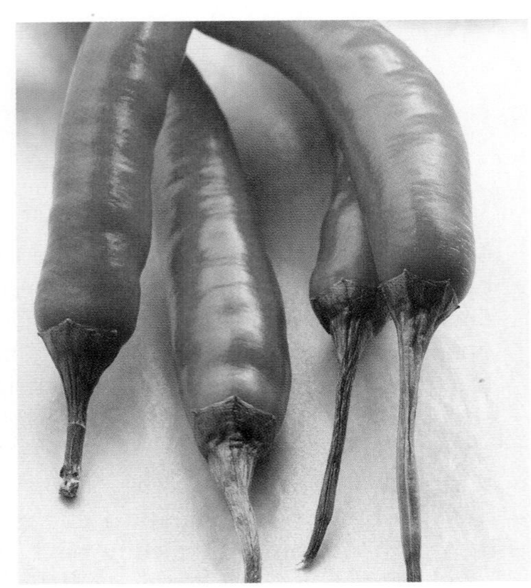

LEARNING OBJECTIVES

After completing this chapter, the student should be able to:

- Define AIDS and HIV and list transmission routes for the virus.
- List nutrition-related complications seen in clients infected with HIV and, for each complication, describe interventions to improve nutritional status.
- Discuss why malnutrition is commonly seen in clients with HIV or AIDS.
- Describe why each client with AIDS needs an individualized nutritional assessment.

Acquired immune deficiency syndrome (AIDS) is a life-threatening disease and a major public health issue. The **human immunodeficiency virus (HIV)** causes AIDS. The impact of this virus on our society is and will continue to be a challenge. This chapter discusses the prevention, diagnosis, and treatment of HIV **infection.** HIV is complicated by the side effects of medications; coinfections with other infections; and disease, wasting; and lipodystrophy. The course of AIDS is commonly complicated by malnutrition. For these reasons, a major portion of this chapter is devoted to the nutritional care of clients infected with HIV.

Human Immunodeficiency Virus

The human immunodeficiency virus attacks both the immune system and the nervous system. **Immunity** refers to resistance to or protection against a specified disease.

When the AIDS virus enters the bloodstream, it begins to attack cells with a specific protein called CD_4 on their surfaces. CD_4 is present on lymphocytes. Lymphocytes are the main source of the body's immune capability, which involves humoral immunity produced by B cells and cell-mediated immunity produced by T cells. CD_4 levels decrease as the HIV disease progresses.

A healthy, uninfected person usually has 500 to 1500 CD_4^+ cells in every microliter of blood. The HIV virus enters the cell, conscripts its DNA, and reprograms it to reproduce the virus. Loss of CD_4 function leaves an individual susceptible to infections and certain cancers. Evidence shows that the AIDS virus may also attack the nervous system, causing damage to the brain.

Acquired Immune Deficiency Syndrome

AIDS is defined by the presence of HIV infection and a low level of white blood cells or T cells of less than 200 cells in every microliter of blood. It is a disease complex characterized by a collapse of the body's natural immunity against disease. Every part of the human body may be affected.

On average, HIV takes about 10 years, without treatment, to progress to AIDS. The survival rate for newly diagnosed clients initiating therapy in 2005 is now estimated to be decades. Many clients still progress to end-stage AIDS because of the development of multidrug-resistant HIV virus or inability to adhere to antiretroviral (medication) therapy (Wassman, Segal-Maurer, and Rubin, 2007).

No Known Cure

Dramatic but expensive treatment advances have changed the health-care community's view of AIDS. The use of highly active antiretroviral therapy (HAART) has decreased mortality rates. However, findings indicate that in the vast majority of patients receiving HAART, who had undetectable levels of HIV-1 RNA in plasma, the virus has not been eradicated. Also, HAART is not a treatment option for much of the world's population. Sadly, the medications are too costly.

Signs and Symptoms

The natural history of HIV infection is divided into three phases:

1. Early symptomatic phase
2. Clinical latency
3. Advanced HIV disease (or AIDS)

Early Symptomatic Phase

An HIV-infected individual may develop an acute flu-like illness, with symptoms appearing about 2 to 6 weeks after exposure to the virus. Typically, the symptoms are not severe enough for the infected individual to seek medical attention.

Clinical Latency

The individual may be **asymptomatic** for years after becoming infected with the virus. About 25% of HIV-infected people do not know they are infected, and the danger lies in their ability to infect other people unknowingly. Even though the person may be symptom-free, viral replication continues. Clients may seek health care with minor infections and wasting syndrome, unaware of their HIV infection.

If the infection is untreated, CD_4^+ cells decline steadily during the latency stage.

Advanced HIV Disease Phase (AIDS)

A diagnosis of AIDS is made whenever a person is HIV infected and has a CD_4 count of less than 200 cells/mm^3 or the client is diagnosed with an AIDS defining illness (Wasserman and Segal-Maurer, 2007). Nutrition-related AIDS defining illnesses include wasting, nutrient malabsorption, and oropharyngeal and esophageal *candidiasis* (thrush).

The Epidemic

The AIDS epidemic started in Africa, and the first cases of the syndrome were described in the United States more than two decades ago. Untreated case fatality rates initially approached 100%. With the introduction of combination or highly active antiretroviral therapy (cART or HAART), the HIV-related death rate has declined 70% since 1995.

The epidemic increasingly affects women, minorities, persons infected through heterosexual contact, and the poor. Gay and bisexual men are still the most severely affected by HIV. These affected groups are usually diagnosed at a later stage of infection when related disease is present and often delay care for themselves because they must care for others or have competing subsistence needs for their time and resources. Genomic Gem 23-1 provides insight into why certain racial and ethnic groups are more severely affected by this virus.

Genomic Gem 23-1
HIV Infections by Race and Ethnicity

The CDC for the first time was able to provide new HIV infections by race/ethnicity in its *Morbidity and Morality Weekly Report* (MMWR), September, 2008. The number of new infections among young, black, gay, and bisexual men was roughly twice that of whites and Hispanic/Latinos. Black men accounted for two-thirds of new infections in 2006.

For some time, the continent of Africa has the highest prevalence of HIV infection in the world. Why would this be so? Sexual behavior, lack of education, family structure, and poverty cannot explain why more than 66% of the world's 33 million people infected with HIV live in sub-Saharan Africa.

Researchers have recently found a mutation in the Duffy antigen receptor expression (DARC). This mutation gives profound protection against some malaria species and became almost universal in the African population (Walton and Rowland-Jones, 2008). Unfortunately, this mutation leads to significantly increased susceptibility to HIV-1 infection in those of African heritage and paradoxically to prolonged survival in HIV-1–infected individuals. This mutation may explain both the high incidence and prevalence of HIV in those of African heritage. Researchers think the gene variant arose tens of thousands of years ago, in response to a deadly strain of malaria.

Complications of HIV Infection

The HIV infection complications explained in this text include opportunistic infections, thrush, tuberculosis, *Pneumocystis* pneumonia, gastrointestinal dysfunction, AIDS dementia complex, gastrointestinal dysfunction, organ dysfunction, wasting, and lipodystrophy. Boxes 23-1 and 23-2 discuss characteristics of AIDS and the common problems these clients experience.

Box 23-1 ■ *Signs and Symptoms of AIDS*

AIDS is characterized by:

- Weakness
- Anorexia
- Diarrhea
- Weight loss
- Fever
- Decreased white blood cell count, or **leukopenia**

Box 23-2 ■ *Conditions Seen in Clients with HIV/AIDS*

Common problems associated with AIDS include:

- Opportunistic infections
- Gastrointestinal dysfunction
- Tumors
- AIDS dementia complex (ADC)
- Organ dysfunction

Opportunistic Infections

Parasitic, bacterial, viral, and fungal organisms are everywhere in our environment. A healthy person's immune system keeps these organisms in check and under control. AIDS places the client at high risk for certain infections, called **opportunistic infections.** Following the guidelines for safe food handling is especially important for this population. Opportunistic infections commonly seen in clients with AIDS include thrush, tuberculosis, and *Pneumocystis* pneumonia.

Thrush

A physical assessment may show signs of **thrush,** a thick whitish coating on the tongue or in the throat that may be accompanied by sore throat. See Figure 23-1. Thrush is a fungal infection that can cause oral ulcers, frequent fevers, and gastrointestinal inflammation. Basic teaching for mouth care by the health educator should include the following information:

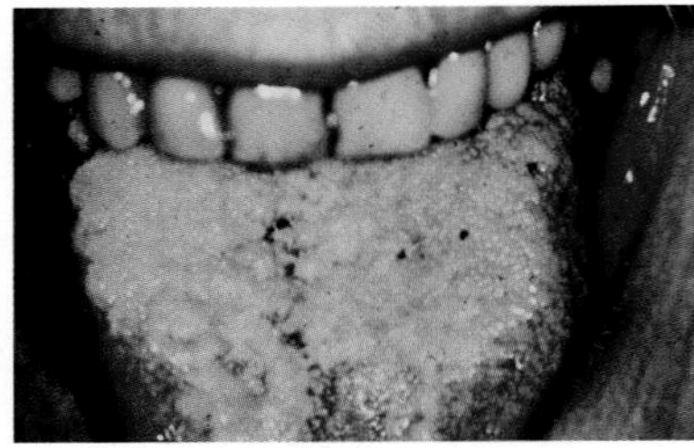

CANDIDIASIS

FIGURE 23-1 Thrush may cause mouth pain and interfere with nutritional intake. A soft diet may be helpful.

- Keep the mouth clean by rinsing with a dilute solution of hydrogen peroxide and water at least three times a day, especially after eating. Instruct clients not to swallow the solution.
- Use a cotton swab instead of a toothbrush if brushing is painful or causes bleeding. Commercial mouthwash may cause discomfort or pain.
- Avoid hot foods.
- Try soft foods, such as scrambled eggs, cottage cheese, mashed potatoes, mashed winter squash, puddings, custards, milk, juices (not citrus), canned fruits such as peaches, pears, and apricots, and bananas.
- Cut meat into small pieces or grind it or blend it.
- Supplement the diet with a complete oral nutritional supplement.
- Use a straw.
- Tilt the head forward or backward to ease swallowing.
- Avoid any food that causes discomfort. Fried, spicy, sour, salty, and sticky foods may not be tolerated, such as chips, nuts, seeds, raw vegetables, peanut butter, pickles, citrus fruits and juices, and tomatoes.

Tuberculosis

Tuberculosis (TB) is spread from person to person through tiny airborne particles. By sharing surroundings with a person who has active pulmonary TB, a susceptible person may inhale the disease-producing bacteria. Fortunately, most people who have inhaled these particles never become contagious or develop active TB. Even a healthy immune system cannot kill all the particles. HIV infection weakens the body's immune system and makes it more likely that the individual who has inhaled TB-related particles will develop active TB.

Pneumocystis Pneumonia

Pneumonia, characterized by shortness of breath, fatigue, and anorexia, is also common in AIDS clients. About 60% of AIDS clients are infected with one type of pneumonia-causing organism, called *Pneumocystis carinii*, hence the name ***Pneumocystis* pneumonia**. The organisms settle in the person's lungs, causing progressively worsening breathing problems and eventually leading to death. Many times clients with this infection are too tired to cook meals.

Gastrointestinal Dysfunction

The gastrointestinal tract is a common site for expression of HIV-related symptoms. The client may feel pain in the mouth or esophagus due to the growth of opportunistic infections. The client may have difficulty swallowing because of open lesions or sores.

AIDS commonly affects both the small and large intestine. The enzymes necessary for digestion and absorption in the wall of the small intestine may be lacking or present in insufficient amounts. Malabsorption may occur with diarrhea. Gut failure may follow. Medications to control these infections also contribute to the gastrointestinal dysfunction.

AIDS Dementia Complex

AIDS dementia complex (ADC) is the most common HIV-caused central nervous system illness associated with AIDS. Forty percent to 50% of adults with AIDS have some neurological dysfunction. Early symptoms of ADC are difficulty in concentration, slowness in thinking and response, and memory impairment. Behavioral symptoms include social withdrawal, apathy, and personality changes. Such symptoms may be interpreted solely as a psychiatric disorder. Motor symptoms include clumsiness of gait, difficulty with fine motor movements, and poor balance and coordination. Clients frequently become so mentally impaired that they cannot procure and prepare their own meals.

Organ Dysfunction

AIDS affects many organs in the body, leading to organ dysfunction. Diseases of the gallbladder, liver, and kidneys are seen in some AIDS clients:

Cholecystitis, inflammation of the gallbladder, can occur in conjunction with certain opportunistic infections seen in AIDS patients.

Hepatomegaly, an enlarged liver, is frequently seen and symptoms include pain, fever, and abnormal liver function test results, especially of the alkaline phosphatase level.

Pancreatitis, inflammation of the pancreas, has also been noted in some infected clients.

AIDS can lead to **end-stage renal failure** within weeks.

Wasting

AIDS wasting syndrome is characterized primarily by involuntary weight loss, consisting of both lean and fat body mass. In spite of treatment with medication, wasting remains a leading AIDS-defining event and is associated with high morbidity and mortality. Early studies have found that death occurred when body weight fell below 66% of ideal body weight due to starvation (Wasserman and Segal-Maurer, 2007). Analysis of body composition, measurement of soft tissue volumes (muscle, fat, and organ), and diagnostic imaging of adipose tissue distribution make it possible to define wasting syndrome in terms of total weight loss and tissue compartment loss.

Wasting may be caused by undernutrition or nutrient malabsorption. The body does not compensate by decreasing resting energy expenditure as it does during starvation in wasting. Thus, kcalorie need remains elevated, and when accompanied by anorexia, the result is a high fatality rate.

Lipodystrophy

Lipodystrophy is a syndrome of peripheral subcutaneous fat loss with visceral fat sparing. Clients who respond well to medication may still present with lipodystrophy syndrome. Metabolic abnormalities in total cholesterol, increased low-density lipoprotein, and increased triglycerides may necessitate that clients modify their diets accordingly.

Box 23-3 describes the signs and symptoms of lipodystrophy.

Treatment

A variety of new medications show some promise of killing or inhibiting the activity of the HIV virus. Clinical Application 23-1 discusses medication

Box 23-3 ■ *Signs and Symptoms of Lipodystrophy*

Characteristics of lipodystrophy:

- Increasing abdominal girth
- Decreasing fat in the extremities and face
- Advent of a buffalo hump
- Breast enlargement in patients with HIV, especially those on HAART with a protease inhibitor
- Increased serum triglyceride levels
- Increased glucose levels
- Increased insulin levels
- Increased blood pressure

23-1

Clinical Application

Medications Used for HIV and AIDS

Drug therapy for clients with HIV has increased in complexity. There are currently four classes of antiretroviral medications: nucleoside reverse transcriptase inhibitors, nonnucleoside reverse transcriptase inhibitors, protease inhibitors, and fusion inhibitors (American Dietetic Association, 2004). Lifelong medication therapy with combinations of these medications may be required for management and presents challenges to nutritional status by introducing potential interactions with food, body metabolism, and side effects. The following table lists common medications used in HIV/AIDS, typical dosing, and food tips.

Protease Inhibitors

MEDICATION	GENERIC NAME	DOSING	FOOD TIPS
Indinavir	Crixivan	bid, every 12 hours tid, every 8 hours	Take on an empty stomach to enhance absorption. Take with a light snack that contains 300 kcal, 6 grams of protein, and 2 grams of fat to reduce stomach upset. Drink at least 1 cup of water or juice (not grapefruit) with each dose. Drink a total of 10 cups of water and/or juice every day to prevent kidney stones.
Ritonavir	Norvir	bid	Take with a full meal. Complications may include diarrhea, lipodystrophy, and elevated lipids. Avoid alcohol.
Saquinavir	Fortovase (Invirase)	bid or tid	Take within 2 hours of a high-fat meal or snack. This will increase the drug's absorption by 5 to 10 times. A high-fat meal should contain about 55 grams of fat. Possible complications include lipodystrophy and elevated lipids.
Nelfinavir	Viracept	tid Doses should not exceed 12 hours	Take with food. Possible complications include diarrhea, lipodystrophy, and elevated lipids.
Didanosine (ddl)	Videx	Once per day	Take on an empty stomach. Do not take with other medications.
Lamivudine (3TC)	Epivir	bid	Take with or without food.
Stavudine (d4T)	Zerit	bid	Take with or without food.
Zalcitabine (ddC)	Hivid	tid	Take with or without food.
Zidovudine (AZT)	Retrovir	bid	Take with food, preferably nonfat. Take 400 IU vitamin E every day to decrease bone marrow suppression.
Abacavir	1592U89	bid	Take with or without food.
Nevirapine	Viramune	bid	No food restriction.
Delavirdine	Efavirenz	Once a day at bedtime	No food restriction.

How are the drugs mentioned in this table combined? Sometimes a protease inhibitor is combined with two nonnucleoside reverse transcriptase inhibitors. For example, Crixivan is combined with AZT and DDL. This requires following a tight schedule. Here is a sample schedule:

6:00 A.M.	Indinavir
7:00 A.M.	Breakfast and AZT
9:00 A.M.	DDL on an empty stomach
11:00 A.M.	Lunch
2:00 P.M.	Indinavir
5:00 P.M.	Dinner and AZT
8:00 P.M.	Snack
10:00 P.M.	Indinavir
12:00 A.M.	DDL on an empty stomach

Other medications may be useful in reversing the nutritional decline and sequelae associated with AIDS: Marinal, dronabinal, and megace have all been shown to have significant efficacy in:

- Appetite stimulation
- Increased kilocalorie intake
- Reversing weight loss
- Improving a client's sense of well-being

Meal plans to support medication regimens include not only meal timing but also carbohydrate, fat, and protein distribution and symptoms management strategies.

treatment for AIDS. Clients with HIV and AIDS take multiple prescribed medications, and almost all need extensive counseling on food and medication interactions. Resistance training may be beneficial for these clients, especially those that are losing lean body mass. Realistically, health-care intervention can only suppress most infections for these clients, not cure them.

Prevention and Counseling

All states and the District of Columbia have specific laws regarding HIV testing. Informed consent (the client or significant other must agree to testing) is required (Huang et al., 2006). Notification of a positive HIV test finding creates a crisis for the individual. A person who has had pretest counseling is more prepared and likely to cope better.

Counseling the individual on how best to fight the virus is important; for example, the HIV-positive individual needs to receive all current immunizations to boost his or her immunity. Behaviors that interfere with wellness and reduce immunity, include:

- Drinking alcohol
- Smoking
- Illegal drug use
- Poor nutrition

They should be discouraged. Adequate rest and exercise all can improve general good health and should be encouraged.

Nutrition and HIV Infection

Nutritional management is both a preventive and a therapeutic treatment in HIV infection. A malnourished client has a limited ability to fight infection. A well-nourished individual infected with the HIV virus is better able to resist opportunistic infections and tolerate the side effects of treatment. Good nutritional status may influence response to medications by:

- Decreasing the incidence of adverse drug reactions
- Providing nutrients for reactions evoked by medications
- Supporting organ functions

One study found the use of a multivitamin supplement delayed the onset of advanced disease and the need for antiretroviral therapy in HIV-positive people (Fawzi et al., 2004). Worldwide, few people who have advanced disease are receiving antiretroviral treatment. Micronutrient supplements have been proposed as a low-cost intervention that may slow the progression of HIV disease. The impact of micronutrient supplementation may be less in the developed nations of the world because the general population is far less likely to be malnourished.

Malnutrition in AIDS Clients

Malnutrition in clients with HIV/AIDS causes a number of physiological alterations that may lead to decreased resistance to infection and is an important predictor of morbidity and mortality. People who are malnourished are six times more likely to die than those who are adequately nourished. A well-balanced diet is essential to optimal immune function. See Box 23-4.

Malabsorption

Diarrhea and malabsorption are probably the major nutrition-related problems for AIDS clients. Diarrhea is also a side effect of antiretroviral medications.

Mucosal atrophy and decreased digestive enzyme activity contribute to the malabsorption and diarrhea seen in persons with AIDS. Carbohydrate and fat malabsorption are frequently seen in AIDS clients with diarrhea. Gastrointestinal problems such as diarrhea may occur in children with HIV infection due to disaccharide intolerance rather than to enteric infection with known pathogens.

Malabsorption of fat, simple sugars, and vitamin B_{12} is known to occur in clients with intestinal infections. AIDS clients who have diarrhea or malabsorption clearly have additional vitamin and mineral needs. Clinicians should measure 25-hydroxy-vitamin D levels (as an indicator of fat-soluble vitamin absorption) and folate or zinc (as an indicator of water-soluble vitamin status; Mason and Roubenoff, 1999).

Box 23-4 ■ *Effects of Malnutrition*

Malnutrition causes numerous physiological alterations within the body. Some of the changes include:

- Increased gut permeability, which allows more alien material to be absorbed into the body
- Decreased intestinal secretions; some of these secretions are necessary for the proper digestion and absorption of food.
- A change in intestinal flora, which may affect the utilization of nutrients
- Hormonal imbalances
- Decreased ability to repair tissue; the body ceases to replace and repair tissue because it lacks the raw materials to do so.

Initially, dietary treatment involves identification of the cause of the diarrhea and a determination of which nutrients the client cannot absorb. The concentration of hydrogen in the breath can be measured after oral lactose or sucrose administration to determine whether the client is intolerant to either of these sugars. An elevated breath hydrogen level implies intolerance, because hydrogen is primarily a product of metabolism of these sugars by colon bacteria.

Fecal microbiological evaluations and intestinal biopsies are used to determine absorptive capability. In some clients infected with HIV, malabsorption of sucrose, maltose, lactose, and fat has been documented, even in the absence of diarrhea.

Clients with a form of carbohydrate intolerance may benefit from either a lactose-restricted or a disaccharide-free diet. A disaccharide-free diet is indicated for severe intolerance to sugar. Sucrose needs to be broken down into glucose and fructose (lactose into glucose and galactose; maltose into glucose and glucose) before absorption is possible.

A disaccharide-free diet excludes most fruits and vegetables and many starches and is nutritionally inadequate. Vitamin C is deficient, and daily supplementation is recommended. Some of these clients may tolerate a small amount of sugar, but they usually need assistance in understanding their tolerance level. A lactose-free diet may be sufficient for clients who are deficient only in lactase.

A low-fat diet may be necessary to control steatorrhea. Several additional meal-planning tips are suggested to promote the client's well-being and to control the malabsorption:

- Fluids should be encouraged to maintain hydration when large fluid volume is lost in stools.
- Yogurt and other foods that contain the *Lactobacillus acidophilus* culture may be helpful if bacteria overgrowth is a problem secondary to long-term anti-infective use.
- Small, frequent meals make the best use of a limited absorptive capacity of the gut.
- A multivitamin supplement is indicated to increase the amount of vitamin available for absorption.
- Oral liquid nutritional supplements may be helpful.
- Aggressive nutritional support such as enteral and parenteral nutrition, if appropriate, should be considered.
- Pancreatric enzymes (Pancrecarb) may be prescribed as indicated.
- Avoidance of sorbital, which is used as a sweetening agent in both sugar-free candies and some medications, has been shown to cause diarrhea and should be avoided.
- Caffeine should be avoided, as it stimulates peristalsis.
- Fiber-containing supplements may be useful.

In some situations, the malabsorption is highly resistant to treatment. Nutritional therapy goals should maximize client comfort. The benefits of overly restricting the client's diet may not suffice to offset the resulting loss in client comfort in an incurable situation.

Increased Nutritional Requirements

Several studies suggest that the resting energy expenditure (REE) is elevated in patients with early HIV infection and increases with subsequent AIDS (Smith and Lowry, 1999). Fever and infection increase kilocaloric, protein, and certain mineral and vitamin requirements.

Historically, dietitians have used the **Harris–Benedict equation** and multiplied the appropriate stress and activity factors to estimate kilocaloric requirements. Many software programs in use are still based on this equaton. The American Dietetic Association in their Evidenced Based Library recommends that kcal needs be measured by indirect calorimetry. If this technology is not available, the second best method for estimating a client's energy need is the Mifflin-St. Jeor equation (www.adaevidencelibrary.com). See Chapter 22.

Hypometabolism

Not all patients with AIDS become hypermetabolic. Studies have indicated that a small percentage of the AIDS population without secondary infection may be hypometabolic and demonstrate a response similar to that seen in starvation (Smith and Lowry, 1999). Hypometabolic patients need a gradual increase in kilocalories and a lower kilocalorie:nitrogen ratio. These patients should also be monitored for refeeding syndrome.

Decreased Food Intake

Anorexia can be a major problem for many clients with AIDS. A poor food intake may be the result of fever, respiratory infections, drug side effects, gastrointestinal complications, oral and esophageal pain, and emotional stress. Clients with AIDS Dementia–Related

Complex (ADC) may experience mechanical problems with eating.

Nutritional Care in AIDS

Manifestations of the HIV virus vary greatly from one client to another. Therefore, nutritional care must be tailored to each client's unique set of symptoms. Quality nutritional care starts with screening.

Screening

Screening HIV-infected clients for nutritional problems is a crucial component of quality client care. Early indicators of decreased nutritional status include decreases in usual body weight, low weight for height, a low albumin level, and a body mass index (BMI) of < 20.

Nutritional assessment of persons living with HIV is important at all stages of the disease to identify the 25% to 35% with inadequate intake who require counseling (Woods et al., 2002). The following should be included in the assessment process:

- A baseline measure of percent body fat and lean body mass to monitor disease progression
- Recent food intake
- Barriers the client may have to safe nutritious food
- Lack of food and poor food choices, which are linked to transmission of HIV infection and a poor response to treatment.

Referral to a social worker is always indicated to address these challenging issues.

Planning Nutrient Delivery

In keeping with the general principle "if the gut works, use it," every effort should be made to feed the client orally. The following dietary modifications to oral intake may be helpful:

- Changing the meal plan, which may resolve the anorexia commonly seen in AIDS clients
- Offering small, frequent feedings
- Serving food cold or at room temperature, which may help some clients consume more kilocalories
- Modifying seasonings and kilocaloric density, which may improve intake
- Modifying texture, which may assist the client with poor chewing ability or oral lesions

If the client is unable to consume sufficient nutrients from table foods, supplemental feedings or other enteral feedings should be considered. The type of malnutrition should influence the food and supplements offered, which the dietitian usually determines.

If the client is unable to consume sufficient nutrients orally and the gut is working, a tube feeding may be considered. Percutaneous endoscopic gastrostomy (PEG) tubes are often used. If the gut is not functioning properly, peripheral parenteral nutrition (PPN) or total parenteral nutrition (TPN) may be considered. The goal should always be to prolong living, not to prolong dying. A client has the right to refuse any alternative-feeding route offered.

Monitoring

To ensure that adequate nutrients are being consumed, body weight, waist circumference, and nutritional intake should be monitored every few weeks along with BMI and percent body fat. The loss of lean tissue central to body metabolism may be present throughout the disease process, regardless of weight maintenance, suggesting that weight is not a good early indicator of declining nutritional status. Throughout this process, health-care workers should maintain a supportive, nonjudgmental approach, which is the key to establishing a trusting relationship.

Client Teaching

An assessment of the client's knowledge level and understanding of an individualized meal plan is appropriate. All AIDS clients need instruction on food safety because low immune system functioning makes them much more susceptible to food-borne illnesses. Education will minimize the likelihood of opportunistic infection. Instructions on dietary modifications including nutrient-dense meals and the use of supplemental feedings are also indicated. See Box 23-5.

Food Faddism and Quackery

Some clients with AIDS are vulnerable to both food faddism and quackery because they become desperate to try anything that arouses hope.

Food faddism is an unusual pattern of food behavior enthusiastically adapted by its adherents.

Food quackery is the promotion for profit of a medical scheme or remedy that is unproved or known to be false.

Box 23-5 ■ *Counseling the Client With HIV and AIDS*

These nutritional principals are important to discuss with AIDS clients soon after the initial diagnosis.

- Review the principles of safe food handling and storage with the client.
- Discuss considering multivitamin and mineral supplement.
- Discourage inappropriate weight loss as many HIV clients lose lean body mass first and fat second. Address prevention, restoration, and maintenance of optimal body composition with emphasis on lean tissue. Encourage physical activity.
- If indicated, encourage more and frequent meals to increase energy intake. Snacks, complete nutritional supplements, and intravenous feedings may be necessary.
- Suggest including soluble-fiber supplementation, which has been shown to be an effective treatment for diarrhea (Brown and Batterham, 2001).
- Discuss potential medication–nutrition interactions.
- Review use of nutrient supplements and potential interactions with nonprescription and herbal supplements.
- Address food and nutrition security issues. Refer to the social worker if the client lacks enough food.

During counseling, evaluate signs and symptoms and tailor counseling to the client's unique needs. In addition, closely monitor the client's blood lipids, triglyceride, glucose, and cholesterol levels and recommend modification of the diet as indicated.

Health-care educators need to carefully balance and consider the danger of unusual food behaviors versus taking away any hope the client may have. Clients may tune out educators if they perceive that their beliefs and feelings are discounted without sensitivity. Some unusual food behaviors are not harmful, and some food behaviors can result in negative health consequences. See Dollars and Sense 23-1.

Follow-Up Care

The nutritional status of a client may depend on appropriate follow-up care. A referral to a community agency, a home health-care program, an outpatient clinic, or a dietitian should be made to provide continuity of care.

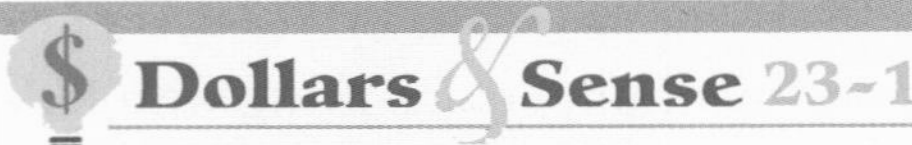

Dollars & Sense 23-1

No Money for Food

The client with limited resources who spends money on dietary supplements and herbal products of limited health benefits and spends very little or no money on food will develop malnutrition.

A reliable desktop reference and carefully chosen Internet sites can help the health educator recommend what is inappropriate. Care must be taken by health educators not to use Internet sites that sell questionable products.

Keystones

- The AIDS epidemic is worldwide.
- Although HAART and treatment with protease inhibitors have reduced mortality rates, no cure has been found for AIDS.
- Transmittal routes include blood-to-blood, perinatal, and sexual contact.
- As health-care professionals, we can all protect ourselves from AIDS by using extreme care when handling blood and equipment that has been in contact with blood and as private individuals by practicing safe sexual behaviors.
- HIV attacks the immune system and leaves its victims defenseless against opportunistic infections.
- AIDS is a disease with many clinical complications.
- Nutritional management is both a preventive and a therapeutic treatment in clients infected with HIV.
- Increased nutrient needs, decreased food intake, and impaired nutrient absorption contribute to the malnutrition seen in AIDS clients.

CASE STUDY 23-1

Ms. S is a 30-year-old woman who acquired HIV from her drug-abusing husband and subsequently infected their son in utero. She could not believe the test results when she was first told. Now she is seeking nutritional information to allow her to increase her chance for a quality life and her son's chance to survive infancy. Her knowledge of basic nutrition is good. She expressed some concern about transportation and has already missed one of her prenatal visits because her husband sold their car for money to buy drugs. She is also unable to go to the grocery store easily. She is 5 ft 6 in. tall and weighs 120 lb. All her laboratory work was within normal limits. Percent body fat is 25%.

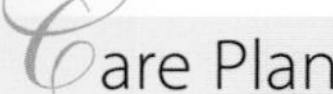

Care Plan

Subjective Data

Lack of information on relationship of nutrition to AIDS ■ Concrete goals established

Objective Data

HIV-positive tests, both mother and infant ■ Percent body fat, 25%

Analysis

Lack of information related to modifying AIDS progression and changing unhealthy home environment

Plan

DESIRED OUTCOMES EVALUATION CRITERIA	ACTIONS/INTERVENTIONS	RATIONALE
Client will verbalize areas in which nutrition could affect AIDS development.	Reinforce need for regular, balanced meals. Emphasize adequate kcalories.	The stress of receiving this diagnosis may impede use of previously learned information.
	Instruct Ms. S to keep home environment clean, especially kitchen, bathroom, and basements, where molds and fungi could thrive.	Organisms that are harmless to persons with normal immune systems can cause opportunistic infections in HIV-infected persons.
	Teach client to monitor herself and her son for changes in health related to food intake or digestion.	Discovering beginning malabsorption problems would permit treatment before malnutrition becomes apparent.
Client will monitor her percent body fat.	Explain the relationships among percent body fat, percent lean body mass, and exercise.	Exercise can prevent a loss of lean body mass.
		Weight can be stable but body fat content can increase.
Client will keep her medical appointments and obtain groceries as needed.	Refer to social worker for help with transportation.	The social worker has knowledge of local available resources.

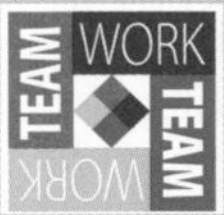

23-1

Social Worker's Note

If the client is an inpatient, the social worker typically writes in the discharge planning section of the medical record. If the client is an outpatient, the social worker typically phones the physician's office directly with a solution to the problem and writes a short note to be placed in the medical record.

Note: I met with the client, who described a sad home situation. We discussed the need for her to remove herself and unborn child from her present environment. I arranged for client to move into a shelter for abused women. She agreed to do this immediately.

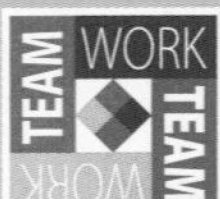

23-2

Dietitian's Notes

The following Dietitian's Notes are representative of the documentation found in a client's medical record.

Subjective: Met with the client, who expressed an interest in making any improvements to her diet. She currently eats three times each day and does not avoid any of the major food groups. She does not take a multivitamin/mineral supplement.

Objective: 5 ft 6 in. Percent body fat 25%; 120 lb

Analysis: Ideal body weight range 117 to 143 lb. Weight in kg is 54.5 kg. Estimated kcal need at 25 to 35 kcal/kg and 54.5 kg equals 1363 to 1907. Estimated protein need at 1.0 to 1.5 grams/kg equals 54.4 to 82 grams. Clients reported food intake based on a 24-hour dietary recall and cross checked with a food frequency showed a kcalorie intake between 1400 and 1600. Her usual protein intake is between 40 and 50 grams per day. We discussed options for the client to increase her protein intake.

Plan: Recommend the addition of one cup of low-fat yogurt or milk per day. Client agreed to do this.

Critical Thinking Questions

1. The client has developed mouth sores from thrush and would like you to arrange for her to have TPN. She claims it is just too painful to eat. What would you recommend?
2. The client's child has been diagnosed HIV positive. During a home visit, you notice the kitchen is filthy. You instruct the client on food safety and sanitation. On a return visit, despite prior instruction on food safety, you notice that the client's kitchen is still not clean. The client claims she is too tired to clean. What do you do?
3. The client went to a health food store and purchased several bottles of vitamin pills and herbal supplements. She believes she can take these in lieu of eating. What should you do?

Chapter Review

1. The health-care worker's best insurance against HIV transmission on the job is:
   a. Frequent hand washing
   b. Universal precautions
   c. Body substance isolation
   d. Adherence to all food safety policies and procedures
2. A client on HAART can partially compensate for fat redistribution syndrome by:
   a. Taking medications as prescribed
   b. Taking supplemental vitamins and minerals
   c. Consuming a low-fat diet
   d. Exercising

Chapter Review—cont'd

3. Compared to wasting, cachexia is:
   a. A slower process
   b. The result of both a protein and kilocalorie deficit
   c. Always the result of a poor food intake
   d. Best treated by the inclusion of 400 additional kilocalories per day
4. Clinicians measure ____ as an indicator of fat-soluble vitamin absorption.
   a. Folate
   b. Zinc
   c. 25-Hydroxy-vitamin D
   d. Glucose
5. Educating an AIDS client about food safety is important:
   a. To minimize the risk of rare tumors
   b. To prevent body fat redistribution
   c. To enhance renal function
   d. To prevent opportunistic infections

Clinical Analysis

1. Mr. Y, a 45-year-old black man, was diagnosed as HIV-positive 1 month ago. His height is 6 ft 0 in. and his weight is 178 lb and stable. He reports no signs or symptoms and has not seen a physician yet. He wants to know what he should eat. As the nurse during this first visit, you might discuss:
   a. The many benefits of HAART
   b. Food safety, exercise, good nutrition, and the importance of follow-up with a physician
   c. The expected outcome and potential complications
   d. Vitamin–mineral supplementation, increased kilocalorie needs, and the treatment for malabsorption
2. Carlos, a 25-year-old Hispanic man, presents with severe diarrhea. He was diagnosed with HIV about 8 years ago. He has five to six watery stools each day that do not appear to be related to his medications. His height is 5 ft 10 in., and his weight is 140 lb (usual weight is 175 lb). He is an inpatient, and the physician has ordered a stool culture but the results are not back. You recommend:
   a. Extra fluids with meals to prevent dehydration
   b. A clear-liquid, complete nutritional supplement
   c. A high-fat and high-fiber diet to provide both kilocalories and bulk to his diet
   d. Six small meals with a milkshake between meals to push kilocalories and protein
3. Dave, a 36-year-old white man, complains of fatigue. He is often too tired to cook and has little interest in food. He lives alone and is on disability. His CD_4 cell count is 400, and his viral load is 100,000. You recommend:
   a. A tube feeding
   b. Referral to a social service agency for a friendly visitor
   c. Meals-on-Wheels
   d. Six small meals daily

24

Nutritional Care of the Terminally Ill

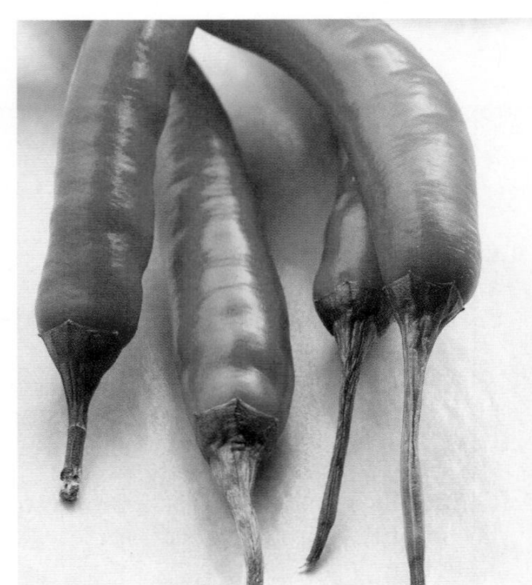

LEARNING OBJECTIVES

After completing this chapter, the student should be able to:

- Differentiate between palliative and curative nutritional care.
- State appropriate nutritional screening questions for the terminally ill client.
- List at least two appropriate dietary management techniques for symptom control for each of the following: anemia, anorexia, bowel obstruction, cachexia, constipation, cough, dehydration, diarrhea, dysgeusia, esophageal reflux, fever, fluid accumulation, hiccups, incontinence, jaundice and hepatic encephalopathy, migraine headache, nausea and vomiting, pruritus, stomatitis, weakness, wounds and pressure sores, and **xerostomia.**
- State appropriate assessment questions for a terminally ill client.
- Discuss the ethical and legal considerations for feeding a terminally ill client.

This chapter discusses clients who have been certified by physicians to be terminally ill. An individual is considered terminally ill if he or she has a medical prognosis of 6 months or less based on the usual disease progression. Although a physician can estimate life expectancy based on disease progression, this is not an exact science. A client diagnosed with a terminal disease may live longer or less long than predicted because the disease may not follow its usual progression. Individuals who have been certified by a physician as terminally ill can elect the Hospice benefit under federal guidelines (www.ncfa.gov/medicaid). Hospice is the major health-care program for the terminally ill in the United States.

Dealing With Death

Our culture emphasizes the enjoyment of life. At the beginning of this century, most people died at home, and many died young. Death was a part of everyday life. In the past 50 years, most people have died in hospitals or long-term care facilities. Often an ambulance is called if a person is dying.

Although health-care workers have received much training on how to reverse the effects of disease, we have received much less training on how to assist our clients with dying. With changes in the health-care system bringing decreased lengths of hospital stays, an increasing number of clients will again be cared for in their homes. Training health-care workers to provide home care for terminally ill clients is becoming essential.

Nutritional and dietary issues are at the center of some ethical questions concerning the care of these clients. Health-care professionals need to address patients' values, goals of care, and preferences with regard to treatment to truly become patient advocates.

The Dying Process

Death is an unavoidable part of the life cycle. Both physiological and psychological changes occur as part of the dying process. The client's age, diagnosis, and physical condition influence physiological changes. Regardless of the underlying disease, cardiopulmonary failure is the final cause of death. Pulmonary and circulatory failure may be gradual or sudden. The major signs and symptoms in the final days and hours of life include:

- Cessation of eating and drinking
- Oliguria and incontinence
- Muscle weakness
- Difficulty in breathing
- Cyanosis
- Decreased mental alertness
- Changes in vital signs.

Hospice team members may describe clients with a terminal diagnosis as actively dying. An actively dying client has a life expectancy of a few hours or a few days. The reason for the actively dying designation is to determine staff needs.

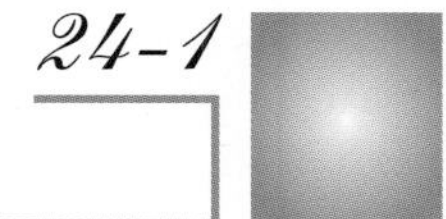

Physiological Response to Fluid Restriction

Young, healthy, active individuals who are deprived of water develop thirst, dry mouth, and headache, followed by fatigue; cognitive impairment occurs as dehydration progresses and becomes severe with abnormal electrolytes, rising blood urea nitrogen, and hemoconcentration. If water is not taken, renal failure is likely.

In terminally ill clients, dehydration results in the same signs and symptoms. However, these metabolic changes may produce a sedative effect on the brain just before death. In cases where the evidence in the case strongly suggests that hydration or feeding does not provide benefit, the healthcare team has a responsibility to explain this to the patient or authorized surrogate, but the patient or authorized surrogate must decide whether to provide hydration (American Dietetic Association, 2008a).

Withholding nutrition has been studied closely and the majority of reports indicate that physiological adaptation allows patients not to suffer from the absence of food (American Dietetic Association, 2008a).

Cessation of Eating and Drinking

Life will soon cease when a client's eating and drinking diminishes critically. One study reported that 8% of clients with cancer completely cease to eat or drink (Feuz and Rapin, 1994). Oral intake dwindles because a client has no desire to eat or because disease prevents digestion. This greatly decreased oral intake is often worrisome to family members.

Health-care workers need to counsel family members that dehydration at this time is believed to have a euphoric effect and is not painful. Clinical Application 24-1 discusses the physiological responses to fluid restriction. Fluids and comfort care such as the following actions can reduce the thirst sensations from dehydration:

- Ice chips
- Lubricating the lips
- Small amounts of food and water

Withholding and minimizing hydration can have the desirable effect of reducing:

- Disturbing oral secretions
- Bronchial secretions
- Need for frequent urination
- Cough from diminished pulmonary congestion

It is unkind to force food or fluids on a client who is actively dying.

Oliguria and Incontinence

Because oral intake is usually decreased for several days before death, urine output is often diminished and may cease. The color of the urine may become very dark. A period of incontinence often precedes the oliguria, and anuria occurs. General fatigue, muscle weakness, and decreased mental acuity are among the reasons for the incontinence. Bedding should be changed as quickly as possible to avoid skin irritation. Death usually occurs within 48 to 72 hours after urine output stops.

Difficulty in Breathing

Most clients have some difficulty breathing before death. Caregivers may become alarmed when they hear a loud, hoarse, and bubbling sound. This sound is caused by the passage of breath through pharyngeal and pulmonary secretions that lodge at the back of the client's throat. Atropine is often administered to decrease the secretions. Elevating the head of the bed, gentle suctioning, and positioning the client on his or her side help maintain a clear airway. All terminally ill clients do not have these sounds with respiration. Some clients experience apnea (a temporary cessation of breathing). A change such as these in breathing is an indicator that life will soon cease.

Cyanosis

Slightly bluish, grayish, or dark purple discoloration of the skin caused by poor oxygenation is called **cyanosis**. The client's feet, legs, hands, and groin feel cold. Many health-care workers believe this is one of the most useful indicators that the end of life is approaching. Slowed circulation and decreased tissue perfusion cause these signs.

Decreased Mental Alertness

The amount of blood reaching the brain, lungs, liver, and kidneys decreases as general circulation slows. Sleepiness, apathy, disorientation, confusion, restlessness, and finally a decreased level of consciousness that frequently progresses to a sleep-like state are among the signs that death is imminent.

Changes in Vital Signs

Signs of impeding death include:

- A decrease in body temperature
- An increase in pulse rate
- A rise and then a decrease in respirations
- A fall in blood pressure

Death occurs when there is no pulse and respiration ceases.

Family members and caregivers of terminally ill clients often express fear at the thought of being alone with an actively dying client. For this reason, health-care workers often remain with the client and their loved ones during this time. Some health-care workers resist working with the terminally ill because they think that they cannot cope with this experience. However, death is not always a painful experience. Health-care workers who share the death experience with a client and the client's family often describe the experience as rewarding and profound.

Palliative versus Curative Care

Palliative care has been defined as the active total care of an individual when curative measures are no longer considered an option by either the medical team or the client. The goal of curative care is arresting the disease. The goal of palliative care is the relief of symptoms to alleviate or ease pain and discomfort. Emphasis in palliative care is placed on addressing:

- Pain
- Loneliness
- Loss of control

These concerns are common in dying clients. Palliative care programs address and include the client and family members in the plan of care.

Hospice dates back to medieval times. During the crusades, travelers needed a place to stop for comfort. The Knights of Hospitallers of the Order of St. John of Jerusalem in the twelfth century sheltered sick and religious pilgrims. They established hospices in England, Germany, Italy, Cyprus, and Rhodes. The soul, the mind, and the spirit were considered as much in need of help as the body.

Around the fifteenth century, anatomic and surgical practices developed. Physicians moved into hospitals that emphasized curative treatments. Monks and nuns remained in cloisters and cared for the people the physicians could not heal, including the disabled, the chronically ill, and the terminally ill.

During the eighteenth and nineteenth centuries, great advances in curative treatments occurred, and hospitals became highly specialized in acute life-threatening situations. Hospitals were less able to offer shelter to people nearing life's end. At the same time, caring for the terminally ill became less a private or religious function and more a public and governmental one.

The modern hospice has its roots in the late nineteenth century, when a place of shelter for the incurably ill was founded in Dublin. The British physician Dr. Cicely Saunders inspired the hospice movement in the United States. Dr. Saunders is noted for her work in pain control and for the founding of St. Christopher's Hospice in London in 1967. The first operational hospice program in the United States was established in New Haven, Connecticut, in the early 1970s.

Hospice philosophy includes the belief that death is a natural aspect of life. Hospice is committed to the philosophy that persons have the right to die in the setting of their choice and to be as comfortable as possible. Central to the hospice philosophy is the idea that palliative care is appropriate when treatment of the client's disease becomes ineffective and irrelevant. Studies suggest that medical care for patients with serious advanced illnesses is characterized by:

- Undertreatment of symptoms
- Conflict about who should make decisions about patient care
- Impairments in caregivers' physical and psychological health
- Depletion of family resources (Morrison and Meier, 2004)

Nutrition Screening

All palliative care begins with the establishment of the goals of care. Studies suggest that what terminally ill patients want is to:

- Have their pain and other symptoms relieved
- Improve their quality of life

- Avoid being a burden to their family
- Have a close relationship with loved ones
- Maintain a sense of control

The goal of palliative nutritional care is to assist the client and caregiver with any food-related concerns. These difficulties may be related to uncomfortable symptoms and attitudes and beliefs held about food. Screening the client with a terminal illness for food-related concerns is the first step. There are major differences between screening a client who is undergoing curative or preventive treatment and screening a terminally ill client who is receiving palliative care.

First, the health-care worker needs to ascertain if the client has any symptoms that may be diminished by nutritional intervention. Second, the attitudes and beliefs of the client or caregiver about food need to be examined. Some clients and their caregivers have difficulty accepting that the terminally ill client frequently eats much less than is needed to sustain life. Box 24-1 is an example of a nutrition screening form for the client with a terminal condition.

Health-care professionals, patients, and family members frequently want to discuss the use of an intravenous or tube feedings in a terminally ill patient during the screening process. The frequency of percutaneous endoscopic gastrostomy (PEG) tube use has increased from 15,000 in 1989 to 123,000 in 1995 (Mallett, Potter, and Heller, 2002).

The use of any artificial feeding should always be considered but is often inconsistent with treatment goals. For example, in the case of a patient with end-stage dementia who has dysphagia, placement of a PEG tube may be considered (Morrison and Meier, 2004). If the treatment goal of the patient is to reduce suffering and enhance the quality of life, a PEG tube is unlikely to meet this goal. The position of the American Dietetic Association is that individuals have the right to request or refuse nutrition and hydration as medical treatment. This refusal includes a PEG tube placement. If death is immient and feeding will not alter the condition, the health-care provider should consider whether or not nutrient support will be burdensome (American Dietetic Association, 2008a).

Assessment

During the nutritional assessment, every question posed to the client or caregiver should have a purpose. Health-care workers generally need to know the results of laboratory tests, diagnostic procedures, physical examinations, and anthropometric measures as well as the level of immune function and food intake information to determine a client's nutritional status, which may have no value in the provision of nutritional care for a terminally ill client, however.

For example, why ask if a client drinks milk? Is it to estimate if the client is meeting the calcium, riboflavin, and vitamin D allowances? If it is determined that the client's milk intake is suboptimal, would anything

Box 24-1 ■ *Sample Nutrition Screening Form**

Name _____ Caregiver's Name _____

Date _____ Diagnosis _____

1. Have you had any concerns about weight changes or food intake?

   No _____ Yes _____ Describe _____

2. For clients on tube feedings or parenteral feedings only: Have your feedings created or increased discomfort, diarrhea, distension, other?

   Type: _____ Amount _____ Infusion rate _____

3. Do you feel your symptoms could be decreased or controlled through dietary change?

   _____ No _____ Yes Describe _____

4. Do you feel diet or nutritional supplement would benefit you or your disease process?

   _____ No _____ Yes Type _____

5. Do you believe that your diet caused your disease or will slow the progression of your disease?

   _____ No _____ Yes Describe _____

6. Do you find eating enhances comfort? _____ No _____ Yes
7. What concerns do you have regarding your diet intake? _____
8. Would you (client or caregiver) like to discuss food-related concerns with the dietitian? _____ No _____ Yes

*For printing, available on DavisPlus.

be done about the inadequacy? If the client has diarrhea with severe abdominal cramping after the ingestion of milk, however, a recommendation to drink lactose-free milk would be appropriate. Unless the client will experience relief from bothersome symptoms, it is best not to recommend behavioral changes that may be difficult for the client to make. On the other hand, if the client expresses concern about the nutritional adequacy of his or her diet, nutrition education is not contraindicated. See Box 24-1.

Intervention and Symptom Control

Box 24-2 describes appropriate dietary management for symptom control for a client with a terminal illness. If a health-care worker feels uncomfortable discussing these issues with the client or lacks the time to counsel the client, a referral to the dietitian is indicated.

Ethical and Legal Considerations

Many of the legal and ethical issues concerning health-care delivery and health-care provider–client relations involve the provision of nutrition and hydration. In the past, before the development of tube feedings and intravenous feedings, the inability to eat and drink by mouth meant death from progressive body wasting. Stopping food or water inevitably leads to death within 14 days from dehydration (Wade, 2001).

Box 24-2 ■ *Dietary Management for Symptom Control*

Anemia

- Recommend a vitamin C source with red meats and iron-fortified foods.
- Discourage use of coffee, tea, and chocolate if the client has gastrointestinal bleeding.
- Recommend a multivitamin supplement if the client desires, but avoid megadose vitamins.

Anorexia

- Discuss practical issues with the client or caregiver, such as food attitudes, social aspects of eating, food preferences, and beliefs about food.
- Encourage concentration on the sensual pleasure of eating, such as table setting, garnishes, smells, and socialization.
- Evaluate the client's desire for a sense of well-being.
- Suggest use of small, frequent feedings.
- Educate the caregiver to recognize early signs of malnutrition and provide protein supplements, make food accessible, and encourage eating as desired by the client and caregiver if the client's prognosis is more than a few weeks.
- Evaluate the client's acceptance of a liquid diet and recommend complete oral nutritional supplements.
- Teach the caregiver that the client has the right to self-determination and may refuse to eat or drink when actively dying. The caregiver should continue to offer nourishment as a sign of love and caring but not harass the client to eat or drink.

Bowel Obstruction

- NPO may be indicated; limited clear liquids may be possible.
- Encourage small meals low in fiber and residue if oral intake is not contraindicated.
- Encourage the client to eat slowly, chew food well, and rest after each meal if oral intake is not contraindicated.
- Recommend dry feedings if oral intake is not contraindicated.
- Recommend avoidance of sugary fatty foods, alcohol, and foods with a strong odor.

Cachexia

- Teach relaxation techniques and encourage use before mealtime.
- Encourage the client and the caregiver to concentrate on the sensual pleasures of eating such as setting an attractive table and plate and using food garnishes and providing an appetizing eating environment by removing bedpans and emesis basin before serving the food.
- Evaluate client for dysgeusia and dysphagia and xerostomia.

Constipation

- Encourage high-fiber foods (bran, whole grains, fruits, vegetables, nuts, and legumes) if an adequate fluid intake can be maintained.
- Instruct the client to avoid high-fiber foods if dehydration or an obstruction is suspected or anticipated.
- Assess the client's fluid intake and recommend an increased intake if needed.
- Recommend taking 1 to 2 ounces of a special recipe with the evening meal: 2 cups applesauce, 2 cups unprocessed bran (All-Bran®), and 1 cup of 100% prune juice. Refrigerate this mixture between uses and discard after 5 days if not used.
- Suggest limiting cheese and high-fat, sugary foods (doughnuts, cakes, pies, cookies) that may be constipating.
- Discontinue calcium and iron supplements if they contribute to constipation.
- Review the client's medications. If the client is taking bulking agents (milk of magnesia, magnesium citrate, Metamucil®, or Golytely®), a large fluid intake is essential. Suggest the client or caregiver mask the taste of these medications in applesauce, mashed potatoes, gravy, orange juice, and nectars.

Cough

- Encourage fluids and ice chips.
- Recommend hard candy, including sour balls.
- Have the client try tea and coffee to dilate pulmonary vessels.

Dehydration

- Encourage intake of fluids such as juices, ice cream, gelatin, custards, puddings, and soups if the client's life expectancy is more than a few days.
- Encourage the client to try creative beverages such as orange sherbet and milkshake.

Box 24-2 ■ *Dietary Management for Symptom Control—cont'd*

- Consider a nasogastric tube feeding for fluid delivery only after a discussion with other team members, client, and caregivers. Plain water and foods high in electrolytes can be delivered via a tube feeding.
- Consider a parenteral line only after a tube feeding is considered and rejected and after an in depth discussion with the team members, client, and family. Client goals, expectations, and quality-of-life issues should all be very carefully considered. Parenteral lines for the delivery of nutrients and water are rarely indicated in terminally ill clients. There is strong clinical, ethical, and legal support for and against the administration of food and water when issues arise regarding what is and is not wanted by the patient and what is or is not warranted by empirical and clinical evidence (ADA, 2002).

Diarrhea

- Consider modification of the diet to omit lactose, gluten, or fat if related to diarrhea.
- Suggest a decrease in dietary fiber content.
- Consider the omission of gas-forming vegetables if an association between the consumption of these foods and diarrhea can be ascertained.
- Consider the use of a low-residue diet.
- Encourage consumption of high-potassium foods (bananas, tomato juice, orange juice, potatoes) if the client is dehydrated.
- Recommend dry feedings (drink fluids 1 hour before or 30 to 60 minutes after meals).
- Encourage intake of medium-chain triglycerides and a diet high in protein and carbohydrates for steatorrhea due to pancreatic insufficiency.
- Consider the use of a complete oral nutritional supplement to provide adequate nutrient composition while helping the client overcome mild-to-moderate malabsorption.
- For copious diarrhea or diarrhea combined with a coccyx decubitus, consider use of a clear-liquid complete nutritional supplement or a predigested oral nutritional supplement.

Disgeusia (abnormal taste)

- Encourage oral care before mealtime.
- Evaluate whether the client experiences a bitter, sweet, or no taste after food consumption.
- If foods taste bitter, encourage consumption of poultry, fish, milk and milk products, and legumes. Recommend the use of marinated meats and poultry in juices or wine. Sour and salty foods are generally not liked when a client experiences a bitter taste. Cook food in a glass or porcelain container to improve taste. Recommend a decreased use of red meats, sour juices, coffee, tea, tomatoes, and chocolate. The use of a modular protein supplement may be helpful if the client's protein intake is suboptimal.
- If foods taste sweet, recommend sour juices, tart foods, lemon juice, vinegar, pickles, spices, herbs, and the use of a modular carbohydrate supplement.
- If food has no taste, recommend foods served at room temperature, highly seasoned foods, and sugary foods.

Dyspnea (difficulty breathing)

- Encourage intake of coffee, tea, carbonated beverages, and chocolate. These foods are bronchodilators that increase blood pressure, dilate pulmonary vessels, increase glomerular filtration rate, and thereby break up and expel pulmonary secretions and fluids.
- Encourage use of a soft diet. Liquids are usually better tolerated than solids. Cold foods are often better accepted than hot foods.
- Recommend small, frequent feedings.
- Encourage ice chips, frozen fruit juices, and popsicles; these are often well accepted.
- Consider the use of a complete high-fat, low-carbohydrate nutritional supplement. This decreases carbon dioxide retention and assists in breathing.

Esophageal Reflux

- Recommend small feedings.
- Discourage consumption of foods that lower esophageal sphincter pressure, such as high-fat foods, chocolate, peppermint, spearmint, and alcohol.
- Encourage the client to sit up while eating and for 1 hour afterward.
- Recommend avoidance of food within 3 hours before bedtime.
- Teach relaxation techniques.

Fever

- Recommend a high fluid intake.
- Consider a tube feeding for severe dehydration to maintain hydration after a discussion with team members. This is not recommended if death is imminent (hours/days).
- Recommend high-protein, high-caloric foods.

Fluid Accumulation

- Recommend a mild sodium restriction (3 to 4 grams/day). Recommend a lower sodium restriction only if this is the wish of the client.
- Discourage a fluid restriction unless the client has significant hyponatremia.
- Provide a list of foods high in protein and potassium.

Hiccups

- Recommend smaller meals and slow eating.
- Discourage the use of a straw.
- Add peppermint to food to decrease gastric distention (Gallagher-Allred, 1989).
- Recommend the client swallow a large teaspoon of granulated sugar.

Hypoglycemia

- Assess the client's and caregiver's knowledge about diabetes and hypoglycemia.
- Determine if the client is truly insulin dependent as part of the admission assessment process. The following suggest true insulin dependence:
  - Introduction of insulin soon after the diagnosis
  - A history of previous ketoacidosis
  - Use of more than one daily dose of insulin for years
- Evaluate the client's expressed desire for extent of medical care. The primary guide for determining the level of nutritional intervention is the wish of the client.
- Determine the last time the client experienced the signs of a hypoglycemic episode. Many of these clients have deficiencies in the counteregulatory hormones, especially epinephrine, and may lapse into a coma without any warning signs. Caregivers need to be informed of this potential complication. Educate the client and/or caregiver on the treatment of hypoglycemia (15–15 rule, "Diet in Diabetes Mellitus and Hypoglycemia").

Continued

Box 24-2 ■ *Dietary Management for Symptom Control—cont'd*

- Monitor the client's blood glucose level. A suitable range for blood sugars would be 127 to 309 mg/dL in the hospice population.
- Encourage consumption of 30 to 50 grams of carbohydrate every 3 hours to prevent starvation ketosis. Each of the following is equal to 30 to 50 grams of carbohydrate: ¾ cup of Carnation Instant Breakfast®, 1 cup of regular gelatin, 1 cup of vanilla ice cream, 1½ cups of ginger ale, 1 cup of orange juice, 1 cup of apple juice.

Incontinence

- Discourage intake of coffee, tea, and carbonated beverages containing caffeine, especially before bedtime.
- Continue to encourage adequate fluid intake.

Jaundice and Hepatic Encephalopathy

- Encourage a high-carbohydrate diet.
- Encourage a protein-restricted diet only if the client desires.
- Specialized oral nutritional supplements for clients with liver disease are often ineffective for the terminally ill but may be beneficial when the client desires to "live long enough to ___________."
- Evaluate for the presence of esophageal varices. If present, provide soft foods.

Nausea and Vomiting

- Discuss practical issues with the client and caregiver such as food attitudes, social aspects of eating, and unpredictable food preferences.
- Recommend the client restrict fluids to 1 hour before or after meals to prevent early satiety.
- Assess if sweet, fried, or fatty foods are poorly tolerated; recommend avoidance if necessary.
- Evaluate if starchy foods such as crackers, breads, potatoes, rice, and pasta are better tolerated. Encourage increased consumption if helpful.
- Encourage the client to eat slowly, chew food well, and rest after each meal as these behaviors may increase food intake.
- Recommend the client avoid offensive odors during food preparation.
- Recommend that the person who has recently experienced severe nausea and vomiting try 1 to 2 bites of food per hour.
- Emphasize the sensual aspects of food, including appearance (serve garnished food on attractive tableware), odor of environment (remove bedpans and emesis basins from room), taste (cater to the client's likes and dislikes), and the importance of companionship during mealtime.
- Recommend the avoidance of food if nausea and vomiting become severe and food makes the client feel worse. Feeding may not be desirable if death is expected within hours or a few days and the effects of partial dehydration or the withdrawal of nutrition support will not adversely alter client comfort.

Migraine Headaches

- Recommend that the client eat at regular intervals. Hunger or missed meals can trigger a migraine headache.
- Recommend that the highly motivated client keep a food diary and record the onset of any headaches. Migraine headaches can be triggered by one or many foods. Common food offenders include many common food additives, processed meats, peanuts and peanut products, soybeans, yeast, chocolate, aged cheeses, seasonings, caffeine, some types of alcohol, and flavorings.

Pruritus (severe itching)

- Recommend avoidance of known allergy foods.
- Encourage fluid intake for clients receiving antihistamines.
- Recommend avoidance of coffee, tea, carbonated beverages containing caffeine, alcohol, and cocoa that can cause vasodilation and itching.

Stomatitis (inflammation of the mouth)

- Consider a multivitamin supplement with folic acid and vitamin B_{12}.
- Recommend avoidance of spicy, acidic, rough, hot, and salty foods.
- Recommend a consistency modification, such as pureed, soft, or liquid.
- Consider the use of a complete nutritional supplement.
- Recommend creamy foods, white sauces, and gravies.
- Consider between-meal supplements, such as milkshakes, eggnogs, and puddings.
- Recommend the caregiver add sugar to acid or salty foods to alter the food's taste.
- Recommend meals be served when the client's pain is under control.
- Recommend good oral care before and after meals.

Weakness

- Recommend a multivitamin–mineral supplement with folic acid, vitamin B_{12}, and iron.
- Encourage high-potassium foods (bananas, cantaloupe, milk, baked winter squash, etc.) if the client vomits easily.
- Recommend a modification in the food's consistency (mechanical soft or full liquid) to decrease the energy cost of eating.

Wounds and Pressure Sores

- Recommend the caregiver cater to the client's food preferences.
- Use of aggressive nutritional support is rarely effective but may be appropriate if the client and family desire quantity. For example, "I want to live and see my ______________________."
- Correct elevated glucose levels to decrease risk of infection.
- Evaluate the use of a multivitamin and mineral supplement that contains zinc and vitamin C. As excess dietary zinc impedes healing, do not routinely recommend a zinc supplement without assessment information.
- Encourage protein and caloric intake equal to estimated needs only if the client desires and is able.
- Encourage the client to dip foods in gravy, margarine, butter, and olive oil to increase calorie intake.

Xerostomia (dry mouth)

- Encourage frequent sips of water, fruit juices, ice chips, popsicles, ice cream, and sherbet.
- Recommend the use of hard candy.
- Consider a modification of food consistency such as soft, mechanical soft, or full liquids.
- Recommend avoidance of extremely hot or cold foods. Foods served at room temperature are generally better tolerated.
- Recommend creamy foods, white sauces, and gravies.
- Encourage the client to dip foods in gravy, margarine, butter, olive oil, coffee, and broth.
- Consider the need for a complete liquid nutritional supplement between meals.

Now a decision needs to be made whether to feed a client. A client may experience a more comfortable death if he or she is slightly dehydrated. On the other hand, efforts to hydrate some clients (not those actively dying) may offer a benefit. This is controversial. Death from dehydration precludes the use of any organs for transplantation (Wade, 2001). Some clients feel a strong need to be an organ donor. Sometimes a client, significant other, or physician thinks that artificial hydration may promote client comfort and prolong life in a given situation.

Perhaps a client's vital signs had been fluctuating and are now stable. Ethicists use rational processes for determining the most morally desirable course of action in the face of conflicting value choices. The process of choosing an ethical course of action involves:

- Medical goals and proportionality
- Client preferences
- Quality of life
- Contextual features

Contextual features are the characteristics of a given situation.

Medical Care Goals and Proportionality

The medical care goals that apply to the client with a terminal illness include:

- Relieving symptoms, pain, and suffering
- Preventing untimely death ("I want to live long enough to....")
- Improving functional status or maintaining compromised status
- Educating and counseling the client and his or her significant others regarding the client's condition and prognosis
- Avoiding harming the client in the course of care
- Promoting health and preventing disease not related to the terminal disease

The physician is responsible for the initial education and counseling of clients regarding their condition and prognosis.

The principle of proportionality is an important ethical consideration in the treatment of terminally ill clients. **Proportionality** means a medical treatment is ethically mandatory to the extent that it is likely to confer greater benefits than burdens to the client. For example, many experts believe that a client who is actively dying and is slightly dehydrated has a more comfortable death. Dehydration has been reported to reduce:

- A client's secretions and excretions
- Breathing problems
- Emesis
- Incontinence

Dehydration can sedate the brain just before death. Greatly diminished oral intake or its cessation is one of the signs that death is imminent. In another context, a client who is terminally ill but whose condition is stable and enjoys many activities of daily living may appreciate or request education on how to maintain hydration. A nutritional intervention is appropriate if the client would receive greater benefits than burdens.

Client Preference

The most important ethical principle to consider is the client's right to self-determination. Some individuals may perceive suffering as an important means of personal growth or a religious experience. Other individuals may hope a miracle cure will be discovered for his or her disease. Others may be ready for and accepting of death. Health-care workers have a responsibility to provide a combination of emotional support and technical nutritional advice on how best to achieve each client's goals.

Quality of Life

The most fundamental goal of medical care is an improvement in the quality of life for those who seek care. If improvement is not possible, a goal of medical care is maintenance of the same quality of life or slowing a decline in quality of life. Oral feeding is part of being human and associated with human dignity. One study found that 92% of all cancer clients could eat or drink until the day they died (Feuz and Rapin, 1994). These clients derived some pleasure from the sensual aspect of food and the socialization that accompanies meals. Food conveys:

- Emotional
- Spiritual
- Sociological, and
- Biological meanings

If food remains enjoyable for a client with a terminal illness, the health-care worker should encourage mealtimes to be shared with loved ones. If eating is not a pleasant experience, however, it should not be overemphasized.

Contextual

Every terminally ill client has his or her own story, with both a history and a future. A client's decision to eat or not to eat is part of his or her narrative. Two examples can illustrate why eating issues should always be given consideration when formulating a care plan.

Client 1 lives in a rooming house without air conditioning; his family does not want to get involved; he does not have cooking facilities; he refuses to eat the meals delivered to him from the Senior Nutrition Center; and he insists that he wants to die at home. Client 1 refuses to eat.

Client 2 lives with his male companion in a beach house; his friend carries him every day to the beach to watch the sunset; meals are prepared for him by his companion and many other neighbors and friends. Client 2 tries to eat a small amount at least six times a day.

The willingness to eat is part of each man's story. The contextual features in a patient's situation often relate to food acceptance. In Client 1's situation, the health-care worker may offer a valuable service by reassuring the client that he will not be abandoned because he refuses to eat. The fear of abandonment is among the most frequently cited apprehensions of dying. Even if a client refuses to eat, health-care workers should remain supportive. The client may change his or her mind. The health-care worker should not consider the rejection of food as a sign of personal or professional failure.

A consideration of a client's medical goals, preferences, quality of life, and contextual features may provide a framework for resolution of ethical dietary issues. Hospice programs have interdisciplinary care teams, and the interdisciplinary team conference is the best arena in which to discuss ethical feeding conflicts.

Legal Issues

The issue of whether to discontinue food and fluid to a client with a terminal illness first emerged in the 1960s. Clients have the legal right to refuse treatment, including artificial feedings. This right is based on the Fourteenth Amendment to the Constitution, which refers to the right to liberty, including the right to be left alone and not invaded or treated against one's will. Courts have recognized that competent adults have the right to refuse treatment, including artificial feeding.

Each state may exert its authority to expand the individual's right to liberty, however, based on other concepts. The preservation of life, the prevention of suicide, the protection of innocent third parties (such as minor children), and the protection of the ethical integrity and professional discretion of the medical profession are among these concepts. Health-care workers need to be familiar with the laws in their individual states and the policies and procedures of the organization for which they work.

They should also know their professional organization's standards of practice. In some states, a charge of battery can be made if a client is fed artificially against his or her wishes. In some states, a charge of negligence can be made if clients are allowed to intentionally starve themselves to death. Situations such as these should be discussed at the interdisciplinary team meeting or brought to the risk manager's attention. (The risk manager is hired by a health-care organization to identify, evaluate, and correct potential risks of injuring clients, staff, visitors, or property.)

With incompetent adult clients, caretakers and family should try to ascertain the client's wishes from past written and oral statements and actions. State laws differ as to whether nutrition and hydration are medically obligatory or medically optional. Some clients may wish for the withdrawal of antibiotics and ventilators but wish to continue nutritional support. This situation may occur when an individual has a PEG tube in place because of an inability to swallow, such as may occur with cancer of the esophagus.

What can health-care workers legally do if the client is incompetent and the family wants the feeding tube removed? What can the health-care worker legally do if family members disagree about whether to have the feeding tube removed? When in doubt, the best advice is to continue to feed the client until the health-care team, the institution's ethics committee, or the facility's risk manager reviews the case. The artificial feeding can be stopped at a future time if the decision is changed, but a deceased person cannot be brought back to life.

Individuals may make their wishes known in writing through advanced directives, such as a living will or durable power of attorney. An **advanced directive** is a signed document in which the client has specified what type of medical care is desired should he or she lose the ability to make decisions. A **durable power of attorney** for health care is a document in which the client gives another person power to make medical treatment and related personal care decisions for him or her. It can be used as an addition to the advanced directive. Health-care workers are responsible for becoming familiar with a client's advanced directive, durable power of attorney, and living will. In the event that a client does not have a written directive, the next of kin or guardian should be consulted about a probable preference for the level of nutritional intervention.

General Considerations

Palliative care does not automatically preclude aggressive nutritional support. The client's informed preference for the level of nutrition intervention is important. If the client wants maximal nutrition support and the policy of the organization is not to provide hyperalimentation or tube feedings for terminally ill clients, the client has the right to be informed of the name of a facility that will provide this service. Artificial feeding generally is not desirable if death is expected within hours or a few days.

The effects of partial dehydration and the withdrawal of nutritional support will not adversely alter the client's comfort. Enteral or parenteral feeding would probably worsen the client's condition, symptoms, or discomfort when shock, pulmonary edema, diarrhea, or aspiration is a potential or actual complication. The client or surrogate needs to be informed of these facts when he or she requests maximal support.

Keystones

- Death is an aspect of life.
- If we want to help the dying, we must examine our own attitudes toward death.
- Treatment for terminally ill clients is palliative.
- The goal of care is symptomatic relief to reduce or alleviate pain.
- Nutritional intervention can frequently alleviate or reduce the pain and suffering of a terminally ill client.
- The use of oral feedings should always be given consideration over tube and parenteral feedings.
- Oral feeding is ordinary care, whereas tube feedings and hyperalimentation are considered by some to be extraordinary care.
- In the United States, the client's expressed desire is the primary guide for determining the extent of nutritional and hydration therapy.
- Our Constitution guarantees clients the right to self-determination.
- Ethical and legal dilemmas should be brought to the attention of the interdisciplinary team, the risk manager, or the facility's ethics committee promptly.
- Artificial feeding should never be stopped unless one of these parties has investigated the situation and made a legal and ethical determination that the feeding should cease.
- Each health-care worker has an obligation to know his or her client's advanced directive, durable power of attorney, and living will documentation.

CASE STUDY 24-1

Ms. Z is a 60-year-old woman who has a diagnosis of amyotrophic lateral sclerosis (ALS), also called Lou Gehrig's disease, with a prognosis of less than 6 months. The client has at least two swallowing impediments. She is unable to dislodge food that collects under her tongue, in cheeks, and on her hard palate. She does not have adequate swallow control (the bolus goes down before she wants it to). Because of these impediments, Ms. Z is unable to tolerate thin liquids, and the maintenance of hydration and aspiration are of concern to the caregiver. Ms. Z is alert, oriented, and highly educated. She saw a television program that led her to believe that a high-protein diet would delay the progression of ALS. She would like instruction on a high-protein diet.

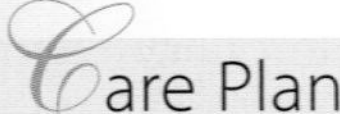

Care Plan

Subjective Data

Client believes a high-protein diet will delay the progression of her ALS. ■ Caregiver is concerned about the danger of aspiration and the maintenance of hydration.

Objective Data

Diagnosis: ALS with a prognosis of less than 6 months ■ Lack of swallowing control

Analysis

Related to lack of desired information about foods high in protein as evidenced by verbal statements. ■ Deficient knowledge related to a lack of understanding of how to increase and/or maintain hydration with the client's swallowing impediments as evidenced by the caregiver's verbal statements

Plan

DESIRED OUTCOMES EVALUATION CRITERIA	ACTIONS/INTERVENTIONS	RATIONALE
The client will indicate how she can incorporate foods high in protein and of semisolid or pureed consistency into her diet.	Refer to dietitian	Because a 70- to 80-g protein diet would most likely not harm the client and would make her feel in control, instruction on the diet is appropriate.
The caregiver will verbalize how to reduce the likelihood of aspiration by following safety precautions for clients with dysphagia.	Discuss feeding issues with the caregiver such as the correct body positioning and eating conditions.	The risk of aspiration is high in clients with dysphagia.
	Eliminate distractions. Position individual in an upright position (90 degrees at the hip) with feet flat on floor. Give semiliquids in very small amounts (syringe) and only after food has been cleared from the mouth. Feed the client very small bites. Encourage several dry swallows between bites of food. If the Adam's apple rises, it is likely the food is being swallowed and not deposited in the cheeks. A wet-sounding voice with a gurgle may mean food is resting on the vocal cords.	

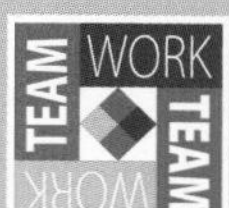

24-1

Dietitian's Notes

The following Dietitian's Notes are representative of the documentation found in a client's medical record.

Subjective: The client requested a high-protein diet because she believes it may delay the progression of her ALS. Client reports an intake of one poached egg, thickened whole milk, one slice of bread softened with gelatin, and one cup of thickend orange juice at breakfast. For lunch patient has ½ banana, ½ a tuna or chicken salad sandwich (bread softened with gelatin the night before). For dinner the client has one-half cup of pureed casserole (beef stew or macaroni and cheese with ½ cup of added pureed vegetables), and a glass of thickened whole milk. She drinks at least three glasses of thickend water each day. She believes she is 5 ft tall and weighs 90 lb. She denies a declining body weight.

Objective: Hospice patient

Analysis: Ideal body weight 90 to 100 lb. Estimated kcalorie needs at actual body weight of 41 kg and 20 to 30 kcal/kg equals 820 to 1230 kcal. Estimated protein needs at 1.2 grams/kg equals 49 grams. Client's reported protein intake is about 55 grams per day and her kcalorie intake is about 1251 kcal per day. Patient is currently eating about 1.1 grams of protein/kg of body weight. Reassured client and her daughter that her current intake is already high in protein and both her stable body weight and reported food intake are within current guidelines. Both were reassured with the assesment.

Plan: No further action is necessary; however, my phone number was provided, and both parties were encouraged to call with any further food-related issues.

Critical Thinking Questions

1. The client's swallowing disorders are becoming more severe. Ms. Z is capable of eating only very small bites of food very slowly. The client's daughter is her caregiver, and she states, "It has been taking me 2 hours to feed my mother each meal. If I go any faster, she chokes. My husband is becoming very resentful and has asked me to make a decision. He says I can't continue to spend all day with my mother and ignore him." What would you say to this caregiver?

2. The caregiver believes the client is still mentally alert and oriented, although the client cannot communicate. The client has progressed to the point where she has lost all motor function. She cannot talk or walk and has lost the use of her hands. The client's physician now believes Ms. Z has an ileus (paralysis of the bowel). Why does this mean the patient cannot be fed orally? What are the treatment options? Who needs to be informed of the treatment options?

Chapter Review

1. A diet prescription consistent with palliative care goals is:
   a. 40 grams of protein for liver failure
   b. Low-cholesterol, low-saturated-fat diet for hyperlipoproteinemia
   c. Gluten-free diet for diarrhea and celiac disease
   d. High-calorie, high-protein diet for anorexia in an actively dying client

2. An appropriate nutritional screening question for a client with a terminal illness is:
   a. "How many times a day do you eat?"
   b. "How much weight have you lost in the past month?"
   c. "Do you look forward to meals?"
   d. "Do you include a green or yellow vegetable in your diet each day?"

Continued

Chapter Review—cont'd

3. The most important ethical principle to consider when a decision must be made about whether or not to feed a client is:
   a. The client's right to self-determination
   b. Proportionality
   c. Medical goals
   d. The client's quality of life
4. Which recommendation would be appropriate for a client with end-stage congestive heart failure who requests dietary advice?
   a. Recommend a low-potassium diet
   b. Recommend a 1000 mL fluid restriction
   c. Monitor the client's fluid intake and output
   d. Recommend a 3- or 4-gram sodium diet
5. The intervention appropriate for a terminally ill client with dyspnea who requests dietary treatment is:
   a. Encourage a high-fiber diet
   b. Consider a high-fat, low-carbohydrate complete nutritional supplement
   c. Recommend fresh fruits, whole grains, and vegetables
   d. Encourage avoidance of caffeine

Clinical Analysis

1. Mr. O is actively dying. Mr. O's wife is concerned because her husband adamantly refuses all food and fluids. The nurse should:
   a. Call the doctor and request an order for a tube feeding
   b. Call the doctor and request an order for an intravenous feeding
   c. Instruct the caregiver to be more creative in the type of food and fluids she gives the client
   d. Counsel the caregiver that oral intake often ceases near the end of life
2. Mrs. P has a diagnoses of brain cancer and insulin-dependent diabetes mellitus and a prognosis of a few days. She and her caregiver have been self-monitoring her blood glucose levels. The caregiver is quite concerned because Mrs. P's blood glucose levels are running between 400 and 500 milligrams per deciliter. Historically, the client claims to have followed her 1200-kcalorie diet faithfully. Recently, her appetite is markedly reduced and her blood glucose levels are elevated (hypermetabolism). The physician has been contacted and refuses to increase the client's insulin further but recommends to Mrs. P's caregiver to stop monitoring the client's blood glucose levels. The nurse should:
   a. Encourage the caregiver to offer Mrs. P frequent sips of clear liquid fruit juices (about 30 grams of carbohydrate every 3 hours)
   b. Encourage the caregiver to continue to offer the client the 1200-kcalorie diet to avoid a hypoglycemic episode
   c. Recommend the caregiver look for a new doctor because obviously the doctor does not know how to treat clients with insulin-dependent diabetes
   d. Contact the hospice medical director and ask for an order to increase the client's insulin
3. Mr. J has a partial bowel obstruction and shows signs of dehydration. He has an order for Metamucil prn. The nurse should immediately recommend:
   a. Eating high-fiber foods such as bran, whole grains, fruits, and vegetables
   b. Discontinuating Metamucil
   c. Increasing the dose of Metamucil
   d. Eating cheese, cakes, pies, cookies, and doughnuts

APPENDIX A

Dietary Reference Intakes for Individuals: Vitamins, Minerals, Macronutrients, and Water: RDAs, AIs, Tolerable Intake Levels

Dietary Reference Intakes (DRIs): Recommended Intakes for Individuals, Vitamins, Vitamins Food and Nutrition Board, Institute of Medicine, National Academies

LIFE-STAGE GROUP	VITAMIN A (mcg/d)[a]	VITAMIN C (mg/d)	VITAMIN D (mcg/d)[b,c]	VITAMIN E (mg/d)[d]	VITAMIN K (mcg/d)	THIAMIN (mg/d)	RIBOFLAVIN (mg/d)	NIACIN (mg/d)[e]	VITAMIN B_6 (mg/d)	FOLATE (mcg/d)[f]	VITAMIN B_{12} (mcg/d)	PANTOTHENIC ACID (mg/d)	BIOTIN (mcg/d)	CHOLINE (mg/d)[g]
Infants														
0–6 mo	400*	40*	5*	4*	2.0*	0.2*	0.3*	2*	0.1*	65*	0.4*	1.7*	5*	125*
7–12 mo	500*	50*	5*	5*	2.5*	0.3*	0.4*	4*	0.3*	80*	0.5*	1.8*	6*	150*
Children														
1–3 yr	300	15	5*	6	30*	0.5	0.5	6	0.5	150	0.9	2*	8*	200*
4–8 yr	400	25	5*	7	55*	0.6	0.6	8	0.6	200	1.2	3*	12*	250*
Males														
9–13 yr	600	45	5*	11	60*	0.9	0.9	12	1.0	300	1.8	4*	20*	375*
14–18 yr	900	75	5*	15	75*	1.2	1.3	16	1.3	400	2.4	5*	25*	550*
19–30 yr	900	90	5*	15	120*	1.2	1.3	16	1.3	400	2.4	5*	30*	550*
31–50 yr	900	90	5*	15	120*	1.2	1.3	16	1.3	400	2.4	5*	30*	550*
51–70 yr	900	90	10*	15	120*	1.2	1.3	16	1.7	400	2.4[h]	5*	30*	550*
>70 yr	900	90	15*	15	120*	1.2	1.3	16	1.7	400	2.4[h]	5*	30*	550*
Females														
9–13 yr	600	45	5*	11	60*	0.9	0.9	12	1.0	300	1.8	4*	20*	375*
14–18 yr	700	65	5*	15	75*	1.0	1.0	14	1.2	400[i]	2.4	5*	25*	400*
19–30 yr	700	75	5*	15	90*	1.1	1.1	14	1.3	400[i]	2.4	5*	30*	425*
31–50 yr	700	75	5*	15	90*	1.1	1.1	14	1.3	400[i]	2.4	5*	30*	425*
51–70 yr	700	75	10*	15	90*	1.1	1.1	14	1.5	400	2.4[h]	5*	30*	425*
>70 yr	700	75	15*	15	90*	1.1	1.1	14	1.5	400	2.4[h]	5*	30*	425*
Pregnancy														
≤18 yr	750	80	5*	15	75*	1.4	1.4	18	1.9	600[j]	2.6	6*	30*	450*
19–30 yr	770	85	5*	15	90*	1.4	1.4	18	1.9	600[j]	2.6	6*	30*	450*
31–50 yr	770	85	5*	15	90*	1.4	1.4	18	1.9	600[j]	2.6	6*	30*	450*
Lactation														
≤18 yr	1200	115	5*	19	75*	1.4	1.6	17	2.0	500	2.8	7*	35*	550*
19–30 yr	1300	120	5*	19	90*	1.4	1.6	17	2.0	500	2.8	7*	35*	550*
31–50 yr	1300	120	5*	19	90*	1.4	1.6	17	2.0	500	2.8	7*	35*	550*

SOURCES: Dietary Reference Intakes for Calcium, Phosphorus, Magnesium, Vitamin D, and Fluoride (1997); Dietary Reference Intakes for Thiamin, Riboflavin, Niacin, Vitamin B_6, Folate, Vitamin B_{12}, Pantothenic Acid, Biotin, and Choline (1998); Dietary Reference Intakes for Vitamin C, Vitamin E, Selenium, and Carotenoids (2000); and Dietary Reference Intakes for Vitamin A, Vitamin K, Arsenic, Boron, Chromium, Copper, Iodine, Iron, Manganese, Molybdenum, Nickel, Silicon, Vanadium, and Zinc (2001). These reports may be accessed via www.nap.edu.

Note: This table (taken from the DRI reports; see www.nap.edu) presents Recommended Dietary Allowances (RDAs) in bold type and Adequate Intakes (AIs) in regular type followed by an asterisk (*). RDAs and AIs may both be used as goals for individual intake. RDAs are set to meet the needs of almost all (97%–98%) individuals in a group. For healthy breastfed infants, the AI is the mean intake. The AI for other life-stage and gender groups is believed to cover needs of all individuals in the group, but lack of data or uncertainty in the data prevent being able to specify with confidence the percentage of individuals covered by this intake.

[a] As retinol activity equivalents (RAEs). 1 RAE = 1 mcg of retinol, 12 mcg of β-carotene, 24 mcg of α-carotene, or 24 mcg of β-cryptoxanthin. To calculate RAEs from REs of provitamin A carotenoids in foods, divide the REs by 2. For preformed vitamin A in foods or supplements and for provitamin A carotenoids in supplements, 1 RE = 1 RAE.

[b] Calciferol 1 mcg calciferol = 40 IU of vitamin D.

[c] In the absence of adequate exposure to sunlight.

[d] As α-tocopherol. α-Tocopherol includes *RRR*-α-tocopherol, the only form of α-tocopherol that occurs naturally in foods, and the *2R*-stereoisometric forms of α-tocopherol (*RRR-*, *RSR-*, *RRS-*, and RSS-α-tocopherol) that occur in fortified foods and supplements. It does not include the *2S*-stereoisometric forms of α-tocopherol (*SRR-*, *SSR-*, *SR-*, and *SSS-* α-tocopherol), also found in fortified foods and supplements.

[e] As niacin equivalents (NE). 1 mg of niacin = 60 mg of tryptophan; 0–6 months = preformed niacin (not NE).

[f] As dietary folate equivalents (DFE). 1 DFE = 1 mcg of food folate = 0.6 mcg of folic acid from fortified food or as a supplement consumed with food = 0.5 mcg of a supplement taken on an empty stomach.

[g] Although AIs have been set for choline, few data assess whether a dietary supply of choline is needed at all stages of the life cycle, and it may be that the choline requirement can be met by endogenous synthesis at some of these stages.

[h] Because 10%–30% of older people may malabsorb food-bound B_{12}, it is advisable for those older than 50 years to meet their RDA mainly by consuming foods fortified with B_{12} or a supplement containing B_{12}.

[i] In view of evidence linking folate intake with neural tube defects in the fetus, it is recommended that all women capable of becoming pregnant consume 400 mcg from supplements or fortified foods in addition to intake of food folate from a varied diet.

[j] It is assumed that women will continue consuming 400 mcg from supplements or fortified food until their pregnancy is confirmed and they enter prenatal care, which ordinarily occurs after the end of the periconceptional period—the critical time for formation of the neural tube.

SOURCE: Tables compiled and copied with permission from Mahon, KL and Escott-Stump, S: Krause's Food, Nutrition, and Diet Therapy, ed 11. Elsevier, Philadelphia, 2004.

Dietary Reference Intakes (DRIs): Recommended Intakes for Individuals, Minerals, Minerals Food and Nutrition Board, Institute of Medicine, National Academies

LIFE-STAGE GROUP	CALCIUM (mg/d)	CHRONIUM (mcg/d)	COPPER (mcg/d)	FLUORIDE (mg/d)	IODINE (mcg/d)	IRON (mg/d)	MAGNESIUM (mg/d)	MANGANESE (mg/d)	MOLYBDENUM (mcg/d)	PHOSPHORUS (mg/d)	SELENIUM (mcg/d)	ZINC (mg/d)
Infants												
0–6 mo	210*	0.2*	200*	0.01*	110*	0.27*	30*	0.003*	2*	100*	15*	2*
7–12 mo	270*	5.5*	220*	0.5*	130*	**11**	75*	0.6*	3*	275*	20*	**3**
Children												
1–3 yr	500*	11*	**340**	0.7*	**90**	**7**	**80**	1.2*	**17**	**460**	**20**	**3**
4–8 yr	800*	15*	**440**	1*	**90**	**10**	**130**	1.5*	**22**	**500**	**30**	**5**
Males												
9–13 yr	1300*	25*	**700**	2*	**120**	**8**	**240**	1.9*	**34**	**1250**	**40**	**8**
14–18 yr	1300*	35*	**890**	3*	**150**	**11**	**410**	2.2*	**43**	**1250**	**55**	**11**
19–30 yr	1000*	35*	**900**	4*	**150**	**8**	**400**	2.3*	**45**	**700**	**55**	**11**
31–50 yr	1000*	35*	**900**	4*	**150**	**8**	**420**	2.3*	**45**	**700**	**55**	**11**
51–70 yr	1200*	30*	**900**	4*	**150**	**8**	**420**	2.3*	**45**	**700**	**55**	**11**
>70 yr	1200*	30*	**900**	4*	**150**	**8**	**420**	2.3*	**45**	**700**	**55**	**11**
Females												
9–13 yr	1300*	21*	**700**	2*	**120**	**8**	**240**	1.6*	**34**	**1250**	**40**	**8**
14–18 yr	1300*	24*	**890**	3*	**150**	**15**	**360**	1.6*	**43**	**1250**	**55**	**9**
19–30 yr	1000*	25*	**900**	3*	**150**	**18**	**310**	1.8*	**45**	**700**	**55**	**8**
31–50 yr	1000*	25*	**900**	3*	**150**	**18**	**320**	1.8*	**45**	**700**	**55**	**8**
51–70 yr	1200*	20*	**900**	3*	**150**	**8**	**320**	1.8*	**45**	**700**	**55**	**8**
>70 yr	1200*	20*	**900**	3*	**150**	**8**	**320**	1.8*	**45**	**700**	**55**	**8**
Pregnancy												
≤18 yr	1300*	29*	**1000**	3*	**220**	**27**	**400**	2.0*	**50**	**1250**	**60**	**12**
19–30 yr	1000*	30*	**1000**	3*	**220**	**27**	**350**	2.0*	**50**	**700**	**60**	**11**
31–50 yr	1000*	30*	**1000**	3*	**220**	**27**	**360**	2.0*	**50**	**700**	**60**	**11**
Lactation												
≤18 yr	1300*	44*	**1300**	3*	**290**	**10**	**360**	2.6*	**50**	**1250**	**70**	**13**
19–30 yr	1000*	45*	**1300**	3*	**290**	**9**	**310**	2.6*	**50**	**700**	**70**	**12**
31–50 yr	1000*	45*	**1300**	3*	**290**	**9**	**320**	2.6*	**50**	**700**	**70**	**12**

SOURCES: Dietary Reference Intakes for Calcium, Phosphorus, Magnesium, Vitamin D, and Fluoride (1997); Dietary Reference Intakes for Thiamin, Riboflavin, Niacin, Vitamin B_6, Folate, Vitamin B_{12}, Pantothenic Acid, Biotin, and Choline (1998); Dietary Reference Intakes for Vitamin C, Vitamin E, Selenium, and Carotenoids (2000); and Dietary Reference Intakes for Vitamin A, Vitamin K, Arsenic, Boron, Chromium, Copper, Iodine, Iron, Manganese, Molybdenum, Nickel, Silicon, Vanadium, and Zinc (2001).

Note: This table presents Recommended Dietary Allowances (RDAs) in bold type and Adequate Intakes (AIs) in ordinary type followed by an asterisk (*). RDAs and AIs may both be used as goals for individual intake. RDAs are set to meet the needs of almost all (97%–98%) individuals in a group. For healthy breastfed infants, the AI is the mean intake. The AI for other life-stage and gender groups is believed to cover needs of all individuals in the group, but lack of data or uncertainty in the data prevent being able to specify with confidence the percentage of individuals covered by this intake.

SOURCE: Tables compiled and copied with permission from Mahon, KL and Escott-Stump, S: Krause's Food, Nutrition, and Diet Therapy, ed 11. Elsevier, Philadelphia, 2004.

Dietary Reference Intakes (DRIs): Tolerable Upper Intake Levels (UL[a]) for Vitamins, Vitamins Food and Nutrition Board, Institute of Medicine, National Academies

LIFE-STAGE GROUP	VITAMIN A (mcg/d)[b]	VITAMIN C (mg/d)	VITAMIN D (mcg/d)	VITAMIN E (mg/d)[c,d]	VITAMIN K	THIAMIN	RIBOFLAVIN	NIACIN (mg/d)[d]	VITAMIN B_6 (mg/d)[d]	FOLATE (mcg/d)[d]	VITAMIN B_{12}	PANTOTHENIC ACID	BIOTIN	CHOLINE (g/d)	CAROTENOIDS[e]
Infants															
0–6 mo	600	ND[f]	25	ND	ND	ND	ND	ND	ND	ND	ND	ND	ND	ND	ND
7–12 mo	600	ND	25	ND	ND	ND	ND	ND	ND	ND	ND	ND	ND	ND	ND
Children															
1–3 yr	600	400	50	200	ND	ND	ND	10	30	300	ND	ND	ND	1.0	ND
4–8 yr	900	650	50	300	ND	ND	ND	15	40	400	ND	ND	ND	1.0	ND
Males, Females															
9–13 yr	1700	1200	50	600	ND	ND	ND	20	60	600	ND	ND	ND	2.0	ND
14–18 yr	2800	1800	50	800	ND	ND	ND	30	80	800	ND	ND	ND	3.0	ND
19–70 yr	3000	2000	50	1000	ND	ND	ND	35	100	1000	ND	ND	ND	3.5	ND
>70 yr	3000	2000	50	1000	ND	ND	ND	35	100	1000	ND	ND	ND	3.5	ND
Pregnancy															
≥18 yr	2800	1800	50	800	ND	ND	ND	30	80	800	ND	ND	ND	3.0	ND
19–50 yr	3000	2000	50	1000	ND	ND	ND	35	100	1000	ND	ND	ND	3.5	ND
Lactation															
18 yr	2800	1800	50	800	ND	ND	ND	30	80	800	ND	ND	ND	3.0	ND
19–50 yr	3000	2000	50	1000	ND	ND	ND	35	100	1000	ND	ND	ND	3.5	ND

SOURCES: Dietary Reference Intakes for Calcium, Phosphorus, Magnesium, Vitamin D, and Fluoride (1997); Dietary Reference Intakes for Thiamin, Riboflavin, Niacin, Vitamin B_6, Folate, Vitamin B_{12}, Pantothenic Acid, Biotin, and Choline (1998); Dietary Reference Intakes for Vitamin C, Vitamin E, Selenium, and Carotenoids (2000); and Dietary Reference Intakes for Vitamin A, Vitamin K, Arsenic, Boron, Chromium, Copper, Iodine, Iron, Manganese, Molybdenum, Nickel, Silicon, Vanadium, and Zinc (2001). These reports may be accessed via www.nap.edu.

[a]UL = The maximum level of daily nutrient intake that is likely to pose no risk of adverse effects. Unless otherwise specified, the UL represents total intake from food, water, and supplements. Due to lack of suitable data, ULs could not be established for vitamin K, thiamin, riboflavin, vitamin B_{12}, pantothenic acid, biotin, or carotenoids. In the absence of ULs, extra caution may be warranted in consuming levels above recommended intakes.

[b]As preformed vitamin A only.

[c]As α-tocopherol; applies to any form of supplemental α-tocopherol.

[d]The ULs for vitamin E, niacin, and folate apply to synthetic forms obtained from supplements, fortified foods, or a combination of the two.

[e]β-Carotene supplements are advised only to serve as a provitamin A source for individuals at risk of vitamin A deficiency.

[f]ND = Not determinable due to lack of data of adverse effects in this age group and concern with regard to lack of ability to handle excess amounts. Source of intake should be from food only to prevent high levels of intake.

SOURCE: Tables compiled and copied with permission from Mahon, KL and Escott-Stump, S: Krause's Food, Nutrition, and Diet Therapy, ed. 11, Elsevier, Philadelphia, 2004.

Dietary Reference Intakes (DRIs): Tolerable Upper Intake Levels (UL[a]) for Minerals, Minerals Food and Nutrition Board, Institute of Medicine, National Academies

LIFE-STAGE GROUP	ARSENIC[b]	BORON (mg/d)	CALCIUM (g/d)	CHROMIUM	COPPER (mcg/d)	FLUORIDE (mg/d)	IODINE (mcg/d)	IRON (mg/d)	MAGNESIUM (mg/d)[c]	MANGANESE (mg/d)	MOLYBDENUM (mcg/d)	NICKEL (mg/d)	PHOSPHORUS (g/d)	SELENIUM (mcg/d)	SILICON[d]	VANADIUM (mg/d)[e]	ZINC (mg/d)
Infants																	
0–6 mo	ND[f]	ND	ND	ND	ND	0.7	ND	40	ND	ND	ND	ND	ND	45	ND	ND	4
7–12 mo	ND	ND	ND	ND	ND	0.9	ND	40	ND	ND	ND	ND	ND	60	ND	ND	5
Children																	
1–3 yr	ND	3	2.5	ND	1000	1.3	200	40	65	2	300	0.2	3	90	ND	ND	7
4–8 yr	ND	6	2.5	ND	3000	2.2	300	40	110	3	600	0.3	3	150	ND	ND	12
Males, Females																	
9–13 yr	ND	11	2.5	ND	5000	10	600	40	350	6	1100	0.6	4	280	ND	ND	23
14–18 yr	ND	17	2.5	ND	8000	10	900	45	350	9	1700	1.0	4	400	ND	ND	34
19–70 yr	ND	20	2.5	ND	10,000	10	1100	45	350	11	2000	1.0	4	400	ND	1.8	40
>70 yr	ND	20	2.5	ND	10,000	10	1100	45	350	11	2000	1.0	3	400	ND	1.8	40
Pregnancy																	
≥18 yr	ND	17	2.5	ND	8000	10	900	45	350	9	1700	1.0	3.5	400	ND	ND	34
19–50 yr	ND	20	2.5	ND	10,000	10	1100	45	350	11	2000	1.0	3.5	400	ND	ND	40
Lactation																	
≥18 yr	ND	17	2.5	ND	8000	10	900	45	350	9	1700	1.0	4	400	ND	ND	34
19–50 yr	ND	20	2.5	ND	10,000	10	1100	45	350	11	2000	1.0	4	400	ND	ND	40

SOURCES: Dietary Reference Intakes for Calcium, Phosphorus, Magnesium, Vitamin D, and Fluoride (1997); Dietary Reference Intakes for Thiamin, Riboflavin, Niacin, Vitamin B_6, Folate, Vitamin B_{12}, Pantothenic Acid, Biotin, and Choline (1998); Dietary Reference Intakes for Vitamin C, Vitamin E, Selenium, and Carotenoids (2000); and Dietary Reference Intakes for Vitamin A, Vitamin K, Arsenic, Boron, Chromium, Copper, Iodine, Iron, Manganese, Molybdenum, Nickel, Silicon, Vanadium, and Zinc (2001). These reports may be accessed via www.nap.edu.

[a]UL = The maximum level of daily nutrient intake that is likely to pose no risk of adverse effects. Unless otherwise specified, the UL represents total intake from food, water, and supplements. Due to lack of suitable data, ULs could not be established for arsenic, chromium, and silicon. In the absence of ULs, extra caution may be warranted in consuming levels above recommended intakes.

[b]Although the UL was not determined for arsenic, there is no justification for adding arsenic to food or supplements.

[c]The ULs for magnesium represent intake from a pharmacologic agent only and do not include intake from food and water.

[d]Although silicon has not been shown to cause adverse effects in humans, there is no justification for adding silicon to supplements.

[e]Although vanadium in food has not been shown to cause adverse effects in humans, there is no justification for adding vanadium to food, and vanadium supplements should be used with caution. The UL is based on adverse effects in laboratory animals, and this data could be used to set a UL for adults but not children and adolescents.

[f]ND = Not determinable due to lack of data of adverse effects in this age group and concern with regard to lack of ability to handle excess amounts. Source of intake should be from food only to prevent high levels of intake.

SOURCE: Tables compiled and copied with permission from Mahon, KL and Escott-Stump, S: Krause's Food, Nutrition, and Diet Therapy, ed. 11, Elsevier, Philadelphia, 2004.

Dietary Reference Intakes (DRIs): Recommended Intakes for Individuals, Macronutrients, Macronutrients Food and Nutrition Board, Institute of Medicine, National Academies

LIFE-STAGE GROUP	PROTEIN		CARBOHYDRATE		FIBER		FAT		n-6 POLYUNSATURATED FATTY ACIDS (LINOLEIC ACID)		n-3 POLYUNSATURATED FATTY ACIDS (α-LINOLENIC ACID)		SATURATED AND *TRANS*-FATTY ACIDS AND CHOLESTEROL	
	RDA/AI g/day[a]	AMDR[b]	RDA/AI g/day	AMDR	RDA/AI g/day	AMDR	RDA/AI g/day	AMDR	RDA/AI g/day	AMDR	RDA/AI g/day	AMDR[d]	RDA/AI g/day[e]	AMDR
Infants														
0–6 mo	9.1	ND[c]	60	ND	ND		31		4.4	ND	0.5	ND	ND	
7–12 mo	13.5	ND	95	ND	ND		30		4.6	ND	0.5	ND	ND	
Children														
1–3 yr	13	5–20	130	45–65	19			30–40	7	5–10	0.7	0.6–1.2		
4–8 yr	19	10–30	130	45–65	25			25–35	10	5–10	0.9	0.6–1.2		
Males														
9–13 yr	34	10–30	130	45–65	31			25–35	12	5–10	1.2	0.6–1.2		
14–18 yr	52	10–30	130	45–65	38			25–35	16	5–10	1.6	0.6–1.2		
19–30 yr	56	10–35	130	45–65	38			20–35	17	5–10	1.6	0.6–1.2		
31–50 yr	56	10–35	130	45–65	38			20–35	17	5–10	1.6	0.6–1.2		
50–70 yr	56	10–35	130	45–65	30			20–35	14	5–10	1.6	0.6–1.2		
>70 yr	56	10–35	130	45–65	30			20–35	14	5–10	1.6	0.6–1.2		
Females														
9–13 yr	34	10–30	130	45–65	26			25–35	10	5–10	1.0	0.6–1.2		
14–18 yr	46	10–30	130	45–65	26			25–35	11	5–10	1.1	0.6–1.2		
19–30 yr	46	10–35	130	45–65	25			20–35	12	5–10	1.1	0.6–1.2		
31–50 yr	46	10–35	130	45–65	25			20–35	12	5–10	1.1	0.6–1.2		
50–70 yr	46	10–35	130	45–65	21			20–35	11	5–10	1.1	0.6–1.2		
>70 yr	46	10–35	130	45–65	21			20–35	11	5–10	1.1	0.6–1.2		
Pregnant														
≤18 yr	71	10–35	175	45–65	28			20–35	13	5–10	1.4	0.6–1.2		
19–30 yr	71	10–35	175	45–65	28			20–35	13	5–10	1.4	0.6–1.2		
31–50 yr	71	10–35		45–65	28			20–35	13	5–10	1.4	0.6–1.2		
Lactation														
≤18 yr	71	10–35	210	45–65	29			20–35	13	5–10	1.3	0.6–1.2		
19–30 yr	71	10–35	210	45–65	29			20–35	13	5–10	1.3	0.6–1.2		
31–50 yr	71	10–35	210	45–65	29			20–35	13	5–10	1.3	0.6–1.2		

Data from Dietary Reference Intakes for Energy, Carbohydrate, Fiber, Fat, Fatty Acids, Cholesterol, Protein, and Amino Acids, The National Academies Press, Washington, DC, 2002.

Note: This table represents Recommended Dietary Allowances (RDAs) in bold type and Adequate Intakes (AIs) in ordinary type. RDAs and AIs may both be used as goals for individual intake. RDAs are set to meet the needs of almost all (97%–98%) individuals in a group. For healthy breastfed infants, the AI is the mean intake. The AI for other life-stage and gender groups is believed to cover the needs of all individuals in the group, but lack of data prevents being able to specify with confidence the percentage of individuals covered by this intake.

[a]Based on 1.5 g/kg per day for infants, 1.1 g/kg per day for 1–3 yr, 0.95 g/kg per day for 4–13 yr, 0.85 g/kg per day for 14–18 yr, 0.8 g/kg per day for adults, and 1.1 g/kg per day for pregnant (using prepregnancy weight) and lactating women.

[b]Acceptable Macronutrient Distribution Range (AMDR) is the range of intake for a particular energy source that is associated with reduced risk of chronic disease while providing intakes of essential nutrients. If an individual has consumed in excess of the AMDR, there is a potential of increasing the risk of chronic diseases and insufficient intakes of essential nutrients.

[c]ND = Not determinable due to lack of data of adverse effects in this age group and concern with regard to lack of ability to handle excess amounts. Source of intake should be from food only to prevent high levels of intake.

[d]Approximately 10% of the total can come from longer-chain, n-3 fatty acids.

[e]Keep intake as low as possible while consuming a nutritionally adequate diet.

SOURCE: Tables compiled and copied with permission from Mahon, KL and Escott-Stump, S: Krause's Food, Nutrition, and Diet Therapy, ed 11. Elsevier, Philadelphia, 2004.

Dietary Reference Intakes for Water, Potassium, Sodium, Chloride, and Sulfate		
Water		
AI	men 19–30 yr	3.7 liters
AI	women 19–30 yr	2.7 liters
Potassium		
AI	4.7 grams	adults
UL	not established	
Sodium		
AI*	1.5 grams/day	younger adults
AI	1.3 grams/day	men and women 50–70 yr
AI	1.2 grams/day	men and women ≥71 yr
UL†	2.3 grams/day	younger adults
Sulfate		
EAR	not established	
UL	not established	
Sulfate requirements are met when intakes include recommended levels for sulfur-containing amino acids		
Chloride		
AI	2.3 grams/day	younger adults
AI	2.0 grams/day	50–70 yr
AI	1.8 grams/day	≥71 yr

*AI does not apply to highly active such as endurance athletes.
†The UL may be lower among certain groups of individuals who are most sensitive to blood pressure effects of increased sodium intake (e.g., older persons, African Americans, and individuals with hypertension, diabetes, or chronic kidney disease). In contrast, for individuals who are unacclimatized to prolonged physical activity in a hot environment, their needs may exceed the UL because of sodium sweat loss.
SOURCE: Institute of Medicine of the National Academies, Dietary References for Energy, Carbohydrate, Fiber, Fat, Fatty Acids, Cholesterol, Protein, and Amino Acids, The National Academy, Washington DC, 2002.

APPENDIX B

Food Exchange List

Within each group, these foods can be exchanged for each other. You can use this list to give yourself more choices.

Vegetables contain 25 calories and 5 grams of carbohydrate. One serving equals:

½ cup	Cooked vegetables (carrots, broccoli, zucchini, cabbage, etc.)
1 cup	Raw vegetables or salad greens
½ cup	Vegetable juice
If you're hungry, eat more fresh or steamed vegetables.	

Fat-Free and Very Lowfat Milk contain 90 calories per serving. One serving equals:

1 cup	Milk, fat-free or 1% fat
¾ cup	Yogurt, plain non fat or low fat
1 cup	Yogurt, artificially sweetened

Very Lean Protein choices have 35 calories and 1 gram of fat per serving. One serving equals:

1 ounce	Turkey breast or chicken breast, skin removed
1 ounce	Fish fillet (flounder, sole, scrod, cod, etc.)
1 ounce	Canned tuna in water
1 ounce	Shellfish (clams, lobster, scallop, shrimp)
¾ cup	Cottage cheese, non fat or low fat
2 each	Egg whites
¼ cup	Egg substitute
1 ounce	Fat-free cheese
½ cup	Beans-cooked (black beans, kidney, chick peas or lentils): count as 1 starch/bread and 1 very lean protein

Fruits contain 15 grams of carbohydrate and 60 calories. One serving equals:

1 small	Apple, banana, orange, nectarine
1 medium	Fresh peach
1	Kiwi
½	Grapefruit
½	Mango
1 cup	Fresh berries (strawberries, raspberries or blueberries)
1 cup	Fresh melon cubes
⅛	Honeydew melon
4 ounces	Unsweetened juice
4 teaspoons	Jelly or jam

Lean Protein choices have 55 calories and 2–3 grams of fat per serving. One serving equals:

1 ounce	Chicken—dark meat, skin removed
1 ounce	Turkey—dark meat, skin removed
1 ounce	Salmon, swordfish, herring
1 ounce	Lean beef (flank steak, London broil, tenderloin, roast beef)*
1 ounce	Veal, roast or lean chop*
1 ounce	Lamb, roast or lean chop*
1 ounce	Pork, tenderloin or fresh ham*
1 ounce	Low fat cheese (3 grams or less of fat per ounce)
1 ounce	Low fat luncheon meats (with 3 grams or less of fat per ounce)
¼ cup	4.5% cottage cheese
2 medium	Sardines

*Limit to 1 or 2 times per week.

Medium Fat Proteins have 75 calories and 5 grams of fat per serving. One serving equals:

1 ounce	Beef (any prime cut), corned beef, ground beef†
1 ounce	Pork chop
1 each	Whole egg (medium)†
1 ounce	Mozzarella cheese
¼ cup	Ricotta cheese
4 ounces	Tofu (note this is a Heart Healthy choice)

†Choose these very infrequently.

Starches contain 15 grams of carbohydrate and 80 calories per serving. One serving equals:

1 slice	Bread (white, pumpernickel, whole wheat, rye)
2 slices	Reduced calorie or "lite" bread
¼ (1 ounce)	Bagel (varies)
½	English muffin
½	Hamburger bun
¾ cup	Cold cereal
⅓ cup	Rice, brown or white, cooked
⅓ cup	Barley or couscous, cooked
⅓ cup	Legumes (dried beans, peas or lentils), cooked
½ cup	Pasta, cooked
½ cup	Bulgar, cooked
½ cup	Corn, sweet potato or green peas
3 ounces	Baked sweet or white potato
¾ ounce	Pretzels
3 cups	Popcorn, hot air popped or microwave (80% light)

Fats contain 45 calories and 5 grams of fat per serving. One serving equals:

1 teaspoon	Oil (vegetable, corn, canola, olive, etc.)
1 teaspoon	Butter
1 teaspoon	Stick margarine
1 teaspoon	Mayonnaise
1 tablespoon	Reduced fat margarine or mayonnaise
1 tablespoon	Salad dressing
1 tablespoon	Cream cheese
2 tablespoons	Lite cream cheese
⅛th	Avocado
8 large	Black olives
10 large	Stuffed green olives
1 slice	Bacon

SOURCE: National Heart, Lung, and Blood Institute, a part of the National Institutes of Health and the U.S. Department of Health and Human Services. http://www.nhlbi.nih.gov/health/public/heart/obesity/lose_wt/fd_exch.htm.

APPENDIX C

Answers to Questions

CHAPTER 1

Chapter Review
1. b 2. d 3. a 4. b 5. c 6. a

Clinical Analysis
1. d 2. a 3. d

CHAPTER 2

Chapter Review
1. b 2. b 3. c 4. a 5. c

Clinical Analysis
1. d 2. b 3. a

CHAPTER 3

Chapter Review
1. b 2. c 3. c 4. d 5. a

Clinical Analysis
1. c 2. d 3. a

CHAPTER 4

Chapter Review
1. c 2. b 3. c 4. b 5. c

Clinical Analysis
1. d 2. a 3. c

CHAPTER 5

Chapter Review
1. a 2. c 3. b 4. b 5. d

Clinical Analysis
1. d 2. c 3. a

CHAPTER 6

Chapter Review
1. c 2. a 3. c 4. b 5. d

Clinical Analysis
1. d 2. d 3. b

CHAPTER 7

Chapter Review
1. c 2. d 3. a 4. a 5. b

Clinical Analysis
1. d 2. c 3. b

CHAPTER 8

Chapter Review
1. b 2. c 3. a 4. d 5. b

Clinical Analysis
1. a 2. b 3. c 4. d

CHAPTER 9

Chapter Review
1. d 2. a 3. c 4. b 5. b

Clinical Analysis
1. a 2. d 3. a

CHAPTER 10

Chapter Review
1. b 2. a 3. c 4. a 5. d

Clinical Analysis
1. c 2. b 3. d

CHAPTER 11

Chapter Review

1. c 2. b 3. c 4. b 5. d

Clinical Analysis

1. d 2. c 3. a

CHAPTER 12

Chapter Review

1. b 2. d 3. b 4. a 5. d

Clinical Analysis

1. b 2. b 3. c

CHAPTER 13

Chapter Review

1. c 2. a 3. d 4. b 5. a

Clinical Analysis

1. b 2. a 3. c

CHAPTER 14

Chapter Review

1. c 2. a 3. c 4. b 5. a

Clinical Analysis

1. c 2. c 3. a

CHAPTER 15

Chapter Review

1. b 2. d 3. c 4. d 5. a

Clinical Analysis

1. c 2. a 3. c

CHAPTER 16

Chapter Review

1. a 2. b 3. d 4. b 5. b

Clinical Analysis

1. a 2. b 3. c

CHAPTER 17

Chapter Review

1. a 2. b 3. d 4. b 5. a

Clinical Analysis

1. c 2. a 3. b

CHAPTER 18

Chapter Review

1. a 2. c 3. d 4. b 5. d

Clinical Analysis

1. b 2. d 3. c

CHAPTER 19

Chapter Review

1. b 2. b 3. d 4. a 5. d

Clinical Analysis

1. c 2. b 3. a

CHAPTER 20

Chapter Review

1. c 2. b 3. d 4. b 5. d

Clinical Analysis

1. a 2. b 3. b

CHAPTER 21

Chapter Review

1. b 2. d 3. c 4. d 5. a

Clinical Analysis

1. c 2. b 3. a

CHAPTER 22

Chapter Review

1. c 2. c 3. b 4. d 5. c

Clinical Analysis

1. c 2. d 3. b

CHAPTER 23

Chapter Review

1. b 2. d 3. a 4. c 5. d

Clinical Analysis

1. b 2. b 3. b

CHAPTER 24

Chapter Review

1. c 2. c 3. a 4. d 5. b

Clinical Analysis

1. d 2. a 3. b

APPENDIX D

Glossary

This glossary contains commonly used terms as well as terms that appear in **boldface** in the book.

Abdominal circumference (girth)— Distance around the trunk at the umbilicus.

Abdominal obesity— Excess body fat located between the chest and pelvis.

Abortifacient— Anything used to cause or induce an abortion.

Absorption— The movement of the end products of digestion from the gastrointestinal tract into the blood and/or lymphatic system.

Accreditation— Process by which a nongovernmental agency recognizes an institution for meeting established criteria of quality.

Acculturation— Process of adopting the values, attitudes, and behaviors of another culture.

Acetone— A ketone body found in urine, which can be due to the excessive breakdown of stored body fat.

Acetylcholine— A chemical necessary for the transmission of nervous impulses.

Acetyl CoA— Important intermediate byproduct in metabolism formed from the breakdown of glucose, fatty acids, and certain amino acids.

Achalasia— Failure of the gastrointestinal muscle fibers to relax where one part joins another.

Achlorhydria— Absence of free hydrochloric acid in the stomach.

Acidosis— Condition that results when the pH of the blood falls below 7.35; may be caused by diarrhea, uremia, diabetes mellitus, respiratory depression, and certain drug therapies.

Acquired immune deficiency syndrome (AIDS)— A disease complex caused by a virus that attacks the immune system and causes neurological disease and permits opportunistic infections and malignancies.

Acrodermatitis enteropathica— Rare autosomal-recessive disease that causes zinc deficiency through an unknown mechanism of absorptive failure; fatal if untreated.

Acute illness— A sickness characterized by rapid onset, severe symptoms, and a short course.

Acute renal failure— Condition that occurs suddenly, in which the kidneys are unable to perform essential functions; usually temporary.

Adaptive thermogenesis— The adjustment in energy expenditure the body makes to a large increase or decrease in kilocalorie intake of several days' duration.

Additive— A substance added to food to increase its flavor, shelf life, and/or characteristics such as texture, color, and aroma.

Adequate Intake (AI)— The average observed or experimentally defined intake by a defined population or subgroup that appears to sustain a defined nutritional state; incorporates information on the reduction of disease risk; may be used as a goal for an individual's nutrient intake if an EAR or RDA cannot be set.

Adipose cells— Cells in the human body that store fat.

Adipose tissue— Tissue containing masses of fat cells.

Adolescence— Time from the onset of puberty until full growth is reached.

ADP (adenosine diphosphate)— A substance present in all cells involved in energy metabolism. Energy is released when molecules of ATP, another compound in cells, release a phosphoric acid chain and become ADP. The opposite chemical reaction of adding the third phosphoric acid group to ADP requires much energy.

Adrenal glands— Small organs on the superior surface of the kidneys that secrete many hormones, including epinephrine (adrenalin) and aldosterone.

Aerobic exercise— Training methods such as running or swimming that require continuous inspired oxygen.

Afferent— Proceeding toward a center, as arteries, veins, lymphatic vessels, and nerves.

Afferent arteriole— Small blood vessel by which blood enters the glomerulus (functional unit of the kidney).

Aflatoxin— A naturally occurring food contaminant produced by some strains of *Aspergillus* molds; found especially on peanuts and peanut products.

AIDS dementia complex (ADC)— A central nervous system disorder caused by the human immunodeficiency virus.

ALA— See Alpha-linolenic acid.

Albumin— A plasma protein responsible for much of the colloidal osmotic pressure of the blood.

Aldosterone— An adrenocorticoid hormone that increases sodium and water retention by the kidneys.

Alimentary canal— The digestive tube extending from the mouth to the anus.

Alkaline phosphatase— An enzyme found in highest concentration in the liver, biliary tract epithelium, and bones; enzyme levels are elevated in liver, bone, and biliary disease.

Alkalosis— Condition that results when the pH of the blood rises above 7.45; may be caused by vomiting, nasogastric suctioning, or hyperventilation.

Allele— One of two or more different genes containing specific inheritable characteristics that occupy corresponding positions (loci) on paired chromosomes; an individual possessing a pair of identical alleles, either dominant or recessive, is homozygous for this gene.

Allergen— Substance that provokes an abnormal, individual hypersensitivity.

Allergy— State of abnormal, individual hypersensitivity to a substance.

Alopecia— Hair loss, especially of the head; baldness.

Alpha-linolenic acid— A polyunsaturated omega-3 fatty acid found in some plants.

Alpha-tocopherol equivalent (α-TE)— The measure of vitamin E; 1 milligram of alpha-tocopherol equivalent equals 1.4 International Units of natural alpha-tocopherol or 1 IU of synthetic vitamin.

Amenorrhea— Absence of menstruation; normally occurs before puberty, after menopause, and during pregnancy and lactation.

Amino acids— Organic compounds that are the building blocks of protein; also the end products of protein digestion.

Amniotic fluid— Albuminous liquid that surrounds and protects the fetus throughout pregnancy.

Amylase— A class of enzymes that splits starches; for example, salivary amylase, pancreatic amylase.

Anabolic phase— The third and last phase of stress; characterized by the building up of body tissue and nutrient stores; also called recovery phase.

Anabolism— The building up of body compounds or tissues by the synthesis of more complex substances from simpler ones; the constructive phase of metabolism.

Anaerobic exercise— A form of physical activity such as weight lifting or sprinting that does not rely on continuous inspired oxygen.

Anaphylaxis— Exaggerated, life-threatening hypersensitivity response to a previously encountered antigen; in severe cases, produces bronchospasm, vascular collapse, and shock.

Anastomosis— The surgical connection between tubular structures.

Anemia— Condition of less-than-normal values for red blood cells or hemoglobin, or both; result is decreased effectiveness in oxygen transport; causes may include inadequate iron intake, malabsorption, and chronic or acute blood loss.

Anencephaly— Congenital absence of the brain; cerebral hemispheres missing or reduced to small masses; fatal within a few weeks.

Angina pectoris— Severe pain and a sense of constriction about the heart caused by lack of oxygen to the heart muscle.

Angiotensin II— End product of complex reaction in response to low blood pressure; effect is vasoconstriction and aldosterone secretion.

Anion— An ion with a negative charge.

Anorexia— Loss of appetite.

Anorexia nervosa— A mental disorder characterized by a 25% loss of usual body weight, an intense fear of becoming obese, and self-starvation.

Anorexia of aging— Loss of appetite in an elderly individual related to physiologic, social, psychological, or medical causes.

Anorexigenic— Causing loss of appetite.

Antagonist— A substance that counteracts the action of another substance.

Anthropometric measurements— Physical measurements of the human body such as height, weight, and skinfold thickness; used to determine body composition and growth.

Anthropometry— The science of measuring the human body.

Antibody— A specific protein developed in the body in response to a substance that the body senses to be foreign.

Anticholinergic— An agent that blocks parasympathetic nerve impulses, thereby causing dry mouth, blurred vision due to dilated pupils, and decreased gastrointestinal and bronchial secretions.

Antidiuretic hormone (ADH)— Hormone formed in the hypothalamus and released from the posterior pituitary in response to blood that is too concentrated; effect is return of water to the bloodstream by the kidney.

Antigen— Protein or oligosaccharide marker on surface of cells; body can detect foreign antigens on organisms, foods, and transplanted tissues.

Anti-insulin antibodies (AIAs)— A protein found to be elevated in persons with insulin-dependent diabetes mellitus.

Antineoplastic drug— A drug that combats tumors.

Antioxidant— A substance that prevents or inhibits the uptake of oxygen; in the body, antioxidants prevent tissue damage; in foods, antioxidants prevent deterioration.

Anuria— A total lack of urine output.

Apoferritin— A protein found in intestinal mucosal cells that combines with iron to form ferritin; it is always found attached to iron in the body.

Apolipoproteins— Protein components of lipoproteins that assist in regulating lipid metabolism; apo A, the primary HDL apoprotein, is inversely related to the risk for developing coronary artery disease.

Appetite— A strong desire for food or for a pleasant sensation, based on previous experience, that causes one to seek food for the purpose of tasting and enjoying.

Aquaporin— Water transport proteins, found in many cell membranes, that serve as water-selective channels and explain the speed at which water moves across cell membranes.

Arachidonic acid— An omega-6 polyunsaturated fatty acid present in peanuts; precursor of prostaglandins.

Ariboflavinosis— Condition arising from a deficiency of riboflavin in the diet.

Aromatic amino acids— Phenylalanine, tryptophan, tyrosine; ratio to branched-chain amino acids altered in liver failure

Arrhythmia— Irregular heartbeat.

Arteriosclerosis— Common arterial disorder characterized by thickening, hardening, and loss of elasticity of the arterial walls; also called "hardening of the arteries."

Arthritis— Inflammatory condition of the joints, usually accompanied by pain and swelling.

Ascites— Accumulation of serous fluid in the peritoneal (abdominal) cavity.

Ascorbic acid— Vitamin C; *ascorbic* literally means "without scurvy."

Ash— The residue that remains after an item is burned; usually refers to the mineral content of the human body.

Aspartame— Artificial sweetener composed of aspartic acid and phenylalanine; 180 times sweeter than sucrose; brand names: Equal, Nutrasweet.

***Aspergillus*—** Genus of molds that produce aflatoxins.

Aspiration— The state whereby a substance has been drawn into the nose, throat, or lungs.

Assessment— An organized procedure to gather pertinent facts.

Astrocyte— A supporting cell of the central nervous system that contributes to the blood-brain barrier.

Asymptomatic— Without symptoms.

Ataxia— Defective muscular coordination, especially seen in voluntary movement attempts.

Atherosclerosis— A form of arteriosclerosis characterized by the deposit of fatty material inside the arteries; major factor contributing to heart disease.

Atom— Smallest particle of an element that has all the properties of the element. An atom consists of the nucleus, which contains protons (positively charged particles), neutrons (particles with no electrical charge), and surrounding electrons (negatively charged particles).

Atopy— Genetic predisposition to develop allergy primarily involving IgE antibodies; a child with two atopic parents has a 75% chance of similar symptoms; a child with one atopic parent has a 50% chance.

ATP (adenosine triphosphate)— Compound in cells, especially muscle cells, that stores energy; when needed, enzymes break off one phosphoric acid group, which releases energy for muscle contraction.

Atrophy— Decrease in size of a normally developed organ or tissue.

Autoimmune disease— A disorder in which the body produces an immunologic response against itself.

Autonomy— Achieving independence; the psychosocial developmental task of the toddler.

Autosomal recessive inheritance— Non–sex-linked pattern of inheritance in which an affected gene must be received from both parents for the individual to be affected; examples: cystic fibrosis, PKU, galactosemia, sickle cell disease.

Avidin— Protein in raw egg white that inhibits the B vitamin biotin.

Bacteria— Single-celled microorganisms that lack a true nucleus; may be either harmless to humans or disease producing.

Balanced diet— One including sufficient foods from each of the major food groups daily; one containing all the essential nutrients in required amounts.

Bariatric surgery— Surgery performed to treat and control obesity.

Barium enema— Series of x-ray studies of the colon used to demonstrate the presence and location of polyps, tumors, diverticula, or positional abnormalities. The client is first administered an enema containing a radio-opaque substance (barium) that enhances visualization when the film is exposed.

Barium swallow— The primary diagnostic tool for direct visualization of the swallowing mechanism is called the *cookie swallow* or *modified barium swallow*. During this procedure, the client consumes three items of different viscosities. Each item contains a contrast medium that allows all phases of the swallowing mechanism to be visualized in x-rays. A physician is always present during this procedure.

Basal ganglia— Four masses of gray matter located in the cerebrum; contribute to the subconscious aspects of voluntary movement; inhibit tremors.

Benign— Not recurrent or progressive; nonmalignant; benign tumor may be life-threatening in crucial tissue such as the brain.

Beriberi— Disease caused by deficiency of vitamin B_1 (thiamin).

Beta-carotene— Carotenoid with the greatest provitamin A activity.

Beta-endorphin— Chemical released in the brain during exercise that produces a state of relaxation.

Bicarbonate— Any salt containing the HCO_3^- anion; blood bicarbonate is a measure of alkali (base) reserve of the body; bicarbonate of soda is sodium bicarbonate ($NaHCO_3$).

Bile— Yellow secretion of the liver that alkalinizes the intestine and breaks large fat globules into smaller ones to facilitate enzyme digestive action.

Binging— Eating to excess; eating from 5,000 to 20,000 kilocalories per day.

Bioavailability— The rate and extent to which an active drug or nutrient or metabolite enters the general circulation, permitting access to the site of action; measured by concentration of the drug in body fluids or by the magnitude of the pharmacologic response.

Bioelectric impedance— Indirect measure of body fatness based on differences in electrical conductivity of fat, muscle, and bone.

Biologic value— Scoring system of how well food proteins can be converted into body protein; eggs are norm of 100% of nitrogen being retained.

Biotin— B-complex vitamin widely available in foods.

Bladder— A body organ, also called the urinary bladder, that receives urine from the kidneys and discharges it through the urethra.

Blood pressure— Force exerted against the walls of blood vessels by the pumping action of the heart.

Blood urea nitrogen (BUN)— The amount of nitrogen present in the blood as urea, often elevated in renal disorders; may be referred to as serum urea nitrogen (SUN).

B-lymphocytes (B-cells)— White blood cells that protect against infection by inducing antibody production; see Humoral immunity.

Body frame size— Designation of a person's skeletal structure as small, medium, or large; used to determine healthy body weight (HBW).

Body image— The mental image a person has of himself or herself.

Body mass index (BMI)— Weight in kilograms divided by the square of height in meters; BMIs of 19 to 24 are considered normal.

Body substance isolation— A situation in which all body fluids should be considered contaminated and treated as such by all health-care workers.

Bolus— A mass of food that is ready to be swallowed or a single dose of feeding or medication.

Bolus feeding— Giving a 4- to 6-hour volume of a tube feeding within a few minutes.

Bomb calorimeter— A device used to measure the energy content of food.

Botulism— An often fatal form of food intoxication caused by the ingestion of food containing poisonous toxins produced by the microorganism *Clostridium botulinum*.

Bowman's capsule— The cuplike top of an individual nephron; functions as a filter in the formation of urine.

Branched-chain amino acids— Leucine, isoleucine, lysine, valine; sometimes used as therapy for hepatic coma.

Buffer— A substance that can react to offset excess acid or excess alkali (base) in a solution; blood buffers include carbonic acid, bicarbonate, phosphates, and proteins, including hemoglobin.

Bulimia— Excessive food intake followed by extreme methods, such as self-induced vomiting and the use of laxatives, to rid the body of the foods eaten.

C-reactive protein (CRP)— An abnormal protein produced by the liver in response to acute inflammation that is strongly associated with future vascular events.

Cachexia— State of malnutrition and wasting seen in chronic conditions such as cancer, AIDS, malaria, tuberculosis, and pituitary disease.

Calcidiol— Inactive form of vitamin D produced by the liver; half-life about 3 weeks; main storage site is the blood.

Calcification— Process in which tissue becomes hardened with calcium deposits; necessary for bone anabolism; pathological in vitamin D toxicity.

Calcitonin— Hormone produced by the thyroid gland that slows the release of calcium from the bone when serum calcium levels are high.

Calcitriol— The activated form of vitamin D, 1,25-dihydroxycholecalciferol.

Calorie— A measurement unit of energy; unit equaling the amount of heat required to raise the temperature of 1 gram of water 1 degree Celsius; laypersons' term for kilocalorie.

Campylobacter— Flagellated, gram-negative bacteria; important cause of diarrheal illnesses.

Candida albicans— Microscopic fungal organism normally present on skin and mucous membranes of healthy people; cause of thrush, vaginitis, opportunistic infections.

Capillary— Minute vessel connecting arteriole and venule; vessel wall acts as semipermeable membrane to exchange substances between blood and lymph and interstitial fluid.

Carbohydrate— Any of a group of organic compounds, including sugar, starch, and cellulose, that contains only carbon, oxygen, and hydrogen.

Carbonic acid— Aqueous solution of carbon dioxide; carbon dioxide in solution or in blood is carbonic acid.

Carcinogen— Any substance or agent that causes the development of or increases the risk of cancer.

Carcinoma— A malignant neoplasm that occurs in epithelial tissue.

Cardia— Upper orifice of the stomach connecting with the esophagus.

Cardiac arrhythmia— Irregular heartbeat.

Cardiac sphincter— Smooth muscle band at the lower end of the esophagus; prevents reflux of stomach contents.

Cardiomyopathy— Disease of heart muscle; may be primary due to unknown cause or secondary to another cardiac disorder or systemic disease.

Carotene— One of several yellow to red antioxidant pigments that are precursors to vitamin A.

Carotenemia— Excess carotene in the blood, producing yellow skin but not discoloring the whites of the eyes.

Carotenoid— Group of more than 500 red, orange, or yellow pigments found in fruits and vegetables, about 50 of which are precursors of vitamin A; includes carotene, which is such a precursor, and lycopene, which is not.

Casein— Principal protein in cow's milk.

Catabolism— The breaking down of body compounds or tissues into simpler substances; the destructive phase of metabolism.

Catalyst— A substance that speeds up a chemical reaction without entering into or being changed by the reaction.

Cataract— Clouding of the lens of the eye.

Cation— An ion with a positive charge.

Cecum— The first portion of the large intestine between the ileum and the ascending colon.

Celiac disease (gluten-sensitive enteropathy)— An intolerance to dietary gluten, which damages the intestine and produces diarrhea and malabsorption.

Cell— The smallest functional unit of structure in all plants and animals.

Cellular immunity— Delayed immune response produced by T-lymphocytes, which mature in the thymus gland; examples of this type of response are rejection of transplanted organs and some autoimmune diseases.

Cerebrovascular accident (CVA)— An abnormal condition in which the brain's blood vessels are occluded by a thrombus, an embolus, or hemorrhage, resulting in damaged brain tissue; stroke.

Chelating agent— A chemical compound that binds metallic ions into a ring structure, inactivating them; used to remove poisonous metals from the body.

Chemical digestion— Digestive process that involves the splitting of complex molecules into simpler forms.

Chemical reaction— The process of combining or breaking down substances to obtain different substances.

Chlorophyll— The green plant pigment necessary for the manufacture of carbohydrates.

Cholecalciferol— Vitamin D_3, formed when the skin is exposed to sunlight; further processed by the liver and kidneys; may be reported as serum 25-hydroxy-cholecalciferol.

Cholecystitis— Inflammation of the gallbladder.

Cholecystokinin— A hormone secreted by the duodenum; stimulates contraction of the gallbladder (releases bile) and the secretion of pancreatic juice.

Cholelithiasis— The presence of gallstones.

Cholestasis— Blockage of the flow of bile; due to liver disease or obstructions in the duct system.

Cholesterol— A fat-like substance made in the human body and found in foods of animal origin; associated with an increased risk of heart disease.

Choline— Vitamin-like organic compound recognized as an essential nutrient; required for normal carbohydrate and fat metabolism and involved in protein metabolism.

Chronic illness— A sickness persisting for a long period that shows little change or a slow progression over time.

Chronic obstructive pulmonary disease (COPD)— A group of chronic diseases with a common characteristic of chronic airflow obstruction.

Chronic renal failure— An irreversible condition in which the kidneys cannot perform vital functions.

Chvostek's sign— Spasm of facial muscles following a tap over the facial nerve in front of the ear; indication of tetany.

Chylomicron— A lipoprotein that carries triglycerides in the bloodstream after meals.

Chyme— The mixture of partly digested food and digestive secretions found in the stomach and small intestine during digestion of a meal.

Chymotrypsin— A protein-splitting enzyme produced by the pancreas; active in the intestine.

Cirrhosis— Chronic disease of the liver in which functioning cells degenerate and are replaced by fibrosed connective tissue.

Client-care conference— A meeting that includes all health-care team members and may include the client or a significant other to review and update the client's nursing care plan.

***Clostridium botulinum*—** An anaerobic (grows without air) organism that produces a poisonous toxin; the cause of botulism.

***Clostridium perfringens*—** A bacterium that produces a poisonous toxin that causes a food intoxication; the symptoms are generally mild and of short duration and include intestinal disorders.

Coenzyme— A substance that combines with an enzyme to activate it.

Cognitive— Referring to or associated with the act of knowing.

Colectomy— Surgical removal of part or all of the colon.

Collagen— Fibrous insoluble protein found in connective tissue.

Collecting tubule— The last segment of the renal tubule; follows the distal convoluted tubule. Several nephrons usually share a single collecting tubule.

Colloidal osmotic pressure (COP)— Pressure produced by plasma and cellular proteins.

Colon— The large intestine from the end of the small intestine to the rectum.

Colostomy— Surgical procedure in which an opening to the large intestine is constructed on the abdomen.

Comorbidity— A disease coexisting with the primary disease.

Complementation— Principle of meal planning advocating combining plant foods within a meal so that it contains all the essential amino acids; now applied to daily intake rather than to single meals.

Complete protein— A protein containing all essential amino acids that humans need; usually found in animal sources such as milk, meat, eggs, and fish.

Complex carbohydrate— A carbohydrate composed of many molecules of $C_6H_{12}O_6$ joined together; polysaccharide; includes starch, glycogen, and fiber.

Compound— Two or more elements united chemically in specific proportions.

Compound fat— Substance obtained when one of the fatty acids joined to the glycerol molecule is replaced by another molecule, such as a protein.

Conditionally essential nutrient— Substance normally manufactured by the body; in certain situations, the body cannot manufacture an optimal amount.

Constipation— Decrease in a person's normal frequency of defecation; stool often hard, dry, or difficult to expel.

Contamination iron— Iron that leaches from cookware into the food; in special circumstances, can become hazardous.

Continuous ambulatory peritoneal dialysis (CAPD)— A form of self-dialysis in which the dialysate is allowed to remain in the abdominal cavity for 4–6 hours before replacement.

Continuous feeding— Enteral feeding in which the formula drips slowly throughout the prescribed time span.

Contraindication— Any circumstance under which treatment should not be given.

Coronary heart disease (CHD)— Disease resulting from the decreased flow of blood through the coronary arteries to the heart muscle.

Coronary occlusion— Blockage of one or more branches of the coronary arteries, which supply the heart muscle with oxygen and nutrients.

Creatine— Nonprotein substance synthesized in the body from arginine, glycine, and methionine; combines with phosphate to form creatine phosphate, which is stored in muscle tissue as an energy source.

Creatinine— Nonprotein nitrogenous end product of creatine metabolism; because creatinine is excreted by the kidneys, serum creatinine levels are used to detect and monitor renal disease and to estimate muscle protein reserves.

Cretinism— A congenital condition resulting from a lack of thyroid secretions; characterized by a stunted and malformed body and arrested mental development.

Crohn's disease— Inflammatory disease appearing in any area of the bowel in which diseased areas can be found alternating with healthy tissue.

Cross-contamination— The spreading of a disease-producing organism from one food, person, or object to another food, person, or object.

Cruciferous— Belonging to a botanical mustard family; includes broccoli, Brussels sprouts, cabbage, cauliflower, kale, kohlrabi, and swiss chard.

Crystalluria— The presence of crystals in the urine; may be caused by the administration of sulfonamides.

Culture— The learned, shared, and transmitted values, beliefs, and norms of a particular group that guides its thinking, decisions, and actions in patterned ways.

Cyanocobalamin— Vitamin B_{12}; essential for proper blood formation.

Cyclical variation— A recurring series of events during a specified period.

Cystic fibrosis— Hereditary disease often affecting the lungs and pancreas in which glandular secretions are abnormally thick.

Cystitis— Inflammation of the bladder.

Cytochrome P450 enzymes— Group of genetically determined enzymes that help to metabolize fat-soluble vitamins, steroids, fatty acids, and other substances and to detoxify drugs and environmental pollutants.

Deamination— Metabolic process whereby nitrogen is removed from an amino acid.

Deciliter (dL)— 100 milliliters or $\frac{1}{10}$ liter.

Decubitus ulcer— A pressure sore on the lower back, such as a bedsore.

Dehiscence— Separation of the edges of a surgical incision.

Delusion— False belief that is firmly maintained despite obvious proof to the contrary.

Dementia— The impairment of intellectual function that usually is progressive and interferes with normal social and occupational activities.

Dental caries— The gradual decay and disintegration of the teeth; a dental cavity is a hole in a tooth caused by dental caries.

Dental plaque— Colorless and transparent gummy mass of microorganisms that grows on the teeth, predisposing them to decay.

Deoxyribonucleic acid (DNA)— Protein substance in the cell nucleus that directs all the cell's activities, including reproduction.

Desirable body weight— A person's body weight as compared with the 1959 Desirable Height/Weight Table.

Desired outcome— The behavioral or physical change in a client that indicates the achievement of a nursing goal.

Development— Gradual process of changing from a simple to a more complex organism; involves psychosocial and physical changes, not only an increase in size.

Dextrose— Another name for the simple sugar glucose.

DHA— See Docosahexaenoic acid.

Diabetes incipidus— Increased water intake and increased urine output resulting from inadequate secretion of antidiuretic hormone (ADH) by the posterior pituitary or by failure of the kidney tubules to respond to ADH; underlying causes can be tumor, surgery, trauma, infection, radiation injury, or congenital anomaly.

Diabetes mellitus— Disease caused by insufficient insulin secretion by the pancreas or insulin resistance by body tissues causing excess glucose in the blood and deranged carbohydrate, fat, and protein metabolism.

Diabetic neuropathy— Degeneration of peripheral nerves occurring in diabetes; possible causes are microscopic changes in blood vessels or metabolic defects in nerve tissue.

Diacetic acid— A ketone body found in the urine, which can be due to the excessive breakdown of stored body fat.

Diagnostic— Relating to scientific and skillful methods to establish the cause and nature of a sick person's illness.

Dialysate— In renal failure, the fluid used to remove or deliver compounds or electrolytes that the failing kidney cannot excrete or retain in proper concentrations.

Dialysis— The process of diffusing blood across a semipermeable membrane to remove toxic materials and to maintain fluid, electrolyte, and acid-base balances in cases of impaired kidney function or absence of the kidneys.

Dialysis dementia— A neurological disturbance seen in clients who have been on dialysis for a number of years.

Diastolic pressure— Pressure exerted against the arteries between heart beats; the lower number of a blood pressure reading.

Dietary fiber— Material in foods, mostly from plants, that the human body cannot break down or digest.

Dietary recall, 24-hour— Description of what a person has eaten for the previous 24 hours.

Dietary Reference Intake (DRI)— Four nutrient-based reference values that can be used for assessing and planning diets for the healthy general population; refer to average daily intakes for 1 or more weeks; include Estimated Average Requirements (EARs), Recommended Dietary Allowances (RDAs), Adequate Intakes (AIs), and Tolerable Upper Intake Levels (ULs).

Dietary status— Description of what a person has been eating; his or her usual intake.

Digestion— The process by which food is broken down mechanically and chemically in the gastrointestinal tract into forms simple enough for intestinal absorption.

Diglyceride— Two fatty acids joined to a glycerol molecule.

Dilutional hyponatremia— Serum sodium that is low, not because of an absolute lack of sodium but because of an excess of water.

Disaccharide— A simple sugar composed of two units of $C_6H_{12}O_6$ joined together; examples include sucrose, lactose, and maltose.

Disulfide linkage— Specific chemical bond joining amino acids; in hair, skin, and nails, holds amino acids in their distinct shapes.

Diverticulitis— Inflammation of a diverticulum.

Diverticulosis— Presence of one or more diverticula.

Diverticulum— A sac or pouch in the walls of a tubular organ; pl., diverticula.

Docosahexaenoic acid (DHA)— a polyunsaturated Omega-3 fatty acid found in fish oils.

Dopamine— Catecholamine synthesized by the adrenals; immediate precursor in the synthesis of norepinephrine.

Double-blind— Technique of scientific investigation in which neither the investigator nor the subject knows what treatment, if any, the subject is receiving.

Double bond— A type of chemical connection in which, for example, a fatty acid has two neighboring carbon atoms, each lacking one hydrogen atom.

Drink— An alcoholic beverage; see Standard drink.

Dual-energy x-ray absorptiometry (DEXA)— Diagnostic test using two x-ray beams to determine body composition; used to measure bone mineral density as an indicator of osteopenia and osteoporosis.

Duct— A structural tube designed to allow secretions to move from one body part to another body part.

Dumping syndrome— A condition in which the contents of the stomach empty too rapidly into the duodenum; mostly occurs in patients who have had gastric resections.

Duodenum— The first part of the small intestine between the stomach and the jejunum.

Dysphoria— A speech disorder characterized by hoarseness.

Dyspnea— Difficulty breathing.

Ebb phase— The first phase in the stress response; the body reduces blood pressure, cardiac output, body temperature, and oxygen consumption to meet increased demands.

Eclampsia— An obstetrical emergency involving hypertension, proteinuria, and convulsions appearing after the twentieth week of pregnancy.

Eczema— Skin inflammation, acute or chronic; caused by external (chemical irritation or microbial invasion) or internal (genetic or psychological) factors.

Edema— The accumulation of excessive amounts of fluid in interstitial spaces.

Edentulous— The state of having no teeth.

Efferent— Directed away from a center; used to describe arteries, veins, lymphatic vessels, and nerves.

Efferent arteriole— Small blood vessel by which blood leaves the nephron.

Efficacy— Ability of a drug to achieve the desired effect.

Eicosapentaenoic acid (EPA)— Omega-3 fatty acid found in fish oils.

Electrocardiogram (ECG)— A graphic record produced by an electrocardiograph that shows the electrical activity of the heart.

Electroencephalogram (EEG)— The record obtained from an electroencephalograph that shows the electrical activity of the brain.

Electrolyte— An element or compound that when dissolved in water separates (dissociates) into ions that are capable of conducting an electrical current; acids, bases, and salts are common electrolytes.

Element— A substance that cannot be separated into simpler parts by ordinary means.

Elemental or "predigested" formula— Formula that contains either partially or totally predigested nutrients.

Embolus— A circulating mass of undissolved matter in a blood or lymphatic vessel; may be composed of tissues, fat globules, air bubbles, clumps of bacteria, or foreign bodies, including pieces of medical devices.

Embryo— A developing infant in the prenatal period between the second and eighth weeks inclusive.

Empty kilocalories— Refers to a food that contains kilocalories and almost no other nutrients.

Emulsification— The physical breaking up of fat into tiny droplets.

Emulsifier— A molecule that attracts both water- and fat-soluble molecules.

Emulsion— One liquid evenly distributed in a second liquid with which it usually does not mix.

Endemic— The constant presence of a disease or infectious agent within a given geographic area; the usual prevalence of a given disease within such an area.

Endogenous— Produced within or caused by factors within the organism.

Endoscope— A device consisting of a tube and an optical system for observing the inside of a hollow organ or cavity.

Endothelium— Flat cells lining blood and lymphatic vessels, the heart, and various body cavities; produce compounds affecting vascular lumen and platelets.

End-stage renal failure— A state in which the kidneys have lost most or all of their ability to maintain internal homeostasis and produce urine.

Energy— The capacity to do work.

Energy balance— A situation in which kilocaloric intake equals kilocaloric output.

Energy expenditure— The amount of fuel the body uses for a specified period.

Energy imbalance— Situation in which kilocalories eaten do not equal the number of kilocalories used for energy.

Energy nutrients— The chemical substances in food that are able to supply fuel; refers collectively to carbohydrate, fat, and protein.

Enrichment— The addition of nutrients previously present in a food but removed during food processing or lost during storage.

Enteral tube feeding— The feeding of a formula by tube into the gastrointestinal tract.

Enteric-coated— A type of drug preparation designed to dissolve in the intestine rather than in the stomach.

Enteritis— Inflammation of the intestines, particularly the small intestine.

Enzyme— Complex protein produced by living cells that acts as a catalyst.

Epidemic— Occurrence in a region of more than the expected number of cases of a communicable disease.

Epilepsy— Disease marked by repetitive abnormal electrical discharges within the brain; signs and symptoms vary with type: partial, generalized, or unclassified.

Epinephrine— Hormone of the adrenal gland; produces the fight-or-flight response.

Epithelial tissue— A type of tissue that forms the outer layer of skin and lines body surfaces opening to the outside; functions include protection, absorption, and secretion.

Ergocalciferol— Vitamin D_2 formed by the action of sunlight on plants.

Ergot poisoning— Poisoning resulting from excessive use of the drug ergot or from the ingestion of grain or grain products infected with the *Claviceps purpurea* fungus.

Erikson, Erik— Psychologist who devised a theory of human development consisting of eight stages of life, each with a psychosocial developmental task to be mastered.

Erosion— Destruction of the surface of a tissue, either on the external surface of the body or internally.

Erythropoietin— Hormone released by the kidney to stimulate red blood cell production.

Esophagostomy— A surgical opening in the esophagus.

Esophagus— A muscular canal extending from the mouth to the stomach.

Essential amino acid— One of the amino acids that cannot be manufactured by the human body; must be obtained from food or artificial feeding.

Essential (primary) hypertension— Elevated blood pressure that develops without apparent cause.

Essential nutrient— A substance found in food that must be present in the diet because the human body lacks the ability to manufacture it in sufficient amounts for optimal health.

Estimated Average Requirement— Intake that meets the estimated nutrient need of 50% of the individuals in a life-stage and gender group; used to set the RDA and to assess or plan the intake of groups.

Ethanol— Grain alcohol; ounces of ethanol in beverages can be estimated with the conversion factors of 0.045 for beer, 0.121 for wine, and 0.409 for liquor.

Ethnocentrism— Belief that one's own view of the world is superior to anyone else's.

Etiology— The cause of a disease.

Evaporative water loss— Insensible water loss through the skin.

Exchange— A defined quantity of food on the American Dietetic and Diabetes Associations' food exchange list or on another, similar exchange list.

Exchange list— A food guide developed by the American Dietetic and Diabetes Associations; often used in clinical practice to aid in meal planning.

Excretion— The elimination of waste products from the body in feces, urine, exhaled air, and perspiration.

Exogenous— Outside the body.

External muscle layer— Muscle layer of the alimentary canal.

External water loss— Water lost to the outside of the body.

Extracellular fluid— Fluid found between the cells and within the blood and lymph vessels.

Extrinsic factor— Vitamin B_{12}, necessary for proper red blood cell development.

Failure to thrive (FTT)— Medical diagnosis for infants who fail to gain weight appropriately or who lose weight; also applied to elderly who lose ability to care for themselves.

Fasting— The state of having had no food or fluid enterally or no parenteral nutrition.

Fasting blood sugar (FBS)— Blood glucose measured in the fasting state; normal values are 70–110 mg per deciliter.

Fat-free mass— Lean body mass plus nonfat components of adipose tissue.

Fatty acid— Part of the structure of a fat.

Fatty liver— Accumulation of lipids in the liver cells; may be reversible if the cause, of which there are many, is removed.

Feedback cycle— Control system of many bodily functions involving the interaction between a stimulus and an effect; in positive feedback, the effect increases the stimulus as uterine contractions increasing oxytocin secretion; in negative feedback, the effect decreases the stimulus as blood levels of thyroid hormone decrease secretion of thyroid-stimulating hormone.

Ferric iron— Oxidized iron, which is less absorbable from the gastrointestinal tract than ferrous iron; abbreviated Fe^{3+}.

Ferritin—An iron-phosphorus-protein complex formed in the intestinal mucosa by the union of ferric iron with apoferritin; the form in which iron is stored in the tissues, mainly in liver, spleen, and bone marrow cells.

Ferrous iron— The more absorbable form of iron for humans; abbreviated Fe^{2+}.

Fetal alcohol syndrome (FAS)— A condition characterized by mental and physical abnormalities in an infant caused by the mother's consumption of alcohol during pregnancy.

Fetus— The human child in utero from the third month until birth; also applicable to the later stages of gestation of other animals.

Fiber, dietary— Material in foods, mostly from plants, that the human body cannot break down or digest.

Fibrin— Insoluble protein formed from fibrinogen by the action of thrombin; forms the meshwork of a blood clot.

Fibrinogen— Protein in blood essential to the clotting process; also called Factor I; see Fibrin.

Filtration— The process of removing particles from a solution by allowing the liquid to pass through a membrane or other partial barrier.

First-degree relative— An individual's parents, siblings, or children.

First pass effect— Process whereby drugs are extensively metabolized by the small intestine or liver enzymes; result is that less drug reaches the systemic circulation.

Flatus— Gas in the digestive tract, averaging 400 to 1200 milliliters per day.

Flavonoids— Nonnutritive antioxidant compounds that occur naturally in certain foods such as onions, apples, tea, and red wine; inhibit oxidation of LDL in laboratory experiments.

Flow phase— The second phase in the stress response; marked by pronounced hormonal changes.

Fluorosis— Condition due to excessive prolonged intake of fluoride; tissues affected are teeth and bones.

Folate— B vitamin necessary for DNA formation and proper red blood cell formation; form occurring in foods and body tissues.

Folic acid— B vitamin necessary for DNA formation and proper red blood cell formation; oxidized form used to fortify foods and in supplements.

Food acceptance record— A checklist that indicates food items accepted or rejected by the client.

Food allergy— Sensitivity to a food that does not cause a negative reaction in most people.

Food faddism— An unusual pattern of food behavior enthusiastically adapted by its adherents.

Food frequency— A usual food intake or a description of what an individual usually eats during a typical day.

Food infection— Infection acquired through contact with food or water contaminated with disease-producing microorganisms.

Food intoxication— An illness caused by the consumption of a food in which bacteria have produced a poisonous toxin.

Food quackery— The promotion for profit of a medical scheme or remedy that is unproven or known to be false.

Food record— A diary of a person's self-reported food intake.

Fortification— Process of adding nutritive substances not naturally occurring in the given food to increase its nutritional value; for example, milk fortified with vitamins A and D.

Free-living— Way of life in which one freely indulges one's appetites and desires, as opposed to living in an institution.

Free radicals— Atoms or molecules that have lost an electron and vigorously pursue its replacement; in doing so, free radicals can damage normal cell constituents.

Fructose— A monosaccharide found in fruits and honey; a simple sugar.

Fundus— Larger part of a hollow organ; the part of the stomach above its attachment to the esophagus.

Galactose— A monosaccharide derived mainly from the breakdown of the sugar in milk, lactose; a simple sugar.

Galactosemia— Lack of an enzyme needed to metabolize galactose; absolute contraindication to breastfeeding.

Gallbladder— A pear-shaped organ on the underside of the liver that concentrates and stores bile.

Gastric bypass— A surgical procedure that routes food around the stomach.

Gastric lipase— An enzyme in the stomach that aids in the digestion of fats.

Gastric stapling— A surgical procedure on the stomach to induce weight loss by reducing the size of the stomach; also known as gastroplasty.

Gastrin— A hormone secreted by the gastric mucosa; stimulates the secretion of gastric juice.

Gastritis— Inflammation of the stomach.

Gastroesophageal reflux (acid-reflux disorder) (GERD)— Regurgitation of stomach contents into the esophagus.

Gastroparesis— Partial paralysis of the stomach.

Gastrostomy— A surgical opening in the stomach.

Gene— Basic unit of heredity; linear segment of deoxyribonucleic acid (DNA) that occupies a specific location on a specific chromosome; provides the instructions for protein synthesis.

Generativity— The seventh of Erikson's developmental stages, in which the middle-aged adult guides the next generation.

Generic name— The name given to a drug by its original developer; usually the same as the official name given to it by the Food and Drug Administration.

Genetic susceptibility— Likelihood of an individual developing a given trait as determined by heredity.

Genomics— The study of an organism's complete set of DNA; regarding nutrition, the study of how different foods may interact with specific genes to increase the risk of common chronic diseases.

Genotype— Total of the hereditary information present in an organism whether or not expressed in the individual's phenotype (see Phenotype).

Geriatrics— Branch of medicine involved in the study and treatment of diseases of the elderly.

Gestation— Time from fertilization of the ovum until birth; in humans, the length of gestation is usually 38–42 weeks.

Gestational diabetes (GDM)— Hyperglycemia and altered carbohydrate, protein, and fat metabolism related to the increased physiological demands of pregnancy.

Globin— The simple protein portion of hemoglobin.

Glomerular filtrate— The fluid that has been passed through the glomerulus.

Glomerular filtration rate (GFR)— An index of kidney function; the amount of filtrate formed each minute in all the nephrons of both kidneys.

Glomerulonephritis— Inflammation of the glomeruli.

Glomerulus— The network of capillaries inside Bowman's capsule.

Glossitis— Inflammation of the tongue.

Glucagon— A hormone secreted by the alpha cells of the pancreas; increases the concentration of glucose in the blood.

Gluconeogenesis— The production of glucose from noncarbohydrate sources such as amino acids and glycerol.

Glucose— A monosaccharide (simple sugar) commonly called the blood sugar; the same as dextrose.

Glucose tolerance test— A test of blood and urine after the patient receives a concentrated dose of glucose; used to diagnose abnormalities of glucose metabolism.

Gluteal-femoral obesity— Excess body fat centered around an individual's buttocks, hips, and thighs.

Gluten— A type of protein found in wheat, rye, and barley; may contaminate oats through processing.

Gluten-sensitive enteropathy (celiac disease)— An intestinal disorder caused by an abnormal response following the consumption of gluten.

Glycemic index— A measure of how much the blood glucose level increases following consumption of a particular food that contains a given amount of carbohydrate.

Glycerol— The backbone of a fat molecule; pharmaceutical preparation is glycerin.

Glycogen— The form in which carbohydrate is stored in liver and muscle.

Glycogenolysis— The breakdown of glycogen.

Glycosuria— Glucose in the urine.

Glycosylated hemoglobin— Hemoglobin to which a glucose group is attached; in diabetes mellitus, if the blood glucose level has not been controlled over the previous 120 days, the glycosylated hemoglobin level is elevated.

Goiter— Enlargement of the thyroid gland characterized by pronounced swelling in the neck.

Goitrogens— Substances that block the absorption of iodine, thereby causing goiter; found in cabbage, rutabaga, and turnips, but only related to goiter in cassava.

Gout— A hereditary metabolic disease that is a form of acute arthritis and is marked by inflammation of the joints.

GRAS List— Food additives categorized by the U.S. Food and Drug Administration to be Generally Recognized As Safe.

Growth— Progressive increase in size of a living thing that entails the synthesis of new protoplasm and multiplication of cells.

Gut failure— Impaired absorption due to structural damage to the small intestine; symptoms include diarrhea, malabsorption, and unsuccessful absorption of oral food.

Half-life— In drug therapy, time required by the body to metabolize or inactivate half the amount of a substance.

Harris-Benedict equation— A formula commonly used to estimate resting energy expenditure in a stressed client.

Health— The state of complete physical, mental, and social well-being, not just the absence of disease or infirmity.

Healthy body weight (HBW)— Estimate of a weight suitable for an individual based on frame size and height and weight tables.

Heart failure— Inability of heart to circulate blood sufficiently to meet body's needs.

Hematocrit— Percentage of total blood volume that is red blood cells; normal levels are 40%–54% for men, 37%–47% for women.

Hematuria— Blood in the urine.

Heme— The iron-containing portion of the hemoglobin molecule.

Heme iron— Iron bound to hemoglobin and myoglobin in meat, fish, and poultry; 10%–30% of the iron in these foods is absorbed.

Hemochromatosis— A genetic disease of iron metabolism in which iron accumulates in the tissues.

Hemodialysis— A method for cleansing the blood of wastes by circulating blood through a machine that contains tubes made of synthetic semipermeable membranes.

Hemoglobin— The iron-carrying pigment of the red blood cells; carries oxygen from the lungs to the tissues.

Hemolysis— Rupture of red blood cells releasing hemoglobin into the plasma; causes include bacterial toxins, chemicals, inappropriate medications, vitamin E deficiency.

Hemolytic anemia— An abnormal reduction in the number of red blood cells due to hemolysis.

Hemosiderin— An iron oxide–protein compound derived from hemoglobin; a storage form of iron.

Hemosiderosis— Condition resulting from excess deposits of hemosiderin, especially in the liver and spleen; caused by destruction of red blood cells, which occurs in diseases such as hemolytic anemia, pernicious anemia, and chronic infection.

Heparin— A chemical, found naturally in many tissues, that inhibits blood clotting by preventing the conversion of prothrombin to thrombin; also given as an anticoagulant medication.

Hepatic portal circulation— A subdivision of the vascular system in which blood from the digestive organs and spleen circulates through the liver before returning to the heart.

Hepatitis— Inflammation of the liver, caused by viruses, drugs, alcohol, or toxic substances.

Heterozygous— Having two different genes, one from each parent, governing a particular trait; the dominant gene will produce the given trait in the individual.

Hiatal hernia— A protrusion of part of the stomach into the chest cavity.

High-density lipoprotein (HDL)— A plasma protein that carries fat in the bloodstream to the tissues or to the liver to be excreted; elevated blood levels are associated with a decreased risk of heart disease.

High-fructose corn syrup (HFCS)— A common food additive used as a sweetener; made from fructose.

Hives (urticaria)— Sudden swelling and itching of skin or mucous membranes, often caused by allergies; if the respiratory tract is involved, may be life-threatening.

Homeostasis— Tendency toward balance in the internal environment of the body, achieved by automatic monitoring and regulating mechanisms.

Homozygous— Having two identical genes, one from each parent, governing a particular trait; necessary condition to produce a disease caused by a recessive gene, such as sickle cell anemia.

Hormone— A substance produced by cells of the body that is released into the bloodstream and carried to target sites to regulate the activity of other cells and organs.

Human immunodeficiency virus (HIV)— The virus that causes AIDS.

Humoral immunity— Development of antibodies to specific antigens by the B-lymphocytes, some of which retain the ability to recognize the antigen if it is encountered again; basis of immunizations.

Humulin— Exact duplicate of human insulin manufactured by altering bacterial DNA.

Hunger— The sensation resulting from a lack of food, characterized by dull or acute pain around the lower part of the chest.

Hydrochloric acid (HCl)— Strong acid secreted by the stomach that aids in protein digestion.

Hydrogenation— The process of adding hydrogen to a fat to make it more highly saturated.

Hydrolysis— A chemical reaction that splits a substance into simpler compounds by the addition of water; in hydrolyzed infant formulas, whole proteins are split into smaller pieces.

Hydrostatic pressure— The pressure created by the pumping action of the heart on the fluid in the blood vessels.

Hyperalimentation— Another name for total parenteral nutrition.

Hyperbilirubinemia— Excessive bilirubin in the blood; bilirubin is produced by the breakdown of red blood cells.

Hypercalcemia— A serum calcium level that is too high; in adults, more than 5.5 milliequivalents per liter.

Hypercholesterolemia— Excessive cholesterol in the blood.

Hyperemesis gravidarum— Severe nausea and vomiting persisting after the fourteenth week of pregnancy of unknown etiology.

Hyperglycemia— An elevated level of glucose in the blood; fasting value above 110 milligrams per deciliter, depending on measuring technique used.

Hyperglycemic hyperosmolar nonketotic syndrome (HHNS)— Life-threatening complication of NIDDM characterized by blood glucose levels greater than 600 milligrams per deciliter, absence of or slight ketosis, profound cellular dehydration, and electrolyte imbalances.

Hyperkalemia— Excessive potassium in the blood; greater than 5.0 milliequivalents per liter of serum in adults.

Hyperlipoproteinemia— Increased lipoproteins and lipids in the blood.

Hypermetabolism— An abnormal increase in the rate at which fuel or kilocalories are burned.

Hypernatremia— An excess of sodium in the blood; greater than 145 milliequivalents per liter of serum in adults.

Hyperparathyroidism— Excessive secretion of parathyroid hormone, causing changes in the bones, kidney, and gastrointestinal tract.

Hyperphosphatemia— Excessive amount of phosphates in the blood; in adults, greater than 4.7 milligrams per 100 milliliters of serum.

Hypertension— Condition of elevated blood pressure; diagnosed if blood pressure is greater than 140/90 on three successive occasions or if person is receiving antihypertensive medication.

Hypertensive disorders of pregnancy— Blood pressure greater than 140 mmHg systolic or greater than 90 mmHg diastolic occurring in pregnancy. Subcategories are chronic hypertension, gestational hypertension, preeclampsia, and eclampsia.

Hypertensive kidney disease— A condition in which vascular or glomerular lesions cause hypertension but not total renal failure.

Hyperthyroidism— Oversecretion of thyroid hormones, which increases the metabolic rate above normal.

Hypertonic— A solution that contains more particles and exerts more osmotic pressure than the plasma.

Hypervitaminosis— Condition caused by excessive intake of vitamins.

Hypocalcemia— A depressed level of calcium in the blood; less than 4.5 milliequivalents per liter of serum in adults.

Hypoglycemia— A depressed level of glucose in the blood; less than 70 milligrams per deciliter.

Hypokalemia— Potassium depletion in the circulating blood; less than 3.5 milliequivalents per liter of serum in adults.

Hyponatremia— Too little sodium per volume of blood; less than 135 milliequivalents per liter of serum in adults.

Hypophosphatemia— Too little phosphate per volume of blood; in adults, less than 2.4 milligrams per 100 milliliters of serum.

Hypothalamus— A portion of the brain that helps to regulate water balance, thirst, body temperature, carbohydrate and fat metabolism, and sleep.

Hypothyroidism— Undersecretion of thyroid hormones; reduces the metabolic rate.

Hypotonic— A solution that contains fewer particles and exerts less osmotic pressure than the plasma does.

Iatrogenic malnutrition— Excessive or deficit intake of one or more nutrients induced by the oversight or omissions of health-care workers.

Ideal body weight— A person's weight as compared with the 1943 Height/Weight Tables.

Identity— The fifth developmental task in Erikson's theory, in which the adolescent decides on an appropriate role.

Idiopathic— Without a recognizable cause.

Ileocecal valve— The valve between the ileum and cecum.

Ileostomy— Surgical procedure in which an opening to the small intestine (ileum) is constructed on the abdomen.

Ileum— The lower portion of the small intestine.

Immune— Produced by, involved in, or concerned with resistance or protection against a specified disease.

Immune system— The organs in the body responsible for fighting off substances interpreted as foreign.

Immunity— The state of being protected from a particular disease, especially an infectious disease.

Immunoglobulin— Blood proteins with known antibody activity; five types of immunoglobulins have been identified: IgA, IgD, IgE, IgG, and IgM.

Immunosuppressive agent— Medication that interferes with the body's ability to fight infection.

Impaired glucose tolerance (IGT)— A type of classification for hyperglycemia; for persons who have a glucose intolerance but do not meet the criteria for classification as having diabetes.

Implantation— Embedding of the fertilized egg in the lining of the uterus 6 or 7 days after fertilization.

Incidence— The frequency of occurrence of any event or condition over a given time and in relation to the population in which it occurs.

Incomplete protein— Protein lacking one or more of the essential amino acids that humans need; found primarily in plant sources such as grains and vegetables; gelatin is an animal product but is an incomplete protein.

Incubation period— The time it takes to show disease symptoms after exposure to the causative organism.

Indication— A circumstance that indicates when a treatment should or can be used.

Indoles— Compounds found in vegetables of the cruciferous family that activate enzymes to destroy carcinogens.

Industry— The fourth stage of development in Erikson's theory in which the school-age child learns to work effectively.

Infant botulism— Neurological toxicity caused by ingestion of *Clostridium botulinum* spores from honey or soil-contaminated foods; infant's intestinal tract flora cannot suppress the spores; also called intestinal botulism.

Infection— Entry and development of parasites or entry and multiplication of microorganisms in the bodies of persons or animals; may or may not cause signs and symptoms.

Initiation— The first step in the cell's becoming cancerous, when physical forces, chemicals, or biologic agents permanently alter the cell's DNA.

Initiative— The third stage of development in Erikson's theory, in which the preschooler learns to set and achieve goals.

Insensible water loss— Water that is lost invisibly through the lungs and skin.

Insoluble— Incapable of being dissolved in a given substance.

Insulin— Hormone secreted by the beta cells of the pancreas in response to an elevated blood glucose level.

Insulin-dependent diabetes mellitus (IDDM)— Type 1 diabetes; persons with this disorder must take insulin to survive.

Insulin resistance— A disorder characterized by elevated levels of both glucose and insulin; thought to be related to a lack of insulin receptors.

Intact feeding— A feeding consisting of nutrients that have not been predigested.

Intact nutrients— Nutrients that have not been predigested.

Intact or "polymeric" formula— An oral or enteral feeding that contains all the essential nutrients in a specified volume.

Integrity— The final stage of Erikson's theory of psychosocial development, in which the older adult learns to look back on his or her life as worthwhile.

Intermittent feeding— Giving a 4- to 6-hour volume of a tube feeding over 20–30 minutes.

Intermittent peritoneal dialysis— Method of dialysis treatment in which the dialysate remains in a patient's abdominal cavity for about 30 minutes and then drains from the body by gravity.

International Unit (IU)— Individually scaled measure of vitamins A, D, and E agreed to by a committee of scientists; largely replaced by finer measures.

Interstitial fluid— Extracellular fluid located between the cells.

Intimacy— The sixth stage of development in Erikson's theory, in which the young adult builds reciprocal, caring relationships.

Intracellular fluid— Fluid located within the cells.

Intravascular fluid— Fluid found in the blood and lymph vessels.

Intravenous— Through a vein.

Intrinsic factor— Specific protein-binding factor secreted by the stomach, necessary for the absorption of vitamin B_{12}.

Invisible fat— Dietary fats that cannot be seen easily; hidden fats in foods such as baked goods, peanut butter, emulsified milk, and so forth.

Ion— An atom or group of atoms carrying an electrical charge; an ion with a positive charge is called a cation; an ion with a negative charge is called an anion.

Ionic bond— A chemical bond formed between atoms by the loss and gain of electrons.

Iron deficiency— State of inadequate iron stores measured by laboratory tests such as serum ferritin and transferrin saturation; may progress to anemia when the person's hemoglobin value drops.

Irrigation— Flushing a prescribed solution through a tube or cavity.

Irritable bowel syndrome— Diarrhea or alternating constipation-diarrhea with no discernible organic cause.

Islet cell antibody— A protein found to be elevated in a person with insulin-dependent diabetes mellitus.

Islets of Langerhans— Clusters of cells in the pancreas including alpha, beta, and delta cells; alpha cells produce glucagon, beta cells produce insulin, and delta cells produce somatostatin.

Isotonic— A solution that has the same osmotic pressure as blood plasma.

Isotretinoin— Vitamin A metabolite used to treat severe acne, requiring strict contraceptive protocols in fertile women because the metabolite can cause birth defects.

Jaundice— Yellowing of skin, whites of eyes, and mucous membranes due to excessive bilirubin in the blood; causes may be obstructed bile duct, liver disease, or hemolysis of red blood cells.

Jejunoileal bypass— A surgical procedure that removes a portion of the small intestine, bypassing about 90% of it.

Jejunostomy— A surgical opening into the jejunum.

Jejunum— The second portion of the small intestine.

Kaposi's sarcoma— A type of cancer often related to the immunocompromised state that accompanies AIDS; characterized by multiple areas of cell proliferation, initially in the skin and eventually in other body sites.

Keshan disease— Deterioration of the heart due to selenium deficiency, but heart failure not reversible by supplementation; named for the province of Keshan, China; fatality rate as high as 80%; in mice, linked to a mutation of an avirulent virus to a virulent one producing myocardial disease; virulent strain then caused heart disease in mice not selenium-deficient.

Keto acid— Amino acid residue left after deamination.

Ketoacidosis— Acidosis due to an excess of ketone bodies.

Ketone bodies— Compounds such as acetone and diacetic acid that are formed when fat is metabolized incompletely.

Ketonuria— The presence of ketone bodies in the urine.

Ketosis— The physical state of the human body with ketones elevated in the blood and present in the urine; one example is diabetic ketoacidosis.

Kilocaloric density— The kilocalories contained in a given volume of a food.

Kilocalorie— A measurement unit of energy; the amount of heat required to raise 1 kilogram of water 1 degree Celsius; often referred to as calories by the general public.

Kilocalorie: nitrogen ratio— A mathematical relationship expressed as the number of kilocalories per gram of nitrogen provided in a feeding.

Kilojoule— A measurement unit of energy; one kilocalorie equals 4.184 kilojoules.

Konzo— An irreversible paralytic disease of the lower extremities caused by consumption of inadequately processed cassava roots that contain cyanide along with a diet deficient in sulphur-based amino acids.

Korsakoff's psychosis— Amnesia, often seen in chronic alcoholism, caused by degeneration of the thalamus due to thiamin deficiency; characterized by loss of short-term memory and inability to learn new skills.

Krebs cycle— A complicated series of reactions that results in the release of energy from carbohydrates, fats, and proteins, also known as the TCA (tricarboxylic acid) cycle.

Kussmaul respirations— Pattern of rapid and deep breathing due to the body's attempt to correct metabolic acidosis by eliminating carbon dioxide through the lungs.

Kwashiorkor— Severe protein deficiency in child after weaning; symptoms include edema, pigmentation changes, impaired growth and development, and liver pathology.

Lactalbumin— Simple soluble protein found in greater concentration in human breast milk than in cow's milk; easily absorbed by the infant.

Lactase— An intestinal enzyme that converts lactose into glucose and galactose.

Lacteal— The central lymph vessel in each villus.

Lactose— A disaccharide found mainly in milk and milk products.

Large intestine— The part of the alimentary canal that extends from the small intestine to the anus.

LCAT deficiency— A lack of LCAT, an enzyme that transports cholesterol from the tissues to the liver for removal from the body.

Lean body mass— Also called fat-free mass; the weight of the body minus the fat content but including essential fats that are associated with the central nervous system, the viscera, the bone marrow, and cell membranes.

Legumes— Plants that have nitrogen-fixing bacteria in their roots; a good alternative to meat as a protein source; examples are dried beans, lentils.

Lesion— Area of diseased or injured tissue.

Leukopenia— Abnormal decrease in the number of white blood corpuscles; usually below 5000 per cubic millimeter.

Life expectancy— The probable number of years that persons of a given age may be expected to live.

Limiting amino acid— Particular essential amino acid lacking or undersupplied in a food that classifies the food as an incomplete protein.

Linoleic acid— An essential fatty acid.

Lipectomy— Surgical removal of adipose tissue.

Lipid— Any one of a group of fats or fat-like substances that are insoluble in water; includes true fats (fatty acids and glycerol), lipoids, and sterols.

Lipoid— Substances resembling fats but containing groups other than glycerol and fatty acids that make up true fats; example: phospholipids.

Lipolysis— The breakdown of adipose tissue for energy.

Lipoprotein— Combination of a protein with lipid components such as cholesterol, phospholipids, and triglycerides.

Lipoprotein lipase— An enzyme that breaks down chylomicrons.

Liposuction— Surgical removal of adipose tissue through a vacuum hose.

Listeriosis— Bacterial infection caused by *Listeria monocytogenes* that is particularly virulent for fetuses; transmitted from the mother to the fetus in utero or through the birth canal; outbreaks associated with raw or contaminated milk, soft cheeses, contaminated vegetables, and ready-to-eat meats; others at risk—the elderly, those with impaired immune systems, and farm workers.

Liver— A digestive organ that aids in the metabolism of all the energy nutrients, screens toxic substances from the blood, manufactures blood proteins, and performs many other important functions.

Loop of Henle— The segment of the renal tubule that follows the proximal convoluted tubule.

Low birth weight (LBW)— Characterizing an infant that weighs less than 2500 g (5.5 lb) at birth.

Low-density lipoprotein (LDL)— A plasma protein containing more cholesterol and triglycerides than protein; elevated blood levels are associated with increased risk of heart disease.

Luminal effect— Drug-induced changes within the intestine that affect the absorption of nutrients and drugs without altering the intestine.

Lycopene— A red pigmented carotenoid with powerful antioxidant functions but no provitamin A activity; found in tomatoes and various berries and fruits.

Lymph— A body fluid collected from the interstitial fluid all over the body and returned to the bloodstream via the lymphatic vessels.

Lymphatic system— All the structures involved in the transportation of lymph from the tissues to the bloodstream.

Lysine— Amino acid often lacking in grains.

Macrocytic anemia— Anemia in which the red blood cells are larger than normal; one characteristic of pernicious anemia also found in folic acid deficiency.

Macrophage— Monocyte (see Fig. 8-13) that has left the circulation and settled in a tissue such as the spleen, lymph nodes, and tonsils; with neutrophils, major phagocytic cells of immune system.

Major minerals— Those present in the body in quantities greater than 5 grams (approximately 1 teaspoonful); humans need at least 100 milligrams daily (approximately 1/50 teaspoonful); also called macrominerals.

Malabsorption— Inadequate movement of digested food from the small intestine into the blood or lymphatic system.

Malignant— Tumor that infiltrates surrounding tissue and spreads to distant sites of the body.

Malnutrition— Poor nutrition; results when the body's cells receive either an excess or a deficiency of one or more nutrients.

Maltase— An intestinal enzyme that converts maltose into glucose.

Maltose— A disaccharide produced when starches are broken down by the body into simpler units; two units of glucose joined together.

Marasmus— Malnutrition due to a protein and kilocalorie deficit.

Mastication— The process of chewing.

Mechanical digestion— The digestive process that involves the physical breaking down of food into smaller pieces.

Megadose— Dose providing 10 times or more of the recommended dietary allowance.

Megaloblastic anemia— Anemia characterized by large immature red blood cells in the bloodstream that cannot carry oxygen properly; occurs in folic acid deficiency and pernicious anemia.

Menaquinone— Vitamin K that is synthesized by intestinal bacteria; also called vitamin K_2.

Meninges— Three membranes covering the brain and spinal cord; from the outside named the dura, arachnoid, and pia maters.

Meningocele— Congenital protrusion of the meninges through a defect in the skull or the spinal column.

Meningoencephalocele— Protrusion of the brain and its coverings through a defect in the skull.

Menkes' disease— Metabolic defect blocking the absorption of copper in the gastrointestinal tract.

Meta-analysis— Statistical procedure for combining data from a number of studies to analyze therapeutic effectiveness.

Metabolic syndrome— Combination of atherosclerotic risk factors, including dyslipidemia, insulin resistance, obesity, and hypertension, that produces an increased risk for CAD.

Metabolism— The sum of all physical and chemical changes that take place in the body; the two fundamental processes involved are anabolism and catabolism.

Metastasis— The "seeding" of cancer cells to distant sites of the body; spread via blood or lymph vessels or by spilling into a body cavity.

Methionine— Amino acid often lacking in legumes.

Microalbuminuria— Small amounts of protein in the urine. Detected by a laboratory using methods more sensitive than traditional urinalysis.

Microgram— One-millionth of a gram or one-thousandth of a milligram; abbreviated mcg or μ.

Micronize— To pulverize a substance into very tiny particles.

Microvilli— Microscopic, hair-like rodlets (resembling bristles on a brush) covering the edge of each villus.

Midarm circumference— Measure of the distance around the middle of the upper arm; used to assess body protein stores.

Mildly obese— Twenty to 40% overweight; 120%–140% healthy body weight.

Milk-alkali syndrome— Condition characterized by high blood calcium and a more alkaline urine that predisposes to the precipitation of calcium in the kidney; caused by ingestion of excessive absorbable alkali and milk; associated with the milk and cream and antacid treatment of peptic ulcers used years ago.

Milliequivalent— Unit of measure used for determining the concentration of electrolytes in solution; expressed as milliequivalents per liter; abbreviated mEq.

Milling— The process of grinding grain into flour.

Milliosmole— Unit of measure for osmotic activity.

Mineral— An inorganic element or compound occurring in nature; in the body, some minerals help regulate bodily functions and are essential to good health.

Mixed malnutrition— The result of a deficiency or excess of more than one nutrient.

Moderately obese— Forty-one to 100% overweight; 141%–200% healthy body weight.

Modified diet— A term used in health-care institutions to mean the food served to a client has been altered or changed from that served to clients on regular diets, usually by physician order.

Modular supplement— A nutritional supplement that contains a limited number of nutrients, usually only one.

Mold— Any of a group of parasitic or other organisms living on decaying matter; fungi.

Molecule— The smallest quantity into which a substance may be divided without loss of its characteristics.

Monoamine oxidase inhibitor (MAO inhibitor)— A class of drugs that may have critical interactions with foods.

Monocyte— White blood cell (see Fig. 8-13) that circulates in the bloodstream for about 24 hours before settling into tissues to become a macrophage; with macrophages, provide a defense against foreign antigens.

Monoglyceride— One fatty acid joined to a glycerol molecule.

Monosaccharide— A simple sugar composed of one unit of $C_6H_{12}O_6$; examples include glucose, fructose, and galactose.

Monounsaturated fat— A lipid in which the majority of fatty acids contain one carbon-to-carbon double bond.

Morbidity— The state of being diseased; number of cases of disease in relation to population.

Mortality— The death rate; number of deaths per unit of population.

Motility— Power to move spontaneously.

Mucosa— A mucous membrane that lines body cavities.

Mucosal effect— Drug-induced changes within the intestine that affect the absorption of drugs or nutrients by damaging the tissues.

Mucus— A thick fluid secreted by the mucous membranes and glands.

Multiparous— Having borne more than one child.

Mutation— Permanent transmissible change in a gene; natural mutation produces evolutionary change in organisms; induced mutation results from exposure to environmental influences such as physical forces, chemicals, or biologic agents.

Mycotoxin— A substance produced by mold growing in food that can cause illness or death when ingested by humans or animals.

Myelin sheath— Fatty covering surrounding the long appendages of some nerves; serves to increase the transmission speed of impulses.

Myocardial infarction (MI)— Area of dead heart muscle; usually the result of coronary occlusion.

Myocardium— The heart muscle.

Myoglobin— A protein located in muscle tissue that contains and stores oxygen.

MyPyramid— USDA food guide balanced by healthy activity; food groups are grains, vegetables, fruits, oils, milk, meat and beans.

Myxedema— A condition that occurs in older children and adults, resulting from hypofunction of the thyroid gland characterized by a drying and thickening of the skin and slowing of physical and mental activity.

Narcolepsy— A chronic condition consisting of recurrent attacks of drowsiness and sleep.

Nasoduodenal tube (ND tube)— A tube inserted via the nose into the duodenum.

Nasogastric tube (NG tube)— A tube inserted via the nose into the stomach.

Nasojejunal tube (NJ tube)— A tube inserted via the nose into the jejunum.

Neoplasm— A new and abnormal formation of tissue (tumor) that grows at the expense of the healthy organism.

Nephritis— General term for inflammation of the kidneys.

Nephron— The structural and functional unit of the kidney.

Nephropathy— A kidney disease characterized by inflammation and degenerative lesions.

Nephrosclerosis— A hardening of the renal arteries; may be caused by arteriosclerosis of the kidney arteries.

Nephrotic syndrome— The end result of a variety of diseases that cause the abnormal passage of plasma proteins into the urine.

Neuropathy— Any disease of the nerves.

NHANES— National Health and Nutrition Examination Survey, a nationally representative cross-sectional survey of civilian noninstitutionalized population of the U.S.; conducted by the Centers for Disease Control's National Center for Health Statistics.

Niacin— A B-vitamin that functions as a coenzyme in the production of energy from glucose; obtained from meat or produced from the amino acid tryptophan, present in milk, eggs, and meat; also called nicotinic acid.

Niacin equivalent (NE)— Measure of niacin activity; equal to 1 milligram of preformed niacin or 60 milligrams of tryptophan.

Night blindness— Vision that is slow to adapt to dim light; caused by vitamin A deficiency or hereditary factors or, in the elderly, by poor circulation.

Nitrogen— Colorless, odorless, tasteless gas forming about 80% of the Earth's air.

Nitrogen balance— The difference between the amount of nitrogen ingested and that excreted each day; when intake is greater, a positive balance exists; when intake is less, a negative balance exists.

Nitrogen-fixing bacteria— Organisms that absorb nitrogen from the air, which, upon the death of the bacteria, is released for legume plants to use in the anabolism of protein.

Nomogram— A chart that shows a relationship between numerical values.

Nonessential— In nutrition, refers to a chemical substance or nutrient the body normally can manufacture.

Nonessential amino acid— Any amino acid that can normally be synthesized by the body in sufficient quantities.

Nonheme iron— Iron that is not bound to hemoglobin or myoglobin; all the iron in plant sources.

Non-insulin-dependent diabetes mellitus (NIDDM)— Type 2 diabetes; insulin resistance commonly occurs; although some persons with this disorder take insulin, it is not necessary for their long-term survival.

Norwalk virus— A causative organism that is responsible for more than 50% of the reported cases of epidemic viral gastroenteropathy. The incubation period ranges from 18 to 72 hours, and the outbreaks are usually self-limiting. Flu-like intestinal symptoms last for 24–48 hours.

Nulliparous— Never having borne a child.

Nursing action (intervention)— Specific care to be administered, including physical and psychological care, teaching, counseling, and referring.

Nursing-bottle syndrome— A condition in which an infant has many dental caries caused by drinking milk or other sweet liquids during sleep.

Nutrient— Chemical substance supplied by food that the body needs for growth, maintenance, and/or repair.

Nutrient density— The concentration of nutrients in a given volume of food compared with the food's kilocalorie content.

Nutrition— The science of food and its relationship to living beings.

Nutrition support service— A team service for clients on enteral and parenteral feedings that assesses, monitors, and counsels these clients.

Nutritional assessment— The evaluation of a client's nutritional status based on a physical examination, anthropometric measurements, laboratory data, and food intake information.

Nutritional status— Condition of the body as it relates to the intake and use of nutrients.

Obese— Body fat content greater than 24% in males or 33% in females.

Obesity— Excessive amount of fat on the body; obesity for women is a fat content greater than 33%; obesity for men is a fat content greater than 24%.

Objective data— Findings verifiable by another through physical assessment or diagnostic tests, also termed signs.

Obligatory excretion— Minimum amount of urine production necessary to keep waste products in solution, amounting to 400–600 milliliters per day.

Oliguria— A decreased output of urine.

Oncogene— Carcinogenic gene that stimulates excessive reproduction of the cell.

Opportunistic infection— Infection caused by normally nonpathogenic organisms in a host with decreased resistance.

Opsin— A protein that combines with vitamin A to form rhodopsin, a chemical in the retina necessary for vision.

Optic nerve— The second cranial nerve, which transmits impulses for the sense of sight.

Oral cavity— The cavity in the skull bounded by the mouth, palate, cheeks, and tongue.

Organ— Somewhat independent body part having specific functions. Examples: stomach, liver.

Orthostatic hypotension— A drop in blood pressure producing dizziness, fainting, or blurred vision when arising from a lying or sitting position or when standing motionless in a fixed position.

Osmolality— Measure of osmotic pressure exerted by the number of dissolved particles per weight of liquid; clinically usually reported as mOsm/kg.

Osmolarity— Measure of osmotic pressure exerted by the number of dissolved particles per volume of liquid; clinically usually reported as mOsm/L.

Osmosis— The movement of water across a semipermeable cell membrane from an area with fewer particles to one with more particles.

Osmotic pressure— The pressure that develops when a concentrated solution is separated from a less-concentrated solution by a semipermeable membrane.

Osteoarthritis— Progressive deterioration of the cartilage in the joints; risk factors are aging, obesity, occupational or athletic abuse of joints, and trauma.

Osteoblasts— Bone cells that build bone.

Osteocalcin— Hormonally regulated calcium-binding protein made almost exclusively by the bone-building cells called osteoblasts; vitamin K facilitates synthesis of osteocalcin.

Osteoclasts— Bone cells that break down bone.

Osteodystrophy— Defective bone formation.

Osteomalacia— Adult form of rickets.

Osteopenia— Bone mineral density 1 to 2.5 standard deviations below the mean of healthy young adults.

Osteoporosis— Bone mineral density more than 2.5 standard deviations below the mean of young adults.

Ostomy— A surgically formed opening to permit passage of urine or bowel contents to the outside.

Overnutrition— The result of an excess of one or more nutrients in the diet.

Overweight— Ten to 20% above healthy body weight; 110%–120% healthy body weight.

Ovum— The egg cell that, after fertilization by a sperm cell, develops into a new individual.

Oxalates— Salts of oxalic acid found in some plant foods; bind with the calcium in the plant, making it unavailable to the body.

Oxidation— The process in which a substance is combined with oxygen.

Oxidative stress— Cellular damage caused by oxygen-derived free radical formation; potential damage can be decreased by antioxidants.

Oxytocin— A hormone produced by the posterior pituitary gland in the brain; effects are uterine contractions and release of milk.

Pancreas— An abdominal gland that secretes enzymes important in the digestion of carbohydrates, fats, and proteins; also secretes the hormones insulin and glucagon.

Pancreatic lipase— An enzyme produced by the pancreas; used in fat digestion.

Pancreatitis— Inflammation of the pancreas.

Pantothenic acid— A B-complex vitamin found in almost all foods; deficiencies from lack of food have not been documented.

Paralytic ileus— A temporary cessation of peristalsis that causes an intestinal obstruction.

Paralytic shellfish poisoning— Disease caused by the consumption of poisonous clams, oysters, mussels, or scallops.

Parasite— An organism that lives within, upon, or at the expense of a living host.

Parathyroid hormone (PTH)— Hormone secreted by the parathyroid glands; regulates calcium and phosphorus metabolism in the body.

Parenteral feeding— A feeding administered by any route other than the gastrointestinal tract.

Paresthesia— Abnormal or unpleasant sensation resulting from nerve injury; described as a feeling of numbness, prickliness, stinging, or burning.

Parietal— Two bones that form the sides and roof of the skull; also two lobes of the cerebrum lying roughly under those bones.

Parity— Condition of having carried a pregnancy to viability (20 weeks or 500-gram birth weight) regardless of whether resulted in a live birth; nulliparous—never carried a child to viability; multiparous—more than once.

Parotid glands— One of the salivary glands of the mouth, located just below and in front of the ears; the mumps virus causes infectious parotitis.

Pectin— Purified carbohydrate obtained from peel of citrus fruits or apple pulp; gels when cooked with sugar at correct pH to thicken jelly and jam; contained in mashed raw apple, applesauce, firm banana; recommended for diarrhea to contribute firmness to stools.

Pellagra— Deficiency disease due to lack of niacin and tryptophan; characterized by the three Ds: dermatitis, diarrhea, and dementia.

Pepsin— An enzyme secreted in the stomach that begins protein digestion.

Pepsinogen— The antecedent of pepsin; activated by hydrochloric acid, a component of gastric juice.

Peptidases— Enzymes that assist in the digestion of protein by reducing the smaller molecules to single amino acids.

Peptide bond— Chemical bond that links two amino acids in a protein molecule.

Percutaneously— Affected through the skin.

Perforated ulcer— Condition in which an ulcer penetrates completely through the stomach or intestinal wall, spilling the organ's contents into the peritoneal cavity.

Perinatal— Period beginning after the 28th week of pregnancy and ending 28 days after birth.

Periodontal disease— Disorder of the gingiva (gums) and the supporting structures of the teeth.

Peripheral parenteral nutrition (PPN)— An intravenous feeding via a vein away from the center of the body.

Peristalsis— A wave-like muscular movement that propels food along the alimentary canal.

Peritoneal dialysis— Method of removing waste products from the blood by injecting the flushing solution into a client's abdomen and using the client's peritoneum as the semipermeable membrane.

Peritoneum— The membrane that covers the internal abdominal organs and lines the abdominal cavity.

Peritonitis— Inflammation of the peritoneal cavity.

Pernicious anemia— Inadequate red blood cell formation due to lack of intrinsic factor from the stomach, which is required for the absorption of vitamin B_{12}; leads to neural deterioration.

Pesticides— A chemical used to kill insects or rodents.

Petechiae— Pinpoint, flat, round, red lesions caused by intradermal or submucosal hemorrhage.

P-glycoprotein— Cell membrane pump influencing cellular uptake and release of chemicals; affects relative susceptibility or resistance of cells to drug therapy.

pH— *Potential of Hydrogen*; a scale representing the relative acidity or alkalinity of a solution; a value of 7 is neutral, less than 7 is acidic, and greater than 7 is alkaline.

Pharmacodynamics— Study of drugs and their actions on living organisms; the clinical effects of the drugs.

Pharmacokinetics— The study of the action of drugs, emphasizing absorption time, duration of effect, distribution in the body, and method of excretion.

Pharynx— Muscular passage between the oral cavity and the esophagus.

Phenotype— Observable properties of an organism; blood type is completely inherited; other phenotypes can be altered by environmental agents.

Phenylalanine— Essential amino acid, which is indigestible if a person lacks a particular enzyme. Accumulation of phenylalanine in the blood can lead to mental retardation.

Phenylketonuria (PKU)— Hereditary disease caused by the body's failure to convert phenylalanine to tyrosine because of a defective enzyme.

Phospholipid— Diglyceride containing phosphorus; primary lipid constituent of cell membranes; examples include lecithin and myelin.

Photosynthesis— Process by which plants containing chlorophyll are able to manufacture carbohydrates from carbon dioxide and water using the sun's energy.

Phylloquinone— Vitamin K_1, found in foods.

Phytic acid— A substance found in grains that forms an insoluble complex with calcium; phytates.

Phytochemicals— Nonnutritive food components that provide medical or health benefits including the prevention or treatment of a disease.

Phytonadione— Synthetic, water-soluble pharmaceutical form of vitamin K_1; can be administered orally or by injection.

Pica— The craving to eat nonfood substances such as clay and starch.

Pitting edema— Usually of the skin of the extremities; firm pressure by a finger produces an indentation that remains for 5 seconds.

Placebo— Drug or treatment used as inactive control in a test of therapy; "placebo effect" attributed to positive response caused by subject's expectations.

Placenta— The organ in the uterus through which the unborn child exchanges carbon dioxide for oxygen and wastes for nourishment; lay term is afterbirth.

Plant sterols— Compounds, structurally similar to cholesterol, that in prescribed amounts interfere with the absorption of cholesterol and thus lower LDL-C levels; marketed as table spreads (butter substitutes) and salad dressings.

Plaque— Accumulation of material; in lining of arteries, lipids obstruct blood flow; on crowns of teeth, forerunner of dental caries and periodontal disease.

Plasma— The liquid portion of the blood including the clotting elements.

Plasma transferrin receptor— Measure of iron status; increases even in mild deficiency; unaffected by inflammation.

Plumbism— Lead poisoning.

Pneumocystis pneumonia— A type of lung infection frequently seen in AIDS patients; caused by the organism *Pneumocystis carinii.*

Polycythemia— Increase in red blood cells (RBCs); may be physiologic due to demand for oxygen-carrying capacity or pathologic as in p. vera, a chronic, life-shortening disorder of unknown etiology involving hematologic stem cells.

Polydipsia— Excessive thirst.

Polymer— A natural or synthetic substance formed by combining two or more molecules of the same substance.

Polymorphism— Occurrence of more than one form in a life cycle; variation in alleles within a species.

Polypeptide— A chain of amino acids linked by peptide bonds that form proteins.

Polyphagia— Excessive appetite.

Polypharmacy— Concurrent use of a large number of drugs, increasing risk of interactions; especially likely in client with many diseases treated by multiple healthcare providers.

Polysaccharide— Complex carbohydrates composed of many units of $C_6H_{12}O_6$ joined together; examples important in nutrition include starch, glycogen, and fiber.

Polyunsaturated fat— A fat in which the majority of fatty acids contain more than one carbon-to-carbon double bond; intake is associated with a decreased risk of heart disease.

Polyuria— Excessive urination.

Positive feedback cycle— Situation in which a condition provokes a response that worsens the condition. Example: low blood pressure due to a failing heart stimulates the kidney to save sodium and water, increasing fluid retention.

Postprandial— Following a meal.

Potable water— Water that is safe for drinking, free of harmful substances.

Potassium pump— Proteins located in cell membranes that provide an active transport mechanism to move potassium ions across a membrane to their area of greater concentration; moves potassium ions into the cells.

Prebiotic— Nondigestible food ingredients that encourage the growth of favorable intestinal microorganisms.

Precursor— A substance from which another substance is derived.

Preeclampsia— Hypertension and proteinuria, appearing after the twentieth week of pregnancy.

Preformed vitamin— A vitamin already in a complete state in ingested foods, as opposed to a provitamin, which requires conversion in the body to be in a complete state.

Pressure ulcer— Tissue breakdown from external force impairing circulation.

Prevalence— The number of cases of a disease or condition present in a specified population at a given time.

Primary amenorrhea— Delay of menarche (initial menstrual period) until after age of 16 or absence of secondary sex characteristics after age 14.

Primary malnutrition— A nutrient deficiency due to poor food choices or a lack of nutritious food to eat.

Principle of complementarity— Combining incomplete-protein foods so that each supplies the amino acids lacking in the other.

Prion— A proteinaceous infectious agent, extremely difficult to destroy; resistant to heat, pressure cooking, ultraviolet light, irradiation, bleach, formaldehyde, and weak acids; even autoclaving at 135 degrees for 18 minutes does not eliminate infectivity.

Probiotic— Live microbial food supplements that improve the microbial balance of the intestine, mainly by reinforcing the intestinal mucosal barrier against harmful agents.

Prognosis— Probable outcome of an illness based on client's condition and natural course of the disease.

Promotion— The second step in a cell turning cancerous, through the action of environmental substances on the altered, initiated gene.

Prostaglandins— Long-chain, unsaturated fatty acids mostly synthesized in the body from arachidonic acid; have hormone-like effects.

Protein— Nutrient necessary for building body tissue; composed of carbon, hydrogen, oxygen, and nitrogen (and sometimes with sulfur, phosphorus, or iron); amino acids represent the basic structure of proteins.

Protein binding sites— Various sites in the body tissues to which drugs may become attached, rendering the drug temporarily inactive.

Protein-calorie malnutrition (PCM)— Condition in which the person's diet lacks both protein and kilocalories.

Proteinuria— Protein in the urine.

Prothrombin— A protein essential to the blood-clotting process; manufactured by the liver using vitamin K.

Protocol— A description of steps to be followed when performing a procedure or providing care for a particular condition.

Proto-oncogene— Gene that in the normal cell stimulates growth and maintenance; when mutated, becomes an oncogene.

Provitamin— Inactive substance that the body converts to an active vitamin.

Provitamin A— Carotenoids that are precursors of vitamin A, the most powerful of which is beta-carotene.

Proximal convoluted tubule— The first segment of the renal tubule.

Psychology— The science of mental processes and their effects on behavior.

Psychosis— Severe mental disturbance with personality derangement and loss of contact with reality.

Psychosocial development— The maturing of an individual in relationships with others and within himself or herself.

Ptyalin— A salivary enzyme that breaks down starch and glycogen to maltose and a small amount of glucose; also known as salivary amylase.

Puberty— The period of life at which the physical ability to reproduce is attained.

Pulmonary— Concerning or involving the lungs.

Pulmonary edema— The accumulation of fluid in the lungs.

Pulse pressure— The difference between systolic and diastolic blood pressure; normally 30–40 mmHg; narrows in insufficient fluid volume and widens in excessive fluid volume.

Purging— The intentional clearing of food out of the human body by vomiting and/or using enemas, laxatives, and/or diuretics.

Purines— One of the end products of the digestion of some nitrogen-containing compounds.

Pyelonephritis— An inflammation of the central portion of the kidney.

Pyloric sphincter— The sphincter muscle guarding the opening between the stomach and small intestine.

Pyridoxine— Pharmaceutical name for vitamin B_6.

Pyruvate— An intermediate in the metabolism of energy nutrients.

Quality assurance— A planned and systematic program for evaluating the quality and appropriateness of services rendered.

Quetelet's Index— Body Mass Index.

Radiologist— Physician with special training in diagnostic imaging and radiation treatments.

Rancid— Having the rank smell and sour taste of stale fat or oil from decomposition.

Rate— The speed or frequency of an event per unit of time.

Rationale— Reason certain actions are likely to achieve a desired outcome; in nursing, ideally based on research indicating a nursing action was effective in similar circumstances.

Rebound scurvy— Vitamin C deficiency produced in a person following cessation of megadosing due to a habitually lessened rate of absorption.

Recessive trait— One that requires two recessive genes for the trait, one from each parent, for the trait to be expressed (to be manifested) in the individual.

Recommended Dietary Allowance— Intake that meets the needs of 97%–98% of the individuals in a life-stage and gender group; intended as a goal for daily intake by individuals, not for assessing adequacy of an individual's nutrient intake.

Rectum— The lower part of the large intestine.

Refeeding— The reintroduction of kilocalories and nutrients into a patient either orally or parenterally.

Refeeding syndrome— A detrimental state that results when a previously severely malnourished person is reintroduced to food and/or nutrients and kilocalories improperly.

Regurgitate— To cause to flow backward, as with an infant "spitting up."

Relative risk— In epidemiological studies, the ratio of the frequency of a certain disorder in groups exposed and groups not exposed to a particular hereditary or environmental factor.

Renal— Pertaining to the kidney.

Renal corpuscle— Refers collectively to both Bowman's capsule and the glomerulus.

Renal exchange lists— A specialized type of exchange list for clients with kidney disease who require restriction of one or more of the following: protein, sodium, phosphorus, and potassium.

Renal osteodystrophy— Defective bone development caused by phosphorus retention, a low or normal serum calcium level, and increased parathyroid activity.

Renal pelvis— A structure inside the kidney that receives urine from the collecting tubules.

Renal threshold— The blood glucose level at which glucose begins to spill into the urine.

Renal tubule— The second major portion of the nephron; appears rope-like.

Renin— An enzyme produced by the kidney that catalyzes the conversion of angiotensinogen to angiotensin I.

Rennin— An enzyme that coagulates milk.

Reservoir— Place that an infectious agent normally lives and multiplies so that it can be transmitted to a susceptible host.

Residue— Trace amount of any substance in a product at the time of sale; substance remaining in the bowel after absorption.

Respiration— The exchange of oxygen and carbon dioxide between a living organism and the environment.

Respirator— A machine used to assist respiration.

Respiratory acidosis— Blood pH less than 7.35 caused by pulmonary disease, characterized by a retention of carbon dioxide.

Respiratory alkalosis— Blood pH greater than 7.45 caused by pulmonary disease, characterized by a loss of carbon dioxide.

Resting energy expenditure (REE)— The amount of fuel the human body uses at rest for a specified period of time; often used interchangeably with basal metabolic rate (BMR).

Retina— Inner lining of eyeball that contains light-sensitive nerve cells; corresponds to film in camera.

Retinoic acid syndrome— Characteristic fetal deformities, including small ears or no ears, abnormal or missing ear canals, brain malformation, and heart defects caused by excessive preformed vitamin A or isotretinoin.

Retinol— One of the active forms of preformed vitamin A.

Retinol Activity Equivalent (RAE)— Measure of vitamin A activity that considers both preformed vitamin A (retinol) and its precursor (carotene); 1 RAE equals 3.3 International Units from animal foods or 20 International Units from plant foods.

Retinopathy— Any disorder of the retina.

Retrolental fibroplasia (RLF)— A disease of the vessels of the retina present in premature infants; often caused by exposure to high postnatal oxygen concentration.

Rhabdomyolysis— Breakdown of muscle fibers resulting in myoglobin in the bloodstream; some components are toxic to kidney and can cause kidney damage.

Rhodopsin— Light-sensitive protein in the retina that contains vitamin A; also called visual purple.

Riboflavin— Coenzyme in the metabolism of protein; also called vitamin B_2.

Ribonucleic acid (RNA)— A substance in the cell nucleus that controls protein synthesis in all living cells.

Rickets— Disease caused by a deficiency of vitamin D that affects the young during the period of skeletal growth, resulting in bones that are abnormally shaped and weak.

Ritter syndrome— An inflammatory skin disease seen in newborns, characterized by pustules that fill with a straw-colored fluid and become encrusted.

Rooting reflex— The infant's natural response to a stroke on its cheek, which turns the head toward that side to nurse.

Rotavirus— Most common cause of infectious enteritis in human infants; survives for long periods on hard surfaces, in contaminated water, and on hands.

Roux-en-Y— A surgical connection between the distal end of the small bowl and another organ such as the stomach.

Rugae— Folds of mucosa of organs such as the stomach.

Salivary amylase— An enzyme that initiates the breakdown of starch in the mouth.

Salivary glands— The glands that secrete saliva into the mouth.

***Salmonella*—** A genus of bacteria responsible for many cases of foodborne illness.

Salmonellosis— A bacterial infection manifested by the sudden onset of headache, abdominal pain, diarrhea, nausea, and vomiting. Fever is almost always present. Contaminated food is the predominant method of transmission.

Sarcoma— A malignant neoplasm that occurs in connective tissue such as muscle or bone.

Satiety— The feeling after consuming food that enough has been eaten; the sensation of satisfaction.

Saturated fat— A fat in which the majority of fatty acids contain no carbon-to-carbon double bonds.

Scurvy— Disease due to deficiency of vitamin C marked by bleeding problems and, later, by bony skeleton changes.

Seasonal variation— Refers to differences during spring, summer, fall, and winter.

Sebaceous gland— Oil-secreting gland of the skin; most sebaceous glands have a hair follicle associated with them.

Secondary diabetes— A World Health Organization (WHO) classification for diabetes when the hyperglycemia occurs as a result of another disorder.

Secondary hypertension— High blood pressure that develops as the result of another condition.

Secondary malnutrition— A nutrient deficiency due to improper absorption and distribution of nutrients.

Secretin— A hormone that stimulates the production of bile by the liver and the secretion of sodium bicarbonate juice by the pancreas.

Self-efficacy— One's belief in his or her ability to perform a task or behavior.

Self-monitoring of blood glucose (SMBG)— A procedure that persons with diabetes follow to test their own blood glucose levels.

Sensible water loss— Visible water loss through perspiration, urine, and feces.

Sensitivity— Characteristic of diagnostic test; the proportion of people correctly identified as having the condition in question; a score of 100% would indicate that all the affected persons were identified by the test.

Sepsis— A condition in which disease-producing organisms are present in the blood.

Serosa— A serous membrane that covers internal organs and lines body cavities.

Serotonin— A body chemical that assists the transmission of nerve impulses; it produces constriction of blood vessels and is thought to be related to sleep.

Serum— The liquid portion of the blood minus the clotting elements.

Serum transferrin— Globulin in the blood that binds and transports iron; level increases in early iron deficiency, before hemoglobin and hematocrit readings drop.

Severely obese— Greater than 100% overweight; also expressed as greater than 201% healthy body weight.

Shelf life— The duration of time a product can remain in storage without deterioration.

***Shigella*—** Organisms causing intestinal disease; spread by fecal-oral transmission from a client or carrier via direct contact or indirectly by contaminated food.

SIADH (Syndrome of Inappropriate Secretion of Antidiuretic Hormone)— Pathological secretion of ADH; result is dilutional hyponatremia.

Signs— See Objective data.

Simple carbohydrate— Composed of one or two units of $C_6H_{12}O_6$; includes the monosaccharides (glucose, fructose, and galactose) and the disaccharides (sucrose, lactose, and maltose).

Simple fat— Lipids that consist of fatty acids or a simple filler such as a hydroxyl (OH) molecule joined to glycerol.

Small for gestational age (SGA)— Infant weighing less at birth than considered normal for the calculated length of the pregnancy.

Small intestine— The part of the alimentary canal between the stomach and the large intestine, where most absorption of nutrients occurs.

Sodium pump— Proteins located in cell membranes that provide an active transport mechanism to move sodium ions across a membrane to their area of greater concentration; moves sodium ions out of the cells and water follows.

Solubility— The ability of one substance to dissolve into another in solution.

Soluble— Able to be dissolved.

Solute— The substance that is dissolved in a solvent.

Solvent— A liquid holding another substance in solution.

Somatostatin— A hormone produced by the delta cells of the islets of Langerhans that inhibits both the release of insulin and the production of glucagon.

Specific gravity— The weight of a substance compared to an equal volume of a standard substance; usual standard for liquids is water; its specific gravity set at 1.000.

Specificity— Characteristic of diagnostic test; the proportion of people correctly identified as not having the condition in question; a score of 100% would indicate that all of the unaffected persons were identified by the test.

Sphincter— A circular band of muscles that constricts a passage.

Spina bifida— Congenital defect in spinal column whereby the vertebrae fail to close; clinical manifestations may or may not include protrusion of the meninges outside the spinal canal.

Spore— A form assumed by some bacteria that is highly resistant to heat, drying, and chemicals.

Sprue— Chronic form of malabsorption syndrome affecting the small intestine; subcategories: tropical and nontropical.

Standard drink— One standard alcoholic beverage; usually 12 ounces of beer, 4 ounces of wine, or 1.5 ounces of liquor.

Staphylococcus aureus— One of the most common species of bacteria, which produces a poisonous toxin. The main reservoir is nose and throat discharge. Food can act as a vehicle for transmission, so proper hand washing is an essential means of control.

Starches— Polysaccharides; many units of $C_6H_{12}O_6$ joined together; complex carbohydrates.

Steatorrhea— The presence of greater than normal amounts of fat in the stool, producing foul-smelling, bulky excrement.

Sterol— Substance related to fats and belonging to the lipoids; for example, cholesterol.

Stimulus control— The identification of cues that precede a behavior and rearranging daily activities to avoid such cues.

Stoma— A surgically created opening in the abdominal wall.

Stomach— The portion of the alimentary canal between the esophagus and small intestine.

Stomatitis— An inflammation of the mouth.

Stress— Any threat to a person's mental or physical well-being.

Stress factor— A number used to predict how much a client's kilocalorie need has increased as a result of a disease state.

Subcutaneously— Beneath the skin.

Subdural hematoma— Collection of blood under the outermost membrane covering the brain and spinal cord; usually resulting from head injury.

Subjective data— Experiences the client reports, also termed symptoms.

Submucosa— Structural layer of the alimentary canal below the mucosa; contains tissues and blood vessels.

Sucrase— An enzyme in the intestinal mucosa that splits sucrose into glucose and fructose.

Sucrose— A disaccharide; one unit of glucose and one unit of fructose joined together; ordinary white table sugar.

Superior vena cava— One of the largest diameter veins in the human body; used to deliver total parenteral nutrition.

Symptoms— See Subjective data.

System— An organized grouping of related structures or parts.

Systolic pressure— Pressure exerted against the arteries when the heart contracts; the upper number of the blood pressure reading.

Tapeworm— A parasitic intestinal worm that is acquired by humans through the ingestion of raw seafood or undercooked beef or pork.

Tardive dyskinesia— Neurological syndrome involving involuntary, slow, rhythmic, movements often seen in the mouth and tongue; side effect of psychotropic drugs, especially phenothiazines.

Target heart rate— Seventy percent of maximum heart rate (number of heartbeats per minute); a person's target heart rate can be objectively determined by a stress test. Individuals can estimate their target heart rate by subtracting their age from 220 and multiplying the difference by 70%. A person's target heart rate is the rate at which the pulse should be maintained for at least 20 minutes during aerobic exercise.

Teratogenic— Capable of causing abnormal development of the embryo; results in a malformed fetus.

Term infant— One born between the beginning of the 38th week through the 42nd week of gestation.

Tetany— Muscle contractions, especially of the wrists and ankles, resulting from low levels of ionized calcium in the blood; causes include parathyroid deficiency, vitamin D deficiency, and alkalosis.

Therapeutic index— Maximum tolerated dose of a drug divided by the minimum curative dose; a narrow index indicates greater potential for adverse side effects.

Thermic effect of exercise (TEE)— The number of kilocalories used above resting energy expenditure as a result of physical activity.

Thermic effect of foods (diet-induced thermogenesis, specific-dynamic action)— The energy cost to extract and utilize the kilocalories and nutrients in foods; the heat produced after eating a meal.

Thiamin— Coenzyme in the metabolism of carbohydrates and fats; vitamin B_1.

Thiaminase— An enzyme in raw fish that destroys thiamin.

Third-space losses— Sequestering of fluid in body cavities such as the chest and abdomen; in the abdominal cavity, it produces ascites.

Thoracic— Pertaining to the chest, or thorax.

Threonine— Essential amino acid often lacking in grains.

Thrombus— A blood clot that obstructs a blood vessel; obstruction of a vessel of the brain or heart is among the most serious effects.

Thrush— An infection caused by the organism *Candida albicans;* characterized by the formation of white patches and ulcers in the mouth and throat.

Thymus— Gland in the chest, above and in front of the heart, that contributes to the immune response, including the maturation of T-lymphocytes.

Thyroid-stimulating hormone (TSH)— A hormone secreted by the pituitary gland that stimulates the thyroid gland to secrete thyroxine and triiodothyronine; thyrotropin.

Thyrotropin-releasing factor (TRF)— Stimulates the secretion of thyroid-stimulating hormone; produced in the hypothalamus.

Thyroxine (T_4)— A hormone secreted by the thyroid gland; increases the rate of metabolism and energy production.

Tissue— A group or collection of similar cells and their similar intercellular substance that acts together in the performance of a particular function.

T-lymphocytes (T-cells)— White blood cells that recognize and fight foreign cells such as cancer; thymic lymphocytes.

Tolerable Upper Intake Level (UL)— Highest average daily intake by an individual that is unlikely to pose risks of adverse health effects in 97%–98% of individuals in specified life-stage and gender group; ordinarily refers to intake from food, fortified food, water, and supplements.

Tolerance level— The highest dose at which a residue causes no ill effects in laboratory animals.

Total parenteral nutrition (TPN)— An intravenous feeding that provides all nutrients known to be required.

Toxoplasmosis— Infection with the protozoan *Toxoplasma gondii;* when infected in utero, infant may suffer mental retardation, blindness, and epilepsy.

Trace minerals— Those present in the body in amounts less than 5 grams; daily intake of less than 100 milligrams needed; also called microminerals or trace elements.

Traction— The process of using weights to draw a part of the body into alignment.

Transcellular fluid— Located in body cavities and spaces; constantly being secreted and absorbed; examples: cerebrospinal fluid, pericardial fluid, pleural fluid.

Transferrin— Protein in the blood that binds and transports iron.

Trauma— A physical injury or wound caused by an external force; an emotional or psychological shock that usually results in disordered behavior.

Triceps skinfold— Measure of skin and subcutaneous tissue over the triceps muscle in the upper arm; used in body fat assessment.

***Trichinella spiralis*—** A worm-like parasite that becomes embedded in the muscle tissue of pork.

Trichinosis— The infestation of *Trichinella spiralis,* a parasitic roundworm, transmitted by eating raw or insufficiently cooked pork.

Triglyceride— Three fatty acids joined to a glycerol molecule.

Triiodothyronine (T_3)— A hormone secreted by the thyroid gland that increases the rate of metabolism and energy production.

Trousseau's sign— Spasms of the forearm and hand upon inflation of the blood pressure cuff; sign of tetany or lack of ionized calcium in the blood.

Trust— First stage of Erikson's theory of psychosocial development, in which the infant learns to rely on those caring for it.

Trypsin— An enzyme formed in the intestine that assists in protein digestion.

Tryptophan— An essential amino acid, often lacking in legumes; serves as provitamin for the production of niacin by the liver.

Tubular reabsorption— The movement of fluid back into the blood from the renal tubule.

Tubule— A small tube or canal.

Tumor suppressor gene— Gene that inhibits growth and division of the cell.

Turgor— Resilience of skin; when pinched, quickly returns to original shape in well-hydrated young person; test for deficient fluid volume that is not reliable for elderly clients.

Type 1 diabetes— Persons with this disorder must take insulin to survive and are prone to ketoacidosis; also called insulin-dependent diabetes mellitus (IDDM) and juvenile diabetes.

Type 2 diabetes— Although some persons with this disorder take insulin, it is not necessary for their survival; also called non–insulin-dependent diabetes (NIDDM) and adult-onset diabetes mellitus.

Tyramine— A monoamine present in various foods that will provoke a hypertensive crisis in persons taking monoamine oxidase (MAO) inhibitors.

Ulcer— An open sore or lesion of the skin or mucous membrane.

Ulcerative colitis— Inflammatory disease of the large intestine that usually begins in the rectum and spreads upward in a continuous pattern.

Ultrasound bone densitometer— Machine that uses sound waves to estimate bone density as a screening test.

Uncomplicated starvation— A food deprivation without an underlying stress state.

Undernutrition— The state that results from a deficiency of one or more nutrients.

Underwater weighing— Most accurate measure of body fatness.

Universal precautions— A list of procedures developed by the Centers for Disease Control for when blood and certain other body fluids should be considered contaminated and treated as such.

Unsaturated fat— A fat in which the majority of fatty acids contain one or more carbon-to-carbon double bonds.

Urea— The chief nitrogenous constituent of urine; the final product, along with CO_2, of protein metabolism.

Uremia— A toxic condition produced by the retention of nitrogen-containing substances normally excreted by the kidneys.

Ureter— The tube that carries urine from the kidney to the bladder.

Urinary calculus— A kidney stone, or deposit of mineral salts.

Urinary tract infection (UTI)— The condition in which disease-producing microorganisms invade a client's bladder, ureter, or urethra.

USDA Dietary Guidelines— Guidelines for health promotion issued by the U.S. Departments of Agriculture and Health and Human Services; revised in 2005.

US Pharmacopeia (USP)— Compendium of standards of strength and purity for drugs; issued and revised periodically by a national committee.

Usual food intake— A description of what a person habitually eats.

Vaginitis— Inflammation of the vagina, most often caused by an infectious agent.

Vasopressin— Antidiuretic hormone; abbreviated ADH.

Ventilation— Process by which gases are moved into and out of the lungs; two aspects of ventilation are inhalation and exhalation.

Very-low-calorie diet (VLCD)— Diet that contains less than 800 kilocalories per day.

Very-low-density lipoprotein (VLDL)— A plasma protein containing mostly triglycerides with small amounts of cholesterol, phospholipid, and protein; transports triglycerides from the liver to tissues.

Villi— Multiple minute projections on the surface of the folds of the small intestine that absorb fluid and nutrients; plural of villus.

Virus— Very small noncellular parasite that is entirely dependent on the nutrients inside host cells for its metabolic and reproductive needs.

Visible fat— Dietary fat that can be easily seen, such as the fat on meat or in oil.

Vitamin— Organic substance needed by the body in very small amounts; yields no energy and does not become part of the body's structure.

Waist-to-Hip Ratio (WHR)— Waist measurement divided by hip measurement; if greater than 0.8 in women or greater than 0.95 in men, indicates increased risk of health problems related to obesity.

Warfarin— Anticoagulant that interferes with the liver's synthesis of vitamin K–dependent clotting factors II, VII, IX, and X.

Water intoxication— Excess intake or abnormal retention of water.

Weight cycling— The repeated gain and loss of body weight.

Wernicke-Korsakoff syndrome— A disorder of the central nervous system resulting from thiamine deletion; often seen in chronic alcoholism; signs and symptoms include motor, sensory, and memory deficits.

Wernicke's encephalopathy— Inflammatory, hemorrhagic, degenerative lesions in several areas of the brain resulting in double vision, involuntary eye movements, lack of muscle coordination, and mental deficits; caused by thiamin deficiency, often seen in chronic alcoholism but also in gastrointestinal tract disease and hyperemesis gravidarum.

Whey— Component of milk; in human milk, contains soluble proteins that are easily digested; major whey protein in breast milk is alpha-lactalbumin, with an amino acid pattern much like that of the body tissues.

Wilson's disease— Rare genetic defect of copper metabolism that permits copper to accumulate in various organs.

Women, Infants, and Children (WIC)— Federal program providing nutrition education and supplemental food to low-income pregnant or breast-feeding women and children up to 5 years of age.

Xerophthalmia— Drying and thickening of the epithelial tissues of the eye; can be caused by vitamin A deficiency.

Xerostomia— Dry mouth caused by decreased salivary secretions.

Yo-yo effect— The repeated loss and gain of body weight.

Zoochemical— Physiologically active ingredient in animals.

APPENDIX E

Bibliography

Chapter 1

American Dietetic Association: Position of the American Dietetic Association: Food insecurity and hunger in the United States. J Am Diet Assoc 106:446, 2006.

American Dietetic Association: Position of the American Dietetic Association: Functional foods. J Am Diet Assoc 104:814, 2004.

Bachman, JL, et al: Sources of food group intakes among the US population 2001–2002. J Am Diet Assoc 108:804, 2008.

Elliott, R, and Ong, TJ: Nutritional genomics. BMJ 324:1438, 2002.

Gottschlich, MM (eds): The A.S.P.E.N. Nutrition Support Core Curriculum: A Case-Study Based Approach—The Adult Patient. American Society For Parenteral and Enteral Nutrition, Silver Spring, MD, 2007.

Kleinman, RE, et al: Diet, breakfast, and academic performance in children. Ann Nutr Metab 46(Suppl 1):24, 2002.

Korol, DL: Enhancing cognitive function across the life span. Ann N Y Acad Sci 959:167, 2002.

Mukamal, KJ, et al: Tea consumption and mortality after acute myocardial infarction. Circulation 105:2476, 2002.

Murphy, SP, and Johnson, RK: The scientific basis of recent US guidance on sugars intake. Am J Clin Nutr. Author reply. Am J Clin Nutr 524, Aug, 2004.

Panel on Macronutrients, Panel on the Definition of Dietary Fiber, Subcommittee on Upper Reference Levels of Nutrients, Subcommittee on Interpretation and Uses of Dietary Reference Intakes, and the Standing Committee on the Scientific Evaluation Dietary Reference Intakes for Energy, Carbohydrate, Fiber, Fat, Fatty Acids, Cholesterol, Protein, and Amino Acids. National Academy Press, Washington, DC, 2002/2005.

U.S. Department of Agriculture, Center for Nutrition Policy and Promotion: MyPyramid. CNPP-14, U.S. Department of Health and Human Services, Washington, DC, April, 2005. Accessed 2009 at: www.health.gov/dietaryguidelines/dga2005/recommendations.

Accessed June 2010 at: www.medterms.com.

Accessed June 2010 at: www.mypyramid.gov.

U.S. Department of Agriculture and U.S. Department of Health and Human Services: Nutrition and Your Health: Dietary Guidelines for Americans 2005, ed 5. Home and Garden Bulletin No. 232, U.S. Department of Health and Human Services, Washington, DC, 2005.

White, JR, et al: Clarifying the role of insulin in type 2 diabetes management. Clin Diabetes 21:1, 2003.

Chapter 2

American Diabetes Association and American Dietetic Association: Exchange Lists for Meal Planning. American Diabetes Association and American Dietetic Association, Alexandria, VA, and Chicago, 1995.

Brown, L, Edwards, J, and Hartwell, H: A taste of the unfamiliar. Understanding the meanings attached to food by international postgraduate students in England. Appetite 54:202, 2010.

Daniels, SR, Khoury, PR, and Morrison, JA: The utility of body mass index as a measure of body fatness in children and adolescents: Differences by race and gender. Pediatrics 99:804, 1997.

Hagey, R: The phenomenon, the explanations and the responses: Metaphors surrounding diabetes in urban Canadian Indians. Soc Sci Med 18:265, 1984.

Harley, K, Stamm, NL, and Eskenazi, B: The effect of time in the U.S. on the duration of breastfeeding in women of Mexican descent. Matern Child Health J 11:119, 2007.

Heymsfield, SB, Nunez, C, and Pietrobelli, A: Bioimpedance analysis: What are the next steps? Nutr Clin Pract 12:201, 1997.

Jackson, LE: Understanding, eliciting and negotiating clients' multicultural health beliefs. Nurse Pract 18:30, 1993.

Jacobs, DO: Bioelectrical impedance analysis: Implications for clinical practice. Nutr Clin Pract 12:204, 1997.

Kovacevich, DS, et al: Nutrition risk classification: A reproducible and valid tool for nurses. Nutr Clin Pract 12:20, 1997.

Metropolitan Life Insurance Company Height-Weight Table. Metropolitan Life, Warwick, RI, 1983.

National Academy of Sciences: Dietary Reference Intakes. Nutr Rev 55:319, 1997a.

National Academy of Sciences: Origin and framework of the development of Dietary Reference Intakes. Nutr Rev 55:332, 1997b.

National Academy of Sciences: Uses of Dietary Reference Intakes. Nutr Rev 55:327, 1997c.

Ordovas, JM, Kaput, J, and Corella, D: Nutrition in the genomics era: Cardiovascular disease risk and the Mediterranean diet. Mol Nutr Food Res 51:1293, 2007.

Shannon, C: Acculturation: Aboriginal and Torres Strait Islander nutrition. Asia Pac J Clin Nutr 11(Suppl 3):S576, 2002.

Shintani, TT, et al: Obesity and cardiovascular risk intervention through the ad libitum feeding of traditional Hawaiian diet. Am J Clin Nutr 53:1647S, 1991.

Shintani, T, et al: Waianae Diet Program: long-term follow-up. Hawaii Med J 58:117, 1999.

Sowattanangoon, N, Kochabhakdi, N, and Petrie, KJ: Buddhist values are associated with better diabetes control in Thai patients. Int J Psychiatry Med 38:481, 2008.
Sun, G, et al: Comparison of multifrequency bioelectrical impedance analysis with dual-energy X-ray absorptiometry for assessment of percentage body fat in a large, healthy population. Am J Clin Nutr 81:74, 2005.
Tengvall, M, et al: Body composition in the elderly: reference values and bioelectrical impedance spectroscopy to predict total body skeletal muscle mass. Clin Nutr 28:52, 2009.
Yates, AA: Dietary reference intakes: Rationale and applications. In Shils, ME, et al (eds): Modern Nutrition in Health and Disease, ed 10. Lippincott Williams & Wilkins, Philadelphia, 2006.

Chapter 3

American Dietetic Association: ADA's nutrition trends survey result. J Am Diet Assoc 102:7(Suppl), 2002.
American Diabetes Association, American Dietetic Association: Exchange lists for meal planning. American Dietetic Association, Alexandria, VA, 2003.
Buchman, JL, et al: Sources of food group intakes among the U.S. population, 2001–2002. J Am Diet Assoc 108:804, 2008.
Duyff, LD: American Dietetic Association Complete Food and Nutrition Guide, ed 2. John Wiley & Sons, Hoboken, NJ, 2002.
Food and Nutrition Board, National Academy of Science, Institute of Medicine: Dietary Reference Intakes for Energy, Carbohydrate, Fiber, Fat, Fatty Acids, Cholesterol, Protein, and Amino Acids. National Academy Press, Washington, DC, 2002.
Fowler, MJ: Classification of diabetes: Not all hypoglycemia is the same. Clin Diabetes 25:74, 2007.
Gottschlich, MM (ed): The A.S.P.E.N. Nutrition Support Core Curriculum: A Case-based Approach—The Adult Patient. American Society for Parenteral and Enteral Nutrition, Silver Spring, MD, 2007.
Holt, R, Roberts, G, and Scully, C: Dental damage, sequelae, and prevention. BMJ 320:1719, 2000.
Korol, DL: Enhancing cognitive function across the life span. Ann N Y Acad Sci 959:167, 2002.
Nielson, SJ, and Popkin, BM: Patterns and trends in food portion sizes, 1977–1998. JAMA 289:450, 2003.
Uhlman, M, and Ridder, K: Nutrition information, questionable serving sizes confuse Americans. The Salt Lake City Tribune, October 20, 2002.
U.S. Department of Agriculture: Continuing survey of food intake by individuals, 1994–1996. Accessed April 2005 at: www.usda.gov.
Accessed June 2008 at: www.aspartame.org.
Accessed January 2010 at: www.cavediabetesjournal.org.

Chapter 4

Agricultural Research Service Dietary Guidelines Committee: Dietary Guidelines for Americans 2000. Accessed at: www.ars.usda.gov/dgac.
American Dietetic Association: International Dietetics & Nutrition Terminology (IDNT) Reference Manual, ed 1. American Dietetic Association, Chicago, 2008.
American Dietetic and Diabetic Associations: Exchange Lists for Meal Planning. American Dietetic Association, Chicago, 2003.
Blundell, JE, Stubbs, J: Diet composition and the control of food intake in humans. In Bray, GA, Bouchard, C (eds): Handbook of Obesity: Etiology and Pathophysiology. Marcel Dekker, New York, 2004.
Caballero, B: A nutrition paradox—underweight and obesity in developing countries. N Engl J Med 352:1514, 2005.
Chanmugan, P, et al: Did fat intake in the United States really decline between 1989–1991 and 1994–1996? J Am Diet Assoc 103:867, 2003.
Cunningham, E, and Marason, W: Should my client's diet contain plant sterol/sterol esters to lower cholesterol? J Am Diet Assoc 102:81, 2002.
Dausch, J: Trans-fatty acids: A regulatory update. J Am Diet Assoc 102:18, 2002.
Doak, CM, et al: The dual burden household and the nutrition transition paradox. Int J Obesity Res 29:129, 2005.
Food and Nutrition Board, Institute of Medicine: Dietary Reference Intakes for Energy, Carbohydrate, Fiber, Fat, Fatty Acids, Cholesterol, Protein, and Amino Acids. National Academy Press, Washington, DC, 2002/2005.
Gottschlich, MM (eds): The A.S.P.E.N. Nutrition Support Core Curriculum: A Case-Based Approach—The Adult Patient. American Society for Parenteral and Enteral Nutrition, Silver Spring, MD, 2007.
Hise, ME, and Brown, JC: Lipids. In The A.S.P.E.N. Nutrition Support Core Curriculum: A Case-Based Approcah—The Adult Patient. American Society for Parenteral and Enteral Nutrition, Silver Spring, MD, 2007.
International Food Information Council (IFIC) and The Food and Drug Administration (FDA): The Benefits of Balance: Managing Fat in Your Diet. International Food Information Council and Food and Drug Administration, Washington, DC, 1998.
Kendler, BS: Recent nutritional approaches to the prevention and therapy of cardiovascular disease. Prog Cardiovasc Nurs 12:3, 1997.
Lichtenstein, AH: Trans fatty acids and hydrogenated fat: What do we know? Nutr Today 30:102, 1995.
Lichtenstein, AH, et al: Dietary fat consumption and health. Nutr Rev 56:53, 1998.
Morris, MC: Consumption of fish and n-3 fatty acids and risk of incident Alzheimer disease. Arcg Neryil 60:940, 2003.
National Institutes of Health, National Heart, Lung, and Blood Institute: Clinical Guidelines on the Identification and Treatment of Overweight and Obesity in Adults. U.S. Department of Health and Human Services, Bethesda, MD, 1998.
Pearson, TA, et al: AHA Guidelines for Primary Prevention of Cardiovascular Disease and Stroke: 2002 Update. Consensus panel guide to comprehensive risk reduction for adult patients without coronary or other vascular diseases. Circulation 106:388, 2002.
Tucker, KL, et al: The combination of high fruit and vegetable and low saturated fat intakes is more protective against mortality in aging men than is either alone: Baltimore longitudinal study of aging. J Nutr 135:556, 2005.
U.S. Department of Agriculture (USDA) and U.S. Department of Health and Human Services. Dietary Guidelines for Americans, ed 4. Extension Bulletin E-2773, Michigan State University, East Lansing, 2001.
U.S. Department of Agriculture: Continuing survey of food intake by individuals, 1994–1996. Accessed at: www.usda.gov/bbnrc/foodsurvey.
U.S. Department of Agriculture: Dietary Guidelines. Accessed at: www.usda.gov/dietaryguidelines/dga2000.
U.S. Department of Agriculture: The food guide pyramid. Accessed at: www.usda.gov/py.
U.S. Department of Agriculture, Center for Nutrition Policy and Health Promotion: Nutrition insights: The role of nuts in a healthy diet. Accessed December 2008 at: www.usda.gov/cnpp.

World Health Organization: Years of healthy life can be increased 5–10 years. Accessed at: www.who.int/mediacentre/releases/pr84/en/print.html.

Wiese, HF, Hansen, AE, and Adam, DJD: Essential fatty acids in infant nutrition. J Nutr 58:345, 1958.

Willett, WC: Diet, nutrition, and the prevention of cancer. In Shils, ME (ed): Modern Nutrition in Health and Disease, ed 9. Williams & Wilkins, Baltimore, 1999.

Chapter 5

American Diabetes Association and American Dietetic Association: Exchange Lists for Meal Planning. American Diabetes Association and American Dietetic Association, Alexandria, VA, and Chicago, 1995.

Bank, A: On the road to gene therapy for beta-thalassemia and sickle cell anemia. Pediatr Hematol Oncol 25:1, 2008.

Bonds, DR: Three decades of innovation in the management of sickle cell disease: The road to understanding the sickle cell disease clinical phenotype. Blood Rev 19:99, 2005.

Carvalho, NF, et al: Severe nutritional deficiencies in toddlers resulting from health food milk alternatives. Pediatrics 107: E46, 2001.

Chang, JC, Ye, L, and Kan, YW: Correction of the sickle cell mutation in embryonic stem cells. Proc Natl Acad Sci U S A 103:1036, 2006.

Denton, I: Getting the konzo prevention message out. Cassava Cyanide Diseases Network News, (10) December 2007.

Diasolua Ngudi, D, Kuo, YH, and Lambein, F: Food safety and amino acid balance in processed cassava "Cossettes." J Agric Food Chem 50:3042, 2002.

Dwyer, AJ, et al: Nutritional status and wound healing in open fractures of the lower limb. Int Orthop 29:251, 2005.

Ferrando, AA, Paddon-Jones, D, and Wolfe, RR. Bedrest and myopathies: Curr Opin Clin Nutr Metab Care 9:410, 2006.

Gambol, PJ: Maternal phenylketonuria and case management implications. J Pediatr Nurs 22:129, 2007.

Gropper, SS, Smith, JL, and Groff, JL: Advanced Nutrition and Human Metabolism, ed 5. Wadsworth, Belmont, CA, 2009.

Hanley, WB: Finding the fertile woman with phenylketonuria. Eur J Obstet Gynecol Reprod Biol 137:131, 2008.

Johnston, PK, and Sabate, J: Nutritional implications of vegetarian diets. In Shils, ME, et al (eds): Modern Nutrition in Health and Disease, ed 10. Lippincott Williams & Wilkins, Philadelphia, 2006.

Katz, KA, et al: Rice nightmare: Kwashiorkor in two Philadelphia-area infants fed Rice Dream beverage. J Am Acad Dermatol 52: S69, 2005.

Koch, R, Moseley, K, and Guttler, F: Tetrahydrobiopterin and maternal PKU. Mol Genet Metab 86:S139, 2005.

Kris-Etherton, P, and Skulas, A: Essential fatty acids and vegetarians: The missing link in long-chain Omega-3 fatty acid recommendations. Nutr MD 31:1, 2005.

Liu, SA, et al: Risk factors for wound infection after surgery in primary oral cavity cancer patients. Laryngoscope 117:166, 2007.

March of Dimes: PKU (Phenylketonuria). March of Dimes, 2007. Accessed April 20, 2008 at: http://www.marchofdimes.com/printableArticles/19695_1219.asp.

Matthews, DE: Proteins and amino acids. In Shils, ME, et al (eds): Modern Nutrition in Health and Disease, ed 10. Lippincott Williams & Wilkins, Philadelphia, 2006.

Phenylketonuria. Merck Manual. Accessed April 20, 2008 at: http://www.merck.com/mmpe/print/sec19/ch296/ch296c.html.

Piercecchi-Marti, MD, et al: Malnutrition, a rare form of child abuse: Diagnostic criteria. J Forensic Sci 51:670, 2006.

U.S. Food and Drug Administration: FDA approves Kuvan for treatment of phenylketonuria (PKU). FDA News December 13, 2007. Accessed April 17, 2008 at: http://www.fda.gov.bbs/topics/NEWS/2007/NEW01761.html.

Venes, D (ed): Tabor's Cyclopedic Medical Dictionary, ed 20. FA Davis, Philadelphia, 2005.

Zurfluh, MR, et al: Molecular genetics of tetrahydrobiopterin-responsive phenylalanine hydroxylase deficiency. Hum Mutat 29:167, 2008.

Chapter 6

American Dietetic Association: International Dietetics and Nutrition Terminolgy Manual. American Dietetic Association, Chicago, 2008.

Food and Nutrition Board, Institute of Medicine: Dietary Reference Intakes for Energy, Carbohydrate, Fiber, Fatty Acids, Cholesterol, Protein, and Amino Acids. National Academy Press, Washington, DC, 2002.

Gropper, SS, and Smith, JL: Advanced Nutrition and Human Metabolism, ed 5. Wadsworth, St. Paul, MN, 2008.

Guthrie, HA: Introductory Nutrition, ed 7. Times Mirror/Mosby College Publishing, St. Louis, 1989.

Hoffer, LJ: Metabolic consequences of starvation. In Shils, ME (ed): Modern Nutrition in Health and Disease, ed 10. Lippincott Williams & Wilkins, Philadelphia, 2006.

Leibel, RL, Rosenbaum, M, and Hirsch, J: Changes in energy expenditure resulting from altered body weight. N Engl J Med 332:621, 1995.

Mahon, KL, and Escott-Stump, S (eds): Krause's Food, Nutrition, & Diet Therapy, ed 12. Elsevier, Philadelphia, 2007.

Roll, BJ, et al: Increasing the portion size of a sandwich increases energy intake. J Am Diet Assoc 104:367, 2004.

Shils, ME (eds): Modern Nutrition in Health and Disease, ed 10. Lippincott Williams & Wilkins, Philadelphia, 2006.

Subcommittee on the 10th Edition of the RDAs, Food and Nutrition Board, Commission of Life Sciences, National Research Council: Recommended Dietary Allowances. National Academy Press, Washington, DC, 1989, pp 24–38.

Swinburn, B: The runaway weight gain train: Too many accelerators, not enough brakes. BMJ 329:736, 2004.

Treuth, MS, et al: Metabolic adaptation to a high-fat and high-carbohydrate diets in children and adolescents. Am J Clin Nutr 77:479, 2003.

U.S. Department of Agriculture: NHANES 2005–2006. Accessed August 2007 at: www.ars.usda.gov/ba/bhnrc/fsrg.

Chapter 7

Akikusa, JD, Garrick, D, and Nash, MC: Scurvy: Forgotten but not gone. J Paediatr Child Health 39:75, 2003.

Armas, LA, Hollis, BW, and Heaney, RP: Vitamin D_2 is much less effective than vitamin D_3 in humans. J Clin Endocrinol Metab 89:5387, 2004.

Ashourian, N, and Mousdicas, N: Pellagra-like dermatitis. N Engl J Med 354:1614, 2006.

Astudillo, L, et al: Development of beriberi heart disease 20 years after gastrojejunostomy [letter]. Am J Med 113:157, 2003.

Bartlett, PC, Morris, JG, Jr, and Spengler, J: Foodborne illness associated with niacin: Report of an outbreak linked to excessive niacin in enriched cornmeal. Public Health Rep 97:258, 1982.

Bingham, AC, Kimura, Y, and Imundo, L: A 16-year-old boy with purpura and leg pain. J Pediatr 142:560, 2003.

Bischoff-Ferrari, HA, et al: Estimation of optimal serum concentrations of 25-hydroxyvitamin D for multiple health outcomes. Am J Clin Nutr 84:18, 2006.

Bischoff-Ferrari, HA, et al: Fracture prevention with vitamin D supplementation: A meta-analysis of randomized controlled trials. JAMA 293:2257, 2005.

Blank, S, et al: An outbreak of hypervitaminosis D associated with the overfortification of milk from a home-delivery dairy. Am J Public Health 85:656, 1995.

Bonet, ML, et al: Vitamin A and the regulation of fat reserves. Cell Mol Life Sci 60:1311, 2003.

Bouillon, R, Norman, AW, and Lips, P: Vitamin D deficiency [letter]. N Engl J Med 357:1980, 2007.

Bourgeois, C, Cervantes-Laurean, D, and Moss, J: Niacin. In Shils, ME, et al (eds): Modern Nutrition in Health and Disease, ed 10. Lippincott Williams & Wilkins, Philadelphia, 2006.

Butterworth, RF: Thiamin. In Shils, ME, et al (eds): Modern Nutrition in Health and Disease, ed 10. Lippincott Williams & Wilkins, Philadelphia, 2006.

Cannell, JJ, et al: Epidemic influenza and vitamin D. Epidemiol Infect 134:1129, 2006.

Carmel, R: Cobalamin (Vitamin B_{12}). In Shils, ME, et al (eds): Modern Nutrition in Health and Disease, ed 10. Lippincott Williams & Wilkins, Philadelphia, 2006a.

Carmel, R: Folic acid. In Shils, ME, et al (eds): Modern Nutrition in Health and Disease, ed 10. Lippincott Williams & Wilkins, Philadelphia, 2006b.

Carvalho, NF: Severe nutritional deficiencies in toddlers resulting from health food milk alternatives. Pediatrics 107:E46, 2001.

Centers for Disease Control and Prevention: Neurologic impairment in children associated with maternal dietary deficiency of cobalamin—Georgia, 2001. MMWR 52:61, 2003. Accessed December 18, 2003 at: http://www.cdc.gov/mmwr/PDF/wk/mm5204.pdf.

Centers for Disease Control and Prevention: Severe malnutrition among young children—Georgia, January 1997–June 1999. MMWR 50:224, 2001. Accessed June 19, 2003 at: http://www.cdc.gov/mmwr/preview/mmwrhtml/nn5012a3.htm.

Chatterjee, M, and Speiser, PW: Pamidronate treatment of hypercalcemia caused by vitamin D toxicity. J Pediatr Endrocrinol Metab 20:1241, 2007.

Chiu, CJ, and Taylor, A: Nutritional antioxidants and age-related cataract and maculopathy. Exp Eye Res 84:229, 2007.

Conversion factors, weights and measures, and metabolic water formation. In Shils, ME, et al (eds): Modern Nutrition in Health and Disease, ed 10. Lippincott Williams & Wilkins, Philadelphia, 2006.

Cyhlarova, E, et al: Niacin skin test response in dyslexia. Prostaglandins Leukot Essent Fatty Acids 77:123, 2007.

Delanghe, JR, et al: Vitamin C deficiency and scurvy are not only a dietary problem but are codetermined by the haptoglobin polymorphism. Clin Chem 53:1397, 2007.

Delcourt, C: Application of nutrigenomics in eye health. Forum Nutr 60:168, 2007.

Delgado-Sanchez, L, Godkar, D, and Niranjan, S: Pellagra: Rekindling of an old flame. Am J Ther 15:173, 2008.

DePaola, DP, et al: Nutrition and dental medicine. In Shils, ME, et al (eds): Modern Nutrition in Health and Disease, ed 10. Lippincott Williams & Wilkins, Philadelphia, 2006.

Dhar, M, Bellevue, R, and Carmel, R: Pernicious anemia with neuropsychiatric dysfunction in a patient with sickle cell anemia treated with folate supplementation. N Engl J Med 348:2204, 2003.

Donahue, SP: Recurrence of idiopathic intracranial hypertension after weight loss: The carrot craver. Am J Ophthalmol 130:850, 2000.

Evans, JR: Antioxidant vitamin and mineral supplements for slowing the progression of age-related macular degeneration. Cochrane Database Syst Rev 2:CD000254, 2006.

Fitzpatrick, S, et al: Vitamin D–deficient rickets: A multifactorial disease. Nutr Rev 58:218, 2000.

Garland, CF, et al: The role of vitamin D in cancer prevention. Am J Public Health 96:252, 2006.

Goodrich, RP, et al: The Mirasol PRT system for pathogen reduction of platelets and plasma: An overview of current status and future trends. Transfus Apher Sci 35:5, 2006.

Gropper, SS, Smith, JL, and Groff, JL: Advanced Nutrition and Human Metabolism, ed 5. Wadsworth, Belmont, CA, 2009.

Harrow, JJ, et al: Diagnostic pitfalls: Case report of scurvy in a man with spinal cord injury. J Spinal Cord Med 26:163, 2003.

Hathcock, JN: Risk assessment for vitamin D. Am J Clin Nutr 85:6, 2007.

Heaney, RP: Barriers to optimizing vitamin D_3 intake for the elderly. J Nutr 130:1123, 2006.

Holick, MF: Vitamin D. In Shils, ME, et al (eds): Modern Nutrition in Health and Disease, ed 10. Lippincott Williams & Wilkins, Philadelphia, 2006.

Holick, MF: Vitamin D deficiency. N Engl J Med 357:266, 2007.

Holick, MF, et al: Vitamin D_2 is as effective as vitamin D_3 in maintaining circulating concentrations of 25-hydroxyvitamin D. J Clin Endocrinol Metab 93:677, 2008.

Huiming, Y, Chaomin, W, and Meng, M: Vitamin A for treating measles in children. Cochrane Database Syst Rev 4:CD001479, 2005.

Jackson, RD, et al: Calcium plus vitamin D supplementation and the risk of fractures. N Engl J Med 354:669, 2006.

Jager, RD, Mieler, WF, and Miller, JW: Age-related macular degeneration. N Engl J Med 358:2602, 2008.

Johnson, MA: If high folic acid aggravates vitamin B_{12} deficiency what should be done about it? Nutr Rev 65:451, 2007.

Johnston, CS, and Bowling, DL: Stability of ascorbic acid in commercially available orange juices. J Am Diet Assoc 102:525, 2002.

Kowalski, TE, et al: Vitamin A hepatotoxicity: A cautionary note regarding 25,000 IU supplements. Am J Med 97:523, 1994.

Kreiter, SR, et al: Nutritional rickets in African American breast-fed infants. J Pediatr 137:153, 2000.

Lamb, E: Vitamin D deficiency presenting acutely in an infant [letter]. BMJ January 30, 1999. Accessed September 15, 1999 at: http://www.bmj.com/cgi/eletters/318/7175/39.

Lerner, V, and Kanevsky, M: Acute dementia with delirium due to vitamin B_{12} deficiency: A case report. Int J Psychiatry Med 32:215, 2002.

Levin, NA, and Greer, KE: Scurvy in an unrepentant carnivore. Cutis 66:39, 2000.

Levine, M, Katz, A, and Padayatty, SJ: Vitamin C. In Shils, ME, et al (eds): Modern Nutrition in Health and Disease, ed 10. Lippincott Williams & Wilkins, Philadelphia, 2006.

Li, Y, and Schellhorn, HE: Vitamin C and human nutrition. Cyberounds Nutrition Conference. Released March 25, 2008. Accessed April 17, 2008 at: http://www.cyberounds.com/conf/nutrition/2008-03-25/index.html.

Linus Pauling Institute: Choline. Accessed May 14, 2008 at: http://lpi.oregonstate.edu/infocenter/othernuts/choline.

Liu, PT, et al: Toll-like receptor triggering of a vitamin D–mediated human antimicrobial response. Science 311:1770. 16 December 2005; accepted 8 February 2006; published online 23 February 2006; 10.1126/Science.1123933.

MacDonald, A, and Forsyth, A: Nutritional deficiencies and the skin. Clin Exp Dermatol 30:388, 2005.
Mark, BL, and Carson, JAS: Vitamin D and autoimmune disease—implications for practice from the multiple sclerosis literature. J Am Diet Assoc 106:418, 2006.
Marra, MV, and Boyar, AP: Position of the American Dietetic Association: nutrient supplementation. J Am Diet Assoc 109:2073, 2009.
McCormick, DB: Riboflavin. In Shils, ME, et al (eds): Modern Nutrition in Health and Disease, ed 10. Lippincott Williams & Wilkins, Philadelphia, 2006.
McLaren, DS, and Frigg, M: Sight and Life Manual on Vitamin A Deficiency Disorders (VADD), ed 2. Sight and Life, Basel, Switzerland, 2001.
Messamore, E, Hoffman, WF, & Janowsky, A: The niacin skin flush abnormality in schizophrenia: a quantitative dose-response study. Schizophr Res 62:251, 2003.
Miksad, R, et al: Hepatic hydrothorax associated with vitamin A toxicity. J Clin Gastroenterol 34:275, 2002.
Milea, D, Cassoux, N, and LeHoang, P: Blindness in a strict vegan [letter]. N Engl J Med 342:897, 2000.
Mills, JL, et al: Low vitamin B_{12} concentrations in patients without anemia: The effect of folic acid fortification of grain. Am J Clin Nutr 77:1474, 2003.
Morse, JW, Morse, SJ, and Patterson, J: Niacin reaction: Common vitamin, uncommon ED diagnosis. Am J Emerg Med 17:320, 1999.
Multivitamins, What to avoid, how to choose. Consumer Reports 71(2):19.
Munger, KL, et al: Serum 25-hydroxyvitamin D levels and risk of multiple sclerosis. JAMA 296:2832, 2006.
National Institutes of Health, Office of Dietary Supplements: Dietary Supplement Fact Sheet: Vitamin D, 2008. Accessed May 21, 2008 at: http://ods.od.nih.gov/factsheets/vitamind.asp.
Nutrition Data-a. Foods highest in folate. Accessed May 9, 2008 at: http://www.nutritiondata.com.
Nutrition Data-b. Foods highest in vitamin B_6. Accessed May 8, 2008 at: http://www.nutritiondata.com.
Ozturk, F, et al: Pellagra: A sporadic pediatric case with a full triad of symptoms. Cutis 68:31, 2001.
Pangan, AL, and Robinson, D: Hemarthrosis as initial presentation of scurvy. J Rheumatol 28:1923, 2001.
Penniston, KL, and Tanumihardjo, SA: The acute and chronic toxic effects of vitamin A. Am J Clin Nutr 83:191, 2006.
Pham, DQ, and Plakogiannis, R: Vitamin E supplementation in Alzheimer's disease, Parkinson's disease, tardive dyskinesia, and cataract: Part 2. Ann Pharmacother 39:1870, 2005a.
Pham, DQ, and Plakogiannis, R. Vitamin E supplementation in cardiovascular disease and cancer prevention: Part 1. Ann Pharmacother 39:1870, 2005b.
Preston, AM, et al: Influence of environmental tobacco smoke on vitamin C status in children. Am J Clin Nutr 77:167, 2003.
Roman, GC: Nutritional disorders of the nervous system. In Shils, ME, et al (eds): Modern Nutrition in Health and Disease, ed 10. Lippincott Williams & Wilkins, Philadelphia, 2006.
Ross, DA: Recommendations for vitamin A supplementation. J Nutr 132:2902S, 2002.
Sen, CK, Khanna, S, and Roy, S: Tocotrienols: Vitamin E beyond tocopherols. Life Sci 78:2088, 2006.
Shah, M, et al: Nutritional rickets still afflict children in north Texas. Tex Med 96:64, 2000.
Stephen, R, and Utecht, T: Scurvy identified in the emergency department: A case report. J Emerg Med 21:235, 2001.
Stroh, C, et al: Vitamin A deficiency (VAD) after a duodenal switch procedure: a case report. Obes Surg 20:397, 2010.
Tamura, Y, et al: Scurvy presenting as painful gait with bruising in a young boy. Arch Pediatr Adolesc Med 7:732, 2000.
Towbin, A, et al: Beriberi after gastric bypass surgery in adolescence. J Pediatr 145:263, 2004.
Traber, MG: Vitamin E. In Shils, ME, et al (eds): Modern Nutrition in Health and Disease, ed 10. Lippincott Williams & Wilkins, Philadelphia, 2006.
Trumbo, PR: Pantothenic acid. In Shils, ME, et al (eds): Modern Nutrition in Health and Disease, ed 10. Lippincott Williams & Wilkins, Philadelphia, 2006.
Van Leeuwen, R, et al: Dietary intake of antioxidants and risk of age-related macular degeneration. JAMA 294:3101, 2005.
Vieth, R: Critique of the considerations for establishing the tolerable upper intake level for vitamin D: Critical need for revision upwards. J Nutr 136:1117, 2006.
Vieth, R: Vitamin D toxicity, policy, and science. J Bone Miner Res 22(Suppl 2):V64, 2007.
Wagner, CL, and Greer, FR: Prevention of rickets and vitamin D deficiency in infants, children, and adolescents. Pediatrics 122:1142, 2008.
Weinstein, M, Babyn, P, and Zlotkin, S: An orange a day keeps the doctor away: Scurvy in the year 2000. Pediatrics 108:E55, 2001.
West, KP, Jr: Vitamin A deficiency disorders in children and women. Food Nutr Bull 24:S78, 2003.
Wolpowitz, D, and Gilchrest, BA: The vitamin D questions: How much do you need and how should you get it? J Am Acad Dermatol 54:301, 2006.
Zeisel, SH, and Niculescu, MD: Choline and phosphatidylcholine. In Shils, ME, et al (eds): Modern Nutrition in Health and Disease, ed 10. Lippincott Williams & Wilkins, Philadelphia, 2006.

Chapter 8

Abernathy, CO, Thomas, DJ, and Calderon, RL: Health effects and risk assessment of arsenic. J Nutr 133:1536S, 2003.
Alexander, J: Selenium. Novartis Found Symp 282:143, 2007.
Almond, CSD, et al: Hyponatremia among runners in the Boston Marathon. N Engl J Med 352:1550, 2005.
American College of Sports Medicine, American Dietetic Association, and Dietitians of Canada: Joint Position Statement: Nutrition and athletic performance. Med Sci Sports Exerc 32:2130, 2000.
American Dental Association: Fluoride and infant formula frequently asked questions. Posted December 15, 2006. Accessed June 5, 2008 at: http://www.ada.org/public/topics/fluoride/infantsformula_faq.asp#2.
American Dental Association: Home water treatment systems. Posted August 7, 2003. Accessed June 5, 2008 at: http://www.ada.org/public/topics/documents/art_water_home.pdf.
Appendix D. In Kleinman, RE (ed): Pediatric Nutrition Handbook, ed 5. American Academy of Pediatrics, Elk Grove Village, IL, 2004.
Asari, R, et al: Hypoparathyroidism after total thyroidectomy: a prospective study. Arch Surg 143:132, 2008.
Bailey, CS, et al: Excessive calcium ingestion leading to milk-alkali syndrome. Ann Clin Biochem 45(Pt)5:527, 2008.
Beall, DP, et al: Milk-alkali syndrome: A historical review and description of the modern version of the syndrome. Am J Med Sci 331:233, 2006.
Borak, J: Neonatal hypothyroidism due to maternal vegan diet. J Pediatr Endocrinol Metab 18:621, 2005.
Burk, RF, and Levander, OA: Selenium. In Shils, ME, et al (eds): Modern Nutrition in Health and Disease, ed 10. Lippincott Williams & Wilkins, Philadelphia, 2006.
Caruso, TJ, Prober, CG, and Gwaltey, JM, Jr: Treatment of naturally acquired common colds with zinc: A structured review. Clin Infect Dis 45:569, 2007.

Centers for Disease Control and Prevention: Childhood lead poisoning associated with tamarind candy and folk remedies—California, 1999–2000. MMWR 51:684, 2002a. Accessed June 25, 2008 at: http://www.cdc.gov/mmwr/preview/mmwrhtml/mm5131a3.htm.

Centers for Disease Control and Prevention: Death of a child after ingestion of a metallic charm—Minnesota, 2006. MMWR 55:340, 2006a. Accessed June 2, 2008 at: http://www.cdc.gov/mmwr/preview/mmwrhtml/mm5512a4.htm.

Centers for Disease Control and Prevention: Deaths associated with hypocalcemia from chelation therapy—Texas, Pennsylvania, and Oregon, 2003–2005. MMWR 55:204, 2006b. Accessed June 25, 2008 at: http://www.cdc.gov/mmwr/preview/mmwrhtml/mm5508a3.htm.

Centers for Disease Control and Prevention: Elevated serum aluminum levels in hemodialysis patients associated with the use of electric pumps—Wyoming, 2007. MMWR 57:689, 2008a. Accessed July 21, 2008 at: http://www.cdc.gov/mmwr/preview/mmwrhtml/mm5725a4.htm?s_cid=mm5725s4_e.

Centers for Disease Control and Prevention: Fatal pediatric lead poisoning—New Hampshire, 2000. MMWR 50:457, 2001a. Accessed June 25, 2008 at: http://www.cdc.gov/mmwr/preview/mmwrhtml/mm5022a1.htm.

Centers for Disease Control and Prevention: Fluoridation Status 2006. National Center for Chronic Disease Prevention and Health Promotion, 2008b. Accessed January 21, 2010 at: http://apps.nccd.cdc.gov/nohss/FluoridationMap.asp?Year=2006.

Centers for Disease Control and Prevention: Heat-related deaths—four states, July–August 2001, and United States, 1979–1999. MMWR 51:567, 2002b. Accessed June 18, 2008 at: http://www.cdc.gov/mmwr/PDF/wk/mm5126.pdf.

Centers for Disease Control and Prevention: Heat-related deaths—United States, 1999–2003. MMWR 55:796, 2006c. Accessed June 18, 2008 at: http://www.cdc.gov/mmwr/preview/mmwrhtml/mm5529a2.htm.

Centers for Disease Control and Prevention: Lead poisoning associated with imported candy and powdered food coloring—California and Michigan. MMWR 47:1041, 1998. Accessed June 25, 2008 at: http://www.cdc.gov/mmwr/preview/mmwrhtml/00055939.htm.

Centers for Disease Control and Prevention: Lead poisoning from ingestion of a toy necklace—Oregon, 2003. MMWR 53:509, 2004. Accessed June 2, 2008 at: http://www.cdc.gov/mmwr/preview/mmwrhtml/mm5323a5.htm.

Centers for Disease Control and Prevention: Populations receiving optimally fluoridated public drinking water—United States, 1992—2006. MMWR 57:737, 2008c. Accessed January 23, 2010 at: http://www.cdc.gov/mmwr/preview/mmwrhtml/mm5727a1.htm.

Centers for Disease Control and Prevention: Recommendations for using fluoride to prevent and control dental caries in the United States. MMWR 50(RR-14):1, 2001b. Accessed January 21, 2010 at: http://www.cdc.gov/mmwr/PDF/RR/RR5014.pdf.

Cerulli, J, et al: Chromium picolinate toxicity. Ann Pharmacother 32:428, 1998.

Chalupka, S: Tainted water on tap. Am J Nurs 105:40, 2005.

Chitambar, CR, and Asok, CA: Nutritional aspects of hematologic diseases. In Shils, ME, et al (eds): Modern Nutrition in Health and Disease, ed 10. Lippincott Williams & Wilkins, Philadelphia, 2006.

Christensen, NK, et al: Juniper ash as a source of calcium in the Navajo diet. J Am Diet Assoc 98:333, 1998.

Chung, RT, Misdraji, MD, and Sahani, DV: Case 33—2006: A 43-year-old man with diabetes, hypogonadism, cirrhosis, arthralgias, and fatigue. N Engl J Med 355:1812, 2006.

Cleveland, LM, et al: Lead hazards for pregnant women and children: Part 1. Am J Nurs 108:40, 2008.

Cuddihy, MT, et al: Osteoporosis intervention following distal forearm fractures: A missed opportunity? Arch Intern Med 152:421, 2002.

Dawson-Hughes, B: Osteoporosis. In Shils, ME, et al (eds): Modern Nutrition in Health and Disease, ed 10. Lippincott Williams & Wilkins, Philadelphia, 2006.

DePaola, DP, et al: Nutrition and dental medicine. In Shils, ME, et al (eds): Modern Nutrition in Health and Disease, ed 10. Lippincott Williams & Wilkins, Philadelphia, 2006.

de Villiers, TJ: Bazedoxifene: a novel selective estrogen receptor modulator for postmenopausal osteoporosis. Climacteric 13:210, 2010.

Dunn, JT: Iodine. In Shils, ME, et al (eds): Modern Nutrition in Health and Disease, ed 10. Lippincott Williams & Wilkins, Philadelphia, 2006.

Fairweather-Tait, SJ, Fox, TE, and Mallilin A: Balti curries and iron. BMJ 310:1368, 1995.

Flynn, MR, and Susi, P: Neurological risks associated wtih manganese exposure from welding operations—a literature review. Int J Hyg Environ Health 212:459, 2009.

Fournier, M: Perfecting your acid-base balancing act. Am Nurse Today 4:17, 2009.

Gade, W, and Robinson, B: CLS meets the aquaporin family: Clinical cases involving aquaporin systems. Clin Lab Sci 19:80, 2006.

Gibson, RS, Donovan, UM, and Heath, A-LM: Dietary strategies to improve the iron and zinc nutriture of young women following a vegetarian diet. Plant Foods Hum Nutr 51:1, 1997.

Griffin, I: Zinc physiology and therapeutics: recent insights. Cyberounds Continuing Education. Released September 15, 2007. Accessed September 13, 2007 at: www.cyberounds.com/images/subpageTitles/confNutrition.png.

Gropper, SS, Smith, JL, and Groff, JL: Advanced Nutrition and Human Metabolism, ed 5. Wadsworth, Belmont, CA, 2009.

Hackley, G, and Katz-Jacobson, A: Lead poisoning in pregnancy: A case study with implications for midwives. J Midwifery Womens Health 48:30, 2003.

Hassan, HA, Netchvolodoff, C, and Raufman, JP: Zinc-induced copper deficiency in a coin swallower. Am J Gastroenterol 95:2975, 2000.

Heaney, RP: Role and importance of calcium in preventing and managing osteoporosis. Medscape Continuing Education, 2006. Accessed April 21, 2006 at: http://www.medscape.com/viewprogram/5237.

Heimburger, DC, McLaren, DS, and Shils, ME: Clinical manifestations of nutrient deficiencies and toxicities: A resume. In Shils, ME, et al (eds): Modern Nutrition in Health and Disease, ed 10. Lippincott Williams & Wilkins, Philadelphia, 2006.

Hibuse, T, et al: Aquaporins and glycerol metabolism. Biochem Biophys Acta 1758:1004, 2006.

Hobson, WL: Bottled, filtered, and tap water use in Latino and Non-Latino children. Arch Pediatr Adolesc Med 161:457, 2007.

Holick, MF, et al: Prevalence of vitamin D inadequacy among postmenopausal North American women receiving osteoporosis therapy. J Clin Endocrinol Metab 90:3215, 2005.

Hsieh, CT, et al: Seizure associated with total parenteral nutrition-related hypermanganesemia. Pediatr Neurol 36:181, 2007.

Hu, H, et al: Increased expression of aquaporin-4 in human traumatic brain injury and brain tumors. J Zhejiang Univ Sci B 6:33, 2005.

Iinuma, Y, et al: Whole-blood manganese levels and brain manganese accumulation in children receiving long-term home parenteral nutrition. Pediatr Surg Int 19:268, 2003.

Institute of Medicine: Dietary Reference Intakes: Electrolytes and water. National Academy of Sciences, Washington, DC, 2004a. Accessed June 9, 2008 at: http://www.iom.edu/Object.File/Master/20/004/0.pdf.

Institute of Medicine: Dietary Reference Intakes: Elements. National Academy of Sciences, Washington, DC, 2001. Accessed June 2, 2008 at: http://www.iom.edu/Object.File/Master/7/294/0.pdf.

Institute of Medicine: Dietary Reference Intakes for Water, Potassium, Sodium Chloride, and Sulfate. National Academy Press, Washington, DC, 2004b. Accessed June 24, 2008 at: http://www.nap.edu/catalog.php?record_id=10925.

Ishibashi, K, Hara, S, and Kondo, S: Aquaporin water channels in mammals. Clin Exp Nephrol 13:107, 2009.

Kafritsa, Y, et al: Long-term outcome of brain manganese deposition in patients on home parenteral nutrition. Arch Dis Child 79:262, 1998.

Kaleita, TA, Kinsbourne, M, and Menkes, JH: A neurobehavioral syndrome after failure to thrive on chloride-deficient formula. Dev Med Child Neurol 33:626, 1991.

Khosia, S and Melton, LJ: Osteopenia. N Engl J Med 356:2293, 2007.

King, JC, and Cousins, RJ: Zinc. In Shils, ME, et al (eds): Modern Nutrition in Health and Disease, ed 10. Lippincott Williams & Wilkins, Philadelphia, 2006.

Knochel, JP: Phosphorus. In Shils, ME, et al (eds): Modern Nutrition in Health and Disease, ed 10. Lippincott Williams & Wilkins, Philadelphia, 2006.

Komarnisky, LA, Christopherson, RJ, and Basu, TK: Sulfur: Its clinical and toxicologic aspects. Nutrition 19:54, 2003.

Lanham-New, SA: Nutritional influences on bone health: An update on current research and clinical implications. Medscape Continuing Education, 2006. Accessed April 9, 2006 at: http://www.medscape.com/viewprogram/5034.

Lewis, AM: Heatstroke in older adults. Am J Nurs 107:52, 2007.

Marra, MV, and Boyar, AP: Position of the American Dietetic Association: nutrient supplementation. J Am Diet Assoc 109:2073, 2009.

Marshall, I: WITHDRAWN: zinc for the common cold. Cochrane Database Syst Rev 3:CD001364, 2006.

Merck Manual: Iron Poisoning. November 2005. Accessed January 28, 2009 at: http://www.merck.com/mmpe/sec21/ch326/ch326i.html?qt=iron%20poisoning&alt=sh.

Meyer, PA, et al: Surveillance for elevated blood lead levels among children—United States, 1997–2001. MMWR 52:SS10, 2003. Accessed November 30, 2003 at: http://www.cdc.gov/mmwr/PDF/ss/ss5210.pdf.

Miller, MB, et al: Pool cue chalk: A source of environmental lead. Pediatrics 97:916, 1996.

Mowad, E, Haddad, I, and Gemmel, DJ: Management of lead poisoning from ingested fishing sinkers. Arch Pediatr Adolesc Med 152:485, 1998.

Natural Resources Defense Council: Bottled water: Pure drink or pure hype? Executive Summary, 1999. Accessed June 17, 2008 at: http://www.nrdc.org/water/drinking/bw/exesum.asp.

Natural Resources Defense Council: What's on tap? Executive Summary, 2003. Accessed June 17, 2008 at: http://www.nrdc.org/water/drinking/uscities/execsum.asp.

Nishiyama, S, et al: Transient hypothyroidism or persistent hyperthyrotropinemia in neonates born to mothers with excessive iodine intake. Thyroid 14:1077, 2004.

Nutrition Fact Sheet: Molybdenum. Northwestern University, 2007. Accessed January 25, 2010 at: http://www.feinberg.northwestern.edu/nutrition/factsheets/molybdenum.html.

Nyenwe, EA, and Dagogo-Jack, S: Recognizing iodine deficiency in iodine-replete environments. N Engl J Med 357:1263, 2007.

O'Brien, KK, et al: Hyponatremia associated with overhydration in U.S. Army trainees. Mil Med 166:405, 2001.

Oh, MS, and Uribarri, J: Electrolytes, water, and acid-base balance. In Shils, ME, et al (eds): Modern Nutrition in Health and Disease, ed 10. Lippincott Williams & Wilkins, Philadelphia, 2006.

Oral therapy for acute diarrhea. In Kleinman, RE (ed): Pediatric Nutrition Handbook, ed 5. American Academy of Pediatrics, Elk Grove Village, IL, 2004.

Phillips, LD: Manual of I.V. Therapeutics, ed 4. FA Davis, Philadelphia, 2005.

Poole, RL, et al: Aluminum exposure from pediatric parenteral nutrition: Meeting the new FDA regulation. JPEN J Parenter Enteral Nutr 32:242, 2008.

Rude, RK, and Shils, ME: Magnesium. In Shils, ME, et al (eds): Modern Nutrition in Health and Disease, ed 10. Lippincott Williams & Wilkins, Philadelphia, 2006.

Sardesai, VM: Molybdenum: An essential trace element. Nutr Clin Pract 8:277, 1993.

Sawka, MN, et al: Exercise and fluid replacement. Med Sci Sports Exerc 39:377, 2007.

Scanlon, VC, and Sanders, T: Essentials of Anatomy and Physiology, ed 5. FA Davis, Philadelphia, 2007.

Schurks, M, Diener, HC, and Goadsby, P: Update on the prophylaxis of migraine. Curr Treat Options Neurol 10:20, 2008.

Shaikh, MG, et al: Transient neonatal hypothyroidism due to a maternal vegan diet. J Pediatr Endocrinol Metab 16:111, 2003.

Shannon, M, and Graef, J: Hazard of lead in infant formula [letter]. N Engl J Med 326:137, 1992.

Speerhas, RA, and Seidner, DL: Measured versus estimated aluminum content of parenteral nutrient solutions. Am J Health Syst Pharm 64:740, 2007.

Stoecker, BJ: Chromium. In Shils, ME, et al (eds): Modern Nutrition in Health and Disease, ed 10. Lippincott Williams & Wilkins, Philadelphia, 2006.

Ulett, K, Wells, B, and Centor, R: Hypercalcemia and acute renal failure in milk-alkali syndrome: a case report. J Hosp Med 5: E18, 2010.

U.S. Food and Drug Administration: Health claim notification for fluoridated water and reduced risk of dental caries. October 14, 2006a. Accessed June 4, 2008 at: http://www.cfsan.fda.gov/~dms/flfluoro.html.

U.S. Food and Drug Administration: Iron-containing supplements and drugs: Label warning statements and unit-dose packaging requirements; removal of regulations for unit-dose packaging requirements for dietary supplements and drugs. Final rule; removal of regulatory provisions in response to court order. Fed Reg 68:59714, 2003. Accessed May 20, 2004 at: http://www.gpoaccess.gov/fr/index.html.

U.S. Food and Drug Administration: Oral sodium phosphate (OSP) products for bowel cleansing. FDA Alert, May 2006b. Accessed June 23, 2008 at: http://www.fda.gov/medwatch/safety/2006/safety06.htm#phosphate.

Vassilev, ZP, et al: Case of elevated blood lead in a South Asian family that has used Sindoor for food coloring. Clin Toxicol (Phila) 43:301, 2005.

Venes, D (ed): Taber's Cyclopedic Medical Dictionary, ed 20. FA Davis, Philadelphia, 2005.

Verkman, AS: Role of aquaporin water channels in eye function. Exp Eye Res 76:137, 2003.

Weaver, CM, and Heaney, RP: Calcium. In Shils, ME, et al (eds): Modern Nutrition in Health and Disease, ed 10. Lippincott Williams & Wilkins, Philadelphia, 2006.

Wood, RJ, and Ronnenberg, AG: Iron. In Shils, ME, et al (eds): Modern Nutrition in Health and Disease, ed 10. Lippincott Williams & Wilkins, Philadelphia, 2006.

Yool, AJ: Aquaporins: Multiple roles in the central nervous system. Neuroscientist 13:470, 2007.

Zhou, Y, and Brittin, HC: Increased iron content of some Chinese foods due to cooking in steel woks. J Am Diet Assoc 94:1153, 1994.

Chapter 9

American Dietetic Association: International Dietetics and Nutrition Terminology Manual. American Dietetic Association, Chicago, 2008.

American Dietetic Association: Manual of Clinical Dietetics, ed 6. American Dietetic Association, Chicago, 2000.

Colaizzo-Anas, T: Nutrient intake, digestion, absorption, and excretion. In Gottschlich, MM, et al (eds): The A.S.P.E.N. Nutrition Support Core Curriculum: A Case-Based Approach—The Adult Patient. American Society for Parenteral and Enteral Nutrition, Silver Spring, MD, 2007.

Duyff, RL: American Dietetic Association Complete Food and Nutrition Guide, ed 3. American Dietetic Association, Hoboken, NJ, 2008.

Galvai, TJ: Dysphagia: Going down and staying down. Am J Nurs 101:37, 2001.

IFIC Foundation: Food sensitivities, allergies, and intolerance: Separating fact from fiction. Food Insight. IFIC Foundation, Washington, DC, 2003.

McCallum, SL: The National Dysphagia Diet: Implementation at a regional rehabilitation center and hospital system. J Am Diet Assoc 103:285, 2003.

Metheny, NA, et al: Tracheobronchial aspiration of gastric contents in critically ill tube-fed patients: Frequency, outcomes, and risk factors. Crit Care Med 34:1007, 2006.

Nelson, JK, et al: Mayo Clinic Diet Manual: A Handbook of Dietary Practice, ed 7. Elsevier Health Science, Philadelphia, 1994.

Raymond, N, Heap, J, and Case, S: The gluten-free diet: An update for health professional. Practical Gastroenterol Sept 2006.

Scanlon, VC, and Sanders, T: Essentials of Anatomy and Physiology, ed 4. FA Davis, Philadelphia, 2003.

Sheikh, A: Food Allergy. BMJ 335:1337, 2002.

Taylor, SL, Hefle, SL, and Munoz-Furlong, A: Food allergies and avoidance diets. Nutr Today 34:15, 1999.

The National Dysphagia Diet Task Force: The National Dysphagia Diet Standardization for Optimal Care. American Dietetic Association, Chicago, 2002.

Chapter 10

Abrams, SA: In utero physiology: Role in nutrient delivery and fetal development for calcium, phosphorus, and vitamin D. Am J Clin Nutr 85:604S, 2007.

Adoptive Breastfeeding Resource Website: Profiles. July 7, 2008. Accessed October 19, 2008 at: http://www.fourfriends.com/abrw/Profiles/profiles.htm.

Allen, LH: Multiple micronutrients in pregnancy and lactation: an overview. Am J Clin Ntr 8(suppl):1206S, 2005.

American Academy of Pediatrics, Committee on Nutrition and Section on Allergy and Immunology: Effects of early nutritional interventions on the development of atopic disease in infants and children: The role of maternal dietary restriction, breastfeeding, timing of introduction of complementary foods, and hydrolyzed formulas. Pediatrics 121:183, 2008.

American Academy of Pediatrics, Section on Breastfeeding: Breastfeeding and the use of human milk. Pediatrics 115:496, 2005.

American Dietetic Association: Position of the American Dietetic Association: Nutrition and lifestyle for a healthy pregnancy outcome. J Am Diet Assoc 108:553, 2008.

American Dietetic Association: Position of the American Dietetic Association: Promoting and supporting breastfeeding. J Am Diet Assoc 105:810, 2005.

Anderson, JW: Diabetes mellitus: Medical nutrition therapy. In Shils, ME, et al (eds): Modern Nutrition in Health and Disease, ed 10. Lippincott Williams & Wilkins, Philadelphia, 2006.

Arora, M: Maternal dietary intake of polyunsaturated fatty acids modifies the relationship between lead levels in bone and breast milk. J Nutr 138:73, 2008.

Baby-Friendly USA: 65 US Baby-friendly Hospitals and Birth Centers as of July 2008, 2006a. Accessed July 30, 2008 at: http://www.babyfriendlyusa.org/eng/03.html.

Baby-Friendly USA: Info for breastfeeding advocates/health care professionals, 2006b. Accessed August 5, 2008 at: http://www.babyfriendlyusa.org/eng/06.html.

Baby-Friendly USA: The ten steps to successful breastfeeding, 2004. Accessed July 30, 2008 at: http://www.babyfriendlyusa.org/eng/10steps.html.

Bamigboye, AA, and Smyth, R: Interventions for varicose veins and leg oedema in pregnancy. Cochrane Database Syst Rev 1: CD001066, 2007.

Blom, HJ, et al: Neural-tube defects and folate: Case far from closed. Nat Rev Neurosci 7:724, 2006.

Boyer, KM, et al: Risk factors for *Toxoplasma gondii* infection in mothers of infants with congenital toxoplasmosis: Implications for prenatal management and screening. Am J Obstet Gynecol 192:564, 2005.

Bracken, MB, et al: Association of maternal caffeine consumption with decrements in fetal growth. Am J Epidemiol 157:456, 2003.

Bradley, CS, et al: Constipation in pregnancy: Prevalence, symptoms, and risk factors. Obstet Gynecol 110:1351, 2007.

Breastfeeding. In Kleinman, RE (ed): Pediatric Nutrition Handbook, ed 5. American Academy of Pediatrics, Elk Grove Village, IL, 2004.

Brown, JE: Nutrition Through the Life Cycle, ed 3. Thomson Wadsworth, Belmont, CA, 2008.

Byrne, J, and Carolan, S: Adverse reproductive outcomes among pregnancies of aunts and (spouses of) uncles in Irish families with neural tube defects. Am J Med Genet A 140:52, 2006.

Camadoo, L, Tibbot, R, and Isaza, F: Maternal vitamin D deficiency associated with neonatal hypocalcaemic convulsions. Nutr J 6:23, 2007.

Centers for Disease Control and Prevention: Alcohol consumption among pregnant and childbearing-aged women—United States, 1991–1999. MMWR 51:273, 2002. Accessed August 18, 2008 at: http://www.cdc.gov/mmwr/preview/mmwrhtml/mm5113a2.htm.

Centers for Disease Control and Prevention: Alcohol consumption among women who are pregnant or who might become pregnant—United States, 2002. MMWR 53:1178, 2004a. Accessed August 19, 2008 at: http://www.cdc.gov/mmwr/preview/mmwrhtml/mm5350a4.htm.

Centers for Disease Control and Prevention: Births: Final data for 2005. Natl Vital Stat Rep 56(6), 2007a. Accessed July 15, 2008 at: http://www.cdc.gov/nchs/data/nvsr56/nvsr56_06.pdf.

Centers for Disease Control and Prevention: Folate status in women of childbearing age, by race/ethnicity—United States, 1999–2000, 2001–2002, and 2003–2004. MMWR 55:1377, 2007b. Accessed July 16, 2008 at: http://www.cdc.gov/mmwr/preview/mmwrhtml/mm5551a.htm.

Centers for Disease Control and Prevention: Guidelines for identifying and referring persons with fetal alcohol syndrome. MMWR 54:1, 2005. Accessed July 2, 2008 at: http://www.cdc.gov/mmwr/PDF/rr/rr5411.pdf.

Centers for Disease Control and Prevention: Multistate outbreak of listeriosis—United States, 2000. MMWR 49:1129, 2000a.

Accessed August 19, 2008 at: http://www.cdc.gov/mmwr/preview/mmwrhtml/mm4950a1.htm.

Centers for Disease Control and Prevention: Neurologic impairment in children associated with maternal dietary deficiency of cobalamin—Georgia, 2001. MMWR 52:61, 2003. Accessed August 19, 2008 at: http://www.cdc.gov/mmwr/preview/mmwrhtml/mm5204a1.htm.

Centers for Disease Control and Prevention: Outbreak of *Listeria monocytogenes* infections associated with pasteurized milk from a local dairy—Massachusetts, 2007. MMWR 57:1097, 2008a. Accessed February 7, 2009 at: http://www.cdc.gov/mmwr/preview/mmwrhtml/mm5740a1.htm.

Centers for Disease Control and Prevention: Outbreak of listeriosis associated with homemade Mexican-style cheese—North Carolina, October 2000–January 2001. MMWR 50:560, 2001a. Accessed August 19, 2008 at: http://www.cdc.gov/mmwr/preview/mmwrhtml/mm5026a3.htm.

Centers for Disease Control and Prevention: Preventing congenital toxoplasmosis. MMWR 49:57, 2000b. Accessed August 19, 2008 at: http://www.cdc.gov/mmwr/preview/mmwrhtml/rr4902a5.htm.

Centers for Disease Control and Prevention: Quick stats: Percentage of women who gained <15 pounds during pregnancy, by age group and race/ethnicity of mother—United States, 2005. MMWR 57:294, 2008b. Accessed July 1, 2008 at: http://www.cdc.gov/mmwr/PDF/wk/mm5711.pdf.

Centers for Disease Control and Prevention: Quick stats: Percentage of women who gained >40 pounds during pregnancy, by race/ethnicity of mother—United States, 1990, 2000, and 2005. MMWR 57:127, 2008c. Accessed July 1, 2008 at: http://www.cdc.gov/mmwr/preview/mmwrhtml/mm5705a7.htm.

Centers for Disease Control and Prevention: Recommendations for the use of folic acid to reduce the number of cases of spina bifida and other neural tube defects. MMWR 41(RR-14):1, 1992.

Centers for Disease Control and Prevention: Trends in wheat-flour fortification with folic acid and iron—Worldwide, 2004 and 2007. MMWR 57:8, 2008d. Accessed July 1, 2008 at: http://www.cdc.gov/mmwr/preview/mmwrhtml/mm5701a4.htm.

Centers for Disease Control and Prevention: Update: Multistate outbreak of listeriosis—United States, 1998–1999. MMWR 47:1117, 1999.

Centers for Disease Control and Prevention: Use of vitamins containing folic acid among women of childbearing age—United States, 2007. MMWR 57:5, 2008e. Accessed July 1, 2008 at: http://www.cdc.gov/mmwr/preview/mmwrhtml/mm5701a3.htm.

Cheetham, TC, et al: A risk management program aimed at preventing fetal exposure to isotretinoin: Retrospective cohort study. J Am Acad Dermatol 55:442, 2006.

Chettle, CC: Food gone bad. Nursing Spectrum Midwestern Edition 9:34, 2008.

Chiossi, G, et al: Hyperemesis gravidarum complicated by Wernicke encephalopathy: Background, case report, and review of the literature. Obstet Gynecol Surv 61:255, 2006.

Chitambar, CR, and Antony, AC: Nutritional aspects of hematologic diseases. In Shils, ME, et al (eds): Modern Nutrition in Health and Disease, ed 10. Lippincott Williams & Wilkins, Philadelphia, 2006.

Conde-Agudelo, A, Rosas-Bermudez, A, and Kafury-Goeta, AC: Birth spacing and risk of adverse perinatal outcomes. JAMA 295:1809, 2006.

Crenshaw, J: Breastfeeding in nonmaternity settings. Am J Nurs 105:40, 2005.

Czeizel, AE, and Dudas, I: Prevention of the first occurrence of neural-tube defects by periconceptional vitamin supplementation. N Engl J Med 327:1832, 1992.

Deglin, JH, and Vallerand, AH: Davis's Drug Guide for Nurses, ed 11. FA Davis, Philadelphia, 2009.

De Marco, P, et al: Current perspectives on the genetic causes of neural tube defects. Neurogenetics 7:201, 2006.

DePaola, DP, et al: Nutrition and dental medicine. In Shils, ME, et al (eds): Modern Nutrition in Health and Disease, ed 10. Lippincott Williams & Wilkins, Philadelphia, 2006.

Dodgson, JE, et al: An ecological perspective of breastfeeding in an indigenous community. J Nurs Scholarsh 34:235, 2002.

Ecker, JL, and Greene, MF: Gestational diabetes—setting limits, exploring treatments. N Engl J Med 358:2061, 2008.

Eerdekens, A, et al: Maternal bariatric surgery: adverse outcomes in neonates. Eur J Pediatr 169:191, 2010.

Eroglu, A, et al: Spontaneous esophageal rupture following severe vomiting in pregnancy. Dis Esophagus 15:242, 2002.

Eventov-Friedman, S, Klinger, G, and Shinwell, ES: Third trimester fetal intracranial hemorrhage owing to vitamin K deficiency associated with hyperemesis gravidarum. J Pediatr Hematol Oncol 31:985, 2009.

Fedorka, PD, and Heasley, SW: Preeclampsia: The little-known truth. Am Nurse 3(2):9, 2008.

Fortinguerra, F, Clavenna, A, and Bonati, M: Psychotropic drug use during breastfeeding: a review of the evidence. Pediatrics 124(4):e547.

Galloway, R, and McGuire, J: Daily versus weekly: How many iron pills do pregnant women need? Nutr Rev 54:318, 1996.

Gibson-Davis, CM, and Brooks-Gunn, J: Couples' immigration status and ethnicity as determinants of breastfeeding. Am J Public Health 96:641, 2006.

Grotegut, CA, et al: Baking soda pica: A case of hypokalemic metabolic alkalosis and rhabdomyolysis in pregnancy. Obstet Gynecol 107:484, 2006.

Haggerty, CL, et al: Association between allelic variants in cytokine genes and preeclampsia. Am J Obstet Gynecol 193:209, 2005.

Hart, JA: Viewpoint: mercury level and fish: Risks vs benefits. Medscape Family Medicine/Primary Care 7(2), October 17, 2005. Accessed March 12, 2009 at: http://www.medscape.com/viewarticle/511382.

Heymann, DL (ed): Control of Communicable Diseases Manual, ed 18. American Public Health Association, Washington, DC, 2004.

Higdon, JV, and Frei, B: Coffee and health: A review of recent human research. Crit Rev Food Sci Nutr 46:101, 2006.

Hill, JB, Yost, NP, and Wendel, GD: Acute renal failure in association with severe hyperemesis gravidarum. Obstet Gynecol 100:1119, 2002.

Holick, MF: Resurrection of vitamin D deficiency and rickets. J Clin Invest 116:2062, 2006.

Hollis, BW: Vitamin D requirement during pregnancy and lactation. J Bone Miner Res 22(Suppl 2):V39, 2007.

Indraccolo, U, et al: Thiamin deficiency and beriberi features in a patient with hyperemesis gravidarum. Nutrition 21:967, 2005.

Ip, S, et al: Breastfeeding and maternal and infant health outcomes in developed countries. U.S. Department of Health and Human Services, Rockville, MD, 2007. Accessed August 12, 2008 at: http://www.ahrq.gov/downloads/pub/evidence/pdf/brfout/brfout.pdf.

Jewell, D, and Young, G: Interventions for nausea and vomiting in early pregnancy. Cochrane Database Syst Rev 4:CD000145, 2003.

Jewell, DJ, and Young, G: Interventions for treating constipation in pregnancy. Cochrane Database Syst Rev 2:CD001142, 2001.

Johnston, RB: Will increasing folic acid in fortified grain products further reduce neural tube defects without causing harm?: Consideration of the evidence. Pediatr Res 63:2, 2007.

Jones, PJH, and Kubow, S: Lipids, sterols, and their metabolites. In Shils, ME, et al (eds): Modern Nutrition in Health and Disease, ed 10. Lippincott Williams & Wilkins, Philadelphia, 2006.

Kanra, MD, et al: Answer to hypotonia: A simple hemogram. J Child Neurol 20:930, 2005.

Karlsson, MK, Ahlborg, HG, and Karlsson, C: Maternity and bone mineral density. Acta Orthop 76:2, 2005.

Kibar, Z, Capra,V, and Gros, P: Toward understanding the genetic basis of neural tube defects. Clin Genet 71:295, 2007.

King, JC, and Cousins, RJ: Zinc. In Shils, ME, et al (eds): Modern Nutrition in Health and Disease, ed 10. Lippincott Williams & Wilkins, Philadelphia, 2006.

Koletzko, B, et al: The roles of long-chain polyunsaturated fatty acids in pregnancy, lactation and infancy: Review of current knowledge and consensus recommendations. J Perinat Med 36:5, 2008.

Latva-Pukkila, U, Isolauri, E, and Laitinen, K: Dietary and clinical impacts of nausea and vomiting during pregnancy. J Hum Nutr Diet 23:69, 2010.

Liang, SG, et al: Pneumomediastinum following esophageal rupture associated with hyperemesis gravidarum. J Obstet Gynaecol Res 28:172, 2002.

Lupton, C, Burd, L, and Harwood, R: Cost of fetal alcohol spectrum disorders. Am J Med Genet C Semin Med Genet 127C:42, 2004.

Ma, FY, and Falkenberg, M: Case reports: Transient osteoporosis of the hip: An atypical case. Clin Orthop Relat Res 445:245, 2006.

Malvasi, A, et al: Possible long-term teratogenic effect of isotretinoin in pregnancy. Eur Rev Med Pharmacol Sci 13:393, 2009.

March of Dimes: Food-borne risks in pregnancy. Professionals and Researchers, May 2006. Accessed July 17, 2008 at: http://www.marchofdimes.com/printableArticles/681_1152.asp.

Martin, I, et al: Neonatal withdrawal syndrome after chronic maternal drinking of mate. Ther Drug Monit 29:127, 2007.

McDowell, MA, Wang, C-Y, and Kennedy-Stephenson, J. Breastfeeding in the United States: Findings from the National Health and Nutrition Examination Surveys 1999-2006. NCHS Data Briefs, no. 5, National Center for Health Statistics, Hyattsville, MD, April 2008. Accessed October 19, 2008 at: http://www.cdc.gov/nchs/data/databriefs/db05.htm.

Mitchell, LE: Epidemiology of neural tube defects. Am J Med Genet C Semin Med Genet 135C:88, 2005.

MRC Vitamin Study Research Group: Prevention of neural tube defects: Results of the Medical Research Council Vitamin Study. Lancet 338:131, 1991.

Nulman, I, et al: Long-term neurodevelopment of children exposed to maternal nausea and vomiting of pregnancy and diclectin. J Pediatr 155:45, 2009.

Nygaard, IH, et al: Does oral magnesium substitution relieve pregnancy-induced leg cramps? Eur J Obstet Gynecol Reprod Biol 141:23, 2008.

Ozgoli, G, Goli, M, and Simbar, M: Effects of ginger capsules on pregnancy, nausea, and vomiting. J Altern Complement Med 15:243, 2009.

Pardi, G, and Cetin, I: Human fetal growth and organ development: 50 years of discoveries. Am J Obstet Gynecol 194:1088, 2006.

Peris, P, et al: Pregnancy associated osteoporosis: The familial effect. Clin Exp Rheumatol 20:697, 2002.

Picciano, MF, and McDonald, SS: Lactation. In Shils, ME, et al (eds): Modern Nutrition in Health and Disease, ed 10. Lippincott Williams & Wilkins, Philadelphia, 2006.

Pitkin, RM: Folate and neural tube defects. Am J Clin Nutr 85(Suppl):285S, 2007.

Purnell, LD, and Paulanka, BJ: Transcultural Health Care, ed 3. FA Davis, Philadelphia, 2008. Accessed August 4, 2008 at: http://davisplus.fadavis.com/purnell/Bonus_Chapters/Ch29.pdf.

Rude, RK, and Shils, ME: Magnesium. In Shils, ME, et al (eds): Modern Nutrition in Health and Disease, ed 10. Lippincott Williams & Wilkins, Philadelphia, 2006.

Saunders, C, et al: Gestational nightblindness among women attending a public maternity hospital in Rio de Janeiro, Brazil. J Health Popul Nutr 22:348, 2004.

Selitsky, T, Chandra, P, and Schiavello, HJ: Wernicke's encephalopathy with hyperemesis and ketoacidosis. Obstet Gynecol 107:486, 2006.

Shannon, M: Severe lead poisoning in pregnancy. Ambul Pediatr 3:37, 2003.

Skjaerven, R, et al: Recurrence of pre-eclampsia across generations: Exploring fetal and maternal genetic components in a population based cohort. BMJ, doi:10.11136/bmj.38555.462685.8F (published 16 September 2005).

State of New Jersey, Department of Health and Senior Services: When not to breastfeed. Last modified April 3, 2009. Accessed January 29, 2010 at: http://www.state.nj.us/health/fhs/wic/nottobreastfeed.shtml.

Tielsch, JM, et al: Maternal night blindness during pregnancy is associated with low birthweight, morbidity, and poor growth in South India. J Nutr 138:787, 2008.

Turner, RE: Nutrition during pregnancy. In Shils, ME, et al (eds): Modern Nutrition in Health and Disease, ed 10. Lippincott Williams & Wilkins, Philadelphia, 2006.

U.S. Department of Agriculture: Nutrition program facts. WIC, 2006. Accessed August 6, 2008 at: http://www.fns.usda.gov/wic/WIC-Fact-Sheet.pdf.

U.S. Department of Health and Human Services and U.S. Environmental Protection Agency: What You Need to Know about Mercury in Fish and Shellfish. March 2004. Accessed August 19, 2008 at: http://www.cfsan.fda.gov/~dms/admehg3.html.

U.S. Food and Drug Administration: FDA Public Health Advisory: Use of codeine by some breastfeeding mothers may lead to life-threatening side effects in nursing babies. August 17, 2007a. Accessed August 13, 2008 at: http://www.fda.gov/cder/drug/advisory/codeine.htm.

U.S. Food and Drug Administration: Information for healthcare professionals: Use of codeine products in nursing mothers, August 17, 2007b. Accessed August 12, 2008 at: http://www.fda.gov/cder/drug/InfoSheets/HCP/codeineHCP.htm.

U.S. Food and Drug Administration: Isotretinoin pregnancy risk management program, September 7, 2007. Accessed July 22, 2008 at: http://www.fda.gov/ohrms/dockets/ac/07/slides/2007-4311s1-05-sponsor-group-backup.ppt.

U.S. Food and Drug Administration: Patient information sheet isotretinoin, November 17, 2005. Accessed July 10, 2008 at: http://www.gda.gov/cder/drug/InfoSheets/patient/IsotretinoinPT.htm.

U.S. Food and Drug Administration: Recalls and safety alerts: Rare side-effect of codeine in nursing mothers. November 2007. Accessed August 13, 2008 at: http://www.accessdata.fda.gov/scripts/cdrh/cfdocs/psn/printer.cfm?id=684.

Wagner, BA, et al: Nutritional management of hyperemesis gravidarum. Nutr Clin Pract 15:65, 2000.

Chapter 11

About FAAN. Food Allergy and Anaphylaxis Network. Undated. Accessed December 10, 2008 at: http://www.foodallergy.org/about.html.

Abrams, SA: In utero physiology: Role in nutrient delivery and fetal development for calcium, phosphorus, and vitamin D. Am J Clin Nutr 85:604S, 2007.

Academy of Breastfeeding Medicine: Protocol #8: Human milk storage information for home use for healthy full-term infants.

Undated. Accessed December 14, 2008 at: http://www.bfmed.org/ace-files/protocol/milkstorage_abm.pdf.

Adolescent nutrition. In Kleinman, RE (ed): Pediatric Nutrition Handbook, ed 5. American Academy of Pediatrics, Elk Grove Village, IL, 2004.

Ambalavanan, N, et al: Vitamin A supplementation for extremely low birth weight infants: Outcome at 18 to 22 months. Pediatrics 115:e249, 2005.

American Academy of Pediatrics Committee on Nutrition: Prevention of pediatric overweight and obesity. Pediatrics 112:424, 2003. Reaffirmed October 2006.

American Academy of Pediatrics Committee on Nutrition: The use and misuse of fruit juice in pediatrics. Pediatrics 107:1210, 2001. Reaffirmed October 2006.

American Academy of Pediatrics Committee on Nutrition and Section on Allergy and Immunology: Effects of early nutritional interventions on the development of atopic disease in infants and children: The role of maternal dietary restriction, breastfeeding, timing of introduction of complementary foods, and hydrolyzed formulas. Pediatrics 121:183, 2008.

American Academy of Pediatrics Section on Breastfeeding: Breast-feeding and the use of human milk. Pediatrics 115:496, 2005.

American Dietetic Association: Pediatric weight management evidence-based nutrition practice guideline. American Dietetic Association, 2008.

American Dietetic Association: Position of the American Dietetic Association: Benchmarks for nutrition programs in child care settings. J Am Diet Assoc 105:979, 2005.

American Dietetic Association: Position of the American Dietetic Association and Dietitians of Canada: Vegetarian diets. J Am Diet Assoc 103:748, 2003. Accessed December 6, 2008 at: http://www.eatright.org.

Appendix K-1. In Kleinman, RE (ed): Pediatric Nutrition Handbook, ed 5. American Academy of Pediatrics, Elk Grove Village, IL, 2004.

Appendix W. In Kleinman, RE (ed): Pediatric Nutrition Handbook, ed 5. American Academy of Pediatrics, Elk Grove Village, IL, 2004.

Arnon, SS, et al: Human botulism immune globulin for the treatment of infant botulism. N Engl J Med 354:462, 2006.

Bahna, SL: Hypoallergenic formulas: Optimal choices for treatment versus prevention. Ann Allergy Asthma Immunol 101:453, 2008.

Ballester, F, et al: Asthma visits to emergency rooms and soybean unloading in the harbors of Valencia and A Coruna, Spain. Am J Epidemiol 149:315, 1999.

Bannon, GA, and Martino-Catt, S: Application of current allergy assessment guidelines to next-generation biotechnology-derived crops. J AOAC Int 90:1492, 2007.

Baroncelli, GI, et al: Osteoporosis in children and adolescents: Etiology and management. Paediatr Drugs 7:295, 2005.

Bay, A, et al: Evaluation of vitamin K deficiency in children with acute and intractable diarrhea. Adv Ther 23:469, 2006.

Beals, KA, and Meyer, NL: Female athlete triad update. Clin Sports Med 26:69, 2007.

Bhatia, J, and Greer, F: Use of soy protein-based formulas in infant feeding. Pediatrics 121:1062, 2008.

Birch, EE, et al: Visual acuity and cognitive outcomes at 4 years of age in a double-blind, randomized trial of long-chain polyunsaturated fatty acid–supplemented infant formula. Early Hum Dev 83:279, 2007.

Bjorksten, B: Genetic and environmental risk factors for the development of food allergy. Curr Opin Allergy Clin Immunol 5:249, 2005.

Blanco, C, et al: Latex allergy: Clinical features and cross-reactivity with fruits. Ann Allergy 73:309, 1994.

Boch, SA, Munoz-Furlong, A, and Sampson, HA: Fatalities due to anaphylactic reactions to foods. J Allergy Clin Immunol 107:191, 2001.

Boch, SA, Munoz-Furlong, A, and Sampson, HA: Further fatalities caused by anaphylactic reactions to food, 2001–2006 [letter]. J Allergy Clin Immunol 119:1016, 2007.

Breastfeeding. In Kleinman, RE (ed): Pediatric Nutrition Handbook, ed 5. American Academy of Pediatrics, Elk Grove Village, IL, 2004.

Brehler, R, et al: "Latex-fruit syndrome": Frequency of cross-reacting IgE antibodies. Allergy 52:404, 1997.

Bren, L: Food labels identify allergens more clearly. FDA Consumer Magazine. March-April 2006. Accessed December 10, 2008 at: http://www.fda.gov/fdac/features/2006/206_foodlabels.html.

Brotanek, JM, et al: Iron deficiency in early childhood in the United States: Risk factors and racial/ethnic disparities. Pediatrics 120:568, 2007.

Brown, JE (ed): Nutrition Through the Life Cycle, ed 3. Thomson Wadsworth, Belmont, CA, 2008.

Buckley, M: Product focus: Some new and important clues to the causes of colic. Br J Community Nurs 5:462, 2000.

Campbell, MK, and Kelsey, KS: The PEACH survey: A nutrition screening tool for use in early intervention programs. J Am Diet Assoc 94:1156, 1994.

Carvalho, NE, et al: Severe nutritional deficiencies in toddlers resulting from health food milk alternatives. Pediatrics 107: E46, 2001.

Casanueva, E, et al: Vitamin C supplementation to prevent premature rupture of the chorioamniotic membranes: A randomized trial. Am J Clin Nutr 81:859, 2005.

Cathey, M, and Gaylord, N: Picky eating: A toddler's approach to mealtime. Pediatr Nurs 30:101, 2004.

Centers for Disease Control and Prevention: Achievements in public health, 1900–1999: Healthier mothers and babies. MMWR 48:849, 1999a. Accessed October 1, 1999 at: http://www.cdc.gov/epo/mmwr/preview/mmwrhtml/mm4838a2.htm.

Centers for Disease Control and Prevention: Breastfeeding trends and updated national health objectives for exclusive breastfeeding—United States, birth years 2000–2004. MMWR 56:760, 2007. Accessed July 28, 2008 at: http://www.cdc.gov/mmwr/preview/mmwrhtml/mm5630a2.htm.

Centers for Disease Control and Prevention: Childhood diarrhea: Messages for parents. 1999b. Accessed October 29, 1999 at: http://www.cdc.gov/od/oc/parents.

Centers for Disease Control and Prevention: Children and teens told by doctors that they were overweight—United States, 1999–2002. MMWR 54:848, 2005a.

Centers for Disease Control and Prevention: Competitive foods and beverages available for purchase in secondary schools—selected sites, United States, 2004. MMWR 54:917, 2005b.

Centers for Disease Control and Prevention: Infant botulism—New York City, 2001–2002. MMWR 52:21, 2003a. Accessed February 25, 2004 at: http://www.cdc.gov/mmwr/preview/mmwrhtml/mm5202a1.htm.

Centers for Disease Control and Prevention: Infant mortality and low birth weight among black and white infants—United States, 1980–2000. MMWR 51:589, 2002. Accessed February 18, 2004 at: http://www.cdc.gov/mmwr/preview/mmwrhtml/mm5127a1.htm.

Centers for Disease Control and Prevention: Managing acute gastroenteritis among children: Oral rehydration, maintenance, and nutritional therapy. MMWR 52:1, 2003b. Accessed May 10, 2005 at: http://www.cdc.gov/mmwr/PDF/RR/RR5216.pdf.

Centers for Disease Control and Prevention: Neurologic impairment in children associated with maternal dietary deficiency of cobalamin—Georgia, 2001. MMWR 52:61, 2003c. Accessed

January 22, 2004 at: http://www.cdc.gov/mmwr/preview/mmwrhtml/mm5204a1.htm.

Centers for Disease Control and Prevention: Prevention of rotavirus gastroenteritis among infants and children. MMWR 55:1, 2006. Accessed December 10, 2008 at: http://www.cdc.gov/mmwr/preview/mmwrhtml/rr5512a1.htm.

Centers for Disease Control and Prevention: QuickStats: Infant, neonatal, and postneonatal annual mortality rates—United States, 1940–2005. MMWR 57:377, 2008.

Chantry, CJ, Howard, CR, and Auinger, MS: Full breastfeeding duration and associated decrease in respiratory tract infection in U.S. children. Pediatrics 117:425, 2006.

Chatoor, I: Feeding disorders in infants and toddlers: Diagnosis and treatment. Child Adolesc Psychiatr Clin N Am 11:163, 2002.

Chen, A, and Rogan, W: Breastfeeding and the risk of postneonatal death in the United States. Pediatrics 113:e435, 2004.

Chitambar, CR, and Antony, AC: Nutritional aspects of hematologic diseases. In Shils, ME, et al (eds): Modern Nutrition in Health and Disease, ed 10. Lippincott Williams & Wilkins, Philadelphia, 2006.

Cinquetti, M, et al: Latex allergy in a child with banana anaphylaxis. Acta Paediatr 84:709, 1995.

Clark, S, et al: Multicenter study of emergency department visits for food allergies. J Allergy Clin Immunol 113:347, 2004.

Complementary feeding. In Kleinman, RE (ed): Pediatric Nutrition Handbook, ed 5. American Academy of Pediatrics, Elk Grove Village, IL, 2004.

Cook, AJ, and Friday, JE: Pyramid servings intakes in the United States 1999–2002, 1 day. Community Nutrition Research Group, Agricultural Research Service. March 2005. Accessed November 30, 2008 at: http://www.ars.usda.gov/sp2UserFiles/Place/12355000/foodlinks/ts_3-0.pdf.

Cordain, L, et al: Acne vulgaris: A disease of Western civilization. Arch Dermatol 138:1584, 2002.

Cormier, E, and Elder, JH: Diet and child behavior problems: Fact or fiction? Pediatr Nurs 33:138, 2007.

Cox, N, and Hinkle, R: Infant botulism. Am Fam Physician 65:1388, 2002.

Crocco, AG, Villasis-Keever, M, and Jadad, AR: Two wrongs don't make a right: Harm aggravated by inaccurate information on the Internet. Pediatrics 109:522, 2002.

Crotteau, CA, Wright, ST, and Eglash, A: Clinical inquiries. What is the best treatment for infants with colic? J Fam Pract 55:634, 2006.

Cruz, NV, and Bahna, SL: Do food or additives cause behavior disorders? Pediatr Ann 35:744, 2006.

Daniels, SR, et al: Overweight in children and adolescents: Pathophysiology, consequences, prevention, and treatment. Circulation 111:1999, 2005.

Davidovici, BB, and Wolf, R: The role of diet in acne: facts and controversies. Clin Dermatol 28:12, 2010.

Davis, MM, et al: Recommendations for prevention of childhood obesity. Pediatrics 120:S229, 2007.

Deglin, JH, and Vallerand, AH (eds): Davis's Drug Guide for Nurses, ed 11. FA Davis, Philadelphia, 2009.

Delbourg, MF, et al: Hypersensitivity to banana in latex-allergens of 33 and 37 kD. Ann Allergy Asthma Immunol 76:321, 1996.

Dennehy, PH: Rotavirus vaccines: An overview. Clin Microbiol Rev 21:198, 2008.

Der, G, Batty, GD, and Deary, IJ: Effect of breast feeding on intelligence in children: Prospective study, sibling pairs analysis, and meta-analysis. BMJ 333:945, 2006.

Dietz, WH, and Robinson, TN: Overweight children and adolescents. N Engl J Med 352:2100, 2005.

Duro, D, et al: Association between infantile colic and carbohydrate malabsorption from fruit juices in infancy. Pediatrics 109:797, 2002.

Failure to thrive. In Kleinman, RE (ed): Pediatric Nutrition Handbook, ed 5. American Academy of Pediatrics, Elk Grove Village, IL, 2004.

Fats and fatty acids. In Kleinman, RE (ed): Pediatric Nutrition Handbook, ed 5. American Academy of Pediatrics, Elk Grove Village, IL, 2004.

Feeding the child. In Kleinman, RE (ed): Pediatric Nutrition Handbook, ed 5. American Academy of Pediatrics, Elk Grove Village, IL, 2004.

Feingold, D, and Hame, SL: Female athlete triad and stress fractures. Orthop Clin North Am 37:575, 2006.

Ferdowsain, HR, and Levin, S: Does diet really affect acne? Skin Therapy Lett 15:1, 2010.

Finkelstein, DM, Hill, EL, and Whitaker, RC: School food environments and policies in US public schools. Pediatrics 122: e251, 2008.

Formanek, R, Jr: Food allergies: When food becomes the enemy. FDA Consumer Magazine July-August, 2001. Revised April 2004. Accessed December 10, 2008 at: http://magazine-directory.com/FDA-Consumer.htm.

Formula feeding of term infants. In Kleinman, RE (ed): Pediatric Nutrition Handbook, ed 5. American Academy of Pediatrics, Elk Grove Village, IL, 2004.

Forste, R, Weiss, J, and Lippincott, E: The decision to breastfeed in the United States: Does race matter? Pediatrics 108:291, 2001.

Fox, AT, et al: Food allergy as a risk factor for nutritional rickets. Pediatr Allergy Immunol 15:566, 2004.

Fry, T: The new "breast from birth" growth charts: An updated version of the paper given at the Primary Care Conference and Exhibition, May 2003. J Fam Health Care 13:124, 2003.

Ganglberger, E: Hev b 8, the Hevea brasiliensis latex profilin, is a cross-reactive allergen of latex, plant foods and pollen. Int Arch Allergy Immunol 125:216, 2001.

Garcia-Careaga, M, Jr, and Kerner, JA, Jr: Gastrointestinal manifestations of food allergies in pediatric patients. Nutr Clin Prac 20:526, 2005.

Garcia-Ortiz, JC, et al: Bronchial asthma induced by hypersensitivity to legumes. Allergol Immunopathol Madr 23:38, 1995.

Gibson-Davis, CM, and Brooks-Gunn, J: Breastfeeding and verbal ability of 3-year-olds in a multicity sample. Pediatrics 118: e1444, 2006.

Gillman, MW, et al: Family dinner and diet quality among older children and adolescents. Arch Fam Med 9:235, 2000.

Goulding, A: Risk factors for fractures in normally active children and adolescents. Med Sport Sci 51:102, 2007.

Gropper, SS, Smith, JL, and Groff, JL: Advanced Nutrition and Human Metabolism, ed 5. Wadsworth, Belmont, CA, 2009.

Gupta, SK: Is colic a gastrointestinal disorder? Curr Opin Pediatr 14:588, 2002.

Hallett, R, Haapanen, LAD, and Teuber, SS: Food allergies and kissing. N Engl J Med 346:1833, 2002.

Hamasha, AA, et al: Oral health behaviors of children in low and high socioeconomic status families. Pediatr Dent 28:310, 2006.

Hampton, T: Genetic link found for premature birth risk. JAMA 296:1713, 2006.

Heird, WC, and Cooper A: Infancy and childhood. In Shils, ME, et al (eds): Modern Nutrition in Health and Disease, ed 10. Lippincott Williams & Wilkins, Philadelphia, 2006.

Henriksen, C, et al: Improved cognitive development among preterm infants attributable to early supplementation of human milk with docosahexaenoic acid and arachidonic acid. Pediatrics 121:1137, 2008.

Henry, MC, and Moss, RL: Neonatal necrotizing enterocolitis. Semin Pediatr Surg 17:98, 2008.

Heymann, DL (ed): Control of Communicable Diseases Manual, ed 18. American Public Health Association, Washington, DC, 2004.

Hill, DJ, et al: Effect of a low-allergen maternal diet on colic among breastfed infants: A randomized controlled trial. Pediatrics 116:e709, 2005.

Hill, JO, Catenacci, VA, and Wyatt, HR: Obesity: etiology. In Shils, ME, et al (eds): Modern Nutrition in Health and Disease, ed 10. Lippincott Williams & Wilkins, Philadelphia, 2006.

Hoecker, JL: Infant botulism: How can it be prevented? May 15, 2010. Accessed May 16, 2010 at http://www.mayoclinic.com/health/infant-botulism/HQ00854.

Hofman, PL, et al: Premature birth and later insulin resistance. N Engl J Med 351:2179, 2004.

Hubbard, D, and Tobias, JD: Intracerebral hemorrhage due to hemorrhagic disease of the newborn and failure to administer vitamin K at birth. South Med J 99:1216, 2006.

Huiras, R: Banking on breast milk. Nursing Spectrum Midwest Edition, June 8, 2007.

Institute of Medicine of the National Academy of Sciences: Nutrition standards for foods in schools: Leading the way toward healthier youth. April 2007. Accessed December 2, 2008 at: http://www.iom.edu/Object.File/Master/42/505/Food%20in%20Schools.pdf.

James, J, et al: Preventing childhood obesity by reducing consumption of carbonated drinks: Cluster randomised controlled trial. BMJ 328:1237, 2004.

Klemola, T, et al: Feeding a soy formula to children with cow's milk allergy: The development of immunoglobulin E–mediated allergy to soy and peanuts. Pediatr Allergy Immunol 16:641, 2005.

Klish, WJ, and Montandon, CM: Nutrition and upper gastrointestinal disorders. In Halpern, SL (ed): Quick Reference to Clinical Nutrition, ed 2. JB Lippincott, Philadelphia, 1987.

Koletzko, B: Long-term consequences of early feeding on later obesity risk. Nestle Nutr Workshop Ser Pediatr Program 58:1, 2006.

Latasa, M, et al: Fruit sensitization in patients with allergy to latex. J Investig Allergol Clin Immunol 5:97, 1995.

Llatser, R, Zambrano, C, and Guillaumet, B: Anaphylaxis to natural rubber latex in a girl with food allergy. Pediatrics 94:736, 1994.

Lo, CW: Human milk: Nutritional properties. In Walker, WA, and Watkins, JB (eds): Nutrition in Pediatrics, ed 2. BC Decker, Hamilton, Ontario, 1997.

Maloney, J, and Nowak-Wegrzyn, A: Educational clinical case series for pediatric allergy and immunology: Allergic proctocolitis, food protein–induced enterocolitis syndrome and allergic eosinophilic gastroenteritis with protein-losing gastroenteropathy as manifestations of non–IgE-mediated cow's milk allergy. Pediatr Allergy Immunol 18:360, 2007.

Mandel, C: The female athlete triad goes 3-dimensional. Presentation at Performance Nutrition for Athletes and Active Individuals. Michigan State University, East Lansing, MI, September 12, 2008.

Marcason, W: Milk consumption and acne—is there a link? J Am Diet Assoc 110:152, 2010.

McCann, D, et al: Food additives and hyperactive behaviour in 3-year-old and 8/9-year-old children in the community: A randomised, double-blinded, placebo-controlled trial. Lancet 370:1560, 2007.

Mello, MM, Studdert, DM, and Brennan, MD: Obesity—the new frontier of public health law. N Engl J Med 354:2601, 2006.

Mennella, JA, Jagnow, CP, and Beauchamp, GK: Prenatal and postnatal flavor learning by human infants. Pediatrics 107: E88, 2001.

Merck Manual: Nutrition. November 2005. Accessed February 6, 2010 at: http://www.merck.com/mmpe/sec19/ch266/ch266c.html?qt=breast%20milk&alt=sh#sec19-ch266-ch266c-51.

Merck Manual: Physical Growth, September 2009. Accessed February 6, 2010 at: http://www.merck.com/mmpe/sec19/ch269/ch269b.html?qt=physical%20growth%20&alt=sh.

Morris, JL, and Zidenberg-Cherr, S: Garden-enhanced nutrition curriculum improves fourth-grade school children's knowledge of nutrition and preferences for some vegetables. J Am Diet Assoc 102:91, 2002.

Neifert, MR: Prevention of breastfeeding tragedies. Pediatr Clin North Am 48:273, 2001.

Nutritional needs of the preterm infant. In Kleinman, RE (ed): Pediatric Nutrition Handbook, ed 5. American Academy of Pediatrics, Elk Grove Village, IL, 2004.

Ogden, C: Prevalence and trends in overweight among US children and adolescents, 1999–2000. JAMA 288:1728, 2002.

Ogden, CL, Carroll, MD, and Flegal, KM: High body mass index for age among US children and adolescents, 2003–2006. JAMA 299:2401, 2008.

Olsen, EM: Failure to thrive: Still a problem of definition. Clin Pediatr (Phila) 45:1, 2006.

Owen, CG, et al: Effect of infant feeding on the risk of obesity across the life course: A quantitative review of published evidence. Pediatrics 115:1367, 2005.

Parry, LL, et al: A systematic review of parental perception of overweight status in children. J Ambul Care Manage 31:253, 2008.

Pedrosa, M, et al: Palatability of hydrolysates and other substitution formulas for cow's milk–allergic children: A comparative study of taste, smell, and texture evaluated by healthy volunteers. J Investig Allergol Clin Immunol 16:351, 2006.

Phan, TG, et al: Passive transfer of nut allergy after liver transplantation. Arch Intern Med 163:237, 2003.

Picciano, MF, and McDonald, SS: Lactation. In Shils, ME, et al (eds): Modern Nutrition in Health and Disease, ed 10. Lippincott Williams & Wilkins, Philadelphia, 2006.

Picciano, MF, et al: Dietary supplement use among infants, children, and adolescents in the United States, 1999–2002. Arch Pediatr Adolesc Med 161:978, 2007.

Polhamus, D, et al: Pediatric Nutrition Surveillance 2006 Report. U.S. Department of Health and Human Services, Centers for Disease Control and Prevention. Atlanta, 2007.

Rampersaud, GC, et al: Breakfast habits, nutritional status, body weight, and academic performance in children and adolescents. J Am Diet Assoc 105:743, 2005.

Ross Laboratories: Pediatric products. Accessed July 28, 2004 at: http://www.ross.com/productHandbook/default.asp.

Ryan, AS: Breastfeeding and the risk of childhood obesity. Coll Antropol 31:19, 2007.

Sachs, M, Dykes, F, and Carter, B: Feeding by numbers: An ethnographic study of how breastfeeding women understand their babies' weight charts. Int Breastfeed J 1:29, 2006.

Sampson, HA, Mendelson, L, and Rosen, JP: Fatal and near-fatal anaphylactic reactions to food in children and adolescents. N Engl J Med 327:380, 1992.

Saraçlar, Y, et al: Latex sensitivity among hospital employees and atopic children. Turk J Pediatr 40:61, 1998.

Schanler, RJ: The low-birth-weight infant. In Walker, WA, and Watkins, JB (eds): Nutrition in Pediatrics, ed 2. BC Decker, Hamilton, Ontario, 1997.

Schnabl, KL, et al: Necrotizing enterocolitis: A multifactorial disease with no cure. World J Gastroenterol 14:2142, 2008.

Schwartz, MB, et al: Examining the nutritional quality of breakfast cereals marketed to children. J Am Diet Assoc 108:702, 2008.

Singh, MB, and Bhalla, PL: Genetic engineering for removing food allergens from plants. Trends Plant Sci 13:257, 2008.

Singhal, A: Does breastfeeding protect from growth acceleration and later obesity? Nestle Nutr Workshop Ser Pediatr Program 60:15, 2007.

Sinn, N: Nutritional and dietary influences on attention deficit hyperactivity disorder. Nutr Rev 66:558, 2008.
Smith, RN, et al: The effect of a low glycemic load diet on acne vulgaris and the fatty acid composition of skin surface triglycerides. J Dermatol Sci 50:41, 2008.
Smith, RN, et al: A low-glycemic-load diet improves symptoms in acne vulgaris patients: A randomized controlled trial. Am J Clin Nutr 86:107, 2007.
Spandorfer, PR, et al: Oral versus intravenous rehydration of moderately dehydrated children: A randomized, controlled trial. Pediatrics 115:295, 2005.
Stevenson, J: Dietary influences on cognitive development and behaviour in children. Proc Nutr Soc 65:361, 2006.
Story, RE: Manifestations of food allergy in infants and children. Pediatr Ann 37:530, 2008.
Taylor, AV, et al: Detection and quantitation of raw fish aeroallergens from an open-air fish market. J Allergy Clin Immunol 105:166, 2000.
Taylor, JA, Geyer, LJ, and Feldman, KW: Use of supplemental vitamin D among infants breastfed for prolonged periods. Pediatrics 125:105, 2010.
Taylor, SL, and Hefle, SL: Food allergies and intolerances. In Shils, ME, et al (eds): Modern Nutrition in Health and Disease, ed 10. Lippincott Williams & Wilkins, Philadelphia, 2006.
Thiboutot, DM, and Strauss, JS: Diet and acne revisited. Arch Dermatol 138:1591, 2002.
Thompson, AM, and Bizzarro, MJ: Necrotizing enterocolitis in newborns: Pathogenesis, prevention and management. Drugs 68:1227, 2008.
Thorp, FK, Pierce, P, and Deedwania, C: Nutrition in the infant and young child. In Halpern, SL (ed): Quick Reference to Clinical Nutrition, ed 2. JB Lippincott, Philadelphia, 1987.
Treuth, MS, and Griffin, IJ: Adolescence. In Shils, ME, et al (eds): Modern Nutrition in Health and Disease, ed 10. Lippincott Williams & Wilkins, Philadelphia, 2006.
Trotman, H, et al: Hypernatraemic dehydration in Jamaican breastfed neonates: A 12-year review in a baby-friendly hospital. Ann Trop Paediatr 24:295, 2004.
U.S. Department of Agriculture: MyPyramid for Kids. September 2005. Accessed December 16, 2008 at: http://teamnutrition.usda.gov/Resources/mpk_poster2.pdf.
U.S. Department of Agriculture, Agricultural Research Service: Nutrient intakes from food: Mean amounts consumer per individual, one day, 2005–2006, 2008a. Accessed August 26, 2008 at: http://www.ars.usda.gov/ba/bhnrc/fsrg.
U.S. Department of Agriculture, Food and Nutrition Service: National school lunch program, July 2008b. Accessed December 2, 2008 at: http://www.fns.usda.gov/cnd/Lunch/AboutLunch/NSLPFactSheet.pdf.
U.S. Department of Agriculture, Food and Nutrition Service: School breakfast program, July 2008c. Accessed December 2, 2008 at: http://www.fns.usda.gov/cnd/breakfast/AboutBfast/SBPFactSheet.pdf.
U.S. Department of Health and Human Services: Healthy People 2010, January 2005. Accessed December 16, 2008 at: http://www.healthypeople.gov/#_TOC471971365.
Van Leeuwen, AM, et al: Davis's Comprehensive Handbook of Laboratory and Diagnostic Tests with Nursing Implications. FA Davis, Philadelphia, 2006.
van Odijk, J, et al: Breastfeeding and allergic disease: A multidisciplinary review of the literature (1966–2001) on the mode of early feeding in infancy and its impact on later atopic manifestations. Allergy 58:833, 2003.
Vitamins. In Kleinman, RE (ed): Pediatric Nutrition Handbook, ed 5. American Academy of Pediatrics, Elk Grove Village, IL, 2004.
Wagner, CL, and Greer, FR: Prevention of rickets and vitamin D deficiency in infants, children, and adolescents. Pediatrics 122:1142, 2008.
Wang, AC, et al: Breastfeeding-associated neonatal hypernatremic dehydration in a medical center: A clinical investigation. Acta Paediatr Taiwan 48:186, 2007.
World Health Organization: WHO child growth standards based on length/height, weight, and age. Acta Paediatr Suppl 450:76, 2006.
Wright, C, and Birks E: Risk factors for failure to thrive: A population-based survey. Child Care Health Dev 26:5, 2000.
Wright, KS, Quinn, TJ, and Carey, GB: Infant acceptance of breast milk after maternal exercise. Pediatrics 109:585, 2002.
Ziegler, EE: Adverse effects of cow's milk in infants. Nestle Nutr Workshop Ser Pediatr Program 60:185, 2007.

Chapter 12

Amella, EJ: Assessing nutrition in older adults. Am J Nurs 108:55, 2008.
Anantharaju, A, Feller, A, and Chedid, A: Aging liver. A review. Gerontology 48:343, 2002.
Ancelin, ML, Christen, Y, and Ritchie, K: Is antioxidant therapy a viable alternative for mild cognitive impairment? Examination of the evidence. Dement Geriatr Cogn Disord 24:1, 2007.
Andersson, I, and Sidenvall, B: Case studies of food shopping, cooking and eating habits in older women with Parkinson's disease. J Adv Nurs 35:69, 2001.
Bales, CW, and Ritchie, CS: The elderly. In Shils, ME, et al (eds): Modern Nutrition in Health and Disease, ed 10. Lippincott Williams & Wilkins, Philadelphia, 2006.
Bellisle, F: Experimental studies of food choices and palatability responses in European subjects exposed to the Umami taste. Asia Pac J Clin Nutr 17(Suppl)1:376, 2008.
Biernacki, C, and Barratt, J: Improving the nutritional status of people with dementia. Br J Nurs 10:1104, 2001.
Bogoch, ER, et al: Effective initiation of osteoporosis diagnosis and treatment for patients with a fragility fracture in an orthopaedic environment. J Bone Joint Surg Am 88:25, 2006.
Bourre, JM: Dietary omega-3 fatty acids and psychiatry: Mood, behaviour, stress, depression, dementia and aging. J Nutr Health Aging 9:31, 2005.
Boyce, JM, and Shone, GR: Effects of ageing on smell and taste. Postgrad Med J 82:239, 2006.
Bradbury, J, et al: Nutrition counseling increases fruit and vegetable intake in the edentulous. J Dent Res 85:463, 2006.
Brown, JE (ed): Nutrition Through the Life Cycle, ed 3. Thomson Wadsworth, Belmont, CA, 2008.
Bush, LA, et al: D-E-N-T-A-L: A rapid self-administered screening instrument to promote referrals for further evaluation in older adults. J Am Geriatr Soc 44:979, 1996.
Castellanos, VH, Marra, MV, and Johnson, P: Enhancement of select foods at breakfast and lunch increases energy intakes of nursing home residents with low meal intakes. J Am Diet Assoc 109:445, 2009.
Centers for Disease Control and Prevention: Hip Fractures Among Older Adults, National Center for Injury Prevention and Control, June 10, 2008a. Accessed September 8, 2008 at: http://www.cdc.gov/ncipc/factsheets/adulthipfx.htm.
Centers for Disease Control and Prevention: Quick stats: Life expectancy ranking at birth, by sex—selected countries and territories, 2004. MMWR 57:346, 2008b. Accessed August 26, 2008 at: http://www.cdc.gov/mmwr/preview/mmwrhtml/mm5713a8.htm.

Centers for Disease Control and Prevention: Trends in strength training—United States, 1998–2004. MMWR 55:769, 2006. Accessed February 9, 2010 at: http://www.cdc.gov/mmwr/preview/mmwrhtml/mm5528a1.htm.

Centers for Disease Control and Prevention and The Merck Company Foundation: Executive Summary. The State of Aging and Health in America 2007. The Merck Company Foundation, Whitehouse Station, NJ, 2007a. Accessed August 26, 2008 at: http://apps.nccd.cdc.gov/saha.

Centers for Disease Control and Prevention and The Merck Company Foundation: Indicator 3: Oral Health: Complete Tooth Loss. The State of Aging and Health in America 2007. The Merck Company Foundation, Whitehouse Station, NJ, 2007b. Accessed August 26, 2008 at: http://apps.nccd.cdc.gov/saha/IndicatorDetails.aspx?IndID=CTL&Gender=N.

Centers for Disease Control and Prevention and The Merck Company Foundation: Indicator 5: No Leisure-Time Physical Activity, The State of Aging and Health in America 2007. The Merck Company Foundation, Whitehouse Station, NJ, 2007c. Accessed August 26, 2008 at: http://apps.nccd.cdc.gov/saha/IndicatorDetails.aspx?IndID=NLT&Gender=N.

Centers for Disease Control and Prevention and The Merck Company Foundation: Indicator 6: Eating 5 Fruits and Vegetables Daily. The State of Aging and Health in America 2007d. The Merck Company Foundation, Whitehouse Station, NJ, 2007. Accessed August 26, 2008 at: http://apps.nccd.cdc.gov/saha/IndicatorDetails.aspx?IndID=FAD&Gender=N&printfriendly=1.

Centers for Medicare & Medicaid Service: MDS Active resident information report: First quarter 2008 G1hA: Physical functioning and structural problems—eating—ADL self-performance. Accessed August 25, 2008 at: http://www.cms.hhs.gov/MDSPubQIandResRep/04_activeresreport.asp?isSubmitted=res3&var=G1hA&date=22.

Centers for Medicare & Medicaid Services: Requirements for paid feeding assistants in long term care facilities final rule. Fed Reg 68:55528, 2003.

Denney, A: Quiet music: An intervention for mealtime agitation? J Gerontol Nurs 23:16, 1997.

DePaola, DP, et al: Nutrition and dental medicine. In Shils, ME, et al (eds): Modern Nutrition in Health and Disease, ed 10. Lippincott Williams & Wilkins, Philadelphia, 2006.

DiMaria-Ghalili, RA, and Guenter, PA: The Mini Nutritional Assessment. Am J Nurs 108:50, 2008.

DIPART (Vitamin D Individual Patient Analysis of Randomized Trials) Group: Patient level pooled analysis of 68,500 patients from seven major vitamin D fracture trials in US and Europe. BMJ 340:b5463.

Doll-Shankaruk, M, Yau, WNC, and Oelke, C: Implementation and effects of a medication pass nutritional supplement program in a long-term care facility: A pilot study. J Gerontol Nurs 34:45, 2008.

Donini, LM, et al: MNA predictive value in the follow-up of geriatric patients. J Nutr Health Aging 7:282, 2003.

Duerr, L: Food security status of older adult home-delivered meals program participants and components of its measurement. J Nutr Elder 26:1, 2006a.

Duerr, L: Prevalence of food insecurity and comprehensiveness of its measurement for older adult congregate meals program participants. J Nutr Elderly 25:121, 2006b.

Duncan, DG, et al: Using dietetic assistants to improve the outcome of hip fracture: A randomised controlled trial of nutritional support in an acute trauma ward. Age Ageing 35:148, 2006.

El Nasser, H: Fewer seniors live in nursing homes. USA Today, September 27, 2007. Accessed August 26, 2008 at: http://www.usatoday.com/news/nation/census/2007-09-27-nursinghomes_N.htm.

Eneroth, M, Olsson, UB, and Thorngren, KG: Nutritional supplementation decreases hip fracture-related complications. Clin Orthop Relat Res 451:212, 2006.

Esiri, MM: Ageing and the brain. J Pathol 211:181, 2007.

Etminan, M, Gill, SS, and Samii, A: Intake of vitamin E, vitamin C, and carotenoids and the risk of Parkinson's disease: A meta-analysis. Lancet Neurol 4:362, 2005.

Evans, BC, Crogan, NL, and Shultz, JA: The meaning of mealtimes. J Gerontol Nurs 31:11, 2005.

Feldstein, AC, et al: An outreach program improved osteoporosis management after a fracture. J Am Geriatr Soc 55:1464, 2007.

Francucci, CM, et al: Role of vitamin K on biochemical markers, bone mineral density, and fracture risk. J Endocrinol Invest 30(Suppl):24, 2007.

Freeman, M: Reconsidering the effects of monosodium glutamate: A literature review. J Am Acad Nurse Pract 18:482, 2006.

Fuller-Thomson, E, and Redmond, M: Falling through the social safety net: Food stamp use and nonuse among older impoverished Americans. Gerontologist 48:235, 2008.

Gankam Kengne, F, et al: Mild hyponatremia and risk of fracture in the ambulatory elderly. QJM 101:583, 2008.

Garrow, D, et al: Feeding alternatives in patients with dementia: Examining the evidence. Clin Gastroenterol Hepatol 5:1372, 2007.

Ghosh, D, Skinner, MA, and Laing, WA: Pharmacogenomics and nutrigenomics: Synergies and differences. Eur J Clin Nutr 61:567, 2007.

Griffin, SO, et al: Effectiveness of fluoride in preventing caries in adults. J Dent Res 86:410, 2007.

Hays, NP, and Roberts, SB: The anorexia of aging in humans. Physiol Behav 88:257, 2006.

Heimburger, DC: Adulthood. In Shils, ME, et al (eds): Modern Nutrition in Health and Disease, ed 10. Lippincott Williams & Wilkins, Philadelphia, 2006.

Hillier, TA, et al: Nulliparity and fracture risk in older women: The study of osteoporotic fractures. J Bone Miner Res 18:893, 2003.

Iwamoto, J, Takeda, T, and Sato, Y: Role of vitamin K_2 in the treatment of postmenopausal osteoporosis. Curr Drug Saf 1:87, 2006.

Janssen, I, and Mark, AE: Elevated body mass index and mortality risk in the elderly. Obes Rev 8:41, 2007.

Jensen, GL, et al: Noncompliance with body weight measurement in tertiary care teaching hospitals. JPEN J Parenter Enteral Nutr 27:89, 2003.

Johnson, LJ, and McCool, AC: Dietary intake and nutritional status of older adult homeless women: A pilot study. J Nutr Elderly 23:1, 2003.

Kamel, HK: Postmenopausal osteoporosis: etiology, current diagnostic strategies, and nonprescription interventions. J Manag Care Pharm 12(suppl S-a):S4, 2006.

Kayser-Jones, J, and Schell, E: The mealtime experience of a cognitively impaired elder: Ineffective and effective strategies. J Gerontol Nurs 23:33, 1997.

Koike, T, et al: External hip protectors are effective for the elderly with higher-than-average risk factors for hip fractures. Osteoporos Int 20:1613, 2009.

Kuo, I, et al: Successful direct intervention for osteoporosis in patients with minimal trauma fractures. Osteoporos Int 18:1633, 2007.

Lesourd, B: Nutritional factors and immunological ageing. Proc Nutr Soc 65:319, 2006.

Majumdar, SR, et al: Persistence, reproducibility, and cost-effectiveness of an intervention to improve the quality of osteoporosis care after a fracture of the wrist: Results of a controlled trial. Osteoporos Int 18:261, 2007.

Mamdani, M, et al: Warfarin therapy and risk of hip fracture among elderly patients. Pharmacotherapy 23:1, 2003.

Martin, JE, and Sheaff, MT: Renal aging. J Pathol 211:198, 2007.
Martini, L, and Wood, RJ: Relative bioavailability of calcium-rich dietary sources in the elderly. Am J Clin Nutr 76:1345, 2002.
Mattes, RD: The chemical senses and nutrition in aging: Challenging old assumptions. J Am Diet Assoc 102:192, 2002.
Mentes, JC, and Iowa-Veterans Affairs Research Consortium: Hydration management protocol. J Gerontol Nurs 26:6, 2000.
Merck Manual of Geriatrics: Caries. September 2005. Accessed February 9, 2010 at: http://www.merck.com/mkgr/mmg/sec13/ch104/ch104b.jsp.
Merck Manual of Geriatrics: Proximal femoral fractures. 2009. Accessed February 9, 2010 at: http://www.merck.com/mkgr/mmg/sec2/ch22/ch22e.jsp.
Miller, N, et al: Hard to swallow: dysphagia in Parkinson's disease. Age Ageing 35:614, 2006.
Morais, JA, Chevalier, S, and Gougeon, R: Protein turnover and requirements in healthy and frail elderly. J Nutr Health Aging 10:272, 2006.
Morgan, SL, and Baggott, JE: Nutrition and diet in rheumatic diseases. In Shils, ME, et al (eds): Modern Nutrition in Health and Disease, ed 10. Lippincott Williams & Wilkins, Philadelphia, 2006.
Morley, JE: Nutrition in the older person. In Shils, ME, et al (eds): Modern Nutrition in Health and Disease, ed 10. Lippincott Williams & Wilkins, Philadelphia, 2006.
Morris, MC: The role of nutrition in Alzheimer's disease: epidemiological evidence. Eur J Neurol 16(Suppl 1):1, 2009.
National Center for Health Statistics: Life expectancy hits record high. February 28, 2005. Accessed August 26, 2008 at: http://www.cdc.gov/nchs/pressroom/05facts/lifexpectancy.htm.
National Institute of Neurological Disorders and Stroke: Parkinson's Disease Backgrounder. October 18, 2004. Accessed August 27, 2008 at: http://ninds.nih.gov/disorders/parkinsons_disease/parkinsons_disease_backgrounder.htm.
Nestle Nutrition Institute: MNA Mini Nutritional Assessment. Undated. Accessed February 9, 2010 at: http://www.mna-elderly.com.
Nord, M, and Kantor, LS: Seasonal variation in food insecurity is associated with heating and cooling costs among low-income elderly Americans. J Nutr 136:2939, 2006.
Opotowsky, AR, Su, BW, and Bilezikian, JP: Height and lower extremity length as predictors of hip fracture: Results of the NHANES I Epidemiologic Follow-up Study. J Bone Miner Res 18:1674, 2003.
Paddon-Jones, D, et al: Role of dietary protein in the sarcopenia of aging. Am J Clin Nutr 87:1562S, 2008.
Peters, R: Ageing and the brain. Postgrad Med J 82:84, 2006.
Quinn, C: The Nutrition Screening Initiative: Meeting the nutritional needs of elders. Orthop Nurs 16:13, 1997.
Raisz, LG: Osteoporosis. Merck Manual, 2008. Accessed August 27, 2008 at: http://www.merck.com/mmpe/sec04/ch036/ch036a.html#sb036_1.
Robinson, SB, and Rosher, RB: Can a beverage cart help improve hydration? Geriatr Nurs 23:208, 2002.
Rubenstein, LZ, et al: Screening for undernutrition in geriatric practice: Developing the Short-Form Mini-Nutritional Assessment (MNA-SF). J Gerontol A Biol Sci Med Sci 56:M366, 2001.
Russell, L: The importance of patients' nutritional status in wound healing. Br J Nurs 10:S42, 2001.
Russell, RM, Rasmussen, H, and Lichtenstein, AH: Modified food guide pyramid for people over 70 years of age. J Nutr 129:751, 1999.
Sen, CK, Khanna, S, and Roy, S: Tocotrienols: Vitamin E beyond tocopherols. Life Sci 78:2088, 2006.
Shahar, DR, et al: The effect of widowhood on weight changes, dietary intake, and eating behavior in the elderly population. J Aging Health 13:189, 2001.
Shils, ME. Changes in weight and height with age. In Shils, ME, et al (eds): Modern Nutrition in Health and Disease, ed 10. Lippincott Williams & Wilkins, Philadelphia, 2006.
Simmons, SF, et al: Family members' preferences for nutrition interventions to improve nursing home residents' oral food and fluid intake. J Am Geriatr Soc 51:69, 2003.
Slemenda, C: Prevention of hip fractures: Risk factor modification. Am J Med 103:65S, 1997.
Soter, A, et al: Accuracy of self-report in detecting taste dysfunction. Laryngoscope 118:611, 2008.
Stockdell, R, and Amella, EJ: The Edinburgh Feeding Evaluation in Dementia Scale. Am J Nurs 108(8):46, 2008.
Stratton, RJ, et al: Enteral nutritional support in prevention and treatment of pressure ulcers: A systematic review and meta-analysis. Ageing Res Rev 4:422, 2005.
Symons, TB, et al: Aging does not impair the anabolic response to a protein-rich meal. Am J Clin Nutr 86:451, 2007.
Travers, SP, and Geran, LC: Bitter-responsive brainstem neurons: characteristics and functions. Physiol Behav 97:592, 2009.
Tully, MW, et al: The Eating Behavior Scale: A simple method of assessing functional ability in patients with Alzheimer's disease. J Gerontol Nurs 23:9, 1997.
Uauy, R, and Dangour, AD: Nutrition in brain development and aging: Role of essential fatty acids. Nutr Rev 64:S24, 2006.
U.S. Census Bureau: Percent of the total population who are 65 years and over. American FactFinder, 2007. Accessed August 26, 2008 at: http://factfinder.census.gov/servlet/GCTTable?_bm=y&-geo_id=01000US&-_box_head_nbr=GCT-T4-R&-ds_name=PEP_2007_EST&-format=US-9Sc.
U.S. Department of Agriculture, Agricultural Research Service: Nutrient intakes from food: Mean amounts consumer per individual, one day, 2005–2006, 2008. Accessed August 26, 2008 at: http://www.ars.usda.gov/ba/bhnrc/fsrg.
Wang, XP, and Ding, HL: Alzheimer's disease: epidemiology, genetics, and beyond. Neurosci Bull 24:105, 2008.
Watson, R, and Green, SM: Feeding and dementia: A systematic literature review. J Adv Nurs 54:86, 2006.
Welch, P, Porter, J, and Endres, J: Efficacy of a medication pass supplement program in long-term care compared to a traditional system. J Nutr Elderly 22:19, 2003.
Wendland, BE, et al: Malnutrition in institutionalized seniors: The iatrogenic component. J Am Geriatr Soc 51:85, 2003.
Wilkins, CH, and Birge, SJ: Prevention of osteoporotic fractures in the elderly. Am J Med 118:1190, 2005.
Williams, AN, and Woessner, KM: Monosodium glutamate "allergy": Menace or myth? Clin Exp Allergy 39:640, 2009.
Winkler, S, et al: Depressed taste and smell in geriatric patients. J Am Dent Assoc 130:1759, 1999.
Winograd, CH, and Brown, EM: Aggressive oral refeeding in hospitalized patients. Am J Clin Nutr 52:967, 1990.
Woo, C, et al: Single-point assessment of warfarin use and risk of osteoporosis in elderly men. J Am Geriatr Soc 56:1171, 2008.

Chapter 13

American Dietetic Association: Pocket Guide for International Dietetics and Nutrition Terminology (IDNT) Reference Manual, ed 1. American Dietetics Association, Chicago, 2008.
American Dietetic Association: Position of the American Dietetic Association: Food and water safety. J Am Diet Assoc 103:1203, 2003.

Centers for Disease Control and Prevention: Preliminary FoodNet data on the incidence of infection with pathogens transmitted commonly through food—10 states, 2006. Accessed August 2008 at: www.cdc.gov/mmwr.

Donnelly, CA: Bovine spongiform encephalopathy in the United States—An epidemiologist's view. N Engl J Med 350:539, 2004.

Food Safety Healthy People 2010. Accessed August 2008 at: http://www.health.gov/healthypeople.

Shils, ME (ed): Modern Nutrition in Health and Disease, ed 10. Lippincott Williams & Wilkins, Philadelphia, 2006.

U.S. Department of Agriculture: Dietary Guidelines for Americans 2005. Accessed August 2008 at: http://www.health.gov/dietaryguidelines/dga2005/toolkit.

U.S. Department of Agriculture: My Pyramid. Accessed August 2008 at: www.MyPyramid.gov.

Venes, D (ed): Taber's Cyclopedic Medical Dictionary, ed 20. FA Davis, Philadelphia, 2005.

Chapter 14

American Dietetic Association: International Dietetics & Nutrition Terminology (IDNT) Reference Manual, ed 1. American Dietetic Association, Chicago, 2008.

American Dietetic Association: Manual of Clinical Dietetics, ed 6. American Dietetic Association, Chicago, 2000.

A.S.P.E.N.: Tube Feeding Misconnections: Fatal Medical Mistakes. Press release April 15, 2008. American Society for Parenteral and Enteral Nutrition, Silver Spring, MD, 2008.

Blouch, AC, and Mueller, C: Enteral and parenteral nutrition support. In Food, Nutrition and Diet Therapy. Elsevier, Philadelphia, 2004.

Butterworth, CE: The skeleton in the hospital closet. Nutr Today 9:8, 1975.

Butterworth, CE, and Blackburn, GL: Hospital malnutrition and how to assess the nutritional status of a patient. Nutr Today 10:8, 1975.

Climent, J: Tube feeding bad for patients with dementia. BMJ 320:335, 2000.

Dupertuis, YM: Physical characteristics of total parenteral nutrition bags significantly affect the stability of vitamins C and B_1: A controlled prospective study. J Parenter Enteral Nutr 26:310, 2002.

Falk, A: Evaluating the effectiveness of a micronutrient assessment tool for long-term total parenteral nutrition patients. Nurs Clin Pract 17:240, 2002.

Gottschlich, MM: The A.S.P.E.N. Nutrition Core Curriculum: A Case-Based Approach—The Adult Patient. American Society for Parenteral and Enteral Nutrition. Silver Spring, MD, 2007.

Healthy People 2010. U.S. Department of Health and Human Services, Washington, DC, 2000.

Metheny, N, and Titler, MG: Assessing placement of feeding tubes. Am J Nurs 101:36, 2001.

Pfau, PR, and Rombeau, JL: Nutrition. Med Clin North Am 84:1209, 2000.

Phillips, LD: Manual of Intravenous Therapy, ed 4. FA Davis, Philadelphia, 2006.

Super, J: Tube feedings making you blue. Drug Therapy Topics. University of Washington Medical Center 32:6, 2003.

U.S. Food and Drug Administration: FDA Public Health Advisory. Reports of Blue Discoloration and Death in Patients Receiving Enteral Feedings Tinted with the Dye, FD&C No. 1. Accessed January 2004 at: http://www.cfsan.fda.gov.

Venes, D (ed): Taber's Cyclopedic Medical Dictionary, ed 20. FA Davis, Philadelphia, 2005.

Vollmann, J, et al: Rethinking the role of tube feeding in patients with advanced dementia [letter]. N Engl J Med 342:1755, 2000.

Chapter 15

Akamine, D, Filho, MK, and Peres, CM: Drug-nutrient interactions in elderly people. Curr Opin Clin Nutr Metab Care 10:304, 2007.

Anderson, GD: Sex differences in drug metabolism: Cytochrome P-450 and uridine diphosphate glucoronosyltransferase. J Gend Specif Med 5:25, 2002.

Atwater, J, Montgomery-Salguero, J, and Roll, DB: The USP Dietary Supplement Verification Program: Helping pharmacists and consumers select dietary supplements. US Pharm 6:61, 2005.

Bass, S, and Marden, E: The new dietary ingredient safety provision of DSHEA: A return to congressional intent. Am J Law Med 31:285, 2005.

Bent, S, et al: Spontaneous bleeding associated with ginkgo biloba: A case report and systematic review of the literature. J Gen Intern Med 20:657, 2005.

Borrione, P, et al: Rhabdomyolysis in a young vegetarian athlete. Am J Phys Med Rehabil 88:951, 2009.

Boullata, J: Natural health product interactions with medication. Nutr Clin Pract 20:33, 2005.

Carlson, J: The role of nutrition in enhancing aerobic training and endurance performance. Presentation at Performance Nutrition for Athletes and Active Individuals. Michigan State University, East Lansing, September 12, 2008.

Centers for Disease Control and Prevention: Lead poisoning associated with ayurvedic medications—five states, 2000–2003. MMWR 53:582, 2004. Accessed August 4, 2004 at: http://www.cdc.gov/mmwr/preview/mmwrhtml/mm5326a3.htm.

Chan, L-N: Drug-nutrient interactions. In Shils, ME, et al (eds): Modern Nutrition in Health and Disease, ed 10. Lippincott Williams & Wilkins, Philadelphia, 2006.

Chen, JJ, Swope, DM, and Dashtipour, K: Comprehensive review of rasagiline, a second-generation monoamine oxidase inhibitor, for the treatment of Parkinson's disease. Clin Ther 29:1825, 2007.

Ciocca, M: Medication and supplement use by athletes. Clin Sports Med 24:719, 2005.

Clauson, KA, Santamarina, ML, and Rutledge, JC: Clinically relevant safety issues associated with St. John's wort product labels. BMC Complement Altern Med 8:42, 2008.

Coderre, K, Faria, C, and Dyer, E: Probable warfarin interaction with menthol cough drops. Pharmacotherapy 30:110, 2010.

Cohen, PJ: Science, politics, and the regulation of dietary supplements: It's time to repeal DSHEA. Am J Law Med 31:175, 2005.

Consumer Lab: About ConsumerLab.com. Accessed February 28, 2010 at: http://www.consumerlab.com/aboutcl.asp.

Consumer Lab: Athletic banned substances screened products. 2008. Accessed February 28, 2010 at: http://www.consumerlab.com/results/Athletic_Banned_Substance_Supplement_Tests_Approved.asp.

Dahan, A, and Altman, H: Food-drug interaction: Grapefruit juice augments drug bioavailability—mechanism, extent and relevance. Eur J Clin Nutr 58:1, 2004.

Dahmer, S, and Schiller, RM: Glucosamine. Am Fam Physician 78:471, 2008.

Das, R, Parajuli, S, and Gupta, S: A rash imposition from a lifestyle omission: A case report of pellagra [letter]. Ulster Med J 75:92, 2006.

Deglin, JH, and Vallerand, AH (eds): Davis's Drug Guide for Nurses, ed 11. FA Davis, Philadelphia, 2009.

Dellow, EL, Unwin, RH, and Honour, JW: Pontefract cakes can be bad for you: Refractory hypertension and liquorice excess. Nephrol Dial Transplant 14:218, 1999.

Dickerson, RN, et al: Vitamin K-independent warfarin resistance after concurrent administration of warfarin and continuous enteral nutrition. Pharmacotherapy 28:308, 2008.

Draves, AH, and Walker SE: Analysis of the hypericin and pseudohypericin content of commercially available St. John's wort preparations. Can J Clin Pharmacol 10:114, 2003.

Drazen, JM: Inappropriate advertising of dietary supplements. N Engl J Med 348:777, 2003.

Duellman, MC, et al: Protein supplement users among high school athletes have misconceptions about effectiveness. J Strength Cond Res 22:1124, 2008.

Elinav, E, and Chajek-Shaul, T: Licorice consumption causing severe hypokalemic paralysis. Mayo Clin Proc 78:767, 2003.

Estes, JD, et al: High prevalence of potentially hepatotoxic herbal supplement use in patients with fulminant hepatic failure. Arch Surg 138:852, 2003.

Franco, V, et al: Role of vitamin K intake in chronic oral anticoagulation: Prospective evidence from observational and randomized protocols. Am J Med 116:651, 2004.

Fugate, SE, and Ramsey, AM: Resistance to oral vitamin K for reversal of overanticoagulation during Crohn's disease relapse. J Thromb Thrombolysis 17:219, 2004.

Gardiner, P, Phillips, R, and Shaughnessy, AF: Herbal and dietary supplement—drug interactions in patients with chronic illnesses. Am Fam Physician 77:73, 2008.

Geyer, H, et al: Analysis of non-hormonal nutritional supplements for anabolic-androgenic steroids—results of an international study. Int J Sports Med 25:124, 2004.

Gilroy, CM, et al: Echinacea and truth in labelling. Arch Intern Med 163:699, 2003.

Grant, P: Warfarin and cranberry juice: An interaction? J Heart Valve Dis 13:25, 2004.

Guay, DR: Rasagiline (TVP-1012): A new selective monoamine oxidase inhibitor for Parkinson's disease. Am J Geriatr Pharmacother 4:330, 2006.

Hespel, P, Maughan, RJ, and Greenhaff, PL: Dietary supplements for football. J Sports Sci 24:749, 2006.

Ingelman-Sundberg, M, et al: Influence of cytochrome P450 polymorphisms on drug therapies: Pharmacogenetic, pharmacoepigenetic and clinical aspects. Pharmacol Ther 116:496, 2007.

Institute of Medicine Committee on the Use of Complementary and Alternative Medicine. Complementary and Alternative Medicine in the United States. National Academy Press, Washington, DC, 2005. Accessed May 13, 2005 at: http://www.nap.edu/openbook/0309092701/html.

Ize-Ludlow, D, et al: Neurotoxicities in infants seen with the consumption of star anise tea. Pediatrics 114:e653, 2004.

Jenkinson, DM, and Harbert, AJ: Supplements and sports. Am Fam Physician 78:1039, 2008.

Juurlink, DN, et al: Drug-induced lithium toxicity in the elderly: A population-based study. J Am Geriatr Soc 52:794, 2004.

Karri, SK, Saper, RB, and Kales, SN: Lead encephalopathy due to traditional medicines. Curr Drug Saf 3:54, 2008.

Kaur, S, et al: Pellagrous dermatitis induced by phenytoin [letter]. Pediatr Dermatol 19:93, 2002.

Kaye, AD, Kucera, I, and Sabar, R: Perioperative anesthesia clinical considerations of alternative medicines. Anesthesiol Clin N America 22:125, 2004.

Kelly, JP, et al: Use of herbal/natural supplements according to racial/ethnic group. J Altern Complement Med 12:555, 61, 2006.

Khor, SP, and Hsu, A: The pharmacokinetics and pharmacodynamics of levodopa in the treatment of Parkinson's disease. Curr Clin Pharmacol 2:234, 2007.

Knudsen, JF, and Sokol, GH: Potential glucosamine-warfarin interaction resulting in increased international normalized ratio: Case report and review of the literature and MedWatch database. Pharmacotherapy 28:540, 2008.

Kobayashi, K, et al: Cerebral hemorrhage associated with vitamin K deficiency in congenital tuberculosis treated with isoniazid and rifampin. Pediatr Infect Dis J 21:1088, 2002.

Lanski, SL, et al: Herbal therapy use in a pediatric emergency department population: Expect the unexpected. Pediatrics 111:981, 2003.

Lee, YH, et al: Effect of glucosamine or chondrotin sulfate on the osteoarthritis progression: a meta-analysis. Rheumatol Int 30:357, 2010.

Li, Z, et al: Cranberry does not affect prothrombin time in male subjects on warfarin. J Am Diet Assoc 106:2057, 2006.

Lilja, JJ, Backman, JT, and Neuvonen, PJ: Effects of daily ingestion of cranberry juice on the pharmacokinetics of warfarin, tizanidine, and midazolam—probes of CYP2C9, CYP1A2, and CYP3A4. Clin Pharmacol Ther 81:833, 2007.

Lin, SH, et al: An unusual cause of hypokalemic paralysis: Chronic licorice ingestion. Am J Med Sci 325:153, 2003.

Linus Pauling Institute: Vitamin D. Oregon State University, January 2008. Accessed October 1, 2008 at: http://lpi.oregonstate.edu/infocenter/vitamins/vitaminD.

Lynch, T, and Price, A: The effect of cytochrome P450 metabolism on drug response, interactions, and adverse effects. Am Fam Physician 76:391, 2007.

Lyon, VB, and Fairley, JA: Anticonvulsant-induced pellagra. J Am Acad Dermatol 46:597, 2002.

Macdermid, PW, and Stannard, SR: A whey-supplemented, high-protein diet versus a high-carbohydrate diet: Effects on endurance cycling performance. Int J Sport Nutr Exerc Metab 16:65, 2006.

Magkos, F, and Kavouras, SA: Caffeine use in sports, pharmacokinetics in man, and cellular mechanisms of action. Crit Rev Food Sci Nutr 45:535, 2005.

Mannel, M: Drug interactions with St. John's wort: Mechanisms and clinical implications. Drug Saf 27:773, 2004.

Mattarello, MJ, et al: Effect of licorice on PTH levels in healthy women. Steroids 71:403, 2006.

McKinnon, BT: FDA safety alert: Hazards of precipitation associated with parenteral nutrition. Nutr Clin Pract 11:59, 1996.

Meisel, C, Johne, A, and Roots, I: Fatal intracerebral mass bleeding associated with Ginkgo biloba and ibuprofen [letter]. Atherosclerosis 167:367, 2003.

MHRA: Cranberry. October 2004, modified February 2008. Accessed September 18, 2008 at: http://www.mhra.gov.uk/PrintPreview/DefaultSP/CON1004343.

Mirtallo, JM: Complications associated with drug and nutrient interactions. J Infus Nurs 27:19, 2004.

Morris, CA, and Avorn, J: Internet marketing of herbal products. JAMA 290:1505, 2003.

Morrow, LE, et al: Acute isoniazid toxicity and the need for adequate pyridoxine supplies. Pharmacotherapy 26:1529, 2006.

Murphy, PA, et al: Interaction of St. John's Wort with oral contrceptives: Effects on the pharmacokinetics of norethindrone and ethinyl estradiol, ovarian activity and breakthrough bleeding. Contraception 71:402, 2005.

Murray, B: The role of salt and glucose replacement drinks in the marathon. Sports Med 37:358, 2007.

Neff, GW, et al: Consumption of dietary supplements in a liver transplant population. Liver Transpl 10:881, 2004.

Nelson, JL, and Robergs, RA: Exploring the potential ergogenic effects of glycerol hyperhydration. Sports Med 37:981, 2007.

Paeng, CH, Sprague, M, and Jackevicius, CA: Interaction between warfarin and cranberry juice. Clin Ther 29:1730, 2007.

Papandreou, D, et al: The ketogenic diet in children with epilepsy. Br J Nutr 95:5, 2006.

Patel, DR, Torres, AD, and Greydanus, DE: Kidneys and sports. Adolesc Med 16:111, 2005.

Peng, CC, et al: Incidence and severity of potential drug—dietary supplement interactions in primary care patients: An exploratory study of 2 outpatient practices. Arch Intern Med 164:630, 2004.

Persky, AM, and Rawson, ES: Safety of creatine supplementation. Subcell Biochem 46:275, 2007.

Petty, HR, et al: Identification of colchicine in placental blood from patients using herbal medicines. Chem Res Toxicol 14:1254, 2001.

Pham, DQ, and Pham, AQ: Interaction potential between cranberry juice and warfarin. Am J Health Syst Pharm 64:490, 2007.

Pittler, MH, and Ernst, E: Clinical effectiveness of garlic (*Allium sativum*). Mol Nutr Food Res 51:1382, 2007.

Rapaport, MH: Dietary restrictions and drug interactions with monoamine oxidase inhibitors: The state of the art. J Clin Psychiatry 68(Suppl 8):42, 2007.

Ray, KK, Dorman, S, and Watson, RDS: Severe hyperkalemia due to the concomitant use of salt substitutes and ACE inhibitors in hypertension: A potentially life threatening interaction. J Hum Hypertens 13:717, 1999.

Rindone, JP, and Murphy, TW: Warfarin-cranberry juice interaction resulting in profound hypoprothrombinemia and bleeding. Am J Ther 13:283, 2006.

Roberge, RJ, et al: Diarrhea-associated over-anticoagulation in a patient taking warfarin: Therapeutic role of cholestyramine. Vet Hum Toxicol 42:351, 2000.

Robinson, DS, and Amsterdam, JD: The selegiline transdermal system in major depressive disorder: A systematic review of safety and tolerability. J Affect Disord 105:15, 2008.

Rodriguez, NR, Di Marco, NM, and Langley, S: American College of Sports Medicine position stand. Nutrition and athletic performance. Med Sci Sports Exerc 41:709, 2009.

Rosener, M, and Dichgans, J: Severe combined degeneration of the spinal cord after nitrous oxide anesthesia in a vegetarian [letter]. J Neurol Neurosurg Psychiatry 60:354, 1996.

Saldanha, LG: The dietary supplement marketplace: Constantly evolving. Nutr Today 42(2):52, 2007.

Saper, RB, et al: Lead, mercury, and arsenic in US- and Indian-manufactured ayurvedic medicines sold via the Internet. JAMA 300:915, 2008.

Sarino, LV, et al: Drug interaction between oral contraceptives and St. John's Wort: appropriateness of advice received from community pharmacists and health food store clerks. J Am Pharm Assoc 47:42, 2007.

Sawka, MN, et al: Exercise and fluid replacement. Med Sci Sports Exerc 39:377, 2007.

Schmidt, LE, and Dalhoff, K: Food-drug interactions. Drugs 62:1481, 2002.

Sehnert, S: Fueling the strength and power athlete. Presentation at Performance Nutrition for Athletes and Active Individuals. Michigan State University, East Lansing, September 12, 2008.

Sica, DA: Interaction of grapefruit juice and calcium channel blockers. Am J Hypertens 19:768, 2006.

Slone Epidemiology Center: Patterns of Medication Use in the United States. Boston University, Boston, 2006. Accessed April 17, 2009 at: http://www.bu.edu/slone/SloneSurvey/AnnualRpt/SloneSurveyWebReport2006.pdf.

Society of Hospital Pharmacists of Hong Kong: Drug–enteral tube feeding interaction. Accessed May 15, 2005 at: http://www.shphk.org.hk/index.php?option=com_content&task=view&id=200&Itemid=38.

Spriet, LL, Perry, CG, and Talanian, JL: Legal pre-event nutritional supplements to assist energy metabolism. Essays Biochem 44:27, 2008.

Srinivasan, VS: Challenges and scientific issues in the standardization of botanicals and their preparations. United States Pharmacopeia's dietary supplement verification program—a public health program. Life Sciences 78:2039, 2006.

Sutter, ME, et al: Selenium toxicity: A case of selenosis caused by a nutritional supplement. Ann Intern Med 148:970, 2008.

Suvarna, R, Pirmohamed, M, and Henderson, L: Possible interaction between warfarin and cranberry juice. BMJ 327:1454, 2003.

Taylor, JR, and Wilt, VM: Probable antagonism of warfarin by green tea. Ann Pharmacother 33:426, 1999.

Thorsteinsdottir, B, Grande, JP, and Garovic, VD: Acute renal failure in a young weight lifter taking multiple food supplements, including creatine monohydrate. J Ren Nutr 16:341, 2006.

U.S. Food and Drug Administration: Claims that can be made for conventional foods and dietary supplements. September 2003, updated May 14, 2009. Accessed February 27, 2010 at: http://www.fda.gov/Food/LabelingNutrition/LabelClaims/ucm111447.htm.

U.S. Food and Drug Administration: FDA issues advisory on star anise "teas." September 10, 2003. Accessed May 13, 2005 at: http://www.fda.gov/bbs/topics/NEWS/2003/NEW00941.html.

U.S. Food and Drug Administration: FDA warns consumers about "Total Body Formula" and "Total Body Mega Formula." March 27, 2008a. Accessed April 17, 2009 at: http://www.fda.gov/bbs/topics/NEWS/2008/NEW01812.html.

U.S. Food and Drug Administration: Intravenous ceftriaxone (marketed as Rocephin and generics) and calcium drug-drug interaction: Potential risk for cardiovascular adverse events in neonates. Postmarket Rev 2(3), 2009a. Accessed February 19, 2010 at: http://www.fda.gov/Drugs/DrugSafety/DrugSafetyNewsletter/ucm189806.htm.

U.S. Food and Drug Administration: KG Enterprises LLC, Inc. issues a voluntary nationwide recall of all Maxidus pills, a product marketed as a dietary supplement. March 31, 2008b. Accessed September 23, 2008 at: http://www.fda.gov/oc/po/firmrecalls/kg03_08.html.

U.S. Food and Drug Administration: Overview of dietary supplements. October 14, 2009b. Accessed February 27, 2010 at: http://www.fda.gov/Food/DietarySupplements/ConsumerInformation/ucm110417.htm.

U.S. Food and Drug Administration: TWC Global LLC, Inc. issues a voluntary nationwide recall of Axcil and Desirin products marketed as dietary supplements. September 12, 2007. Accessed September 23, 2008 at: http://www.fda.gov/oc/po/firmrecalls/twcglobal09_07.html.

Whitt, KN, et al: Cholestatic liver injury associated with whey protein and creatine supplements. Semin Liver Dis 28:226, 2008.

Williams, MH: Sports nutrition. In Shils, ME, et al (eds): Modern Nutrition in Health and Disease, ed 10. Lippincott Williams & Wilkins, Philadelphia, 2006.

Chapter 16

American Dietetic and Diabetic Associations: Exchange Lists for Meal Planning. American Dietetic Association, Chicago, 2003.

American Psychiatric Association Work Group on Eating Disorders: Practice guidelines for the treatment of patients and eating disorders (revision). Am J Psychiatry 157(Suppl 1):1, 2000.

Atkinson, R: Evaluation of implementation and effect of primary school based interventions to reduce the risk factors for obesity. BMJ 232:1027, 2001
Blundell, JE, Stubbs, J: Diet composition and the control of food intake in humans. In Bray, GA, Blouchard, C (eds): Handbook of Obesity: Etiology and Pathophysiology. Marcel Dekker, New York, 2004.
Bouchard, C: Inhibition of food intake by inhibitors of fatty acid synthase. N Engl J Med 343:1888, 2000.
Canning, H, and Mayer, J: Obesity: Its possible effect on college acceptance. N Engl J Med 275:1172, 1966.
Centers for Disease Control and Prevention: Disease conditions. Accessed June 2010 at: http://www.cdc.gov/DiseasesConditions.
Centers for Disease Control and Prevention: Obesity trends 1965–2007. Accessed August 2009 at: http://www.cdc.gov/nccdphp/dnpa/obesity/trends.
Fontaine, KR, et al: Years of life lost due to obesity. JAMA 289:187, 2003.
Forbes, GB: Body composition. In Shils, ME, et al (eds): Modern Nutrition in Health and Disease, ed 10. Lippincott Williams & Wilkins, Philadelphia, 2006.
Foreyt, JP: Lifestyle approaches to the IRS. Accessed February 2004 at: http://www.medscape.com/viewarticle/467200-3.
Fruhbeck, G: Chilhood obesity: Time for action not complacency. BMJ 320:328, 2000.
Gortmaker, SL, et al: Social and economic consequences of overweight in adolescence and young adulthood. N Engl J Med 329:1008, 1993.
Haines, PS, et al: Weekend eating in the United States is linked to greater energy, fat, and alcohol intake. Obes Res 11:945, 2003.
Huse, P, and Lucas, AR: Behavioral disorders affecting food intake: Anorexia nervosa, bulimia nervosa, and other psychiatric conditions. In Shils, ME, et al (eds): Modern Nutrition in Health and Disease, ed 10. Lippincott Williams & Wilkins, Philadelphia, 2006.
Keyes, A, et al: The Biology of Human Starvation, 2 vols. University of Minnesota Press, Minneapolis, 1950.
Lowell, BB, and Spiegelman, BM: Toward a molecular understanding of adaptive thermogenesis. Nature 404:652, 2000.
Ludwig, DS, et al: Dietary fiber, weight gain, and cardiovascular disease risk factors in young adults. JAMA 282:1539, 1999.
National Institutes of Health and National Heart, Lung, and Blood Institute: Clinical Guidelines on the Identification, Evaluation, and Treatment of Overweight and Obesity in Adults. NIH, Bethesda, MD, June 1998.
Polivy, J: Psychological consequences of food restriction. J Am Diet Assoc 96:589, 1996.
Poston, WS, II, et al: Challenges in obesity management. South Med J 8:710, 1998.
Saltzman, E: Low carbohydrate and high-protein diets for treatment of obesity, 2004–2005. Accessed June 2010 at: http://www.cyberrounds.com.
Samaras, K, et al: Genetic and environmental influences on total-body and central abdominal fat: The effect of physical activity in twin females. Ann Intern Med 130:873, 1999.
Shisslak, CM, Crago, M, and Estesil, S: The spectrum of eating disturbances. Int J Eat Disord 18:209, 1995
Stentz, CA, et al: Effects of the amount of exercise on body weight, body composition, and measures of central obesity. Arch Intern Med 164:1, 2004.
Stunkard, AJ: A history of binge eating. In Fairbanks, CG, and Wilson, GT (eds): Binge Eating, Assessment, and Treatment. Guilford Press, New York, 1993.
Stunkard, AJ, and Burt, V: Obesity and body image II: Age of onset of disturbances in the body image. Am J Psychiatry 123:1443, 1967.
Stunkard, AJ, and Mendelson, M: Disturbances in body image of some obese persons. J Am Diet Assoc 38:328, 1961.
U.S. Department of Agriculture (USDA): Steps to a healthier you. Accessed June 2010 at: www.MyPyramid.gov.
Van Itallie, TB: Obesity. In Jeejeebhoy, KN (ed): Current Therapy in Nutrition. BC Decker, Toronto, Canada, 1988.
Venes, D (ed): Taber's Cyclopedic Medical Dictionary, ed 20. FA Davis, Philadelphia, 2005.
Wast, RV: The female athlete: The triad of disordered eating, amenorrhea, and osteoporosis. Sports Med 2:63, 1998.
Wilding, J: Science, medicine, and the future: Obesity treatment. BMJ 315:997, 1997.
Yunsheng, MA, et al: Association between eating patterns and obesity in a free-living US adult population. Epidemiology 158:85, 2003.
Zerbe, KJ: Anorexia nervosa: When the pursuit of bodily perfection becomes a killer. Postgrad Med 1:161, 1999.

Chapter 17

American Diabetes Association: Diagnosis and classification of diabetes mellitus. Diabetes Care 28:237, 2005.
American Diabetes Association: 2008 Nutrition recommendations and interventions for diabetes. Diabetes Care 31:S61, 2008
American Diabetes Association: Accessed 2008 at: www.diabetes.org/home.
American Dietetic Association: Basic Carbohydrate Counting. American Dietetic Association, Chicago, 2003.
American Dietetic Association: International Dietetics and Nutrition Terminology (IDNT) Reference Manual. American Dietetic Association, Chicago, 2008.
American Dietetic Association: Total diet approach to communicating food and nutrition information. Position paper. American Dietetic Association, Chicago, 2008
Centers for Disease Control and Prevention: National Diabetes Fact Sheet, 2007. Accessed January 2010 at: http://www.cdc.gov/health/diabetes.
Diabetes Control and Complication Trial Group: The effect of intensive treatment of diabetes on the development and progression of long-term complications in insulin-dependent diabetes mellitus. N Engl J Med 329:977, 1998.
Diabetes Control and Complication Trial Group: Influence of intensive treatment on quality-of-life outcomes in the diabetes control and complications trial. Diabetes Care 19:195, 1993.

Chapter 18

Aglony, M, Acevedo, M, and Ambrosio, G: Hypertension in adolescents. Expert Rev Cardiovasc Ther 7:1595, 2009.
Ambrose, JA, and Barua, RS: The pathophysiology of cigarette smoking and cardiovascular disease: An update. J Am Coll Cardiol 43:1731, 2004.
American Diabetes Association and American Dietetic Association: Exchange Lists for Meal Planning. American Diabetes Association and American Dietetic Association, Alexandria, VA, and Chicago, 1995.
American Dietetic Association: Disorders of lipid metabolism evidence-based nutrition practice guideline. 2008a.
American Dietetic Association: Heart failure evidence-based nutrition practice guideline. 2008b.
American Dietetic Association: Hypertension evidence-based nutrition practice guideline. 2008c.

American Heart Association: Fish and omega-3 fatty acids. 2008. Accessed October 13, 2008 at: http://www.americanheart.org/presenter.jhtml?identifier=4632.

American Heart Association: Health disparities fact sheet. May 2008. Accessed October 15, 2008 at: http://www.americanheart.org/downloadable/heart/1221236162767Disparities%20Fact%20Sheet%205-08%20FINAL.pdf.

American Heart Association: Iron and heart disease. 2000. Accessed June 5, 2000 at: http://www.americanheart.org/Heart_and_Stroke_A_Z_Guide/iron.html.

American Heart Association and American Stroke Association: Heart Disease and Stroke Statistics. 2008. Accessed October 17, 2008 at: http://www.americanheart.org/downloadable/heart1200078608862HS_stats%202008.pdf.

Appel, LJ, et al: ASH Position Paper: Dietary approaches to lower blood pressure. J Clin Hypertens 11:358, 2009.

Appel, LJ, et al: A clinical trial of the effects of dietary patterns on blood pressure. N Engl J Med 336:1117, 1997.

Appel, LJ, and Anderson, CAM: Compelling evidence for public health action to reduce salt intake. N Engl J Med 362:650, 2010.

Arnett, DK: Relevance of genetics and genomics for prevention and treatment of cardiovascular disease: A scientific statement from the American Heart Association Council on Epidemiology and Prevention, the Stroke Council, and the Functional Genomics and Translational Biology Interdisciplinary Working Group. Circulation 115:2878, 2007. Accessed October 14, 2008 at: http://circ.ahajournals.org.cgi/content/full/115/22/2878.

Barker, DJP: Fetal origins of cardiovascular disease. Ann Med 31(Suppl 1):3, 1999.

Bonita, JS, et al: Coffee and cardiovascular disease: In vitro, cellular, animal, and human studies. Pharmacol Res 55:187, 2007.

Bonomini, F, et al: Atherosclerosis and oxidative stress. Histol Histopathol 23:381, 2008.

Brown, JE: Nutrition Through the Life Cycle, ed 3. Thomson Wadsworth, Belmont, CA, 2008.

Brunzell, JD: Hypertriglyceridemia. N Engl J Med 357:1009, 2007.

Centers for Disease Control and Prevention: Disparities in screening for and awareness of high blood cholesterol—United States, 1999–2002. MMWR 54:117, 2005a. Accessed October 10, 2008 at: http://www.cdc.gov/mmwr/preview/mmwrhtml/mm5405a2.htm.

Centers for Disease Control and Prevention: Heart disease fact sheet. July 1, 2008. Accessed October 8, 2008 at: http://www.cdc.gov/DHDSP/library/fs_heart_disease.htm.

Centers for Disease Control and Prevention: Heart failure fact sheet. January 25, 2010. Accessed March 3, 2010 at: http://www.cdc.gov/print.do?url=http://www.cdc.gov/dhdsp/library/fs_heart_failure.htm.

Centers for Disease Control and Prevention: Stroke fact sheet. June 25, 2008. Accessed October 8, 2008 at: http://www.cdc.gov/DHDSP/library/fs_stroke.htm.

Centers for Disease Control and Prevention: Trends in cholesterol screening and awareness of high blood cholesterol—United States, 1991–2003. MMWR 54:865, 2005b. Accessed March 5, 2010 at: http://www.cdc.gov/mmwr/preview/mmwrhtml/mm5435a2.htm.

Cornelis, MC, et al: Coffee, CYP1A2 genotype, and risk of myocardial infarction. JAMA 295:1135, 2006.

Cornelis, MC, and El-Sohemy, A: Coffee, caffeine, and coronary heart disease. Curr Opin Clin Nutr Metab Care 10:745, 2007.

Daniels, SR, and Greer, FR: Lipid screening and cardiovascular health in childhood. Pediatrics 122:198, 2008.

Davis, BC, and Kris-Etherton, PM: Achieving optimal essential fatty acid status in vegetarians: Current knowledge and practical implications. Am J Clin Nutr 78:640S, 2003.

Delanghe, JR, et al: Vitamin C deficiency and scurvy are not only a dietary problem but are codetermined by the haptoglobin polymorphism. Clin Chem 53:1397, 2007.

Dietary Management of Hyperlipoproteinemias. A Handbook for Physicians and Dietitians. U.S. Department of Health, Education, and Welfare, Bethesda, MD, 1980.

Din, JN, Newby, DE, and Flapan, AD: Omega 3 fatty acids and cardiovascular disease—fishing for a natural treatment. BMJ 328:30, 2004.

Ding, EL, and Mozaffarian, D: Optimal dietary habits for the prevention of stroke. Semin Neurol 26:11, 2006.

Eriksson, JG: The role of genes in growth and later health. Nestle Nutr Workshop Ser Pediatr Program 61:69, 2008.

Expert Panel on Detection, Evaluation, and Treatment of High Blood Cholesterol in Adults: Executive summary of the third report of the Expert Panel on Detection, Evaluation, and Treatment of High Blood Cholesterol in Adults (Adult Treatment Panel III). JAMA 285:2486, 2001.

Fauci, AS, et al: Harrison's Principles of Internal Medicine Companion Handbook. McGraw-Hill, New York, 1998.

Fonseca, C: Diagnosis of heart failure in primary care. Heart Fail Rev 11:95, 2006.

George, MG, et al: Paul Coverdell National Acute Stroke Registry surveillance—four states, 2005–2007. MMWR 58/SS-7, 2009. Accessed March 3, 2010 at: http://www.cdc.gov/mmwr/PDF/ss/ss5807.pdf.

Godfrey, KM, and Barker, DJ: Fetal programming and adult health. Public Health Nutr 4:611, 2001.

Goldberg, AC: Dyslipidemias. Merck Manual, September 2008. Accessed March 7, 2010 at: http://www.merck.com/mmpe/sec12/ch159/ch159b.html?qt=cholesterol%20goals&alt=sh#sec12-ch159-ch159b-1292.

Greenberg, JA, et al: Caffeinated beverage intake and the risk of heart disease mortality in the elderly: A prospective analysis. Am J Clin Nutr 85:392, 2007.

Gropper, SS, Smith, JL, and Groff, JL: Advanced Nutrition and Human Metabolism, ed 5. Wadsworth, Belmont, CA, 2009.

Grundy, SM: Nutrition in the management of disorders of serum lipids and lipoproteins. In Shils, ME, et al (eds): Modern Nutrition in Health and Disease, ed 10. Lippincott Williams & Wilkins, Philadelphia, 2006.

Grundy, SM, et al: Implications of recent clinical trials for the National Cholesterol Education Program Adult Treatment Panel III guidelines. Circulation 110:227, 2004.

Hausenloy, DJ, and Yellon, DM: Targeting residual cardiovascular risk: Raising high-density lipoprotein cholesterol levels. Heart 94:706, 2008.

He, FJ, et al: Fruit and vegetable consumption and stroke: Meta-analysis of cohort studies. Lancet 367:320, 2006.

Hofman, PL, Jackson, WE, and Knight, DB: Premature birth and later insulin resistance. N Engl J Med 351:2179, 2004.

Holvoet, P: Relations between metabolic syndrome, oxidative stress and inflammation and cardiovascular disease. Verh K Acad Geneeskd Belg 70:193, 2008.

Horowitz, CR, Rein, SB, and Leventhal, H: A story of maladies, misconceptions and mishaps: Effective management of heart failure. Soc Sci Med 58:631, 2004.

Klipstein-Grosbusch, K, et al: Dietary iron and risk of myocardial infarction in the Rotterdam Study. Am J Epidemiol 149:421, 1999.

Kotchen, TA, and Kotchen, JM: Nutrition, diet, and hypertension. In Shils, ME, et al (eds): Modern Nutrition in Health and Disease, ed 10. Lippincott Williams & Wilkins, Philadelphia, 2006.

Lichtenstein, AH, et al: Diet and lifestyle recommendations revision 2006: A scientific statement from the American Heart Association Nutrition Committee. Circulation 114:82, 2006.

Lopez-Garcia, E, et al: Coffee consumption and coronary heart disease in men and women: A prospective cohort study. Circulation 113:2045, 2006.

Love, JA, and Prusa, KJ: Nutrient composition and sensory attributes of cooked ground beef: Effects of fat content, cooking method, and water rinsing. J Am Diet Assoc 92:1367, 1992.

Matsuura, E, et al: Oxidation of LDL and its clinical implication. Autoimmun Rev 7:558, 2008.

Melanson, SF: Measurement of organochlorines in commercial over-the-counter fish oil preparations: Implications for dietary and therapeutic recommendations for omega-3 fatty acids and a review of the literature. Arch Pathol Lab Med 129:74, 2005.

Mukamal, K: Alcohol intake and noncoronary cardiovascular diseases. Ann Epidemiol 17(5):S8, 2007.

National Center for Health Statistics: Deaths, percent of total deaths, and death rates for the 15 leading causes of death: United States and each state, 2005. June 16, 2008. Accessed October 8, 2008 at: http://www.cd.gov/nchs/data/dvs/LCWK9_2005.pdf.

National High Blood Pressure Education Program Working Group on High Blood Pressure in Children and Adolescents: Fourth report on the diagnosis, evaluation, and treatment of high blood pressure in children and adolescents. Pediatrics 114:555, 2004. Accessed September 8, 2004 at: http://pediatrics.appublications.org/cgi/content/full/114/2/S2/555.

National Institutes of Health: The DASH diet. Press Release, April 3, 1997. Accessed May 30, 2000 at: http://www.nih.gov/news/pr/apr97/Dash.htm.

Nygard, O, et al: Plasma homocysteine levels and mortality in patients with coronary artery disease. N Engl J Med 337:230, 1997.

O'Callaghan, P: Homocysteine—is it the end of the line? Br J Cardiol 14:69, 2007.

Parikh, A, Lipsitz, SR, and Natarajan, S: Association between a DASH-like diet and mortality in adults with hypertension: findings from a population-based follow-up study. Am J Hypertens 22:409, 2009.

Patel, MD, and Thompson, PD: Phytosterols and vascular disease. Atherosclerosis 186:12, 2006.

Qureshi, AI, et al: Prevalence and trends of prehypertension and hypertension in United States: National Health and Nutrition Examination Surveys 1976 to 2000. Med Sci Monit 11:CR403-9.

Rader, DJ: Illuminating HDL—is it still a viable therapeutic target? N Engl J Med 357:2180, 2007.

Refsum, H, et al: Facts and recommendations about total homocysteine determinations: An expert opinion. Clin Chem 50:3, 2004.

Renaud, S, and Gueguen, R: The French paradox and wine drinking. Novartis Found Symp 216:208, 1998.

Salonen, JT, et al: High stored iron levels are associated with excess risk of myocardial infarction in Eastern Finnish men. Circulation 86:803, 1992.

Scanlon, VC, and Sanders T: Essentials of Anatomy and Physiology, ed 5. FA Davis, Philadelphia, 2007.

Schnell, ZB, Van Leeuwen, AM, and Kranpitz, TR (eds): Davis's Comprehensive Handbook of Laboratory and Diagnostic Tests with Nursing Implications. FA Davis, Philadelphia, 2003.

Serra-Majem, L, et al: How could changes in diet explain changes in coronary heart disease mortality in Spain? The Spanish paradox. Am J Clin Nutr 61(Suppl):1351S, 1995.

Sofi, F, et al: Coffee consumption and risk of coronary heart disease: A meta-analysis. Nutr Metab Cardiovasc Dis 17:209, 2007.

Sperling, MA: Prematurity—a window of opportunity? N Engl J Med 351:2229, 2004.

Tanne, D, et al: Elevated homocysteine in heart patients linked with higher stroke risk. Stroke 34 February 21. Rapid access issue, 2003. Accessed August 16, 2004 at: http://www.americanheart.org/presenter.jhtml?identifier=3008854.

Theuwissen, E, and Mensink, RP: Water-soluble dietary fibers and cardiovascular disease. Physiol Behav 94:285, 2008.

Thies, F, et al: Association of n-3 polyunsaturated fatty acids with stability of atherosclerotic plaques: A randomized controlled trial. Lancet 361:477, 2003.

Tuomainen, TP, et al: Association between body iron stores and the risk of acute myocardial infarction in men. Circulation 97:1461, 1998.

Tzonou, A, et al: Dietary iron and coronary heart disease risk: A study from Greece. Am J Epidemiol 147:161, 1998.

U.S. Department of Health and Human Services: The Seventh Report of the Joint National Committee on Prevention, Detection, Evaluation, and Treatment of High Blood Pressure. National Institutes of Health, Washington, DC, 2003. Accessed August 10, 2004 at: http://www.nhlbi.nih.gov/guidelines/hypertension/express.pdf.

U.S. Food and Drug Administration: FDA allows foods containing psyllium to make health claim on reducing risk of heart disease. U.S. Department of Health and Human Services, Rockville, MD, February 17, 1998. Accessed October 13, 2008 at: http://www.fda.gov/bbs/topics/ANSWERS/ANS00850.html.

U.S. Food and Drug Administration: FDA announces qualified health claims for omega-3 fatty acids. U.S. Department of Health and Human Services, Rockville, MD, September 8, 2004. Accessed October 13, 2008 at: http://www.fda.gov/bbs/topics/news/2004/NEW01115.html.

U.S. Food and Drug Administration: FDA approves new health claim for soy protein and coronary heart disease. U.S. Department of Health and Human Services, Rockville, MD, October 20, 1999. Accessed October 13, 2008 at: http://www.fda.gov/bbs/topics/ANSWERS/ANS00980.html.

Varughese, S: Management of acute decompensated heart failure. Crit Care Nurs Q 30:94, 2007.

Vasan, RS, et al: Plasma homocysteine and risk for congestive heart failure in adults without prior myocardial infarction. JAMA 289:1251, 2003.

Vollset, SE, et al: Plasma total homocysteine and cardiovascular and noncardiovascular mortality: The Hordaland Homocysteine Study. Am J Clin Nutr 74:130, 2001.

Wierzbicki, AS: Homocysteine and cardiovascular disease: a review of the evidence. Diab Vasc Dis Res 4:143, 2007.

Chapter 19

American Diabetes Association: Nephropathy in diabetes: Position statement. Diabetes Care 27:S79, 2004.

American Dietetic Association: International Dietetics and Nutrition Terminology (IDNT) Reference Manual, ed 1. American Dietetic Association, Chicago, 2008.

American Dietetic Association: Position of the American Dietetic Association: Vegetarian diets. J Am Diet Assoc 97:1317, 1997.

Beto, JA, and Bansal, VK: Medical nutrition therapy in chronic kidney failure: Integrating clinical practice guidelines. J Am Diet Assoc 104:404, 2004.

Carter, S: From the editor's desk. Renal Nutrition Forum, Vol. 23, No. 4. Renal Practice Group/American Dietetic Association. Rancho Sante, CA, 2004.

Inman, JI: A Clinical Guide to the Nutritional Care of the Renal Patient. New England Center for Nutrition Education, Stoughton, MA, 1999.

Kontiokari, T, et al: Randomised trial of cranberry lingoberry juice and lactobacillus GG drink for prevention of urinary tract infections in women. BMJ 322:1571, 2001.

Kopple, JD: Renal, diet and the kidney. In Shils, ME, et al (eds): Modern Nutrition in Health and Disease, ed 10. Lippincott Williams & Wilkins, Philadelphia, 2006.

Kugler, C, Vlaminck, H, and Maes, AH: Nonadherence with diet and fluid restrictions among adults having hemodialysis. J Nurs Sch 37:25, 2005.

Kuhlmann, MK, et al: Malnutrition in hemodialysis patients: Self-assessment, medical evaluations, and "verifiable" parameters. Med Klin 1:13, 1997.

Massey, LK: Dietary influences on urinary oxalate and risk of kidney stones. Front Biosci 8:S584, 2003.

Monsen, ER: Meeting the challenge of the renal diet. J Am Diet Assoc 93:6, 1993.

Moore, MC: Mosby's Pocket Guide to Nutrition and Care, ed 6. Mosby Year Book, St. Louis, 2009.

National Kidney Foundation: K/DOQI Clinical Practice Guidelines for Chronic Kidney Disease: Evaluation, classification and stratification. Am J Kidney Dis 39(Suppl 1):S1, 2002.

National Kidney Foundation: K/DOQI Clinical Practice Guidelines for Nutrition in Children with CKD: 2008 Update. Am J Kidney Dis 53(Suppl 2):S11, 2009.

Pennington, JA, and Souglass, JA: Bowers and Churches Food Values of Portions Commonly Used, ed 18. Lippincott Williams & Wilkins, Baltimore, 2004.

Rubin, HR, et al: Patient ratings of dialysis care with peritoneal dialysis vs. hemodialysis. JAMA 291:697, 2004.

Scanlon, VD, and Sanders, T: Essentials of Anatomy and Physiology, ed 4. FA Davis, Philadelphia, 2003.

Venes, D (ed): Taber's Cyclopedic Medical Dictionary, ed 21. FA Davis, Philadelphia, 2010.

Weaver, CM, and Heaney, RP: Calcium. In Shils, ME, et al (eds): Modern Nutrition in Health and Disease, ed 9. Williams & Wilkins, Baltimore, 1999.

Chapter 20

Abou-Assi, S, Craig, K, and O'Keefe, SJ: Hypocaloric jejunal feeding is better than total parenteral nutrition in acute pancreatitis: Results of a randomized comparative study. Am J Gastroenterol 97:2255, 2002.

American Society of Anesthesiologists Task Force on Preoperative Fasting: Practice guidelines for preoperative fasting and the use of pharmacologic agents to reduce the risk of pulmonary aspiration: Application to healthy patients undergoing elective procedures. Anesthesiology 90:896, 1999. Accessed March 22, 2009 at: http://www.asahq.org/publicationsAndServices/NPO.pdf.

Au, DH, et al: Alcohol screening scores and risk of hospitalizations for GI conditions in men. Alcohol Clin Exp Res 31:443, 2007.

Beattie, RM, et al: Inflammatory bowel disease. Arch Dis Child 91:426, 2006.

Bentz, S, et al: Clinical relevance of IgG antibodies against food antigens in Crohn's disease: a double-blind cross-over diet intervention study. Digestion 81:252, 2010.

Bostwick, JM, and Seaman, JS: Hospitalized patients and alcohol: Who is being missed? Gen Hosp Psychiatry 26:59, 2004.

Boyle, MP: Adult cystic fibrosis. JAMA 298:1787, 2007.

Brady, M, et al: Preoperative fasting for preventing perioperative complications in children. Cochrane Database Syst Rev 4: CD005285, 2009.

Brady, M, Kinn, S, and Stuart, P: Preoperative fasting for adults to prevent perioperative complications. Cochrane Database Syst Rev 4:CD005285, 2003.

Brown, AC, and Roy, M: Does evidence exist to include diet therapy in the treatment of Crohn's disease? Expert Rev Gastroenterol Hepatol 4:191, 2010.

Cabada, MM, and White, AC, Jr: Travelers' diarrhea: An update on susceptibility, prevention, and treatment. Curr Gastroenterol Rep 10:473, 2008.

Cabre, E, and Gassull, MA: Nutrition in liver disease. Curr Opin Clin Nutr Metab Care 8:545, 2005.

Calder, PC: Polyunsaturated fatty acids, inflammatory processes and inflammatory bowel diseases. Mol Nutr Food Res 52:885, 2008.

Centers for Disease Control and Prevention: Acute hepatitis C virus infections attributed to unsafe injection practices at an endoscopy clinic—Nevada, 2007. MMWR 57:513, 2008a. Accessed November 8, 2008 at: http://www.cdc.gov/mmwr/preview/mmwrhtml/mm5719a2.htm.

Centers for Disease Control and Prevention: Alcohol-attributable deaths and years of potential life lost—United States, 2001. MMWR 53:866, 2004. Accessed November 9, 2008 at: http://www.cdc.gov/mmwr/preview/mmwrhtml/mm5337a2.htm.

Centers for Disease Control and Prevention: Surveillance for acute viral hepatitis—United States, 2006. MMWR 57:1, 2008b. Accessed November 8, 2008 at: http://www.cdc.gov/mmwr/preview/mmwrhtml/ss5702a1.htm.

Centers for Disease Control and Prevention: Transmission of hepatitis B virus among persons undergoing blood glucose monitoring in long-term-care facilities—Mississippi, North Carolina, and Los Angeles County, California, 2003–2004. MMWR 54:220, 2005. Accessed June 2, 2005 at: http://www.cdc.gov/mmwr/preview/mmwrhtml/mm5409a2.htm.

Charoenkwan, K, Phillipson, G, and Vutyavanich, T: Early versus delayed (traditional) oral fluids and food for reducing complications after major abdominal gynaecologic surgery. Cochrane Database Syst Rev 4:CD004508, 2007.

Chiba, M, et al: Lifestyle-related disease in Crohn's disease: relapse prevention by a semi-vegetarian diet. World J Gastroenterol 16:2484, 2010.

Chiossi, G, et al: Hyperemesis gravidarum complicated by Wernicke encephalopathy: Background, case report, and review of the literature. Obstet Gynecol Surv 61:255, 2006.

Cohen, S: Peptic ulcer disease. Merck Manual, 2007. Accessed November 1, 2008 at: http://www.merck.com/mmpe/sec02/ch013/ch013e.html?qt=pepticpercent20ulcer&alt=sh.

Collin, P, and Reunala, T: Recognition and management of the cutaneous manifestations of celiac disease: A guide for dermatologists. Am J Clin Dermatol 4:13, 2003.

Cooper, A, and Heird, WC: Nutritional management of infants and children with specific diseases or other conditions. In Shils, ME, et al (eds): Modern Nutrition in Health and Disease, ed 10. Lippincott Williams & Wilkins, Philadelphia, 2006.

Cordoba, J, et al: Normal protein diet for episodic hepatic encephalopathy: Results of a randomized study. J Hepatol 41:38, 2004.

Cottone, M, Orlando, A, and Modesto, I: Postoperative maintenance therapy for inflammatory bowel disease. Curr Opin Gastroenterol 22:377, 2006.

Deglin, JH, and Vallerand, AH: Davis's Drug Guide for Nurses, ed 11. FA Davis, Philadelphia, 2009.

Despins, LA, Kivlahan, C, and Cox, KR: Acute pancreatitis. Am J Nurs 105(11):54, 2005.

Douglas, LC, and Sanders, ME: Probiotics and prebiotics in dietetics practice. J Am Diet Assoc 108:510, 2008.

Drumm, ML, et al: Genetic modifiers of lung disease in cystic fibrosis. N Engl J Med 353:1443, 2005.

DuPont, HL: Travelers' diarrhea: Antimicrobial therapy and chemoprevention. Nat Clin Pract Gastroenterol Hepatol 2:191, 2005.

Feetham, S, Thomson, EJ, and Hinshaw, AS: Nursing leadership in genomics for health and society. J Nurs Sch 37:102, 2005.

Fujiwara, Y, et al: Association between dinner-to-bed time and gastroesophageal reflux disease. Am J Gastroenterol 100:2633, 2005.

Gaby, AR: Nutritional approaches to prevention and treatment of gallstones. Altern Med Rev 14:258, 2009.

Gentilcore, D, et al: Postprandial hypotension—novel insights into pathophysiology and therapeutic implications. Curr Vasc Pharmacol 4:161, 2006.

Gillen, D, and McColl, KE: Gastroduodenal disease, *Helicobacter pylori*, and genetic polymorphisms. Clin Gastroenterol Hepatol 3:1180, 2005.

Green, PH, and Jabri, B: Celiac disease. Annu Rev Med 57:207, 2006.

Griffiths, AM: Inflammatory bowel disease. In Shils, ME, et al (eds): Modern Nutrition in Health and Disease, ed 10. Lippincott Williams & Wilkins, Philadelphia, 2006.

Haussinger, D, and Gorg, B: Interaction of oxidative stress, astrocyte swelling and cerebral ammonia toxicity. Curr Opin Clin Nutr Metab Care 13:87, 2010.

Hegazi, RAF, and O'Keefe, SJD: Nutritional immunomodulation of acute pancreatitis. Curr Gastroenterol Rep 9:99, 2007.

Heidelbaugh, JJ, and Sherbondy, M: Cirrhosis and chronic liver failure: Part II. Complications and treatment. Am Fam Physician 74:767, 2006.

Heymann, DL (ed): Control of Communicable Diseases Manual, ed 18. American Public Health Association, Washington, DC, 2004.

Hinson, JA, Roberts, DW, and James, LP: Mechanisms of acetaminophen-induced liver necrosis. Handb Exp Pharmacol 2010(196):369, 2010.

Holecek, M: Three targets of branched-chain amino acid supplementation in the treatment of liver disease. Nutrition 26:482, 2010.

Intagliata, N, and Koch, KL: Gastroparesis in type 2 diabetes mellitus: Prevalence, etiology, diagnosis, and treatment. Curr Gastroenterol Rep 9:270, 2007.

Ioannidis, O, Lavrentieva, A, and Botsios, D: Nutrition support in acute pancreatitis. JOP 9:375, 2008.

Jacobson, BC, et al: Body-mass index and symptoms of gastroesophageal reflux in women. N Engl J Med 354:2340, 2006.

Jadallah, KA, and Khader, YS: Celiac disease in patient with presumed irritable bowel syndrome: a case-finding study. World J Gastroenterol 15:5321, 2009.

Joachim, G: Responses of people with inflammatory bowel disease to foods consumed. Gastroenterol Nurs 23:160, 2000.

Jones, MP: The role of psychosocial factors in peptic ulcer disease: Beyond *Helicobacter pylori* and NSAIDs. J Psychosom Res 60:407, 2006.

Jowett, SL, et al: Dietary beliefs of people with ulcerative colitis and their effect on relapse and nutrient intake. Clin Nutr 23:161, 2004a.

Jowett, SL, et al: Influence of dietary factors on the clinical course of ulcerative colitis: A prospective cohort study. Gut 53:1479, 2004b.

Kim, MN, et al: The effects of probiotics on PPI-triple therapy for *Helicobacter pylori* eradication. Helicobacter 13:261, 2008.

Kivi, M, and Tindberg, Y: *Helicobacter pylori* occurrence and transmission: A family affair? Scand J Infect Dis 38:407, 2006.

Kliegman, RM, and Willoughby, RE: Prevention of necrotizing enterocolitis with probiotics. Pediatrics 115:171, 2005.

Koo, HL, and DuPont, HL: Current and future developments in travelers' diarrhea therapy. Expert Rev Anti Infect Ther 4:417, 2006.

Korzenik, JR: Case closed? Diverticulitis: Epidemiology and fiber. J Clin Gastroenterol 40:S112, 2006.

Kudsk, KA, and Sacks, GS: Nutrition in the care of the patient with surgery, trauma, and sepsis. In Shils, ME, et al (eds): Modern Nutrition in Health and Disease, ed 10. Lippincott Williams & Wilkins, Philadelphia, 2006.

Lacy, BE: Update on the diagnosis and treatment of chronic constipation and irritable bowel syndrome. Medscape CME. November 15, 2007. Accessed November 4, 2008 at: http://www.medscape.com/viewprogram/8145_pnt.

Leenen, CH, and Dieleman, LA: Inulin and oligofructose in chronic inflammatory bowel disease. J Nutr 137:2572S, 2007.

Lieber, CS: Nutrition in liver disorders and the role of alcohol. In Shils, ME, et al (eds): Modern Nutrition in Health and Disease, ed 10. Lippincott Williams & Wilkins, Philadelphia, 2006.

Lin, HC, et al: Oral probiotics reduce the incidence and severity of necrotizing enterocolitis in very low birth weight infants. Pediatrics 115:1, 2005.

Lomax, AR, and Calder, PC: Probiotics, immune function, infection and inflammation: a review of the evidence from studies conducted in humans. Curr Pharm Des 15:1428, 2009.

Longacre, AV, and Garcia-Tsao, G: A commonsense approach to esophageal varices. Clin Liver Dis 10:613, 2006.

Magee, FA, et al: Contribution of dietary protein to sulfide production in the large intestine: An in vitro and a controlled feeding study in humans. Am J Clin Nutr 72:1488, 2000.

Malozemoff, W, and Gentlemen, B: When dinner's done—postprandial hypotension in older adults. Nursing Spectrum Midwest 5:18, 2004.

Matarese, LE, et al: Short bowel syndrome: Clinical guidelines for nutrition management. Nutr Clin Pract 20:493, 2005.

McCabe, H: Riboflavin deficiency in cystic fibrosis: Three case reports. J Hum Nutr Diet 14:365, 2001.

McClave, SA, et al: Nutrition support in acute pancreatitis: a systematic review of the literature. JPEN J 30:143, 2006.

Medical News Today: Five states step up efforts to screen newborns for cystic fibrosis. July 16, 2008. Accessed November 11, 2008 at: http://www.medicalnewstoday.com/articles/115074.php.

Musher, DM, and Musher, BL: Contagious acute gastrointestinal infections. N Engl J Med 351:2417, 2004.

National Digestive Diseases Information Clearinghouse: Crohn's disease. National Institute of Diabetes and Digestive and Kidney Diseases, 2006a. Accessed November 6, 2008 at: http://digestive.niddk.nih.gov/ddiseases/pubs/crohns/.

National Digestive Diseases Information Clearinghouse: Irritable bowel syndrome. National Institute of Diabetes and Digestive and Kidney Diseases, September 2007. Accessed November 2, 2008 at: http://digestive.niddk.nih.gov/ddiseases/pubs/ibs/.

National Digestive Diseases Information Clearinghouse: Ulcerative colitis. National Institute of Diabetes and Digestive and Kidney Diseases, 2006b. Accessed November 7, 2008 at: http://digestive.niddk.nih.gov/ddiseases/pubs/colitis/.

O'Brien, CP: The CAGE questionnaire for detection of alcoholism. JAMA 300:2054, 2008.

Ogershok, PR, et al: Wernicke encephalopathy in nonalcoholic patients. Am J Med Sci 323:107, 2002.

Ohge, H, et al: Association between fecal hydrogen sulfide production and pouchitis. Dis Colon Rectum 48:469, 2005.

O'Sullivan, M, and O'Morain, C: Nutrition in inflammatory bowel disease. Best Pract Res Clin Gastroenterol 20:561, 2006.

Pandol, S, and Cohen, H: Chronic pancreatitis: Diagnosis and management. Cyberounds Gastroenterology Conference. Released January 22, 2007. Accessed October 21, 2008 at: http://www.cyberounds.com/conf/gastroenterology/2007-01-08/print.html.

Park, W, and Vaezi, MF: Etiology and pathogenesis of achalasia: The current understanding. Am J Gastroenterol 100:1404, 2005.

Parkman, HP, Hasler, WL, and Fisher, RS: American Gastroenterological Association medical position statement: Diagnosis and treatment of gastroparesis. Gastroenterology 127:1589, 2004.

Parrish, CR: The clinician's guide to short bowel syndrome. Prac Gastroenterol 29(9):67, 2005.

Petrov, MS, and Zagainov, VE: Influence of enteral versus parenteral nutrition on blood glucose control in acute pancreatitis: A systematic review. Clin Nutr 26:514, 2007.

Pezzilli, R: Etiology of chronic pancreatitis: has it changed in the last decade? World J Gastroenterol 15:4737, 2009.

Raimondo, M, and Scolapio, JS: Nutrition in pancreatic disorders. In Shils, ME, et al (eds): Modern Nutrition in Health and Disease, ed 10. Lippincott Williams & Wilkins, Philadelphia, 2006.

Rowan, FE, et al: Sulphate-reducing bacteria and hydrogen sulphide in the aetiology of ulcerative colitis. Br J Surg 96:151, 2009.

Sakorafas, GH, Milingos, D, and Peros, G: Asymptomatic cholelithiasis: Is cholecystectomy really needed? A critical reappraisal 15 years after the introduction of laparoscopic cholecystectomy. Dig Dis Sci 52:1313, 2007.

Sartor, RB: Probiotic therapy of intestinal inflammation and infections. Curr Opin Gastroenterol 21:44, 2005.

Shaffer, EA: Epidemiology and risk factors for gallstone disease: Has the paradigm changed in the 21st century? Curr Gastroenterol Rep 7:132, 2005.

Shaffer, EA: Gallstone disease: Epidemiology of gallbladder stone disease. Best Pract Res Clin Gastroenterol 20:981, 2006.

Shamir, R, Phillip, M, and Levine, A: Growth retardation in pediatric Crohn's disease: Pathogenesis and interventions. Inflamm Bowel Dis 13:620, 2007.

Sheu, BS, et al: Pretreatment with *Lactobacillus-* and *Bifidobacterium*-containing yogurt can improve the efficacy of quadruple therapy in eradicating residual *Helicobacter pylori* infection after failed triple therapy. Am J Clin Nutr 83:864, 2006.

Singh, E, and Redfield, D: Prophylaxis for travelers' diarrhea. Curr Gastroenterol Rep 11:297, 2009.

Smith, MM: Emergency: Variceal hemorrhage from esophageal varices associated with alcoholic liver disease. Am J Nurs 110(2):32, 2010.

Smothers, BA, Yahr, HT, and Ruhl, CE: Detection of alcohol use disorders in general hospital admissions in the United States. Arch Intern Med 164:749, 2004.

Stenson, WF: The esophagus and stomach. In Shils, ME, et al (eds): Modern Nutrition in Health and Disease, ed 10. Lippincott Williams & Wilkins, Philadelphia, 2006.

Strate, LL, et al: Nut, corn, and popcorn consumption and the incidence of diverticular disease. JAMA 300:907, 2008.

Suckling, B, Johnson, MM, and Chin, R, Jr: Nutrition, respiratory function, and disease. In Shils, ME, et al (eds): Modern Nutrition in Health and Disease, ed 10. Lippincott Williams & Wilkins, Philadelphia, 2006.

Tilg, H, and Kaser, A: Diet and relapsing ulcerative colitis: Take off the meat? Gut 53:1399, 2004.

Tsai, CJ, et al: Frequent nut consumption and decreased risk of cholecystectomy in women. Am J Clin Nutr 80:76, 2004a.

Tsai, CJ, et al: A prospective cohort study of nut consumption and the risk of gallstone disease in men. Am J Epidemiol 160:961, 2004b.

Tsiaousi, ET, et al: Malnutrition in end stage liver disease: Recommendations and nutritional support. J Gastroenterol Hepatol 23:527, 2008.

Vandenplas, Y, et al: Probiotics in infectious diarrhoea in children: Are they indicated? Eur J Pediatr 166:1211, 2007.

Vanderpool, C, Yan, F, Polk, DB: Mechanisms of probiotic action: Implications for therapeutic applications in inflammatory bowel diseases. Inflamm Bowel Dis 14:1585, 2008.

Vandewoude, MF: Fibre-supplemented tube feeding in the hospitalised elderly. Age Ageing 34:120, 2005.

Wang, GJ, et al: Acute pancreatitis: etiology and common pathogenesis. World J Gastroenterol 15:1427, 2009.

Wang, KY, et al: Effects of ingesting *Lactobacillus-* and *Bifidobacterium*-containing yogurt in subjects with colonized *Helicobacter pylori*. Am J Clin Nutr 80:737, 2004.

Wheeler, C, et al: An outbreak of hepatitis A associated with green onions. N Engl J Med 353:890, 2005.

Willcutts, K, Scarano, K, and Eddins, CW: Ostomies and fistulas: A collaborative approach. Prac Gastroenterol 29(11):63, 2005.

Williams, LS, and Hopper, PD: Understanding Medical Surgical Nursing, ed 3. FA Davis, Philadelphia, 2007.

Williams, NT: Probiotics. Am J Health Syst Pharm 67:449, 2010.

Wolvers, D, et al: Guidance for substantiating the evidence for beneficial effects of probiotics: prevention and management of infectons by probiotics. J Nutr 140:698S, 2010.

Yates, J: Traveler's diarrhea. Am Fam Physician 71:2095, 2005.

Zar, S, et al: Food-specific IgG4 antibody–guided exclusion diet improves symptoms and rectal compliance in irritable bowel syndrome. Scand J Gastroenterol 40:800, 2005.

Chapter 21

Abayomi, J: A study to investigate women's experiences of radiation enteritis following radiotherapy for cervical cancer. J Hum Nutr Diet 18:353, 2005.

Albert-Puleo, M: Physiological effects of cabbage with reference to its potential as a dietary cancer-inhibitor and its use in ancient medicine. J Ethnopharmacol 9:261, 1983.

Alpha-tocopherol, Beta-carotene Cancer Prevention Study Group: Effect of vitamin E and beta-carotene on the incidence of lung cancer and other cancers in male smokers. N Engl J Med 330:1029, 1994.

American Cancer Society: Cancer Facts and Figures 2010. American Cancer Society, Atlanta, 2010. Accessed June 2, 2010 at: http://www.cancer.org/downloads/STT/Cancer_Facts_and_Figures_2010.pdf.

American Cancer Society: Cancer Facts and Figures 2008. American Cancer Society, Atlanta, 2008. Accessed November 17, 2008 at: http://www.cancer.org/downloads/STT/2008CAFFfinalsecured.pdf.

American Institute for Cancer Research: Caveat grilling debate. Newsletter 6:1, 2002.

American Institute for Cancer Research: Experts reissue warning about grilling. May 23, 2005. Accessed May 25, 2005 at: http://www.aicr.org/press/pubsearchdetail.lasso?index=2026.

American Institute for Cancer Research: The New American Plate. AICR, Washington, DC, 2000. Accessed May 25, 2005 at: http://www.aicr.org/publications/brochures/online/nap.pdf.

Amling, CL: Relationship between obesity and prostate cancer. Curr Opin Urol 15:167, 2005.

Ansari, MS, and Ansari, S: Lycopene and prostate cancer. Future Oncol 1:425, 2005.

Baracos, VE: Cancer-associated cachexia and underlying biological mechanisms. Annu Rev Nutr 26:435, 2006.

Birt, DF: Phytochemicals and cancer prevention: From epidemiology to mechanism of action. J Am Diet Assoc 106:20, 2006.

Buckland, G, et al: Adherence to a Mediterranean diet and risk of gastric adenocarcinoma within the European Prospective Investigation into Cancer and Nutrition (EPIC) cohort study. Am J Clin Nutr 91:381, 2010.

Burstein, HJ, and Schwartz, RS: Molecular origins of cancer. N Engl J Med 358:527, 2008.

Caire-Juvera, G, et al: Vitamin A and retinol intakes and the risk of fractures among participants of the Women's Health Initiative Observational Study. Am J Clin Nutr 89:323, 2009.

Carmichael, AR: Obesity and prognosis of breast cancer. Obes Rev 7:333, 2006.

Cerully, JL, Klein, WM, and McCaul, JD: Lack of acknowledgment of fruit and vegetable recommendations among nonadherent individuals: Associations with information processing and cancer cognitions. J Health Commun 11(Suppl 1):103, 2006.

Chan, JM, et al: Diet after diagnosis and the risk of prostate cancer progression, recurrence, and death (United States). Cancer Causes Control 17:199, 2006.

Chiou, HL, et al: NAT2 fast acetylator genotype is associated with an increased risk of lung cancer among never-smoking women in Taiwan. Cancer Lett 223:93, 2005.

Da Costa, KA, et al: Choline deficiency increases lymphocyte apoptosis and DNA damage in humans. Am J Clin Nutr 84:88, 2006.

Dong, LM, et al: Genetic susceptibility to cancer. JAMA 299:2423, 2008.

Doyle, C, et al: Nutrition and physical activity during and after cancer treatment: An American Cancer Society Guide for informed choices. CA Cancer J Clin 56:323, 2006. Accessed November 21, 2008 at: http://caonline.amcancersoc.org/cgi/content/full/56/2323.

Esper, DH, and Harb, WA: The cancer cachexia syndrome: A review of metabolic and clinical manifestations. Nutr Clin Pract 20:369, 2005.

Fitzgerald, N: Nutrition knowledge, food label use, and food intake patterns among Latinas with and without type 2 diabetes. J Am Diet Assoc 108:960, 2008.

Foerster, SB, et al: California's "5 a Day—for Better Health" campaign: An innovative population-based effort to effect large-scale dietary change. Am J Prev Med 11:124, 1995.

Giovannucci, E, et al: Risk factors for prostate cancer incidence and progression in the health professionals follow-up study. Int J Cancer 121:1571, 2007.

Go, VL, et al: Nutrient-gene interaction: Metabolic genotype-phenotype relationship. J Nutr 135:3016S, 2005.

Graham-Maar, RC, et al: Elevated vitamin A intake and serum retinol in preadolescent children with cystic fibrosis. Am J Clin Nutr 84:174, 2006.

Haydon, AM, et al: Effect of physical activity and body size on survival after diagnosis with colorectal cancer. Gut 55:62, 2006.

Heaney, RP: Calcium, dairy products, and osteoporosis. J Am Coll Nutr 19:83S, 2000.

Hofmann, T, et al: Modulation of detoxification enzymes by watercress: In vitro and in vivo investigations in human peripheral blood cells. Eur J Nutr 48:483, 2009.

Hsing, AW, Sakoda, LC, and Chua, S, Jr: Obesity, metabolic syndrome, and prostate cancer. Am J Clin Nutr 86:s843, 2007.

Isaacson, C: The change of the staple diet of black South Africans from sorghum to maize (corn) is the cause of the epidemic of squamous carcinoma of the oesophagus. Med Hypotheses 64:658, 2005.

Kamat, AM, and Lamm, DL: Chemoprevention of bladder cancer. Urol Clin North Am 29:157, 2002.

Kandala, V, and Playfor, S: Massive tongue swelling following the use of synthetic saliva. Paediatr Anaesth 13:827, 2003.

Kavanaugh, CJ, Trumbo, RP, and Ellwood, KC: The U.S. Food and Drug Administration's evidence-based review for qualified health claims: Tomatoes, lycopene, and cancer. J Natl Cancer Inst 99:1074, 2007.

Kirsh, VA, et al: A prospective study of lycopene and tomato product intake and risk of prostate cancer. Cancer Epidemiol Biomarkers Prev 15:92, 2006.

Kushi, LH, et al: American Cancer Society Guidelines on nutrition and physical activity for cancer prevention: Reducing risk of cancer healthy food choices and physical activity. CA Cancer J Clin 56:254, 2006. Accessed November 18, 2008 at: http://caonline.amcancersoc.org/cgi/content/full/56/254.

Larsson, SC, Bergkvist, L, and Wolk, A: Processed meat consumption, dietary nitrosamines and stomach cancer risk in a cohort of Swedish women. Int J Cancer 119:915, 2006.

Li, FP, and Pawlish, K: Cancers in Asian-Americans and Pacific Islanders: Migrant studies. Chinese American Medical Society. Undated. Accessed November 22, 2008 at: http://www.camsociety.org/issues/fredli.htm.

Lynn, A, et al: Cruciferous vegetables and colo-rectal cancer. Proc Nutr Soc 65:135, 2006.

Martin, KR: Using nutrigenomics to evaluate apoptosis as a preemptive target in cancer prevention. Curr Cancer Drug Targets 7:438, 2007.

McGough, C, et al: Role of nutritional intervention in patients treated with radiotherapy for pelvic malignancy. Br J Cancer 90:2278, 2004.

Meyerhardt, JA, et al: Association of dietary patterns with cancer recurrence and survival in patients with stage III colon cancer. JAMA 298:754, 2007.

Meyerhardt, JA, et al: Physical activity and survival after colorectal cancer diagnosis. J Clin Oncol 24:3527, 2006.

Milner, JA: Nutrition and cancer: Essential elements for a roadmap. Cancer Lett 269:189, 2008.

Modesitt, SC, and van Nagell, JR, Jr: The impact of obesity on the incidence and treatment of gynecologic cancers: a review. Obstet Gynecol Surv 60:683, 2005.

MRC Vitamin Study Research Group: Prevention of neural tube defects: Results of the Medical Research Council Vitamin Study. Lancet 338:131, 1991.

Muscaritoli, M, et al: New strategies to overcome cancer cachexia: From molecular mechanisms to the "Parallel Pathway." Asia Pac J Clin Nutr 17(Suppl 1):387, 2008.

Omenn, GS, et al: The Beta-Carotene and Retinol Efficacy Trial (CARET) for chemoprevention of lung cancer in high risk populations: Smokers and asbestos-exposed workers. Cancer Res 54:2038S, 1994.

Omenn, GS, et al: Risk factors for lung cancer and for intervention effects in CARET, the Beta-Carotene and Retinol Efficacy Trial. J Natl Cancer Inst 98:1550, 1996.

Pierce, JP, et al: Influence of a diet very high in vegetables, fruit, and fiber and low in fat on prognosis following treatment for breast cancer: The Women's Healthy Eating and Living (WHEL) randomized trial. JAMA 298:289, 2007.

Rathkopf, D, and Schwartz, GK: Molecular basis of carcinogenesis. In Shils, ME, et al (eds): Modern Nutrition in Health and Disease, ed 10. Lippincott Williams & Wilkins, Philadelphia, 2006.

Redlich, CA, et al: Effect of supplementation with beta-carotene and vitamin A on lung nutrient levels. Cancer Epidemiol Biomarkers Prev 7:211, 1998.

Reszka, E, Wasowicz, W, and Gromadzinska, J: Genetic polymorphism of xenobiotic metabolizing enzymes, diet, and cancer susceptibility. Br J Nutr 96:609, 2006.

Salmon, CP, et al: Minimization of heterocyclic amines and thermal inactivation of *Escherichia coli* in fried ground beef. J Nat Cancer Inst 92:1773, 2000.

Schattner, M, and Shike, M: Nutrition support of the patient with cancer. In Shils, ME, et al (eds): Modern Nutrition in Health and Disease, ed 10. Lippincott Williams & Wilkins, Philadelphia, 2006.

Sloane, D: Cancer epidemiology in the United States: Racial, social, and economic factors. Methods Mol Biol 471:65, 2009.

Stan, SD, et al: Bioactive food components and cancer risk reduction. J Cell Biochem 104:339, 2008.

Terry, MB, et al: Alcohol metabolism, alcohol intake, and breast cancer risk: A sister-set analysis using the Breast Cancer Family Registry. Breast Cancer Res Treat 106:281, 2007.

Tomlinson, SS: Dietary and lifestyle factors associated with breast cancer rates. J Am Acad Phys Assist 7:622, 1994.

Tsugane, S, and Sasazuki, S: Diet and the risk of gastric cancer: Review of epidemiological evidence. Gastric Cancer 10:75, 2007.

U.S. Preventive Services Task Force: Vitamin supplementation to prevent cancer and cardiovascular disease. U.S. Department of Health and Human Services, Rockville, MD, 2003. Accessed November 21, 2008 at: http://www.ahrq.gov/clinic/uspstf/uspsvita.htm.

Velentzis, LS, et al: Do phytoestrogens reduce the risk of breast cancer and breast cancer recurrence? What clinicians need to know. Eur J Cancer 44:1799, 2008.

Vij, U, and Kumar, A: Phyto-oestrogens and prostatic growth. Natl Med J India 17:22, 2004.

Wiggenraad, RG: Prophylactic gastrostomy placement and early tube feeding may limit loss of weight during chemoradiotherapy for advanced head and neck cancer: A preliminary study. Clin Otolaryngol 32:384, 2007.

Willett, WC, and Giovannucci, E: Epidemiology of diet and cancer risk. In Shils, ME, et al (eds): Modern Nutrition in Health and Disease, ed 10. Lippincott Williams & Wilkins, Philadelphia, 2006.

Wood, CE, et al: Effects of soybean glyceollins and estradiol in postmenopausal female monkeys. Nutr Cancer 56:74, 2006.

Zhou, W, et al: Vitamin D is associated with improved survival in early-stage non-small cell lung cancer patients. Cancer Epidemiol Biomarkers Prev 14:2303, 2005.

Chapter 22

Ajemian, MS, et al: Routine fiberoptic endoscopic evaluation of swallowing following prolonged intubation: Implications for management. Arch Surg 136:437, 2001.

American Dietetic Association: International Dietetics and Nutrition Terminology Reference Manual, ed 1. American Dietetic Association, Chicago, 2008.

American Dietetic Association: Manual of Clinical Dietetics, ed 6. American Dietetic Association, Chicago, 2000.

Bray, GA: Afferent signals regulating food intake. Proc Nutr Soc 59:373, 2000.

Brown, SE, and Light, RW: What is now known about protein-energy depletion: When COPD patients are malnourished. J Respir Dis May:36, 1983.

Cresci, GA, et al: Trauma, surgery, and burns. In Gottschlich, MM (ed): The A.S.P.E.N. Nutrition Support Core Curriculum: A Case-Based Approach—The Adult Patient. American Society for Parenteral and Enteral Nutrition. Silver Spring, MD, 2007.

Demling, RH, and DeSanti, L: Involuntary weight loss and protein-energy malnutrition: Diagnosis and treatment. Accessed May 2005 at: www.medscape.com.

Frankenfield, D, Smith, JS, and Cooney, RN: Validation of 2 approaches to predicting resting energy metabolic rate in critically ill patients. JPEN J Parenter Enter Nutr 28:4, 2004.

Gottschlich, MM (ed): The A.S.P.E.N. Nutrition Support Core Curriculum: A Case-Based Approach—The Adult Patient. American Society for Parenteral and Enteral Nutrition. Silver Spring, MD, 2007.

Gramlich, L, et al: Does enteral nutrition compared to parenteral nutrition result in better outcomes in critically ill adult patient? A systematic review of the literature. Nutrition 10:843, 2004.

Ireton-Jones, C, Jones, JD: Improved equation for predicting energy expenditure in patients: The Ireton-Jones equations. Nutr Clinical Pract 17:29-31, 2002.

Laaban, JP, Kouchakji, B, Dore, MF, et al: Nutritional status of patients with chronic obstructive pulmonary disease and acute respiratory failure. Chest 103:1362, 1993.

Mason, J, and Epstein, S: Nutritional management of the patient with acute respiratory failure. Accessed May 2005 at: www.cyberounds.com.

Mechanick, JL, and Brett, EM: Nutrition and the chronically critically ill patient. Curr Opin Clin Nut Metab Care 8:33, 2005.

Mueller, DH: Medical nutrition therapy for pulmonary disease. In Mahon, K, and Escott-Stump, S (eds): Food, Nutrition, and Diet Therapy, ed 11. Saunders, Philadelphia, 2004.

Peters, JA, Thomas-Peters, CD: Nutritional assessment of patients with respiratory disease. In Wilkens, RI, Sheldon, RI, Krider, SI (eds): Clinical Assessment in Respiratory Care, ed 5. Elsevier Mosby, St. Louis, 2005.

Schwartz DB, DiMaria, RA: Pulmonary and cardiac failure. In Gottschlich, MM (ed): A.S.P.E.N. Nutrition Support Core Curriculum: A Case-Based Approach—The Adult Patient. American Society for Parenteral and Enteral Nutrition. Silver Spring, MD, 2007.

Skipper, A: Dietitian's Handbook of Enteral and Parenteral Nutrition, ed 2. Aspen Publishing, Gaithersburg, MD, 1998.

Society of Critical Care Medicine: Critical Care Statistics in the United States. Society of Critical Care Medicine, Des Plains, IL, 2006.

Steckmiller, JK, Cowan, L, and Johns, P: Wound healing. In Gottschlich, MM (ed): The A.S.P.E.N. Nutrition Support Core Curriculum: A Case-Based Approach—The Adult Patient. American Society for Parenteral and Enteral Nutrition. Silver Spring, MD, 2007.

Thomas, CL (ed): Taber's Cyclopedic Medical Dictionary, ed 18. FA Davis, Philadelphia, 1997.

Van den Berg, G, et al: Intensive insulin therapy in critically ill patients. N Engl J Med 345:1359, 2001.

Venes, D (ed): Taber's Cyclopedic Medical Dictionary, ed 20. FA Davis, Philadelphia, 2005.

Accessed November 2008 at: www.adaevidencelibrary.com.

Accessed November 2008 at: www.nhlbi.nih.gov/health/dci/Diseases/Copd.

Winkler, MF, and Malone, AM: Medical nutrition therapy for metabolic stress: Sepsis, trauma, burns, and surgery. In Mahon, K, and Escott-Stump, S (eds): Food, Nutrition, and Diet Therapy. Saunders, Philadelphia, 2004, p 1062.

Chapter 23

American Dietetic Association: Manual of Clinical Dietetics, ed 6. American Dietetic Association, Chicago, 2000.

American Dietetic Association: Position of the American Dietetic Association: Addressing world hunger, malnutrition, and food insecurity. J Am Diet Assoc 103:1046, 2003.

American Dietetic Association: Position of the American Dietetic Association: Food insecurity and hunger in the United States. J Am Diet Assoc 106:446, 2006.

American Dietetic Association: Position of the American Dietetic and Canadian Dietetic Associations: Nutrition intervention in the care of persons with human immunodeficiency virus. J Am Diet Assoc 104:1425, 2004.

Batterham, M: Lipodystrophy—A Side Effect of Protease Inhibitor Therapy. Positive Communications: A publication of the HIV/AIDS Dietetic Practice Group. American Dietetic Association, Chicago, 1998.

Batterham, M, Brown, D, and Garcia, R: Nutritional management of HIV/AIDS in the era of highly active antiretroviral therapy: A review. Aust J Nutr Diet 58:211, 2001.

Benatar, SR: Health care reform and crisis of HIV and AIDS in South Africa. N Engl J Med 351:81, 2004.

Brown, D, and Batterham, M: Nutritional management in the era of highly active antiretroviral therapy: A review of treatment strategy. Aust J Nutr Diet 58:224, 2001.
Centers for Disease Control and Prevention: Health, United States, 2004. Atlanta. Accessed September 2008 at: http://www.cdc.gov/nchs/data/hus04trend.
Fawzi, W, et al: A randomized trial of multivitamin supplements and HIV disease progression and mortality. N Engl J Med 351:23, 2004.
HIV/AIDS in the era of highly active antiretroviral therapy: A review. Aust J Nutr Diet 58:211, 2001.
Huang, L, et al: Intensive care of patients with HIV infection. N Engl J Med 335:173, 2006.
Hunt, CA, and Billing, NA: A service evaluation to determine the effectiveness of current dietary advice in teaching human immunodeficiency virus–associated weight loss and to highlight service improvements. J Hum Nutr Diet 15:391, 2008.
Mason, J, and Roubenoff, R: Nutritional issues of clinical concern in HIV patients. Accessed July 28, 1999 at: http://www.cyberounds.com/conferences/0499/conference.html.
Ott, M, et al: Early changes of body composition in human immunodeficiency virus–infected patients: Tetrapolar body impedance and analysis indicates significant malnutrition. Am J Clin Nutr 57:15, 1993.
Smith, MK, and Lowry, SF: The hypermetabolic state. In Shils, ME, et al (eds): Modern Nutrition in Health and Disease, ed 9. Williams & Wilkins, Baltimore, 1999.
Solomons, NE: International priorities for clinical and therapeutic nutrition in the context of public relations. In Shils, ME, et al (eds): Modern Nutrition in Health and Disease, ed 9. Williams & Wilkins, Baltimore, 1999.
Steinbrook, R: The AIDS epidemic in 2004. N Engl J Med 351:115, 2004.
Trujillo, EB, et al: Assessment of nutritional status, nutrient intake, and nutrition support in AIDS patients. J Am Diet Assoc 92:477, 1992.
Ungvarski, PJ, and Flaskerud, JH: HIV/AIDS: A Guide to Primary Care Management. WB Saunders, Philadelphia, 1999.
Viral load tests. Accessed May 2000 at: www.aidsinfonyc.org.
Walton, RT, and Rowland-Jones, S: HIV and chemokine binding to RBC-DARC matters. Cell Hosts Microbes 4:3, 2008.
Wasserman, PJ, and Segal-Maurer, S: Human immunodeficiency virus (HIV). In Gottschlich, MM (ed): The A.S.P.E.N. Nutrition Core Support Curriculium: A Case-Based Approach—The Adult Patient. American Society for Parenteral and Enteral Nutrition. Silver Spring, MD, 2007.
Woods, MN, et al: Nutrient intake and body weight in a large HIV cohort that includes women and minorities. J Am Diet Assoc 102:203, 2002.
Accessed August 2008 at: www.todaysdietitian.com/+dauo8newsletter.
Accessed September 2008 at: www.mmwr.gov.

Chapter 24

American Dietetic Association: Position of the American Dietetic Association: Ethical and legal issues in nutrition, hydration, and feeding. J Am Diet Assoc 108:873, 2008a.
American Dietetic Association: Pocket Guide for International Dietetics and Nutrition Terminology (IDNT) Reference Manual, ed 1. American Dietetic Association, Chicago, 2008b.
American Dietetic Association: Pocket Guide for International Dietetics and Nutrition Terminology (IDNT) Reference Manual, ed 1. American Dietetic Association, Chicago, 2008c.
Gottschlich, MM (ed): The A.S.P.E.N. Nutrition Support Core Curriculum: A Case-Based Approach—The Adult Patient. American Society for Parenteral and Enteral Nutrition, Silver Spring, MD, 2007.
Maillet, JO, Potter, RL, and Heller, LH: Position of the American Dietetic Association: Ethical and legal issues in nutrition, hydration, and feeding. J Am Diet Assoc 102:716, 2002.
Morrison, RS, and Meier, DE: Clinical practice: Palliative care. N Engl J Med 350:2582, 2004.

Index

Note: Page numbers followed by *f* refer to figures; page numbers followed by *t* refer to tables.

A

B

C

G

H

I

M

N

Q

R

S

T

U

V

W

X

Y

Z